CRC Handbook of Tables for Probability and Statistics

Second Edition

Editor
William H. Beyer, Ph.D.
Professor
Department of Mathematics
University of Akron
Akron, Ohio

CRC Press, Inc.
Boca Raton, Florida

Direct all inquiries to CRC Press, Inc., 2000 Corporate Blvd., N.W., Boca Raton, Florida, 33431.

Formerly the Chemical Rubber Co.
Second Printing, 1974
Third Printing, 1976
Fourth Printing, 1979
Fifth Printing, 1981
Sixth Printing, 1983
Seventh Printing, 1985

International Standard Book Number 0-8493-0692-2
Former International Book Number 0-8719-692-7

Library of Congress Card Number 66-17301
Printed in the United States

Preface

Statistics is an important component of scientific reasoning, as well as an integral part of academics, business, and technology. As viewed by the late Sir Ronald Fisher, statistics is the key technology of the present day. Practicing statisticians and scientists working in diverse fields need an authoritative reference handbook of statistical tables developed to "aid" in the investigation and solution of many of today's challenging problems. This book has been compiled and arranged to meet the needs of these users of statistics.

This Second Edition of the Handbook of tables for Probability and Statistics brings together in a logically arranged, documented, and readily usable form an extensive collection of relatively standard statistical tables. The general arrangement of the First Edition has been retained. Many of the tables have been expanded and increased in effectiveness. All tables have been corrected of all errors detected. Examples of expanded tables are:

Individual Terms of the Binomial Distribution
Cumulative Terms of the Binomial Distribution
Confidence Limits for Proportions
Tests of Significance in 2 × 2 Contingency Tables
Critical Values for Testing Outliers
Critical Values of U in the Mann-Whitney Test
Distribution of the Total Number-of-Runs Test
Number of Combinations

Included in the expository section of the Handbook (Part I) is a completely rewritten section on descriptive statistics.

Additional tables and graphs which enhance the importance of this Second Edition are:

Summary of Significance Tests
Summary of Confidence Intervals
Table of Signs for Calculating Effects in Factorial Designs up to Six Factors
Operating Characteristic (OC) Curves for Tests on the Mean and Standard Deviation(s) of Normal Distributions
Cochran's Test for the Homogeneity of Variances
Percentage Points of the Maximum F-Ratio
Confidence Limits for σ Based on Mean Range
Critical Values for Duncan's New Multiple Range Test
Critical Values for Rank-Sum Tests for Dispersion
Cumulative Sum Control Charts (CSCC)
Logarithms of the Binomial Coefficients

Preparation of this enlarged Second Edition has been possible only through the participation of recognized authorities who have taken time from their busy schedules to interpret their thoughts into writing. The Editor has been fortunate indeed to secure the aid of a well coordinated and specially selected advisory board. The names of members of the advisory board are presented in the forefront of this handbook. The Editor is most grateful to them for their continued cooperation and for their invaluable contributions.

The Editor gratefully acknowledges the authors, editors, and publishers who gave permission to reproduce these tables. Reference to the sources of material used in this handbook is indicated in the acknowledgment section. It is quite possible that proper credit has not always been given. Regrets and apologies are offered to the authors of such material.

To the many users of the current edition who sent in suggestions for alterations and additions, the Editorial Staff extends a special thanks. It is hoped that those interested will continue to send in suggestions and comments to assist in the continuous improvement of the contents.

William H. Beyer
April, 1968

Advisory Board

Editor and Chairman

Acknowledgments

Acknowledgment is made to the following authors, editors, and publishers whose material has been used in this Handbook of tables for Probability and Statistics, and for which permission has been received.

American Society for Testing Materials STP-15C;
 ASTM Manual on Quality Control of Materials (1951)
  XI.1—Factors for Computing Control Limits

American Statistical Association, Journal of
 Vol. 55 (1960) 723–731, H. L. Harter
  II.8—Circular Error Probabilities
 Vol. 32 (1937) 349–386, W. E. Ricker
  III.6—Confidence Limits for the Expected Value of a Poisson Distribution
 Vol. 41 (1946) 557–566, W. J. Dixon and A. M. Mood
  X.1—Critical Values for the Sign Test
 Vol. 46 (1951) 68–78, F. J. Massey, Jr.
 Vol. 47 (1952) 425–441, Z. W. Birnbaum
  X.7—Critical Values for the Kolmogorov-Smirnov One-Sample Statistic
 Vol. 47 (1952) 583–621, W. H. Kruskal and W. A. Wallis
  X.9—Kruskal-Wallis One-Way Analysis of Variance by Ranks
 Vol. 55 (1960) 428–445, S. Siegel and J. W. Tukey
  X.10—Critical Values for a Sum of Ranks Procedure for Relative Spread in Unpaired Samples

Bargmann, Rolf E.
 Department of Statistics
 University of Georgia
 Athens, Georgia
  Part I. "General Linear Model"

Biometrika Trustees; E. S. Pearson and H. O. Hartley,
 Cambridge University Press
 Biometrika
  Vol. 40 (1953) 74–86, R. Latscha
   III.11—Tests of Significance in 2 × 2 Contingency Tables
  Vol. 38 (1951) 112–130, E. S. Pearson and H. O. Hartley
   VI.2—Power Functions of the Analysis-of-Variance Tests
  Vol. 39 (1952) 422–424, H. A. David
   VI.6—Percentage Points of the Maximum F-Ratio
  Vol. 48 (1961) 151–165, H. L. Harter
   VII.1—Expected Values of Order Statistics from a Standard Normal Population
  Vol. 32 (1942) 301–310, E. S. Pearson and H. O. Hartley
   VII.6—Simple Estimates in Small Samples
  Vol. 34 (1947) 41–67, E. Lord
   VIII.4—Substitute t-Ratios

 Biometrika Tables for Statisticians
  Vol. 1 (1962) 114–121 II.10—Probit Analysis
  Vol. 1 (1962) 204–205 III.5 —Confidence Limits for Proportions

Vol. 1 (1962) 234–235 III.7 —Various Functions of p and $q = 1 - p$
Vol. 1 (1962) 142–155 III.10—Percentage Points of the Beta Distribution
Vol. 1 (1962) 188–193 III.11—Tests of Significance in 2×2 Contingency Tables
Vol. 1 (1962) 135 IV.2 —Power Function of the t-Test
Vol. 1 (1962) 130–131 V.1 —Percentage Points, Chi-Square Distribution
Vol. 1 (1962) 157–163 VI.1 —Percentage Points, F-Distribution
Vol. 1 (1962) 166–171 VIII.1 —Probability Integral of the Range
Vol. 1 (1962) 165 VIII.2 —Percentage Points, Distribution of the Range
Vol. 1 (1962) 176–177 VIII.3 —Percentage Points, Studentized Range
Vol. 1 (1962) 138 IX.1 —Percentage Points, Distribution of the Correlation Coefficient when $\rho = 0$
Vol. 1 (1962) 140–141 IX.2 —Confidence Limits for the Population Correlation Coefficient
Vol. 1 (1962) 139 IX.3 —The Transformation $z = \tanh^{-1} r$ for the Correlation Coefficient
Vol. 1 (1962) 211 X.13—Critical Values of Kendall's Rank Correlation Coefficient
Vol. 1 (1962) 165 XI.2 —Percentage Points of the Distribution of the Mean Deviation

BIOMETRICS
Vol. 11 (1955) 1–42, D. B. Duncan
VIII.4 —Critical Values for Duncan's New Multiple Range Test

THE CHEMICAL RUBBER CO.
CRC Standard Mathematical Tables, 15th Edition, S. M. Selby
II.1 —The Normal Probability Function and Related Functions
II.3 —Factors for Computing Probable Errors
II.4 —Probability of Occurrence of Deviations
III.1 —Individual Terms, Binomial Distribution
III.2 —Cumulative Terms, Binomial Distribution
III.3 —Individual Terms, Poisson Distribution
III.4 —Cumulative Terms, Poisson Distribution
XII.4 —Random Units
XIII.1 —Miscellaneous Constants
XIII.2 —Numerical Constants
XIII.3 —Radians to Degrees, Minutes and Seconds
XIII.4 —Natural Functions for Angles in Radians
XIII.10—Reciprocals of Factorials and Their Logarithms
Handbook of Mathematical Tables, 3rd Edition, S. M. Selby
Part I —Finite Differences
XIII.5 —Squares, Cubes and Roots
XIII.6 —Exponential Functions
XIII.7 —Six-Place Logarithms
XIII.8 —Natural or Naperian Logarithms
XIII.9 —Factorials and Their Logarithms
XIII.11—Powers of Numbers
XIII.12—Sums of Powers of Integers
XIII.14—Gamma Function
Handbook of Chemistry and Physics, 48th Edition, R. C. Weast
XIII.13—Integrals

DAVID, HERBERT A.
Department of Biostatistics
University of North Carolina
Chapel Hill, North Carolina
VIII.7—Analysis of Variance Based on Range

INSTITUTE OF EDUCATIONAL RESEARCH
Indiana University, Bloomington, Indiana
Vol. 1, No. 2 (1953), D. Auble
X.4—Critical Values of U in the Wilcoxon (Mann-Whitney) Two Sample Statistic

KRAMER, CLYDE Y.
Professor of Statistics
Virginia Agricultural Experiment Station
Virginia Polytechnic Institute
Blacksburg, Virginia
Part I—Simplified Computations for Multiple Regression

LEDERLE LABORATORIES
Some Rapid Approximate Statistical Procedures (1964) 20–28, F. Wilcoxon and R. A. Wilcox
X.2—Critical Values of T in the Wilcoxon Matched-Pairs Signed-Ranks Test
X.5—Critical Values for the Wilcoxon Rank Sum Test

MATHEMATICAL STATISTICS, ANNALS OF, D. L. BURKHOLDER, EDITOR
Vol. 17 (1946) 178–197, C. D. Ferris, F. E. Grubbs, and C. L. Weaver
II.5—Operating Characteristic (OC) Curves for a Test on the Mean of a Normal Distribution with Known Standard Deviation
Vol. 31 (1960) 619–624, M. Zelen and N. C. Severo
II.6—Bivariate Normal Probabilities
Vol. 31 (1960) 625–642, D. L. Heck
II.9—Charts of Upper 1%, 2.5% and 5% Points of the Distribution of the Largest Characteristic Root
Vol. 17 (1946) 178–197, C. D. Ferris, F. E. Grubbs, and C. L. Weaver
IV.5—Operating Characteristic (OC) Curves for a Test on the Mean of a Normal Distribution with Unknown Standard Deviation
V.4—Operating Characteristic (OC) Curves for a Test on the Standard Deviation of a Normal Distribution
VI.4—Operating Characteristic (OC) Curves for a Test on the Standard Deviations of Two Normal Distributions
Vol. 27 (1956) 427–451, A. E. Sarhan, B. G. Greenberg
VII.2—Variances and Covariances of Order Statistics
Vol. 22 (1951) 68–78, W. J. Dixon
VII.4—Critical Values for Testing Outliers
Vol. 17 (1946) 377–408, F. Mosteller
VII.5—Percentile Estimates in Large Samples
Vol. 31 (1960) 1122–1147, H. L. Harter
VIII.2—Percentage Points, Distribution of the Range
VIII.3—Percentage Points, Studentized Range
Vol. 20 (1949a) 257–267, J. E. Walsh
VIII.5—Substitute t-Ratios
Vol. 21 (1950) 112–116, R. F. Link
VIII.6—Substitute F-Ratio
Vol. 18 (1947) 50–60, H. B. Mann, D. R. Whitney
X.3—Probabilities for the Wilcoxon (Mann-Whitney) Two-Sample Statistic
Vol. 14 (1943) 66–87, C. Eisenhart and F. C. Swed
X.6—Distribution of the Total Number-of-Runs Test
Vol. 23 (1952) 435–441, F. J. Massey, Jr.
X.8—Critical Values for the Kolmogorov-Smirnov Two Sample Statistic
Vol. 31 (1960), 1178–1179, R. A. Bradley and A. Ansari
X.11—Significant Values for a Rank-Sum Test for Dispersion
Vol. 9 (1938) 133–148, E. G. Olds and Vol. 20 (1949) 117–118, E. G. Olds
X.12—Critical Values of Spearman's Rank Correlation Coefficient

MCGRAW-HILL BOOK COMPANY
Handbook of Probability and Statistics with Tables, R. S. Burington and D. C. May
(1953) 102–105 11.7—Circular Normal Probabilities
Selected Techniques of Statistical Analysis, C. Eisenhart, M. W. Hastay, W. A. Wallis
(1947) 102–107 II.2—Tolerance Factors for Normal Distributions
(1947) 284–309 V.3—Number of Observations for the Comparison of a Population Variance With a Standard Value Using the Chi-Square Test

VI.3—Number of Observations Required for the Comparison of Two Population Variances Using the F-Test
(1947) 390–391 VI.5—Cochran's Test for the Homogeneity of Variances
Introduction to Statistical Analysis, 2nd Edition, W. J. Dixon, F. J. Massey, Jr.
(1957) 405–407 VII.6—Simple Estimates in Small Samples

OLIVER AND BOYD, LTD., EDINBURGH, SCOTLAND
Design and Analysis of Industrial Experiments, O. L. Davies
Research Vol. 1 (1948) 520–525
(1956) 606–607 IV.3—Number of Observations for t-Test of Mean
(1956) 609–610 IV.4—Number of Observations for t-Test of Difference Between Two Means
(1956) 613–614 V.3—Number of Observations for the Comparison of a Population Variance With a Standard Value Using the Chi-Square Test
Statistical Tables for Biological, Agricultural, and Medical Research, R. A. Fisher, F. Yates
The Literary Executor of the Late Sir Ronald Fisher, F.R.S., Cambridge, Dr. Frank Yates, F.R.S., Rothamstead and Messrs. Oliver and Boyd, Ltd., Edinburgh, Scotland
(1938) 46 IV.1—Percentage Points, Student's t-Distribution
(1938) 98–103 XII.8—Orthogonal Polynomials

THE ROYAL SOCIETY, LONDON, ENGLAND
Royal Society Mathematical Tables
Vol. 3 (1954) 2 XII.2—Number of Combinations

SPRINGER-VERLAG NEW YORK, INC.
Fünfstellige Funktionentafeln (1930), Hayashi, K.
XII.1—Number of Permutations

STANFORD UNIVERSITY PRESS
Tables of the Hypergeometric Probability Distribution, G. J. Lieberman and D. B. Owen
(1961) III.8—Hypergeometric Distribution

STATISTICAL PUBLISHING SOCIETY, CALCUTTA, INDIA
Sankhya
Vol. 4 (1940) 551–558 S. K. Banerjee, K. R. Nair
VII.3—Confidence Intervals for Medians

VIRGINIA POLYTECHNIC INSTITUTE, R. E. BARGMANN, J. E. WHITE
"Some Contributions to the Evaluation of Pearsonian Distribution Functions"
Research sponsored by the National Institutes of Health, Epidemiology, and Biometry, Technical Report No. 1 (1960)
XII.9—Percentage Points of Pearson Curves

WRIGHT AIR DEVELOPMENT CENTER, WRIGHT-PATTERSON AFB
WADC Technical Report 58–484, H. L. Harter, D. S. Clemm, and G. H. Guthrie
Vol. II (1959) VIII.4—Critical Values for Duncan's New Multiple Range Test

JOHN WILEY & SONS, INC.
Contributions to Order Statistics, A. E. Sarhan and B. G. Greenberg
(1962) 116 VIII.8—Confidence Intervals for σ Based on Mean Range
Experimental Designs, W. G. Cochran, G. M. Cox
(1957) Part I—Plans for Design of Experiments
Statistical Tables and Formulas, A. Hald
(1952) 66–69 III.5—Confidence Limits for Proportions
(1952) 44–45 V.2—Percentage Points, Chi-Square Over Degrees of Freedom Distribution
Statistics and Experimental Design, N. L. Johnson, F. C. Leone
Vol. 1 (1964) 412 X.12—Critical Values of Spearman's Rank Correlation Coefficient
Vol. 1 (1964) 320–341 XI.3—Cumulative Sum Control Charts

Contents

Part II—NORMAL DISTRIBUTION

GREEK ALPHABET

Greek letter	Greek name	English equivalent	Greek letter	Greek name	English equivalent
Α α	Alpha	a	Ν ν	Nu	n
Β β	Beta	b	Ξ ξ	Xi	x
Γ γ	Gamma	g	Ο ο	Omicron	ŏ
Δ δ	Delta	d	Π π	Pi	p
Ε ϵ	Epsilon	ĕ	Ρ ρ	Rho	r
Ζ ζ	Zeta	z	Σ σ ς	Sigma	s
Η η	Eta	ē	Τ τ	Tau	t
Θ θ ϑ	Theta	th	Υ υ	Upsilon	u
Ι ι	Iota	i	Φ ϕ φ	Phi	ph
Κ κ	Kappa	k	Χ χ	Chi	ch
Λ λ	Lambda	l	Ψ ψ	Psi	ps
Μ μ	Mu	m	Ω ω	Omega	ō

I. Probability and Statistics

DESCRIPTIVE STATISTICS

a) Ungrouped Data

The formulas of this section designated as *a*) apply to a random sample of size n, denoted by x_i, $i = 1, 2, \ldots, n$.

b) Grouped Data

The formulas of this section designated as *b*) apply to data grouped into a frequency distribution having class marks x_i, $i = 1, 2, \ldots, k$, and corresponding class frequencies f_i, $i = 1, 2, \ldots, k$. The total number of observations given by

$$n = \sum_{i=1}^{k} f_i$$

In the formulas that follow, c denotes the width of the class interval, x_o denotes one of the class marks taken to be the computing origin, and $u_i = \frac{x_i - x_o}{c}$. Then coded class marks are obtained by replacing the original class marks with the integers $\ldots, -3, -2, -1, 0, 1, 2, 3, \ldots$ where 0 corresponds to class mark x_o in the original scale.

Mean (Arithmetic Mean)

a) $\bar{x} = \frac{1}{n}\sum_{i=1}^{n} x_i = x_1 + x_2 + \cdots + x_n$

b.1) $\bar{x} = \frac{1}{n}\sum_{i=1}^{k} f_i x_i = \frac{f_1x_1 + f_2x_2 + \cdots + f_kx_k}{n}$

If data is coded

b.2) $\bar{x} = x_o + c\frac{\sum_{i=1}^{k} f_i u_i}{n}$

Weighted Mean (Weighted Arithmetic Mean)

If with each value x_i is associated a weighting factor $w_i \geq 0$, then $\sum_{i=1}^{n} w_i$ is the total weight, and

a) $\bar{x} = \frac{\sum_{i=1}^{n} w_i x_i}{\sum_{i=1}^{n} w_i} = \frac{w_1x_1 + w_2x_2 + \cdots + w_nx_n}{w_1 + w_2 + \cdots + w_n}$

Geometric Mean

a) G.M. $= \sqrt[n]{x_1 \cdot x_2 \cdots x_n}$

In logarithmic form

$$\log\,(\text{G.M.}) = \frac{1}{n}\sum_{i=1}^{n} \log x_i = \frac{\log x_1 + \log x_2 + \cdots + \log x_n}{n}$$

b) $\text{G.M.} = \sqrt[n]{x_1^{f_1} \cdot x_2^{f_2} \cdots x_k^{f_k}}$

In logarithmic form

$$\log\,(\text{G.M.}) = \frac{1}{n}\sum_{i=1}^{k} f_i \log x_i = \frac{f_1 \log x_1 + f_2 \log x_2 + \cdots + f_k \log x_k}{n}$$

Harmonic Mean

a) $$\text{H.M.} = \frac{n}{\sum_{i=1}^{n} \frac{1}{x_i}} = \frac{n}{\frac{1}{x_1} + \frac{1}{x_2} + \cdots + \frac{1}{x_n}}$$

b) $$\text{H.M.} = \frac{n}{\sum_{i=1}^{k} \frac{f_i}{x_i}} = \frac{n}{\frac{f_1}{x_1} + \frac{f_2}{x_2} + \cdots + \frac{f_k}{x_k}}$$

Relation Between Arithmetic, Geometric, and Harmonic Mean

$\text{H.M.} \leq \text{G.M.} \leq \bar{x}$, (Equality sign holds only if all sample values are identical.)

Mode

a) A mode M_o of a sample of size n is a value which occurs with greatest frequency, i.e., it is the most common value. A mode may not exist, and even if it does exist it may not be unique.

b) $$M_o = L + C\,\frac{\Delta_1}{\Delta_1 + \Delta_2},$$

where L is the lower class boundary of the modal class (class containing the mode),
Δ_1 is the excess of modal frequency over frequency of next lower class,
Δ_2 is the excess of modal frequency over frequency of next higher class.

Median

a) If the sample is arranged in ascending order of magnitude, then the median M_d is given by the $\frac{n+1}{2}$ *nd* value. When n is odd, the median is the middle value of the set of ordered data; when n is even, the median is usually taken as the mean of the two middle values of the set of ordered data.

b) $$M_d = L + c\,\frac{\frac{n}{2} - F_c}{f_m},$$

where L is lower class boundary of median class (class containing the median),
F_c is the sum of the frequencies of all classes lower than the median class,
f_m is the frequency of the median class.

Empirical Relation Between Mean, Median, and Mode

Mean-Mode = 3 (Mean-Median)

Quartiles

a) If the data is arranged in ascending order of magnitude, the jth quartile Q_j, $j = 1, 2,$ or 3, is given by the $\frac{j(n+1)}{4}$ th value. It may be necessary to interpolate between successive values.

b) The jth quartile Q_j, $j = 1, 2,$ or 3, is obtained from formula *b*) for the median by counting $\frac{jn}{4}$ cases starting at the bottom of the distribution.

Deciles

a) If the sample is arranged in ascending order of magnitude, the jth decile D_j, $j = 1, 2, \ldots,$ or 9, is given by the $\frac{j(n+1)}{10}$ th value. It may be necessary to interpolate between successive values.

b) The jth decile D_j, $j = 1, 2, \ldots,$ or 9, is obtained from formula *b*) for the median by counting $\frac{jn}{10}$ cases starting at the bottom of the distribution.

Percentiles

a) If the sample is arranged in ascending order of magnitude, the jth percentile P_j, $j = 1, 2, \ldots,$ or 99 is given by the $\frac{j(n+1)}{100}$ th value. It may be necessary to interpolate between successive values.

b) The jth percentile P_j, $j = 1, 2, \ldots,$ or 99, is obtained from formulas *b*) for the median by counting $\frac{jn}{100}$ cases starting at the bottom of the distribution.

Mean Deviation

a) $$\text{M.D.} = \frac{1}{n}\sum_{i=1}^{n} |x_i - \bar{x}|$$

or

$$\text{M.D.} = \frac{1}{n}\sum_{i=1}^{n} |x_i - M_d|$$

where $\bar{x}$ is the mean and M_d is the median of the sample.

b) $$\text{M.D.} = \frac{1}{n}\sum_{i=1}^{k} f_i|x_i - \bar{x}|$$

or

$$\text{M.D.} = \frac{1}{n}\sum_{i=1}^{k} f_i|x_i - M_d|$$

where $\bar{x}$ is the mean and M_d the median of the sample.

Standard Deviation

a) $s = \sqrt{\dfrac{\sum_{i=1}^{n} (x_i - \bar{x})^2}{n-1}}$, where $\bar{x}$ is the mean of the sample.

For computational purposes,

$$s = \sqrt{\frac{\sum_{i=1}^{n} x_i^2 - n\bar{x}^2}{n-1}}$$

$$s = \sqrt{\frac{n \sum_{i=1}^{n} x_i^2 - \left(\sum_{i=1}^{n} x_i\right)^2}{n(n-1)}}$$

b) $s = \sqrt{\dfrac{\sum_{i=1}^{k} f_i(x_i - \bar{x})^2}{n-1}}$, where $\bar{x}$ is the mean of the sample.

For computational purposes

$$s = \sqrt{\frac{\sum_{i=1}^{k} f_i x_i^2 - n\bar{x}^2}{n-1}}$$

$$s = \sqrt{\frac{n \sum_{i=1}^{k} f_i x_i^2 - \left(\sum_{i=1}^{k} f_i x_i\right)^2}{n(n-1)}}$$

If data is coded,

$$s = c\sqrt{\frac{n \sum_{i=1}^{k} f_i u_i^2 - \left(\sum_{i=1}^{k} f_i u_i\right)^2}{n(n-1)}}$$

Variance

The variance is the square of the standard deviation.

Range

The range of a set of values is the difference between the largest and smallest values in the set.

Root Mean Square

a) $\text{R.M.S.} = \dfrac{1}{n} \sum_{i=1}^{n} x_i^2$

b) $\text{R.M.S.} = \dfrac{1}{n} \sum_{i=1}^{k} f_i x_i^2$

Interquartile Range

$$Q_3 - Q_1,$$

where Q_1 and Q_3 are the first and third quartiles.

Quartile Deviation (Semi-Interquartile Range)

$$\frac{Q_3 - Q_1}{2},$$

where Q_1 and Q_3 are the first and third quartiles.

Coefficient of Variation

$$V = \frac{100s}{\bar{x}},$$

where $\bar{x}$ is the mean and s the standard deviation of the sample.

Coefficient of Quartile Variation

$$V = 100\,\frac{Q_3 - Q_1}{Q_3 + Q_1},$$

where Q_1 and Q_3 are the first and third quartiles.

Standardized Variable (Standard Scores)

$$z = \frac{x_i - \bar{x}}{s},$$

where $\bar{x}$ is the mean and s the standard deviation of the sample.

Moments

a) The rth moment about the origin is given by

$$m'_r = \frac{1}{n}\sum_{i=1}^{n} x_i^{\,r}$$

The rth moment about the mean $\bar{x}$ is given by

$$m_r = \frac{1}{n}\sum_{i=1}^{n} (x_i - \bar{x})^r$$

If $\sum_{i=1}^{n} (x_i - \bar{x})^r$ is expanded by use of the binomial theorem, moments about the mean may be expressed in terms of moments about the origin.

b) The rth moment about the origin is given by

$$m'_r = \frac{1}{n}\sum_{i=1}^{k} f_i x_i^{\,r}$$

The rth moment about the mean $\bar{x}$ is given by

$$m_r = \frac{1}{n}\sum_{i=1}^{k} f_i (x_i - \bar{x})^r$$

If $\sum_{i=1}^{k} f_i(x_i - \bar{x})^r$ is expanded by use of the binomial theorem, moments about the mean may be expressed in terms of moments about the origin.

If data is coded

$$m'_r = c^r \frac{\sum_{i=1}^{k} f_i u_i^r}{n}$$

Coefficient of Skewness

$$\alpha_3 = \frac{m_3}{(m_2)^{3/2}},$$

where m_2 and m_3 are the second and third moments about the mean of the sample.

Coefficient of Momental Skewness

$$\frac{\alpha_3}{2} = \frac{m_3}{2(m_2)^{3/2}},$$

where m_2 and m_3 are the second and third moments about the mean of the sample.

Pearson's First Coefficient of Skewness

$$S_{k_1} = \frac{3(\bar{x} - M_o)}{s},$$

where $\bar{x}$ is the mean, M_o the mode, and s the standard deviation of the sample.

Pearson's Second Coefficient of Skewness

$$S_{k_2} = \frac{3(\bar{x} - M_d)}{s},$$

where $\bar{x}$ is the mean, M_d the median, and s the standard deviation of the sample.

Quartile Coefficient of Skewness

$$S_{k_Q} = \frac{Q_3 - 2Q_2 + Q_1}{Q_3 - Q_1},$$

where Q_1, Q_2, and Q_3 are the first, second, and third quartiles.

Coefficient of Kurtosis

$$\alpha_4 = \frac{m_4}{(m_2)^2},$$

where m_2 and m_4 are the second and fourth moments about the mean of the sample.

Coefficient of Excess (Kurtosis)

$$\alpha_4 - 3 = \frac{m_4}{(m_2)^2} - 3,$$

where m_2 and m_4 are the second and fourth moments about the mean of the sample.

Sheppards Corrections for Grouping

Let all class intervals be of equal length c. If the distribution of x has a high order of contact with the x-axis at both tails, (i.e., if the distribution of x has tails which are very nearly tangent to the x-axis), one may improve the grouped data approximation to the variance by adding Sheppard's correction $-\frac{c^2}{12}$. Thus

$$\text{corrected variance} = \text{grouped data variance} - \frac{c^2}{12}$$

Analogous corrections for grouped data sample moments

$$m'_r = \frac{1}{n}\sum_{i=1}^{k} f_i x_i^r \qquad \text{and} \qquad m_r = \frac{1}{n}\sum_{i=1}^{k} f_i(x_i - \bar{x})^r$$

yield improved estimates m'_{r_c} and m_{r_c} given by

$$m'_{1_c} = m'_1 \qquad m_{1_c} = m_1$$

$$m'_{2_c} = m'_2 - \frac{c^2}{12} \qquad m_{2_c} = m_2 - \frac{c^2}{12}$$

$$m'_{3_c} = m'_3 - \frac{c^2}{4} m'_1 \qquad m_{3_c} = m_3$$

$$m'_{4_c} = m'_4 - \frac{c^2}{2} m'_1 + \frac{7c^4}{240} \qquad m_{4_c} = m_4 - \frac{c^2}{2} m_2 + \frac{7c^4}{240}$$

Curve Fitting, Regression, and Correlation

The following formulas apply to a set of n ordered pairs $\{(x_i,y_i)\}$, $i = 1, 2, \ldots, n$. The assumptions of normal regression analysis are that the x's are fixed variables, and the y's are independent random variables having normal distributions with common variance σ^2. The assumptions of normal correlation analysis are that $\{(x_i,y_i)\}$ constitute a random sample from a bivariate normal population.

Curve Fitting

1. Polynomial Function

$$y = b_0 + b_1 x + b_2 x^2 + \cdots + b_m x^m$$

For a polynomial function fit by the method of least squares, the values of $b_o, b_1, \ldots, b_m$ are obtained by solving the system of $m + 1$ normal equations

$$nb_o + b_1\Sigma x_i + b_2\Sigma x_i^2 + \cdots + b_m\Sigma x_i^m = \Sigma y_i$$
$$b_o\Sigma x_i + b_i\Sigma x_i^2 + b_2\Sigma x_i^3 + \cdots + b_m\Sigma x_i^{m+1} = \Sigma x_i y_i$$
$$\cdots\cdots\cdots\cdots\cdots\cdots\cdots\cdots\cdots\cdots\cdots\cdots$$
$$b_o\Sigma x_i^m + b_1\Sigma x_i^{m+1} + b_2\Sigma x_i^{m+2} + \cdots + b_m\Sigma x_i^{2m} = \Sigma x_i^m y_i$$

2. Straight Line

$$y = b_0 + b_1 x$$

For a straight line fit by the method of least squares, the values b_o and b_1 are obtained by solving the normal equations

$$nb_0 + b_1\Sigma x_i = \Sigma y_i$$
$$b_0\Sigma x_i + b_1\Sigma x_i^2 = \Sigma x_i y_i$$

The solutions of these normal equations are

$$b_1 = \frac{n\Sigma x_i y_i - (\Sigma x_i)(\Sigma y_i)}{n\Sigma x_i^2 - (\Sigma x_i)^2}$$

$$b_0 = \frac{\Sigma y_i}{n} - b_1\frac{\Sigma x_i}{n} = \bar{y} - b_1\bar{x}$$

3. Exponential Curve

$$y = ab^x$$

or

$$\log y = \log a + (\log b)x$$

For an exponential curve fit by the method of least squares, the values log a and log b are obtained by fitting a straight line to the set of ordered pairs $\{(x_i, \log y_i)\}$.

4. Power Function

$$y = ax^b$$

or

$$\log y = \log a + b \log x$$

For a power function fit by the method of least squares, the values log a and b are obtained by fitting a straight line to the set or ordered pairs $\{(\log x_i, \log y_i)\}$.

Regression and Correlation

1. Simple Linear Regression.

For a regression of y on x

$$E(y/x) = \beta_0 + \beta_1 x,$$

where $E(y/x)$ is the mean of the distribution of y for a given x.

Standard Error of Estimate

$$s_e = \sqrt{\frac{\Sigma[y_i - (b_0 + b_1 x_i)]^2}{n-2}},$$

where b_0 and b_1 are given by

$$b_1 = \frac{n\Sigma x_i y_i - (\Sigma x_i)(\Sigma y_i)}{n\Sigma x_i^2 - (\Sigma x_i)^2}$$

$$b_0 = \frac{\Sigma y_i}{n} - b_1 \frac{\Sigma x_i}{n} = \bar{y} - b_1 \bar{x}$$

2. Correlation.

An estimate of the population correlation coefficient ρ is given by

$$r = \frac{\Sigma(x_i - \bar{x})(y_i - \bar{y})}{\sqrt{[\Sigma(x_i - \bar{x})^2][\Sigma(y_i - \bar{y})^2]}}$$

or by the computing formula

$$r = \frac{n\Sigma x_i y_i - (\Sigma x_i)(\Sigma y_i)}{\sqrt{[n\Sigma x_i^2 - (\Sigma x_i)^2][n\Sigma y_i^2 - (\Sigma y_i)]^2}}$$

For grouped data

$$r = \frac{n\Sigma f x_i y_i - (\Sigma f_x x_i)(\Sigma f_y y_i)}{\sqrt{[n\Sigma f_x x_i^2 - (\Sigma f_x x_i)^2][n\Sigma f_y y_i^2 - (\Sigma f_y y_i)^2]}}$$

where f_x and f_y denote the frequencies corresponding to the class marks x and y, and f denotes the frequency of the corresponding cell of the correlation table.

If the data is coded

$$r = \frac{n\Sigma f uv - (\Sigma f_u u)(\Sigma f_v v)}{\sqrt{[n\Sigma f_u u^2 - (\Sigma f_u u)^2][n\Sigma f_v v^2 - (\Sigma f_v v)^2]}}$$

where the u's and v's are coded class marks. The frequencies f_u and f_v are defined analogous to f_x and f_y.

BASIC CONCEPTS FOR ALGEBRA OF SETS

I. *Algebra of Sets*

1. A set is a collection or an aggregate of objects, called "the elements of the set". If a is an element of set A, we write $a \in A$. If not then $a \notin A$. If a set contains only the element a, we denote it by $\{a\}$.
2. The *null set,* denoted by ϕ, is the set which has no elements.
3. Two sets A and B are called "equal",* written $A = B$ if (1) every element of A is an element of B and (2) every element of B is an element of A.
4. If every element of set A is an element of set B, we call set A a "subset" of set B, written $A \subset B$ (or $B \supset A$). By convention $\phi \subset A$ for every set A.
5. If $A \subset B$ and if $B \subset A$, then A is called an *improper* subset of B—also $A = B$ by (3). If $A \subset B$ and if B includes at least one element which is not an element of A, then A is a *proper* subset of B. The symbol $\subset$ is sometimes used to mean *proper* inclusion, with $\subseteq$ meaning inclusion as defined above. $\neq \subset$ is sometimes also used for proper inclusion.
6. If all of the elements under consideration are elements of a universal set I, then for all sets A, $A \subset I$.
7. The set A', called the *complementary* set of A (relative to I), is the set which contains all the elements of I which are not elements of A.
8. Two binary operations on sets are $\cup$ and $\cap$. $A \cup B$, called the *union* (sometimes called the *join*) of sets A and B is the set of all elements which are elements of A or of B or of both. $A \cap B$, called the *intersection* (sometimes called the *meet*) of sets A and B is the set of all elements which are elements of *both* A *and* B.
9. Some properties of sets involving these relations:

   For all sets A, B, C in a universal set I. Only in those rules explicitly involving I, or those using complementation (which is defined in terms of I) is it necessary to assume that $A, B, C, \ldots$, lie in a universal set.

A. (Closure)
- A_1: There is a unique set $A \cup B$
- A_2: There is a unique set $A \cap B$

B. (Commutative Laws)
- B_1: $A \cup B = B \cup A$
- B_2: $A \cap B = B \cap A$

C. (Associative Laws)
- C_1: $(A \cup B) \cup C = A \cup (B \cup C)$
- C_2: $(A \cap B) \cap C = A \cap (B \cap C)$

D. (Distributive Laws)
- D_1: $A \cup (B \cap C) = (A \cup B) \cap (A \cup C)$
- D_2: $A \cap (B \cup C) = (A \cap B) \cup (A \cap C)$

E. (Idempotent Laws)
- E_1: $A \cup A = A$
- E_2: $A \cap A = A$

F. Properties of I and ϕ
- F_1: $A \cap I = A$
- F_2: $A \cup \phi = A$
- F_3: $A \cap \phi = \phi$
- F_4: $A \cup I = I$

* This equality, as well as ordinary equality between numbers, is a special case of an *equivalence relation.* In general, an equivalence relation is any relation with the following three properties:
1. Reflexive Law: $A = A$.
2. Symmetric Law: If $A = B$, then $B = A$.
3. Transitive Law: If $A = B$ and $B = C$, then $A = C$.

G. Properties of $\subset$.

G_1: $A \subset (A \cup B)$
G_2: $(A \cap B) \subset A$
G_3: $A \subset I$
G_4: $\phi \subset A$
G_5: If $A \subset B$, then $A \cup B = B$
If $B \subset A$, then $A \cap B = B$

H. Properties of $'$.

H_1: For every set A, there is a unique set A'
H_2: $A \cup A' = I$
H_3: $A \cap A' = \phi$
H_4: $(A \cup B)' = A' \cap B'$
H_5: $(A \cap B)' = A' \cup B'$

I. *Duality*

If we interchange $\left\{\begin{matrix} \cup \text{ and } \cap \\ \phi \text{ and } I \\ \subset \text{ and } \supset \end{matrix}\right\}$ in any correct formula we obtain another correct formula.

J. The above Algebra of Sets is a representation of a *Boolean* Algebra, which may be defined:

Undefined concepts: Set H of elements $a, b, c, \ldots$
2 binary operations $\oplus$, $\otimes$

Postulates for all $a, b, c,$ of H

P_1: $a \oplus b \in H$; P_1': $a \otimes b \in H$
P_2: $a \oplus b = b \oplus a$; P_2': $a \otimes b = b \otimes a$
P_3: $(a \oplus b) \oplus c = a \oplus (b \oplus c)$;
P_3': $(a \otimes b) \otimes c = a \otimes (b \otimes c)$
P_4: $a \oplus (b \otimes c) = (a \oplus b) \otimes (a \oplus c)$
P_4': $a \otimes (b \oplus c) = (a \otimes b) \oplus (a \otimes c)$
P_5: There exists an element Z in H, such that for every element a of H, $a \oplus Z = a$
P_5': There exists an element U in H, such that for every element a of H, $a \otimes U = a$
P_6: For every element a of H, there exists an element a' such that $a \oplus a' = U$ and $a \otimes a' = Z$

PROBABILITY

Definitions

A sample space S associated with an experiment is a set S of elements such that any outcome of the experiment corresponds to one and only one element of the set. An event E is a subset of a sample space S. An element in a sample space is called a sample point or a simple event (Unit subset of S).

Definition of Probability

If an experiment can occur in n mutually exclusive and equally likely ways, and if exactly m of these ways correspond to an event E, then the probability of E is given by

$$P(E) = \frac{m}{n}.$$

If E is a subset of S, and if to each unit subset of S, a non-negative number, called its probability, is assigned, and if E is the union of two or more different simple events, then the probability of E, denoted by $P(E)$, is the sum of the probabilities of those simple events whose union is E.

Marginal and Conditional Probability

Suppose a sample space S is partioned into rs disjoint subsets where the general subset is denoted by $E_i \cap F_j$. Then the marginal probability of E_i is defined as

$$P(E_i) = \sum_{j=1}^{s} P(E_i \cap F_j)$$

and the marginal probability of F_j is defined as

$$P(F_j) = \sum_{i=1}^{r} P(E_i \cap F_j) .$$

The conditional probability of E_i, given that F_j has occurred, is defined as

$$P(E_i/F_j) = \frac{P(E_i \cap F_j)}{P(F_j)}, \qquad P(F_j) \neq 0$$

and that of F_j, given that E_i has occurred, is defined as

$$P(F_j/E_i) = \frac{P(E_i \cap F_j)}{P(E_i)}, \qquad P(E_i) \neq 0 .$$

Probability Theorems

1. If ϕ is the null set, $P(\phi) = 0$.
2. If S is the sample space, $P(S) = 1$.
3. If E and F are two events

$$P(E \cup F) = P(E) + P(F) - P(E \cap F).$$

4. If E and F are mutually exclusive events,

$$P(E \cup F) = P(E) + P(F).$$

5. If E and E' are complementary events,

$$P(E) = 1 - P(E').$$

6. The conditional probability of an event E, given an event F, is denoted by $P(E/F)$ and is defined as

$$P(E/F) = \frac{P(E \cap F)}{P(F)},$$

where $P(F) \neq 0$.
7. Two events E and F are said to be independent if and only if

$$P(E \cap F) = P(E) \cdot P(F).$$

E is said to be statistically independent of F if $P(E/F) = P(E)$ and $P(F/E) = P(F)$.
8. The events $E_1, E_2, \ldots, E_n$ are called mutually independent for all combinations if and only if every combination of these events taken any number at a time is independent.

9. *Bayes Theorem.*

If $E_1, E_2, \ldots, E_n$ are n mutually exclusive events whose union is the sample space S, and E is any arbitrary event of S such that $P(E) \neq 0$, then

$$P(E_k/E) = \frac{P(E_k) \cdot P(E/E_k)}{\sum_{j=1}^{n} [P(E_j) \cdot P(E/E_j)]}$$

EXAMPLE: Two unbiased six sided dice, one red and one green, are tossed and the number of dots appearing on their upper faces is observed.

The sample space S consists of 36 elements, i.e.

$$S = \{(1, 1), (1, 2), \ldots, (6, 5), (6, 6)\}\ .$$

1. What is the probability of throwing a seven, denoted by the event A?

$$A = \{(1, 6)\} \cup \{(2, 5)\} \cup \{(3, 4)\} \cup \{(4, 3)\} \cup \{(5, 2)\} \cup \{(6, 1)\}$$
$$P(A) = \tfrac{1}{36} + \tfrac{1}{36} + \tfrac{1}{36} + \tfrac{1}{36} + \tfrac{1}{36} + \tfrac{1}{36} = \tfrac{1}{6}$$

2. What is the probability of throwing a seven or a ten? Denote by A the event "throwing a 7" and by B the event "throwing a ten" .

$$P(A) = \tfrac{1}{6} \qquad P(A \cup B) = P(A) + P(B)$$
$$P(B) = \tfrac{1}{12} \qquad\qquad = \tfrac{1}{6} + \tfrac{1}{12}$$
$$= \tfrac{1}{4}$$

3. What is the probability that the red die shows a number less than or equal to three and the green die shows a number greater than or equal to five? Denote by C the event "red die shows number ≤ 3" and by D the event "green die shows number ≥ 5" .

$$C \cap D = \{(1, 5), (2, 5), (3, 5), (1, 6), (2, 6), (3, 6)\}$$
$$P(C \cap D) = \tfrac{6}{36} = \tfrac{1}{6}$$

Note:

$$P(C) = \tfrac{18}{36} = \tfrac{1}{2}$$
$$P(D) = \tfrac{12}{36} = \tfrac{1}{3}$$
$$P(C) \cdot P(D) = \tfrac{1}{2} \cdot \tfrac{1}{3} = \tfrac{1}{6}$$

Thus $P(C \cap D) = P(C) \cdot P(D)$ and events C and D are independent.

4. What is the probability that the green die shows a one, given that the sum of the numbers on the two dice is less than four? Denote by E the event "green die shows 1" and by F the event "sum of numbers on dice <4" .

$$E = \{(1, 1), (1, 2), (1, 3), (1, 4), (1, 5), (1, 6)\}$$
$$F = \{(1, 1), (1, 2), (2, 1)\}$$
$$E \cap F = \{(1, 1), (1, 2)\}$$
$$P(E/F) = \frac{P(E \cap F)}{P(F)} = \frac{\frac{2}{36}}{\frac{3}{36}} = \tfrac{2}{3}$$

5. What is the probability that the sum of the numbers on the two dice is not seven?

$$P(A) = \tfrac{1}{6}$$
$$P(A') = 1 - \tfrac{1}{6} = \tfrac{5}{6}$$

Random Variable

A function whose domain is a sample space S and whose range is some set of real numbers is called a random variable, denoted by **X**. The function **X** transforms sample points of S into points on the x-axis. **X** will be called a discrete random variable if it is a random variable that assumes only a finite or denumerable number of values on the x-axis.

X will be called a continuous random variable if it assumes a continuum of values on the x-axis.

Probability Function (Discrete Case)

The random variable X will be called a discrete random variable if there exists a function f such that $f(x_i) \geq 0$ and $\sum_i f(x_i) = 1$ for $i = 1, 2, 3, \ldots$ and such that for any event E,

$$P(E) = P[\mathbf{X} \text{ is in } E] = \sum_E f(x)$$

where $\sum_E$ means sum $f(x)$ over those values x_i that are in E and where $f(x) = P[\mathbf{X} = x]$. The probability that the value of X is some real number x, is given by $f(x) = P[\mathbf{X} = x]$, where f is called the probability function of the random variable X.

Cumulative Distribution Function (Discrete Case)

The probability that the value of a random variable X is less than or equal to some real number x is defined as

$$\begin{aligned} F(x) &= P(\mathbf{X} \leq x) \\ &= \Sigma f(x_i), \qquad -\infty < x < \infty, \end{aligned}$$

where the summation extends over those values of i such that $x_i \leq x$.

Probability Density (Continuous Case)

The random variable X will be called a continuous random variable if there exists a function f such that $f(x) \geq 0$ and $\int_{-\infty}^{\infty} f(x)\,dx = 1$ for all x in interval $-\infty < x < \infty$ and such that for any event E

$$P(E) = P(\mathbf{X} \text{ is in } E) = \int_E f(x)\,dx.$$

$f(x)$ is called the probability density of the random variable X. The probability that X assumes any given value of x is equal to zero and the probability that it assumes a value on the interval from a to b, including or excluding either end point, is equal to

$$\int_a^b f(x)\,dx.$$

Cumulative Distribution Function (Continuous Case)

The probability that the value of a random variable X is less than or equal to some real number x is defined as

$$\begin{aligned} F(x) &= P(\mathbf{X} \leq x), \qquad -\infty < x < \infty \\ &= \int_{-\infty}^{x} f(x)\,dx. \end{aligned}$$

From the cumulative distribution, the density, if it exists, can be found from

$$f(x) = \frac{dF(x)}{dx}.$$

From the cumulative distribution

$$\begin{aligned} P(a \leq \mathbf{X} \leq b) &= P(\mathbf{X} \leq b) - P(\mathbf{X} \leq a) \\ &= F(b) - F(a) \end{aligned}$$

Mathematical Expectation

A. EXPECTED VALUE

Let **X** be a random variable with density $f(x)$. Then the expected value of **X**, $E(\mathbf{X})$, is defined to be

$$E(\mathbf{X}) = \sum_x xf(x)$$

if **X** is discrete and

$$E(\mathbf{X}) = \int_{-\infty}^{\infty} xf(x)\,dx$$

if **X** is continuous. The expected value of a function g of a random variable **X** is defined as

$$E[g(\mathbf{X})] = \sum_x g(x) \cdot f(x)$$

if **X** is discrete and

$$E[g(\mathbf{X})] = \int_{-\infty}^{\infty} g(x) \cdot f(x)\,dx$$

if **X** is continuous.

Theorems

1. $E[a\mathbf{X} + b\mathbf{Y}] = aE(\mathbf{X}) + bE(\mathbf{Y})$
2. $E[\mathbf{X} \cdot \mathbf{Y}] = E(\mathbf{X}) \cdot E(\mathbf{Y})$ if **X** and **Y** are statistically independent.

B. MOMENTS

a. Moments About the Origin. The moments about the origin of a probability distribution are the expected values of the random variable which has the given distribution. The rth moment of **X**, usually denoted by ν_r, is defined as

$$\mu'_r = E[\mathbf{X}^r] = \sum_x x^r f(x)$$

if **X** is discrete and

$$\mu'_r = E[\mathbf{X}^r] = \int_{-\infty}^{\infty} x^r f(x)\,dx$$

if **X** is continuous.

The first moment, μ'_1, is called the mean of the random variable **X** and is usually denoted by μ.

b. Moments About the Mean. The rth moment about the mean, usually denoted by μ_r, is defined as

$$\mu_r = E[(\mathbf{X} - \mu)^r] = \sum_x (x - \mu)^r f(x)$$

if **X** is discrete and

$$\mu_r = E[(\mathbf{X} - \mu)^r] = \int_{-\infty}^{\infty} (x - \mu)^r f(x)\,dx$$

if **X** is continuous.

The second moment about the mean, μ_2, is given by

$$\mu_2 = E[(\mathbf{X} - \mu)^2] = \mu'_2 - (\mu'_1)^2 = \mu'_2 - \mu^2$$

and is called the variance of the random variable **X**, and is denoted by σ^2. The square root of the variance, σ, is called the standard deviation.

Theorems

1. $\sigma^2_{c\mathbf{X}} = c^2\sigma^2_{\mathbf{X}}$
2. $\sigma^2_{c+\mathbf{X}} = \sigma^2_{\mathbf{X}}$
3. $\sigma^2_{a\mathbf{X}+b} = a^2\sigma^2_{\mathbf{X}}$

c. Factorial Moments. The rth factorial moment of a probability distribution is defined as

$$\mu'_{(r)} = E[\mathbf{X}^{[r]}] = \sum_x x^{[r]} f(x)$$

if $\mathbf{X}$ is discrete and

$$\mu'_{(r)} = E[\mathbf{X}^{[r]}] = \int_{-\infty}^{\infty} x^{[r]} f(x)\, dx$$

if $\mathbf{X}$ is continuous, where the symbol $x^{[r]}$ denotes the factorial expression

$$x^{[r]} = x(x-1)(x-2)\cdots(x-r+1),\ r = 1, 2, 3, \ldots .$$

C. Generating Functions

a. Moment Generating Functions. The moment generating function (m.g.f.) of the random variable $\mathbf{X}$ is defined as

$$m_{\mathbf{x}}(t) = E(e^{t\mathbf{X}}) = \sum_x e^{tx} f(x)$$

if $\mathbf{X}$ is discrete and

$$m_{\mathbf{x}}(t) = E(e^{t\mathbf{X}}) = \int_{-\infty}^{\infty} e^{tx} f(x)\, dx$$

if $\mathbf{X}$ is continuous.
$E(e^{t\mathbf{X}})$ is the expected value of $e^{t\mathbf{X}}$. If $m_{\mathbf{x}}(t)$ and its derivatives exist, $|t| < h^2$, the rth moment about the origin is

$$\mu'_r = m_{\mathbf{x}}^{(r)}(0), \qquad r = 0, 1, 2, \ldots$$

where $m_{\mathbf{x}}^{(r)}(0)$ is the rth derivative of $m_{\mathbf{x}}(t)$ with respect to t, evaluated at $t = 0$. For

$$\begin{aligned} m_{\mathbf{x}}(t) &= E(e^{t\mathbf{X}}) \\ &= E\left[1 + \mathbf{X}t + \frac{(\mathbf{X}t)^2}{2!} + \cdots\right] \\ &= 1 + \mu'_1 t + \mu'_2 \frac{t^2}{2!} + \cdots . \end{aligned}$$

Thus, the moments μ'_r appear as coefficients of $\frac{t^r}{r!}$, and $m_x(t)$ may be regarded as generating the moments μ'_r. The moments μ_r may be generated by the generating function

$$M_{\mathbf{x}}(t) = E[e^{t(\mathbf{X}-\mu)}] = e^{-\mu t} E(e^{t\mathbf{X}}) = e^{-\mu t} m_{\mathbf{x}}(t) .$$

b. Factorial Moment Generating Function. The factorial moment generating function is defined as

$$E(t^{\mathbf{X}}) = \sum_x t^x f(x) \qquad \text{(probability generating function)}$$

if $\mathbf{X}$ is discrete and

$$E(t^{\mathbf{X}}) = \int_{-\infty}^{\infty} t^x f(x)\, dx$$

if $\mathbf{X}$ is continuous.

The rth factorial moment is obtained from the factorial moment generating function by differentiating it r times with respect to t and then evaluating the result when $t = 1$.

Theorems

1. If c is a constant, the m.g.f. of $c + \mathbf{X}$ is $e^{ct} m_{\mathbf{x}}(t)$.
2. If c is a constant, the m.g.f. of $c\mathbf{X}$ is $m_{\mathbf{x}}(ct)$.

3. If $\mathbf{Y} = \sum_{i=1}^{n} \mathbf{X}_i$, and $m_x(t)$ is the m.g.f. of $\mathbf{X}_i$, where $\mathbf{X}_1, \ldots, \mathbf{X}_n$ is a random sample from $f(x)$, then the m.g.f. of $\mathbf{Y}$ is $[m_x(t)]^n$.

D. Cumulant Generating Function

Let $m_x(t)$ be a m.g.f. If $\ln m_x(t)$ can be expanded in the form

$$c(t) = \ln m_x(t) = \kappa_1 t + \kappa_2 \frac{t^2}{2!} + \kappa_3 \frac{t^3}{3!} + \cdots + \kappa_r \frac{t^r}{r!} + \cdots,$$

then $c(t)$ is called the cumulant generating function (semi-invariant generating function) and κ_r are called the cumulants (semi-invariants) of a distribution.

$$\kappa_r = c^{(r)}(0)$$

where $c^{(r)}(0)$ is the rth derivative of $c(t)$ with respect to t evaluated at $t = 0$.

E. Characteristic Functions

The characteristic function of a distribution is defined as

$$\phi(t) = E(e^{it\mathbf{X}}) = \sum_x e^{itx} \cdot f(x)$$

if $\mathbf{X}$ is discrete and

$$\phi(t) = E(e^{it\mathbf{X}}) = \int_{-\infty}^{\infty} e^{itx} \cdot f(x)\, dx$$

if $\mathbf{X}$ is continuous.
Here t is a real number, $i^2 = -1$, and $e^{it\mathbf{X}} = \cos(t\mathbf{X}) + i \sin(t\mathbf{X})$. The characteristic function also generates moments, if they exist for

$$i^r \mu_r' = \phi^{(r)}(0)$$

where $\phi^{(r)}(0)$ is the rth derivative of $\phi(t)$ with respect to t evaluated at $t = 0$.

Multivariate Distributions

A. Discrete Case

The k-dimensional random variable $(\mathbf{X}_1, \mathbf{X}_2, \ldots, \mathbf{X}_k)$ is a k-dimensional discrete random variable if it assumes values only at a finite or denumerable number of points $(x_1, x_2, \ldots, x_k)$. Define

$$P[\mathbf{X}_1 = x_1, \mathbf{X}_2 = x_2, \ldots, \mathbf{X}_k = x_k] = f(x_1, x_2, \ldots, x_k)$$

for every value that the random variable can assume. $f(x_1, x_2, \ldots, x_k)$ is called the joint density of the k-dimensional random variable. If E is any subset of the set of values that the random variable can assume, then

$$P(E) = P[(\mathbf{X}_1, \mathbf{X}_2, \ldots, \mathbf{X}_k) \text{ is in } E] = \sum_E f(x_1, x_2, \ldots, x_k)$$

where the sum is over all those points in E. The cumulative distribution is defined as

$$F(x_1, x_2, \ldots, x_k) = \sum_{x_1} \sum_{x_2} \cdots \sum_{x_k} f(x_1, x_2, \ldots, x_k).$$

B. Continuous Case

The k random variables $\mathbf{X}_1, \mathbf{X}_2, \ldots, \mathbf{X}_k$ are said to be jointly distributed if there exists a function f such that $f(x_1, x_2, \ldots, x_k) \geq 0$ for all $-\infty < x_i < \infty$,

$i = 1, 2, \ldots, k$ and such that for any event E

$$P(E) = P[(\mathbf{X}_1, \mathbf{X}_2, \ldots, \mathbf{X}_k) \text{ is in } E] = \int_E f(x_1, x_2, \ldots, x_k)\, dx_1\, dx_2 \cdots dx_k.$$

$f(x_1, x_2, \ldots, x_k)$ is called the joint density of the random variables $\mathbf{X}_1, \mathbf{X}_2, \ldots, \mathbf{X}_k$.

The cumulative distribution is defined as

$$F(x_1, x_2, \ldots, x_k) = \int_{-\infty}^{x_1} \int_{-\infty}^{x_2} \cdots \int_{-\infty}^{x_k} f(x_1, x_2, \ldots, x_k)\, dx_k \cdots dx_2\, dx_1 .$$

Given the cumulative distribution, the density may be found by

$$f(x_1, x_2, \ldots, x_k) = \frac{\partial}{\partial x_1} \cdot \frac{\partial}{\partial x_2} \cdots \frac{\partial}{\partial x_k} F(x_1, x_2, \ldots, x_k) .$$

Moments

The rth moment of $\mathbf{X}_i$, say, is defined as

$$E(\mathbf{X}_i^r) = \sum_{x_1} \sum_{x_2} \cdots \sum_{x_k} x_i^r f(x_1, x_2, \ldots, x_k)$$

if the $\mathbf{X}_i$ are discrete and

$$E(\mathbf{X}_i^r) = \int_{-\infty}^{\infty} \int_{-\infty}^{\infty} \cdots \int_{-\infty}^{\infty} x_i^r f(x_1, x_2, \ldots, x_k)\, dx_k \cdots dx_2\, dx_1$$

if the $\mathbf{X}_i$ are continuous.

Joint moments about the origin are defined as

$$E(\mathbf{X}_1^{r_1} \mathbf{X}_2^{r_2} \cdots \mathbf{X}_k^{r_k})$$

where $r_1 + r_2 + \cdots + r_k$ is the order of the moment.

Joint moments about the mean are defined as

$$E[(\mathbf{X}_1 - \mu_1)^{r_1} (\mathbf{X}_2 - \mu_2)^{r_2} \cdots (\mathbf{X}_k - \mu_k)^{r_k}].$$

Marginal and Conditional Distributions

If the random variables $\mathbf{X}_1, \mathbf{X}_2, \ldots, \mathbf{X}_k$ have the joint density function $f(x_1, x_2, \ldots, x_k)$, then the marginal distribution of the subset of the random variables, say, $\mathbf{X}_1. \mathbf{X}_2, \ldots, \mathbf{X}_p$ $(p < k)$, is given by

$$g(x_1, x_2, \ldots, x_p) = \sum_{x_{p+1}} \sum_{x_{p+2}} \cdots \sum_{x_k} f(x_1, x_2, \ldots, x_k)$$

if the X's are discrete, and

$$g(x_1, x_2, \ldots, x_p) = \int_{-\infty}^{\infty} \int_{-\infty}^{\infty} \cdots \int_{-\infty}^{\infty} f(x_1, x_2, \ldots, x_k)\, dx_{p+1} \cdots dx_{k-1}\, dx_k$$

if the X's are continuous.

The conditional distribution of a certain subset of the random variables is the joint distribution of this subset under the condition that the remaining variables are given certain values. The conditional distribution of $\mathbf{X}_1, \mathbf{X}_2, \ldots, \mathbf{X}_p$ given $\mathbf{X}_{p+1}, \mathbf{X}_{p+2}, \ldots, \mathbf{X}_k$ is

$$h(x_1, x_2, \ldots, x_p | x_{p+1}, x_{p+2}, \ldots, x_k) = \frac{f(x_1, x_2, \ldots, x_k)}{g(x_{p+1}, x_{p+2}, \ldots, x_k)}$$

if $g(x_{p+1}, x_{p+2}, \ldots, x_k) \neq 0$.

The variance σ_{ii} of $\mathbf{X}_i$ and the covariance σ_{ij} of $\mathbf{X}_i$ and $\mathbf{X}_j$ are given by

$$\sigma_{ii} = \sigma_i^2 = E[(\mathbf{X}_i - \mu_i)^2]$$

and

$$\sigma_{ij} = \rho_{ij}\sigma_i\sigma_j = E[(\mathbf{X}_i - \mu_i)(\mathbf{X}_j - \mu_j)]$$

where ρ_{ij} is the correlation coefficient and σ_i and σ_j are the standard deviations of $\mathbf{X}_i$ and $\mathbf{X}_j$.

A joint m.g.f. is defined as

$$m(t_1, t_2, \ldots, t_k) = E[e^{t_1\mathbf{X}_1 + t_2\mathbf{X}_2 + \cdots + t_k\mathbf{X}_k}]$$

if it exists for all values of t_i such that $|t_i| < h^2$.

The rth moment of $\mathbf{X}_i$ may be obtained by differentiating the m.g.f. r times with respect to t_i and then evaluating the result when all t's are set equal to zero. Similarly, a joint moment would be found by differentiating the m.g.f. r_1 times with respect to t_1, $\ldots$, r_k times with respect to t_k, and then evaluating the result when all t's are set equal to zero.

Probability Distributions

A. Discrete Case

1. *Discrete Uniform Distribution.* If the random variable $\mathbf{X}$ has a probability function given by

$$P(\mathbf{X} = x) = f(x) = \frac{1}{n}, \qquad x = x_1, x_2, \ldots, x_n,$$

then the variable $\mathbf{X}$ is said to possess a discrete uniform distribution.

Properties

When $x_i = i$ for $i = 1, 2, \ldots,$ and n

$$\text{Mean} = \mu = \frac{n+1}{2}$$

$$\text{Variance} = \sigma^2 = \frac{n^2 - 1}{12}$$

$$\text{Standard Deviation} = \sigma = \sqrt{\frac{n^2 - 1}{12}}$$

$$\text{Moment Generating Function} = m_x(t) = \frac{e^t(1 - e^{nt})}{n(1 - e^t)}$$

2. *Binomial Distribution.* If the random variable $\mathbf{X}$ has a probability function given by

$$P(\mathbf{X} = x) = f(x) = \binom{n}{x} \theta^x (1 - \theta)^{n-x}, \qquad x = 0, 1, 2, \ldots, n$$

where

$$\binom{n}{x} = \frac{n!}{x!(n - x)!},$$

then the variable $\mathbf{X}$ is said to possess a binomial distribution. $f(x)$ is the general term of the expansion of $[\theta + (1 - \theta)]^n$.

Properties

$$\text{Mean} = \mu = n\theta$$

$$\text{Variance} = \sigma^2 = n\theta(1 - \theta)$$

$$\text{Standard Deviation} = \sigma = \sqrt{n\theta(1 - \theta)}$$

$$\text{Moment Generating Function} = m_{\mathbf{x}}(t) = [\theta e^t + (1 - \theta)]^n$$

3. *Geometric Distribution.* If the random variable **X** has a probability function given by

$$P(\mathbf{X} = x) = f(x) = \theta(1 - \theta)^{x-1}, \qquad x = 1, 2, 3, \ldots,$$

then the variable **X** is said to possess a geometric distribution.

Properties

$$\text{Mean} = \mu = \frac{1}{\theta}$$

$$\text{Variance} = \sigma^2 = \frac{1 - \theta}{\theta^2}$$

$$\text{Standard Deviation} = \sigma = \sqrt{\frac{1 - \theta}{\theta^2}}$$

$$\text{Moment Generating Function} = m_x(t) = \frac{\theta e^t}{1 - e^t(1 - \theta)}$$

4. *Multinomial Distribution.* If a set of random variables $\mathbf{X}_1, \mathbf{X}_2, \ldots, \mathbf{X}_n$ has a probability function given by

$$P(\mathbf{X}_1 = x_1, \mathbf{X}_2 = x_2, \ldots, \mathbf{X}_n = x_n) = f(x_1, x_2, \ldots, x_n) = \frac{N!}{\prod_{i=1}^{n} x_i!} \prod_{i=1}^{n} \theta_i^{x_i}$$

where x_i are positive integers and each $\theta_i > 0$ for $i = 1, 2, \ldots, n$ and

$$\sum_{i=1}^{n} \theta_i = 1, \qquad \sum_{i=1}^{n} x_i = N,$$

then the joint distribution of $\mathbf{X}_1, \mathbf{X}_2, \ldots, \mathbf{X}_n$ is called the multinomial distribution. $f(x_1, x_2, \ldots, x_n)$ is the general term of the expansion of $(\theta_1 + \theta_2 + \cdots + \theta_n)^N$.

Properties

$$\text{Mean of } \mathbf{X}_i = \mu_i = N\theta_i$$

$$\text{Variance of } \mathbf{X}_i = \sigma_i^2 = N\theta_i(1 - \theta_i)$$

$$\text{Covariance of } \mathbf{X}_i \text{ and } \mathbf{X}_j = \sigma_{ij}^2 = -N\theta_i\theta_j$$

$$\text{Joint Moment Generating Function} = (\theta_1 e^{t_1} + \cdots + \theta_n e^{t_n})^N$$

5. *Poisson Distribution.* If the random variable **X** has a probability function given by

$$P(\mathbf{X} = x) = f(x) = \frac{e^{-\lambda}\lambda^x}{x!}, \qquad \lambda > 0,\ x = 0, 1, \ldots,$$

then the variable **X** is said to possess a Poisson distribution.

Properties

$$\text{Mean} = \mu = \lambda$$

$$\text{Variance} = \sigma^2 = \lambda$$

$$\text{Standard Deviation} = \sigma = \sqrt{\lambda}$$

$$\text{Moment Generating Function} = m_x(t) = e^{\lambda(e^t - 1)}$$

6. *Hypergeometric Distribution.* If the random variable **X** has a probability function given by

$$P(\mathbf{X} = x) = f(x) = \frac{\binom{k}{x}\binom{N-k}{n-x}}{\binom{N}{n}}, \qquad x = 0, 1, 2, \ldots, [n, k],$$

where $[n, k]$ means the smaller of the two numbers n, k, then the variable $\mathbf{X}$ is said to possess a hypergeometric distribution.

Properties

$$\text{Mean} = \mu = \frac{kn}{N}$$

$$\text{Variance} = \sigma^2 = \frac{k(N-k)n(N-n)}{N^2(N-1)}$$

$$\text{Standard Deviation} = \sigma = \sqrt{\frac{k(N-k)n(N-n)}{N^2(N-1)}}$$

7. *Negative Binomial Distribution*. If the random variable $\mathbf{X}$ has a probability function given by

$$P(\mathbf{X} = x) = f(x) = \binom{x+r-1}{r-1}\theta^r(1-\theta)^x, \qquad x = 0, 1, 2, \ldots;$$

then the variable $\mathbf{X}$ is said to possess a negative binomial distribution, known also as the Pascal or Pólya distribution.

Properties

$$\text{Mean} = \mu = \frac{r}{\theta}$$

$$\text{Variance} = \sigma^2 = \frac{r}{\theta}\left(\frac{1}{\theta} - 1\right) = \frac{r(1-\theta)}{\theta^2}$$

$$\text{Standard Deviation} = \sigma = \sqrt{\frac{r}{\theta}\left(\frac{1}{\theta} - 1\right)} = \sqrt{\frac{r(1-\theta)}{\theta^2}}$$

$$\text{Moment Generating Function} = m_x(t) = e^{tr}\theta^r[1 - (1-\theta)e^t]^{-r}$$

B. Continuous Case

1. *Uniform Distribution*. A random variable $\mathbf{X}$ is said to be distributed as the uniform distribution if the density function is given by

$$f(x) = \frac{1}{\beta - \alpha}, \qquad \alpha < x < \beta,$$

where α and β are parameters with $\alpha < \beta$.

Properties

$$\text{Mean} = \mu = \frac{\alpha + \beta}{2}$$

$$\text{Variance} = \sigma^2 = \frac{(\beta - \alpha)^2}{12}$$

$$\text{Standard Deviation} = \sigma = \sqrt{\frac{(\beta - \alpha)^2}{12}}$$

$$\text{Moment Generating Function} = m_x(t) = \frac{2}{(\beta - \alpha)t}\sin\left[\frac{(\beta - \alpha)t}{2}\right]e^{\frac{\alpha+\beta}{2}t}$$

2. *Normal Distribution*. A random variable $\mathbf{X}$ is said to be normally distributed if its density function is given by

$$f(x) = \frac{1}{\sqrt{2\pi}\,\sigma}e^{-(x-\mu)^2/2\sigma^2}, \qquad -\infty < x < \infty$$

where μ and σ are parameters, called the mean and the standard deviation or the random variable $\mathbf{X}$, respectively.

Properties

$$\text{Mean} = \mu$$
$$\text{Variance} = \sigma^2$$
$$\text{Standard Deviation} = \sigma$$
$$\text{Moment Generating Function} = m_{\mathbf{x}}(t) = e^{t\mu + \frac{\sigma^2 t^2}{2}}$$

Cumulative Distribution

$$F(x) = \int_{-\infty}^{x} \frac{1}{\sqrt{2\pi}\,\sigma} e^{-(x-\mu)^2/2\sigma^2}\, dx$$

Set $y = \dfrac{x-\mu}{\sigma}$ to obtain the cumulative standard normal.

3. *Gamma Distribution.* A random variable **X** is said to be distributed as the gamma distribution if the density function is given by

$$f(x) = \frac{1}{\Gamma(\alpha+1)\beta^{\alpha+1}} x^{\alpha} e^{-x/\beta}, \qquad 0 < x < \infty$$

where α and β are parameters with $\alpha > -1$ and $\beta > 0$.

Properties

$$\text{Mean} = \mu = \beta(\alpha+1)$$
$$\text{Variance} = \sigma^2 = \beta^2(\alpha+1)$$
$$\text{Standard Deviation} = \sigma = \beta\sqrt{\alpha+1}$$
$$\text{Moment Generating Function} = m_{\mathbf{x}}(t) = (1-\beta t)^{-(\alpha+1)}, \qquad t < \frac{1}{\beta}.$$

4. *Exponential Distribution.* A random variable **X** is said to be distributed as the exponential distribution if the density function is given by

$$f(x) = \frac{1}{\theta} e^{-x/\theta}, \qquad x > 0$$

where θ is a parameter and $\theta > 0$.

Properties

$$\text{Mean} = \mu = \theta$$
$$\text{Variance} = \sigma^2 = \theta^2$$
$$\text{Standard Deviation} = \sigma = \sqrt{\theta^2}$$
$$\text{Moment Generating Function} = m_x(t) = (1-\theta t)^{-1}$$

5. *Beta Distribution.* A random variable **X** is said to be distributed as the beta distribution if the density function is given by

$$f(x) = \frac{\Gamma(\alpha+\beta+2)}{\Gamma(\alpha+1)\Gamma(\beta+1)} x^{\alpha}(1-x)^{\beta}, \qquad 0 < x < 1$$

where α and β are parameters with $\alpha > -1$ and $\beta > -1$.

Properties

$$\text{Mean} = \mu = \frac{\alpha+1}{\alpha+\beta+2}$$

$$\text{Variance} = \sigma^2 = \frac{(\alpha+1)(\beta+1)}{(\alpha+\beta+2)^2(\alpha+\beta+3)}$$

$$r\text{th moment about the origin} = \nu_r = \frac{\Gamma(\alpha+\beta+2)\Gamma(\alpha+r+1)}{\Gamma(\alpha+\beta+r+2)\Gamma(\alpha+1)}.$$

Sampling Distributions

Population—A finite or infinite set of elements of a random variable **X**.

Random Sample—If the random variables $\mathbf{X}_1, \mathbf{X}_2, \ldots, \mathbf{X}_n$ have a joint density,

$$g(x_1, x_2, \ldots, x_n) = f(x_1)f(x_2) \cdots f(x_n)$$

where the density of each $\mathbf{X}_i$ is $f(x)$, then $\mathbf{X}_1, \mathbf{X}_2, \ldots, \mathbf{X}_n$ is said to be a random sample of size n from the population with density $f(x)$.

Sampling Distributions

A random sample is selected from a population in which the form of the probability function is known, and from the joint density of the random variables a distribution, called the sampling distribution, of a function of the random variables is derived.

1. *Chi-Square Distribution.* If $\mathbf{Y}_1, \mathbf{Y}_2, \ldots, \mathbf{Y}_n$ are normally and independently distributed with mean 0 and variance 1, then

$$\chi^2 = \sum_{i=1}^{n} \mathbf{Y}_i^2$$

is distributed as Chi-Square (χ^2) with n degrees of freedom. The density function is given by

$$f(\chi^2) = \frac{(\chi^2)^{\frac{1}{2}(n-2)}}{2^{\frac{n}{2}}\Gamma\left(\frac{n}{2}\right)} e^{-\chi^2/2}, \qquad 0 < \chi^2 < \infty .$$

Proportioo

$$\text{Mean} = \mu = n$$
$$\text{Variance} = \sigma^2 = 2n$$

Reproductive Property of χ^2 - Distribution

If $\chi_1^2, \chi_2^2, \ldots, \chi_k^2$ are independently distributed according to χ^2 - distributions with $n_1, n_2, \ldots, n_k$ degrees of freedom, respectively, then $\sum_{j=1}^{k} \chi_j^2$ is distributed according to a χ^2 - distribution with $n = \sum_{j=1}^{k} n_j$ degrees of freedom.

2. *Snedecor's F-Distribution.* If a random variable **X** is distributed as χ^2 with m degrees of freedom (χ_m^2) and a random variable **Y** is distributed as χ^2 with n degrees of freedom (χ_n^2) and if **X** and **Y** are independent, then $F = \dfrac{\mathbf{X}/m}{\mathbf{Y}/n}$ is distributed as Snedecor's F with m and n degrees of freedom, denoted by $F(m, n)$. The density function of the F-distribution is given by

$$f(F) = \frac{\Gamma\left(\frac{m+n}{2}\right)\left(\frac{m}{n}\right)^{m/2} F^{(m-2)/2}}{\Gamma\left(\frac{m}{2}\right)\Gamma\left(\frac{n}{2}\right)\left(1 + \frac{m}{n}F\right)^{(m+n)/2}}, \qquad 0 < F < \infty .$$

Properties

$$\text{Mean} = \mu = \frac{n}{n-2}, \qquad n > 2$$

$$\text{Variance} = \sigma^2 = \frac{2n^2(m+n-2)}{m(n-2)^2(n-4)}, \qquad n > 4\ .$$

The transformation $w = \dfrac{mF/n}{1 + \dfrac{mF}{n}}$ transforms the F-density into a Beta density.

3. *Student's t-Distribution.* If a random variable **X** is normally distributed with mean 0 and variance σ^2, and if $\mathbf{Y}^2/\sigma^2$ is distributed as χ^2 with n degrees of freedom and if **X** and **Y** are independent, then

$$t = \frac{\mathbf{X}\sqrt{n}}{\mathbf{Y}}$$

is distributed as Student's t with n degrees of freedom. The density function is given by

$$f(t) = \frac{\Gamma\left(\dfrac{n+1}{2}\right)}{\sqrt{n\pi}\,\Gamma\left(\dfrac{n}{2}\right)\left(1 + \dfrac{t^2}{n}\right)^{\frac{1}{2}(n+1)}}, \qquad -\infty < t < \infty\ .$$

Properties

$$\text{Mean} = \mu = 0$$

$$\text{Variance} = \sigma^2 = \frac{n}{n-2}, \qquad n > 2\ .$$

SUMMARY OF SIGNIFICANCE TESTS: TESTING FOR THE VALUE OF A SPECIFIED PARAMETER

Hypothesis	Conditions	Test Statistic	Distribution of Test Statistic	Critical Region	Table in Handbook	Sample Size
1. $\mu = \mu_0$	Known σ	$z = \dfrac{(\bar{x} - \mu_0)\sqrt{n}}{\sigma}$	Normal	$z > z_\alpha$ if we wish to reject when $\mu > \mu_0$ $z < -z_\alpha$ if we wish to reject when $\mu < \mu_0$ $\|z\| > z_{\alpha/2}$ if we wish to reject when $\mu \neq \mu_0$	II.1 II.1 II.1	II.5 *c*) and *d*) II.5 *c*) and *d*) II.5 *a*) and *b*)
2. $\mu = \mu_0$	Unknown σ	$t = \dfrac{(\bar{x} - \mu_0)\sqrt{n}}{s}$	Student's t – with $(n - 1)$ d.f.	$t > t_{\alpha;n-1}$ if we wish to reject when $\mu > \mu_0$ $t < -t_{\alpha;n-1}$ if we wish to reject when $\mu < \mu_0$ $\|t\| > t_{\alpha/2;n-1}$ if we wish to reject when $\mu \neq \mu_0$	IV.1 IV.1 IV.1	IV.5 *c*) and *d*) IV.5 *c*) and *d*) IV.5 *a*) and *b*)
3. $\sigma = \sigma_0$		$\chi^2 = \dfrac{(n - 1)s^2}{\sigma_0^2}$	χ^2 with $n - 1$ d.f.	$\chi^2 > \chi^2_{\alpha;n-1}$ if we wish to reject when $\sigma > \sigma_0$ $\chi^2 < \chi^2_{1-\alpha;n-1}$ if we wish to reject when $\sigma < \sigma_0$ $\chi^2 < \chi^2_{1-\alpha/2;n-1}$ or $\chi^2 > \chi^2_{\alpha/2;n-1}$ if we wish to reject when $\sigma \neq \sigma_0$	V.1 V.1 V.1	V.4 *c*) and *d*) V.4 *e*) and *f*) V.4 *a*) and *b*)
4. $\theta = \theta_0$	Large sample. (For small samples, exact tests are based on tables of binomial probabilities)	$z = \dfrac{\frac{x}{n} - \theta_0}{\sqrt{\dfrac{\theta_0(1 - \theta_0)}{n}}}$ Continuity correction: Replace x in numerator of formula with $x - \frac{1}{2}$ or $x + \frac{1}{2}$, whichever makes z numerically smallest.	Normal	$z > z_\alpha$ if we wish to reject when $\theta > \theta_0$ $z < -z_\alpha$ if we wish to reject when $\theta < \theta_0$ $\|z\| > -z_{\alpha/2}$ if we wish to reject when $\theta \neq \theta_0$	II.1 II.1 II.1	II.5 *c*) and *d*) II.5 *c*) and *d*) II.5 *a*) and *b*)

SUMMARY OF SIGNIFICANCE TESTS: COMPARISON OF TWO POPULATIONS

Hypothesis	Conditions	Test Statistic	Distribution of Test Statistic	Critical Region	Table in Handbook	Sample Size
1. $\mu_x = \mu_y$	Known σ_x and σ_y	$z = \dfrac{\bar{x} - \bar{y}}{\sqrt{\dfrac{\sigma_x^2}{n_x} + \dfrac{\sigma_y^2}{n_y}}}$	Normal	$z > z_\alpha$ if we wish to reject when $\mu_x > \mu_y$ $z < -z_\alpha$ if we wish to reject when $\mu_x < \mu_y$ $\lvert z\rvert > z_{\alpha/2}$ if we wish to reject when $\mu_x \neq \mu_y$	II.1 II.1 II.1	II.5 *c*) and *d*) II.5 *c*) and *d*) II.5 *a*) and *b*)
2. $\mu_x = \mu_y$	Unknown σ_x and σ_y $\sigma_x = \sigma_y$	$t = \dfrac{\bar{x} - \bar{y}}{\sqrt{\dfrac{(n_x - 1)s_x^2 + (n_y - 1)s_y^2}{n_x + n_y - 2}}\sqrt{\dfrac{1}{n_x} + \dfrac{1}{n_y}}}$	Student's t-with $n - 1$ d.f.	$t > t_{\alpha;n_x+n_y-2}$ if we wish to reject when $\mu_x > \mu_y$ $t < -t_{\alpha;n_x+n_y-2}$ if we wish to reject when $\mu_x < \mu_y$ $\lvert t\rvert > t_{\alpha/2;n_x+n_y-2}$ if we wish to reject when $\mu_x \neq \mu_y$	IV.1 IV.1 IV.1	IV.5 *c*) and *d*) IV.5 *c*) and *d*) IV.5 *a*) and *b*)
3. $\mu_x = \mu_y$	Unknown σ_x and σ_y $\sigma_x \neq \sigma_y$	$t = \dfrac{\bar{x} - \bar{y}}{\sqrt{\dfrac{s_x^2}{n_x} + \dfrac{s_y^2}{n_y}}}$	Student's t-with ν d.f.	$t > t_{\alpha;\nu}$ if we wish to reject when $\mu_x > \mu_y$ $t < -t_{\alpha;\nu}$ if we wish to reject when $\mu_x < \mu_y$ $\lvert t\rvert > t_{\alpha/2;\nu}$ if we wish to reject when $\mu_x \neq \mu_y$ where d.f. ν is given by closest integer to $\nu = -2 + \dfrac{\left(\dfrac{s_x^2}{n_x} + \dfrac{s_y^2}{n_y}\right)^2}{\dfrac{\left(\dfrac{s_x^2}{n_x}\right)^2}{n_x + 1} + \dfrac{\left(\dfrac{s_y^2}{n_y}\right)^2}{n_y + 1}}$	IV.1 IV.1 IV.1	IV.5 *c*) and *d*) IV.5 *c*) and *d*) IV.5 *a*) and *b*)
4. $\mu_x = \mu_y$	Correlated pairs	$t = \dfrac{\bar{d}\sqrt{n}}{s_d}$ where $d_i = x_i - y_i$	Student's t-with $n - 1$ d.f.	$t > t_{\alpha;n-1}$ if we wish to reject when $\mu_x > \mu_y$ $t < -t_{\alpha;n-1}$ if we wish to reject when $\mu_x < \mu_y$ $\lvert t\rvert > t_{\alpha/2;n-1}$ if we wish to reject when $\mu_x \neq \mu_y$	IV.1 IV.1 IV.1	IV.5 *c*) and *d*) IV.5 *c*) and *d*) IV.5 *a*) and *b*)
5. $\sigma_x^2 = \sigma_y^2$		$F = \dfrac{s_x^2}{s_y^2}$ In a two-sided test, put larger mean square in the numerator	F with $n_x - 1$ and $n_y - 1$ d.f.	$F > F_{\alpha;n_x-1,n_y-1}$ if we wish to reject when $\sigma_x > \sigma_y$ $F > F_{\alpha/2;n_x-1,n_y-1}$ if $s_x^2 > s_y^2$ and we wish to reject when $\sigma_x \neq \sigma_y$ $F > F_{\alpha/2;n_y-1,n_x-1}$ if $s_x^2 < s_y^2$ and we wish to reject when $\sigma_x \neq \sigma_y$	VI.1 VI.1 VI.1	VI.4 *c*) and *d*) VI.4 *c*) and *d*) VI.4 *a*) and *b*)
6. $\theta_1 = \theta_2$	Large sample	$z = \dfrac{\dfrac{x_1}{n_1} - \dfrac{x_2}{n_2}}{\sqrt{\dfrac{\dfrac{x_1}{n_1}\left(1 - \dfrac{x_1}{n_1}\right)}{n_1} + \dfrac{\dfrac{x_2}{n_2}\left(1 - \dfrac{x_2}{n_2}\right)}{n_2}}}$ Continuity Correction: Replace x in numerator of formula with $x - \frac{1}{2}$ or $x + \frac{1}{2}$, whichever makes z numerically smallest.	Normal	$z > z_\alpha$ if we wish to reject when $\theta_1 > \theta_2$ $z < -z_\alpha$ if we wish to reject when $\theta_1 < \theta_2$ $\lvert z\rvert > z_{\alpha/2}$ if we wish to reject when $\theta_1 \neq \theta_2$	II.1 II.1 II.1	II.5 *c*) and *d*) II.5 *c*) and *d*) II.5 *a*) and *b*)

SUMMARY OF CONFIDENCE INTERVALS

Parameter	Conditions	Point Estimate	Confidence Interval	Table in Handbook
1. μ	Known σ	$\bar{x}$	$\bar{x} - z_{\alpha/2}\frac{\sigma}{\sqrt{n}} < \mu < \bar{x} + z_{\alpha/2}\frac{\sigma}{\sqrt{n}}$	Normal
2. μ	Unknown σ	$\bar{x}$	$\bar{x} - t_{\alpha/2}\frac{s}{\sqrt{n}} < \mu < \bar{x} + t_{\alpha/2}\frac{s}{\sqrt{n}}$	Student's t with $n - 1$ d.f.
3. $\mu_x - \mu_y$	$\sigma_x = \sigma_y$ known	$\bar{x} - \bar{y}$	$\bar{x} - \bar{y} - z_{\alpha/2}\sqrt{\frac{\sigma_x^2}{n_x} + \frac{\sigma_y^2}{n_y}} < \mu_x - \mu_y < \bar{x} - \bar{y} + z_{\alpha/2}\sqrt{\frac{\sigma_x^2}{n_x} + \frac{\sigma_y^2}{n_y}}$	Normal
4. $\mu_x - \mu_y$	$\sigma_x = \sigma_y$ unknown	$\bar{x} - \bar{y}$	$\bar{x} - \bar{y} - t_{\alpha/2}\frac{\sqrt{(n_x - 1)s_x^2 + (n_y - 1)s_y^2}}{\sqrt{\frac{n_x n_y(n_x + n_y - 2)}{n_x + n_y}}} < \mu_x - \mu_y < \bar{x} - \bar{y} + t_{\alpha/2}\frac{\sqrt{(n_x - 1)s_x^2 + (n_y - 1)s_y^2}}{\sqrt{\frac{n_x n_y(n_x + n_y - 2)}{n_x + n_y}}}$	Student's t with $n_x + n_y - 2$ d.f.
5. $\mu_d = \mu_x - \mu_y$	Correlated pairs σ_x and σ_y unknown	$\bar{d} = \bar{x} - \bar{y}$	$\bar{d} - t_{\alpha/2}\frac{\sigma_d}{\sqrt{n}} < \mu_d < \bar{d} + t_{\alpha/2}\frac{\sigma_d}{\sqrt{n}}$	Student's t with $n - 1$ d.f.
6. σ		s	$\sqrt{\frac{(n-1)s^2}{\chi^2_{\alpha/2;n-1}}} < \sigma < \sqrt{\frac{(n-1)s^2}{\chi^2_{1-\alpha/2;n-1}}}$	χ^2 with $n - 1$ d.f.
7. $\frac{\sigma_x^2}{\sigma_y^2}$		$\frac{s_x^2}{s_y^2}$	$\frac{s_x^2}{s_y^2}\frac{1}{F_{\alpha/2;n_x-1,n_y-1}} < \frac{\sigma_x^2}{\sigma_y^2} < \frac{s_x^2}{s_y^2}\frac{1}{F_{1-\alpha/2;n_x-1,n_y-1}}$	F with $n_x - 1$ and $n_y - 1$ d.f.
8. θ	Large sample	$\frac{x}{n}$	$\frac{x}{n} - z_{\alpha/2}\sqrt{\frac{\frac{x}{n}\left(1 - \frac{x}{n}\right)}{n}} < \theta < \frac{x}{n} + z_{\alpha/2}\sqrt{\frac{\frac{x}{n}\left(1 - \frac{x}{n}\right)}{n}}$	Normal
9. $\theta_1 - \theta_2$	Large sample	$\frac{x_1}{n_1} - \frac{x_2}{n_2}$	$\frac{x_1}{n_1} - \frac{x_2}{n_2} - z_{\alpha/2}\sqrt{\frac{\frac{x_1}{n_1}\left(1 - \frac{x_1}{n_1}\right)}{n_1} + \frac{\frac{x_2}{n_2}\left(1 - \frac{x_2}{n_2}\right)}{n_2}} < \theta_1 - \theta_2 < \frac{x_1}{n_1} - \frac{x_2}{n_2} + z_{\alpha/2}\sqrt{\frac{\frac{x_1}{n_1}\left(1 - \frac{x_1}{n_1}\right)}{n_1} + \frac{\frac{x_2}{n_2}\left(1 - \frac{x_2}{n_2}\right)}{n_2}}$	Normal

ANALYSIS OF VARIANCE (ANOVA) TABLES

The analysis of variance (ANOVA) table containing the sum of squares, degrees of freedom, mean square, expectations, etc., present the initial analysis in a compact form. This kind of tabular representation is customarily used to set out the results of analysis of variance calculations. Appropriate ANOVA tables for various experimental design models are presented here. In the tables, the use of "dot notation" indicates a summing over all observations in the population, i.e., when summing over a suffix, that suffix is replaced by a dot. Small letters refer to observations, whereas capital letters refer to observation totals.

ANALYSIS OF VARIANCE AND EXPECTED MEAN SQUARES FOR THE ONE-WAY CLASSIFICATION

Model: $y_{ij} = \mu + \alpha_i + \epsilon_{ij} \qquad (i = 1, 2, \ldots, k; j = 1, 2, \ldots, n_i)$

Source of Variation	Degrees of Freedom	Sum of Squares	Mean Square	Test Statistic
Between groups	$k - 1$	$S_1 = \sum_i n_i(\bar{y}_{i.} - \bar{y}_{..})^2 = \sum_i \left(\frac{Y_{i.}^2}{n_i}\right) - \frac{Y_{..}^2}{n_.}$	$s_1^2 = \frac{S_1}{k-1}$	$F = \frac{s_1^2}{s_e^2}$
Within groups	$n_. - k$	$S_e = \sum_i \sum_j (\bar{y}_{ij} - \bar{y}_{i.})^2 = \sum_i \sum_j y_{ij}^2 - \sum_i \left(\frac{Y_{i.}^2}{n_i}\right)$	$s_e^2 = \frac{S_e}{n_. - k}$	
Total	$n_. - 1$	$S = \sum_i \sum_j (y_{ij} - \bar{y}_{..})^2 = \sum_i \sum_j y_{ij}^2 - \frac{Y_{..}^2}{n_.}$		

Source of Variation	Degrees of Freedom	Mean Square	Expected Mean Square for Fixed Model	Expected Mean Square for Random Model
Between groups	$k - 1$	s_1^2	$\sigma^2 + \frac{\sum_i n_i\alpha_i^2}{k-1}$	$\sigma^2 + \frac{1}{k-1}\left(n_. - \frac{\sum n_i^2}{n_.}\right)\sigma_\alpha^2$
Within groups	$n_. - k$	s_e^2	σ^2	σ^2
Total	$n_. - 1$			

Notation:

$$Y_{i.} = \sum_j y_{ij}; \quad Y_{..} = \sum_i \sum_j y_{ij}; \quad \bar{y}_{i.} = \frac{1}{n_i}\sum_j y_{ij} = \frac{1}{n_i} Y_{i.};$$

$$n_. = \sum_i n_i; \quad \bar{y}_{..} = \frac{1}{n_.}\sum_i \sum_j y_{ij} = \frac{Y_{..}}{n_.}$$

ANALYSIS OF VARIANCE AND EXPECTED MEAN SQUARES FOR THE TWO-WAY CLASSIFICATION WITH ONE OBSERVATION PER CELL

Model: $y_{ij} = \mu + \alpha_i + \beta_j + \epsilon_{ij} \quad (i = 1, 2, \ldots c; j = 1, 2, \ldots, r)$

Source of Variation	Degrees of Freedom	Sum of Squares	Mean Square	Test Statistic
Column effects	$c - 1$	$SSC = \frac{\sum_i Y_{i.}^2}{r} - \frac{Y_{..}^2}{cr}$	$s_1^2 = \frac{SSC}{c-1}$	$\frac{s_1^2}{s_e^2}$
Row effects	$r - 1$	$SSR = \frac{\sum_j Y_{.j}^2}{c} - \frac{Y_{..}^2}{cr}$	$s_2^2 = \frac{SSR}{r-1}$	$\frac{s_2^2}{s_e^2}$
Error	$(c - 1)(r - 1)$	$SSE = SST - SSC - SSR$	$s_e^2 = \frac{SSE}{(c-1)(r-1)}$	
Total	$cr - 1$	$SST = \sum_i \sum_j y_{ij}^2 - \frac{Y_{..}^2}{cr}$		

Source of Variation	Degrees of Freedom	Mean Square	Expected Mean Square for: Fixed Model	Mixed Model (α)	Random Model
Column effects	$c - 1$	s_1^2	$\sigma^2 + r\left(\frac{\sum_i \alpha_i^2}{c-1}\right)$	$\sigma^2 + r\left(\frac{\sum_i \alpha_i^2}{c-1}\right)$	$\sigma^2 + r\sigma_\alpha^2$
Row effects	$r - 1$	s_2^2	$\sigma^2 + c\left(\frac{\sum_j \beta_j^2}{r-1}\right)$	$\sigma^2 + c\sigma_\beta^2$	$\sigma^2 + c\sigma_\beta^2$
Error	$(c - 1)(r - 1)$	s_e^2	σ^2	σ^2	σ^2
Total	$cr - 1$				

ANALYSIS OF VARIANCE AND EXPECTED MEAN SQUARES FOR NESTED CLASSIFICATIONS WITH UNEQUAL SAMPLES

Model: $y_{iju} = \mu + \alpha_i + \delta_{ij} + \epsilon_{iju}$ $(i = 1, 2, \ldots, k; j = 1, 2, \ldots, n_i; u = 1, 2, \ldots, n_{ij})$

Source of Variation	Degrees of Freedom	Sum of Squares	Mean Square	Expected Mean Square for Fixed Model (α, δ)
Between main groups	$k - 1$	$S_1 = \sum_i \frac{Y_{i..}^2}{n_{i.}} - \frac{Y_{...}^2}{n_{..}}$	$s_1^2 = \frac{S_1}{k-1}$	$\sigma^2 + \frac{\sum_i n_{i.}\alpha_i^2}{k-1}$
Subgroups within main groups (experimental error)	$\sum_i n_i - k$	$S_2 = \sum_i \sum_j \frac{Y_{ij.}^2}{n_{ij}} - \sum_i \frac{Y_{i..}^2}{n_{i.}}$	$s_2^2 = \frac{S_2}{\sum_i n_i - k}$	$\sigma^2 + \frac{\sum_i \sum_j n_{ij}\delta_{ij}^2}{\sum_i n_i - k}$
Within subgroups (sampling error)	$n_{..} - \sum_i n_i$	$S_e = \sum_i \sum_j \sum_u y_{iju}^2 - \sum_i \sum_j \frac{Y_{ij.}^2}{n_{ij}}$	$s_e^2 = \frac{S_3}{n_{..} - \sum_i n_i}$	σ^2
Total	$n_{..} - 1$	$S = \sum_i \sum_j \sum_u y_{iju}^2 - \frac{Y_{...}^2}{n_{..}}$		

Source of Variation	Degrees of Freedom	Mean Square	Expected Mean Square for		
			Mixed Model (α)	Mixed Model (δ)	Random Model
Between main groups	$k - 1$	s_1^2	$\sigma^2 + b\sigma_\delta^2 + \frac{\sum_i n_{i.}\alpha_i^2}{k-1}$	$\sigma^2 + c\delta_\alpha^2$	$\sigma^2 + b\sigma_\delta^2 + c\sigma_\alpha^2$
Experimental error	$\sum_i n_i - k$	s_2^2	$\sigma^2 + a\sigma_\delta^2$	$\sigma^2 + \frac{\sum_i \sum_j n_{ij}\delta_{ij}^2}{\sum_i n_i - k}$	$\sigma^2 + a\sigma_\delta^2$
Sampling error	$n_{..} - \sum_i n_i$	s_e^2	σ^2	σ^2	σ^2
Total	$n_{..} - 1$				

where

$$\begin{cases} a = \dfrac{n_{..} - \sum_i \dfrac{\sum_j n_{ij}^2}{n_{i.}}}{\sum_i n_i - k} \\[2ex] b = \dfrac{\sum_i \dfrac{\sum_j n_{ij}^2}{n_{i.}} - \dfrac{\sum_i \sum_j n_{ij}^2}{n_{..}}}{k - 1} \\[2ex] c = \dfrac{n_{..} - \dfrac{\sum_i n_{i.}^2}{n_{..}}}{k - 1} \end{cases}$$

ANALYSIS OF VARIANCE AND EXPECTED MEAN SQUARES FOR NESTED CLASSIFICATIONS WITH EQUAL SAMPLES

Model: $y_{iju} = \mu + \alpha_i + \delta_{ij} + \epsilon_{iju}$ $(i = 1, 2, \ldots, k;\ j = 1, 2, \ldots, n;\ u = 1, 2, \ldots, r)$

Source of Variation	Degrees of Freedom	Sum of Squares	Mean Square	Expected Mean Square for Fixed Model (α, δ)
Between main groups	$k - 1$	$S_1 = \sum_i \frac{Y_{i..}^2}{nr} - \frac{Y_{...}^2}{knr}$	$s_1^2 = \frac{S_1}{k-1}$	$\sigma^2 + nr\frac{\sum_i \alpha_i^2}{k-1}$
Experimental error	$k(n - 1)$	$S_2 = \frac{\sum_i \sum_j Y_{ij.}^2}{r} - \frac{\sum_i Y_{i.}^2}{nr}$	$s_2^2 = \frac{S_2}{k(n-1)}$	$\sigma^2 + r\frac{\sum_i \sum_j \delta_{ij}^2}{k(n-1)}$
Sampling error	$kn(r - 1)$	$S_e = \sum_i \sum_j \sum_u y_{iju}^2 - \frac{\sum_i \sum_j Y_{ij.}^2}{r}$	$s_e^2 = \frac{S_e}{kn(r-1)}$	σ^2
Total	$knr - 1$	$S = \sum_i \sum_j \sum_u y_{iju}^2 - \frac{Y_{...}^2}{knr}$		

Source of Variation	Degrees of Freedom	Mean Square	Expected Mean Square for		
			Mixed Model (α)	Mixed Model (δ)	Random Model
Between main groups	$k - 1$	s_1^2	$\sigma^2 + r\sigma_\delta^2 + nr\left(\frac{\sum \alpha_i^2}{k-1}\right)$	$\sigma^2 + nr\sigma_\alpha^2$	$\sigma^2 + r\sigma_\delta^2 + nr\sigma_\alpha^2$
Experimental error	$k(n - 1)$	s_2^2	$\sigma^2 + r\sigma_\delta^2$	$\sigma^2 + \frac{r\sum_i \sum_j \delta_{ij}^2}{k(n-1)}$	$\sigma^2 + r\sigma_\delta^2$
Sampling error	$kn(r - 1)$	s_e^2	σ^2	σ^2	σ^2
Total	$knr - 1$				

where

$$a = b = r$$
$$c = nr$$

ANALYSIS OF VARIANCE AND EXPECTED MEAN SQUARES FOR A FIXED MODEL TWO-FACTOR FACTORIAL EXPERIMENT IN A ONE-WAY CLASSIFICATION DESIGN

Model: $y_{iju} = \mu + \alpha_i + \beta_j + (\alpha\beta)_{ij} + \epsilon_{iju}$ $(i = 1, 2, \ldots, c; j = 1, 2, \ldots, r; u = 1, 2, \ldots, n)$

Source of Variation	Degrees of Freedom	Sum of Squares	Mean Square	Expected Mean Square for Fixed Model [α, β, $(\alpha\beta)$]
Treatment combinations	$cr - 1$	$SSTr$	$s_0^2 = \dfrac{SSTr}{cr-1}$	$\sigma^2 + n\dfrac{\sum_i^c\sum_j^r(\mu_{ij}-\mu)^2}{cr-1}$
Factor A	$c - 1$	SSA	$s_1^2 = \dfrac{SSA}{c-1}$	$\sigma^2 + rn\dfrac{\sum_i^c \alpha_i^2}{c-1}$
Factor B	$r - 1$	SSB	$s_2^2 = \dfrac{SSB}{r-1}$	$\sigma^2 + cn\dfrac{\sum_j^r \beta_j^2}{r-1}$
Interaction	$(c-1)(r-1)$	$SSAB = SSTr - SSA - SSB$	$s_3^2 = \dfrac{SSAB}{(c-1)(r-1)}$	$\sigma^2 + n\dfrac{\sum_i^c\sum_j^r(\alpha\beta)_{ij}^2}{(c-1)(r-1)}$
Within (error)	$cr(n-1)$	$SSW = SST - SSTr$	$s_e^2 = \dfrac{SSW}{cr(n-1)}$	σ^2
Total	$crn - 1$	SST		

where

$$SSTr = \frac{\sum_i^c\sum_j^r Y_{ij.}^2}{n} - \frac{Y_{...}^2}{crn} \qquad SSA = \frac{\sum_i^c Y_{i..}^2}{rn} - \frac{Y_{...}^2}{crn}$$

$$SSB = \frac{\sum_j^r Y_{.j.}^2}{cn} - \frac{Y_{...}^2}{crn} \qquad SST = \sum_i^c\sum_j^r\sum_u^n y_{iju}^2 - \frac{Y_{...}^2}{crn}$$

$$Y_{ij.} = \sum_u^n y_{iju} \qquad Y_{i..} = \sum_j^r\sum_u^n y_{iju} \qquad Y_{.j.} = \sum_i^c\sum_u^n y_{iju}$$

Source of Variation	Mean Square	Expected Mean Square for	
		Random Model	Mixed Model (α)
Factor A	$s_1^2 = \dfrac{SSA}{c-1}$	$\sigma^2 + n\sigma_{\alpha\beta}^2 + rn\sigma_\alpha^2$	$\sigma^2 + n\sigma_{\alpha\beta}^2 + rn\dfrac{\sum_i \alpha_i^2}{c-1}$
Factor B	$s_2^2 = \dfrac{SSB}{r-1}$	$\sigma^2 + n\sigma_{\alpha\beta}^2 + cn\sigma_\beta^2$	$\sigma^2 + cn\sigma_\beta^2$
Interaction	$s_3^2 = \dfrac{SSAB}{(c-1)(r-1)}$	$\sigma^2 + n\sigma_{\alpha\beta}^2$	$\sigma^2 + n\sigma_{\alpha\beta}^2$
Within (error)	$s_e^2 = \dfrac{SSW}{cr(n-1)}$	σ^2	σ^2
Total	$s_5^2 = \dfrac{SST}{crn-1}$		

ANALYSIS OF VARIANCE AND EXPECTED MEAN SQUARES FOR A THREE-FACTOR FACTORIAL EXPERIMENT IN A COMPLETELY RANDOMIZED DESIGN

Model: $y_{ijku} = \mu + \alpha_i + \beta_j + \gamma_k + (\alpha\beta)_{ij} + (\alpha\gamma)_{ik} + (\beta\gamma)_{jk} + (\alpha\beta\gamma)_{ijk} + \epsilon_{ijku}$
$(i = 1, 2, \ldots, c; j = 1, 2, \ldots, r; k = 1, 2, \ldots, l; u = 1, 2, \ldots, n)$

Source of Variation	Degrees of Freedom	Sum of Squares	Mean Square	Expected Mean Square for *Fixed Model*
Factor A	$c - 1$	SSA	s_1^2	$\sigma^2 + rln \dfrac{\sum_i \alpha_i^2}{c-1}$
Factor B	$r - 1$	SSB	s_2^2	$\sigma^2 + cln \dfrac{\sum_j \beta_j^2}{r-1}$
Factor C	$l - 1$	SSC	s_3^2	$\sigma^2 + crn \dfrac{\sum_k \gamma_k^2}{l-1}$
Interaction $A \times B$	$(c - 1)(r - 1)$	$SSAB$	s_4^2	$\sigma^2 + ln \dfrac{\sum_i \sum_j (\alpha\beta)_{ij}^2}{(c-1)(r-1)}$
Interaction $A \times C$	$(c - 1)(l - 1)$	$SSAC$	s_5^2	$\sigma^2 + rn \dfrac{\sum_i \sum_k (\alpha\beta)_{ik}^2}{(c-1)(l-1)}$
Interaction $B \times C$	$(r - 1)(l - 1)$	$SSBC$	s_6^2	$\sigma^2 + cn \dfrac{\sum_j \sum_k (\beta\gamma)_{jk}^2}{(r-1)(l-1)}$
Interaction $A \times B \times C$	$(c - 1)(r - 1)(l - 1)$	$SSABC$	s_7^2	$\sigma^2 + n \dfrac{\sum_i \sum_j \sum_k (\alpha\beta\gamma)_{ijk}^2}{(c-1)(r-1)(l-1)}$
Within (error)	$crl(n - 1)$	SSE	s_e^2	σ^2
Total	$crln - 1$	SST		

where

$$SST = \sum_i \sum_j \sum_k \sum_u y_{ijku}^2 - \frac{Y_{....}^2}{crln}$$

$$SSA = \frac{\sum_i Y_{i...}^2}{rln} - \frac{Y_{....}^2}{crln}$$

$$SSB = \frac{\sum_j Y_{.j..}^2}{cln} - \frac{Y_{....}^2}{crln}$$

$$SSC = \frac{\sum_k Y_{..k.}^2}{crn} - \frac{Y_{....}^2}{crln}$$

$$SSTr(ABC) = \frac{\sum_i \sum_j \sum_k Y_{ijk.}^2}{n} - \frac{Y_{....}^2}{crln}$$

$$SSTr(AB) = \frac{\sum_i \sum_j Y_{ij..}^2}{ln} - \frac{Y_{....}^2}{crln}$$

$$SSTr(AC) = \frac{\sum_i \sum_k Y^2_{i.k.}}{rn} - \frac{Y^2_{....}}{crln}$$

$$SSTr(BC) = \frac{\sum_j \sum_k Y^2_{.jk.}}{cn} - \frac{Y^2_{....}}{crln}$$

$$SSAB = SSTr(AB) - SSA - SSB$$
$$SSAC = SSTr(AC) - SSA - SSC$$
$$SSBC = SSTr(BC) - SSB - SSC$$
$$SSABC = SSTr(ABC) - SSA - SSB - SSC - SSAB - SSAC - SSBC$$
$$SSE = SST - SSTr(ABC)$$

Source of Variation	Mean Square	Expected Mean Square for the Random Model	Expected Mean Square for the Mixed Model (α)	Expected Mean Square for the Mixed Model (α, β)
Factor A	$s_1^2 = \frac{SSA}{c-1}$	$\sigma^2 + n\sigma^2_{\alpha\beta\gamma} + ln\sigma^2_{\alpha\beta} + rn\sigma^2_{\alpha\gamma} + rln\sigma^2_{\alpha}$	$\sigma^2 + n\sigma^2_{\alpha\beta\gamma} + ln\sigma^2_{\alpha\beta} + rn\sigma^2_{\alpha\gamma} + rln\frac{\sum_i \alpha_i^2}{c-1}$	$\sigma^2 + rn\sigma^2_{\alpha\gamma} + rln\frac{\sum_i \alpha_i^2}{c-1}$
Factor B	$s_2^2 = \frac{SSB}{r-1}$	$\sigma^2 + n\sigma^2_{\alpha\beta\gamma} + ln\sigma^2_{\alpha\beta} + cn\sigma^2_{\beta\gamma} + cln\sigma^2_{\beta}$	$\sigma^2 + cn\sigma^2_{\beta\gamma} + cln\sigma^2_{\beta}$	$\sigma^2 + cn\sigma^2_{\beta\gamma} + cln\frac{\sum_j \beta_j^2}{r-1}$
Factor C	$s_3^2 = \frac{SSC}{l-1}$	$\sigma^2 + n\sigma^2_{\alpha\beta\gamma} + rn\sigma^2_{\alpha\gamma} + cn\sigma^2_{\beta\gamma} + crn\sigma^2_{\gamma}$	$\sigma^2 + cn\sigma^2_{\beta\gamma} + crn\sigma^2_{\gamma}$	$\sigma^2 + crn\sigma^2_{\gamma}$
$A \times B$	$s_4^2 = \frac{SSAB}{(c-1)(r-1)}$	$\sigma^2 + n\sigma^2_{\alpha\beta\gamma} + ln\sigma^2_{\alpha\beta}$	$\sigma^2 + n\sigma^2_{\alpha\beta\gamma} + ln\sigma^2_{\alpha\beta}$	$\sigma^2 + n\sigma^2_{\alpha\beta\gamma} + ln\frac{\sum_i \sum_j (\alpha\beta)^2_{ij}}{(c-1)(r-1)}$
$A \times C$	$s_5^2 = \frac{SSAC}{(c-1)(l-1)}$	$\sigma^2 + n\sigma^2_{\alpha\beta\gamma} + rn\sigma^2_{\alpha\gamma}$	$\sigma^2 + n\sigma^2_{\alpha\beta\gamma} + rn\sigma^2_{\alpha\gamma}$	$\sigma^2 + rn\sigma^2_{\alpha\gamma}$
$B \times C$	$s_6^2 = \frac{SSBC}{(r-1)(l-1)}$	$\sigma^2 + n\sigma^2_{\alpha\beta\gamma} + cn\sigma^2_{\beta\gamma}$	$\sigma^2 + cn\sigma^2_{\beta\gamma}$	$\sigma^2 + cn\sigma^2_{\beta\gamma}$
$A \times B \times C$	$s_7^2 = \frac{SSABC}{(c-1)(r-1)(l-1)}$	$\sigma^2 + n\sigma^2_{\alpha\beta\gamma}$	$\sigma^2 + n\sigma^2_{\alpha\beta\gamma}$	$\sigma^2 + n\sigma^2_{\alpha\beta\gamma}$
Within (error)	$s_e^2 = \frac{SSE}{crl(n-1)}$	σ^2	σ^2	σ^2
Total	$s_9^2 = \frac{SST}{crln-1}$			

ANALYSIS OF VARIANCE AND EXPECTED MEAN SQUARES FOR A $t \times t$ LATIN SQUARE

Model: $y_{ij(k)} = \mu + \alpha_i + \beta_j + \gamma_{(k)} + \epsilon_{ij(k)}$ $(i = 1, 2, \ldots, t;\ j = 1, 2, \ldots, t;\ k = 1, 2, \ldots, t)$

Source of Variation	Degrees of Freedom	Sum of Squares	Mean Square	Expected Mean Square for Fixed Model
Columns	$t-1$	$SSC = \frac{\sum_i Y_{i..}^2}{t} - \frac{Y_{...}^2}{t^2}$	$s_1^2 = \frac{SSC}{t-1}$	$\sigma^2 + t\frac{\sum_i \alpha_i^2}{t-1}$
Rows	$t-1$	$SSR = \frac{\sum_j Y_{.j.}^2}{t} - \frac{Y_{...}^2}{t^2}$	$s_2^2 = \frac{SSR}{t-1}$	$\sigma^2 + t\frac{\sum_j \beta_j^2}{t-1}$
Treatments	$t-1$	$SSTr = \frac{\sum_k Y_{..(k)}^2}{t} - \frac{Y_{...}^2}{t^2}$	$s_3^2 = \frac{SSTr}{t-1}$	$\sigma^2 + t\frac{\sum_k \gamma_k^2}{t-1}$
Error	$(t-1)(t-2)$	$SSE = SST - SSC - SSR - SSTr$	$s_e^2 = \frac{SSE}{(t-1)(t-2)}$	σ^2
Total	t^2-1	$SST = \sum_i \sum_j y_{ij(k)}^2 - \frac{Y_{...}^2}{t^2}$		

Source of Variation	Mean Square	Expected Mean Square for		
		Random Model	Mixed Model (γ)	Mixed Model (α, γ)
Columns	$s_1^2 = \frac{SSC}{t-1}$	$\sigma^2 + t\sigma_\alpha^2$	$\sigma^2 + t\sigma_\alpha^2$	$\sigma^2 + t\frac{\sum_i \alpha_i^2}{t-1}$
Rows	$s_2^2 = \frac{SSR}{t-1}$	$\sigma^2 + t\sigma_\beta^2$	$\sigma^2 + t\sigma_\beta^2$	$\sigma^2 + t\sigma_\beta^2$
Treatments	$s_3^2 = \frac{SSTr}{t-1}$	$\sigma^2 + t\sigma_\gamma^2$	$\sigma^2 + t\frac{\sum_k \gamma_k^2}{t-1}$	$\sigma^2 + t\frac{\sum_k \gamma_k^2}{t-1}$
Error	$s_e^2 = \frac{SSE}{(t-1)(t-2)}$	σ^2	σ^2	σ^2

ANALYSIS OF VARIANCE FOR A GRAECO-LATIN SQUARE

Model: $y_{ijuk} = \mu + \alpha_i + \beta_j + \gamma_u + \delta_k + \epsilon_{ijuk}$ $(i, j, u, k = 1, 2, \ldots, n)$

Source of Variation	Degrees of Freedom	Sum of Squares	Mean Square
Factor I (Rows)	$n - 1$	$S_1 = \dfrac{\sum_i Y^2_{i\ldots}}{n} - \dfrac{Y^2_{\ldots\ldots}}{n^2}$	$s_1^2 = \dfrac{S_1}{n-1}$
Factor II (Columns)	$n - 1$	$S_2 = \dfrac{\sum_j Y^2_{.j..}}{n} - \dfrac{Y^2_{\ldots\ldots}}{n^2}$	$s_2^2 = \dfrac{S_2}{n-1}$
Factor III (Latin Letters)	$n - 1$	$S_3 = \dfrac{\sum_u Y^2_{..u.}}{n-1} - \dfrac{Y^2_{\ldots\ldots}}{n^2}$	$s_3^2 = \dfrac{S_3}{n-1}$
Factor IV (Greek Letters)	$n - 1$	$S_4 = \dfrac{\sum_k Y^2_{\ldots k}}{n} - \dfrac{Y^2_{\ldots\ldots}}{n^2}$	$s_4^2 = \dfrac{S_4}{n-1}$
Residual	$(n-1)(n-3)$	S_e = difference	$s_e^2 = \dfrac{S_e}{(n-1)(n-3)}$
Total	$n^2 - 1$	$S = \sum_i \sum_j y^2_{ijuk} - \dfrac{Y^2_{\ldots\ldots}}{n^2}$	

ANALYSIS OF VARIANCE FOR A YOUDEN SQUARE

Model: $y_{iju} = \mu + \alpha_i + \beta_j + \gamma_u + \epsilon_{iju}$
$(i = 1, 2, \ldots, b;\ j = 1, 2, \ldots, t(= b);\ u = 1, 2, \ldots, k(<t))$

Source of Variation	Degrees of Freedom	Sum of Squares	Mean Square
Blocks (crude)		$S_1 = \sum_i \dfrac{Y^2_{i..}}{k} - \dfrac{Y^2_{\ldots}}{bk}$	
Treatments (adjusted)	$t - 1$	$S_2 = \dfrac{t-1}{bk^2(k-1)} \sum_j \left(kY^2_{.j.} - \sum_{i(j)} Y^2_{i..}\right)$	$s_1^2 = \dfrac{S_2}{t-1}$
Treatments (crude)		$S_3 = \sum_j \dfrac{Y^2_{.j.}}{r} - \dfrac{Y^2_{\ldots}}{tr}$	
Blocks (adjusted)	$b - 1$	$S_4 = \dfrac{b-1}{bk^2(k-1)} \sum_i \left(rY^2_{i..} - \sum_{j(i)} Y^2_{.j.}\right)$	$s_2^2 = \dfrac{S_4}{b-1}$
Factor II (γ)	$k - 1$	$S_5 = \dfrac{\sum_u Y^2_{..u}}{k} - \dfrac{Y^2_{\ldots}}{bk}$	$s_3^2 = \dfrac{S_5}{k-1}$
Residual	$bk - t - b - k + 2$	$S_e = S - (S_1 + S_2 + S_5)$ $= S - (S_3 + S_4 + S_5)$	$s_e^2 = \dfrac{S_e}{bk - t - b - k + 2}$
Total	$bk - 1$	$S = \sum_i \sum_j y^2_{iju} - \dfrac{Y^2_{\ldots}}{bk}$	

(Note that $S_1 + S_2 = S_3 + S_4$)

ANALYSIS OF VARIANCE FOR BALANCED INCOMPLETE BLOCK (BIB)

Model: $y_{iju} = \mu + \alpha_i + \beta_j + \epsilon_{iju}$ $(i = 1, 2, \ldots, b; j = 1, 2, \ldots, t; u = n_{ij})$

Source of Variation	Degrees of Freedom	Sum of Squares	Mean Square
Blocks	$b - 1$	$S_1 = \dfrac{\sum_i Y_{i..}^2}{k} - \dfrac{Y_{...}^2}{bk}$	$s_1^2 = \dfrac{S_1}{b-1}$
Treatments (adjusted)	$t - 1$	$S_2 = \dfrac{t-1}{bk^2(k-1)} \sum_j \left[kY_{.j.} - \sum_{i(j)} Y_{i..} \right]^2$	$s_2^2 = \dfrac{S_2}{t-1}$
Residual	$bk - t - b + 1$	S_e = difference	$s_e^2 = \dfrac{S_e}{bk - t - b + 1}$
Total	$bk - 1$	$S = \sum_i \sum_j y_{iju}^2 - \dfrac{Y_{...}^2}{bk}$	

where

t = number of treatment levels
b = number of blocks
k = number of treatment levels per block
r = number of replications of each treatment level
λ = number of blocks in which any given pair of treatment levels appear together
$bk = tr$
$r(k - 1) = \lambda(t - 1)$

GENERAL LINEAR MODEL

by Dr. Rolf E. Bargmann

1. NOTATION

A matrix will be denoted by bold-face capital letters, e.g., if **A** has m rows and n columns, we may often specify $\mathbf{A} = \mathbf{A}(m \times n)$

$$\mathbf{A} = \begin{bmatrix} a_{11} & a_{12} & \cdots & a_{1n} \\ a_{21} & a_{22} & \cdots & a_{2n} \\ \cdot & \cdot & \cdots & \cdot \\ a_{m1} & a_{m2} & \cdots & a_{mn} \end{bmatrix}.$$

$\mathbf{A}'$ denotes the transpose of **A**.
$(\mathbf{A})_{ij} = a_{ij}$ denotes the element in the i'th row and j'th column of **A**.
I denotes the identity matrix.
$\mathbf{D}_x$ denotes a diagonal matrix. The subscript indicates the terms in the diagonal.
$\tilde{\mathbf{T}}$, $\tilde{\mathbf{U}}$, i.e., any matrix with a tilde (˜) above it will denote a lower triangular matrix.

A column vector will be denoted in general, by a lower-case bold-face letter, e.g.,

$$\mathbf{x}, \mathbf{y}, \mathbf{j}, \boldsymbol{\beta}, \boldsymbol{\xi};\ \mathbf{x} = \begin{bmatrix} x_1 \\ x_2 \\ \cdot \\ \cdot \\ \cdot \\ x_r \end{bmatrix}.$$

Occasionally, capital bold-face letters represent column vectors. Examples are as follows:

T (vector of treatment totals)
B (vector of Block totals).

A lower case letter with a prime denotes a row vector, e.g.,

$$\mathbf{x}' = [x_1 \quad x_2 \quad x_3 \quad \cdots \quad x_p] \ .$$

2. THE GENERAL LINEAR MODEL

2.1. The Simple Regression Model

$$y_i = \alpha + \beta x_i + e_i \ ,$$

where x_i is a fixed concomitant variable whose values are assumed to be known before an experiment is performed and is not subject to chance. Let E denote the expectation operator, var and cov the (population) variances and covariances, respectively.

$E(e_i) = 0$, var $(e_i) = \sigma^2$, cov $(e_i,e_j) = 0$, i.e., $E(y_i) = \alpha + \beta x_i$.

If we write

$$\begin{aligned} y_1 &= \alpha + \beta x_1 + e_1 \\ y_2 &= \alpha + \beta x_2 + e_2 \\ &\cdot \quad \cdot \quad \cdot \\ y_n &= \alpha + \beta x_n + e_n \ , \end{aligned}$$

we can write, in matrix form

$$\begin{bmatrix} y_1 \\ y_2 \\ y_3 \\ \cdot \\ y_n \end{bmatrix} = \begin{bmatrix} 1 & x_1 \\ 1 & x_2 \\ 1 & x_3 \\ \cdot & \cdot \\ 1 & x_n \end{bmatrix} \begin{bmatrix} \alpha \\ \beta \end{bmatrix} + \begin{bmatrix} e_1 \\ e_2 \\ e_3 \\ \cdot \\ e_n \end{bmatrix}$$

$$\mathbf{y} = \mathbf{A} \quad \boldsymbol{\xi} + \mathbf{e} \ ,$$

where **A** is the design matrix and can be also written in the form

$$\mathbf{A} = [\underset{(1)}{\mathbf{j}} \ , \ \underset{(1)}{\mathbf{x}}](n).$$

The numbers in parentheses denote the order of the matrix.

j is a column vector containing all ones.
x is a column vector of all concomitant observations.

The simple regression model is frequently written in the form

$$y_i = \mu + \beta(x_i - \bar{x}) + e_i \ ,$$

where $\mu = \alpha + \beta\bar{x}$.

This, too, can be written in the general linear model form

$$\begin{bmatrix} y_1 \\ y_2 \\ \cdot \\ \cdot \\ \cdot \\ y_n \end{bmatrix} = \begin{bmatrix} 1 & (x_1 - \bar{x}) \\ 1 & (x_2 - \bar{x}) \\ \cdot & \cdot \\ \cdot & \cdot \\ \cdot & \cdot \\ 1 & (x_n - \bar{x}) \end{bmatrix} \begin{bmatrix} \mu \\ \beta \end{bmatrix} + \begin{bmatrix} e_1 \\ e_2 \\ \cdot \\ \cdot \\ \cdot \\ e_n \end{bmatrix}$$

$$\mathbf{y} = \mathbf{A} \quad \boldsymbol{\xi} + \mathbf{e} \ ,$$

where $\mathbf{A} = [\mathbf{j}, (\mathbf{x} - \bar{x}\mathbf{j})]$.

2.2. Multiple Regression Model

$$y_i = \beta_0 + \beta_1 x_{1i} + \beta_2 x_{2i} + \beta_3 x_{3i} + \cdots \beta_k x_{ki} + e_i \ .$$

Assumption: $E(e_i) = 0$,

$$\text{var}\ (y_i) = \text{var}\ (e_i) = \sigma^2,$$
$$\text{cov}\ (y_i, y_j) = 0\ .$$

If we write

$$\begin{aligned} y_1 &= \beta_0 + \beta_1 x_{11} + \beta_2 x_{21} + \beta_3 x_{31} + \cdots \beta_k x_{k1} + e_1 \\ y_2 &= \beta_0 + \beta_1 x_{12} + \beta_2 x_{22} + \beta_3 x_{32} + \cdots \beta_k x_{k2} + e_2 \\ &\cdot \\ &\cdot \qquad \cdot \quad \cdot \quad \cdot \\ &\cdot \\ y_n &= \beta_0 + \beta_n x_{1n} + \beta_2 x_{2n} + \beta_3 x_{3n} + \cdots \beta_k x_{kn} + e_n \ , \end{aligned}$$

we can write

$$\begin{bmatrix} y_1 \\ y_2 \\ \cdot \\ y_n \end{bmatrix} = \begin{bmatrix} 1 & x_{11} & x_{21} & x_{31} & \cdots & x_{k1} \\ 1 & x_{12} & x_{22} & x_{32} & \cdots & x_{k2} \\ \cdot & \cdot & \cdot & \cdot & \cdots & \cdot \\ 1 & x_{1n} & x_{2n} & x_{3n} & \cdots & x_{kn} \end{bmatrix} \begin{bmatrix} \beta_0 \\ \beta_1 \\ \beta_2 \\ \beta_3 \\ \cdot \\ \beta_k \end{bmatrix} + \begin{bmatrix} e_1 \\ e_2 \\ e_3 \\ \cdot \\ e_n \end{bmatrix}$$

$$\mathbf{y} \quad = \quad \mathbf{A} \quad \boldsymbol{\xi} \ + \ e\ ,$$

where $\mathbf{A} = [\underset{(1)}{\mathbf{j}}, \ \underset{(k)}{\mathbf{X}}](n)$, and **X** denotes the matrix of all observations on all concomitant variables.

2.3. One-way Classification Analysis of Variance

Model

$$y_{ij} = \mu + \tau_i + e_{ij}$$

where μ = general effect
τ_i = treatment effects
e_{ij} = experimental error,
v treatments with effects $\tau_1, \tau_2, \ldots, \tau_v$; $j = 1, 2, 3, \ldots n_i$.

$$\begin{aligned} y_{11} &= \mu + \tau_1 && + e_{11} \\ y_{12} &= \mu + \tau_1 && + e_{12} \\ &\cdot \quad \cdot && \cdot \\ y_{1n_1} &= \mu + \tau_1 && + e_{1n_1} \\ \hline y_{21} &= \mu \quad + \tau_2 && + e_{21} \\ &\cdot \quad \cdot && \cdot \\ y_{2n_2} &= \mu \quad + \tau_2 && + e_{2n_2} \\ \hline &\cdot \quad \cdot \quad \cdot && \cdot \\ \hline y_{v1} &= \mu && + \tau_v + e_{v1} \\ &\cdot \quad \cdot && \cdot \quad \cdot \\ y_{vn_v} &= \mu && + \tau_v + e_{vn_v}\ . \end{aligned}$$

We can again write this

$$
\begin{bmatrix} y_{11} \\ y_{12} \\ \cdot \\ y_{1n_1} \\ \hline y_{21} \\ \cdot \\ y_{2n_2} \\ \hline \cdot \\ \hline y_{v1} \\ y_{v2} \\ \cdot \\ y_{vn_v} \end{bmatrix}
=
\begin{bmatrix}
1 & 1 & 0 & 0 & \cdots & 0 & 0 \\
1 & 1 & 0 & 0 & \cdots & 0 & 0 \\
\cdot & \cdot & \cdot & \cdot & \cdots & \cdot & \cdot \\
1 & 1 & 0 & 0 & \cdots & 0 & 0 \\ \hline
1 & 0 & 1 & 0 & \cdots & 0 & 0 \\
\cdot & \cdot & \cdot & \cdot & \cdots & \cdot & \cdot \\
1 & 0 & 1 & 0 & \cdots & 0 & 0 \\ \hline
\cdot & \cdot & \cdot & \cdot & \cdots & \cdot & \cdot \\ \hline
1 & 0 & 0 & 0 & \cdots & 0 & 1 \\
1 & 0 & 0 & 0 & \cdots & 0 & 1 \\
\cdot & \cdot & \cdot & \cdot & \cdots & \cdot & \cdot \\
1 & 0 & 0 & 0 & & 0 & 1
\end{bmatrix}
\begin{bmatrix} \mu \\ \tau_1 \\ \tau_2 \\ \cdot \\ \tau_v \end{bmatrix}
+ \mathbf{e}
$$

$$
\mathbf{y} \quad = \quad \mathbf{A} \quad \boldsymbol{\xi} \quad + \mathbf{e}\,.
$$

The design matrix **A** can be written

$$
\mathbf{A} = [\underset{(1)}{\mathbf{j}}, \underset{(v)}{\mathbf{A}_\tau}](n),
$$

where

$$
\mathbf{A}_\tau = \begin{matrix} (n_1) \\ (n_2) \\ \cdot \\ (n_v) \end{matrix}
\begin{bmatrix}
\mathbf{j} & \mathbf{0} & \mathbf{0} & \cdots & \mathbf{0} \\
\mathbf{0} & \mathbf{j} & \mathbf{0} & \cdots & \mathbf{0} \\
\cdot & \cdot & \cdot & \cdots & \cdot \\
\mathbf{0} & \mathbf{0} & \mathbf{0} & \cdots & \mathbf{j}
\end{bmatrix}
$$

and the parameter vector can also be written

$$
\boldsymbol{\xi} = \begin{bmatrix} \mu \\ \boldsymbol{\tau} \end{bmatrix}.
$$

2.4. Two-way Classification (Two Factors Factorial)

Model

$$
y_{ijk} = \mu + \alpha_i + \beta_j + \delta_{ij} + e_{ijk}\,,
$$

where μ = general effect
α_i = factor A effects (usually row effects)
β_j = factor B effects (usually column effects)
δ_{ij} = interaction effects.

For example:

$$
\begin{bmatrix} \mathbf{y}_{11} \\ \mathbf{y}_{12} \\ \mathbf{y}_{13} \\ \mathbf{y}_{21} \\ \mathbf{y}_{22} \\ \mathbf{y}_{23} \end{bmatrix}
=
\begin{matrix} (n_{11}) \\ (n_{12}) \\ (n_{13}) \\ (n_{21}) \\ (n_{22}) \\ (n_{23}) \end{matrix}
\begin{bmatrix}
\mathbf{j} & \mathbf{j} & \mathbf{0} & \mathbf{j} & \mathbf{0} & \mathbf{0} & \mathbf{j} & \mathbf{0} & \mathbf{0} & \mathbf{0} & \mathbf{0} & \mathbf{0} \\
\mathbf{j} & \mathbf{j} & \mathbf{0} & \mathbf{0} & \mathbf{j} & \mathbf{0} & \mathbf{0} & \mathbf{j} & \mathbf{0} & \mathbf{0} & \mathbf{0} & \mathbf{0} \\
\mathbf{j} & \mathbf{j} & \mathbf{0} & \mathbf{0} & \mathbf{0} & \mathbf{j} & \mathbf{0} & \mathbf{0} & \mathbf{j} & \mathbf{0} & \mathbf{0} & \mathbf{0} \\
\mathbf{j} & \mathbf{0} & \mathbf{j} & \mathbf{j} & \mathbf{0} & \mathbf{0} & \mathbf{0} & \mathbf{0} & \mathbf{0} & \mathbf{j} & \mathbf{0} & \mathbf{0} \\
\mathbf{j} & \mathbf{0} & \mathbf{j} & \mathbf{0} & \mathbf{j} & \mathbf{0} & \mathbf{0} & \mathbf{0} & \mathbf{0} & \mathbf{0} & \mathbf{j} & \mathbf{0} \\
\mathbf{j} & \mathbf{0} & \mathbf{j} & \mathbf{0} & \mathbf{0} & \mathbf{j} & \mathbf{0} & \mathbf{0} & \mathbf{0} & \mathbf{0} & \mathbf{0} & \mathbf{j}
\end{bmatrix}
\begin{bmatrix} \mu \\ \alpha_1 \\ \alpha_2 \\ \beta_1 \\ \beta_2 \\ \beta_3 \\ \delta_{11} \\ \delta_{12} \\ \delta_{13} \\ \delta_{21} \\ \delta_{22} \\ \delta_{23} \end{bmatrix}
+ \mathbf{e}
$$

$$
\mathbf{y} \quad = \quad \mathbf{A} \quad \boldsymbol{\xi} \quad + \mathbf{e}\,.
$$

2.5. Analysis of Covariance

Analysis of covariance is equivalent to analysis of variance with one or more concomitant variables added.

For simplicity, let us take one-way classification and one concomitant variable.

Model

$$y_{ij} = \mu + \tau_i + \beta x_{ij} + e_{ij} \ .$$

As a vector equation, this model reads

$$\begin{array}{lllllll}
y_{11} & = \mu + \tau_1 & & & + \beta x_{11} & + e_{11} \\
y_{12} & = \mu + \tau_1 & & & + \beta x_{12} & + e_{12} \\
\cdot & \cdot \quad \cdot & & & \cdot & \cdot \\
y_{1n_1} & = \mu + \tau_1 & & & + \beta x_{1n_1} & + e_{1n_1} \\
\hline
y_{21} & = \mu & + \tau_2 & & + \beta x_{21} & + e_{21} \\
\cdot & \cdot & \cdot & & \cdot & \cdot \\
y_{2n_2} & = \mu & + \tau_2 & & + \beta x_{2n_2} & + e_{2n_2} \\
\hline
y_{31} & = \mu & & + \tau_3 & + \beta x_{31} & + e_{31} \\
\cdot & \cdot & & \cdot & \cdot & \cdot \\
y_{3n_3} & = \mu & & + \tau_3 & + \beta x_{3n_3} & + e_{3n_3}
\end{array}$$

Let $\mathbf{x}_1$, $\mathbf{x}_2$, and $\mathbf{x}_3$ denote the concomitant observations in each group, then

$$\begin{bmatrix} y_{11} \\ y_{12} \\ \cdot \\ \cdot \\ \cdot \\ y_{1n_1} \\ y_{21} \\ \cdot \\ \cdot \\ \cdot \\ y_{2n_2} \\ y_{31} \\ \cdot \\ \cdot \\ \cdot \\ y_{3n_3} \end{bmatrix} = \begin{bmatrix} \mathbf{j} & \mathbf{j} & \mathbf{0} & \mathbf{0} & \mathbf{x}_1 \\ \mathbf{j} & \mathbf{0} & \mathbf{j} & \mathbf{0} & \mathbf{x}_2 \\ \mathbf{j} & \mathbf{0} & \mathbf{0} & \mathbf{j} & \mathbf{x}_3 \end{bmatrix} \begin{bmatrix} \mu \\ \tau_1 \\ \tau_2 \\ \tau_3 \\ \beta \end{bmatrix} + \mathbf{e}$$

$$\mathbf{y} \quad = \quad \mathbf{A} \quad \boldsymbol{\xi} \ + \mathbf{e} \ .$$

With the above illustrations, it is clear that we can write a great variety of models in the general linear model form

$$\mathbf{y} = \mathbf{A}\boldsymbol{\xi} + \mathbf{e} \ .$$

3. SUMMARY OF RULES FOR MATRIX OPERATIONS

3.1. Let $E(\mathbf{y}) = \boldsymbol{\mu}$, var $(\mathbf{y}) = \boldsymbol{\Sigma}$, a symmetric matrix containing all possible variances and covariances. Then, $E(\mathbf{My}) = \mathbf{M}\boldsymbol{\mu}$, var $(\mathbf{My}) = \mathbf{M\Sigma M'}$, for any conforming matrix $\mathbf{M}$. $E(\mathbf{y'M}) = \boldsymbol{\mu}'\mathbf{M}$, var $(\mathbf{y'M}) = \mathbf{M'\Sigma M}$.

3.2. Partitioning of Determinants

$$\begin{vmatrix} \mathbf{A} & \mathbf{B} \\ \mathbf{C} & \mathbf{D} \end{vmatrix} = |\mathbf{A}|\ |\mathbf{D} - \mathbf{CA}^{-1}\mathbf{B}| \text{ if } \mathbf{A}^{-1} \text{ exists} \ .$$

$$= |\mathbf{D}|\ |\mathbf{A} - \mathbf{BD}^{-1}\mathbf{C}| \text{ if } \mathbf{D}^{-1} \text{ exists} \ .$$

3.3. Inverse of a Partitioned Matrix

$$\begin{bmatrix} \mathbf{A} & \mathbf{B} \\ \mathbf{C} & \mathbf{D} \end{bmatrix}^{-1} = \begin{bmatrix} \mathbf{X} & \mathbf{Y} \\ \mathbf{Z} & \mathbf{U} \end{bmatrix}$$

$$\begin{aligned} \text{where } \mathbf{X} &= [\mathbf{A} - \mathbf{B}\mathbf{D}^{-1}\mathbf{C}]^{-1} \\ \mathbf{U} &= [\mathbf{D} - \mathbf{C}\mathbf{A}^{-1}\mathbf{B}]^{-1} \\ \mathbf{Y} &= -\mathbf{A}^{-1}\mathbf{B}\mathbf{U} \\ \mathbf{Z} &= -\mathbf{D}^{-1}\mathbf{C}\mathbf{X}\,. \end{aligned}$$

3.3.1. *Symmetric Case*

$$\begin{bmatrix} \mathbf{A}_{11} & \mathbf{A}_{12} \\ \mathbf{A}_{12}' & \mathbf{A}_{22} \end{bmatrix}^{-1} = \begin{bmatrix} \mathbf{A}^{11} & \mathbf{A}^{12} \\ (\mathbf{A}^{12})' & \mathbf{A}^{22} \end{bmatrix}$$

$$\begin{aligned} \text{where } \mathbf{A}^{11} &= [\mathbf{A}_{11} - \mathbf{A}_{12}\mathbf{A}_{22}^{-1}\mathbf{A}_{12}']^{-1} \\ \mathbf{A}^{22} &= [\mathbf{A}_{22} - \mathbf{A}_{12}'\mathbf{A}_{11}^{-1}\mathbf{A}_{12}]^{-1} \\ \mathbf{A}^{12} &= -\mathbf{A}^{11}\mathbf{A}_{12}\mathbf{A}_{22}^{-1} \\ \text{or } \mathbf{A}^{12} &= -\mathbf{A}_{11}^{-1}\mathbf{A}_{12}\mathbf{A}^{22}\,. \end{aligned}$$

Computational steps: Order the sets in such a way that $\mathbf{A}_{22}$ is the smaller matrix.

a. Obtain $\mathbf{A}_{22}^{-1}$
b. Multiply $\mathbf{A}_{12}\mathbf{A}_{22}^{-1}$
c. Obtain $\mathbf{A}_{12}\mathbf{A}_{22}^{-1}\mathbf{A}_{12}'$
d. Obtain $\mathbf{A}_{11} - \mathbf{A}_{12}\mathbf{A}_{22}^{-1}\mathbf{A}_{12}'$
e. Invert the matrix in *d.*; thus obtain $\mathbf{A}^{11}$
f. Obtain $\mathbf{A}^{11}\mathbf{A}_{12}\mathbf{A}_{22}^{-1}$ by multiplying matrices from steps *e.* and *b.*
g. Change all signs in *f.*; thus obtain $\mathbf{A}^{12}$.
h. Obtain $(\mathbf{A}^{12})'$ by transposing *g.*
i. Obtain $\mathbf{A}_{12}'\mathbf{A}^{12}$, the latter factor from *g.*
j. Obtain $\mathbf{I} - \mathbf{A}_{12}'\mathbf{A}^{12}$, i.e., change all signs in off-diagonal elements of the matrix in step *i.* and complement diagonal elements to 1.
k. Obtain $\mathbf{A}_{22}^{-1}[\mathbf{I} - \mathbf{A}_{12}'\mathbf{A}^{12}]$, i.e., premultiply the matrix in *j.* by $\mathbf{A}_{22}^{-1}$ obtained in step *a.* This is $\mathbf{A}^{22}$.

3.4. Characteristic Roots

a. ch $(\mathbf{AB})$ = ch $(\mathbf{BA})$ except, possibly, for zero roots.
b. Corollary: tr $(\mathbf{AB})$ = tr $(\mathbf{BA})$.
c. If ch $(\mathbf{A}) = \lambda_i$, ch $(\mathbf{A}^{-1}) = 1/\lambda_i$, and ch $(\mathbf{I} \pm \mathbf{A}) = 1 \pm \lambda_i$.

3.5. Differentiation

3.5.1. *Definitions:*

Let f be a scalar function of $x_1, x_2, \ldots x_p$.
Then $\partial f/\partial \mathbf{x}$ denotes a column vector whose ith element is $\partial f/\partial x_i$.
Let f be a scalar function of $x_{11}, x_{12} \ldots x_{1q}, x_{21}, x_{22} \ldots x_{2q}, \ldots x_{p1}, x_{p2}, \ldots x_{pq}$. Then $\partial f/\partial \mathbf{X}$ denotes a matrix whose (i, j) element is $\partial f/\partial x_{ij}$. Note that, in this definition, x_{ij} denotes the element in the i'th row and j'th column of $\mathbf{X}$. If there are any functional relations between the elements of $\mathbf{X}$ (as, for instance, in a symmetric matrix) these relations will be *disregarded* in the above definition. In other words, x_{ij} denotes the variable in the i'th row and j'th column of $\mathbf{X}$, and x_{ji} denotes that in the j'th row and i'th column. If the two happen to be identical, a new symbol will be in order. For example, if $x_{ij} = x_{ji} = y_{ij}$, say, $\partial f/\partial y_{ij} = \partial f/\partial x_{ij} \cdot \partial x_{ij}/\partial y_{ij} + \partial f/\partial x_{ji} \cdot \partial x_{ji}/\partial y_{ij} = \partial f/\partial x_{ij} + \partial f/\partial x_{ji} = (\partial f/\partial \mathbf{X})_{ij} + (\partial f/\partial \mathbf{X})_{ji}$. Here, y_{ij} is the symbol for that distinct variable which occurs in two places in $\mathbf{X}$.

If $y_1, y_2, \ldots y_p$ are functions of x, $\partial\mathbf{y}'/\partial x$ denotes the row vector whose i'th element is $\partial y_i/\partial x$.

If $y_{11}, y_{12}, \ldots y_{1q}, y_{21}, \ldots y_{2q}, \ldots y_{p1}, \ldots y_{pq}$ are functions of x, $\partial\mathbf{Y}/\partial x$ denotes the matrix whose (i,j) element is $\partial y_{ij}/\partial x$.

If each of the quantities $y_1, y_2, \ldots y_q$ is a function of the variables $x_1, x_2, \ldots x_p$, $\partial\mathbf{y}'/\partial\mathbf{x}$ denotes a matrix of order (pxq) whose (i,j) element is $\partial y_j/\partial x_i$. *Note the interchange of subscripts.*

3.5.2. *Rules:*

1. $\partial(\mathbf{x}'\mathbf{x})/\partial\mathbf{x} = 2\mathbf{x}$
2. $\partial(\mathbf{x}'\mathbf{Q}\mathbf{x})/\partial\mathbf{x} = \mathbf{Q}\mathbf{x} + \mathbf{Q}'\mathbf{x}$
3. $\partial(\mathbf{x}'\mathbf{Q}\mathbf{x})/\partial\mathbf{x} = 2\mathbf{Q}\mathbf{x}$ if $\mathbf{Q}$ is symmetric.
4. $\partial(\mathbf{a}'\mathbf{x})/\partial\mathbf{x} = \mathbf{a}$
5. $\partial(\mathbf{a}'\mathbf{Q}\mathbf{x})/\partial\mathbf{x} = \mathbf{Q}'\mathbf{a}$
6. $\partial \operatorname{tr}(\mathbf{A}\mathbf{X})/\partial\mathbf{X} = \mathbf{A}'$
7. $\partial \operatorname{tr}(\mathbf{X}\mathbf{A})/\partial\mathbf{X} = \mathbf{A}'$
8. $\partial \log|\mathbf{X}|/\partial\mathbf{X} = (\mathbf{X}')^{-1}$, if $\mathbf{X}$ is square and nonsingular.
9. "Chain Rule No. 1": $\partial\mathbf{y}'/\partial\mathbf{x} = \partial\mathbf{z}'/\partial\mathbf{x} \cdot \partial\mathbf{y}'/\partial\mathbf{z}$.
10. $\partial(\mathbf{x}'\mathbf{A})/\partial\mathbf{x} = \mathbf{A}$
11. If $\mathbf{e} = \mathbf{b} - \mathbf{A}'\mathbf{x}$, $\partial(\mathbf{e}'\mathbf{e})/\partial\mathbf{x} = \partial\mathbf{e}'/\partial\mathbf{x} \cdot \partial(\mathbf{e}'\mathbf{e})/\partial\mathbf{e}$ (according to rule 9), $= -2\mathbf{A}'\mathbf{e}$ (by rules 10 and 1).
12. "Chain Rule No. 2": If the scalar z is related to a scalar x through variables y_{ij} $(i = 1, 2, \cdots p; j = 1, 2 \cdots q)$,

$$\partial z/\partial x = \operatorname{tr}\,[\partial z/\partial\mathbf{Y} \cdot \partial\mathbf{Y}'/\partial x]$$

or

$$\partial z/\partial x = \operatorname{tr}\,[\partial z/\partial\mathbf{Y}' \cdot \partial\mathbf{Y}/\partial x]$$

This chain rule is correct regardless of any functional relationships which may exist between the elements of $\mathbf{Y}$.

3.6. Some Additional Definitions and Rules

$\mathbf{j}$ denotes a column vector, each element of which is 1. Hence $\mathbf{j}'\mathbf{A}$ is a row vector whose elements are the column sums of $\mathbf{A}$, and $\mathbf{A}\mathbf{j}$ denotes a column vector whose elements are the row sums of $\mathbf{A}$. $\mathbf{j}'\mathbf{A}\mathbf{j}$ denotes the sum of all elements in the matrix $\mathbf{A}$.

$\mathbf{I}$ denotes the identity matrix. If the order must be stated it will be added in parentheses. Hence $\mathbf{I}(p)$ denotes a $(p \times p)$ identity matrix.

If a tilde (~) is placed above a matrix, the matrix is assumed to be triangular. For definiteness, the untransposed matrix

$$\tilde{\mathbf{T}} = \begin{bmatrix} t_{11} & 0 & 0 & \cdots & 0 \\ t_{21} & t_{22} & 0 & \cdots & 0 \\ t_{31} & t_{32} & t_{33} & \cdots & 0 \\ \cdot & \cdot & \cdot & \cdots & \cdot \\ t_{p1} & t_{p2} & t_{p3} & \cdots & t_{pp} \end{bmatrix}$$

is a "lower" triangular matrix, whereas the transposed matrix

$$\tilde{\mathbf{T}}' = \begin{bmatrix} t_{11} & t_{21} & t_{31} & \cdots & t_{p1} \\ 0 & t_{22} & t_{32} & \cdots & t_{p2} \\ 0 & 0 & t_{33} & \cdots & t_{p3} \\ \cdot & \cdot & \cdot & \cdots & \cdot \\ 0 & 0 & 0 & \cdots & t_{pp} \end{bmatrix}$$

is an "upper" triangular matrix.

If $\tilde{\mathbf{T}}$ is lower triangular, so is $\tilde{\mathbf{T}}^{-1}$.

If $\mathbf{Q}$ is a symmetric, positive-definite matrix, we can find, uniquely, a real matrix $\tilde{\mathbf{T}}$, such that $\mathbf{Q} = \tilde{\mathbf{T}}\tilde{\mathbf{T}}'$, provided we let the diagonal elements of $\tilde{\mathbf{T}}$ be positive. This matrix and its inverse can be readily obtained from the forward Doolittle solution. If, in each cycle, we divide each element of the next-to-last row (the row which is immediately above the one beginning with unity) by the square-root of the "leading" (first) element, we obtain $\tilde{\mathbf{T}}'$ on the left and $\tilde{\mathbf{T}}^{-1}$ on the right-hand side.

If $\mathbf{Q}$ is a $(p \times p)$, symmetric, positive-semidefinite matrix of rank r, the matrix $\tilde{\mathbf{T}}$ obtained in the above manner will have zeros to the right of the r'th column. $\mathbf{Q}$ can then be represented as

$$\mathbf{Q} = \begin{matrix} (r) \\ (p-r) \end{matrix} \overset{(r)}{\begin{bmatrix} \tilde{\mathbf{T}}_1 \\ \mathbf{T}_2 \end{bmatrix}} [\underset{(r)}{\tilde{\mathbf{T}}_1'} \quad , \quad \underset{(p-r)}{\mathbf{T}_2'}],$$

where, of course, only $\tilde{\mathbf{T}}_1$ is triangular. This is an important computational device in connection with rule 3.4.a. on characteristic roots. For, if the largest root of $\mathbf{AB}$ is desired, where both $\mathbf{A}$ and $\mathbf{B}$ are symmetric, but $\mathbf{A}$ is of low rank, we can obtain the representation

$$\mathbf{A} = \begin{matrix} (r) \\ (p-r) \end{matrix} \underset{(r)}{\begin{bmatrix} \tilde{\mathbf{T}}_1 \\ \mathbf{T}_2 \end{bmatrix}} [\tilde{\mathbf{T}}_1' \ , \ \mathbf{T}_2']$$

by the forward Doolittle solution. Then, by 3.4.a., $\text{ch}\,(\mathbf{AB}) = \text{ch}\left([\tilde{\mathbf{T}}_1' \ , \ \mathbf{T}_2']\mathbf{B}\begin{bmatrix} \tilde{\mathbf{T}}_1 \\ \mathbf{T}_2 \end{bmatrix}\right)$, and the matrix in parentheses is of small order and symmetric.

$\mathbf{D}_u$ denotes a diagonal matrix whose non-zero elements are $u_1, u_2 \cdots u_p$.

4. PRINCIPLE OF MINIMIZING QUADRATIC FORMS AND GAUSS MARKOV THEOREM

4.1. Some Remarks on Multivariate Distributions

In univariate situation, suppose we have a random variable x, such that

$$E(x) = \mu$$
$$\text{var}\,(x) = \sigma^2 .$$

If we want to find a random variable y, such that

$$E(y) = 0 \quad \text{and} \quad \text{var}\,(y) = 1 ,$$

i.e., we are to find y such that it has mean 0 and variance 1, we perform the "standardization"

$$y = \frac{x - \mu}{\sigma} .$$

We also recall that, if y is normally distributed,

$$y^2 = \frac{(x-\mu)^2}{\sigma^2} = \chi^2 \text{ with 1 d.f} .$$

In multivariate situations, we have random variables $\mathbf{x}$ such that

$$E(\mathbf{x}) = \boldsymbol{\mu} \quad \text{and} \quad \text{var}\,(\mathbf{x}) = \boldsymbol{\Sigma}$$

and we wish to find $\mathbf{y}$ such that

$$E(\mathbf{y}) = \mathbf{0} \quad \text{and} \quad \text{var}\,(\mathbf{y}) = \mathbf{I} .$$

To obtain this, we will proceed as follows: Let

$$\boldsymbol{\Sigma} = \boldsymbol{\Gamma}\boldsymbol{\Gamma}',$$

where $\boldsymbol{\Gamma}$ is a lower triangular matrix, which, given $\boldsymbol{\Sigma}$, can be obtained conveniently as a by-product of the forward Doolittle analysis. Then,

$$\boldsymbol{\Sigma}^{-1} = (\boldsymbol{\Gamma}')^{-1}\boldsymbol{\Gamma}^{-1} .$$

Now, let

$$\begin{aligned} y &= \boldsymbol{\Gamma}^{-1}(\mathbf{x} - \boldsymbol{\mu}) \\ E(\mathbf{y}) &= \boldsymbol{\Gamma}^{-1}E(\mathbf{x} - \boldsymbol{\mu}) = \mathbf{0} \end{aligned}$$

and

$$\begin{aligned} \text{var}\,(\mathbf{y}) &= \boldsymbol{\Gamma}^{-1}\,\text{var}\,(\mathbf{x} - \boldsymbol{\mu})(\boldsymbol{\Gamma}')^{-1} \\ &= \boldsymbol{\Gamma}^{-1}\,\text{var}\,(\mathbf{x})(\boldsymbol{\Gamma}')^{-1} \\ &= \boldsymbol{\Gamma}^{-1}\Sigma(\boldsymbol{\Gamma}')^{-1} \\ &= \boldsymbol{\Gamma}^{-1}\boldsymbol{\Gamma}\boldsymbol{\Gamma}'(\boldsymbol{\Gamma}')^{-1} = \mathbf{I} . \end{aligned}$$

Hence $\mathbf{y}$ is of the desired standard form. Then

$$\begin{aligned} \mathbf{y}'\mathbf{y} &= (\mathbf{x}' - \boldsymbol{\mu}')(\Gamma^{-1})'\Gamma^{-1}(\mathbf{x} - \boldsymbol{\mu}) \\ &= (\mathbf{x}' - \boldsymbol{\mu}')\Sigma^{-1}(\mathbf{x} - \boldsymbol{\mu}) . \end{aligned}$$

This is called the "*Standard Quadratic Form*".

Since it is equal to the sum-of-squares of p standard variables, it will be distributed as χ^2 with p degrees of freedom, if $\mathbf{x}$ has the multivariate normal distribution.

4.2. The Principle of Least Squares

Recall that the General Linear Model is

$$\mathbf{y} = \mathbf{A}\boldsymbol{\xi} + \mathbf{e} .$$

On the assumption, for the time being that $\mathbf{A}$ is of full rank, the "least squares" approach tells us to estimate $\boldsymbol{\xi}$ in such a way that the sum of squares of errors is minimized. Then, $\mathbf{e}'\mathbf{e}$ is the desired sum of squares and

$$\begin{aligned} \mathbf{e} &= \mathbf{y} - \mathbf{A}\boldsymbol{\xi} \\ \mathbf{e}' &= \mathbf{y}' - \boldsymbol{\xi}'\mathbf{A}' \\ \mathbf{e}'\mathbf{e} &= (\mathbf{y}' - \boldsymbol{\xi}'\mathbf{A}')(\mathbf{y} - \mathbf{A}\boldsymbol{\xi}) \\ \frac{\partial(\mathbf{e}'\mathbf{e})}{\partial\boldsymbol{\xi}} &= -2\mathbf{A}'(\mathbf{y} - \mathbf{A}\boldsymbol{\xi}) . \end{aligned}$$

Setting this equal to zero, we obtain

$$\begin{aligned} \mathbf{A}'(\mathbf{y} - \mathbf{A}\hat{\boldsymbol{\xi}}) &= \mathbf{0} \\ (\mathbf{A}'\mathbf{A})\hat{\boldsymbol{\xi}} &= \mathbf{A}'\mathbf{y} . \end{aligned}$$

These are called the *Normal Equations* for the estimation of $\boldsymbol{\xi}$.

4.3. Minimum Variance Unbiased Estimates

The minimum variance, unbiased, linear estimate of $\boldsymbol{\xi}$ is obtained by the application of a very general form of the *Gauss Markov Theorem*:

Let

$$\begin{aligned} \mathbf{y} &= \mathbf{A}\boldsymbol{\xi} + \mathbf{e} \\ E(\mathbf{e}) &= \mathbf{0} \\ \text{var}\,(\mathbf{y}) &= \text{var}\,(\mathbf{e}) = \sigma^2\mathbf{V} \end{aligned}$$

where $\mathbf{V}$ is a matrix (square, symmetric, non-singular) of order $(n \times n)$ with known elements. That is to say that variances of y_i (regardless of i) and covariances between y_i and y_j are known except for an arbitrary scalar multiplier applied to all of them. Then the best linear estimate of an arbitrary linear function $\mathbf{l}'\boldsymbol{\xi}$ is equal to $\mathbf{l}'\hat{\boldsymbol{\xi}}$ where $\hat{\boldsymbol{\xi}}$ minimizes the quadratic form

$$\mathbf{e}'\mathbf{V}^{-1}\mathbf{e} \ .$$

Since

$$E(\mathbf{e}) = \mathbf{0}$$

and

$$\text{var}\ (\mathbf{e}) = \text{var}\ (\mathbf{y}) = \sigma^2\mathbf{V} \ ,$$

the standard quadratic form of $\mathbf{e}$ would be

$$(\mathbf{e}' - [E(\mathbf{e})'])[\text{var}\ (\mathbf{e})]^{-1}(\mathbf{e} - [E(\mathbf{e})]) = (\mathbf{e}' - \mathbf{0}')[\sigma^2\mathbf{V}]^{-1}(\mathbf{e} - \mathbf{0})$$
$$= \frac{1}{\sigma^2}\mathbf{e}'\mathbf{V}^{-1}\mathbf{e} \ .$$

Minimizing this expression is equivalent to minimizing

$$\mathbf{e}'\mathbf{V}^{-1}\mathbf{e} \ .$$

Hence, the statement, "The best linear estimate of an arbitrary function $\mathbf{l}'\boldsymbol{\xi}$ is equal to $\mathbf{l}'\hat{\boldsymbol{\xi}}$ where $\hat{\boldsymbol{\xi}}$ is obtained by minimizing the quadratic form $\mathbf{e}'\mathbf{V}^{-1}\mathbf{e}$", as made in the Gauss-Markov Theorem is, in fact, equivalent to the statement . . . where $\hat{\boldsymbol{\xi}}$ is obtained by minimizing the standard quadratic form due to error. The Normal Equations in this general case are $\mathbf{A}'\mathbf{V}^{-1}\mathbf{A}\hat{\boldsymbol{\xi}} = \mathbf{A}'\mathbf{V}^{-1}\mathbf{y}$.

5. GENERAL LINEAR HYPOTHESIS OF FULL RANK

In this section, we shall discuss, with illustrations, the problem of testing hypotheses about certain parameters and also derive some necessary distribution in connection with testing hypotheses.

5.1. Notation

In general, a null hypothesis will be stated as

$$\mathbf{C}\boldsymbol{\xi} = \mathbf{k} \ ,$$

where $\mathbf{C} = \mathbf{C}(n_h \times m)$, $(n_h \leq m)$, is called the hypothesis matrix and is of rank n_h.

$\boldsymbol{\xi}$ is an $(m \times 1)$ column vector of parameters as defined in the general linear model.

$\mathbf{k}$ is a vector of n_h known elements, usually equal to $\mathbf{0}$.

n_h is called *degrees of freedom due to hypothesis*. Actually it is the number of rows in the hypothesis matrix $\mathbf{C}$. In other words, it is the number of nonredundant statements embodied in the null hypothesis.

n_e is called the *degrees of freedom due to error* and is equal to the number of observations minus the effective number of parameters.

It is important to keep in mind that in stating a composite hypothesis, we should *never* make:

(1) contradicting statements such as,

$$H_0\colon \beta_1 = \beta_2 \quad \text{and} \quad \beta_1 = 2\beta_2 \text{ simultaneously}$$

(2) redundant statements such as,

$$H_0\colon \tau_1 = \tau_2 \quad \text{and} \quad 3\tau_1 = 3\tau_2 \ .$$

5.2. Simple Linear Regression

Model

$$y_i = \mu + \beta x_i + e_i$$

$$\text{parameter vector } \xi = \begin{bmatrix} \mu \\ \beta \end{bmatrix}$$

EXAMPLE 1

$$H_0: \mu = 0$$
$$\text{Alt.}: \mu \neq 0$$

General linear hypothesis

$$[1,0] \begin{bmatrix} \mu \\ \beta \end{bmatrix} = 0$$
$$\mathbf{C} \quad \xi \quad = 0\,, \qquad n_h = 1$$

EXAMPLE 2

$$H_0: \beta = 0$$
$$\text{Alt.}: \beta \neq 0$$
$$[0,1] \begin{bmatrix} \mu \\ \beta \end{bmatrix} = 0$$
$$\mathbf{C} \quad \xi \quad = 0\,, \qquad n_h = 1$$

EXAMPLE 3

$$H_0: \mu = 0,\ \beta = 0 \text{ simultaneously}$$
$$\text{Alt.}: \text{At least one of the } \mu \text{ and } \beta \neq 0$$
$$\begin{bmatrix} 1 & 0 \\ 0 & 1 \end{bmatrix} \begin{bmatrix} \mu \\ \beta \end{bmatrix} = \begin{bmatrix} 0 \\ 0 \end{bmatrix}$$
$$\mathbf{C} \quad \xi \quad = \quad \mathbf{0}\,, \qquad n_h = 2$$

EXAMPLE 4

$$H_0: \mu = \beta$$
$$\text{Alt.}: \mu \neq \beta$$
$$[1,-1] \begin{bmatrix} \mu \\ \beta \end{bmatrix} = 0\,, \qquad n_h = 1$$

5.3. Analysis of Variance, One-way Classification

$$y_{ij} = \mu + \tau_i + e_{ij} \qquad (i = 1, 2, 3 \cdots v)$$
$$\text{Parameter vector } \xi' = [\mu, \tau_1, \tau_2, \tau_3, \ldots \tau_v]$$

EXAMPLE 1

$$H_0: \tau_1 = \tau_2 = \tau_3 = \cdots = \tau_v$$
$$\text{Alt.}: \tau_r \neq \tau_s \qquad \text{for at least one pair}$$

Keep in mind that we must not make redundant statements. Here we have $(v - 1)$ rows in the hypothesis matrix. i.e. $n_h = v - 1$

$$(v-1)\underbrace{\begin{bmatrix} 0 & 1 & -1 & 0 & 0 & \cdots & 0 \\ 0 & 1 & 0 & -1 & 0 & \cdots & 0 \\ 0 & 1 & 0 & 0 & -1 & \cdots & 0 \\ \cdot & \cdot & & \cdot & \cdot & & \cdot \\ 0 & 1 & 0 & 0 & 0 & \cdots & -1 \end{bmatrix}}_{(v+1)} \begin{bmatrix} \mu \\ \tau_1 \\ \tau_2 \\ \tau_3 \\ \cdot \\ \cdot \\ \cdot \\ \tau_v \end{bmatrix} = \begin{bmatrix} 0 \\ 0 \\ 0 \\ 0 \\ \cdot \\ \cdot \\ \cdot \\ 0 \end{bmatrix} (v-1)$$
$$\mathbf{C} \qquad\qquad \xi \quad = \quad \mathbf{0}$$

EXAMPLE 2

H_0: $\tau_1 = \tau_2 = \tau_3 = \cdots = \tau_v = 0$
Alt.: At least one $\tau \neq 0$

$$(v)\begin{bmatrix} 0 & 1 & 0 & 0 & 0 & \cdots & 0 \\ 0 & 0 & 1 & 0 & 0 & \cdots & 0 \\ 0 & 0 & 0 & 1 & 0 & \cdots & 0 \\ \cdot & & \cdot & & \cdot & \cdot & \cdot \\ 0 & 0 & 0 & 0 & 0 & \cdots & 1 \end{bmatrix}_{(v+1)} \begin{bmatrix} \mu \\ \tau_1 \\ \tau_2 \\ \tau_3 \\ \cdot \\ \cdot \\ \cdot \\ \tau_v \end{bmatrix} = \begin{bmatrix} 0 \\ 0 \\ 0 \\ \cdot \\ \cdot \\ \cdot \\ 0 \end{bmatrix} (v)$$

$$\mathbf{C} \qquad \boldsymbol{\xi} = \mathbf{0}$$

n_h = number of rows in C and is equal to v .

EXAMPLE 3. For simplicity, let us take $i = 1, 2, 3, 4$

H_0: $-\tau_1 + 2\tau_2 - \tau_3 = 0$ (Quadratic contrast of three effects)
Alt.: Quadratic contrast $\neq 0$

$$[0 \quad -1 \quad +2 \quad -1 \quad 0] \begin{bmatrix} \mu \\ \tau_1 \\ \tau_2 \\ \tau_3 \\ \tau_4 \end{bmatrix} = 0$$

$$\mathbf{C} \qquad \boldsymbol{\xi} = \mathbf{0}$$

5.4. Multiple Linear Regression

$$y_i = \mu + \beta_1 x_{1i} + \beta_2 x_{2i} + \beta_3 x_{3i} + \cdots \beta_k x_{ki} + e_i$$
parameter vector $\boldsymbol{\xi}' = [\mu, \beta_1, \beta_2, \beta_3, \ldots \beta_k]$

EXAMPLE 1

H_0: $\beta_1 = 0$
Alt.: $\beta_1 \neq 0$

$$[0,1,0,0 \cdots 0] \begin{bmatrix} \mu \\ \beta_1 \\ \beta_2 \\ \beta_3 \\ \cdot \\ \beta_k \end{bmatrix} = 0$$

$$\mathbf{C} \qquad \boldsymbol{\xi} = \mathbf{0}, \qquad n_h = 1.$$

EXAMPLE 2

H_0: $\beta_1 = \beta_2 = \beta_3 = \cdots = \beta_k = 0$
Alt.: At least one $\beta \neq 0$

$$(k)\begin{bmatrix} 0 & 1 & 0 & 0 & \cdots & 0 \\ 0 & 0 & 1 & 0 & \cdots & 0 \\ 0 & 0 & 0 & 1 & \cdots & 0 \\ \cdot & & \cdot & & \cdot & \cdot \\ 0 & 0 & 0 & 0 & \cdots & 1 \end{bmatrix}_{(k+1)} \begin{bmatrix} \mu_1 \\ \beta_2 \\ \beta_3 \\ \beta_4 \\ \cdot \\ \cdot \\ \cdot \\ \beta_k \end{bmatrix} = 0$$

$$\mathbf{C} \qquad \boldsymbol{\xi} = \mathbf{0}, \qquad n_h = k.$$

EXAMPLE 3

H_0: $\beta_1 = 0, \beta_3 = 0$ simultaneously
Alt.: At least one of β_1 and $\beta_3 \neq 0$

$$\underset{\mathbf{C}}{\begin{bmatrix} 0 & 1 & 0 & 0 & \cdots & 0 \\ 0 & 0 & 0 & 1 & \cdots & 0 \end{bmatrix}} \underset{\boldsymbol{\xi}}{\begin{bmatrix} \mu \\ \beta_1 \\ \beta_2 \\ \beta_3 \\ \cdot \\ \cdot \\ \cdot \\ \beta_k \end{bmatrix}} = \underset{\mathbf{0}}{\begin{bmatrix} 0 \\ 0 \end{bmatrix}} ; \qquad n_h = 2 .$$

5.5. Randomized Blocks

$$y_{ij} = \mu + \tau_i + \beta_j + e_{ij}$$

where μ is the general effect
τ_i are the treatment effects $(i = 1, 2, 3)$
β_j are the block effects $(j = 1, 2, 3, 4)$
e_{ij} is the experimental error

$$\text{parameter vector } \boldsymbol{\xi}' = [\mu,\tau_1,\tau_2,\tau_3,\beta_1,\beta_2,\beta_3,\beta_4]$$

EXAMPLE 1

H_0: $\tau_1 = \tau_2 = \tau_3$ (all treatments effects are equal)
Alt.: At least one pair $\tau_r \neq \tau_s$

$$\underset{\mathbf{C}}{\begin{bmatrix} 0 & 1 & -1 & 0 & 0 & 0 & 0 & 0 \\ 0 & 1 & 0 & -1 & 0 & 0 & 0 & 0 \end{bmatrix}} \underset{\boldsymbol{\xi}}{\begin{bmatrix} \mu \\ \tau_1 \\ \tau_2 \\ \tau_3 \\ \beta_1 \\ \beta_2 \\ \beta_3 \\ \beta_4 \end{bmatrix}} = \underset{\mathbf{0}}{\begin{bmatrix} 0 \\ 0 \end{bmatrix}} ; \qquad n_h = 2 .$$

EXAMPLE 2

H_0: $-\tau_1 + 2\tau_2 - \tau_3 = 0$ (quadratic contrast)
Alt.: Quadratic contrast $\neq 0$

$$\underset{\mathbf{C}}{[0 \quad -1 \quad 2 \quad -1 \quad 0 \quad 0 \quad 0 \quad 0]} \underset{\boldsymbol{\xi}}{\begin{bmatrix} \mu \\ \tau_1 \\ \tau_2 \\ \tau_3 \\ \beta_1 \\ \beta_2 \\ \beta_3 \\ \beta_4 \end{bmatrix}} = \mathbf{0} ; \qquad n_h = 1 .$$

From the above illustrations, it can be seen that we can write a great variety of tests in the form of the General Linear Hypothesis provided that we make no redundant hypothesis statements.

5.6. Quadratic Form due to Hypothesis

So far we have discussed only the model of full rank. i.e., in the normal equations,

$$\mathbf{A'A\hat{\xi} = A'y} \ ,$$

(A′A) has an inverse. We shall continue to assume this model throughout this chapter. Recall the General Linear Model

$$\mathbf{y = A\xi + e}$$

$$E(\mathbf{y}) = \mathbf{A\xi} \quad \text{and} \quad \text{var}\ (\mathbf{y}) = \sigma^2\mathbf{I} \ .$$

We then have the normal equations,

$$\mathbf{A'A\hat{\xi} = A'y} \ .$$

The estimate of $\boldsymbol{\xi}$ is

$$\hat{\boldsymbol{\xi}} = \mathbf{(A'A)^{-1}A'y} \ ,$$

and the variance of the estimate is

$$\begin{aligned} \text{var}\ (\hat{\boldsymbol{\xi}}) &= \mathbf{(A'A)^{-1}}\ \text{var}\ \mathbf{(A'y)(A'A)^{-1}} \\ &= \mathbf{(A'A)^{-1}A'}\ \text{var}\ \mathbf{(y)A(A'A)^{-1}} \\ &= \sigma^2\mathbf{(A'A)^{-1}A'A(A'A)^{-1}} \\ &= \sigma^2\mathbf{(A'A)^{-1}} \ . \end{aligned}$$

This is the expression for the variance-covariance matrix of the estimates of $\boldsymbol{\xi}$. Now suppose that we have a null hypothesis

$$H_0\colon \mathbf{C\xi = 0} \ .$$

We have an unbiased estimate of $\mathbf{C\xi}$ namely $\mathbf{C\hat{\xi}}$, i.e., under the null hypothesis,

$$\begin{aligned} E(\mathbf{C\hat{\xi}}) &= \mathbf{C\xi = 0} \\ \text{var}\ (\mathbf{C\hat{\xi}}) &= \mathbf{C}\ \text{var}\ (\hat{\boldsymbol{\xi}})\mathbf{C'} \\ &= \sigma^2\mathbf{C(A'A)^{-1}C'}, \\ [\text{var}\ (\mathbf{C\hat{\xi}})]^{-1} &= \frac{1}{\sigma^2}\mathbf{[C(A'A)^{-1}C']^{-1}} \ . \end{aligned}$$

Thus, under the null hypothesis, the standard quadratic form is

$$\frac{1}{\sigma^2}\mathbf{\hat{\xi}'C'[C(A'A)^{-1}C']^{-1}C\hat{\xi}} \ .$$

The expression, $\mathbf{\hat{\xi}'C'[C(A'A)^{-1}C']^{-1}C\hat{\xi}}$, is called the *sum of squares due to hypothesis*, usually denoted by SSH. If $\mathbf{y}$ has the multivariate normal distribution, SSH/σ^2 is distributed as χ^2 with n_h degrees of freedom, since it is a standard quadratic form.

5.7. Sum of Squares due to Error

Recall the general linear model

$$\mathbf{y = A\xi + e} \ .$$

Let us define $\mathbf{\hat{e} = y - A\hat{\xi}}$, the error of estimation. Then, $\sum_{i=1}^{n} \hat{e}_i^2 = \mathbf{\hat{e}'\hat{e}}$ is called the sum of squares of errors of estimation. It is customarily denoted by SSE

$$\begin{aligned} \text{SSE} = \mathbf{\hat{e}'\hat{e}} &= \mathbf{(y' - \hat{\xi}'A')(y - A\hat{\xi})} \\ &= \mathbf{y'y - \hat{\xi}'A'y - y'A\hat{\xi} + \hat{\xi}'A'A\xi} \\ &= \mathbf{y'y - \hat{\xi}'A'y - y'A\hat{\xi} + \hat{\xi}'A'y} \\ &= \mathbf{y'y - y'A\hat{\xi}} \ , \end{aligned}$$

where **y'y** is the sum of squares over all observations.
A'y is the column vector on the right hand side of the normal equations.
$\hat{\boldsymbol{\xi}}$ is a column vector whose elements are the estimates of $\boldsymbol{\xi}$.

In words, SSE is obtained by subtracting from the sum of squares of all observations, the scalar product of the vector of estimates of $\boldsymbol{\xi}$ and the vector on the right-hand side of the normal equations.

It should be noted that SSE can depend only on the model, and is determined once the model is stated; it is entirely independent of any hypothesis which may be stated or tested.

If **y** is normally distributed, SSE/σ^2 has the χ^2 distribution with n_e degrees of freedom. It is independent of any SSH.

5.8. Summary

We have the general linear model

$$\mathbf{y} = \mathbf{A}\boldsymbol{\xi} + \mathbf{e}$$
$$E(\mathbf{y}) = \mathbf{A}\boldsymbol{\xi} \; .$$

We assume that the model is of full rank, that is, **A'A** is non-singular and thus has an inverse. If we further assume that

$$\text{var}\,(\mathbf{y}) = \sigma^2\mathbf{I} \; ,$$

that is, homoscedasticity plus independence, we will have the normal equations

$$(\mathbf{A'A})\hat{\boldsymbol{\xi}} = \mathbf{A'y}$$

and we can obtain the estimate of $\boldsymbol{\xi}$ by

$$\hat{\boldsymbol{\xi}} = (\mathbf{A'A})^{-1}\mathbf{A'y} \; .$$

Again, if we further assume that the elements of **y** are normally distributed, we may test the following hypothesis:

$$H_0\text{: } \mathbf{C}\boldsymbol{\xi} = \mathbf{0}$$
$$\text{Alt.: } \mathbf{C}\boldsymbol{\xi} = \mathbf{n} \qquad (\neq \mathbf{0})$$

This hypothesis matrix has n_h rows and, if we avoid inconsistency and redundancies in the statement of the hypothesis, n_h will be the "degrees of freedom due to hypothesis".

5.9. Computational Procedure for Testing a Hypothesis

In testing a hypothesis, proceed as follows:

(1) Obtain SSH, the so called "sum of squares due to hypothesis" from the formula

$$\text{SSH} = \hat{\boldsymbol{\xi}}'\mathbf{C}'[\mathbf{C}(\mathbf{A'A})^{-1}\mathbf{C}']^{-1}\mathbf{C}\hat{\boldsymbol{\xi}} \; .$$

(2) Obtain SSE, the "sum of squares due to error" from

$$\text{SSE} = \sum_{\text{all}} y_i^2 - \mathbf{y'A}\hat{\boldsymbol{\xi}} \; .$$

(3) Introduce n_e, the "degrees of freedom due to error" which equals n (sample size) minus effective number of parameters in the model.

(4) Then, if H_0 is true

$$\frac{\text{SSH}/n_h}{\text{SSE}/n_e} = \text{F}_{(n_h, n_e)} \; .$$

5.10. Regression Significance Test

Suppose that we have the general linear model

$$\mathbf{y} = \mathbf{A}\boldsymbol{\xi} + \mathbf{e}$$
$$E(\mathbf{y}) = \mathbf{A}\boldsymbol{\xi} \quad \text{and} \quad \text{var}(\mathbf{y}) = \sigma^2\mathbf{I} \ .$$

Under this model, we have the normal equations

$$\mathbf{A}'\mathbf{A}\hat{\boldsymbol{\xi}} = \mathbf{A}'\mathbf{y}$$
$$\text{SSE} = \mathbf{y}'\mathbf{y} - \mathbf{y}'\mathbf{A}\hat{\boldsymbol{\xi}}$$
$$\text{where } \hat{\boldsymbol{\xi}} = (\mathbf{A}'\mathbf{A})^{-1}\mathbf{A}'\mathbf{y} \ .$$

Now, suppose that our hypothesis is of such a nature that we can easily write the reduced model under the assumption that H_0 is true.

$$\mathbf{y} = \mathbf{A}\boldsymbol{\xi} + \mathbf{e}^*$$
$$\text{subject to the condition } \mathbf{C}\boldsymbol{\xi} = \mathbf{0} \ .$$

Analogously, after estimating $\boldsymbol{\xi}$ in the above model (reduced model) we may write

$$\text{SSE (reduced)} = \mathbf{y}'\mathbf{y} - \mathbf{y}'\mathbf{A}\hat{\boldsymbol{\xi}}$$

where $\hat{\boldsymbol{\xi}}$ is the estimate of $\boldsymbol{\xi}$ in the reduced model. We can then find the sum of squares due to that hypothesis by obtaining

SSE (reduced) and subtracting SSE (the original or general model), i.e.,

$$\text{SSH} = \text{SSE (reduced)} - \text{SSE}.$$

5.11. Alternate Form of the Distribution

$\dfrac{\text{SSE}}{\text{SSE} + \text{SSH}}$ has the Beta distribution with parameters $(n_{e/2}, n_{h/2})$.

The beta tests are *lower-tail* tests, i.e., we reject H_0 if the value of the observed ratio is *smaller* than the tabulated one, i.e.,

$$\text{rejection region } \beta < \text{constant}.$$

Actually in the tables, percentage points of β are stated as

$$\beta(a,b),$$

where $a = 2$ (second parameter)

$b = 2$ (first parameter).

Hence, read those tables simply as $\beta(n_h, n_e)$

$$\frac{\text{SSE}}{\text{SSE (reduced)}} = \beta\left(\frac{n_e}{2}, \frac{n_h}{2}\right) \quad \text{(usual notation)}$$
$$= \beta^*(n_h, n_e) \quad \text{(Tables for Beta percentage points)}$$
$$= I\left(\frac{n_e}{2}, \frac{n_h}{2}\right) \quad \text{(Tables of the Incomplete Beta Function).}$$

6. GENERAL LINEAR MODEL OF LESS THAN FULL RANK

So far we have restricted our discussion to models of full rank in the General Linear Model. In practice, many design models are not initially of this form. Models not of full rank are sometimes called singular models.

If, in the General Linear Model

$$\mathbf{y} = \mathbf{A}\boldsymbol{\xi} + \mathbf{e} \ ,$$

with normal equations

$$\mathbf{A}'\mathbf{A}\hat{\boldsymbol{\xi}} = \mathbf{A}'\mathbf{y}$$

the rank of the design matrix **A** is less than m ($r < m$) then ($\mathbf{A}'\mathbf{A}$) would be singular and has no inverse. We must examine the system to see whether a solution exists. We wish to find functions of the ξ_i's for which unbiased estimates exist.

6.1. Estimable Function and Estimability

Let us estimate a function $\mathbf{l}'\boldsymbol{\xi}$, i.e., find $\mathbf{c}'\mathbf{y} = \mathbf{l}'\hat{\boldsymbol{\xi}}$ such that the expectation

$$E(\mathbf{c}'\mathbf{y}) = \mathbf{l}'\boldsymbol{\xi} \text{ for all } \boldsymbol{\xi} \ ,$$

and var ($\mathbf{c}'\mathbf{y}$) = minimum, i.e., we would like to find a linear function of the y_i's such that

$$E(\mathbf{c}'\mathbf{y}) = \mathbf{l}'\boldsymbol{\xi} \ ,$$

where $\mathbf{l}'$ is a given vector of "weights". The constraints of unbiasedness are

$$\begin{aligned} E(\mathbf{c}'\mathbf{y}) &= \mathbf{l}'\boldsymbol{\xi} \\ \mathbf{c}'E(\mathbf{y}) &= \mathbf{l}'\boldsymbol{\xi} \\ \mathbf{c}'\mathbf{A}\boldsymbol{\xi} &= \mathbf{l}'\boldsymbol{\xi} \qquad \text{for all } \boldsymbol{\xi}\text{, hence,} \\ \mathbf{c}'\mathbf{A} &= \mathbf{l}' \\ \mathbf{c}'\mathbf{A} - \mathbf{l}' &= \mathbf{0} \ . \end{aligned}$$

Hence, we are minimizing

$$\text{var } (\mathbf{c}'\mathbf{y}) \text{ subject to the constraints } \mathbf{c}'\mathbf{A} = \mathbf{l}'$$

where var ($\mathbf{c}'\mathbf{y}$) = $\sigma^2\mathbf{c}'\mathbf{c}$.

The criterion function Φ is then

$$\Phi = \tfrac{1}{2}\mathbf{c}'\mathbf{c} - [\mathbf{c}'\mathbf{A} - \mathbf{l}']\boldsymbol{\lambda}$$

$$\frac{\partial\Phi}{\partial\mathbf{c}} = \mathbf{c} - \mathbf{A}\boldsymbol{\lambda} \ .$$

Setting the derivative equal to zero, we obtain

$$\mathbf{A}\boldsymbol{\lambda} = \hat{\mathbf{c}} \tag{6.1.1}$$

Premultiplying by $\mathbf{A}'$, we have

$$\mathbf{A}'\mathbf{A}\boldsymbol{\lambda} = \mathbf{A}'\hat{\mathbf{c}} \ ,$$

which is equal to **l** under our constraints.

Hence,

$$\mathbf{A}'\mathbf{A}\boldsymbol{\lambda} = \mathbf{l} \ . \tag{6.1.2}$$

(6.1.1) and (6.1.2) are called "conjugate normal equations". If **A** has rank r ($<m$) we can always select r columns which form a "basis" and take the remaining ($m - r$) columns as an extension. The latter columns are linear combinations of the former.

In the model

$$\mathbf{y} = \mathbf{A}\boldsymbol{\xi} + \mathbf{e}$$

let us order the elements in $\boldsymbol{\xi}$ as well as the columns in **A** in such a way that

$$\boldsymbol{\xi}' = [\underset{(r)}{\boldsymbol{\xi}_1'} \ , \ \underset{(m-r)}{\boldsymbol{\xi}_2'}]$$

and

$$\mathbf{A} = [\underset{(r)}{\mathbf{A}_1} \ , \ \underset{(m-r)}{\mathbf{A}_2}](r)$$

and that $\mathbf{A}_1$ is a basis of $\mathbf{A}$. The columns of $\mathbf{A}_2$ must then be linear combinations of those in $\mathbf{A}_1$. We may express this fact formally by saying there exists

$$\mathbf{Q}(r \times \overline{m-r}) \qquad \text{such that} \qquad \mathbf{A}_2 = \mathbf{A}_1\mathbf{Q} \ .$$

Suppose

$$\begin{aligned} \mathbf{A}_2 &= \mathbf{A}_1 Q \\ \mathbf{A}_1'\mathbf{A}_2 &= \mathbf{A}_1'\mathbf{A}_1 Q \\ \mathbf{Q} &= (\mathbf{A}_1'\mathbf{A}_1)^{-1}\mathbf{A}_1'\mathbf{A}_2 \ . \end{aligned}$$

This is one of the ways to determine $\mathbf{Q}$ when $\mathbf{A}_1$ and $\mathbf{A}_2$ are given. Usually, however, we would try to find $\mathbf{Q}$ by inspection.

Now,

$$\begin{aligned} \mathbf{A} &= [\underset{(r)}{\mathbf{A}_1} \ , \ \underset{(m-r)}{\mathbf{A}_2}](r) \\ &= [\mathbf{A}_1, \mathbf{A}_1\mathbf{Q}] = \mathbf{A}_1[\underset{(r)}{\mathbf{I}} \qquad \underset{(m-r)}{\mathbf{Q}}](r) \end{aligned}$$

(6.1.2) can be written as

$$\begin{bmatrix} \mathbf{A}_1' \\ \mathbf{Q}'\mathbf{A}_1' \end{bmatrix} [\mathbf{A}_1 \ , \ \mathbf{A}_1\mathbf{Q}]\boldsymbol{\lambda} = \begin{bmatrix} \mathbf{A}_1'\mathbf{A}_1 & \mathbf{A}_1'\mathbf{A}_1\mathbf{Q} \\ \mathbf{Q}'\mathbf{A}_1'\mathbf{A}_1 & \mathbf{Q}'\mathbf{A}_1'\mathbf{A}_1\mathbf{Q} \end{bmatrix} \boldsymbol{\lambda} = \begin{bmatrix} \mathbf{l}_1 \\ \mathbf{l}_2 \end{bmatrix} \begin{matrix} (r) \\ (m-r) \end{matrix} \ .$$

Expanding we have

(6.1.3) $$[\mathbf{A}_1'\mathbf{A}_1, \mathbf{A}_1'\mathbf{A}_1\mathbf{Q}]\boldsymbol{\lambda} = \mathbf{l}_1$$

(6.1.4) $$[\mathbf{Q}'\mathbf{A}_1'\mathbf{A}_1, \mathbf{Q}'\mathbf{A}_1'\mathbf{A}_1\mathbf{Q}]\boldsymbol{\lambda} = \mathbf{l}_2 \ .$$

Premultiply (6.1.3) by $\mathbf{Q}'$ and obtain

$$[\mathbf{Q}'\mathbf{A}_1'\mathbf{A}_1, \mathbf{Q}'\mathbf{A}_1'\mathbf{A}_1\mathbf{Q}]\boldsymbol{\lambda} = \mathbf{Q}'\mathbf{l}_1 \ .$$

For consistency of the equation system, the condition

$$\mathbf{l}_2 = \mathbf{Q}'\mathbf{l}_1$$

must be met.

That is to say, in the function $\mathbf{l}'\boldsymbol{\xi}$, $\mathbf{l}'$ cannot be chosen arbitrarily but must be of the form

$$\mathbf{l}' = [\underset{(r)}{\mathbf{l}_1'} \ , \ \underset{(m-r)}{\mathbf{l}_2'}] \ , \quad \text{where}$$

(6.1.5) $$\mathbf{l}_2' = \mathbf{l}_1'\mathbf{Q} \ .$$

Only an $\mathbf{l}$ satisfying this relation can be used in the construction of a function which admits of a linear unbiased (and mathematically consistent) estimate.

(6.1.5) is called the condition of "estimability" of a linear function. Hence, we will call a function $\mathbf{l}'\boldsymbol{\xi}$ *estimable* if $\mathbf{l}'$ can be written as

$$[\mathbf{l}_1', \mathbf{l}_2'] \ ,$$

where $\mathbf{l}_2'$ is related to $\mathbf{l}_1'$ in the same way as $\mathbf{A}_2$ to $\mathbf{A}_1$.

We may then define that a parametric function is said to be linearly *estimable* if there exists a linear combination of the observations whose expected value is equal to the function, i.e., if there exists an unbiased estimate.

Now, if the function $\mathbf{l}'\boldsymbol{\xi}$ is estimable, (6.1.3) can be written as

$$(\mathbf{A}_1'\mathbf{A}_1)[\mathbf{I},\mathbf{Q}]\boldsymbol{\lambda} = \mathbf{l}_1 \ .$$

Notice that $\mathbf{l}_2$ may be disregarded since it is determined by the relation $\mathbf{l}_2 = \mathbf{Q}'\mathbf{l}_1$, hence,

$$[\mathbf{I},\mathbf{Q}]\boldsymbol{\lambda} = (\mathbf{A}_1'\mathbf{A}_1)^{-1}\mathbf{l}_1 \ . \tag{6.1.6}$$

The first conjugate normal equations (6.1.1) stated

$$\mathbf{A}\boldsymbol{\lambda} = \hat{\mathbf{c}}$$

or,

$$[\mathbf{A}_1,\mathbf{A}_2]\boldsymbol{\lambda} = \hat{\mathbf{c}}$$
$$\mathbf{A}_1[\mathbf{I},\mathbf{Q}]\boldsymbol{\lambda} = \hat{\mathbf{c}} \ .$$

Inserting (6.1.6), we obtain

$$\mathbf{A}_1(\mathbf{A}_1'\mathbf{A}_1)^{-1}\mathbf{l}_1 = \hat{\mathbf{c}} \ .$$

Hence,

$$\hat{\mathbf{c}}'\mathbf{y} = \widehat{\mathbf{l}'\boldsymbol{\xi}} = \mathbf{l}_1'(\mathbf{A}_1'\mathbf{A}_1)^{-1}\mathbf{A}_1'\mathbf{y} \ ,$$

which is of the same form as in the non-singular case, except that $\mathbf{A}$ has been replaced by its basis $\mathbf{A}_1$ and in $\mathbf{l}$ we consider only the first r elements, i.e., $\mathbf{l}_1$.

Hence, the normal equations in the Least Squares approach, i.e.,

$$\mathbf{A}'\mathbf{A}\hat{\boldsymbol{\xi}} = \mathbf{A}'\mathbf{y}$$

can be used formally in the reduced statement

$$(\mathbf{A}_1'\mathbf{A}_1)\hat{\boldsymbol{\xi}}_1 = \mathbf{A}_1'\mathbf{y} \ .$$

6.2. General Linear Hypothesis Model of Less Than Full Rank

We have the general linear model

$$\begin{aligned}
\mathbf{y} &= \mathbf{A}\boldsymbol{\xi} + \mathbf{e} \\
&= [\mathbf{A}_1,\mathbf{A}_2]\begin{bmatrix}\boldsymbol{\xi}_1 \\ \boldsymbol{\xi}_2\end{bmatrix} + \mathbf{e} \\
&= [\mathbf{A}_1,\mathbf{A}_1\mathbf{Q}]\begin{bmatrix}\boldsymbol{\xi}_1 \\ \boldsymbol{\xi}_2\end{bmatrix} + \mathbf{e} \\
&= \mathbf{A}_1\boldsymbol{\xi}_1 + \mathbf{A}_1\mathbf{Q}\boldsymbol{\xi}_2 + \mathbf{e} \\
&= \mathbf{A}_1(\boldsymbol{\xi}_1 + \mathbf{Q}\boldsymbol{\xi}_2) + \mathbf{e} \ .
\end{aligned}$$

Hence, we may write the general linear model in the form $\mathbf{y} = \mathbf{A}_1\boldsymbol{\xi}^* + \mathbf{e}$, where $\boldsymbol{\xi}^* = \boldsymbol{\xi}_1 + \mathbf{Q}\boldsymbol{\xi}_2$.

6.2.1. *Sum of Squares Due to Error and Its Distribution*

Notice that $\mathbf{e}$ has not been changed in this model, hence we can set up the normal equations

$$(\mathbf{A}_1'\mathbf{A}_1)\hat{\boldsymbol{\xi}}^* = \mathbf{A}_1'\mathbf{y}.$$

$$\begin{aligned}
\text{SSE} = \mathbf{e}'\mathbf{e} &= \mathbf{y}'\mathbf{y} - \mathbf{y}'\mathbf{A}_1\hat{\boldsymbol{\xi}}^* \\
&= \mathbf{y}'\mathbf{y} - \mathbf{y}'\mathbf{A}_1(\mathbf{A}_1'\mathbf{A}_1)^{-1}\mathbf{A}_1'\mathbf{y}
\end{aligned}$$

Then, as before

$$\frac{\text{SSE}}{\sigma^2} = \chi^2(n-r) \qquad \text{where } r \text{ is the rank of } \mathbf{A},$$

and replaces m in the non-singular model. The "effective" number of parameters in the singular model is only r, the remaining $(m - r)$ parameters are determined in terms of the first r by the estimability condition.

6.2.2. *Sum of Squares Due to Hypothesis and Its Distribution*

Suppose that we wish to test

$$H_0 \colon \mathbf{C}\boldsymbol{\xi} = \mathbf{0} \;,$$

where $C = [\underset{(r)}{\mathbf{C}_1} \;,\; \underset{(m-r)}{\mathbf{C}_2}]$.

Then $\mathbf{C}\boldsymbol{\xi} = \mathbf{0}$ implies that

$$[\mathbf{C}_1, \mathbf{C}_2] \begin{bmatrix} \boldsymbol{\xi}_1 \\ \boldsymbol{\xi}_2 \end{bmatrix} = \begin{bmatrix} \mathbf{0} \\ \mathbf{0} \end{bmatrix}.$$

Each row on the left-hand side must represent an estimable function, hence, we must have

$$\mathbf{C}_2 = \mathbf{C}_1\mathbf{Q} \;.$$

This is called the condition of "testability", i.e., if

$$\mathbf{C} = \begin{bmatrix} \mathbf{c}_2' \\ \mathbf{c}_1' \\ \cdot \\ \cdot \\ \cdot \\ \mathbf{c}_{n_h}' \end{bmatrix},$$

where $(\mathbf{c}_i'\boldsymbol{\xi})$ is an estimable function $(i = 1, 2, \ldots, n_h)$. Then the null hypothesis

$$H_0 \colon \mathbf{C}_1\boldsymbol{\xi}_1 + \mathbf{C}_2\boldsymbol{\xi}_2 = \mathbf{0}$$

can be written as

$$\mathbf{C}_1\boldsymbol{\xi}_1 + \mathbf{C}_1\mathbf{Q}\boldsymbol{\xi}_2 = \mathbf{0}$$

or simply $\mathbf{C}_1\boldsymbol{\xi}^* = \mathbf{0}$, where $\boldsymbol{\xi}^* = (\boldsymbol{\xi}_1 + \mathbf{Q}\boldsymbol{\xi}_2)$. Hence, we can formally state that a null hypothesis

$$H_0 \colon \mathbf{C}\boldsymbol{\xi} = \mathbf{0}$$

is "*testable*" if $\mathbf{C}\boldsymbol{\xi}$ consists of n_h estimable functions, i.e., if $\mathbf{C}_2 = \mathbf{C}_1\mathbf{Q}$, where $\mathbf{C} = [\mathbf{C}_1, \mathbf{C}_2]$. Consequently,

$$\text{SSH} = \hat{\boldsymbol{\xi}}^{*\prime}\mathbf{C}_1'[\mathbf{C}_1(\mathbf{A}_1'\mathbf{A}_1)^{-1}\mathbf{C}_1']^{-1}\mathbf{C}_1\hat{\boldsymbol{\xi}}^* \;,$$

where $\hat{\boldsymbol{\xi}}^* = (\mathbf{A}_1'\mathbf{A}_1)^{-1}\mathbf{A}_1\mathbf{y}$.

As before

$$\frac{\text{SSH}}{\sigma^2} = \chi^2_{(n_h)} \;.$$

Again, if the null-hypothesis is true, we have the test statistic F

$$\frac{\text{MSH}/n_h}{\text{MSE}/n_e} = \text{F}_{(n_h, n_e)} \;.$$

6.3. Constraints and Conditions

If the model is singular, of rank $r < m$, $(m - r)$ constraints on the $\hat{\xi}_i$'s (the estimates) may be arbitrarily introduced, for example:

(6.3.1) $$\hat{\xi}_{r+1} = 0, \ldots, \hat{\xi}_m = 0$$

or

(6.3.2) $$\sum_{i=1}^{m} \hat{\xi}_i = 0, \; \sum_{i=1}^{m} n_i\hat{\xi}_i = 0 \;.$$

This is called *reparametrizing* the model. The constraining functions are fairly arbitrary, but they *must not be estimable* functions, otherwise the resulting model will still be singular.

In effect, this is done by deletion of the last $(m - r)$ rows and columns of $\mathbf{A'A}$ and the last $(m - r)$ elements of $\mathbf{A'y}$, for constraints of the type (6.3.1), or by adding a constant to all elements of $\mathbf{A'A}$, for constraints of the type (6.3.2). This has no effect on the value of estimable functions, or test statistics.

An entirely different situation prevails if we place conditions on the *parameters* of a model, especially on interactions. In the two-way classification model

$$E(y_{ijk}) = \mu + \alpha_i + \beta_j + \delta_{ij}$$

one usually specifies

$$\sum_i n_{ij}\delta_{ij} = 0 \qquad \text{for all } j\text{'s}$$

and

$$\sum_j n_{ij}\delta_{ij} = 0 \qquad \text{for all } i\text{'s} \ ,$$

where n_{ij} denotes the number of observations in the (i, j) cell. These are sometimes called *natural constraints* (they are neither *natural* nor *constraints*). They simply represent a set of *conditions* or *assumptions* on the interactions, minimizing this effect (making SSH for interaction a minimum). After introducing these conditions, one still has a singular model, which can be made nonsingular by introduction of the arbitrary constraints

$$\sum_i \hat{\alpha}_i = 0, \sum_j \hat{\beta}_j = 0 \ .$$

(Note the carets, for estimates). One could introduce the different assumptions,

$$\text{All } \alpha_i\text{'s} = 0$$
$$\text{All } \beta_j\text{'s} = 0$$

and would have a simple one-way classification model, quite different from the previous one. A classical example is the following. Suppose some organic substance is attacked by sulphuric acid or by sodium hydroxide.

		NaOH −	NaOH +
H_2SO_4	−	0	4
	+	6	0

Using, formally, the minimizing interaction conditions, one would obtain effect estimates as means of rows and columns

H_2SO_4	absent: 2	present: 3
NaOH	absent: 3	present: 2

and make the ridiculous inference that sodium hydroxide, by itself, has an inhibiting effect. The correct parametric model in this case would be

μ	$\mu + \beta$
$\mu + \alpha$	$\mu + \alpha + \beta + \delta$

,

i.e., interaction occurs only if both substances are present. This leads to the estimation

$$\hat{\mu} = 0$$
$$\hat{\alpha} = 6$$
$$\hat{\beta} = 4$$
$$\hat{\delta} = -10 ,$$

which is the appropriate neutralization model.

It is usually quite easy to decide whether a constraint or a condition is involved. The (model-changing) *conditions* are required whenever a hierarchy of effects is present (main effects, interactions, higher-order interactions), while constraints (with no effect on the model) can be introduced within the same kinds of effects (row effect estimates adding to zero, column effect estimates adding to zero). The sum of squares due to a given hypothesis is a good indicator of the situation. If it changes by the introduction of two different sets of combinations, they are *conditions*, and must be determined in accordance with plausibility of the physical model. If it stays the same, they are usually *constraints on the estimates*, and thus arbitrary, without effect on the model.

SIMPLIFIED COMPUTATIONS FOR MULTIPLE REGRESSION

by Dr. Clyde Y. Kramer

The following method is especially suited for a research problem which has several dependent variables with one set of independent variables. It allows the worker to decide which dependent variables are explained by regression with the least time and work. Regression coefficients and their variances are not usually wanted unless the regression is significant. This procedure eliminates the need of calculating these quantities when prediction is not good enough to be useful.

The main advantages of this method are:

(a) the numbers of digits to the left of the decimal points of the elements of the sums of squares and sums of products matrix are adjusted to be one or zero which permits the use of a uniform number of decimal places in the calculations;
(b) the multiple correlation coefficient and entries for the analysis of variance table for multiple regression can be found without computing the regression coefficients and the inverse of the sums of squares and sums of products matrix;
(c) the additional reduction due to any regression variable over that obtained for previous ones is obtainable for every regression variable;
(d) the research worker can fit only those regression variables that add a significant additional reduction if he so desires;
(e) time or work is not lost if one wishes to obtain the regression coefficients and their variances; and
(f) numerous checks are employed on the calculations that are required.

Algebraic Procedure

For simplicity, this method will be illustrated by considering four independent variables (x_1, x_2, x_3, x_4), and one dependent variable, (y). First compute and record the sums of squares and sums of products in the following manner:

$$\text{(1)} \quad \begin{matrix} a_{11} & a_{12} & a_{13} & a_{14} & a_{1y} \\ & a_{22} & a_{23} & a_{24} & a_{2y} \\ & & a_{33} & a_{34} & a_{3y} \\ & & & a_{44} & a_{4y} \\ & & & & a_{yy} \end{matrix}$$

where

$$a_{ii} = \sum_{\alpha=1}^{n} x_{i\alpha}^2 - \frac{\left(\sum_{\alpha=1}^{n} x_{i\alpha}\right)^2}{n},$$

$$a_{ij} = \sum_{\alpha=1}^{n} x_{i\alpha}x_{j\alpha} - \frac{\left(\sum_{\alpha=1}^{n} x_{i\alpha}\right)\left(\sum_{\alpha=1}^{n} x_{j\alpha}\right)}{n},$$

$$a_{iy} = \sum_{\alpha=1}^{n} x_{i\alpha}y_{\alpha} - \frac{\left(\sum_{\alpha=1}^{n} x_{i\alpha}\right)\left(\sum_{\alpha=1}^{n} y_{\alpha}\right)}{n},$$

$$a_{yy} = \sum_{\alpha=1}^{n} y_{\alpha}^2 - \frac{\left(\sum_{\alpha=1}^{n} y_{\alpha}\right)^2}{n},$$

$i = j = 1, 2, 3, 4$, and n is the number of observations.

The first feature of this method is that the sum of squares for the dependent variable, a_{yy}, is recorded as the last entry of the column containing the sums of products of the dependent variable with the independent variables. The addition of a_{yy} to the last column results in a square matrix. This feature will be utilized to adjust the number of digits preceding the decimal points in the elements of the above matrix. The residual sum of squares is also obtained directly by adding the term a_{yy} to the last column of (1).

Then, in order to simplify the calculations, make the diagonal terms (a_{11}, a_{22}, a_{33}, a_{44}, a_{yy}) lie between 0.1 and 10 by pre- and post-multiplying (1) by a diagonal matrix of powers of ten which is as follows:

$$(2) \qquad \begin{bmatrix} 10^{q_1} & 0 & 0 & 0 & 0 \\ 0 & 10^{q_2} & 0 & 0 & 0 \\ 0 & 0 & 10^{q_3} & 0 & 0 \\ 0 & 0 & 0 & 10^{q_4} & 0 \\ 0 & 0 & 0 & 0 & 10^{p} \end{bmatrix}.$$

This will also result in the sums of products having at most one digit before the decimal points, thus allowing a uniform number of decimal places in all future calculations. The values of the q_i's and p are determined as follows:

Consider only a diagonal term and in it the largest *even* number of places through which the decimal point must be shifted (left or right) to make that term be a number between 0.1 and 10. Then divide this even number by two to get the applicable value of q_1 or p. For example, if $a_{11} = 8{,}238.93$, q_1 would be -2; if $a_{33} = 2{,}213{,}922.00$, q_3 would be -3; and if $a_{yy} = 5{,}098{,}35$, p would be -2.

After pre- and post-multiplying (1) by (2), which in effect is accomplished by adding the q_i's and p according to the term we are adjusting and shifting the decimal point the number of places indicated by the sum, we obtain a matrix of a^*'s. If, as in the above paragraph, $q_1 = -2$ and $p = -2$, we would shift the decimal point of a_{11} four places to the left and the decimal point of a_{1y} four places to the left, etc.

The work sheet will look as follows:

$$
(3)\qquad
\begin{array}{ccccc}
a^*_{11} & a^*_{12} & a^*_{13} & a^*_{14} & a^*_{1y} \\
 & a^*_{22} & a^*_{23} & a^*_{24} & a^*_{2y} \\
 & & a^*_{33} & a^*_{34} & a^*_{3y} \\
 & & & a^*_{44} & a^*_{4y} \\
 & & & & a^*_{yy}
\end{array}
$$

where $a^*_{ii} = 10^{2q_i}a_{ii}$, $a^*_{ij} = 10^{(q_i+q_j)}\, a_{ij}$; $a^*_{iy} = 10^{(q_i+p)}\, a_{iy}$, and $a^*_{yy} = 10^{2p}a_{yy}$. The matrix (3) is then reduced by the Abbreviated Doolittle Method after calculating a^*_{ic}, which is the sum of the terms in the ith row *including* the terms in the ith row omitted because of symmetry. The column of a^*_{ic}'s is used to provide checks on the calculations required to reduce (3).

Since a_{yy} is the total sum of squares used in an analysis of variance table for a multiple regression problem, when we reduce (3) by the Abbreviated Doolittle Method, the term resulting from a^*_{yy} is used to compute the residual sum of squares after fitting all the x_i's. In fact, this sum of squares is readily calculated by multiplying the term resulting from a^*_{yy} by 10^{-2p}.

Algebraic Procedure for the Forward Solution of the Abbreviated Doolittle Method

The work sheet should now look like:

$$
(4)\qquad
\begin{array}{ccccc|c}
a^*_{11} & a^*_{12} & a^*_{13} & a^*_{14} & a^*_{1y} & a^*_{1c} \\
 & a^*_{22} & a^*_{23} & a^*_{24} & a^*_{2y} & a^*_{2c} \\
 & & a^*_{33} & a^*_{34} & a^*_{3y} & a^*_{3c} \\
 & & & a^*_{44} & a^*_{4y} & a^*_{4c} \\
 & & & & a^*_{yy} & a^*_{yc}
\end{array}
$$

We then compute the following from (4):

$$
(5)\qquad
\begin{array}{ccccc|c|l}
 & & & & & & \text{Check Column} \\
A_{11} & A_{12} & A_{13} & A_{14} & A_{1y} & A_{1c} & \\
B_{11} & B_{12} & B_{13} & B_{14} & B_{1y} & B_{1c} & \Sigma B_{1j}(j = 1, 2, 3, 4, y) \\
\hline
 & A_{22} & A_{23} & A_{24} & A_{2y} & A_{2c} & \Sigma A_{2j}(j = 2, 3, 4, y) \\
 & B_{22} & B_{23} & B_{24} & B_{2y} & B_{2c} & \Sigma B_{2j}(j = 2, 3, 4, y) \\
\hline
 & & A_{33} & A_{34} & A_{3y} & A_{3c} & \Sigma A_{3j}(j = 3, 4, y) \\
 & & B_{33} & B_{34} & B_{3y} & B_{3c} & \Sigma B_{3j}(j = 3, 4, y) \\
\hline
 & & & A_{44} & A_{4y} & A_{4c} & \Sigma A_{4j}(j = 4, y) \\
 & & & B_{44} & B_{4y} & B_{4c} & \Sigma B_{4j}(j = 4, y) \\
\hline
 & & & & A_{yy} & A_{yc} & A_{yy}
\end{array}
$$

TABLE I

Source	d.f.	S.S.	M.S.	F
Regression	4	$a_{yy} - 10^{-2p}A_{yy}$	$\dfrac{a_{yy} - 10^{-2p}A_{yy}}{4}$	$\dfrac{\text{M.S. (Regression)}}{\text{M.S. (Residual)}}$
Residual	$n - 5$	$10^{-2p}A_{yy}$	$\dfrac{10^{-2p}A_{yy}}{n-5}$	
Total	$n - 1$	a_{yy}		

where $A_{1j} = a^*_{1j}$
$B_{1j} = A_{1j}/A_{11}$
$A_{2j} = a^*_{2j} - A_{12}B_{1j}$
$B_{2j} = A_{2j}/A_{22}$
$A_{3j} = a^*_{3j} - A_{13}B_{1j} - A_{23}B_{2j}$
$B_{3j} = A_{3j}/A_{33}$
$A_{4j} = a^*_{4j} - A_{14}B_{1j} - A_{24}B_{2j} - A_{34}B_{3j}$
$B_{4j} = A_{4j}/A_{44}$
$A_{yj} = a^*_{yj} - A_{1y}B_{1j} - A_{2y}B_{2j} - A_{3y}B_{3j} - A_{4y}B_{4j}$.

After completing the calculations for each row of (5), we compute the term indicated in the check column and compare it with the A_{ic} or B_{ic} term associated with it. If these do not agree within one of the last two decimal places, a mistake has been made, and the last row should be checked before proceeding.

Tests of Significance

We now have all the values needed to compute R^2 and the entries for the analysis of variance table. R^2 is computed by

(6) $$R^2 = \frac{a_{yy} - 10^{-2p}A_{yy}}{a_{yy}} .$$

The analysis of variance table for regression due to fitting all the x_i's is set up as in Table I. If one wishes to test the significance of the additional reduction due to any regression variable over that obtained for previous ones, the analysis of variance shown in Table II can be set up.

In fact, if the research worker is only interested in fitting those independent variables that add a significant reduction to the regression sum of squares, this can be accomplished by modifying the above. First we compute (4) in the usual way; then the first two rows of (5).

TABLE II

Source	d.f.	S.S.	M.S.	F
Regression due to x_1	1	$10^{-2p}A_{1y}B_{1y} = A$	A	$\frac{A}{\text{M.S. (Residual)}}$
Additional reduction due to x_2 over x_1	1	$10^{-2p}A_{2y}B_{2y} = B$	B	$\frac{B}{\text{M.S. (Residual)}}$
Additional reduction due to x_3 over x_1 and x_2	1	$10^{-2p}A_{3y}B_{3y} = C$	C	$\frac{C}{\text{M.S. (Residual)}}$
Additional reduction due to x_4 over x_1, x_2 and x_3	1	$10^{-2p}A_{4y}B_{4y} = D$	D	$\frac{D}{\text{M.S. (Residual)}}$
Residual	$n - 5$	$10^{-2p}A_{yy}$	$\frac{10^{-2p}A_{yy}}{n - 5}$	
Total	$n - 1$	a_{yy}		

Now we compute an F-ratio where

(7) $$F = \frac{10^{-2p}A_{1y}B_{1y}}{\dfrac{(a_{yy} - 10^{-2p}A_{1y}B_{1y})}{n - 2}} .$$

If this F-ratio which has one and $(n - 2)$ degrees of freedom is significant, we proceed to the next two rows of (5); if it is not significant, we delete the first row of (4), which has the effect of throwing out x_1. If at any time the residual sum of squares is reduced enough that $10^{-2p}A_{1y}B_{1y}$ would be significant, the variable x_1 can be brought back into (4) in another position. If this does not happen, it is left out of the analysis. To see if the added reduction due to x_3 is significant we compute

$$F = \frac{10^{-2p}A_{3y}B_{3y}}{\dfrac{\left(a_{yy} - 10^{-2p}\sum_{i=1}^{3} A_{iy}B_{iy}\right)}{n-4}} \quad (8)$$

We would then proceed as above, if this F-ratio with one and $(n - 4)$ degrees of freedom were significant.

If the above F-tests are not significant, or if the analysis of Table I is not significant, the research worker will be able to stop here because the regression coefficients and their variances will not be required. If, however, the F-test in Table I was significant and the regression coefficients are required, we would proceed as follows.

First a set of modified regression coefficients, b^*_i, are calculated by

$$\begin{aligned} b^*_4 &= B_{4y} \\ b^*_3 &= B_{3y} - b^*_4B_{34} \\ b^*_2 &= B_{2y} - b^*_3B_{23} - b^*_4B_{24} \\ b^*_1 &= B_{1y} - b^*_2B_{12} - b^*_3B_{13} - b^*_4B_{14}\,. \end{aligned} \quad (9)$$

The required set of regression coefficients, b_i, are then computed from (9) and (2) using

$$\begin{aligned} b_1 &= 10^{(q_1-p)}b^*_1 \\ b_2 &= 10^{(q_2-p)}b^*_2 \\ b_3 &= 10^{(q_3-p)}b^*_3 \\ b_4 &= 10^{(q_4-p)}b^*_4\,. \end{aligned} \quad (10)$$

At this stage, we can make a further check on our calculations since $\sum_{i=1}^{4} b_ia_{iy} = a_{yy} - 10^{-2p}A_{yy}$, which is the regression sum of squares in Table I.

To obtain the variances of the b_i's we must obtain the diagonal terms of the inverse of the first four rows and columns of (1). These terms are obtained by first computing the inverse of (4) by the backward solution of the Abbreviated Doolittle Method.

Backward Solution of the Abbreviated Doolittle Method

The inverse of (4) is computed and recorded in the following manner:

$$\begin{matrix} c^*_{11} & c^*_{12} & c^*_{13} & c^*_{14} \\ & c^*_{22} & c^*_{23} & c^*_{24} \\ & & c^*_{33} & c^*_{34} \\ & & & c^*_{44} \end{matrix} \quad (11)$$

where

$$\begin{aligned} c^*_{44} &= 1/A_{44} \\ c^*_{34} &= -c^*_{44}B_{34} \\ c^*_{24} &= -c^*_{34}B_{23} - c^*_{44}B_{24} \\ c^*_{14} &= -c^*_{24}B_{12} - c^*_{34}B_{13} - c^*_{44}B_{14}\,. \end{aligned}$$

At this point another check is applied by computing $\sum_{i=1}^{4} a^*_{i4}c^*_{i4}$, which should be approximately one.

$$c^*_{33} = 1/A_{33} - c^*_{34}B_{34}$$
$$c^*_{23} = -c^*_{33}B_{23} - c^*_{34}B_{24}$$
$$c^*_{13} = -c^*_{23}B_{12} - c^*_{33}B_{13} - c^*_{34}B_{14} \ .$$

One should now check to see that $\sum_{i=1}^{4} a^*_{i3}c^*_{i3}$ is approximately one.

$$c^*_{22} = 1/A_{22} - c^*_{23}B_{23} - c^*_{24}B_{24}$$
$$c^*_{12} = -c^*_{22}B_{12} - c^*_{23}B_{13} - c^*_{24}B_{14} \ .$$

Again check to see if $\sum_{i=1}^{4} a^*_{i2}c^*_{i2}$ is approximately one.

$$c^*_{11} = 1/A_{11} - c^*_{12}B_{12} - c^*_{13}B_{13} - c^*_{14}B_{14} \ .$$

The last check is that $\sum_{i=1}^{4} a^*_{i1}c^*_{i1}$ should be approximately one.

In the above it is obvious because of symmetry that $a^*_{ij} = a^*_{ji}$ and $c^*_{ij} = c^*_{ji}$. Now to obtain the variances of the regression coefficients, we require c_{11}, c_{22}, c_{33}, c_{44} . These are calculated by

(12) $$c_{ii} = 10^{2q_i}c^*_{ii} \ .$$

The variance of b_i is then obtained by multiplying c_{ii} times the residual mean square.

PLANS FOR DESIGN OF EXPERIMENTS

In this section, tables of combinatorial patterns usable as experimental designs are presented. No attempt is made to develop these patterns from first principles nor to discuss the choice of patterns or their applicability in experimental situations. These selected patterns are abridged from a more numerous set of patterns presented in the text *Experimental Designs* by Cochran and Cox (1957). The plan numbers refer to those in Cochran and Cox.

Plan 4.1 Selected latin squares

3 × 3

A	B	C
B	C	A
C	A	B

4 × 4

1

A	B	C	D
B	A	D	C
C	D	B	A
D	C	A	B

2

A	B	C	D
B	C	D	A
C	D	A	B
D	A	B	C

3

A	B	C	D
B	D	A	C
C	A	D	B
D	C	B	A

4

A	B	C	D
B	A	D	C
C	D	A	B
D	C	B	A

5 × 5

A	B	C	D	E
B	A	E	C	D
C	D	A	E	B
D	E	B	A	C
E	C	D	B	A

6 × 6

A	B	C	D	E	F
B	F	D	C	A	E
C	D	E	F	B	A
D	A	F	E	C	B
E	C	A	B	F	D
F	E	B	A	D	C

7 × 7

A	B	C	D	E	F	G
B	C	D	E	F	G	A
C	D	E	F	G	A	B
D	E	F	G	A	B	C
E	F	G	A	B	C	D
F	G	A	B	C	D	E
G	A	B	C	D	E	F

8 × 8

A	B	C	D	E	F	G	H
B	C	D	E	F	G	H	A
C	D	E	F	G	H	A	B
D	E	F	G	H	A	B	C
E	F	G	H	A	B	C	D
F	G	H	A	B	C	D	E
G	H	A	B	C	D	E	F
H	A	B	C	D	E	F	G

9 × 9

A	B	C	D	E	F	G	H	I
B	C	D	E	F	G	H	I	A
C	D	E	F	G	H	I	A	B
D	E	F	G	H	I	A	B	C
E	F	G	H	I	A	B	C	D
F	G	H	I	A	B	C	D	E
G	H	I	A	B	C	D	E	F
H	I	A	B	C	D	E	F	G
I	A	B	C	D	E	F	G	H

10 × 10

A	B	C	D	E	F	G	H	I	J
B	C	D	E	F	G	H	I	J	A
C	D	E	F	G	H	I	J	A	B
D	E	F	G	H	I	J	A	B	C
E	F	G	H	I	J	A	B	C	D
F	G	H	I	J	A	B	C	D	E
G	H	I	J	A	B	C	D	E	F
H	I	J	A	B	C	D	E	F	G
I	J	A	B	C	D	E	F	G	H
J	A	B	C	D	E	F	G	H	I

11 × 11

A	B	C	D	E	F	G	H	I	J	K
B	C	D	E	F	G	H	I	J	K	A
C	D	E	F	G	H	I	J	K	A	B
D	E	F	G	H	I	J	K	A	B	C
E	F	G	H	I	J	K	A	B	C	D
F	G	H	I	J	K	A	B	C	D	E
G	H	I	J	K	A	B	C	D	E	F
H	I	J	K	A	B	C	D	E	F	G
I	J	K	A	B	C	D	E	F	G	H
J	K	A	B	C	D	E	F	G	H	I
K	A	B	C	D	E	F	G	H	I	J

12 × 12

A	B	C	D	E	F	G	H	I	J	K	L
B	C	D	E	F	G	H	I	J	K	L	A
C	D	E	F	G	H	I	J	K	L	A	B
D	E	F	G	H	I	J	K	L	A	B	C
E	F	G	H	I	J	K	L	A	B	C	D
F	G	H	I	J	K	L	A	B	C	D	E
G	H	I	J	K	L	A	B	C	D	E	F
H	I	J	K	L	A	B	C	D	E	F	G
I	J	K	L	A	B	C	D	E	F	G	H
J	K	L	A	B	C	D	E	F	G	H	I
K	L	A	B	C	D	E	F	G	H	I	J
L	A	B	C	D	E	F	G	H	I	J	K

Plan 4.2 Graeco-latin squares

3 × 3

A_{1}	B_{3}	C_{2}
B_{2}	C_{1}	A_{3}
C_{3}	A_{2}	B_{1}

4 × 4

A_{1}	B_{3}	C_{4}	D_{2}
B_{2}	A_{4}	D_{3}	C_{1}
C_{3}	D_{1}	A_{2}	B_{4}
D_{4}	C_{2}	B_{1}	A_{3}

5 × 5

A_{1}	B_{3}	C_{5}	D_{2}	E_{4}
B_{2}	C_{4}	D_{1}	E_{3}	A_{5}
C_{3}	D_{5}	E_{2}	A_{4}	B_{1}
D_{4}	E_{1}	A_{3}	B_{5}	C_{2}
E_{5}	A_{2}	B_{4}	C_{1}	D_{3}

7 × 7

A_{1}	B_{5}	C_{2}	D_{6}	E_{3}	F_{7}	G_{4}
B_{2}	C_{6}	D_{3}	E_{7}	F_{4}	G_{1}	A_{5}
C_{3}	D_{7}	E_{4}	F_{1}	G_{5}	A_{2}	B_{6}
D_{4}	E_{1}	F_{5}	G_{2}	A_{6}	B_{3}	C_{7}
E_{5}	F_{2}	G_{6}	A_{3}	B_{7}	C_{4}	D_{1}
F_{6}	G_{3}	A_{7}	B_{4}	C_{1}	D_{5}	E_{2}
G_{7}	A_{4}	B_{1}	C_{5}	D_{2}	E_{6}	F_{3}

8 × 8

A_{1}	B_{5}	C_{2}	D_{3}	E_{7}	F_{4}	G_{8}	H_{6}
B_{2}	A_{8}	G_{1}	F_{7}	H_{3}	D_{6}	C_{5}	E_{4}
C_{3}	G_{4}	A_{7}	E_{1}	D_{2}	H_{5}	B_{6}	F_{8}
D_{4}	F_{3}	E_{6}	A_{5}	C_{8}	B_{1}	H_{7}	G_{2}
E_{5}	H_{1}	D_{8}	C_{4}	A_{6}	G_{3}	F_{2}	B_{7}
F_{6}	D_{7}	H_{4}	B_{8}	G_{5}	A_{2}	E_{3}	C_{1}
G_{7}	C_{6}	B_{3}	H_{2}	F_{1}	E_{8}	A_{4}	D_{5}
H_{8}	E_{2}	F_{5}	G_{6}	B_{4}	C_{7}	D_{1}	A_{3}

9 × 9

A_{1}	B_{3}	C_{2}	D_{7}	E_{9}	F_{8}	G_{4}	H_{6}	I_{5}
B_{2}	C_{1}	A_{3}	E_{8}	F_{7}	D_{9}	H_{5}	I_{4}	G_{6}
C_{3}	A_{2}	B_{1}	F_{9}	D_{8}	E_{7}	I_{6}	G_{5}	H_{4}
D_{4}	E_{6}	F_{5}	G_{1}	H_{3}	I_{2}	A_{7}	B_{9}	C_{8}
E_{5}	F_{4}	D_{6}	H_{2}	I_{1}	G_{3}	B_{8}	C_{7}	A_{9}
F_{6}	D_{5}	E_{4}	I_{3}	G_{2}	H_{1}	C_{9}	A_{8}	B_{7}
G_{7}	H_{9}	I_{8}	A_{4}	B_{6}	C_{5}	D_{1}	E_{3}	F_{2}
H_{8}	I_{7}	G_{9}	B_{5}	C_{4}	A_{6}	E_{2}	F_{1}	D_{3}
I_{9}	G_{8}	H_{7}	C_{6}	A_{5}	B_{4}	F_{3}	D_{2}	E_{1}

11 × 11

A_{1}	B_{7}	C_{2}	D_{8}	E_{3}	F_{9}	G_{4}	H_{10}	I_{5}	J_{11}	K_{6}
B_{2}	C_{8}	D_{3}	E_{9}	F_{4}	G_{10}	H_{5}	I_{11}	J_{6}	K_{1}	A_{7}
C_{3}	D_{9}	E_{4}	F_{10}	G_{5}	H_{11}	I_{6}	J_{1}	K_{7}	A_{2}	B_{8}
D_{4}	E_{10}	F_{5}	G_{11}	H_{6}	I_{1}	J_{7}	K_{2}	A_{8}	B_{3}	C_{9}
E_{5}	F_{11}	G_{6}	H_{1}	I_{7}	J_{2}	K_{8}	A_{3}	B_{9}	C_{4}	D_{10}
F_{6}	G_{1}	H_{7}	I_{2}	J_{8}	K_{3}	A_{9}	B_{4}	C_{10}	D_{5}	E_{11}
G_{7}	H_{2}	I_{8}	J_{3}	K_{9}	A_{4}	B_{10}	C_{5}	D_{11}	E_{6}	F_{1}
H_{8}	I_{3}	J_{9}	K_{4}	A_{10}	B_{5}	C_{11}	D_{6}	E_{1}	F_{7}	G_{2}
I_{9}	J_{4}	K_{10}	A_{5}	B_{11}	C_{6}	D_{1}	E_{7}	F_{2}	G_{8}	H_{3}
J_{10}	K_{5}	A_{11}	B_{6}	C_{1}	D_{7}	E_{2}	F_{8}	G_{3}	H_{9}	I_{4}
K_{11}	A_{6}	B_{1}	C_{7}	D_{2}	E_{8}	F_{3}	G_{9}	H_{4}	I_{10}	J_{5}

12 × 12

A_{1}	B_{12}	C_{6}	D_{7}	I_{5}	J_{4}	K_{10}	L_{11}	E_{9}	F_{8}	G_{2}	H_{3}
B_{2}	A_{11}	D_{5}	C_{8}	J_{6}	I_{3}	L_{9}	K_{12}	F_{10}	E_{7}	H_{1}	G_{4}
C_{3}	D_{10}	A_{8}	B_{5}	K_{7}	L_{2}	I_{12}	J_{9}	G_{11}	H_{6}	E_{4}	F_{1}
D_{4}	C_{9}	B_{7}	A_{6}	L_{8}	K_{1}	J_{11}	I_{10}	H_{12}	G_{5}	F_{3}	E_{2}
E_{5}	F_{4}	G_{10}	H_{11}	A_{9}	B_{8}	C_{2}	D_{3}	I_{1}	J_{12}	K_{6}	L_{7}
F_{6}	E_{3}	H_{9}	G_{12}	B_{10}	A_{7}	D_{1}	C_{4}	J_{2}	I_{11}	L_{5}	K_{8}
G_{7}	H_{2}	E_{12}	F_{9}	C_{11}	D_{6}	A_{4}	B_{1}	K_{3}	L_{10}	I_{8}	J_{5}
H_{8}	G_{1}	F_{11}	E_{10}	D_{12}	C_{5}	B_{3}	A_{2}	L_{4}	K_{9}	J_{7}	I_{6}
I_{9}	J_{8}	K_{2}	L_{3}	E_{1}	F_{12}	G_{6}	H_{7}	A_{5}	B_{4}	C_{10}	D_{11}
J_{10}	I_{7}	L_{1}	K_{4}	F_{2}	E_{11}	H_{5}	G_{8}	B_{6}	A_{3}	D_{9}	C_{12}
K_{11}	L_{6}	I_{4}	J_{1}	G_{3}	H_{10}	E_{8}	F_{5}	C_{7}	D_{2}	A_{12}	B_{9}
L_{12}	K_{5}	J_{3}	I_{2}	H_{4}	G_{9}	F_{7}	E_{6}	D_{8}	C_{1}	B_{11}	A_{10}

INDEX TO PLANS OF FACTORIAL EXPERIMENTS CONFOUNDED IN RANDOMIZED INCOMPLETE BLOCKS

a. Designs with which any number of replicates may be used

Type	Number of treat-ments	Number of units per block	Interactions confounded in a single replicate*	Plan
2^3	8	4	*ABC*	6.1
2^4	16	8	*ABCD*	6.2
2^4	16	4	*AB*, *ACD*, *BCD*	6.4
2^5	32	8	*ABC*, *ADE*, *BCDE*	6.5
2^6	64	16	*ABCD*, *ABEF*, *CDEF*	6.3
2^6	64	8	*ABC*, *CDE*, *ADF*, *BEF*, *ABDE*, *BCDF*, *ACEF*	6.6
3^3	27	9	*ABC* ($\frac{3}{4}$)	6.7
3^4	81	9	*ABC*, *ABD*, *ACD*, *BCD*, all ($\frac{3}{4}$)	6.8
4^2	16	4	*AB* ($\frac{2}{3}$)	6.12
4×2^2	16	8	*ABC* ($\frac{2}{3}$)	6.13

* The fractions in parentheses give the relative information on the comparisons which are confounded. Where no fraction is given, the comparison is completely confounded.

b. Balanced designs

Type	Number of treat-ments	Units per block	Number of replicates for a balanced design	Interactions confounded and relative information (in parentheses)*	Plan
2^4	16	4	$6n$†	All two-factor ($\frac{5}{6}$); all three factor ($\frac{1}{2}$)	6.4
2^5	32	8	$5n$	All three-factor ($\frac{4}{5}$); all four-factor ($\frac{4}{5}$)	6.5
2^6	64	8	$10n$	All three-factor ($\frac{4}{5}$); all four-factor ($\frac{4}{5}$)	6.6
3^3	27	9	$4n$	All three-factor ($\frac{3}{4}$)	6.7
3^4	81	9	$4n$	All three-factor ($\frac{3}{4}$)	6.8
3×2^2	12	6	$3n$‡	*BC* ($\frac{8}{9}$), *ABC* ($\frac{5}{9}$)	6.9
3×2^3	24	6	$3n$‡	*BC*, *BD*, *CD*, all ($\frac{8}{9}$); *ABC*, *ABD*, *ACD*, all ($\frac{5}{9}$)	6.10
$3^2 \times 2$	18	6	$4n$	*AB* ($\frac{7}{8}$), *ABC* ($\frac{5}{8}$)	6.11
4^2	16	4	$3n$	*AB* ($\frac{2}{3}$)	6.12
4×2^2	16	8	$3n$	*ABC* ($\frac{2}{3}$)	6.13
$4 \times 3 \times 2$	24	12	$9n$‡	*AC* ($\frac{26}{27}$), *ABC* ($\frac{23}{27}$)	6.14

* The factors *ABC* · · · are read from the left; thus the *BC* interaction in a 3×2^2 design is the interaction between the 2 factors at 2 levels.

† The symbol "$6n$" denotes that the number of replicates should be a multiple of 6.

‡ In these cases only the balanced design is recommended.

CONFOUNDED DESIGNS FOR OTHER FACTORIAL EXPERIMENTS

Type	Units per block	Number of replicates	Interactions confounded	Reference
$3^2 \times 2^2$	12	$2n$	AB ($\frac{7}{8}$); $ABCD$ ($\frac{5}{8}$)	6.6
$3^3 \times 2$	18	$2n$	ABC, $ABCD$	6.6
$3^3 \times 2$	6	$2n$	AB, AC, BC ($\frac{7}{8}$), ABD, ACD, BCD, ABC	6.1
4×3^2	12	$2n$	BC ($\frac{7}{8}$), ABC	6.6
$4^2 \times 2$	16	Any	ABC	6.6
$4^2 \times 3$	12	$3n$	AB ($\frac{26}{27}$), ABC	6.6
4^3	16	Any	ABC	6.7
4×2^3	8	$3n$	ABC, ABD, ACD	6.6
4^4	16	Any	ABC, ABD, ACD, BCD	6.7
5^2	5	$4n$	AB ($\frac{3}{4}$)	6.8
5×2^2	10	$5n$	BC ($\frac{24}{25}$), ABC	6.6
5^3	25	Any	ABC	6.8

Plan 6.1 2^3 factorial, blocks of 4 units

Rep. I, *ABC* confounded

abc	*ab*
a	*ac*
b	*bc*
c	(1)

Plan 6.2 2^4 factorial, blocks of 8 units

Rep. I, *ABCD* confounded

a	(1)
b	*ab*
c	*ac*
d	*bc*
abc	*ad*
abd	*bd*
acd	*cd*
bcd	*abcd*

Plan 6.3 2^6 factorial, blocks of 16 units

Rep. I, *ABCD, ABEF, CDEF* confounded

a	*c*	*ab*	*ac*
b	*d*	*cd*	*ad*
acd	*abc*	(1)	*bc*
bcd	*abd*	*abcd*	*bd*
ce	*ae*	*ace*	*abe*
de	*be*	*ade*	*cde*
abce	*acde*	*bce*	*e*
abde	*bcde*	*bde*	*abcde*
cf	*af*	*acf*	*abf*
df	*bf*	*adf*	*cdf*
abcf	*acdf*	*bcf*	*f*
abdf	*bcdf*	*bdf*	*abcdf*
aef	*cef*	*abef*	*acef*
bef	*def*	*cdef*	*adef*
acdef	*abcef*	*ef*	*bcef*
bcdef	*abdef*	*abcdef*	*bdef*

Plan 6.4 Balanced group of sets for 2^4 factorial, blocks of 4 units

Two-factor interactions are confounded in 1 replication and three-factor interactions are confounded in 3 replications. The columns are the blocks.

Rep. I, *AB*, *ACD*, *BCD* confounded

(1)	*ab*	*a*	*b*
abc	*c*	*bc*	*ac*
abd	*d*	*bd*	*ad*
cd	*abcd*	*acd*	*bcd*

Rep. II, *AC*, *ABD*, *BCD*

(1)	*ac*	*a*	*c*
abc	*b*	*bc*	*ab*
acd	*d*	*cd*	*ad*
bd	*abcd*	*abd*	*bcd*

Rep. III, *AD*, *ABC*, *BCD*

(1)	*ad*	*a*	*d*
abd	*b*	*bd*	*ab*
acd	*c*	*cd*	*ac*
bc	*abcd*	*abc*	*bcd*

Rep. IV, *BC*, *ABD*, *ACD*

(1)	*bc*	*b*	*c*
abc	*a*	*ac*	*ab*
bcd	*d*	*cd*	*bd*
ad	*abcd*	*abd*	*acd*

Rep. V, *BD*, *ABC*, *ACD*

(1)	*bd*	*b*	*d*
abd	*a*	*ad*	*ab*
bcd	*c*	*cd*	*bc*
ac	*abcd*	*abc*	*acd*

Rep. VI, *CD*, *ABC*, *ABD*

(1)	*cd*	*c*	*d*
acd	*a*	*ad*	*ac*
bcd	*b*	*bd*	*bc*
ab	*abcd*	*abc*	*abd*

Plan 6.5 Balanced group of sets for 2^5 factorial, blocks of 8 units

Three- and four-factor interactions are confounded in 1 replication.

Rep. I, *ABC*, *ADE*, *BCDE* confounded

(1)	*ab*	*a*	*b*
bc	*ac*	*abc*	*c*
abd	*d*	*bd*	*ad*
acd	*bcd*	*be*	*abcd*
abe	*e*	*ce*	*ae*
ace	*bce*	*ade*	*abce*
de	*abde*	*abcde*	*bde*
bcde	*acde*	*cd*	*cde*

Rep. II, *ABD*, *BCE*, *ACDE*

(1)	*ab*	*a*	*b*
ad	*bd*	*d*	*abd*
abc	*c*	*bc*	*ac*
bcd	*acd*	*abcd*	*cd*
abe	*e*	*be*	*ae*
bde	*ade*	*abde*	*de*
ce	*abce*	*ace*	*bce*
acde	*bcde*	*cde*	*abcde*

Rep. III, *ACE*, *BCD*, *ABDE*

(1)	*ac*	*a*	*c*
ae	*ce*	*e*	*ace*
abc	*b*	*bc*	*ab*
bce	*abe*	*abce*	*be*
acd	*d*	*cd*	*ad*
cde	*ade*	*acde*	*de*
bd	*abcd*	*abd*	*bcd*
abde	*bcde*	*bde*	*abcde*

Rep. IV, *ACD*, *BDE*, *ABCE*

(1)	*ad*	*a*	*d*
ac	*cd*	*c*	*acd*
abd	*b*	*bd*	*ab*
bcd	*abc*	*abcd*	*bc*
ade	*e*	*de*	*ae*
cde	*ace*	*acde*	*ce*
be	*abde*	*abe*	*bde*
abce	*bcde*	*bce*	*abcde*

Rep. V, *ABE*, *CDE*, *ABCD*

(1)	*ae*	*a*	*e*
ab	*be*	*b*	*abe*
ace	*c*	*ce*	*ac*
bce	*abc*	*abce*	*bc*
ade	*d*	*de*	*ad*
bde	*abd*	*abde*	*bd*
cd	*acde*	*acd*	*cde*
abcd	*bcde*	*bcd*	*abcde*

Plan 6.6 Balanced group of sets for 2^6 factorial, blocks of 8 units

All three- and four-factor interactions are confounded in 2 replications.

Rep. I, *ABC*, *CDE*, *ADF*, *BEF*, *ABDE*, *BCDF*, *ACEF* confounded

abc	*a*	*b*	(1)	*bc*	*ac*	*c*	*ab*
bd	*cd*	*abcd*	*acd*	*abd*	*d*	*ad*	*bcd*
ae	*abce*	*ce*	*bce*	*e*	*abe*	*be*	*ace*
cde	*bde*	*ade*	*abde*	*acde*	*bcde*	*abcde*	*de*
cf	*bf*	*af*	*abf*	*acf*	*bcf*	*abcf*	*f*
adf	*abcdf*	*cdf*	*bcdf*	*df*	*abdf*	*bdf*	*acdf*
bef	*cef*	*abcef*	*acef*	*abef*	*ef*	*aef*	*bcef*
abcdef	*adef*	*bdef*	*def*	*bcdef*	*acdef*	*cdef*	*abdef*

Rep. II, *ABD*, *DEF*, *BCF*, *ACE*, *ABEF*, *ACDF*, *BCDE*

abd	*b*	*a*	(1)	*ad*	*bd*	*d*	*ab*
cd	*ac*	*bc*	*abc*	*bcd*	*acd*	*abcd*	*c*
be	*abde*	*de*	*ade*	*e*	*abe*	*ae*	*bde*
ace	*cde*	*abcde*	*bcde*	*abce*	*ce*	*bce*	*acde*
af	*df*	*abdf*	*bdf*	*abf*	*f*	*bf*	*adf*
bcf	*abcdf*	*cdf*	*acdf*	*cf*	*abcf*	*acf*	*bcdf*
def	*aef*	*bef*	*abef*	*bdef*	*adef*	*abdef*	*ef*
abcdef	*bcef*	*acef*	*cef*	*acdef*	*bcdef*	*cdef*	*abcef*

Rep. III, *ABE*, *BDF*, *ACD*, *CEF*, *ADEF*, *BCDE*, *ABCF*

bc	*a*	*ac*	(1)	*abc*	*ab*	*b*	*c*
acd	*bd*	*bcd*	*abd*	*cd*	*d*	*ad*	*abcd*
abe	*ce*	*e*	*ace*	*be*	*bce*	*abce*	*ae*
de	*abcde*	*abde*	*bcde*	*ade*	*acde*	*cde*	*bde*
af	*bcf*	*bf*	*abcf*	*f*	*cf*	*acf*	*abf*
bdf	*acdf*	*adf*	*cdf*	*abdf*	*abcdf*	*bcdf*	*df*
cef	*abef*	*abcef*	*bef*	*acef*	*aef*	*ef*	*bcef*
abcdef	*def*	*cdef*	*adef*	*bcdef*	*bdef*	*abdef*	*acdef*

Rep. IV, *ABF*, *CDF*, *ADE*, *BCE*, *ABCD*, *BDEF*, *ACEF*

ac	*a*	*b*	(1)	*c*	*abc*	*bc*	*ab*
bd	*bcd*	*acd*	*abcd*	*abd*	*d*	*ad*	*cd*
bce	*be*	*ae*	*abe*	*abce*	*ce*	*ace*	*e*
ade	*acde*	*bcde*	*cde*	*de*	*abde*	*bde*	*abcde*
abf	*abcf*	*cf*	*bcf*	*bf*	*af*	*f*	*acf*
cdf	*df*	*abdf*	*adf*	*acdf*	*bcdf*	*abcdf*	*bdf*
ef	*cef*	*abcef*	*acef*	*aef*	*bef*	*abef*	*bcef*
abcdef	*abdef*	*def*	*bdef*	*bcdef*	*acdef*	*cdef*	*adef*

Rep. V, *ACF*, *BCD*, *ADE*, *BEF*, *ABDF*, *CDEF*, *ABCE*

ab	*a*	*bc*	(1)	*b*	*ac*	*c*	*abc*
bcd	*cd*	*abd*	*acd*	*abcd*	*d*	*ad*	*bd*
ce	*bce*	*ae*	*abce*	*ace*	*be*	*abe*	*e*
ade	*abde*	*cde*	*bde*	*de*	*abcde*	*bcde*	*acde*
acf	*abcf*	*f*	*bcf*	*cf*	*abf*	*bf*	*af*
df	*bdf*	*acdf*	*abdf*	*adf*	*bcdf*	*abcdf*	*cdf*
bef	*ef*	*abcef*	*aef*	*abef*	*cef*	*acef*	*bcef*
abcdef	*acdef*	*bdef*	*cdef*	*bcdef*	*adef*	*def*	*abdef*

Rep. VI, *ABC*, *BDE*, *ADF*, *CEF*, *ACDE*, *BCDF*, *ABEF*
Interchange *B* and *C* in replication I
Rep. VII, *ABF*, *DEF*, *BCD*, *ACE*, *ABDE*, *ACDF*, *BCEF*
Interchange *F* and *D* in replication II
Rep. VIII, *ABE*, *BDF*, *CDE*, *ACF*, *ADEF*, *ABCD*, *BCEF*
Interchange *A* and *E* in replication III
Rep. IX, *ABD*, *CDF*, *AEF*, *BCE*, *ABCF*, *BDEF*, *ACDE*
Interchange *F* and *D* in replication IV
Rep. X, *AEF*, *BDE*, *ACD*, *BCF*, *ABDF*, *CDEF*, *ABCE*
Interchange *E* and *C* in replication V

Plan 6.7 Balanced group of sets for 3^3 factorial, blocks of 9 units

ABC confounded

Rep. I, *ABC(W)**			Rep. II, *ABC(X)*			Rep. III, *ABC(Y)*			Rep. IV, *ABC(Z)*		
a	*b*	*c*	*a*	*b*	*c*	*a*	*b*	*c*	*a*	*b*	*c*
000	100	200	000	100	200	000	100	200	000	100	200
110	210	010	110	210	010	210	010	110	210	010	110
220	020	120	220	020	120	120	220	020	120	220	020
101	201	001	201	001	101	101	201	001	201	001	101
211	011	111	011	111	211	011	111	211	111	211	011
021	121	221	121	221	021	221	021	121	021	121	221
202	002	102	102	202	002	202	002	102	102	202	002
012	112	212	212	012	112	112	212	012	012	112	212
122	222	022	022	122	222	022	122	222	222	022	122

* Yates' notation.

Plan 6.8 Balanced group of sets for 3^4 factorial, blocks of 9 units

Three-factor interactions confounded

Rep. I, *ABC* I, *ABD* III, *ACD* IV, *BCD* II confounded

0000	0011	0022	0012	0020	0001	0021	0002	0010
1011	1022	1000	1020	1001	1012	1002	1010	1021
2022	2000	2011	2001	2012	2020	2010	2021	2002
0121	0102	0110	0100	0111	0122	0112	0120	0101
1102	1110	1121	1111	1122	1100	1120	1101	1112
2110	2121	2102	2122	2100	2111	2101	2112	2120
0212	0220	0201	0221	0202	0210	0200	0211	0222
1220	1201	1212	1202	1210	1221	1211	1222	1200
2201	2212	2220	2210	2221	2202	2222	2200	2211

Rep. II, *ABC* II, *ABD* IV, *ACD* I, *BCD* III

0000	0022	0011	0021	0010	0002	0012	0001	0020
1022	1011	1000	1010	1002	1021	1001	1020	1012
2011	2000	2022	2002	2021	2010	2020	2012	2001
0112	0101	0120	0100	0122	0111	0121	0110	0102
1101	1120	1112	1122	1111	1100	1110	1102	1121
2120	2112	2101	2111	2100	2122	2102	2121	2110
0221	0210	0202	0212	0201	0220	0200	0222	0211
1210	1202	1221	1201	1220	1212	1222	1211	1200
2202	2221	2210	2220	2212	2201	2211	2200	2222

Rep. III, *ABC* IV, *ABD* I, *ACD* II, *BCD* I

0000	0021	0012	0022	0010	0001	0011	0002	0020
1021	1012	1000	1010	1001	1022	1002	1020	1011
2012	2000	2021	2001	2022	2010	2020	2011	2002
0122	0110	0101	0111	0102	0120	0100	0121	0112
1110	1101	1122	1102	1120	1111	1121	1112	1100
2101	2122	2110	2120	2111	2102	2112	2100	2121
0211	0202	0220	0200	0221	0212	0222	0210	0201
1202	1220	1211	1221	1212	1200	1210	1201	1222
2220	2211	2202	2212	2200	2221	2201	2222	2210

Rep. IV, *ABC* III, *ABD* II, *ACD* III, *BCD* IV

0000	0012	0021	0011	0020	0002	0022	0001	0010
1012	1021	1000	1020	1002	1011	1001	1010	1022
2021	2000	2012	2002	2011	2020	2010	2022	2001
0111	0120	0102	0122	0101	0110	0100	0112	0121
1120	1102	1111	1101	1110	1122	1112	1121	1100
2102	2111	2120	2110	2122	2101	2121	2100	2112
0222	0201	0210	0200	0212	0221	0211	0220	0202
1201	1210	1222	1212	1221	1200	1220	1202	1211
2210	2222	2201	2221	2200	2212	2202	2211	2220

Plan 6.9 Balanced group of sets for 3 × 2² factorial, blocks of 6 units

BC, *ABC* confounded

Rep. I		Rep. II		Rep. III	
a	*b*	*a*	*b*	*a*	*b*
001	000	000	001	000	001
010	011	011	010	011	010
100	101	101	100	100	101
111	110	110	111	111	110
200	201	200	201	201	200
211	210	211	210	210	211

Plan 6.10 Balanced group of sets for 3 × 2³ factorial, blocks of 6 units

BC, *BD*, *CD*
ABC, *ABD*, *ACD* confounded

Rep. I				Rep. II				Rep. III			
a	*b*	*c*	*d*	*a*	*b*	*c*	*d*	*a*	*b*	*c*	*d*
0100	0000	0001	0010	0010	0001	0000	0100	0001	0010	0100	0000
0011	0111	0110	0101	0101	0110	0111	0011	0110	0101	0011	0111
1010	1001	1000	1100	1001	1010	1100	1000	1100	1000	1001	1010
1101	1110	1111	1011	1110	1101	1011	1111	1011	1111	1110	1101
2001	2010	2100	2000	2100	2000	2001	2010	2010	2001	2000	2100
2110	2101	2011	2111	2011	2111	2110	2101	2101	2110	2111	2011

Plan 6.11 Balanced group of sets for 3² × 2 factorial, blocks of 6 units

AB, *ABC* confounded

Rep. I			Rep. II			Rep. III			Rep. IV		
a	*b*	*c*	*a*	*b*	*c*	*a*	*b*	*c*	*a*	*b*	*c*
100	200	000	200	000	100	100	200	000	200	000	100
210	010	110	010	110	210	010	110	210	110	210	010
020	120	220	120	220	020	220	020	120	020	120	220
201	001	101	101	201	001	201	001	101	101	201	001
011	111	211	211	011	111	111	211	011	011	111	211
121	221	021	021	121	221	021	121	221	221	021	121

Plan 6.12 Balanced group of sets for 4^2 factorial, blocks of 4 units

AB confounded

Rep. I				Rep. II				Rep. III			
a	*b*	*c*	*d*	*a*	*b*	*c*	*d*	*a*	*b*	*c*	*d*
33	32	31	30	33	30	32	31	33	31	32	30
22	23	20	21	21	22	20	23	20	22	21	23
10	11	12	13	12	11	13	10	11	13	10	12
01	00	03	02	00	03	01	02	02	00	03	01

Plan 6.13 Balanced group of sets for 4×2^2 factorial, blocks of 8 units

ABC confounded

Rep. I		Rep. II		Rep. III	
a	*b*	*a*	*b*	*a*	*b*
000	001	000	001	000	001
011	010	011	010	011	010
100	101	101	100	101	100
111	110	110	111	110	111
201	200	201	200	200	201
210	211	210	211	211	210
301	300	300	301	301	300
310	311	311	310	310	311

Plan 6.14 Balanced group of sets for $4 \times 3 \times 2$ factorial, blocks of 12 units

A'C, A'BC confounded

Rep. I		Rep. II		Rep. III	
a	*b*	*a*	*b*	*a*	*b*
000	001	001	000	001	000
011	010	010	011	011	010
021	020	021	020	020	021
100	101	101	100	101	100
111	110	110	111	111	110
121	120	121	120	120	121
201	200	200	201	200	201
210	211	211	210	210	211
220	221	220	221	221	220
301	300	300	301	300	301
310	311	311	310	310	311
320	321	320	321	321	320

A''C, A''BC

Rep. IV		Rep. V		Rep. VI	
a	*b*	*a*	*b*	*a*	*b*
001	000	000	001	000	001
010	011	011	010	010	011
020	021	020	021	021	020
100	101	101	100	101	100
111	110	110	111	111	110
121	120	121	120	120	121
200	201	201	200	201	200
211	210	210	211	211	210
221	220	221	220	220	221
301	300	300	301	300	301
310	311	311	310	310	311
320	321	320	321	321	320

$$A' = a_3 + a_2 - a_1 - a_0$$
$$A'' = a_3 - a_2 - a_1 + a_0$$
$$A''' = a_3 - a_2 + a_1 - a_0$$

A'''C, A'''BC

Rep. VII		Rep. VIII		Rep. IX	
a	*b*	*a*	*b*	*a*	*b*
000	001	001	000	001	000
011	010	010	011	011	010
021	020	021	020	020	021
101	100	100	101	100	101
110	111	111	110	110	111
120	121	120	121	121	120
200	201	201	200	201	200
211	210	210	211	211	210
221	220	221	220	220	221
301	300	300	301	300	301
310	311	311	310	310	311
320	321	320	321	321	320

INDEX TO PLANS FOR 2^n FACTORIALS IN FRACTIONAL REPLICATION

No. of factors	Fraction of a rep.	Size of expt.	Size of block	Two-factor interactions: Total	Two-factor interactions: Max. no. estimable	Error d.f.: 2-factors used as error	Error d.f.: 2-factors estimated	Plan no.
4	1/2	8	8	6	3*	3	0	6A.1‡
5	1/4	8	8	10	2*	2	0	6A.2‡
	1/2	16	16	10	10	10	0	6A.3‡
			8	10	9	9	0	6A.3‡
			4	10	7	7	0	6A.3‡
6	1/8	8	8	15	1*	1	0	6A.4‡
	1/4	16	16	15	7*	9	2	6A.5‡
			8	15	7*	8	1	6A.5‡
			4	15	6*	6	0	6A.5‡
	1/2	32	32	15	15	25	10	6A.6
			16	15	15	24	9	6A.6
			8	15	14	22	8	6A.6
			4	15	12	18	6	6A.6
7	1/16	8	8	21	0	0	0	6A.7‡
	1/8	16	16	21	7*	8	1	6A.9‡
			8	21	7*	7	0	6A.9‡
			4	21	4*	5	1	6A.8‡
	1/4	32	32	21	18†	24	6	6A.11
			16	21	18†	23	5	6A.11
			8	21	17†	21	4	6A.11
			4	21	14†	17	3	6A.10
	1/2	64	64	21	21	56	35	6A.13
			32	21	21	55	34	6A.13
			16	21	21	53	32	6A.13
			8	21	21	49	28	6A.13
			4	21	15	41	26	6A.12
8	1/16	16	16	28	7*	7	0	6A.14‡
			8	28	6*	6	0	6A.14‡
			4	28	4*	4	0	6A.14‡
	1/8	32	32	28	20†	23	3	6A.15‡
			16	28	19†	22	3	6A.15‡
			8	28	17†	20	3	6A.15‡
			4	28	13	16	3	6A.15‡
	1/4	64	64	28	28	55	27	6A.16
			32	28	28	54	26	6A.16
			16	28	28	52	24	6A.16
			8	28	26	48	22	6A.16
			4	28	21	40	19	6A.16
	1/2	128	128	28	28	119	91	6A.17
			64	28	28	118	90	6A.17
			32	28	28	116	88	6A.17
			16	28	28	112	84	6A.17
			8	28	26	104	78	6A.17

* All these interactions have other 2-factor interactions as aliases, and are estimable only if the aliases can be considered negligible. See plans for details.

† Some of the interactions have other 2-factor interactions as aliases. See plans for details.

‡ Except in unusual circumstances, only main effects can be estimated with this design.

Plan 6A.1 2^4 factorial in 8 units ($\frac{1}{2}$ replicate)

Defining contrast: $ABCD$

Estimable 2-factor interactions: $AB = CD$, $AC = BD$, $AD = BC$.

	Effects	d.f.
(1)		
ab	Effects	d.f.
ac	Main	4
ad	2-factor	3
bc		
bd	Total	7
cd		
abcd		

Plan 6A.2 2^5 factorial in 8 units ($\frac{1}{4}$ replicate)

Defining contrasts: ABE, CDE, $ABCD$

Main effects have 2-factors as aliases. The only estimable 2-factors are $AC = BD$ and $AD = BC$.

	Effects	d.f.
(1)		
ab	Effects	d.f.
cd	Main	5
ace	2-factor	2
bce		
ade	Total	7
bde		
abcd		

Plan 6A.3 2^5 factorial in 16 units ($\frac{1}{2}$ replicate)

Defining contrast: $ABCDE$

Blocks of 4 units

Estimable 2-factors: All except CD, CE, DE (confounded with blocks).

Blocks (1)	(2)	(3)	(4)	Effects	d.f.
				Block	3
(1)	*ac*	*ae*	*ad*	Main	5
ab	*bc*	*be*	*bd*	2-factor	7
acde	*de*	*cd*	*ce*		
bcde	*abde*	*abcd*	*abce*	Total	15

CD, CE, DE confounded.

Blocks of 8 units

Estimable 2-factors: All except DE.

Combine blocks 1 and 2; and blocks 3 and 4. DE confounded.

Effects	d.f.
Block	1
Main	5
2-factor	9
Total	15

Blocks of 16 units

Estimable 2-factors: All.

Combine blocks 1–4.

Effects	d.f.
Main	5
2-factor	10
Total	15

Plan 6A.4 2^6 factorial in 8 units ($\frac{1}{8}$ replicate)

Defining contrasts: *ACE, ADF, BCF, BDE, ABCD, ABEF, CDEF*

Main effects have 2-factors as aliases. The only estimable 2-factor is the set $AB = CD = EF$.

(1)
acf
ade
bce
bdf
abcd
abef
cdef

Effects	d.f.
Main	6
2-factor ($AB = CD = EF$)	1
Total	7

Plan 6A.5 2^6 factorial in 16 units ($\frac{1}{4}$ replicate)

Defining contrasts: *ABCE, ABDF, CDEF*

Blocks of 4 units

Estimable 2-factors: The alias sets $AC = BE$, $AD = BF$, $AE = BC$, $AF = BD$, $CD = EF$, $CF = DE$.

Blocks	(1)	(2)	(3)	(4)
	(1)	*acd*	*ab*	*acf*
	abce	*aef*	*ce*	*ade*
	abdf	*bcf*	*df*	*bcd*
	cdef	*bde*	*abcdef*	*bef*

Effects	d.f.
Block	3
Main	6
2-factor	6
Total	15

AB, ACF, BCF confounded.

Blocks of 8 units

Estimable 2-factors: Same as in blocks of 4 units, plus the set $AB = CE = DF$.

Combine blocks 1 and 2; and blocks 3 and 4. *ACF* confounded.

Effects	d.f.
Block	1
Main	6
2-factor	7
3-factor	1
Total	15

Blocks of 16 units

Estimable 2-factors: Same as in blocks of 8 units.

Combine blocks 1–4.

Effects	d.f.
Main	6
2-factor	7
3-factor	2
Total	15

Plan 6A.6 2^6 factorial in 32 units ($\frac{1}{2}$ replicate)

Defining contrast: *ABCDEF*

Blocks of 4 units

Estimable 2-factors: All except *AE, BF,* and *CD* (confounded with blocks).

Blocks	(1)	(2)	(3)	(4)	(5)	(6)	(7)	(8)
	(1)	*ab*	*ac*	*bc*	*ae*	*af*	*ad*	*bd*
	abef	*ef*	*de*	*df*	*bf*	*be*	*ce*	*cf*
	acde	*acdf*	*abdf*	*acef*	*cd*	*abcd*	*abcf*	*abce*
	bcdf	*bcde*	*bcef*	*abde*	*abcdef*	*cdef*	*bdef*	*adef*

AE, BF, CD, ABC, ABD, ACF, ADF confounded.

Effects	d.f.
Block	7
Main	6
2-factor	12
Higher order	6
Total	31

Blocks of 8 units

Estimable 2-factors: All except *CD*.

Combine blocks 1 and 2; blocks 3 and 4; blocks 5 and 6; and blocks 7 and 8. *CD, ABC, ABD* confounded.

Effects	d.f.
Block	3
Main	6
2-factor	14
Higher order	8
Total	31

Blocks of 16 units

Estimable 2-factors: All.

Estimable 3-factors: *ABC* = *DEF* is lost by confounding. The others are in alias pairs, e.g., *ABD* = *CEF*.

Combine blocks 1–4; and blocks 5–8. *ABC* confounded.

Effects	d.f.
Block	1
Main	6
2-factor	15
3-factor	9
Total	31

Blocks of 32 units

Estimable 2-factors: All.

Estimable 3-factors: These are arranged in 10 alias pairs.

Combine blocks 1–8.

Effects	d.f.
Main	6
2-factor	15
3-factor	10
Total	31

Plan 6A.7 2^7 factorial in 8 units ($\frac{1}{16}$ replicate)

Defining contrasts: *ABG, ACE, ADF, BCF, BDE, CDG, EFG, ABCD, ABEF, ACFG, ADEG, BCEG, BDFG, CDEF, ABCDEFG*

Main effects have 2-factors as aliases. No 2-factors are estimable.

(1)
abcd
abef
acfg
adeg
bceg
bdfg
cdef

Effects	d.f.
Main	7
Total	7

Plan 6A.8 2^7 factorial in 16 units ($\frac{1}{8}$ replicate)

Defining contrasts: *ABCD, ABEF, ACEG, ADFG, BCFG, BDEG, CDEF*

Blocks of 4 units

Estimable 2-factors: Only the alias sets *AE* = *BF* = *CG*; *AF* = *BE* = *DG*; *AG* = *CE* = *DF*; *BG* = *DE* = *CF*.

Blocks (1)	(2)	(3)	(4)
(1)	*abg*	*acf*	*ade*
efg	*cdg*	*bdf*	*bce*
abcd	*abef*	*aceg*	*adfg*
abcdefg	*cdef*	*bdeg*	*bcfg*

AB = *CD* = *EF*,
AC = *BD* = *EG*,
AD = *BC* = *FG* confounded.

Effects	d.f.
Block	3
Main	7
2-factor	4
Higher order	1
Total	15

Plan 6A.9 2^7 factorial in 16 units ($\frac{1}{8}$ replicate)

Defining contrasts: *ABCD, ABEF, ACEG, ADFG, BCFG, BDEG, CDEF*

Blocks of 8 units

Estimable 2-factors: Same as in blocks of 4 units, plus the alias sets $AB = CD = EF$, $AC = BD = EG$, $AD = BC = FG$.

Blocks (1)	(2)
(1)	*abg*
abcd	*acf*
abef	*ade*
aceg	*bce*
adfg	*bdf*
bcfg	*cdg*
bdeg	*efg*
cdef	*abcdefg*

Effects	d.f.
Block	1
Main	7
2-factor	7
Total	15

ABG confounded.

Blocks of 16 units

Estimable 2-factors: Same as in blocks of 8 units.

Combine blocks 1 and 2 of the plan for blocks of 8 units.

Effects	d.f.
Main	7
2-factor	7
Higher order	1
Total	15

Plan 6A.10 2^7 factorial in 32 units ($\frac{1}{4}$ replicate)

Defining contrasts: *ABCDE, ABCFG, DEFG*

Blocks of 4 units

Estimable 2-factors: *AB, AC, BC,* and $DF = EG$ are lost by confounding. All other 2-factors are estimable, except that $DE = FG$ and $DG = EF$, so that members of these alias pairs cannot be separated.

Blocks (1)	(2)	(3)	(4)	(5)	(6)	(7)	(8)
(1)	*de*	*ab*	*cdg*	*ac*	*bdg*	*bc*	*adg*
defg	*fg*	*cdf*	*cef*	*bdf*	*bef*	*adf*	*aef*
abcdf	*abcdg*	*ceg*	*abde*	*beg*	*acde*	*aeg*	*bcfg*
abceg	*abcef*	*abdefg*	*abfg*	*acdefg*	*acfg*	*bcdefg*	*bcde*

Effects	d.f.
Block	7
Main	7
2-factor	14
Higher order	3
Total	31

AB, AC, BC, $DF = EG$, *ADG, BDG, CDG* confounded.

Plan 6A.11 2^7 factorial in 32 units ($\frac{1}{4}$ replicate)

Defining contrasts: *ABCDE, ABCFG, DEFG*

Blocks of 8 units

Estimable 2-factors: All except $DF = EG$ (confounded with blocks). However, $DE = FG$ and $DG = EF$ are alias pairs which cannot be separated.

Blocks (1)	(2)	(3)	(4)
(1)	*bdg*	*ab*	*de*
bc	*bef*	*ac*	*fg*
adf	*cef*	*bdf*	*adg*
aeg	*abfg*	*beg*	*aef*
defg	*acfg*	*cdf*	*bcde*
abcdf	*abde*	*ceg*	*bcfg*
abceg	*acde*	*acdefg*	*abcdg*
bcdefg	*cdg*	*abdefg*	*abcef*

Effects	d.f.
Block	3
Main	7
2-factor	17
Higher order	4
Total	31

$DF = EG$, *ADE, AEF* confounded.

Blocks of 16 units

Estimable 2-factors: All, except that *DE* = *FG*, *DG* = *EF*, and *DF* = *EG* are alias pairs.

Combine blocks 1 and 2; and blocks 3 and 4. *AEF* confounded.

Effects	d.f.
Block	1
Main	7
2-factor	18
Higher order	5
Total	31

Blocks of 32 units

Estimable 2-factors: Same as in blocks of 16 units.

Combine blocks 1–4.

Effects	d.f.
Main	7
2-factor	18
Higher order	6
Total	31

Plan 6A.12 2^7 factorial in 64 units ($\frac{1}{2}$ replicate)

Defining contrast: *ABCDEFG*

Blocks of 4 units

Estimable 2-factors: All except *AB*, *AC*, *BC*, *EF*, *EG*, and *FG* (confounded with blocks).

Blocks (1)	(2)	(3)	(4)	(5)	(6)	(7)	(8)
(1)	*ab*	*ac*	*bc*	*ae*	*be*	*ce*	*abce*
abcd	*cd*	*bd*	*ad*	*bcde*	*acde*	*abde*	*de*
defg	*abdefg*	*acdefg*	*bcdefg*	*adfg*	*bdfg*	*cdfg*	*abcdfg*
abcefg	*cefg*	*befg*	*aefg*	*bcfg*	*acfg*	*abfg*	*fg*

(9)	(10)	(11)	(12)	(13)	(14)	(15)	(16)
af	*bf*	*cf*	*abcf*	*ef*	*abef*	*acef*	*bcef*
bcdf	*acdf*	*abdf*	*df*	*abcdef*	*cdef*	*bdef*	*adef*
adeg	*bdeg*	*cdeg*	*abcdeg*	*dg*	*abdg*	*acdg*	*bcdg*
bceg	*aceg*	*abeg*	*eg*	*abcg*	*cg*	*bg*	*ag*

Effects	d.f.
Block	15
Main	7
2-factor	15
Higher order	26
Total	63

AB, *AC*, *BC*, *EF*, *EG*, *FG*, *ADE*, *ADF*, *ADG*, *BDE*, *BDF*, *BDG*, *CDE*, *CDF*, *CDG* confounded.

Plan 6A.13 2^7 factorial in 64 units ($\frac{1}{2}$ replicate)

Defining contrast: *ABCDEFG*

Blocks of 8 units

Estimable 2-factors: All.

Estimable 3-factors: All except *ABC*, *ADE*, *AFG*, *BDF*, *BEG*, *CDG*, *CEF* (confounded with blocks).

Blocks (1)	(2)	(3)	(4)	(5)	(6)	(7)	(8)
(1)	*bc*	*ac*	*ab*	*ag*	*af*	*ae*	*ad*
abdg	*de*	*df*	*dg*	*bd*	*be*	*bf*	*bg*
abef	*fg*	*eg*	*ef*	*ce*	*cd*	*cg*	*cf*
acdf	*abdf*	*abde*	*acde*	*abcf*	*abcg*	*abcd*	*abce*
aceg	*abeg*	*abfg*	*acfg*	*adef*	*adeg*	*adfg*	*aefg*
bcde	*acdg*	*bcdg*	*bcdf*	*befg*	*bdfg*	*bdeg*	*bdef*
bcfg	*acef*	*bcef*	*bceg*	*cdfg*	*cefg*	*cdef*	*cdeg*
defg	*bcdefg*	*acdefg*	*abdefg*	*abcdeg*	*abcdef*	*abcefg*	*abcdfg*

Effects	d.f.
Block	7
Main	7
2-factor	21
3-factor	28
Total	63

Blocks of 16 units

Estimable 2-factors: All.

Estimable 3-factors: All except *ABC, ADE, AFG* (confounded).

Combine blocks 1 and 2; blocks 3 and 4; blocks 5 and 6; and blocks 7 and 8.

Effects	d.f.
Block	3
Main	7
2-factor	21
Higher order	32
Total	63

Blocks of 32 units

Estimable 2-factors: All.

Estimable 3-factors: All except *ABC* (confounded).

Combine blocks 1–4; and blocks 5–8.

Effects	d.f.
Block	1
Main	7
2-factor	21
3-factor	34
Total	63

Blocks of 64 units

Estimable 2-factors: All.

Estimable 3-factors: All.

Combine blocks 1–8.

Effects	d.f.
Main	7
2-factor	21
3-factor	35
Total	63

Plan 6A.14 2^8 factorial in 16 units ($\frac{1}{16}$ replicate)

Defining contrasts: *ABCD, ABEF, ABGH, ACEH, ACFG, ADEG, ADFH, BCEG, BCFH, BDEH, BDFG, CDEF, CDGH, EFGH, ABCDEFGH.*

Blocks of 4 units

Estimable 2-factors: Only the 4 alias sets $AE = BF = CH = DG$; $AF = BE = CG = DH$; $AG = BH = CF = DE$; $AH = BG = CE = DF$. Except in special circumstances, only main effects are estimable.

Blocks (1)	(2)	(3)	(4)
(1)	*abef*	*adeg*	*aceh*
abcd	*abgh*	*adfh*	*acfg*
efgh	*cdef*	*bceg*	*bdeh*
abcdefgh	*cdgh*	*bcfh*	*bdfg*

AB, AC, AD confounded.

Effects	d.f.
Block	3
Main	8
2-factor	4
Total	15

Blocks of 8 units

Estimable 2-factors: As in blocks of 4 units, plus the alias sets $AC = BD = EH = FG$; $AD = BC = EG = FH$.

Combine blocks 1 and 2; and blocks 3 and 4. *AB* confounded.

Effects	d.f.
Block	1
Main	8
2-factor	6
Total	15

Blocks of 16 units

Estimable 2-factors: As in blocks of 8 units, plus the alias set $AB = CD = EF = GH$.

Combine blocks 1–4.

Effects	d.f.
Main	8
2-factor	7
Total	15

Plan 6A.15 2^8 factorial in 32 units ($\frac{1}{8}$ replicate)

Defining contrasts: *BCDH, BDFG, CFGH, ABCEF, ABEGH, ACDEG, ADEFH*

Blocks of 4 units

Estimable 2-factors: All interactions of *A* and of *E*. All other 2-factors are lost by confounding.

Blocks (1)	(2)	(3)	(4)	(5)	(6)	(7)	(8)
(1)	*abd*	*dgh*	*cdf*	*afg*	*ach*	*bcg*	*bfh*
ae	*bde*	*abcf*	*abgh*	*efg*	*ceh*	*adfh*	*acdg*
abcdfgh	*cfgh*	*bcef*	*begh*	*bcdh*	*bdfg*	*defh*	*cdeg*
bcdefgh	*acefgh*	*adegh*	*acdef*	*abcdeh*	*abdefg*	*abceg*	*abefh*

BD, BF, BH, CF, DF, DH, FH and their aliases confounded.

Effects	d.f.
Block	7
Main	8
2-factor	13
Higher order	3
Total	31

Blocks of 8 units

Estimable 2-factors: All interactions of *A* and of *E*, and the alias pairs *BC* = *DH*, *BF* = *DG*, *BG* = *DF*, *BH* = *CD*.

Combine blocks 1 and 2; blocks 3 and 4; blocks 5 and 6; and blocks 7 and 8. *BD*, *CF*, *FH* confounded.

Effects	d.f.
Block	3
Main	8
2-factor	17
Higher order	3
Total	31

Blocks of 16 units

Estimable 2-factors: As in blocks of 8 units, plus the alias sets *CG* = *FH*, *BD* = *CH* = *FG*.

Combine blocks 1–4; and blocks 5–8. *CF* confounded.

Effects	d.f.
Block	1
Main	8
2-factor	19
Higher order	3
Total	31

Blocks of 32 units

Estimable 2-factors: All interactions of *A* and of *E*, plus the alias sets *BC* = *DH*, *BF* = *DG*, *BG* = *DF*, *BH* = *CD*, *CG* = *FH*, *CF* = *GH*, *BD* = *CH* = *FG*.

Combine blocks 1–8.

Effects	d.f.
Main	8
2-factor	20
Higher order	3
Total	31

Plan 6A.16 2^8 factorial in 64 units ($\frac{1}{4}$ replicate)

Defining contrasts: *ABCEG*, *ABDFH*, *CDEFGH*

Blocks of 4 units

Estimable 2-factors: All except *AF*, *AH*, *BC*, *BG*, *CG*, *DE*, *FH* (confounded with blocks).

Blocks	(1)	(2)	(3)	(4)	(5)	(6)	(7)	(8)
	(1)	*adg*	*ach*	*beh*	*eg*	*fh*	*bef*	*acf*
	adefh	*abce*	*bfg*	*abdf*	*bcd*	*ade*	*abdh*	*bgh*
	bcdeg	*efgh*	*cdef*	*cdgh*	*adfgh*	*abcg*	*cdfg*	*cdeh*
	abcfgh	*bcdfh*	*abdegh*	*acefg*	*abcefh*	*bcdefgh*	*acegh*	*abdefg*

(9)	(10)	(11)	(12)	(13)	(14)	(15)	(16)
ab	*ce*	*afg*	*df*	*acd*	*cg*	*dh*	*agh*
cfgh	*bdg*	*bch*	*aeh*	*abeg*	*bde*	*aef*	*bcf*
acdeg	*acdfh*	*degh*	*bcefg*	*cefh*	*abfh*	*bcegh*	*defg*
bdefh	*abefgh*	*abcdef*	*abcdgh*	*bdfgh*	*acdefgh*	*abcdfg*	*abcdeh*

Effects	d.f.
Block	15
Main	8
2-factor	21
Higher order	19
Total	63

AF, *AH*, *BC*, *BG*, *CG*, *DE*, *FH*, *ACD*, *ADG*, *BEF*, *BEH*, *CDF*, *CEF*, *DFG*, *EFG* confounded.

Blocks of 8 units

Estimable 2-factors: All except *BC* and *FH* (confounded with blocks).

Combine blocks 1 and 2; blocks 3 and 4; blocks 5 and 6; blocks 7 and 8; blocks 9 and 10; blocks 11 and 12; blocks 13 and 14; and blocks 15 and 16. *BC*, *FH*, *ACD*, *BEF*, *BEH*, *CEF*, *DFG* confounded.

Effects	d.f.
Block	7
Main	8
2-factor	26
Higher order	22
Total	63

Blocks of 16 units

Estimable 2-factors: All.

Combine blocks 1–4; blocks 5–8; blocks 9–12; and blocks 13–16. *ACD*, *BEF*, *DFG* confounded.

Effects	d.f.
Block	3
Main	8
2-factor	28
Higher order	24
Total	63

Blocks of 32 units

Estimable 2-factors: All.

Combine blocks 1–8; and blocks 9–16. *ACD* confounded.

Effects	d.f.
Block	1
Main	8
2-factor	28
Higher order	26
Total	63

Blocks of 64 units

Estimable 2-factors: All.

Combine blocks 1–16.

Effects	d.f.
Main	8
2-factor	28
Higher order	27
Total	63

Plan 6A.17 2^8 factorial in 128 units ($\frac{1}{2}$ replicate)

Defining contrast: *ABCDEFGH*

For blocks of 8 units, see end of plan.

Blocks of 16 units

Estimable 2-factors: All

Estimable 3-factors: All.

Blocks (1)	(2)	(3)	(4)	(5)	(6)	(7)	(8)
(1)	*acfh*	*fh*	*ac*	*af*	*ch*	*ah*	*cf*
abcd	*bdfh*	*abcdfh*	*bd*	*bcdf*	*abdh*	*bcdh*	*abdf*
adeg	*abefgh*	*abefgh*	*abeg*	*defg*	*begh*	*degh*	*befg*
bceg	*cdefgh*	*bcefgh*	*cdeg*	*abcefg*	*acdegh*	*abcegh*	*acdefg*
adfh	*ab*	*ad*	*abfh*	*dh*	*bf*	*df*	*bh*
bcfh	*cd*	*bc*	*cdfh*	*abch*	*acdf*	*abcf*	*acdh*
efgh	*aceg*	*eg*	*acefgh*	*aegh*	*cefg*	*aefg*	*cegh*
abcdefgh	*bdeg*	*abcdeg*	*bdefgh*	*bcdegh*	*abdefg*	*bcdefg*	*abdegh*
abgh	*ef*	*abfg*	*eh*	*bfgh*	*ae*	*bg*	*aefh*
aceh	*adfg*	*acef*	*adgh*	*cefh*	*dg*	*ce*	*dfgh*
bdeh	*bcfg*	*bdef*	*bcgh*	*abdefh*	*abcg*	*abde*	*abcfgh*
cdgh	*abcdef*	*cdfg*	*abcdeh*	*acdfgh*	*bcde*	*acdg*	*bcdefh*
abef	*gh*	*abeh*	*fg*	*be*	*afgh*	*befh*	*ag*
acfg	*adeh*	*acgh*	*adef*	*cg*	*defh*	*cfgh*	*de*
bdfg	*bceh*	*bdgh*	*bcef*	*abdg*	*abcefh*	*abdfgh*	*abce*
cdef	*abcdgh*	*cdeh*	*abcdfg*	*acde*	*bcdfgh*	*acdefh*	*bcdg*

Effects	d.f.
Block	7
Main	8
2-factor	28
3-factor	56
Higher order	28
Total	127

ABCD, ABEF, ACFG, ADEG, BCEG, BDFG, CDEF confounded.

Blocks of 32 units

Estimable 2-factors: All.

Estimable 3-factors: All.

Combine blocks 1 and 2; blocks 3 and 4; blocks 5 and 6; and blocks 7 and 8. *ABCD, ABEF, CDEF* confounded.

Effects	d.f.
Block	3
Main	8
2-factor	28
3-factor	56
Higher order	32
Total	127

Blocks of 64 units

Estimable 2-factors: All.

Estimable 3-factors: All.

Combine blocks 1–4; and blocks 5–8. *ABCD* confounded.

Effects	d.f.
Block	1
Main	8
2-factor	28
3-factor	56
Higher order	34
Total	127

Blocks of 128 units

Estimable 2-factors: All.

Estimable 3-factors: All.

Combine blocks 1–8.

Effects	d.f.
Main	8
2-factor	28
3-factor	56
Higher order	35
Total	127

Blocks of 8 units

Estimable 2-factors. All except *EG* and *FH* (confounded). Start with the plan for blocks of 32 units. The first 4 rows of blocks 1 and 2 form the first block of 8 units: i.e., this block contains 1, *abcd, adeg, bceg, acfh, bdfh, abefgh, cdefgh*. Similarly, rows 5–8 of blocks 1 and 2 give the second block, rows 9–12 the third and rows 13–16 the fourth. The remaining 12 blocks are formed likewise from blocks 3 and 4; blocks 5 and 6; and blocks 7 and 8.

Effects	d.f.
Block	15
Main	8
2-factor	26
Higher order	78
Total	127

Plan 6A.18 3^4 factorial in 27 units ($\frac{1}{3}$ replicate)

Defining contrasts: 2 d.f. from $ABCD$, equivalent to putting $D = ABC(Y)$

Blocks of 9 units

Estimable 2-factors: 16 of the 24 d.f. are clear. $CD(I)$ is lost by confounding. Also $AB(J) = CD(J)$; $AC(I) = BD(I)$; $AD(I) = BC(I)$.

Blocks (1)	(2)	(3)
0000	0021	0012
0122	0110	0101
0211	0202	0220
1022	1010	1001
1111	1102	1120
1200	1221	1212
2011	2002	2020
2100	2121	2112
2222	2210	2201

Effects	d.f.
Block	2
Main	8
2-factor	16
Total	26

If all interactions of D are negligible, the analysis may be written:

Effects	d.f.
Block	2
Main	8
AB, AC, BC	12
Error (from interactions of D)	4
Total	26

Blocks of 27 units

Estimable 2-factors: As in blocks of 9 units, plus $CD(I)$.

Combine blocks 1, 2, and 3. See section 6A.32 for analysis of variance.

Plan 6A.19 3^5 factorial in 81 units ($\frac{1}{3}$ replicate)

Defining contrasts: 2 d.f. from *ABCDE*

Blocks of 9 units

Estimable 2-factors: All except *AE*(*J*), which is confounded with blocks.

Blocks	(1)	(2)	(3)	(4)	(5)	(6)	(7)	(8)	(9)
ab	*cde*	*cde*	*cde*	*cde*	*cde*	*cde*	*cde*	*cde*	*cde*
00	000	201	102	120	021	222	111	012	210
10	122	020	221	212	110	011	200	101	002
20	211	112	010	001	202	100	022	220	121
01	110	011	212	200	101	002	221	122	020
11	202	100	001	022	220	121	010	211	112
21	021	222	120	111	012	210	102	000	201
02	220	121	022	010	211	112	001	202	100
12	012	210	111	102	000	201	120	021	222
22	101	002	200	221	122	020	212	110	011

Effects	d.f.
Block	8
Main	10
2-factor	38
Higher order	24
Total	80

Blocks of 27 units

Estimable 2-factors: All.

Combine blocks 1–3; blocks 4–6; blocks 7–9.

Effects	d.f.
Block	2
Main	10
2-factor	40
Higher order	28
Total	80

Blocks of 81 units

Estimable 2-factors: All.

Combine blocks 1–9.

Effects	d.f.
Main	10
2-factor	40
Higher order	30
Total	80

Plan 6A.20 4×2^4 factorial in 32 units ($\frac{1}{2}$ replicate)

Defining contrast: A''' *BCDE*

Blocks of 8 units

Estimable 2-factors: All except *DE* (confounded with blocks).

Blocks	(1)	(2)	(3)	(4)
ab	*cde*	*cde*	*cde*	*cde*
00	100	010	111	001
01	011	101	000	110
10	011	101	000	110
11	100	010	111	001
20	111	001	100	010
21	000	110	011	101
30	000	110	011	101
31	111	001	100	010

Effects	d.f.
Block	3
Main	7
2-factor	17
Higher order	4
Total	31

Blocks of 16 units

Estimable 2-factors: All.

Combine blocks 1, 2; and blocks 3, 4.

Effects	d.f.
Block	1
Main	7
2-factor	18
Higher order	5
Total	31

Blocks of 32 units

Estimable 2-factors: All.

Combine blocks 1, 2, 3, and 4.

Effects	d.f.
Main	7
2-factor	18
Higher order	6
Total	31

INDEX TO PLANS, INCOMPLETE BLOCK DESIGNS

t	*k*	*r*	*b*	λ†	*E*	Plan.	Type
4	2	3	6	1	.67	11.1	V
	3	3	4	2	.89	*	V
5	2	4	10	1	.62	11.2	V
	3	6	10	3	.83	11.1a	V
	4	4	5	3	.94	*	V
6	2	5	15	1	.60	11.3	I
	3	5	10	2	.80	11.4	III
	3	10	20	4	.80	11.5	I
	4	10	15	6	.90	11.6	II
	5	5	6	4	.96	*	V
7	2	6	21	1	.58	11.2a	II
	3	3	7	1	.78	11.7	V
	4	4	7	2	.88	11.8	V
	6	6	7	5	.97	*	V
8	2	7	28	1	.57	11.9	I
	4	7	14	3	.86	11.10	I
	7	7	8	6	.98	*	V
9	2	8	36	1	.56	11.3a	II
	4	8	18	3	.84	11.11	II
	5	10	18	5	.90	11.12	II
	6	8	12	5	.94	11.13	II
	8	8	9	7	.98	*	IV
10	2	9	45	1	.56	11.14	I
	3	9	30	2	.74	11.15	II
	4	6	15	2	.83	11.16	III
	5	9	18	4	.89	11.17	III
	6	9	15	5	.93	11.18	III
	9	9	10	8	.99	*	IV
11	2	10	55	1	.55	11.4a	II
	5	5	11	2	.88	11.19	IV
	6	6	11	3	.92	11.20	IV
	10	10	11	9	.99	*	IV
13	3	6	26	1	.72	11.21	II
	4	4	13	1	.81	11.22	IV
	9	9	13	6	.96	11.23	IV
15	3	7	35	1	.71	11.24	I
	7	7	15	3	.92	11.25	IV
	8	8	15	4	.94	11.26	IV
16	6	6	16	2	.89	11.27	IV
	6	9	24	3	.89	11.28	II
	10	10	16	6	.96	11.29	IV
19	3	9	57	1	.70	11.30	II
	9	9	19	4	.94	11.31	IV
	10	10	19	5	.95	11.32	IV
21	3	10	70	1	.70	11.33	I
	5	5	21	1	.84	11.34	IV
	7	10	30	3	.90	11.35	III
25	4	8	50	1	.78	11.36	II
	9	9	25	3	.93	11.37	IV
28	4	9	63	1	.78	11.38	I
	7	9	36	2	.89	11.39	III
31	6	6	31	1	.86	11.40	IV
	10	10	31	3	.93	11.41	IV
37	9	9	37	2	.91	11.42	IV
41	5	10	82	1	.82	11.43	II
57	8	8	57	1	.89	11.44	IV
73	9	9	73	1	.90	11.45	IV
91	10	10	91	1	.91	11.46	IV

† Number of times that two treatments appear together in the same block.

* These plans are constructed by forming all possible combinations of the *t* numbers in groups of size *k*. The number of blocks *b* serves as a check that no group has been missed.

Plan 11.1 $t = 4, k = 2, r = 3, b = 6, \lambda = 1, E = .67$, **Type V**

Block	Rep. I		Block	Rep. II		Block	Rep. III	
(1)	1	2	(3)	1	2	(5)	1	4
(2)	3	4	(4)	2	4	(6)	2	3

Plan 11.2 $t = 5, k = 2, r = 4, b = 10, \lambda = 1, E = .62$, **Type V**

Block	Reps. I and II		Block	Reps. III and IV	
(1)	1	2	(6)	1	4
(2)	3	4	(7)	2	3
(3)	2	5	(8)	3	5
(4)	1	3	(9)	1	5
(5)	4	5	(10)	2	4

Plan 11.1a $t = 5, k = 3, r = 6, b = 10, \lambda = 3, E = .83$, **Type V**

Block	Reps. I, II, and III			Block	Reps. IV, V, and VI		
(1)	1	2	3	(6)	1	2	4
(2)	1	2	5	(7)	1	3	4
(3)	1	4	5	(8)	1	3	5
(4)	2	3	4	(9)	2	3	5
(5)	3	4	5	(10)	2	4	5

Plan 11.3 $t = 6, k = 2, r = 5, b = 15, \lambda = 1, E = .60$, **Type I**

Block	Rep. I		Block	Rep. II		Block	Rep. III		Block	Rep. IV		Block	Rep. V	
(1)	1	2	(4)	1	3	(7)	1	4	(10)	1	5	(13)	1	6
(2)	3	4	(5)	2	5	(8)	2	6	(11)	2	4	(14)	2	3
(3)	5	6	(6)	4	6	(9)	3	5	(12)	3	6	(15)	4	5

Plan 11.4 $t = 6, k = 3, r = 5, b = 10, \lambda = 2, E = .80$, **Type III**

Block				Block			
(1)	1	2	5	(6)	2	3	4
(2)	1	2	6	(7)	2	3	5
(3)	1	3	4	(8)	2	4	6
(4)	1	3	6	(9)	3	5	6
(5)	1	4	5	(10)	4	5	6

Plan 11.5 $t = 6, k = 3, r = 10, b = 20, \lambda = 4, E = .80$, **Type I**

Block	Rep. I			Block	Rep. II			Block	Rep. III			Block	Rep. IV			Block	Rep. V		
(1)	1	2	3	(3)	1	2	4	(5)	1	2	5	(7)	1	2	6	(9)	1	3	4
(2)	4	5	6	(4)	3	5	6	(6)	3	4	6	(8)	3	4	5	(10)	2	5	6

Block	Rep. VI			Block	Rep. VII			Block	Rep. VIII			Block	Rep. IX			Block	Rep. X		
(11)	1	3	5	(13)	1	3	6	(15)	1	4	5	(17)	1	4	6	(19)	1	5	6
(12)	2	4	6	(14)	2	4	5	(16)	2	3	6	(18)	2	3	5	(20)	2	3	4

Plan 11.6 $t = 6, k = 4, r = 10, b = 15, \lambda = 6, E = .90$, **Type II**

Block	Reps. I and II		Reps. III and IV		Reps. V and VI		Reps. VII and VIII		Reps. IX and X
(1)	1 2 3 4	(4)	1 2 3 5	(7)	1 2 3 6	(10)	1 2 4 5	(13)	1 2 5 6
(2)	1 4 5 6	(5)	1 2 4 6	(8)	1 3 4 5	(11)	1 3 5 6	(14)	1 3 4 6
(3)	2 3 5 6	(6)	3 4 5 6	(9)	2 4 5 6	(12)	2 3 4 6	(15)	2 3 4 5

Plan 11.2a $t = 7, k = 2, r = 6, b = 21, \lambda = 1, E = .58$, **Type II**

Block	Reps. I and II		Reps. III and IV		Reps. V and VI
(1)	1 2	(8)	1 3	(15)	1 4
(2)	2 6	(9)	2 4	(16)	2 3
(3)	3 4	(10)	3 5	(17)	3 6
(4)	4 7	(11)	4 6	(18)	4 5
(5)	1 5	(12)	5 7	(19)	2 5
(6)	5 6	(13)	1 6	(20)	6 7
(7)	3 7	(14)	2 7	(21)	1 7

Plan 11.7 $t = 7, k = 3, r = 3, b = 7, \lambda = 1, E = .78$, **Type V**

Block							
(1)	1 2 4	(3)	3 4 6	(5)	5 6 1	(7)	7 1 3
(2)	2 3 5	(4)	4 5 7	(6)	6 7 2		

Plan 11.8 $t = 7, k = 4, r = 4, b = 7, \lambda = 2, E = .88$, **Type V**

Block							
(1)	3 5 6 7	(3)	1 2 5 7	(5)	2 3 4 7	(7)	2 4 5 6
(2)	1 4 6 7	(4)	1 2 3 6	(6)	1 3 4 5		

Plan 11.9 $t = 8, k = 2, r = 7, b = 28, \lambda = 1, E = .57$, **Type I**

Block	Rep. I		Rep. II		Rep. III		Rep. IV
(1)	1 2	(5)	1 3	(9)	1 4	(13)	1 5
(2)	3 4	(6)	2 8	(10)	2 7	(14)	2 3
(3)	5 6	(7)	4 5	(11)	3 6	(15)	4 7
(4)	7 8	(8)	6 7	(12)	5 8	(16)	6 8

	Rep. V		Rep. VI		Rep. VII
(17)	1 6	(21)	1 7	(25)	1 8
(18)	2 4	(22)	2 6	(26)	2 5
(19)	3 8	(23)	3 5	(27)	3 7
(20)	5 7	(24)	4 8	(28)	4 6

Plan 11.10 $t = 8, k = 4, r = 7, b = 14, \lambda = 3, E = .86$, **Type I**

Block	Rep. I		Rep. II		Rep. III		Rep. IV
(1)	1 2 3 4	(3)	1 2 7 8	(5)	1 3 6 8	(7)	1 4 6 7
(2)	5 6 7 8	(4)	3 4 5 6	(6)	2 4 5 7	(8)	2 3 5 8

	Rep. V		Rep. VI		Rep. VII
(9)	1 2 5 6	(11)	1 3 5 7	(13)	1 4 5 8
(10)	3 4 7 8	(12)	2 4 6 8	(14)	2 3 6 7

Plan 11.3a $t = 9, k = 2, r = 8, b = 36, \lambda = 1, E = .56$, **Type II**

Block	Reps. I and II			Reps. III and IV			Reps. V and VI			Reps. VII and VIII	
(1)	1	2	(10)	1	3	(19)	1	4	(28)	1	5
(2)	2	8	(11)	2	5	(20)	2	6	(29)	2	4
(3)	3	4	(12)	3	6	(21)	2	3	(30)	3	8
(4)	4	7	(13)	4	9	(22)	4	5	(31)	4	6
(5)	5	6	(14)	5	8	(23)	5	7	(32)	3	5
(6)	1	6	(15)	6	7	(24)	6	8	(33)	6	9
(7)	3	7	(16)	1	7	(25)	7	9	(34)	2	7
(8)	8	9	(17)	4	8	(26)	1	8	(35)	7	8
(9)	5	9	(18)	2	9	(27)	3	9	(36)	1	9

Plan 11.11 $t = 9, k = 4, r = 8, b = 18, \lambda = 3, E = .84$, **Type II**

Block	Reps. I, II, III, and IV									Reps. V, VI, VII, and VIII									
(1)	1	4	6	7	(6)	4	5	6	9	(10)	1	2	5	7	(15)	1	3	6	8
(2)	2	6	8	9	(7)	2	3	6	7	(11)	2	3	5	6	(16)	4	6	7	8
(3)	1	3	8	9	(8)	2	4	5	8	(12)	3	4	7	9	(17)	3	4	5	8
(4)	1	2	3	4	(9)	3	5	7	9	(13)	1	2	4	9	(18)	2	7	8	9
(5)	1	5	7	8						(14)	1	5	6	9					

Plan 11.12 $t = 9, k = 5, r = 10, b = 18, \lambda = 5, E = .90$, **Type II**

Block	Reps. I, II, III, IV, and V											Reps. VI, VII, VIII, IX, and X										
(1)	1	2	3	7	8	(6)	2	4	5	6	7	(10)	1	2	3	5	9	(15)	3	5	6	7	8
(2)	1	2	4	6	8	(7)	1	3	6	7	9	(11)	1	2	5	6	8	(16)	1	4	7	8	9
(3)	2	3	5	8	9	(8)	1	4	5	8	9	(12)	1	3	4	5	6	(17)	3	4	6	8	9
(4)	2	3	4	6	9	(9)	5	6	7	8	9	(13)	2	3	4	7	8	(18)	1	2	6	7	9
(5)	1	3	4	5	7							(14)	2	4	5	7	9						

Plan 11.13 $t = 9, k = 6, r = 8, b = 12, \lambda = 5, E = .94$, **Type II**

Block	Reps. I and II							Reps. III and IV					
(1)	1	2	4	5	7	8	(4)	1	2	5	6	7	9
(2)	2	3	5	6	8	9	(5)	1	3	4	5	8	9
(3)	1	3	4	6	7	9	(6)	2	3	4	6	7	8
	Reps. V and VI							Reps. VII and VIII					
(7)	1	3	5	6	7	8	(10)	4	5	6	7	8	9
(8)	1	2	4	6	8	9	(11)	1	2	3	4	5	6
(9)	2	3	4	5	7	9	(12)	1	2	3	7	8	9

Plan 11.14 $t = 10, k = 2, r = 9, b = 45, \lambda = 1, E = .56$, **Type I**

Block	Rep. I			Rep. II			Rep. III			Rep. IV			Rep. V	
(1)	1	2	(6)	1	3	(11)	1	4	(16)	1	5	(21)	1	6
(2)	3	4	(7)	2	7	(12)	2	10	(17)	2	8	(22)	2	9
(3)	5	6	(8)	4	8	(13)	3	7	(18)	3	10	(23)	3	8
(4)	7	8	(9)	5	9	(14)	5	8	(19)	4	9	(24)	4	10
(5)	9	10	(10)	6	10	(15)	6	9	(20)	6	7	(25)	5	7

	Rep. VI			Rep. VII			Rep. VIII			Rep. IX	
(26)	1	7	(31)	1	8	(36)	1	9	(41)	1	10
(27)	2	6	(32)	2	3	(37)	2	4	(42)	2	5
(28)	3	9	(33)	4	6	(38)	3	5	(43)	3	6
(29)	4	5	(34)	5	10	(39)	6	8	(44)	4	7
(30)	8	10	(35)	7	9	(40)	7	10	(45)	8	9

Plan 11.15 $t = 10, k = 3, r = 9, b = 30, \lambda = 2, E = .74$, **Type II**

Block	Reps. I, II, and III				Reps. IV, V, and VI				Reps. VII, VIII, and IX		
(1)	1	2	3	(11)	1	2	4	(21)	1	3	5
(2)	2	5	8	(12)	2	3	6	(22)	2	6	7
(3)	3	4	7	(13)	3	4	8	(23)	3	8	9
(4)	1	4	6	(14)	4	5	9	(24)	2	4	10
(5)	5	7	8	(15)	1	5	7	(25)	3	5	6
(6)	4	6	9	(16)	6	8	9	(26)	1	6	8
(7)	1	7	9	(17)	3	7	10	(27)	2	7	9
(8)	2	8	10	(18)	1	8	10	(28)	4	7	8
(9)	3	9	10	(19)	2	5	9	(29)	1	9	10
(10)	5	6	10	(20)	6	7	10	(30)	4	5	10

Plan 11.16 $t = 10, k = 4, r = 6, b = 15, \lambda = 2, E = .83$, **Type III**

Block														
(1)	1	2	3	4	(6)	1	6	8	10	(11)	3	5	9	10
(2)	1	2	5	6	(7)	2	3	6	9	(12)	3	6	7	10
(3)	1	3	7	8	(8)	2	4	7	10	(13)	3	4	5	8
(4)	1	4	9	10	(9)	2	5	8	10	(14)	4	5	6	7
(5)	1	5	7	9	(10)	2	7	8	9	(15)	4	6	8	9

Plan 11.17 $t = 10, k = 5, r = 9, b = 18, \lambda = 4, E = .89$, **Type III**

Block																	
(1)	1	2	3	4	5	(7)	1	4	5	6	10	(13)	2	5	6	8	10
(2)	1	2	3	6	7	(8)	1	4	8	9	10	(14)	2	6	7	9	10
(3)	1	2	4	6	9	(9)	1	5	7	9	10	(15)	3	4	6	7	10
(4)	1	2	5	7	8	(10)	2	3	4	8	10	(16)	3	4	5	7	9
(5)	1	3	6	8	9	(11)	2	3	5	9	10	(17)	3	5	6	8	9
(6)	1	3	7	8	10	(12)	2	4	7	8	9	(18)	4	5	6	7	8

Plan 11.18 $t = 10, k = 6, r = 9, b = 15, \lambda = 5, E = .93$, **Type III**

Block																				
(1)	1	2	4	5	8	9	(6)	2	3	4	6	8	10	(11)	1	4	5	7	8	10
(2)	5	6	7	8	9	10	(7)	1	2	6	7	9	10	(12)	1	2	3	5	7	10
(3)	2	4	5	6	9	10	(8)	1	3	5	6	8	9	(13)	2	3	5	6	7	8
(4)	1	2	4	6	7	8	(9)	1	2	3	8	9	10	(14)	1	3	4	5	6	10
(5)	3	4	7	8	9	10	(10)	2	3	4	5	7	9	(15)	1	3	4	6	7	9

Plan 11.4a $t = 11, k = 2, r = 10, b = 55, \lambda = 1, E = .55$, **Type II**

Block	Reps. I and II		Block	Reps. III and IV		Block	Reps. V and VI		Block	Reps. VII and VIII		Block	Reps. IX and X	
(1)	1	2	(12)	1	3	(23)	1	4	(34)	1	5	(45)	1	6
(2)	2	11	(13)	2	6	(24)	2	3	(35)	2	9	(46)	2	5
(3)	3	10	(14)	3	5	(25)	3	7	(36)	3	6	(47)	3	4
(4)	4	5	(15)	4	10	(26)	4	6	(37)	2	4	(48)	4	7
(5)	5	6	(16)	5	9	(27)	5	10	(38)	5	7	(49)	5	8
(6)	6	7	(17)	6	8	(28)	6	9	(39)	6	10	(50)	6	11
(7)	1	7	(18)	2	7	(29)	7	11	(40)	7	8	(51)	7	10
(8)	3	8	(19)	1	8	(30)	2	8	(41)	4	8	(52)	8	9
(9)	4	9	(20)	7	9	(31)	1	9	(42)	9	11	(53)	3	9
(10)	9	10	(21)	10	11	(32)	8	10	(43)	1	10	(54)	2	10
(11)	8	11	(22)	4	11	(33)	5	11	(44)	3	11	(55)	1	11

Plan 11.19 $t = 11, k = 5, r = 5, b = 11, \lambda = 2, E = .88$, **Type IV**

Block						Block						Block					
(1)	1	2	3	5	8	(5)	5	6	7	9	1	(9)	9	10	11	2	5
(2)	2	3	4	6	9	(6)	6	7	8	10	2	(10)	10	11	1	3	6
(3)	3	4	5	7	10	(7)	7	8	9	11	3	(11)	11	1	2	4	7
(4)	4	5	6	8	11	(8)	8	9	10	1	4						

Plan 11.20 $t = 11, k = 6, r = 6, b = 11, \lambda = 3, E = .92$, **Type IV**

Block							Block							Block						
(1)	4	6	7	9	10	11	(5)	2	3	4	8	10	11	(9)	1	3	4	6	7	8
(2)	1	5	7	8	10	11	(6)	1	3	4	5	9	11	(10)	2	4	5	7	8	9
(3)	1	2	6	8	9	11	(7)	1	2	4	5	6	10	(11)	3	5	6	8	9	10
(4)	1	2	3	7	9	10	(8)	2	3	5	6	7	11							

Plan 11.21 $t = 13, k = 3, r = 6, b = 26, \lambda = 1, E = .72$, **Type II**

Block	Reps. I, II, and III			Block				Block	Reps. IV, V, and VI			Block			
(1)	1	3	9	(8)	3	8	10	(14)	2	5	6	(21)	9	12	13
(2)	2	4	10	(9)	4	9	11	(15)	3	6	7	(22)	1	10	13
(3)	3	5	11	(10)	5	10	12	(16)	4	7	8	(23)	1	2	11
(4)	4	6	12	(11)	6	11	13	(17)	5	8	9	(24)	2	3	12
(5)	5	7	13	(12)	1	7	12	(18)	6	9	10	(25)	3	4	13
(6)	1	6	8	(13)	2	8	13	(19)	7	10	11	(26)	1	4	5
(7)	2	7	9					(20)	8	11	12				

Plan 11.22 $t = 13, k = 4, r = 4, b = 13, \lambda = 1, E = .81$, **Type IV**

Block					Block					Block				
(1)	1	2	4	10	(6)	6	7	9	2	(11)	11	12	1	7
(2)	2	3	5	11	(7)	7	8	10	3	(12)	12	13	2	8
(3)	3	4	6	12	(8)	8	9	11	4	(13)	13	1	3	9
(4)	4	5	7	13	(9)	9	10	12	5					
(5)	5	6	8	1	(10)	10	11	13	6					

Plan 11.23 $t = 13, k = 9, r = 9, b = 13, \lambda = 6, E = .96$, **Type IV**

Block										Block									
(1)	3	5	6	7	8	9	11	12	13	(8)	1	2	3	5	6	7	10	12	13
(2)	1	4	6	7	8	9	10	12	13	(9)	1	2	3	4	6	7	8	11	13
(3)	1	2	5	7	8	9	10	11	13	(10)	1	2	3	4	5	7	8	9	12
(4)	1	2	3	6	8	9	10	11	12	(11)	2	3	4	5	6	8	9	10	13
(5)	2	3	4	7	9	10	11	12	13	(12)	1	3	4	5	6	7	9	10	11
(6)	1	3	4	5	8	10	11	12	13	(13)	2	4	5	6	7	8	10	11	12
(7)	1	2	4	5	6	9	11	12	13										

Plan 11.24 $t = 15, k = 3, r = 7, b = 35, \lambda = 1, E = .71$, **Type I**

Block	Rep. I				Rep. II				Rep. III				Rep. IV		
(1)	1	2	3	(6)	1	4	5	(11)	1	6	7	(16)	1	8	9
(2)	4	8	12	(7)	2	8	10	(12)	2	9	11	(17)	2	13	15
(3)	5	10	15	(8)	3	13	14	(13)	3	12	15	(18)	3	4	7
(4)	6	11	13	(9)	6	9	15	(14)	4	10	14	(19)	5	11	14
(5)	7	9	14	(10)	7	11	12	(15)	5	8	13	(20)	6	10	12

Block	Rep. V				Rep. VI				Rep. VII		
(21)	1	10	11	(26)	1	12	13	(31)	1	14	15
(22)	2	12	14	(27)	2	5	7	(32)	2	4	6
(23)	3	5	6	(28)	3	9	10	(33)	3	8	11
(24)	4	9	13	(29)	4	11	15	(34)	5	9	12
(25)	7	8	15	(30)	6	8	14	(35)	7	10	13

Plan 11.25 $t = 15, k = 7, r = 7, b = 15, \lambda = 3, E = .92$, **Type IV**

See incomplete latin squares Plan 13.7; randomize units in blocks ignoring replications.

Plan 11.26 $t = 15, k = 8, r = 8, b = 15, \lambda = 4, E = .94$, **Type IV**

See incomplete latin squares Plan 13.8; randomize units in blocks ignoring replications.

Plan 11.27 $t = 16, k = 6, r = 6, b = 16, \lambda = 2, E = .89$, **Type IV**

See incomplete latin squares Plan 13.9; randomize units in blocks ignoring replications.

Plan 11.28 $t = 16, k = 6, r = 9, b = 24, \lambda = 3, E = .89$, **Type II**

Block	Reps. I, II, and III							Reps. IV, V, and VI							Reps. VII, VIII, and IX					
(1)	1	2	5	6	11	12	(9)	1	3	6	8	13	15	(17)	1	4	5	8	10	11
(2)	3	4	7	8	9	10	(10)	2	4	5	7	14	16	(18)	2	3	6	7	9	12
(3)	5	6	9	10	13	14	(11)	5	7	9	11	13	15	(19)	5	8	9	12	13	16
(4)	7	8	11	12	15	16	(12)	6	8	10	12	14	16	(20)	1	4	6	7	13	16
(5)	1	2	9	10	15	16	(13)	2	4	6	8	9	11	(21)	1	4	9	12	14	15
(6)	3	4	11	12	13	14	(14)	1	3	5	7	10	12	(22)	6	7	10	11	14	15
(7)	1	2	7	8	13	14	(15)	2	4	10	12	13	15	(23)	2	3	10	11	13	16
(8)	3	4	5	6	15	16	(16)	1	3	9	11	14	16	(24)	2	3	5	8	14	15

Plan 11.29 $t = 16, k = 10, r = 10, b = 16, \lambda = 6, E = .96$, **Type IV**

See incomplete latin squares Plan 13.10; randomize units in blocks ignoring replications.

Plan 11.30 $t = 19, k = 3, r = 9, b = 57, \lambda = 1, E = .70$, **Type II**

See extended incomplete latin squares Plan 13.15a; randomize units in blocks ignoring replications.

Plan 11.31 $t = 19, k = 9, r = 9, b = 19, \lambda = 4, E = .94$, **Type IV**

See incomplete latin squares Plan 13.11; randomize units in blocks ignoring replications.

Plan 11.32 $t = 19, k = 10, r = 10, b = 19, \lambda = 5, E = .95$, **Type IV**

See incomplete latin squares Plan 13.12; randomize units in blocks ignoring replications.

Plan 11.33 $t = 21, k = 3, r = 10, b = 70, \lambda = 1, E = .70$, **Type I**

Block	Rep. I	Block	Rep. II	Block	Rep. III	Block	Rep. IV	Block	Rep. V
(1)	1 2 3	(8)	1 4 15	(15)	1 5 17	(22)	1 6 9	(29)	1 7 21
(2)	4 5 6	(9)	2 5 11	(16)	2 4 14	(23)	2 7 16	(30)	2 13 17
(3)	7 8 9	(10)	3 9 16	(17)	3 7 11	(24)	3 8 21	(31)	3 10 18
(4)	10 11 12	(11)	6 17 20	(18)	6 10 19	(25)	4 17 19	(32)	4 8 11
(5)	13 14 15	(12)	7 12 19	(19)	8 16 20	(26)	5 10 13	(33)	5 16 19
(6)	16 17 18	(13)	8 13 18	(20)	9 15 18	(27)	11 15 20	(34)	6 12 15
(7)	19 20 21	(14)	10 14 21	(21)	12 13 21	(28)	12 14 18	(35)	9 14 20

Block	Rep. VI	Block	Rep. VII	Block	Rep. VIII	Block	Rep. IX	Block	Rep. X
(36)	1 8 10	(43)	1 11 18	(50)	1 12 20	(57)	1 13 19	(64)	1 14 16
(37)	2 18 19	(44)	2 10 20	(51)	2 6 8	(58)	2 9 12	(65)	2 15 21
(38)	3 15 17	(45)	3 5 12	(52)	3 14 19	(59)	3 4 20	(66)	3 6 13
(39)	4 12 16	(46)	4 9 13	(53)	4 18 21	(60)	5 8 14	(67)	4 7 10
(40)	5 9 21	(47)	6 16 21	(54)	5 7 15	(61)	6 7 18	(68)	5 18 20
(41)	6 11 14	(48)	7 14 17	(55)	9 10 17	(62)	10 15 16	(69)	8 12 17
(42)	7 13 20	(49)	8 15 19	(56)	11 13 16	(63)	11 17 21	(70)	9 11 19

Plan 11.34 $t = 21, k = 5, r = 5, b = 21, \lambda = 1, E = .84$, **Type IV**

See incomplete latin squares Plan 13.13; randomize units in blocks ignoring replications.

Plan 11.35 $t = 21, k = 7, r = 10, b = 30, \lambda = 3, E = .90$, **Type III**

Block								Block							
(1)	2	5	10	11	17	19	20	(16)	2	7	10	13	18	20	21
(2)	3	6	11	12	18	20	21	(17)	3	1	11	14	19	21	15
(3)	4	7	12	13	19	21	15	(18)	4	2	12	8	20	15	16
(4)	5	1	13	14	20	15	16	(19)	5	3	13	9	21	16	17
(5)	6	2	14	8	21	16	17	(20)	6	4	14	10	15	17	18
(6)	7	3	8	9	15	17	18	(21)	7	5	8	11	16	18	19
(7)	1	4	9	10	16	18	19	(22)	1	2	4	8	9	11	21
(8)	3	4	8	13	17	19	20	(23)	2	3	5	9	10	12	15
(9)	4	5	9	14	18	20	21	(24)	3	4	6	10	11	13	16
(10)	5	6	10	8	19	21	15	(25)	4	5	7	11	12	14	17
(11)	6	7	11	9	20	15	16	(26)	5	6	1	12	13	8	18
(12)	7	1	12	10	21	16	17	(27)	6	7	2	13	14	9	19
(13)	1	2	13	11	15	17	18	(28)	7	1	3	14	8	10	20
(14)	2	3	14	12	16	18	19	(29)	1	2	3	4	5	6	7
(15)	1	6	9	12	17	19	20	(30)	8	9	10	11	12	13	14

Plan 11.36 $t = 25, k = 4, r = 8, b = 50, \lambda = 1, E = .78$, **Type II**

See extended incomplete latin squares Plan 13.16a; randomize units in blocks ignoring replications.

Plan 11.37 $t = 25, k = 9, r = 9, b = 25, \lambda = 3, E = .93$, **Type IV**

See incomplete latin squares Plan 13.1a; randomize units in blocks ignoring replications.

Plan 11.38 $t = 28, k = 4, r = 9, b = 63, \lambda = 1, E = .78$, **Type I**

Block	Rep. I				Block	Rep. II				Block	Rep. III			
(1)	28	1	10	19	(8)	28	2	11	20	(15)	28	3	12	21
(2)	2	9	13	16	(9)	3	1	14	17	(16)	4	2	15	18
(3)	3	8	11	18	(10)	4	9	12	10	(17)	5	1	13	11
(4)	4	7	23	24	(11)	5	8	24	25	(18)	6	9	25	26
(5)	5	6	20	27	(12)	6	7	21	19	(19)	7	8	22	20
(6)	12	17	22	25	(13)	13	18	23	26	(20)	14	10	24	27
(7)	14	15	21	26	(14)	15	16	22	27	(21)	16	17	23	19

Block	Rep. IV				Block	Rep. V				Block	Rep. VI			
(22)	28	4	13	22	(29)	28	5	14	23	(36)	28	6	15	24
(23)	5	3	16	10	(30)	6	4	17	11	(37)	7	5	18	12
(24)	6	2	14	12	(31)	7	3	15	13	(38)	8	4	16	14
(25)	7	1	26	27	(32)	8	2	27	19	(39)	9	3	19	20
(26)	8	9	23	21	(33)	9	1	24	22	(40)	1	2	25	23
(27)	15	11	25	19	(34)	16	12	26	20	(41)	17	13	27	21
(28)	17	18	24	20	(35)	18	10	25	21	(42)	10	11	26	22

Block	Rep. VII				Block	Rep. VIII				Block	Rep. IX			
(43)	28	7	16	25	(50)	28	8	17	26	(57)	28	9	18	27
(44)	8	6	10	13	(51)	9	7	11	14	(58)	1	8	12	15
(45)	9	5	17	15	(52)	1	6	18	16	(59)	2	7	10	17
(46)	1	4	20	21	(53)	2	5	21	22	(60)	3	6	22	23
(47)	2	3	26	24	(54)	3	4	27	25	(61)	4	5	19	26
(48)	18	14	19	22	(55)	10	15	20	23	(62)	11	16	21	24
(49)	11	12	27	23	(56)	12	13	19	24	(63)	13	14	20	25

Plan 11.39 $t = 28, k = 7, r = 9, b = 36, \lambda = 2, E = .89$, **Type III**

Block								Block							
(1)	4	7	8	9	14	23	28	(19)	4	8	11	17	19	21	25
(2)	1	5	9	10	11	15	24	(20)	1	13	14	18	23	25	26
(3)	6	8	13	15	16	18	21	(21)	2	4	5	6	16	22	23
(4)	7	12	13	17	22	24	25	(22)	3	4	10	11	12	14	18
(5)	4	10	16	17	20	26	27	(23)	1	9	14	16	17	19	22
(6)	2	11	18	19	22	26	28	(24)	1	2	4	13	20	24	28
(7)	1	3	6	12	19	23	27	(25)	3	5	8	17	23	24	26
(8)	2	3	5	14	20	21	25	(26)	5	6	7	10	19	25	28
(9)	1	2	8	10	12	16	25	(27)	1	6	7	8	11	20	26
(10)	2	3	6	9	11	13	17	(28)	9	10	13	19	20	21	23
(11)	4	5	12	13	15	19	26	(29)	2	8	14	15	19	24	27
(12)	3	7	16	18	19	20	24	(30)	3	9	15	16	25	26	28
(13)	6	10	14	21	22	24	26	(31)	5	8	9	12	18	20	22
(14)	11	15	20	22	23	25	27	(32)	11	12	16	21	23	24	28
(15)	1	5	17	18	21	27	28	(33)	1	3	4	7	15	21	22
(16)	2	7	9	12	21	26	27	(34)	5	7	11	13	14	16	27
(17)	3	8	10	13	22	27	28	(35)	4	6	9	18	24	25	27
(18)	6	12	14	15	17	20	28	(36)	2	7	10	15	17	18	23

Plan 11.40 $t = 31, k = 6, r = 6, b = 31, \lambda = 1, E = .86$, **Type IV**

See incomplete latin squares Plan 13.13; randomize units in blocks ignoring replications.

Plan 11.41 $t = 31, k = 10, r = 10, b = 31, \lambda = 3, E = .93$, **Type IV**

See incomplete latin squares Plan 13.2a; randomize units in blocks ignoring replications.

Plan 11.42 $t = 37, k = 9, r = 9, b = 37, \lambda = 2, E = .91$, **Type IV**

See incomplete latin squares Plan 13.15; randomize units in blocks ignoring replications.

Plan 11.43 $t = 41, k = 5, r = 10, b = 82, \lambda = 1, E = .82$, **Type III**

See extended latin squares Plan 13.17a; randomize units in blocks ignoring replications.

Plan 11.44 $t = 57, k = 8, r = 8, b = 57, \lambda = 1, E = .89$, **Type IV**

See incomplete latin squares Plan 13.3a; randomize units in blocks ignoring replications.

Plan 11.45 $t = 73, k = 9, r = 9, b = 73, \lambda = 1, E = .90$, **Type IV**

See incomplete latin squares Plan 13.4a; randomize units in blocks ignoring replications.

Plan 11.46 $t = 91, k = 10, r = 10, b = 91, \lambda = 1, E = .91$, **Type IV**

See incomplete latin squares Plan 13.5a; randomize units in blocks ignoring replications.

INDEX TO PLANS, INCOMPLETE LATIN SQUARES

t	k	r	b	λ	E	Plan	Type†
3	3	6	6	6	1.00	2LS	
	3	9	9	9	1.00	3LS	
	5	5	3	5	.96	13.16	III
	5	10	6	10	.96	13.16	IIa
	7	7	3	7	.08	13.17	IV
	8	8	3	8	.98	13.18	III
	10	10	3	10	.99	13.19	IV
4	3	3	4	2	.89	*	II
	3	6	8	4	.89	**	Ia
	3	9	12	6	.89	**	Ia
	4	8	8	8	1.00	2LS	
	5	5	4	5	.96	13.20	IV
	5	10	8	10	.96	13.20	IIa
	7	7	4	7	.98	13.21	III
	9	9	4	9	.99	13.22	IV
5	2	4	10	1	.67	13.6a	II
	3	6	10	3		13.7a	II
	4	4	5	3	.94	*	II
	4	8	10	6	.94	**	Ia
	5	10	10	10	1.00	2LS	
	6	6	5	6	.97	13.23	IV
	9	9	5	9	.99	13.24	III
6	5	5	6	4	.96	*	II
	5	10	12	8	.96	**	Ia
	7	7	6	7	.98	13.25	IV
7	2	6	21	1	.58	13.8a	V
	3	3	7	1	.78	13.1	II
	3	9	21	3	.78	13.1	Ia
	4	4	7	2	.88	13.2	II
	4	8	14	4	.88	13.2	Ia
	6	6	7	5	.97	*	II
	8	8	7	8	.98	13.26	IV
8	7	7	8	6	.98	*	II
9	2	8	36	1	.56	13.9a	V
	4	8	18	3	.84	13.10a	V
	5	10	18	5	.90	13.11a	V
	8	8	9	7	.98	*	II

t	k	r	b	λ	E	Plan	Type†
10	3	9	30	2	.74	13.12a	V
	9	9	10	8	.99	*	II
11	2	10	55	1	.55	13.13a	V
	5	5	11	2	.88	13.3	I
	6	6	11	3	.92	13.4	I
	10	10	11	9	.99	*	II
13	3	6	26	1	.72	13.14a	V
	4	4	13	1	.81	13.5	I
	9	9	13	6	.95	13.6	I
15	7	7	15	3	.92	13.7	I
	8	8	15	4	.94	13.8	I
16	6	6	16	2	.89	13.9	I
	10	10	16	6	.96	13.10	I
19	3	9	57	1	.70	13.15a	V
	9	9	19	4	.94	13.11	I
	10	10	19	5	.95	13.12	I
21	5	5	21	1	.84	13.13	I
25	4	8	50	1	.78	13.16a	V
	9	9	25	3	.93	13.1a	I
31	6	6	31	1	.86	13.14	I
	10	10	31	3	.93	13.2a	I
37	9	9	37	2	.91	13.15	I
41	5	10	82	1	.82	13.17a	V
57	8	8	57	1	.89	13.3a	I
73	9	9	73	1	.90	13.4a	I
91	10	10	91	1	.91	13.5a	I

* Constructed from a $t \times t$ latin square by omission of the last column.

** By repetition of the plan for $r = t - 1$, which is constructed by taking a $t \times t$ latin square and omitting the last column.

† This refers to the method of analysis. For types I, Ia, II, IIa, and V, see section 13.2; for types III and IV, see section 13.3.

Plan 13.1 $t = 7, k = 3, r = 3, b = 7, \lambda = 1, E = .78$, **Type II**

Block	Reps. I	II	III
(1)	7	1	3
(2)	1	2	4
(3)	2	3	5
(4)	3	4	6
(5)	4	5	7
(6)	5	6	1
(7)	6	7	2

Plan 13.2 $t = 7, k = 4, r = 4, b = 7, \lambda = 2, E = .88$, **Type II**

Block	Reps. I	II	III	IV
(1)	3	5	6	7
(2)	4	6	7	1
(3)	5	7	1	2
(4)	6	1	2	3
(5)	7	2	3	4
(6)	1	3	4	5
(7)	2	4	5	6

Plan 13.3 $t = 11, k = 5, r = 5, b = 11, \lambda = 2, E = .88$, **Type I**

Block	I	II	III	IV	V
(1)	1	2	3	4	5
(2)	7	1	6	10	3
(3)	9	8	1	6	2
(4)	11	9	7	1	4
(5)	10	11	5	8	1
(6)	8	7	2	3	11
(7)	2	6	4	11	10
(8)	6	3	11	5	9
(9)	3	4	10	9	8
(10)	5	10	9	2	7
(11)	4	5	8	7	6

Plan 13.4 $t = 11, k = 6, r = 6, b = 11, \lambda = 3, E = .92$, **Type I**

Block	I	II	III	IV	V	VI
(1)	6	7	8	9	10	11
(2)	5	8	4	11	2	9
(3)	4	5	7	3	11	10
(4)	3	10	2	6	5	8
(5)	2	3	9	7	4	6
(6)	1	6	10	4	9	5
(7)	9	1	3	5	8	7
(8)	8	2	1	10	7	4
(9)	7	11	5	1	6	2
(10)	11	4	6	8	1	3
(11)	10	9	11	2	3	1

Plan 13.5 $t = 13, k = 4, r = 4, b = 13, \lambda = 1, E = .81$, **Type I**

Block	I	II	III	IV
(1)	13	1	3	9
(2)	1	2	4	10
(3)	2	3	5	11
(4)	3	4	6	12
(5)	4	5	7	13
(6)	5	6	8	1
(7)	6	7	9	2
(8)	7	8	10	3
(9)	8	9	11	4
(10)	9	10	12	5
(11)	10	11	13	6
(12)	11	12	1	7
(13)	12	13	2	8

Plan 13.6 $t = 13, k = 9, r = 9, b = 13, \lambda = 6, E = .95$, **Type I**

Block	I	II	III	IV	V	VI	VII	VIII	IX
(1)	2	5	6	7	9	10	11	12	13
(2)	3	6	7	8	10	11	12	13	1
(3)	4	7	8	9	11	12	13	1	2
(4)	5	8	9	10	12	13	1	2	3
(5)	6	9	10	11	13	1	2	3	4
(6)	7	10	11	12	1	2	3	4	5
(7)	8	11	12	13	2	3	4	5	6
(8)	9	12	13	1	3	4	5	6	7
(9)	10	13	1	2	4	5	6	7	8
(10)	11	1	2	3	5	6	7	8	9
(11)	12	2	3	4	6	7	8	9	10
(12)	13	3	4	5	7	8	9	10	11
(13)	1	4	5	6	8	9	10	11	12

Plan 13.7 $t = 15, k = 7, r = 7, b = 15, \lambda = 3, E = .92$, **Type I**

Block	I	II	III	IV	V	VI	VII
(1)	13	8	12	6	7	1	9
(2)	5	14	10	7	12	2	8
(3)	15	12	11	5	8	3	6
(4)	12	11	6	9	2	4	14
(5)	4	5	8	1	14	9	15
(6)	11	9	7	2	13	15	5
(7)	1	2	3	4	5	6	7
(8)	2	3	1	13	15	14	12
(9)	8	6	4	15	10	13	2
(10)	10	4	5	11	1	12	13
(11)	9	13	14	10	6	5	3
(12)	14	7	13	3	4	8	11
(13)	7	15	9	12	3	10	4
(14)	3	1	2	8	9	11	10
(15)	6	10	15	14	11	7	1

Plan 13.8 $t = 15, k = 8, r = 8, b = 15, \lambda = 4, E = .94$, **Type I**

Block	I	II	III	IV	V	VI	VII	VIII
(1)	11	4	2	5	10	3	14	15
(2)	4	1	3	15	13	11	6	9
(3)	9	2	14	4	7	1	10	13
(4)	15	3	1	10	8	13	7	5
(5)	7	13	10	12	11	2	3	6
(6)	6	10	12	1	4	14	8	3
(7)	12	9	13	14	15	10	11	8
(8)	10	11	9	7	6	8	5	4
(9)	5	14	7	3	1	9	12	11
(10)	8	15	6	2	3	7	9	14
(11)	1	7	11	8	2	4	15	12
(12)	2	6	15	9	5	12	1	10
(13)	13	8	5	11	14	6	2	1
(14)	14	5	4	6	12	15	13	7
(15)	3	12	8	13	9	5	4	2

Plan 13.9 $t = 16, k = 6, r = 6, b = 16, \lambda = 2, E = .89$, **Type I**

Block	I	II	III	IV	V	VI
(1)	1	2	3	4	5	6
(2)	2	7	8	9	10	1
(3)	3	1	13	7	11	12
(4)	4	8	1	11	14	15
(5)	5	12	14	1	16	9
(6)	6	10	15	13	1	16
(7)	7	14	2	16	15	3
(8)	8	16	12	2	4	13
(9)	9	15	11	5	13	2
(10)	10	11	6	12	2	14
(11)	11	4	16	3	9	10
(12)	12	3	10	15	8	5
(13)	13	6	9	14	3	8
(14)	14	13	5	10	7	4
(15)	15	9	4	6	12	7
(16)	16	5	7	8	6	11

Plan 13.10 $t = 16, k = 10, r = 10, b = 16, \lambda = 6, E = .96$, **Type I**

Reps.

Block	I	II	III	IV	V	VI	VII	VIII	IX	X
(1)	8	7	9	10	11	12	13	14	15	16
(2)	3	4	5	13	16	11	12	6	14	15
(3)	9	2	4	5	6	8	10	15	16	14
(4)	2	6	3	7	5	10	9	16	12	13
(5)	6	8	2	3	4	7	15	10	13	11
(6)	4	5	14	8	3	9	7	2	11	12
(7)	1	10	11	4	13	5	6	12	8	9
(8)	5	1	15	6	14	3	11	9	7	10
(9)	16	3	1	14	12	6	4	8	10	7
(10)	7	13	16	1	15	4	3	5	9	8
(11)	12	14	7	15	1	2	8	13	6	5
(12)	14	11	13	16	9	1	2	7	4	6
(13)	10	15	12	2	7	16	1	11	5	4
(14)	11	12	6	9	8	15	16	1	2	3
(15)	13	16	8	11	10	14	5	3	1	2
(16)	15	9	10	12	2	13	14	4	3	1

Plan 13.11 $t = 19, k = 9, r = 9, b = 19, \lambda = 4, E = .94$, **Type I**

Reps.

Block	I	II	III	IV	V	VI	VII	VIII	IX
(1)	1	2	3	4	5	6	7	8	9
(2)	14	1	2	3	4	12	11	10	13
(3)	17	16	1	2	15	10	6	5	11
(4)	12	13	16	1	2	7	18	15	8
(5)	9	10	12	16	1	3	17	19	7
(6)	8	11	13	19	17	1	3	6	18
(7)	7	18	11	14	16	19	1	4	5
(8)	6	9	17	12	14	18	15	1	4
(9)	5	8	9	10	13	15	19	14	1
(10)	13	5	14	9	18	2	16	3	17
(11)	10	6	7	15	19	14	2	18	3
(12)	18	17	5	8	12	4	10	2	19
(13)	19	4	15	7	9	17	13	11	2
(14)	2	19	6	11	8	9	14	16	12
(15)	3	15	10	18	11	8	4	9	16
(16)	4	3	19	5	6	16	12	13	15
(17)	15	7	8	17	3	11	5	12	14
(18)	16	14	4	6	7	13	8	17	10
(19)	11	12	18	13	10	5	9	7	6

Plan 13.12 $t = 19, k = 10, r = 10, b = 19, \lambda = 5, E = .95$, **Type I**

	Reps.									
Block	I	II	III	IV	V	VI	VII	VIII	IX	X
(1)	10	11	12	13	14	15	16	17	18	19
(2)	19	5	6	7	8	9	15	16	17	18
(3)	18	19	3	4	7	8	9	12	13	14
(4)	14	17	19	11	4	5	6	9	10	3
(5)	13	2	15	14	18	4	5	6	11	8
(6)	12	14	2	10	15	7	4	5	9	16
(7)	15	13	17	2	12	6	8	10	3	9
(8)	16	10	11	19	2	3	7	13	8	5
(9)	11	16	18	17	6	2	3	4	12	7
(10)	1	8	10	15	11	19	12	7	4	6
(11)	17	1	8	9	16	12	13	11	5	4
(12)	6	15	1	16	9	14	11	3	7	13
(13)	5	6	14	1	3	10	18	8	16	12
(14)	4	7	5	3	1	13	17	18	15	10
(15)	7	12	13	5	19	1	2	14	6	17
(16)	8	9	7	18	10	17	1	2	14	11
(17)	9	4	16	6	13	18	10	1	19	2
(18)	3	18	9	12	5	11	19	15	2	1
(19)	2	3	4	8	17	16	14	19	1	15

Plan 13.13 $t = 21, k = 5, r = 5, b = 21, \lambda = 1, E = .84$, **Type I**

	Reps.						Reps.				
Block	I	II	III	IV	V		I	II	III	IV	V
(1)	21	1	4	14	16	(12)	11	12	15	4	6
(2)	1	2	5	15	17	(13)	12	13	16	5	7
(3)	2	3	6	16	18	(14)	13	14	17	6	8
(4)	3	4	7	17	19	(15)	14	15	18	7	9
(5)	4	5	8	18	20	(16)	15	16	19	8	10
(6)	5	6	9	19	21	(17)	16	17	20	9	11
(7)	6	7	10	20	1	(18)	17	18	21	10	12
(8)	7	8	11	21	2	(19)	18	19	1	11	13
(9)	8	9	12	1	3	(20)	19	20	2	12	14
(10)	9	10	13	2	4	(21)	20	21	3	13	15
(11)	10	11	14	3	5						

Plan 13.1a $t = 25, k = 9, r = 9, b = 25, \lambda = 3, E = .93$, **Type I**

Block	I	II	III	IV	V	VI	VII	VIII	IX
					Reps.				
(1)	1	2	3	4	5	6	7	8	9
(2)	2	4	9	10	24	17	15	22	12
(3)	3	24	8	23	18	21	13	4	10
(4)	4	22	25	8	20	12	11	3	19
(5)	5	15	17	18	8	11	2	13	20
(6)	6	8	12	13	1	14	24	25	15
(7)	7	16	5	22	3	10	25	15	13
(8)	8	10	11	16	6	22	23	1	17
(9)	9	13	20	5	12	23	1	21	22
(10)	10	19	14	12	16	2	8	5	21
(11)	11	18	19	24	10	1	5	9	25
(12)	12	6	10	25	7	18	20	2	23
(13)	13	11	4	9	23	25	14	16	2
(14)	14	3	7	17	11	5	12	23	24
(15)	15	20	21	1	14	7	10	11	4
(16)	16	17	18	7	13	19	4	12	1
(17)	17	14	13	20	19	3	9	10	6
(18)	18	9	22	14	25	8	21	17	7
(19)	19	7	23	15	9	20	16	24	8
(20)	20	5	16	6	4	24	22	14	18
(21)	21	12	6	11	15	9	3	18	16
(22)	22	21	24	19	2	13	6	7	11
(23)	23	1	2	3	22	15	18	19	14
(24)	24	25	1	2	21	16	17	20	3
(25)	25	23	15	21	17	4	19	6	5

Plan 13.14 $t = 31, k = 6, r = 6, b = 31, \lambda = 1, E = .86$, **Type I**

Block	I	II	III	IV	V	VI
			Reps.			
(1)	31	1	3	8	12	18
(2)	1	2	4	9	13	19
(3)	2	3	5	10	14	20
(4)	3	4	6	11	15	21
(5)	4	5	7	12	16	22
(6)	5	6	8	13	17	23
(7)	6	7	9	14	18	24
(8)	7	8	10	15	19	25
(9)	8	9	11	16	20	26
(10)	9	10	12	17	21	27
(11)	10	11	13	18	22	28
(12)	11	12	14	19	23	29
(13)	12	13	15	20	24	30
(14)	13	14	16	21	25	31
(15)	14	15	17	22	26	1
(16)	15	16	18	23	27	2
(17)	16	17	19	24	28	3
(18)	17	18	20	25	29	4
(19)	18	19	21	26	30	5
(20)	19	20	22	27	31	6
(21)	20	21	23	28	1	7
(22)	21	22	24	29	2	8
(23)	22	23	25	30	3	9
(24)	23	24	26	31	4	10
(25)	24	25	27	1	5	11
(26)	25	26	28	2	6	12
(27)	26	27	29	3	7	13
(28)	27	28	30	4	8	14
(29)	28	29	31	5	9	15
(30)	29	30	1	6	10	16
(31)	30	31	2	7	11	17

Plan 13.2a $t = 31, k = 10, r = 10, b = 31, \lambda = 3, E = .93$, **Type I**

	Reps.									
Block	I	II	III	IV	V	VI	VII	VIII	IX	X
(1)	1	2	4	8	9	11	15	16	18	28
(2)	2	3	12	9	10	17	16	19	5	22
(3)	3	4	20	10	17	13	6	18	11	23
(4)	4	5	7	11	12	21	18	14	19	24
(5)	5	6	1	12	13	8	19	20	15	25
(6)	6	7	13	16	14	9	20	21	2	26
(7)	7	1	15	14	8	10	21	17	3	27
(8)	8	11	17	25	16	23	29	7	26	5
(9)	9	12	24	29	27	18	1	26	17	6
(10)	10	13	18	19	29	25	2	27	28	7
(11)	11	14	22	26	19	20	3	28	29	1
(12)	12	8	27	23	20	29	4	22	21	2
(13)	13	9	29	28	21	15	5	23	24	3
(14)	14	10	25	22	15	16	24	29	6	4
(15)	15	24	26	5	2	27	11	10	30	20
(16)	16	25	6	30	3	28	12	11	27	21
(17)	17	26	28	7	30	22	13	12	4	15
(18)	18	27	23	1	5	30	14	13	22	16
(19)	19	28	30	2	6	14	8	24	23	17
(20)	20	22	8	3	7	24	9	30	25	18
(21)	21	23	10	4	1	26	30	25	9	19
(22)	22	21	11	17	24	1	25	2	31	13
(23)	23	15	3	18	25	2	26	31	12	14
(24)	24	16	19	31	26	3	27	4	13	8
(25)	25	17	14	27	31	4	28	5	20	9
(26)	26	18	5	21	28	31	22	6	8	10
(27)	27	19	31	15	22	6	23	9	7	11
(28)	28	20	16	24	23	7	31	1	10	12
(29)	29	30	2	6	4	5	7	3	1	31
(30)	30	31	9	13	11	12	10	8	14	29
(31)	31	29	21	20	18	19	17	15	16	30

Plan 13.16 $t = 3, k = 5, r = 5, b = 3, \lambda = 5, E = .96$, **Type III**

	Reps.				
Block	I	II	III	IV	V
(1)	1	2	3	2	3
(2)	2	3	1	1	2
(3)	3	1	2	3	1

Plan 13.17 $t = 3, k = 7, r = 7, b = 3, \lambda = 7, E = .98$, **Type IV**

	Reps.						
Block	I	II	III	IV	V	VI	VII
(1)	1	2	3	1	2	3	1
(2)	2	3	1	3	1	2	2
(3)	3	1	2	2	3	1	3

Plan 13.18 $t = 3, k = 8, r = 8, b = 3, \lambda = 8, E = .98$, **Type III**

Block	Reps. I	II	III	IV	V	VI	VII	VIII
(1)	1	2	3	1	2	3	1	2
(2)	2	3	1	3	1	2	2	3
(3)	3	1	2	2	3	1	3	1

Plan 13.19 $t = 3, k = 10, r = 10, b = 3, \lambda = 10, E = .99$, **Type IV**

Block	Reps. I	II	III	IV	V	VI	VII	VIII	IX	X
(1)	1	2	3	1	2	3	1	2	3	1
(2)	2	3	1	3	1	2	2	3	1	3
(3)	3	1	2	2	3	1	3	1	2	2

Plan 13.20 $t = 4, k = 5, r = 5, b = 4, \lambda = 5, E = .96$, **Type IV**

Block	Reps. I	II	III	IV	V
(1)	1	2	3	4	1
(2)	2	3	4	1	4
(3)	3	4	1	2	3
(4)	4	1	2	3	2

Plan 13.21 $t = 4, k = 7, r = 7, b = 4, \lambda = 7, E = .98$, **Type III**

Block	Reps. I	II	III	IV	V	VI	VII
(1)	1	2	3	4	1	2	3
(2)	2	1	4	3	3	4	1
(3)	3	4	1	2	4	3	2
(4)	4	3	2	1	2	1	4

Plan 13.22 $t = 4, k = 9, r = 9, b = 4, \lambda = 9, E = .99$, **Type IV**

Block	Reps. I	II	III	IV	V	VI	VII	VIII	IX
(1)	1	2	3	4	1	2	3	4	1
(2)	2	1	4	3	3	4	1	2	4
(3)	3	4	1	2	4	3	2	1	2
(4)	4	3	2	1	2	1	4	3	3

Plan 13.23 $t = 5, k = 6, r = 6, b = 5, \lambda = 6, E = .97$, **Type IV**

Block	Reps. I	II	III	IV	V	VI
(1)	1	2	3	4	5	1
(2)	2	4	5	3	1	3
(3)	3	1	2	5	4	4
(4)	4	5	1	2	3	2
(5)	5	3	4	1	2	5

Plan 13.24 $t = 5, k = 9, r = 9, b = 5, \lambda = 9, E = .99$, **Type III**

Block	Reps. I	II	III	IV	V	VI	VII	VIII	IX
(1)	1	2	3	4	5	1	2	3	4
(2)	2	3	4	5	1	4	5	1	2
(3)	3	4	5	1	2	2	3	4	5
(4)	4	5	1	2	3	5	1	2	3
(5)	5	1	2	3	4	3	4	5	1

Plan 13.25 $t = 6, k = 7, r = 7, b = 6, \lambda = 7, E = .98$, **Type IV**

Block	I	II	III	IV	V	VI	VII
(1)	1	2	3	4	5	6	1
(2)	2	3	6	1	4	5	3
(3)	3	6	2	5	1	4	5
(4)	4	5	1	2	6	3	4
(5)	5	1	4	6	3	2	6
(6)	6	4	5	3	2	1	2

Plan 13.26 $t = 7, k = 8, r = 8, b = 7, \lambda = 8, E = .98$, **Type IV**

Block	I	II	III	IV	V	VI	VII	VIII
(1)	1	2	3	4	5	6	7	1
(2)	2	5	1	7	6	4	3	3
(3)	3	6	7	2	4	1	5	7
(4)	4	7	5	6	3	2	1	6
(5)	5	4	2	3	1	7	6	5
(6)	6	3	4	1	7	5	2	4
(7)	7	1	6	5	2	3	4	2

EXTENDED INCOMPLETE LATIN SQUARES

Plan 13.6a $t = 5, k = 2, r = 4, b = 10, \lambda = 1, E = .67$, **Type II**

Block	I	II
(1)	1	2
(2)	2	5
(3)	3	4
(4)	4	1
(5)	5	3

Block	III	IV
(6)	1	3
(7)	2	4
(8)	3	2
(9)	4	5
(10)	5	1

Plan 13.7a $t = 5, k = 3, r = 6, b = 10, \lambda = 3, E = .83$, **Type II**

Block	I	II	III
(1)	1	2	3
(2)	2	1	5
(3)	3	4	2
(4)	4	5	1
(5)	5	3	4

Block	IV	V	VI
(6)	1	2	4
(7)	2	3	5
(8)	3	4	1
(9)	4	5	2
(10)	5	1	3

Plan 13.8a $t = 7, k = 2, r = 6, b = 21, \lambda = 1, E = .58$, **Type V**

Block	I	II
(1)	1	2
(2)	2	6
(3)	3	4
(4)	4	7
(5)	5	1
(6)	6	5
(7)	7	3

Block	III	IV
(8)	1	3
(9)	2	4
(10)	3	5
(11)	4	6
(12)	5	7
(13)	6	1
(14)	7	2

Block	V	VI
(15)	1	4
(16)	2	3
(17)	3	6
(18)	4	5
(19)	5	2
(20)	6	7
(21)	7	1

Plan 13.9a $t = 9, k = 2, r = 8, b = 36, \lambda = 1, E = .56$, **Type V**

Block	I	II
(1)	1	2
(2)	2	8
(3)	3	4
(4)	4	7
(5)	5	6
(6)	6	1
(7)	7	3
(8)	8	9
(9)	9	5

Block	III	IV
(10)	1	3
(11)	2	5
(12)	3	6
(13)	4	9
(14)	5	8
(15)	6	7
(16)	7	1
(17)	8	4
(18)	9	2

Block	V	VI
(19)	1	4
(20)	2	6
(21)	3	2
(22)	4	5
(23)	5	7
(24)	6	8
(25)	7	9
(26)	8	1
(27)	9	3

Block	VII	VIII
(28)	1	5
(29)	2	4
(30)	3	8
(31)	4	6
(32)	5	3
(33)	6	9
(34)	7	2
(35)	8	7
(36)	9	1

Plan 13.10a $t = 9, k = 4, r = 8, b = 18, \lambda = 3, E = .84$, **Type V**

Block	I	II	III	IV	Block	V	VI	VII	VIII
(1)	1	4	6	7	(10)	1	2	5	7
(2)	2	6	8	9	(11)	2	3	6	5
(3)	3	8	9	1	(12)	3	4	7	9
(4)	4	1	3	2	(13)	4	9	2	1
(5)	5	7	1	8	(14)	5	1	9	6
(6)	6	9	4	5	(15)	6	8	1	3
(7)	7	3	2	6	(16)	7	6	4	8
(8)	8	2	5	4	(17)	8	5	3	4
(9)	9	5	7	3	(18)	9	7	8	2

Plan 13.11a $t = 9, k = 5, r = 10, b = 18, \lambda = 5, E = .90$, **Type V**

Block	I	II	III	IV	V	Block	VI	VII	VIII	IX	X
(1)	1	2	3	7	8	(10)	1	2	3	5	9
(2)	2	6	8	4	1	(11)	2	6	5	1	8
(3)	3	8	5	9	2	(12)	3	5	1	4	6
(4)	4	3	9	2	6	(13)	4	3	2	8	7
(5)	5	1	7	3	4	(14)	5	7	9	2	4
(6)	6	4	2	5	7	(15)	6	8	7	3	5
(7)	7	9	1	6	3	(16)	7	4	8	9	1
(8)	8	5	4	1	9	(17)	8	9	4	6	3
(9)	9	7	6	8	5	(18)	9	1	6	7	2

Plan 13.12a $t = 10, k = 3, r = 9, b = 30, \lambda = 2, E = .74$, **Type V**

Block	I	II	III	Block	IV	V	VI	Block	VII	VIII	IX
(1)	1	2	3	(11)	1	2	4	(21)	1	3	5
(2)	2	5	8	(12)	2	3	6	(22)	2	7	6
(3)	3	7	4	(13)	3	4	8	(23)	3	8	9
(4)	4	1	6	(14)	4	9	5	(24)	4	2	10
(5)	5	8	7	(15)	5	7	1	(25)	5	6	3
(6)	6	4	9	(16)	6	8	9	(26)	6	1	8
(7)	7	9	1	(17)	7	10	3	(27)	7	9	2
(8)	8	10	2	(18)	8	1	10	(28)	8	4	7
(9)	9	3	10	(19)	9	5	2	(29)	9	10	1
(10)	10	6	5	(20)	10	6	7	(30)	10	5	4

Plan 13.13a $t = 11, k = 2, r = 10, b = 55, \lambda = 1, E = .55$, **Type V**

Block	Reps. I	II		Reps. III	IV		Reps. V	VI
(1)	1	2	(12)	1	3	(23)	1	4
(2)	2	11	(13)	2	6	(24)	2	3
(3)	3	10	(14)	3	5	(25)	3	7
(4)	4	5	(15)	4	10	(26)	4	6
(5)	5	6	(16)	5	9	(27)	5	10
(6)	6	7	(17)	6	8	(28)	6	9
(7)	7	1	(18)	7	2	(29)	7	11
(8)	8	3	(19)	8	1	(30)	8	2
(9)	9	4	(20)	9	7	(31)	9	1
(10)	10	9	(21)	10	11	(32)	10	8
(11)	11	8	(22)	11	4	(33)	11	5

	Reps. VII	VIII		Reps. IX	X
(34)	1	5	(45)	1	6
(35)	2	9	(46)	2	5
(36)	3	6	(47)	3	4
(37)	4	2	(48)	4	7
(38)	5	7	(49)	5	8
(39)	6	10	(50)	6	11
(40)	7	8	(51)	7	10
(41)	8	4	(52)	8	9
(42)	9	11	(53)	9	3
(43)	10	1	(54)	10	2
(44)	11	3	(55)	11	1

Plan 13.14a $t = 13, k = 3, r = 6, b = 26, \lambda = 1, E = .72$, **Type V**

Block	Reps. I	II	III		Reps. I	II	III
(1)	1	3	9	(8)	8	10	3
(2)	2	4	10	(9)	9	11	4
(3)	3	5	11	(10)	10	12	5
(4)	4	6	12	(11)	11	13	6
(5)	5	7	13	(12)	12	1	7
(6)	6	8	1	(13)	13	2	8
(7)	7	9	2				

	Reps. IV	V	VI		Reps. IV	V	VI
(14)	2	6	5	(21)	9	13	12
(15)	3	7	6	(22)	10	1	13
(16)	4	8	7	(23)	11	2	1
(17)	5	9	8	(24)	12	3	2
(18)	6	10	9	(25)	13	4	3
(19)	7	11	10	(26)	1	5	4
(20)	8	12	11				

Plan 13.15a $t = 19, k = 3, r = 9, b = 57, \lambda = 1, E = .70$, **Type V**

Block	Reps. I	II	III	Block	Reps. IV	V	VI	Block	Reps. VII	VIII	IX
(1)	1	7	11	(20)	2	3	14	(39)	4	6	9
(2)	2	8	12	(21)	3	4	15	(40)	5	7	10
(3)	3	9	13	(22)	4	5	16	(41)	6	8	11
(4)	4	10	14	(23)	5	6	17	(42)	7	9	12
(5)	5	11	15	(24)	6	7	18	(43)	8	10	13
(6)	6	12	16	(25)	7	8	19	(44)	9	11	14
(7)	7	13	17	(26)	8	9	1	(45)	10	12	15
(8)	8	14	18	(27)	9	10	2	(46)	11	13	16
(9)	9	15	19	(28)	10	11	3	(47)	12	14	17
(10)	10	16	1	(29)	11	12	4	(48)	13	15	18
(11)	11	17	2	(30)	12	13	5	(49)	14	16	19
(12)	12	18	3	(31)	13	14	6	(50)	15	17	1
(13)	13	19	4	(32)	14	15	7	(51)	16	18	2
(14)	14	1	5	(33)	15	16	8	(52)	17	19	3
(15)	15	2	6	(34)	16	17	9	(53)	18	1	4
(16)	16	3	7	(35)	17	18	10	(54)	19	2	5
(17)	17	4	8	(36)	18	19	11	(55)	1	3	6
(18)	18	5	9	(37)	19	1	12	(56)	2	4	7
(19)	19	6	10	(38)	1	2	13	(57)	3	5	8

Plan 13.16a $t = 25, k = 4, r = 8, b = 50, \lambda = 1, E = .78$, **Type V**

Block	Reps. I	II	III	IV	Block	Reps. V	VI	VII	VIII
(1)	1	2	6	25	(26)	1	3	11	19
(2)	2	3	7	21	(27)	2	4	12	20
(3)	3	4	8	22	(28)	3	5	13	16
(4)	4	5	9	23	(29)	4	1	14	17
(5)	5	1	10	24	(30)	5	2	15	18
(6)	6	7	11	5	(31)	6	8	16	24
(7)	7	8	12	1	(32)	7	9	17	25
(8)	8	9	13	2	(33)	8	10	18	21
(9)	9	10	14	3	(34)	9	6	19	22
(10)	10	6	15	4	(35)	10	7	20	23
(11)	11	12	16	10	(36)	11	13	21	4
(12)	12	13	17	6	(37)	12	14	22	5
(13)	13	14	18	7	(38)	13	15	23	1
(14)	14	15	19	8	(39)	14	11	24	2
(15)	15	11	20	9	(40)	15	12	25	3
(16)	16	17	21	15	(41)	16	18	1	9
(17)	17	18	22	11	(42)	17	19	2	10
(18)	18	19	23	12	(43)	18	20	3	6
(19)	19	20	24	13	(44)	19	16	4	7
(20)	20	16	25	14	(45)	20	17	5	8
(21)	21	22	1	20	(46)	21	23	6	14
(22)	22	23	2	16	(47)	22	24	7	15
(23)	23	24	3	17	(48)	23	25	8	11
(24)	24	25	4	18	(49)	24	21	9	12
(25)	25	21	5	19	(50)	25	22	10	13

MAIN EFFECT AND INTERACTIONS IN 2^2, 2^3, 2^4, 2^5, AND 2^6 FACTORIAL DESIGNS

EFFECT	2^2	2^3		2^4				2^5
TREATMENT COMBINATIONS	T A B AB	C AC BC ABC	D AD BD ABD	CD ACD BCD ABCD	E AE BE ABE	CE ACE BCE ABCE	DE ADE BDE ABDE	CDE ACDE BCDE ABCDE
(1)	+−−+	−++−	−++−	+−−+	−++−	+−−+	+−−+	−++−
a	++−−	−−++	−−++	++−−	−−++	++−−	++−−	−−++
b	+−+−	−+−+	−+−+	+−+−	−+−+	+−+−	+−+−	−+−+
ab	++++	−−−−	−−−−	++++	−−−−	++++	++++	−−−−
c	+−−+	+−−+	−++−	−++−	−++−	−++−	+−−+	+−−+
ac	++−−	++−−	−−++	−−++	−−++	−−++	++−−	++−−
bc	+−+−	+−+−	−+−+	−+−+	−+−+	−+−+	+−+−	+−+−
abc	++++	++++	−−−−	−−−−	−−−−	−−−−	++++	++++
d	+−−+	−++−	+−−+	−++−	−++−	+−−+	−++−	+−−+
ad	++−−	−−++	++−−	−−++	−−++	++−−	−−++	++−−
bd	+−+−	−+−+	+−+−	−+−+	−+−+	+−+−	−+−+	+−+−
abd	++++	−−−−	++++	−−−−	−−−−	++++	−−−−	++++
cd	+−−+	+−−+	+−−+	+−−+	−++−	−++−	−++−	−++−
acd	++−−	++−−	++−−	++−−	−−++	−−++	−−++	−−++
bcd	+−+−	+−+−	+−+−	+−+−	−+−+	−+−+	−+−+	−+−+
abcd	++++	++++	++++	++++	−−−−	−−−−	−−−−	−−−−
e	+−−+	−++−	−++−	+−−+	+−−+	−++−	−++−	+−−+
ae	++−−	−−++	−−++	++−−	++−−	−−++	−−++	++−−
be	+−+−	−+−+	−+−+	+−+−	+−+−	−+−+	−+−+	+−+−
abe	++++	−−−−	−−−−	++++	++++	−−−−	−−−−	++++
ce	+−−+	+−−+	−++−	−++−	+−−+	+−−+	−++−	−++−
ace	++−−	++−−	−−++	−−++	++−−	++−−	−−++	−−++
bce	+−+−	+−+−	−+−+	−+−+	+−+−	+−+−	−+−+	−+−+
abce	++++	++++	−−−−	−−−−	++++	++++	−−−−	−−−−
de	+−−+	−++−	+−−+	−++−	+−−+	−++−	+−−+	−++−
ade	++−−	−−++	++−−	−−++	++−−	−−++	++−−	−−++
bde	+−+−	−+−+	+−+−	−+−+	+−+−	−+−+	+−+−	−+−+
abde	++++	−−−−	++++	−−−−	++++	−−−−	++++	−−−−
cde	+−−+	+−−+	+−−+	+−−+	+−−+	+−−+	+−−+	+−−+
acde	++−−	++−−	++−−	++−−	++−−	++−−	++−−	++−−
bcde	+−+−	+−+−	+−+−	+−+−	+−+−	+−+−	+−+−	+−+−
abcde	++++	++++	++++	++++	++++	++++	++++	++++

MAIN EFFECT AND INTERACTIONS IN 2^2, 2^3, 2^4, 2^5, AND 2^6 FACTORIAL DESIGNS

2^6

F AF BF ABF	CF ACF BCF ABCF	DF ADF BDF ABDF	CDF ACDF BCDF ABCDF	EF AEF BEF ABEF	CEF ACEF BCEF ABCEF	DEF ADEF BDEF ABDEF	CDEF ACDEF BCDEF ABCDEF
−++−	+−−+	+−−+	−++−	+−−+	−++−	−++−	+−−+
−−++	++−−	++−−	−−++	++−−	−−++	−−++	++−−
−+−+	+−+−	+−+−	−+−+	+−+−	−+−+	−+−+	+−+−
−−−−	++++	++++	−−−−	++++	−−−−	−−−−	++++
−++−	−++−	+−−+	+−−+	+−−+	+−−+	−++−	−++−
−−++	−−++	++−−	++−−	++−−	++−−	−−++	−−++
−+−+	−+−+	+−+−	+−+−	+−+−	+−+−	−+−+	−+−+
−−−−	−−−−	++++	++++	++++	++++	−−−−	−−−−
−++−	+−−+	−++−	+−−+	+−−+	−++−	+−−+	−++−
−−++	++−−	−−++	++−−	++−−	−−++	++−−	−−++
−+−+	+−+−	−+−+	+−+−	+−+−	−+−+	+−+−	−+−+
−−−−	++++	−−−−	++++	++++	−−−−	++++	−−−−
−++−	−++−	−++−	−++−	+−−+	+−−+	+−−+	+−−+
−−++	−−++	−−++	−−++	++−−	++−−	++−−	++−−
−+−+	−+−+	−+−+	−+−+	+−+−	+−+−	+−+−	+−+−
−−−−	−−−−	−−−−	−−−−	++++	++++	++++	++++
−++−	+−−+	+−−+	−++−	−++−	+−−+	+−−+	−++−
−−++	++−−	++−−	−−++	−−++	++−−	++−−	−−++
−+−+	+−+−	+−+−	−+−+	−+−+	+−+−	+−+−	−+−+
−−−−	++++	++++	−−−−	−−−−	++++	++++	−−−−
−++−	−++−	+−−+	+−−+	−++−	−++−	+−−+	+−−+
−−++	−−++	++−−	++−−	−−++	−−++	++−−	++−−
−+−+	−+−+	+−+−	+−+−	−+−+	−+−+	+−+−	+−+−
−−−−	−−−−	++++	++++	−−−−	−−−−	++++	++++
−++−	+−−+	−++−	+−−+	−++−	+−−+	−++−	+−−+
−−++	++−−	−−++	++−−	−−++	++−−	−−++	++−−
−+−+	+−+−	−+−+	+−+−	−+−+	+−+−	−+−+	+−+−
−−−−	++++	−−−−	++++	−−−−	++++	−−−−	++++
−++−	−++−	−++−	−++−	−++−	−++−	−++−	−++−
−−++	−−++	−−++	−−++	−−++	−−++	−−++	−−++
−+−+	−+−+	−+−+	−+−+	−+−+	−+−+	−+−+	−+−+
−−−−	−−−−	−−−−	−−−−	−−−−	−−−−	−−−−	−−−−

MAIN EFFECT AND INTERACTIONS IN 2^2, 2^3, 2^4, 2^5, AND 2^6 FACTORIAL DESIGNS

EFFECT	2^2	2^3		2^4				2^5
	T A B AB	C AC BC ABC	D AD BD ABD	CD ACD BCD ABCD	E AE BE ABE	CE ACE BCE ABCE	DE ADE BDE ABDE	CDE ACDE BCDE ABCDE
TREATMENT COMBINATIONS								
f	+ − − +	− + + −	− + + −	+ − − +	− + + −	+ − − +	+ − − +	− + + −
af	+ + − −	− − + +	− − + +	+ + − −	− − + +	+ + − −	+ + − −	− − + +
bf	+ − + −	− + − +	− + − +	+ − + −	− + − +	+ − + −	+ − + −	− + − +
abf	+ + + +	− − −	− − − −	+ + + +	− − − −	+ + + +	+ + + +	− − − −
cf	+ − − +	+ − − +	− + + −	− + + −	− + + −	− + + −	+ − − +	+ − − +
acf	+ + − −	+ + − −	− − + +	− − + +	− − + +	− − + +	+ + − −	+ + − −
bcf	+ − + −	+ − + −	− + − +	− + − +	− + − +	− + − +	+ − + −	+ − + −
abcf	+ + + +	+ + + +	− − − −	− − − −	− − − −	− − − −	+ + + +	+ + + +
df	+ − − +	− + + −	+ − − +	− + + −	− + + −	+ − − +	− + + −	+ − − +
adf	+ + − −	− − + +	+ + − −	− − + +	− − + +	+ + − −	− − + +	+ + − −
bdf	+ − + −	− + − +	+ − + −	− + − +	− + − +	+ − + −	− + − +	+ − + −
abdf	+ + + +	− − − −	+ + + +	− − − −	− − − −	+ + + +	− − − −	+ + + +
cdf	+ − − +	+ − − +	+ − − +	+ − − +	− + + −	− + + −	− + + −	− + + −
acdf	+ + − −	+ + − −	+ + − −	+ + − −	− − + +	− − + +	− − + +	− − + +
bcdf	+ − + −	+ − + −	+ − + −	+ − + −	− + − +	− + − +	− + − +	− + − +
abcdf	+ + + +	+ + + +	+ + + +	+ + + +	− − − −	− − − −	− − − −	− − − −
ef	+ − − +	− + + −	− + + −	+ − − +	+ − − +	− + + −	− + + −	+ − − +
acf	+ + − −	− − + +	− − + +	+ + − −	+ + − −	− − + +	− − + +	+ + − −
bef	+ − + −	− + − +	− + − +	+ − + −	+ − + −	− + − +	− + − +	+ − + −
abef	+ + + +	− − − −	− − − −	+ + + +	+ + + +	− − − −	− − − −	+ + + +
cef	+ − − +	+ − − +	− + + −	− + + −	+ − − +	+ − − +	− + + −	− + + −
acef	+ + − −	+ + − −	− − + +	− − + +	+ + − −	+ + − −	− − + +	− − + +
bcef	+ − + −	+ − + −	− + − +	− + − +	+ − + −	+ − + −	− + − +	− + − +
abcef	+ + + +	+ + + +	− − − −	− − − −	+ + + +	+ + + +	− − − −	− − − −
def	+ − − +	− + + −	+ − − +	− + + −	+ − − +	− + + −	+ − − +	− + + −
adef	+ + − −	− − + +	+ + − −	− − + +	+ + − −	− − + +	+ + − −	− − + +
bdef	+ − + −	− + − +	+ − + −	− + − +	+ − + −	− + − +	+ − + −	− + − +
abdef	+ + + +	− − − −	+ + + +	− − − −	+ + + +	− − − −	+ + + +	− − − −
cdef	+ − − +	+ − − +	+ − − +	+ − − +	+ − − +	+ − − +	+ − − +	+ − − +
acdef	+ + − −	+ + − −	+ + − −	+ + − −	+ + − −	+ + − −	+ + − −	+ + − −
bcdef	+ − + −	+ − + −	+ − + −	+ − + −	+ − + −	+ − + −	+ − + −	+ − + −
abcdef	+ + + +	+ + + +	+ + + +	+ + + +	+ + + +	+ + + +	+ + + +	+ + + +

MAIN EFFECT AND INTERACTIONS IN 2^2, 2^3, 2^4, 2^5, AND 2^6 FACTORIAL DESIGNS

2^6

F	AF	BF	ABF	CF	ACF	BCF	ABCF	DF	ADF	BDF	ABDF	CDF	ACDF	BCDF	ABCDF	EF	AEF	BEF	ABEF	CEF	ACEF	BCEF	ABCEF	DEF	ADEF	BDEF	ABDEF	CDEF	ACDEF	BCDEF	ABCDEF
+	−	−	+	−	+	+	−	−	+	+	−	+	−	−	+	−	+	+	−	+	−	−	+	+	−	−	+	−	+	+	−
+	+	−	−	−	−	+	+	−	−	+	+	+	+	−	−	−	−	+	+	+	+	−	−	+	+	−	−	−	−	+	+
+	−	+	−	−	+	−	+	−	+	−	+	+	−	+	−	−	+	−	+	+	−	+	−	+	−	+	−	−	+	−	+
+	+	+	+	−	−	−	−	−	−	−	−	+	+	+	+	−	−	−	−	+	+	+	+	+	+	+	+	−	−	−	−
+	−	−	+	+	−	−	+	−	+	+	−	−	+	+	−	−	+	+	−	−	+	+	−	+	−	−	+	+	−	−	+
+	+	−	−	+	+	−	−	−	−	+	+	−	−	+	+	−	−	+	+	−	−	+	+	+	+	−	−	+	+	−	−
+	−	+	−	+	−	+	−	−	+	−	+	−	+	−	+	−	+	−	+	−	+	−	+	+	−	+	−	+	−	+	−
+	+	+	+	+	+	+	+	−	−	−	−	−	−	−	−	−	−	−	−	−	−	−	−	+	+	+	+	+	+	+	+
+	−	−	+	−	+	+	−	+	−	−	+	−	+	+	−	−	+	+	−	+	−	−	+	−	+	+	−	+	−	−	+
+	+	−	−	−	−	+	+	+	+	−	−	−	−	+	+	−	−	+	+	+	+	−	−	−	−	+	+	+	+	−	−
+	−	+	−	−	+	−	+	+	−	+	−	−	+	−	+	−	+	−	+	+	−	+	−	−	+	−	+	+	−	+	−
+	+	+	+	−	−	−	−	+	+	+	+	−	−	−	−	−	−	−	−	+	+	+	+	−	−	−	−	+	+	+	+
+	−	−	+	+	−	−	+	+	−	−	+	+	−	−	+	−	+	+	−	−	+	+	−	−	+	+	−	−	+	+	−
+	+	−	−	+	+	−	−	+	+	−	−	+	+	−	−	−	−	+	+	−	−	+	+	−	−	+	+	−	−	+	+
+	−	+	−	+	−	+	−	+	−	+	−	+	−	+	−	−	+	−	+	−	+	−	+	−	+	−	+	−	+	−	+
+	+	+	+	+	+	+	+	+	+	+	+	+	+	+	+	−	−	−	−	−	−	−	−	−	−	−	−	−	−	−	−
+	−	−	+	−	+	+	−	−	+	+	−	+	−	−	+	+	−	−	+	−	+	+	−	−	+	+	−	+	−	−	+
+	+	−	−	−	−	+	+	−	−	+	+	+	+	−	−	+	+	−	−	−	−	+	+	−	−	+	+	+	+	−	−
+	−	+	−	−	+	−	+	−	+	−	+	+	−	+	−	+	−	+	−	−	+	−	+	−	+	−	+	+	−	+	−
+	+	+	+	−	−	−	−	−	−	−	−	+	+	+	+	+	+	+	+	−	−	−	−	−	−	−	−	+	+	+	+
+	−	−	+	+	−	−	+	−	+	+	−	−	+	+	−	+	−	−	+	+	−	−	+	−	+	+	−	−	+	+	−
+	+	−	−	+	+	−	−	−	−	+	+	−	−	+	+	+	+	−	−	+	+	−	−	−	−	+	+	−	−	+	+
+	−	+	−	+	−	+	−	−	+	−	+	−	+	−	+	+	−	+	−	+	−	+	−	−	+	−	+	−	+	−	+
+	+	+	+	+	+	+	+	−	−	−	−	−	−	−	−	+	+	+	+	+	+	+	+	−	−	−	−	−	−	−	−
+	−	−	+	−	+	+	−	+	−	−	+	−	+	+	−	+	−	−	+	−	+	+	−	+	−	−	+	−	+	+	−
+	+	−	−	−	−	+	+	+	+	−	−	−	−	+	+	+	+	−	−	−	−	+	+	+	+	−	−	−	−	+	+
+	−	+	−	−	+	−	+	+	−	+	−	−	+	−	+	+	−	+	−	−	+	−	+	+	−	+	−	−	+	−	+
+	+	+	+	−	−	−	−	+	+	+	+	−	−	−	−	+	+	+	+	−	−	−	−	+	+	+	+	−	−	−	−
+	−	−	+	+	−	−	+	+	−	−	+	+	−	−	+	+	−	−	+	+	−	−	+	+	−	−	+	+	−	−	+
+	+	−	−	+	+	−	−	+	+	−	−	+	+	−	−	+	+	−	−	+	+	−	−	+	+	−	−	+	+	−	−
+	−	+	−	+	−	+	−	+	−	+	−	+	−	+	−	+	−	+	−	+	−	+	−	+	−	+	−	+	−	+	−
+	+	+	+	+	+	+	+	+	+	+	+	+	+	+	+	+	+	+	+	+	+	+	+	+	+	+	+	+	+	+	+

FINITE DIFFERENCES

Uniform interval h.

If a function $f(x)$ is tabulated at a uniform interval h, that is, for arguments given by $x_n = x_0 + nh$, where n is an integer, then the function $f(x)$ may be denoted by f_n.

This can be generalized so that for all values of p, and in particular for $0 \leqq p \leqq 1$,

$$f(x_0 + ph) = f(x_p) = f_p \,,$$

where the argument designated x_0 can be chosen quite arbitrarily.

The notation $x = a(h)b(H)C$ means that the arguments run from a to b inclusive at the uniform interval h and thereafter continue to C at the uniform interval H.

The statement $f(x)$ $4D$ means that the function $f(x)$ is to be tabulated and the answer rounded off to four places of decimals.

The statement $f(x)$ $5S$ means that the function $f(x)$ is to be tabulated with the answer being rounded off to five significant figures.

The following table lists and defines the standard operators used in numerical analysis.

Symbol	Function	Definition
E	Displacement	$Ef_p = f_{p+1}$
Δ	Forward difference	$\Delta f_p = f_{p+1} - f_p$
∇	Backward difference	$\nabla f_p = f_p - f_{p-1}$
$\wedge\!\!\!\backslash$	Divided difference	See page 119
δ	Central difference	$\delta f_p = f_{p+\frac{1}{2}} - f_{p-\frac{1}{2}}$
μ	Average	$\mu f_p = \frac{1}{2}(f_{p+\frac{1}{2}} + f_{p-\frac{1}{2}})$
Δ^{-1}	Backward sum	$\Delta^{-1}f_p = \Delta^{-1}f_{p-1} + f_{p-1}$
∇^{-1}	Forward sum	$\nabla^{-1}f_p = \nabla^{-1}f_{p-1} + f_p$
δ^{-1}	Central sum	$\delta^{-1}f_p = \delta^{-1}f_{p-1} + f_{p-\frac{1}{2}}$
D	Differentiation	$Df_p = \dfrac{d}{dx}f(x) = \dfrac{1}{h}\cdot\dfrac{d}{dp}f_p$
$I(=D^{-1})$	Integration	$If_p = \int^{x_p} f(x)dx = h\int^{p} f_p dp$
$J(=\Delta D^{-1})$	Definite integration	$Jf_p = h\int_p^{p+1} f_p dp$

I, Δ^{-1}, ∇^{-1} and δ^{-1} all imply the existence of an arbitrary constant which is determined by the initial conditions of the problem.

Where no confusion can arise the f can be omitted as, for example in writing Δ_p for Δf_p.

Higher differences are formed by successive operations, e.g.,

$$\begin{aligned}\Delta^2 f_p &= \Delta_p^2 \\ &= \Delta \cdot \Delta_p \\ &= \Delta(f_{p+1} - f_p) \\ &= \Delta_{p+1} - \Delta_p \\ &= f_{p+2} - f_{p+1} - f_{p+1} + f_p \,.\end{aligned}$$

Thus $\Delta_p^2 = f_{p+2} - 2f_{p+1} + f_p$.

Note that $f_p \equiv \Delta_p^0 \equiv \nabla_p^0 \equiv \delta_p^0$.

The disposition of the differences and sums relative to the function values is as shown (the arguments are omitted in these cases in the interests of clarity). In manuscript working double spacing is recommended.

Forward difference scheme

Δ_{-1}^{-2}		f_{-2}		Δ_{-3}^{2}	
	Δ_{-1}^{-1}		Δ_{-2}		Δ_{-3}^{3}
Δ_{0}^{-2}		f_{-1}		Δ_{-2}^{2}	
	Δ_{0}^{-1}		Δ_{-1}		Δ_{-2}^{3}
Δ_{1}^{-2}		f_{0}		Δ_{-1}^{2}	
	Δ_{1}^{-1}		Δ_{0}		Δ_{-1}^{3}
Δ_{2}^{-2}		f_{1}		Δ_{0}^{2}	
	Δ_{2}^{-1}		Δ_{1}		Δ_{0}^{3}
Δ_{3}^{-2}		f_{2}		Δ_{1}^{2}	

Backward difference scheme

∇_{-3}^{-2}		f_{-2}		∇_{-1}^{2}	
	∇_{-2}^{-1}		∇_{-1}		∇_{0}^{3}
∇_{-2}^{-2}		f_{-1}		∇_{0}^{2}	
	∇_{-1}^{-1}		∇_{0}		∇_{1}^{3}
∇_{-1}^{-2}		f_{0}		∇_{1}^{2}	
	∇_{0}^{-1}		∇_{1}		∇_{2}^{3}
∇_{0}^{-2}		f_{1}		∇_{2}^{2}	
	∇_{1}^{-1}		∇_{2}		∇_{3}^{3}
∇_{1}^{-2}		f_{2}		∇_{3}^{2}	

Central difference scheme

δ_{-2}^{-2}		f_{-2}		δ_{-2}^{2}		δ_{-2}^{4}
	$\delta_{-1\frac{1}{2}}^{-1}$		$\delta_{-1\frac{1}{2}}$		$\delta_{-1\frac{1}{2}}^{3}$	
δ_{-1}^{-2}		f_{-1}		δ_{-1}^{2}		δ_{-1}^{4}
	$\delta_{-\frac{1}{2}}^{-1}$		$\delta_{-\frac{1}{2}}$		$\delta_{-\frac{1}{2}}^{3}$	
δ_{0}^{-2}		f_{0}		δ_{0}^{2}		δ_{0}^{4}
	$\delta_{\frac{1}{2}}^{-1}$		$\delta_{\frac{1}{2}}$		$\delta_{\frac{1}{2}}^{3}$	
δ_{1}^{-2}		f_{1}		δ_{1}^{2}		δ_{1}^{4}
	$\delta_{1\frac{1}{2}}^{-1}$		$\delta_{1\frac{1}{2}}$		$\delta_{1\frac{1}{2}}^{3}$	
δ_{2}^{-2}		f_{2}		δ_{2}^{2}		δ_{2}^{4}

In the forward difference scheme the subscripts are seen to move forward into the difference table and no fractional subscripts occur. In the backward difference scheme the subscripts lie on diagonals slanting backwards into the table while in the central difference scheme the subscripts maintain their position and the odd order subscripts are fractional.

All three however are merely alternative ways of labeling the same numerical quantities as any difference is the result of subtracting the number diagonally above it in the preceding column from that diagonally below it in the preceding column or, alternatively, it is the sum of the number diagonally above it in the subsequent column with that immediately above it in its own column.

In general $\Delta_{p-\frac{1}{2}n}^{n} \equiv \delta_{p}^{n} \equiv \nabla_{p+\frac{1}{2}n}^{n}$.

If a polynomial of degree r is tabulated exactly i.e., without any round-off errors, then the rth differences are constant.

Tabulate $f(x)3D$ for $x = -.4\ (.2)\ .8$ where $f(x) = x^3 - .3x^2 + .07x - .123$.

x	f	δ	δ^2	δ^3	δ^4
$-.4$	$-.263$				
		106			
$-.2$	$-.157$		-72		
		34		48	
$+0$	$-.123$		-24		0
		10		48	
.2	$-.113$		$+24$		0
		34		48	
.4	$-.079$		72		0
		106		48	
.6	$+.027$		120		
		226			
.8	.253				

Had the function been rounded off to two places of decimals then the third differences would not have been constant. The differences are conventionally expressed in units of the least significant decimal as shown. This obviates the need to write down non-significant zeros. In any well tabulated function the differences decrease in magnitude.

The effect of an error term e in any function value is superimposed upon the difference table in a manner shown in the following table:

f	δ	δ^2	δ^3	δ^4	δ^5
0		0		0	
	0		0		$+1e$
0		0		$+1e$	
	0		$+1e$		$-5e$
0		$+1e$		$-4e$	
	$+1e$		$-3e$		$+10e$
$+e$		$-2e$		$+6e$	
	$-1e$		$+3e$		$-10e$
0		$+1e$		$-4e$	
	0		$-1e$		$+5e$
0		0		$+1e$	
	0		0		$-1e$
0		0		0	

In particular since round-off can contribute an error of half a unit (of the least significant decimal) in the function values, reference to the table of binomial coefficients will show that the maximum effect of this upon the twelfth differences (say) is $924(\frac{1}{2}) = 462$. This could give trouble if the problem does not require this to be multiplied by a small constant and is in fact one of the reasons why numerical differentiation is unreliable.

The following table enables the simpler operators to be expressed in terms of the others:

	E	Δ	δ, μ	∇
E	—	$1 + \Delta$	$1 + \mu\delta + \frac{1}{2}\delta^2$	$(1 - \nabla)^{-1}$
Δ	$E - 1$	—	$\mu\delta + \frac{1}{2}\delta^2$	$\nabla(1 - \nabla)^{-1}$
δ	$E^{\frac{1}{2}} - E^{-\frac{1}{2}}$	$\Delta(1 + \Delta)^{-\frac{1}{2}}$	$2(\mu^2 - 1)^{\frac{1}{2}}$	$\nabla(1 - \nabla)^{-\frac{1}{2}}$
∇	$-E^{-1}$	$\Delta(1 + \Delta)^{-1}$	$\mu\delta - \frac{1}{2}\delta^2$	—
μ	$\frac{1}{2}(E^{\frac{1}{2}} + E^{-\frac{1}{2}})$	$\frac{1}{2}(2 + \Delta)(1 + \Delta)^{-\frac{1}{2}}$	$(1 + \frac{1}{4}\delta^2)^{\frac{1}{2}}$	$\frac{1}{2}(2 - \nabla)(1 - \nabla)^{-\frac{1}{2}}$

In addition to the above there are other identities by means of which the above table can be extended, viz.,

$$E = e^{hD} = \Delta\nabla^{-1}$$

$$\mu = E^{-\frac{1}{2}} + \tfrac{1}{2}\delta = E^{\frac{1}{2}} - \tfrac{1}{2}\delta = \cosh(\tfrac{1}{2}hD)$$

$$\delta = E^{-\frac{1}{2}}\Delta = E^{\frac{1}{2}}\nabla = (\Delta\nabla)^{\frac{1}{2}} = 2\sinh(\tfrac{1}{2}hD) .$$

Note the emergence of Taylor's series from

$$\begin{aligned} f_p &= E^p f_0 \\ &= e^{phD} f_0 \\ &= f_0 + phDf_0 + \frac{1}{2!} p^2h^2D^2f_0 + \cdots . \end{aligned}$$

FUNCTION BUILD-UP FROM DIFFERENCES

Backward differences will be used here since the notation is simpler in this case.

If a function is tabulated as far as f_0 say, then the difference table can be built up. Assuming the differences up to and including ∇_0'' have been formed, if ∇_1'' is known it follows from the definition of backward differences that f_1 can be found from

$$f_1 = f_0 + \nabla_0 + \nabla_0^2 + \nabla_0^3 + \nabla_0^4 + \cdots + \nabla_0^{n-1} + \nabla_1^n .$$

For example, in the cubic tabulated earlier if we take $x_0 = .8$ then $f_0 = .253$ and f_1 can be built-up using the above scheme as follows:

$$\begin{aligned} f_1 &= .253 + (226 + 120 + 48)(10^{-3}) \\ &= .647 \end{aligned}$$

INTERPOLATION

Finite difference interpolation entails taking a given set of points and fitting a function to them. This function is usually a polynomial, although it is rarely found explicitly as such. Central differences formulae are in general to be preferred to those involving either forward or backward differences, although the latter may be essential at the extremities of a table where the central differences may not extend far enough.

The most useful of the central differences formulae are those of *Bessel* and *Everett*, the latter particularly so since it only utilizes even order differences. Nevertheless all central difference formulae stopping at the same difference are equivalent.

Notation used:

$$\Delta_{-m_r}^r \equiv \delta_{(r/2)-m_r}^r \equiv \nabla_{r-m_r}^r$$

$$p = \frac{x - x_0}{h} = 1 - q \quad (\text{usually } 0 \leq p \leq 1) .$$

Any number of finite difference interpolation formulae can be obtained from the following schematic (shown for central differences only, but easily extensible by the above identities):

$$\begin{aligned} y_r &= \sum_{r=0} \binom{p + m_{r-1}}{r} \cdot \delta_{(r/2)-m_r}^r \\ &= f_{-m_0} + \binom{p + m_0}{1} \delta_{\frac{1}{2}-m_1} + \binom{p + m_1}{2} \delta_{1-m_2}^2 + \binom{p + m_2}{3} \delta_{1\frac{1}{2}-m_3}^3 \cdots , \end{aligned}$$

where the m_r are integers so chosen that the binomial coefficient term $\binom{p + m_{r-1}}{r}$ contains all the linear factors occurring in the preceding term $\binom{p + m_{r-2}}{r - 1}$. Obviously $m_{r+1} = m_r$ or $1 + m_r$.

Further formulae are obtained by taking linear combinations of the formulae obtained from the above schematic, or by using the standard identity transformations upon chosen terms of one of the formulae.

Another way of obtaining interpolation formulae is to apply the standard identity transformations to the operator E in the operational form of the interpolation formula, viz., $f_p = E^p f_0$.

Newton's forward formula

$$f_p = f_0 + p\Delta_0 + \frac{1}{2!} p(p - 1)\Delta_0^2 + \frac{1}{3!} p(p - 1)(p - 2)\Delta_0^3 \cdots \quad 0 \leq p \leq 1$$

Newton's backward formula

$$f_p = f_0 + p\nabla_0 + \frac{1}{2!}p(p+1)\nabla_0^2 + \frac{1}{3!}p(p+1)(p+2)\nabla_0^3 \cdots \qquad 0 \leqq p \leqq 1$$

Gauss' forward formula

$$f_p = f_0 + p\delta_{\frac{1}{2}} + G_2\delta_0^2 + G_3\delta_{\frac{1}{2}}^3 + G_4\delta_0^4 + G_5\delta_{\frac{1}{2}}^5 \cdots \qquad 0 \leqq p \leqq 1$$

Gauss' backward formula

$$f_p = f_0 + p\delta_{-\frac{1}{2}} + G_2^*\delta_0^2 + G_3\delta_{-\frac{1}{2}}^3 + G_4^*\delta_0^4 + G_5\delta_{-\frac{1}{2}}^5 \cdots \qquad 0 \leqq p \leqq 1$$

In the above $G_{2n} = \binom{p+n-1}{2n}$

$$G_{2n}^* = \binom{p+n}{2n}$$

$$G_{2n+1} = \binom{p+n}{2n+1} .$$

Stirling's formula

$$f_p = f_0 + \tfrac{1}{2}p(\delta_{\frac{1}{2}} + \delta_{-\frac{1}{2}}) + \tfrac{1}{2}p^2\delta_0^2 + S_3(\delta_{\frac{1}{2}}^3 + \delta_{-\frac{1}{2}}^3) + S_4\delta_0^4 + \cdots \qquad -\tfrac{1}{2} \leqq p \leqq \tfrac{1}{2}$$

Steffenson's formula

$$f_p = f_0 + \tfrac{1}{2}p(p+1)\delta_{\frac{1}{2}} - \tfrac{1}{2}(p-1)p\delta_{-\frac{1}{2}} + (S_3 + S_4)\delta_{\frac{1}{2}}^3 + (S_3 - S_4)\delta_{-\frac{1}{2}}^3 \cdots -\tfrac{1}{2} \leqq p \leqq \tfrac{1}{2}.$$

In the above $S_{2n+1} = \frac{1}{2}\binom{p+n}{2n+1}$

$$S_{2n+2} = \frac{p}{2n+2}\binom{p+n}{2n+1}$$

$$S_{2n+1} + S_{2n+2} = \binom{p+n+1}{2n+2}$$

$$S_{2n+1} - S_{2n+2} = -\binom{p+n}{2n+2}$$

Bessel's formula

$$f_p = f_0 + p\delta_{\frac{1}{2}} + B_2(\delta_0^2 + \delta_1^2) + B_3\delta_{\frac{1}{2}}^3 + B_4(\delta_0^4 + \delta_1^4) + B_5\delta_{\frac{1}{2}}^5 + \cdots \qquad 0 \leqq p \leqq 1$$

Everett's formula

$$f_p = (1-p)f_0 + pf_1 + E_2\delta_0^2 + F_2\delta_1^2 + E_4\delta_0^4 + F_4\delta_1^4 + E_6\delta_0^6 + F_6\delta_1^6 + \cdots \qquad 0 \leqq p \leqq 1$$

The coefficients in the above two formulae are related to each other and to the coefficients in the Gaussian formulae by the identities

$$\begin{aligned} B_{2n} &\equiv \tfrac{1}{2}G_{2n} \equiv \tfrac{1}{2}(E_{2n} + F_{2n}) \\ B_{2n+1} &\equiv G_{2n+1} - \tfrac{1}{2}G_{2n} \equiv \tfrac{1}{2}(F_{2n} - E_{2n}) \\ E_{2n} &\equiv G_{2n} - G_{2n+1} \equiv B_{2n} - B_{2n+1} \\ F_{2n} &\equiv G_{2n+1} \equiv B_{2n} + B_{2n+1} \end{aligned}$$

Also for $q \equiv 1 - p$ the following symmetrical relationships hold:

$$\begin{aligned} B_{2n}(p) &\equiv B_{2n}(q) \\ B_{2n+1}(p) &\equiv -B_{2n+1}(q) \\ E_{2n}(p) &\equiv F_{2n}(q) \\ F_{2n}(p) &\equiv E_{2n}(q) \end{aligned}$$

as can be seen from the tables of these coefficients.

COEFFICIENTS—BESSELS FORMULA

p	B_2	B_3	B_4	B_5	B_6	B_7	$(1-p)$
0.00	−0.000000	0.0000000	0.000000	−0.000000	−0.00000	0.00000	1.00
0.01	2475	8085	415	81	8	1	0.99
0.02	4900	15680	825	158	17	2	0.98
0.03	7275	22795	1230	231	25	3	0.97
0.04	9600	29440	1631	300	33	4	0.96
0.05	−0.011875	0.0035625	0.002026	−0.000365	−0.00041	0.00005	0.95
0.06	14100	41360	2416	425	49	6	0.94
0.07	16275	46655	2801	482	57	7	0.93
0.08	18400	51520	3180	534	64	8	0.92
0.09	20475	55965	3552	583	72	8	0.91
0.10	−0.022500	0.0060000	0.003919	−0.000627	−0.00080	0.00009	0.90
0.11	24475	63635	4279	667	87	10	0.89
0.12	26400	66880	4632	704	94	10	0.88
0.13	28275	69745	4979	737	101	11	0.87
0.14	30100	72240	5310	766	109	11	0.86
0.15	−0.031875	0.0074375	0.005651	−0.000791	−0.00115	0.00012	0.85
0.16	33600	76160	5976	813	122	12	0.84
0.17	35275	77605	6294	831	129	12	0.83
0.18	36900	78720	6604	845	135	12	0.82
0.19	38475	79515	6906	856	142	13	0.81
0.20	−0.040000	0.0080000	0.007200	−0.000864	−0.00148	0.00013	0.80
0.21	41475	80185	7486	868	154	13	0.79
0.22	42900	80080	7763	870	160	13	0.78
0.23	44275	79695	8033	868	165	13	0.77
0.24	45600	79040	8293	862	171	13	0.76
0.25	−0.046875	0.0078125	0.008545	−0.000554	−0.00176	0.00013	0.75
0.26	48100	76960	8788	844	181	12	0.74
0.27	49275	75555	9022	830	186	12	0.73
0.28	50400	73920	9247	814	191	12	0.72
0.29	51475	72065	9462	795	196	12	0.71
0.30	−0.052500	0.0070000	0.009669	−0.000773	−0.00200	0.00011	0.70
0.31	53475	67735	9866	750	204	11	0.69
0.32	54400	65280	10053	724	208	11	0.68
0.33	55275	62645	10231	696	212	10	0.67
0.34	56100	59840	10399	666	216	10	0.66
0.35	−0.056875	0.0056875	0.010557	−0.000633	−0.00219	0.00009	0.65
0.36	57600	53760	10706	600	222	9	0.64
0.37	58275	50505	10844	564	225	8	0.63
0.38	58900	47120	10973	527	228	8	0.62
0.39	59475	43615	11092	488	231	7	0.61
0.40	−0.060000	0.0040000	0.011200	−0.000448	−0.00233	0.00007	0.60
0.41	60475	36285	11298	407	235	6	0.59
0.42	60900	32480	11386	364	237	5	0.58
0.43	61275	28595	11464	321	239	5	0.57
0.44	61600	24640	11532	277	240	4	0.56
0.45	−0.061875	0.0020625	0.011589	−0.000232	−0.00241	0.00003	0.55
0.46	62100	16560	11635	186	242	3	0.54
0.47	62275	12455	11672	140	243	2	0.53
0.48	62400	8320	11698	94	244	1	0.52
0.49	62475	4165	11714	47	244	1	0.51
0.50	−0.062500	0.0000000	0.011719	−0.000000	−0.00244	0.00000	0.50
$(1-p)$	B_2	$-B_3$	B_4	$-B_5$	B_6	$-B_7$	p

Bessel's formula (unmodified)

(a) $f_p = f_0 + p\delta_{\frac{1}{2}} + B_2(\delta_0^2 + \delta_1^2) + B_3\delta_{\frac{1}{2}}^3 + B_4(\delta_0^4 + \delta_1^4) + B_5\delta_{\frac{1}{2}}^5 + B_6(\delta_0^6 + \delta_1^6) + B_7\delta_{\frac{1}{2}}^7 + \cdots.$

The end terms can be neglected, i.e., they contribute less than half a unit in the last place of decimals, if the differences are less than the values shown in the following list:

Neglect	$B_7\delta_{\frac{1}{2}}^7$ if	$\delta^7 < 3500$
	$B_6(\delta_0 + \delta_1)$	$\delta^6 < 100$
	$B_5\delta_{\frac{1}{2}}^5$	$\delta^5 < 500$
	$B_4(\delta_0^4 + \delta_1^4)$	$\delta^4 < 20$
	$B_3\delta_{\frac{1}{2}}^3$	$\delta^3 < 60$
	$B_2(\delta_0^2 + \delta_1^2)$	$\delta^2 < 4$

A powerful simplification is that of throwback. If the higher differences are less than a specified value they can be combined with the lower order ones as follows:

If $\delta^6 < 10{,}000$ use $\delta_m^4 \equiv \delta^4 - 0.20697\delta^6$

and if $\delta^6 < 1{,}000$* use $\delta_m^4 \equiv \delta^4 - 0.2\delta^6$
in the modified form of Bessel's formula

(b) $f_p = f_0 + p\delta_{\frac{1}{2}} + B_2(\delta_0^2 + \delta_1^2) + B_3\delta_{\frac{1}{2}}^3 + B_4(\delta_{m0}^4 + \delta_{m1}^4) + B_5\delta_{\frac{1}{2}}^5.$

If $\delta^4 < 1{,}000$ and $\delta^6 < 1{,}000$* use $\delta_m^2 \equiv \delta^2 - 0.18393\delta^4 + 0.03808\delta^6$
and if $\delta^4 < 1{,}000$* use $\delta_m^2 \equiv \delta^2 - 0.18393\delta^4$
in the modified form of Bessel's formula

(c) $f_p = f_0 + p\delta_{\frac{1}{2}} + B_2(\delta_{m0}^2 + \delta_{m1}^2) + B_3\delta_{\frac{1}{2}}^3.$

Everett's formula (unmodified)

(a) $f_p = (1 - p)f_0 + pf_1 + E_2\delta_0^2 + F_2\delta_1^2 + E_4\delta_0^4 + F_4\delta_1^4 + E_6\delta_0^6 + F_6\delta_1^6 + \cdots.$

As with Bessel's formula, end terms can be neglected as follows:

Neglect	$E_6\delta_0^6 + F_6\delta_1^6$ if	$\delta^6 < 100$
	$E_4\delta_0^4 + F_4\delta_1^4$	$\delta^4 < 20$
	$E_2\delta_0^2 + F_2\delta_1^2$	$\delta^2 < 4$

The corresponding throwback formulae are

(b) $f_p = (1 - p)f_0 + pf_1 + E_2\delta_0^2 + F_2\delta_1^2 + E_4\delta_{m0}^4 + F_4\delta_{m1}^4,$
where $\delta_m^4 \equiv \delta^4 - 0.20697\delta^6$ providing $\delta^6 < 10{,}000$*
or $\delta_m^4 \equiv \delta^4 - 0.2\delta^6$ providing $\delta^6 < 1{,}000$*;
(c) $f_p = (1 - p)f_0 + pf_1 + E_2\delta_{m0}^4 + F_2\delta_{m1}^2$
where $\delta_m^2 \equiv \delta^2 - 0.18393\delta^4 + 0.03808\delta^6$ if $\delta^4, \delta^6 < 1{,}000$*.

---

* Higher even order differences are negligible. Throwback involving odd order differences is of little practical use.

COEFFICIENTS—EVERETTS FORMULA

p	E_2	F_2	E_4	F_4	E_6	F_6	$(1-p)$
0.00	−0.000000	−0.0000000	0.000000	0.000000	−0.00000	−0.00000	1.00
0.01	32835	16665	496	33	9	7	0.99
0.02	64680	33320	983	67	19	14	0.98
0.03	95545	49955	1461	100	28	21	0.97
0.04	125440	66560	1931	133	37	29	0.96
0.05	−0.0154375	−0.0083125	0.002391	0.001661	−0.00046	−0.00036	0.95
0.06	182360	99640	2842	199	55	43	0.94
0.07	209405	116095	3283	232	64	50	0.93
0.08	235520	132480	3714	264	72	57	0.92
0.09	260715	148785	4135	297	80	64	0.91
0.10	−0.0285000	−0.0165000	0.004546	0.003292	−0.00089	−0.00070	0.90
0.11	308385	181115	4946	361	97	77	0.89
0.12	330880	197120	5336	393	105	84	0.88
0.13	352495	213005	5716	424	112	91	0.87
0.14	373240	228760	6085	455	120	97	0.86
0.15	−0.0393125	−0.0244375	0.006442	0.004860	−0.00127	−0.00104	0.85
0.16	412160	259840	6789	516	134	110	0.84
0.17	430355	275145	7125	546	141	117	0.83
0.18	447720	290280	7449	576	148	123	0.82
0.19	464265	305235	7762	605	154	129	0.81
0.20	−0.0480000	−0.0320000	0.008064	0.006336	−0.00161	−0.00135	0.80
0.21	494935	334565	8354	662	167	141	0.79
0.22	509080	348920	8633	689	172	147	0.78
0.23	522445	363055	8900	716	178	153	0.77
0.24	535040	376960	9156	743	184	158	0.76
0.25	−0.0546875	−0.0390625	0.009399	0.007690	−0.00189	−0.00164	0.75
0.26	557960	404040	9632	794	194	169	0.74
0.27	568305	417195	9852	819	199	174	0.73
0.28	577920	430080	10060	843	203	179	0.72
0.29	586815	442685	10257	867	207	184	0.71
0.30	−0.0595000	−0.0455000	0.010442	0.008895	−0.00212	−0.00189	0.70
0.31	602485	467015	10615	912	215	193	0.69
0.32	609280	478720	10777	933	219	198	0.68
0.33	615395	490105	10927	954	222	202	0.67
0.34	620840	501160	11065	973	226	206	0.66
0.35	−0.0625625	−0.0511875	0.011191	0.009924	−0.00229	−0.00210	0.65
0.36	629760	522240	11305	1011	231	213	0.64
0.37	633255	532245	11408	1028	234	217	0.63
0.38	636120	541880	11500	1045	236	220	0.62
0.39	638365	551135	11580	1060	238	223	0.61
0.40	−0.0640000	−0.0560000	0.011648	0.010752	−.00240	−0.00226	0.60
0.41	641035	568465	11705	1089	241	229	0.59
0.42	641480	576520	11751	1102	242	232	0.58
0.43	641345	584155	11785	1114	243	234	0.57
0.44	640640	591360	11808	1125	244	236	0.56
0.45	−0.0639375	−0.0598125	0.011820	0.011357	−0.00245	−0.00238	0.55
0.46	637560	604440	11822	1145	245	240	0.54
0.47	635205	610295	11812	1153	245	241	0.53
0.48	632320	615680	11792	1160	245	242	0.52
0.49	628915	620585	11760	1167	245	243	0.51
0.50	−0.0625000	−0.0625000	0.011719	0.011719	−0.00244	−0.00244	0.50
$(1-p)$	F_2	E_2	F_4	E_4	F_6	E_6	p

Generalized Throwback

Using 0.184 instead of the more precise value of 0.18393 we obtain a very simple but nevertheless accurate interpolation formulae

$$f \equiv (1-p)f_0 + pf_1 + E_2\delta^2_{m0} + F_2\delta^2_{m1} + P_4\theta^4_0 + Q_4\theta^4_1,$$

where $\delta^2_m \equiv \delta^2 - 0.184\delta^4 + 0.03882\delta^6 - 0.0083\delta^8 + 0.0019\delta^{10}$

and $100\theta^4 \equiv \delta^4 - 0.27838\delta^6 + 0.0685\delta^8 - 0.0168\delta^{10}$

and $P_4 \equiv 100(E_4 + 0.184E_2)$; $\quad Q_4 \equiv 100(F_4 + 0.184F_2)$.

Symmetric formulae for interpolation to halves (sub-tabulation to halves)

When $p = \frac{1}{2}$ is substituted into Bessel's interpolation formula the odd coefficients B_{2n+1} all become zero and the resulting formula is

$$f_{\frac{1}{2}} = \left(1 - \frac{1}{8}\delta^2 + \frac{3}{128}\delta^4 - \frac{5}{1024}\delta^6 + \frac{35}{32768}\delta^8 - \cdots\right)\mu f_{\frac{1}{2}}.$$

If this is truncated after one, two, three terms etc. the following formulae and error terms are obtained:

	Error
$f_{\frac{1}{2}} = \frac{1}{2}(f_0 + f_1)$	$\frac{-1}{8}\mu\delta^2_{\frac{1}{2}}$
$f_{\frac{1}{2}} = (-f_{-1} + 9f_0 + 9f_1 - f_2)/16$	$\frac{+3}{128}\mu\delta^4_{\frac{1}{2}}$
$f_{\frac{1}{2}} = (3f_{-2} - 25f_{-1} + 150f_0 + 150f_1 - 25f_2 + 3f_3)/256$	$\frac{-5}{1024}\mu\delta^6_{\frac{1}{2}}$
$f_{\frac{1}{2}} = (-5f_{-3} + 49f_{-2} - 245f_{-1} + 1225f_0 + 1225f_1 - 245f_2 + 49f_3 - 5f_4)/2048$	$\frac{+35}{32768}\mu\delta^8_{\frac{1}{2}}$

Similarly, unsymmetric formulae for subtabulation to halves can be obtained from Newton's formula by substituting $p = \frac{1}{2}$ and truncating, e.g.,

$$f_{\frac{1}{2}} = \left(1 + \frac{1}{2}\Delta - \frac{1}{8}\Delta^2 + \frac{1}{16}\Delta^3 - \frac{5}{128}\Delta^4 + \frac{7}{256}\Delta^5 \cdots\right)f_0$$

	Error
$f_{\frac{1}{2}} = (3f_0 + 6f_1 - f_2)/8$	$\frac{+1}{16}\Delta^3_0$
$f_{\frac{1}{2}} = (5f_0 + 15f_1 - 5f_2 + f_3)/16$	$\frac{-5}{128}\Delta^4_0$
$f_{\frac{1}{2}} = (35f_0 + 140f_1 - 70f_2 + 28f_3 - 5f_4)/128$	$\frac{+7}{256}\Delta^5_0$

The formula obtained by considering the first two terms only of the series is identical with the first one derived from Bessel's formula.

Interpolation techniques which do not require the function to be tabulated for equal interval of the argument

a) Lagrangian Polynomials

The interpolated value is obtained from a set of points which bridge the required point. The nearer the argument of the required value is to the center of the range of arguments of the function values used the better.

For an odd number of points
$$f(x) = \sum_{r=-n}^{n} L_r f_r \,.$$

For an even number of points
$$f(x) = \sum_{r=-n}^{n+1} L_r f_r \,.$$

The interpolating polynomial is of degree $2n$ in the first case and $2n + 1$ in the second. Further, it must pass through the given points $f_{-n}, f_{1-n}, f_{2-n}, \cdots, f_n$ or f_{1+n} as the case may be.

The coefficient L_r associated with the function value f_r is given by

$$L_r = \frac{(x - x_{-n})(x - x_{1-n}) \cdots (x - x_{r-1})(x - x_{r+1}) \cdots (x - x_{n-1})(x - x_n)}{(x_r - x_{-n})(x_r - x_{1-n}) \cdots (x_r - x_{r-1})(x_r - x_{r+1}) \cdots (x_r - x_{n-1})(x_r - x_n)}$$

for the first case with an additional factor $(x - x_{1+n})/(x_r - x_{1+n})$ in the second.

The error involved is equal to the $(2n + 2)$th. derivative, at some point in the range, multiplied by

$$(x - x_{-n})(x - x_{1-n}) \cdots (x - x_{1-n})/(2n + 2)!$$

in the case of the even number of points, and the $(2n + 1)$th. derivative, again at some point in the range, multiplied by

$$(x - x_{-n})(x - x_{1-n}) \cdots (x - x_n)/(2n + 1)!$$

in the other case.

In both cases the multipliers are functions which oscillate with an amplitude which increases substantially as the argument of the required point departs from the center of the range. When the arguments are spaced at equal intervals h and the point x is nearer to x_0 than to the other points, then $L_r(p)$ can be tabulated for $p = (x - x_0)/h$.

If the degree of the approximating polynomial is known the method is very powerful, otherwise it is best avoided.

b) Divided differences

The layout of a divided difference table is similar to that of an ordinary finite difference table.

x_{-1}	f_{-1}		Λ^2_{-1}		Λ^4_{-1}
		$\Lambda_{-\frac{1}{2}}$		$\Lambda_{-\frac{1}{2}}$	
x_0	f_0		Λ^2_0		Λ^4_0
		$\Lambda_{\frac{1}{2}}$		$\Lambda^3_{\frac{1}{2}}$	
x_1	f_1		Λ^2_1		Λ^4_1

where the Λ's are defined as follows:

$$\Lambda_r^0 \equiv f_r, \qquad \Lambda_{r+\frac{1}{2}} \equiv (f_{r+1} - f_r)/(x_{r+1} - x_r),$$

and in general
$$\Lambda_r^{2n} \equiv (\Lambda_{r+\frac{1}{2}}^{2n-1} - \Lambda_{r-\frac{1}{2}}^{2n-1})/(x_{r+n} - x_{r-n})$$

and
$$\Lambda_{r+\frac{1}{2}}^{2n+1} \equiv (\Lambda_{r+1}^{2n} - \Lambda_r^{2n})/(x_{r+1+n} - x_{r-n}).$$

Divided differences can with advantage be replaced by adjusted divided differences.

c) *Adjusted divided differences*

These differences are a modified form of the above and, when the interval of tabulation becomes constant, they reduce to ordinary central differences. Formulae analogous to all the existing formulae involving forward, central and backward differences can be obtained by means of Sheppard's rules which are stated below.

x_{-1}	p_{-1}	f_{-1}		$\overset{\xi}{\delta}{}_{-1}^2$		$\overset{\xi}{\delta}{}_{-1}^4$
			$\overset{\xi}{\delta}_{-\frac{1}{2}}$		$\overset{\xi}{\delta}{}_{-\frac{1}{2}}^3$	
x_0	p_0	f_0		$\overset{\xi}{\delta}{}_0^2$		$\overset{\xi}{\delta}{}_0^4$
			$\overset{\xi}{\delta}_{\frac{1}{2}}$		$\overset{\xi}{\delta}{}_{\frac{1}{2}}^3$	
x_1	p_1	f_1		$\overset{\xi}{\delta}{}_1^2$		$\overset{\xi}{\delta}{}_1^4$
			$\overset{\xi}{\delta}_{1\frac{1}{2}}$		$\overset{\xi}{\delta}{}_{1\frac{1}{2}}^3$	
x_2	p_2	f_2		$\overset{\xi}{\delta}{}_2^2$		$\overset{\xi}{\delta}{}_2^4$

where h is the total range of arguments divided by the number of intervals in that range, the result being rounded to a suitable figure and $x_k \cong p_k \cdot h$ or $(x/h)_k = p_k + w_k$ where the w's are used to shift the origin, if necessary, and to round-off the p's.

Define
$$\overset{\xi}{\delta}_r \equiv \frac{1}{(p_{r+\frac{1}{2}} - p_{r-\frac{1}{2}})}(f_{r+\frac{1}{2}} - f_{r-\frac{1}{2}})$$

and
$$\overset{\xi}{\delta}{}_r^2 \equiv \frac{2}{(p_{r+1} - p_{r-1})}(\overset{\xi}{\delta}_{r+\frac{1}{2}} - \overset{\xi}{\delta}_{r-\frac{1}{2}}).$$

In general
$$\overset{\xi}{\delta}{}_r^{2n+1} \equiv \frac{2n+1}{(p_{r+\frac{1}{2}+n} - p_{r-\frac{1}{2}-n})}(\overset{\xi}{\delta}{}_{r+\frac{1}{2}}^{2n} - \overset{\xi}{\delta}{}_{r-\frac{1}{2}}^{2n}),$$

$$\overset{\xi}{\delta}{}_r^{2n} \equiv \frac{2n}{(p_{r+n} - p_{r-n})}(\overset{\xi}{\delta}{}_{r+\frac{1}{2}}^{2n-1} - \overset{\xi}{\delta}{}_{r+\frac{1}{2}}^{2n-1}).$$

The formula will be in the form

$$f(x) = f_0 + \sum_{r=1}^{N}\left\{\prod (p - p_j \cdot) \frac{\overset{\xi}{\delta}{}_s^r}{r!}\right\},$$

where the product part of each term of the formula consists of r factors and the p_j's and s are chosen as follows:

a) When $r = 1$, $j = 0$ and $s = +\frac{1}{2}$, or $-\frac{1}{2}$, thereafter:—

b) r is increased by unity and s is either increased or decreased by $\frac{1}{2}$. Thus the p's, involved in the new divided difference of the series, are all those which are necessary for the computation of the divided difference used in the *preceding term* plus one more added either to the beginning or to the end of the set.

c) The product part of the term consists of factors $(p - p_j)$ such that all the p's necessary for the evaluation of the *previous* divided difference are involved. For example, Gauss' forward difference interpolation formula in terms of adjusted divided differences is obtained by following the path shown below

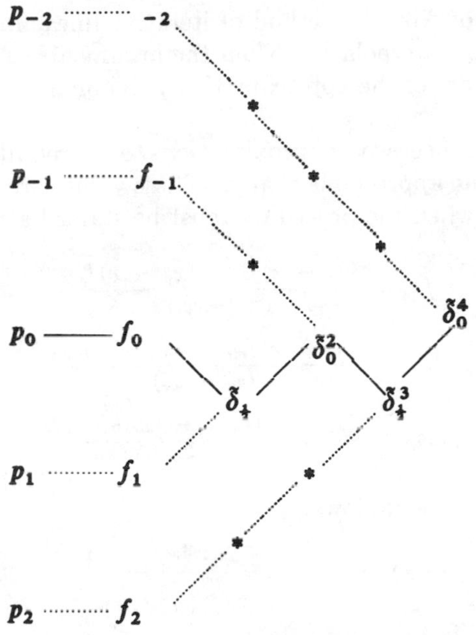

The solid line indicates the path chosen through the difference table.

$$f(x) = f_0 + (p - p_0)\delta_{\frac{1}{2}} + \frac{1}{2!}\cdot(p - p_0)(p - p_1)\delta_0^2 + \frac{1}{3!}\cdot(p - p_0)(p - p_1)(p - p_{-1})\delta_{\frac{1}{2}}^3$$
$$+ \frac{1}{4!}\cdot(p - p_0)(p - p_1)(p - p_{-1})(p - p_2)\delta_0^4 \cdots.$$

Similarly Gauss' backward difference interpolation formula is

$$f(x) = f_0 + (p - p_0)\delta_{-\frac{1}{2}} + \frac{1}{2!}\cdot(p - p_0)(p - p_{-1})\delta_0^2 + \frac{1}{3!}\cdot(p - p_0)(p - p_{-1})(p - p_1)\delta_{-\frac{1}{2}}^3$$
$$+ \frac{1}{4!}\cdot(p - p_0)(p - p_{-1})(p - p_1)(p - p_{-2})\delta_0^4 \cdots,$$

and Stirling's formula is

$$f(x) = f_0 + \frac{(p - p_0)}{2}[\delta_{\frac{1}{2}} + \delta_{-\frac{1}{2}}] + \frac{1}{2!}\cdot\frac{(p - p_0)}{2}[(p - p_{-1}) + (p - p_1)]\delta_0^2$$
$$+ \frac{1}{3!}\cdot\frac{(p - p_1)(p - p_0)(p - p_{-1})}{2}[\delta_{\frac{1}{2}}^3 + \delta_{-\frac{1}{2}}^3]$$
$$+ \frac{1}{4!}\cdot\frac{(p - p_1)(p - p_0)(p - p_{-1})}{2}[(p - p_{-2}) + (p - p_2)]\delta_0^4 \cdots.$$

Replacing the odd order differences, in Gauss' forward formula, by combinations of the previous even order differences the formula analogous to Everett's is obtained, i.e.,

$$f(x) = \left[1 - \frac{(p - p_0)}{(p_1 - p_0)}\right] f_0 + \frac{1(p - p_0)}{(p_1 - p_0)} f_1 - \frac{1}{2!} \frac{(p - p_0)(p - p_1)(p - p_2)}{(p_2 - p_{-1})} \delta_0^2$$
$$+ \frac{1}{2!} \frac{(p - p_0)(p - p_1)(p - p_{-1})}{(p_2 - p_{-1})} \delta_1^2 - \cdots .$$

d) Iterative linear interpolation

Neville's modification of Aiken's method of iterative linear interpolation is one of the most powerful methods of interpolation when the arguments are unevenly spaced as no prior knowledge of the order of the approximating polynomial is necessary nor is a difference table required.

The values obtained are successive approximations to the required result and the process terminates when there is no appreciable change. These values are of course useless if a new interpolation is required when the procedure must be started afresh.

Defining
$$f_{r,s} \equiv \frac{(x_s - x)f_r - (x_r - x)f_s}{(x_s - x_r)}$$
$$f_{r,s,t} \equiv \frac{(x_t - x)f_{r,s} - (x_r - x)f_{s,t}}{(x_t - x_r)}$$
$$f_{r,s,t,u} \equiv \frac{(x_u - x)f_{r,s,t} - (x_r - x)f_{s,t,u}}{(x_u - x_r)},$$

the computation is laid out as follows:

x_{-1}	$(x_{-1} - x)$	f_{-1}			
			$f_{-1,0}$		
x_0	$(x_0 - x)$	f_0		$f_{-1\,0,1}$	
			$f_{0,1}$		$f_{-1\,0\,1,2}$
x_1	$(x_1 - x)$	f_1		$f_{0,1,2}$	
			$f_{1,2}$		
x_2	$(x_2 - x)$	f_2			

As the iterates tend to their limit the common leading figures can be omitted.

e) Gauss' trigonometric interpolation formula

This is of greatest value when the function is periodic, i.e., a Fourier series expansion is possible.

$$f(x) = \sum_{r=0}^{n} C_r f_r ,$$

where $C_r = N_r(x)/N_r(x_r)$ and

$$N_r(x) = \left[\sin \frac{(x - x_0)}{2}\right]\left[\sin \frac{(x - x_1)}{2}\right] \cdots \left[\sin \frac{(x - x_{r-1})}{2}\right]$$
$$\left[\sin \frac{(x - x_{r+1})}{2}\right] \cdots \left[\sin \frac{(x - x_n)}{2}\right].$$

This is similar to the Lagrangian formula.

f) Reciprocal differences

These are used when the quotient of two polynomials will give a better representation of the interpolating function than a simple polynomial expression.

A convenient layout is as shown below:

$$\begin{array}{cccccc}
x_{-1} & f_{-1} & & & & \\
 & & \rho_{-\frac{1}{2}} & & & \\
x_0 & f_0 & & \overset{2}{\rho}_0 & & \\
 & & \rho_{\frac{1}{2}} & & \overset{3}{\rho}_{\frac{1}{2}} & \\
x_1 & f_1 & & \overset{2}{\rho}_1 & & \overset{4}{\rho}_1 \\
 & & \rho_{1\frac{1}{2}} & & \overset{3}{\rho}_{1\frac{1}{2}} & \\
x_2 & f_2 & & \overset{2}{\rho}_2 & & \\
 & & \rho_{2\frac{1}{2}} & & & \\
x_3 & f_3 & & & &
\end{array}$$

where
$$\rho_{r+\frac{1}{2}} \equiv \frac{x_{r+1} - x_r}{f_{r+1} - f_r}$$

and
$$\overset{2}{\rho}_r \equiv \frac{x_{r+1} - x_{r-1}}{f_{r+\frac{1}{2}} - f_{r-\frac{1}{2}}} + f_r$$

In general
$$\overset{2n+1}{\rho}_{r+\frac{1}{2}} \equiv \frac{x_{r+n+1} - x_{r-n}}{\overset{2n}{\rho}_{r+1} - \overset{2n}{\rho}_r} + \overset{2n-1}{\rho}_{r+\frac{1}{2}}$$

$$\overset{2n}{\rho}_r \equiv \frac{x_{r+n} - x_{r-n}}{\overset{2n-1}{\rho}_{r+\frac{1}{2}} - \overset{2n-1}{\rho}_{r-\frac{1}{2}}} + \overset{2n-2}{\rho}_r .$$

The interpolation formula is expressed in the form of a continued fraction expansion.

The expansion corresponding to Newton's forward difference interpolation formula, in the sense of the differences involved, is

$$f(x) = f_0 + \cfrac{(x - x_0)}{\rho_{\frac{1}{2}} + \cfrac{(x_2 - x_1)}{\rho_1 - f_0 + \cfrac{(x - x_2)}{\overset{3}{\rho}_{1\frac{1}{2}} - \rho_{\frac{1}{2}} + \cfrac{(x_4 - x_3)}{\overset{4}{\rho}_2 - \overset{2}{\rho}_1 + \cfrac{(x - x_4)}{\text{etc.}}}}}}$$

while that corresponding to Gauss' forward formula is

$$f(x) = f_0 + \cfrac{(x - x_0)}{\rho_{\frac{1}{2}} + \cfrac{(x_2 - x_1)}{\overset{2}{\rho}_0 - f_0 + \cfrac{(x_3 - x_{-1})}{\overset{3}{\rho}_{\frac{1}{2}} - \rho_{\frac{1}{2}} + \cfrac{(x_4 - x_2)}{\overset{4}{\rho}_0 - \overset{2}{\rho}_0 + \cfrac{(x - x_{-2})}{\text{etc.}}}}}}$$

Inverse interpolation

Any method of interpolation which does not require the arguments to be evenly spaced will be satisfactory, by simply interchanging the roles of the arguments and the function values.

Alternative (i) Sub-tabulate the function until linear interpolation is adequate and simple ratio and proportion will yield the result.

Alternative (ii) Find an approximate value for p from

$$p \cong (f_p - f_0)/(f_1 - f_0)$$

and then iterate using *any* of the standard interpolation formulae;
e.g., Bessel

$$p = [f_p - f_0 - B_2(\delta_0^2 + \delta_1^2) - B_3\delta_{\frac{1}{2}}^3 - \cdots \text{etc.}]/\delta_{\frac{1}{2}}$$

where the Bessel's coefficients on the right hand side are evaluated for the approximate p.

Everrett

$$p = [f_p - f_0 - E_2\delta_0^2 - F_2\delta_1^2 - E_4\delta^4 - F_4\delta_0^4 \cdots]/\delta_{\frac{1}{2}}$$

Newton forward

$$p = [f_p - f_0 - \frac{1}{2!}p(p-1)\Delta_0^2 - \frac{1}{3!}p(p-1)(p-2)\Delta_0^3 \cdots]/\Delta_0$$

Newton backward

$$p = [f_p - f_0 - \frac{1}{2!}p(p+1)\nabla_0^2 - \frac{1}{3!}p(p+1)(p+2)\nabla_0^3 \cdots]/\nabla_0 .$$

Note that the divisors are in fact identical.

II. Normal Distribution

II.1 THE NORMAL PROBABILITY FUNCTION AND RELATED FUNCTIONS

This table gives values of:

a) $f(x)$ = the probability density of a standardized random variable

$$= \frac{1}{\sqrt{2\pi}} e^{-\frac{1}{2}x^2}$$

For negative values of x, one uses the fact that $f(-x) = f(x)$.

b) $F(x)$ = the cumulative distribution function of a standardized normal random variable

$$= \int_{-\infty}^{x} \frac{1}{\sqrt{2\pi}} e^{-\frac{1}{2}t^2}\, dt$$

For negative values of x, one uses the relationship $F(-x) = 1 - F(x)$. Values of x corresponding to a few special values of $F(x)$ are given in a separate table following the main table. (See page 124.)

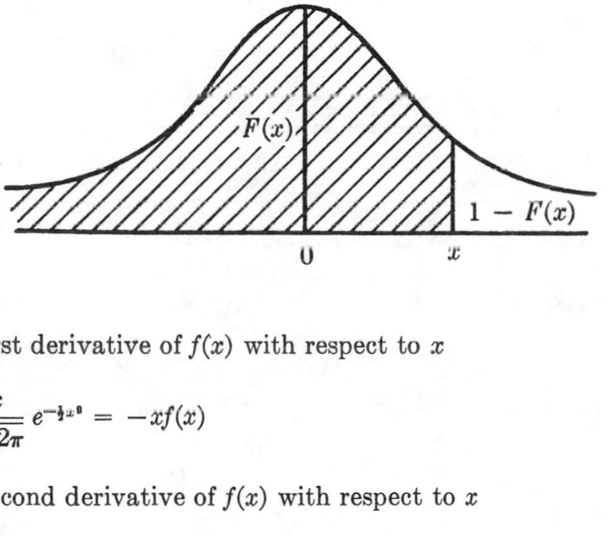

c) $f'(x)$ = the first derivative of $f(x)$ with respect to x

$$= -\frac{x}{\sqrt{2\pi}} e^{-\frac{1}{2}x^2} = -xf(x)$$

d) $f''(x)$ = the second derivative of $f(x)$ with respect to x

$$= \frac{(x^2 - 1)}{\sqrt{2\pi}} e^{-\frac{1}{2}x^2} = (x^2 - 1)f(x)$$

e) $f'''(x)$ = the third derivative of $f(x)$ with respect to x

$$= \frac{3x - x^3}{\sqrt{2\pi}} e^{-\frac{1}{2}x^2} = (3x - x^3)f(x)$$

f) $f^{iv}(x)$ = the fourth derivative of $f(x)$ with respect to x

$$= \frac{x^4 - 6x^2 + 3}{\sqrt{2\pi}} e^{-\frac{1}{2}x^2} = (x^4 - 6x^2 + 3)f(x)$$

It should be noted that other probability integrals can be evaluated by the use of these tables. For example,

$$\int_0^x f(t)dt = \tfrac{1}{2}\,\text{erf}\left(\frac{x}{\sqrt{2}}\right),$$

where $\text{erf}\left(\frac{x}{\sqrt{2}}\right)$ represents the error function associated with the normal curve.

To evaluate erf (2.3) one proceeds as follows: Since $\frac{x}{\sqrt{2}} = 2.3$, one finds $x = (2.3)(\sqrt{2}) = 3.25$. In the entry opposite $x = 3.25$, the value 0.9994 is given. Subtracting 0.5000 from the tabular value, one finds the value 0.4994. Thus erf (2.3) = 2(0.4994) = 0.9988.

NORMAL DISTRIBUTION AND RELATED FUNCTIONS

x	$F(x)$	$1 - F(x)$	$f(x)$	$f'(x)$	$f''(x)$	$f'''(x)$	$f^{\text{iv}}(x)$
.00	.5000	.5000	.3989	−.0000	−.3989	.0000	1.1968
.01	.5040	.4960	.3989	−.0040	−.3989	.0120	1.1965
.02	.5080	.4920	.3989	−.0080	−.3987	.0239	1.1956
.03	.5120	.4880	.3988	−.0120	−.3984	.0359	1.1941
.04	.5160	.4840	.3986	−.0159	−.3980	.0478	1.1920
.05	.5199	.4801	.3984	−.0199	−.3975	.0597	1.1894
.06	.5239	.4761	.3982	−.0239	−.3968	.0716	1.1861
.07	.5279	.4721	.3980	−.0279	−.3960	.0834	1.1822
.08	.5319	.4681	.3977	−.0318	−.3951	.0952	1.1778
.09	.5359	.4641	.3973	−.0358	−.3941	.1070	1.1727
.10	.5398	.4602	.3970	−.0397	−.3930	.1187	1.1671
.11	.5438	.4562	.3965	−.0436	−.3917	.1303	1.1609
.12	.5478	.4522	.3961	−.0475	−.3904	.1419	1.1541
.13	.5517	.4483	.3956	−.0514	−.3889	.1534	1.1468
.14	.5557	.4443	.3951	−.0553	−.3873	.1648	1.1389
.15	.5596	.4404	.3945	−.0592	−.3856	.1762	1.1304
.16	.5636	.4364	.3939	−.0630	−.3838	.1874	1.1214
.17	.5675	.4325	.3932	−.0668	−.3819	.1986	1.1118
.18	.5714	.4286	.3925	−.0707	−.3798	.2097	1.1017
.19	.5753	.4247	.3918	−.0744	−.3777	.2206	1.0911
.20	.5793	.4207	.3910	−.0782	−.3754	.2315	1.0799
.21	.5832	.4168	.3902	−.0820	−.3730	.2422	1.0682
.22	.5871	.4129	.3894	−.0857	−.3706	.2529	1.0560
.23	.5910	.4090	.3885	−.0894	−.3680	.2634	1.0434
.24	.5948	.4052	.3876	−.0930	−.3653	.2737	1.0302
.25	.5987	.4013	.3867	−.0967	−.3625	.2840	1.0165
.26	.6026	.3974	.3857	−.1003	−.3596	.2941	1.0024
.27	.6064	.3936	.3847	−.1039	−.3566	.3040	0.9878
.28	.6103	.3897	.3836	−.1074	−.3535	.3138	0.9727
.29	.6141	.3859	.3825	−.1109	−.3504	.3235	0.9572
.30	.6179	.3821	.3814	−.1144	−.3471	.3330	0.9413
.31	.6217	.3783	.3802	−.1179	−.3437	.3423	0.9250
.32	.6255	.3745	.3790	−.1213	−.3402	.3515	0.9082
.33	.6293	.3707	.3778	−.1247	−.3367	.3605	0.8910
.34	.6331	.3669	.3765	−.1280	−.3330	.3693	0.8735
.35	.6368	.3632	.3752	−.1313	−.3293	.3779	0.8556
.36	.6406	.3594	.3739	−.1346	−.3255	.3864	0.8373
.37	.6443	.3557	.3725	−.1378	−.3216	.3947	0.8186
.38	.6480	.3520	.3712	−.1410	−.3176	.4028	0.7996
.39	.6517	.3483	.3697	−.1442	−.3135	.4107	0.7803
.40	.6554	.3446	.3683	−.1473	−.3094	.4184	0.7607
.41	.6591	.3409	.3668	−.1504	−.3051	.4259	0.7408
.42	.6628	.3372	.3653	−.1534	−.3008	.4332	0.7206
.43	.6664	.3336	.3637	−.1564	−.2965	.4403	0.7001
.44	.6700	.3300	.3621	−.1593	−.2920	.4472	0.6793
.45	.6736	.3264	.3605	−.1622	−.2875	.4539	0.6583
.46	.6772	.3228	.3589	−.1651	−.2830	.4603	0.6371
.47	.6808	.3192	.3572	−.1679	−.2783	.4666	0.6156
.48	.6844	.3156	.3555	−.1707	−.2736	.4727	0.5940
.49	.6879	.3121	.3538	−.1734	−.2689	.4785	0.5721
.50	.6915	.3085	.3521	−.1760	−.2641	.4841	0.5501

NORMAL DISTRIBUTION AND RELATED FUNCTIONS

x	$F(x)$	$1 - F(x)$	$f(x)$	$f'(x)$	$f''(x)$	$f'''(x)$	$f^{iv}(x)$
.50	.6915	.3085	.3521	−.1760	−.2641	.4841	.5501
.51	.6950	.3050	.3503	−.1787	−.2592	.4895	.5279
.52	.6985	.3015	.3485	−.1812	−.2543	.4947	.5056
.53	.7019	.2981	.3467	−.1837	−.2493	.4996	.4831
.54	.7054	.2946	.3448	−.1862	−.2443	.5043	.4605
.55	.7088	.2912	.3429	−.1886	−.2392	.5088	.4378
.56	.7123	.2877	.3410	−.1920	−.2341	.5131	.4150
.57	.7157	.2843	.3391	−.1933	−.2289	.5171	.3921
.58	.7190	.2810	.3372	−.1956	−.2238	.5209	.3691
.59	.7224	.2776	.3352	−.1978	−.2185	.5245	.3461
.60	.7257	.2743	.3332	−.1999	−.2133	.5278	.3231
.61	.7291	.2709	.3312	−.2020	−.2080	.5309	.3000
.62	.7324	.2676	.3292	−.2041	−.2027	.5338	.2770
.63	.7357	.2643	.3271	−.2061	−.1973	.5365	.2539
.64	.7389	.2611	.3251	−.2080	−.1919	.5389	.2309
.65	.7422	.2578	.3230	−.2099	−.1865	.5411	.2078
.66	.7454	.2546	.3209	−.2118	−.1811	.5431	.1849
.67	.7486	.2514	.3187	−.2136	−.1757	.5448	.1620
.68	.7517	.2483	.3166	−.2153	−.1702	.5463	.1391
.69	.7549	.2451	.3144	−.2170	−.1647	.5476	.1164
.70	.7580	.2420	.3123	−.2186	−.1593	.5486	.0937
.71	.7611	.2389	.3101	−.2201	−.1538	.5495	.0712
.72	.7642	.2358	.3079	−.2217	−.1483	.5501	.0487
.73	.7673	.2327	.3056	−.2231	−.1428	.5504	.0265
.74	.7704	.2296	.3034	−.2245	−.1373	.5506	.0043
.75	.7734	.2266	.3011	−.2259	−.1318	.5505	−.0176
.76	.7764	.2236	.2989	−.2271	−.1262	.5502	−.0394
.77	.7794	.2206	.2966	−.2284	−.1207	.5497	−.0611
.78	.7823	.2177	.2943	−.2296	−.1153	.5490	−.0825
.79	.7852	.2148	.2920	−.2307	−.1098	.5481	−.1037
.80	.7881	.2119	.2897	−.2318	−.1043	.5469	−.1247
.81	.7910	.2090	.2874	−.2328	−.0988	.5456	−.1455
.82	.7939	.2061	.2850	−.2337	−.0934	.5440	−.1660
.83	.7967	.2033	.2827	−.2346	−.0880	.5423	−.1862
.84	.7995	.2005	.2803	−.2355	−.0825	.5403	−.2063
.85	.8023	.1977	.2780	−.2363	−.0771	.5381	−.2260
.86	.8051	.1949	.2756	−.2370	−.0718	.5358	−.2455
.87	.8078	.1922	.2732	−.2377	−.0664	.5332	−.2646
.88	.8106	.1894	.2709	−.2384	−.0611	.5305	−.2835
.89	.8133	.1867	.2685	−.2389	−.0558	.5276	−.3021
.90	.8159	.1841	.2661	−.2395	−.0506	.5245	−.3203
.91	.8186	.1814	.2637	−.2400	−.0453	.5212	−.3383
.92	.8212	.1788	.2613	−.2404	−.0401	.5177	−.3559
.93	.8238	.1762	.2589	−.2408	−.0350	.5140	−.3731
.94	.8264	.1736	.2565	−.2411	−.0299	.5102	−.3901
.95	.8289	.1711	.2541	−.2414	−.0248	.5062	−.4066
.96	.8315	.1685	.2516	−.2416	−.0197	.5021	−.4228
.97	.8340	.1660	.2492	−.2417	−.0147	.4978	−.4387
.98	.8365	.1635	.2468	−.2419	−.0098	.4933	−.4541
.99	.8389	.1611	.2444	−.2420	−.0049	.4887	−.4692
1.00	.8413	.1587	.2420	−.2420	.0000	.4839	−.4839

NORMAL DISTRIBUTION AND RELATED FUNCTIONS

x	$F(x)$	$1 - F(x)$	$f(x)$	$f'(x)$	$f''(x)$	$f'''(x)$	$f^{iv}(x)$
1.00	.8413	.1587	.2420	−.2420	.0000	.4839	−.4839
1.01	.8438	.1562	.2396	−.2420	.0048	.4790	−.4983
1.02	.8461	.1539	.2371	−.2419	.0096	.4740	−.5122
1.03	.8485	.1515	.2347	−.2418	.0143	.4688	−.5257
1.04	.8508	.1492	.2323	−.2416	.0190	.4635	−.5389
1.05	.8531	.1469	.2299	−.2414	.0236	.4580	−.5516
1.06	.8554	.1446	.2275	−.2411	.0281	.4524	−.5639
1.07	.8577	.1423	.2251	−.2408	.0326	.4467	−.5758
1.08	.8599	.1401	.2227	−.2405	.0371	.4409	−.5873
1.09	.8621	.1379	.2203	−.2401	.0414	.4350	−.5984
1.10	.8643	.1357	.2179	−.2396	.0458	.4290	−.6091
1.11	.8665	.1335	.2155	−.2392	.0500	.4228	−.6193
1.12	.8686	.1314	.2131	−.2386	.0542	.4166	−.6292
1.13	.8708	.1292	.2107	−.2381	.0583	.4102	−.6386
1.14	.8729	.1271	.2083	−.2375	.0624	.4038	−.6476
1.15	.8749	.1251	.2059	−.2368	.0664	.3973	−.6561
1.16	.8770	.1230	.2036	−.2361	.0704	.3907	−.6643
1.17	.8790	.1210	.2012	−.2354	.0742	.3840	−.6720
1.18	.8810	.1190	.1989	−.2347	.0780	.3772	−.6792
1.19	.8830	.1170	.1965	−.2339	.0818	.3704	−.6861
1.20	.8849	.1151	.1942	−.2330	.0854	.3635	−.6926
1.21	.8869	.1131	.1919	−.2322	.0890	.3566	−.6986
1.22	.8888	.1112	.1895	−.2312	.0926	.3496	−.7042
1.23	.8907	.1093	.1872	−.2303	.0960	.3425	−.7094
1.24	.8925	.1075	.1849	−.2293	.0994	.3354	−.7141
1.25	.8944	.1056	.1826	−.2283	.1027	.3282	−.7185
1.26	.8962	.1038	.1804	−.2273	.1060	.3210	−.7224
1.27	.8980	.1020	.1781	−.2262	.1092	.3138	−.7259
1.28	.8997	.1003	.1758	−.2251	.1123	.3065	−.7291
1.29	.9015	.0985	.1736	−.2240	.1153	.2992	−.7318
1.30	.9032	.0968	.1714	−.2228	.1182	.2918	−.7341
1.31	.9049	.0951	.1691	−.2216	.1211	.2845	−.7361
1.32	.9066	.0934	.1669	−.2204	.1239	.2771	−.7376
1.33	.9082	.0918	.1647	−.2191	.1267	.2697	−.7388
1.34	.9099	.0901	.1626	−.2178	.1293	.2624	−.7395
1.35	.9115	.0885	.1604	−.2165	.1319	.2550	−.7399
1.36	.9131	.0869	.1582	−.2152	.1344	.2476	−.7400
1.37	.9147	.0853	.1561	−.2138	.1369	.2402	−.7396
1.38	.9162	.0838	.1539	−.2125	.1392	.2328	−.7389
1.39	.9177	.0823	.1518	−.2110	.1415	.2254	−.7378
1.40	.9192	.0808	.1497	−.2096	.1437	.2180	−.7364
1.41	.9207	.0793	.1476	−.2082	.1459	.2107	−.7347
1.42	.9222	.0778	.1456	−.2067	.1480	.2033	−.7326
1.43	.9236	.0764	.1435	−.2052	.1500	.1960	−.7301
1.44	.9251	.0749	.1415	−.2037	.1519	.1887	−.7274
1.45	.9265	.0735	.1394	−.2022	.1537	.1815	−.7243
1.46	.9279	.0721	.1374	−.2006	.1555	.1742	−.7209
1.47	.9292	.0708	.1354	−.1991	.1572	.1670	−.7172
1.48	.9306	.0694	.1334	−.1975	.1588	.1599	−.7132
1.49	.9319	.0681	.1315	−.1959	.1604	.1528	−.7089
1.50	.9332	.0668	.1295	−.1943	.1619	.1457	−.7043

NORMAL DISTRIBUTION AND RELATED FUNCTIONS

x	$F(x)$	$1 - F(x)$	$f(x)$	$f'(x)$	$f''(x)$	$f'''(x)$	$f^{iv}(x)$
1.50	.9332	.0668	.1295	−.1943	.1619	.1457	−.7043
1.51	.9345	.0655	.1276	−.1927	.1633	.1387	−.6994
1.52	.9357	.0643	.1257	−.1910	.1647	.1317	−.6942
1.53	.9370	.0630	.1238	−.1894	.1660	.1248	−.6888
1.54	.9382	.0618	.1219	−.1877	.1672	.1180	−.6831
1.55	.9394	.0606	.1200	−.1860	.1683	.1111	−.6772
1.56	.9406	.0594	.1182	−.1843	.1694	.1044	−.6710
1.57	.9418	.0582	.1163	−.1826	.1704	.0977	−.6646
1.58	.9429	.0571	.1145	−.1809	.1714	.0911	−.6580
1.59	.9441	.0559	.1127	−.1792	.1722	.0846	−.6511
1.60	.9452	.0548	.1109	−.1775	.1730	.0781	−.6441
1.61	.9463	.0537	.1092	−.1757	.1738	.0717	−.6368
1.62	.9474	.0526	.1074	−.1740	.1745	.0654	−.6293
1.63	.9484	.0516	.1057	−.1723	.1751	.0591	−.6216
1.64	.9495	.0505	.1040	−.1705	.1757	.0529	−.6138
1.65	.9505	.0495	.1023	−.1687	.1762	.0468	−.6057
1.66	.9515	.0485	.1006	−.1670	.1766	.0408	−.5975
1.67	.9525	.0475	.0989	−.1652	.1770	.0349	−.5891
1.68	.9535	.0465	.0973	−.1634	.1773	.0290	−.5806
1.69	.9545	.0455	.0957	−.1617	.1776	.0233	−.5720
1.70	.9554	.0446	.0940	−.1599	.1778	.0176	−.5632
1.71	.9564	.0436	.0925	−.1581	.1779	.0120	−.5542
1.72	.9573	.0427	.0909	−.1563	.1780	.0065	−.5452
1.73	.9582	.0418	.0893	−.1546	.1780	.0011	−.5360
1.74	.9591	.0409	.0878	−.1528	.1780	−.0042	−.5267
1.75	.9599	.0401	.0863	−.1510	.1780	−.0094	−.5173
1.76	.9608	.0392	.0848	−.1492	.1778	−.0146	−.5079
1.77	.9616	.0384	.0833	−.1474	.1777	−.0196	−.4983
1.78	.9625	.0375	.0818	−.1457	.1774	−.0245	−.4887
1.79	.9633	.0367	.0804	−.1439	.1772	−.0294	−.4789
1.80	.9641	.0359	.0790	−.1421	.1769	−.0341	−.4692
1.81	.9649	.0351	.0775	−.1403	.1765	−.0388	−.4593
1.82	.9656	.0344	.0761	−.1386	.1761	−.0433	−.4494
1.83	.9664	.0336	.0748	−.1368	.1756	−.0477	−.4395
1.84	.9671	.0329	.0734	−.1351	.1751	−.0521	−.4295
1.85	.9678	.0322	.0721	−.1333	.1746	−.0563	−.4195
1.86	.9686	.0314	.0707	−.1316	.1740	−.0605	−.4095
1.87	.9693	.0307	.0694	−.1298	.1734	−.0645	−.3995
1.88	.9699	.0301	.0681	−.1281	.1727	−.0685	−.3894
1.89	.9706	.0294	.0669	−.1264	.1720	−.0723	−.3793
1.90	.9713	.0287	.0656	−.1247	.1713	−.0761	−.3693
1.91	.9719	.0281	.0644	−.1230	.1705	−.0797	−.3592
1.92	.9726	.0274	.0632	−.1213	.1697	−.0832	−.3492
1.93	.9732	.0268	.0620	−.1196	.1688	−.0867	−.3392
1.94	.9738	.0262	.0608	−.1179	.1679	−.0900	−.3292
1.95	.9744	.0256	.0596	−.1162	.1670	−.0933	−.3192
1.96	.9750	.0250	.0584	−.1145	.1661	−.0964	−.3093
1.97	.9756	.0244	.0573	−.1129	.1651	−.0994	−.2994
1.98	.9761	.0239	.0562	−.1112	.1641	−.1024	−.2895
1.99	.9767	.0233	.0551	−.1096	.1630	−.1052	−.2797
2.00	.9772	.0228	.0540	−.1080	.1620	−.1080	−.2700

NORMAL DISTRIBUTION AND RELATED FUNCTIONS

x	$F(x)$	$1 - F(x)$	$f(x)$	$f'(x)$	$f''(x)$	$f'''(x)$	$f^{iv}(x)$
2.00	.9773	.0227	.0540	−.1080	.1620	−.1080	−.2700
2.01	.9778	.0222	.0529	−.1064	.1609	−.1106	−.2603
2.02	.9783	.0217	.0519	−.1048	.1598	−.1132	−.2506
2.03	.9788	.0212	.0508	−.1032	.1586	−.1157	−.2411
2.04	.9793	.0207	.0498	−.1016	.1575	−.1180	−.2316
2.05	.9798	.0202	.0488	−.1000	.1563	−.1203	−.2222
2.06	.9803	.0197	.0478	−.0985	.1550	−.1225	−.2129
2.07	.9808	.0192	.0468	−.0969	.1538	−.1245	−.2036
2.08	.9812	.0188	.0459	−.0954	.1526	−.1265	−.1945
2.09	.9817	.0183	.0449	−.0939	.1513	−.1284	−.1854
2.10	.9821	.0179	.0440	−.0924	.1500	−.1302	−.1765
2.11	.9826	.0174	.0431	−.0909	.1487	−.1320	−.1676
2.12	.9830	.0170	.0422	−.0894	.1474	−.1336	−.1588
2.13	.9834	.0166	.0413	−.0879	.1460	−.1351	−.1502
2.14	.9838	.0162	.0404	−.0865	.1446	−.1366	−.1416
2.15	.9842	.0158	.0396	−.0850	.1433	−.1380	−.1332
2.16	.9846	.0154	.0387	−.0836	.1419	−.1393	−.1249
2.17	.9850	.0150	.0379	−.0822	.1405	−.1405	−.1167
2.18	.9854	.0146	.0371	−.0808	.1391	−.1416	−.1086
2.19	.9857	.0143	.0363	−.0794	.1377	−.1426	−.1006
2.20	.9861	.0139	.0355	−.0780	.1362	−.1436	−.0927
2.21	.9864	.0136	.0347	−.0767	.1348	−.1445	−.0850
2.22	.9868	.0132	.0339	−.0754	.1333	−.1453	−.0774
2.23	.9871	.0129	.0332	−.0740	.1319	−.1460	−.0700
2.24	.9875	.0125	.0325	−.0727	.1304	.1467	.0626
2.25	.9878	.0122	.0317	−.0714	.1289	−.1473	−.0554
2.26	.9881	.0119	.0310	−.0701	.1275	−.1478	−.0484
2.27	.9884	.0116	.0303	−.0689	.1260	−.1483	−.0414
2.28	.9887	.0113	.0297	−.0676	.1245	−.1486	−.0346
2.29	.9890	.0110	.0290	−.0664	.1230	−.1490	−.0279
2.30	.9893	.0107	.0283	−.0652	.1215	−.1492	−.0214
2.31	.9896	.0104	.0277	−.0639	.1200	−.1494	−.0150
2.32	.9898	.0102	.0270	−.0628	.1185	−.1495	−.0088
2.33	.9901	.0099	.0264	−.0616	.1170	−.1496	−.0027
2.34	.9904	.0096	.0258	−.0604	.1155	−.1496	.0033
2.35	.9006	.0094	.0252	−.0593	.1141	−.1495	.0092
2.36	.9909	.0091	.0246	−.0581	.1126	−.1494	.0149
2.37	.9911	.0089	.0241	−.0570	.1111	−.1492	.0204
2.38	.9913	.0087	.0235	−.0559	.1096	−.1490	.0258
2.39	.9916	.0084	.0229	−.0548	.1081	−.1487	.0311
2.40	.9918	.0082	.0224	−.0538	.1066	−.1483	.0362
2.41	.9920	.0080	.0219	−.0527	.1051	−.1480	.0412
2.42	.9922	.0078	.0213	−.0516	.1036	−.1475	.0461
2.43	.9925	.0075	.0208	−.0506	.1022	−.1470	.0508
2.44	.9927	.0073	.0203	−.0496	.1007	−.1465	.0554
2.45	.9929	.0071	.0198	−.0486	.0992	−.1459	.0598
2.46	.9931	.0069	.0194	−.0476	.0978	−.1453	.0641
2.47	.9932	.0068	.0189	−.0467	.0963	−.1446	.0683
2.48	.9934	.0066	.0184	−.0457	.0949	−.1439	.0723
2.49	.9936	.0064	.0180	−.0448	.0935	−.1432	.0762
2.50	.9938	.0062	.0175	−.0438	.0920	−.1424	.0800

NORMAL DISTRIBUTION AND RELATED FUNCTIONS

x	$F(x)$	$1 - F(x)$	$f(x)$	$f'(x)$	$f''(x)$	$f'''(x)$	$f^{iv}(x)$
2.50	.9938	.0062	.0175	−.0438	.0920	−.1424	.0800
2.51	.9940	.0060	.0171	−.0429	.0906	−.1416	.0836
2.52	.9941	.0059	.0167	−.0420	.0892	−.1408	.0871
2.53	.9943	.0057	.0163	−.0411	.0878	−.1399	.0905
2.54	.9945	.0055	.0158	−.0403	.0864	−.1389	.0937
2.55	.9946	.0054	.0155	−.0394	.0850	−.1380	.0968
2.56	.9948	.0052	.0151	−.0386	.0836	−.1370	.0998
2.57	.9949	.0051	.0147	−.0377	.0823	−.1360	.1027
2.58	.9951	.0049	.0143	−.0369	.0809	−.1350	.1054
2.59	.9952	.0048	.0139	−.0361	.0796	−.1339	.1080
2.60	.9953	.0047	.0136	−.0353	.0782	−.1328	.1105
2.61	.9955	.0045	.0132	−.0345	.0769	−.1317	.1129
2.62	.9956	.0044	.0129	−.0338	.0756	−.1305	.1152
2.63	.9957	.0043	.0126	−.0330	.0743	−.1294	.1173
2.64	.9959	.0041	.0122	−.0323	.0730	−.1282	.1194
2.65	.9960	.0040	.0119	−.0316	.0717	−.1270	.1213
2.66	.9961	.0039	.0116	−.0309	.0705	−.1258	.1231
2.67	.9962	.0038	.0113	−.0302	.0692	−.1245	.1248
2.68	.9963	.0037	.0110	−.0295	.0680	−.1233	.1264
2.69	.9964	.0036	.0107	−.0288	.0668	−.1220	.1279
2.70	.9965	.0035	.0104	−.0281	.0656	−.1207	.1293
2.71	.9966	.0034	.0101	−.0275	.0644	−.1194	.1306
2.72	.9967	.0033	.0099	−.0269	.0632	−.1181	.1317
2.73	.9968	.0032	.0096	−.0262	.0620	−.1168	.1328
2.74	.9969	.0031	.0093	−.0256	.0608	−.1154	.1338
2.75	.9970	.0030	.0091	−.0250	.0597	−.1141	.1347
2.76	.9971	.0029	.0088	−.0244	.0585	−.1127	.1356
2.77	.9972	.0028	.0086	−.0238	.0574	−.1114	.1363
2.78	.9973	.0027	.0084	−.0233	.0563	−.1100	.1369
2.79	.9974	.0026	.0081	−.0227	.0552	−.1087	.1375
2.80	.9974	.0026	.0079	−.0222	.0541	−.1073	.1379
2.81	.9975	.0025	.0077	−.0216	.0531	−.1059	.1383
2.82	.9976	.0024	.0075	−.0211	.0520	−.1045	.1386
2.83	.9977	.0023	.0073	−.0206	.0510	−.1031	.1389
2.84	.9977	.0023	.0071	−.0201	.0500	−.1017	.1390
2.85	.9978	.0022	.0069	−.0196	.0490	−.1003	.1391
2.86	.9979	.0021	.0067	−.0191	.0480	−.0990	.1391
2.87	.9979	.0021	.0065	−.0186	.0470	−.0976	.1391
2.88	.9980	.0020	.0063	−.0182	.0460	−.0962	.1389
2.89	.9981	.0019	.0061	−.0177	.0451	−.0948	.1388
2.90	.9981	.0019	.0060	−.0173	.0441	−.0934	.1385
2.91	.9982	.0018	.0058	−.0168	.0432	−.0920	.1382
2.92	.9982	.0018	.0056	−.0164	.0423	−.0906	.1378
2.93	.9983	.0017	.0055	−.0160	.0414	−.0893	.1374
2.94	.9984	.0016	.0053	−.0156	.0405	−.0879	.1369
2.95	.9984	.0016	.0051	−.0152	.0396	−.0865	.1364
2.96	.9985	.0015	.0050	−.0148	.0388	−.0852	.1358
2.97	.9985	.0015	.0048	−.0144	.0379	−.0838	.1352
2.98	.9986	.0014	.0047	−.0140	.0371	−.0825	.1345
2.99	.9986	.0014	.0046	−.0137	.0363	−.0811	.1337
3.00	.9987	.0013	.0044	−.0133	.0355	−.0798	.1330

NORMAL DISTRIBUTION AND RELATED FUNCTIONS

x	$F(x)$	$1 - F(x)$	$f(x)$	$f'(x)$	$f''(x)$	$f'''(x)$	$f^{iv}(x)$
3.00	.9987	.0013	.0044	−.0133	.0355	−.0798	.1330
3.01	.9987	.0013	.0043	−.0130	.0347	−.0785	.1321
3.02	.9987	.0013	.0042	−.0126	.0339	−.0771	.1313
3.03	.9988	.0012	.0040	−.0123	.0331	−.0758	.1304
3.04	.9988	.0012	.0039	−.0119	.0324	−.0745	.1294
3.05	.9989	.0011	.0038	−.0116	.0316	−.0732	.1285
3.06	.9989	.0011	.0037	−.0113	.0309	−.0720	.1275
3.07	.9989	.0011	.0036	−.0110	.0302	−.0707	.1264
3.08	.9990	.0010	.0035	−.0107	.0295	−.0694	.1254
3.09	.9990	.0010	.0034	−.0104	.0288	−.0682	.1243
3.10	.9990	.0010	.0033	−.0101	.0281	−.0669	.1231
3.11	.9991	.0009	.0032	−.0099	.0275	−.0657	.1220
3.12	.9991	.0009	.0031	−.0096	.0268	−.0645	.1208
3.13	.9991	.0009	.0030	−.0093	.0262	−.0633	.1196
3.14	.9992	.0008	.0029	−.0091	.0256	−.0621	.1184
3.15	.9992	.0008	.0028	−.0088	.0249	−.0609	.1171
3.16	.9992	.0008	.0027	−.0086	.0243	−.0598	.1159
3.17	.9992	.0008	.0026	−.0083	.0237	−.0586	.1146
3.18	.9993	.0007	.0025	−.0081	.0232	−.0575	.1133
3.19	.9993	.0007	.0025	−.0079	.0226	−.0564	.1120
3.20	.9993	.0007	.0024	−.0076	.0220	−.0552	.1107
3.21	.9993	.0007	.0023	−.0074	.0215	−.0541	.1093
3.22	.9994	.0006	.0022	−.0072	.0210	−.0531	.1080
3.23	.9994	.0006	.0022	−.0070	.0204	−.0520	.1066
3.24	.9994	.0006	.0021	−.0068	.0199	−.0509	.1053
3.25	.9994	.0006	.0020	−.0066	.0194	−.0499	.1039
3.26	.9994	.0006	.0020	−.0064	.0189	−.0488	.1025
3.27	.9995	.0005	.0019	−.0062	.0184	−.0478	.1011
3.28	.9995	.0005	.0018	−.0060	.0180	−.0468	.0997
3.29	.9995	.0005	.0018	−.0059	.0175	−.0458	.0983
3.30	.9995	.0005	.0017	−.0057	.0170	−.0449	.0969
3.31	.9995	.0005	.0017	−.0055	.0166	−.0439	.0955
3.32	.9995	.0005	.0016	−.0054	.0162	−.0429	.0941
3.33	.9996	.0004	.0016	−.0052	.0157	−.0420	.0927
3.34	.9996	.0004	.0015	−.0050	.0153	−.0411	.0913
3.35	.9996	.0004	.0015	−.0049	.0149	−.0402	.0899
3.36	.9996	.0004	.0014	−.0047	.0145	−.0393	.0885
3.37	.9996	.0004	.0014	−.0046	.0141	−.0384	.0871
3.38	.9996	.0004	.0013	−.0045	.0138	−.0376	.0857
3.39	.9997	.0003	.0013	−.0043	.0134	−.0367	.0843
3.40	.9997	.0003	.0012	−.0042	.0130	−.0359	.0829
3.41	.9997	.0003	.0012	−.0041	.0127	−.0350	.0815
3.42	.9997	.0003	.0012	−.0039	.0123	−.0342	.0801
3.43	.9997	.0003	.0011	−.0038	.0120	−.0334	.0788
3.44	.9997	.0003	.0011	−.0037	.0116	−.0327	.0774
3.45	.9997	.0003	.0010	−.0036	.0113	−.0319	.0761
3.46	.9997	.0003	.0010	−.0035	.0110	−.0311	.0747
3.47	.9997	.0003	.0010	−.0034	.0107	−.0304	.0734
3.48	.9997	.0003	.0009	−.0033	.0104	−.0297	.0721
3.49	.9998	.0002	.0009	−.0032	.0101	−.0290	.0707
3.50	.9998	.0002	.0009	−.0031	.0098	−.0283	.0694

NORMAL DISTRIBUTION AND RELATED FUNCTIONS

x	$F(x)$	$1 - F(x)$	$f(x)$	$f'(x)$	$f''(x)$	$f'''(x)$	$f^{iv}(x)$
3.50	.9998	.0002	.0009	−.0031	.0098	−.0283	.0694
3.51	.9998	.0002	.0008	−.0030	.0095	−.0276	.0681
3.52	.9998	.0002	.0008	−.0029	.0093	−.0269	.0669
3.53	.9998	.0002	.0008	−.0028	.0090	−.0262	.0656
3.54	.9998	.0002	.0008	−.0027	.0087	−.0256	.0643
3.55	.9998	.0002	.0007	−.0026	.0085	−.0249	.0631
3.56	.9998	.0002	.0007	−.0025	.0082	−.0243	.0618
3.57	.9998	.0002	.0007	−.0024	.0080	−.0237	.0606
3.58	.9998	.0002	.0007	−.0024	.0078	−.0231	.0594
3.59	.9998	.0002	.0006	−.0023	.0075	−.0225	.0582
3.60	.9998	.0002	.0006	−.0022	.0073	−.0219	.0570
3.61	.9998	.0002	.0006	−.0021	.0071	−.0214	.0559
3.62	.9999	.0001	.0006	−.0021	.0069	−.0208	.0547
3.63	.9999	.0001	.0005	−.0020	.0067	−.0203	.0536
3.64	.9999	.0001	.0005	−.0019	.0065	−.0198	.0524
3.65	.9999	.0001	.0005	−.0019	.0063	−.0192	.0513
3.66	.9999	.0001	.0005	−.0018	.0061	−.0187	.0502
3.67	.9999	.0001	.0005	−.0017	.0059	−.0182	.0492
3.68	.9999	.0001	.0005	−.0017	.0057	−.0177	.0481
3.69	.9999	.0001	.0004	−.0016	.0056	−.0173	.0470
3.70	.9999	.0001	.0004	−.0016	.0054	−.0168	.0460
3.71	.9999	.0001	.0004	−.0015	.0052	−.0164	.0450
3.72	.9999	.0001	.0004	−.0015	.0051	−.0159	.0440
3.73	.9999	.0001	.0004	−.0014	.0049	−.0155	.0430
3.74	.9999	.0001	.0004	−.0014	.0048	−.0150	.0420
3.75	.9999	.0001	.0004	−.0013	.0046	−.0146	.0410
3.76	.9999	.0001	.0003	−.0013	.0045	−.0142	.0401
3.77	.9999	.0001	.0003	−.0012	.0043	−.0138	.0392
3.78	.9999	.0001	.0003	−.0012	.0042	−.0134	.0382
3.79	.9999	.0001	.0003	−.0012	.0041	−.0131	.0373
3.80	.9999	.0001	.0003	−.0011	.0039	−.0127	.0365
3.81	.9999	.0001	.0003	−.0011	.0038	−.0123	.0356
3.82	.9999	.0001	.0003	−.0010	.0037	−.0120	.0347
3.83	.9999	.0001	.0003	−.0010	.0036	−.0116	.0339
3.84	.9999	.0001	.0003	−.0010	.0034	−.0113	.0331
3.85	.9999	.0001	.0002	−.0009	.0033	−.0110	.0323
3.86	.9999	.0001	.0002	−.0009	.0032	−.0107	.0315
3.87	.9999	.0001	.0002	−.0009	.0031	−.0104	.0307
3.88	.9999	.0001	.0002	−.0008	.0030	−.0100	.0299
3.89	1.0000	.0000	.0002	−.0008	.0029	−.0098	.0292
3.90	1.0000	.0000	.0002	−.0008	.0028	−.0095	.0284
3.91	1.0000	.0000	.0002	−.0008	.0027	−.0092	.0277
3.92	1.0000	.0000	.0002	−.0007	.0026	−.0089	.0270
3.93	1.0000	.0000	.0002	−.0007	.0026	−.0086	.0263
3.94	1.0000	.0000	.0002	−.0007	.0025	−.0084	.0256
3.95	1.0000	.0000	.0002	−.0006	.0024	−.0081	.0250
3.96	1.0000	.0000	.0002	−.0006	.0023	−.0079	.0243
3.97	1.0000	.0000	.0002	−.0006	.0022	−.0076	.0237
3.98	1.0000	.0000	.0001	−.0006	.0022	−.0074	.0230
3.99	1.0000	.0000	.0001	−.0006	.0021	−.0072	.0224
4.00	1.0000	.0000	.0001	−.0005	.0020	−.0070	.0218

x	1.282	1.645	1.960	2.326	2.576	3.090
$F(x)$	.90	.95	.975	.99	.995	.999
$2[1 - F(x)]$	.20	.10	.05	.02	.01	.002

II.2 TOLERANCE FACTORS FOR NORMAL DISTRIBUTIONS

This table gives factors K such that the probability is γ that at least a proportion P of the distribution will be included between $\bar{x} - Ks$ and $\bar{x} + Ks$, where $\bar{x}$ and s are estimates of the mean and standard deviation computed from a sample of size N. Values of K are given for $P = 0.75, 0.90, 0.95, 0.99, 0.999$ and $\gamma = 0.75, 0.90, 0.95, 0.99$ and for various values of N. For example, if $\bar{x} = 10.0$ and $s = 1.0$, $N = 16$, the interval $\bar{x} \pm Ks = 10.0 \pm 3.812(1.0) = 10.0 \pm 3.812$, or the interval 6.188 to 13.812 will contain 99% of the population with confidence coefficient 0.95. The values of K are computed assuming that the observations are from normal populations.

TOLERANCE FACTORS FOR NORMAL DISTRIBUTIONS

$\lambda = 0.75$

N \ P	0.75	0.90	0.95	0.99	0.999	N \ P	0.75	0.90	0.95	0.99	0.999
2	4.498	6.301	7.414	9.531	11.920	55	1.249	1.785	2.127	2.795	3.571
3	2.501	3.538	4.187	5.431	6.844	60	1.243	1.778	2.118	2.784	3.556
4	2.035	2.892	3.431	4.471	5.657	65	1.239	1.771	2.110	2.773	3.543
5	1.825	2.599	3.088	4.033	5.117	70	1.235	1.765	2.104	2.764	3.531
6	1.704	2.429	2.889	3.779	4.802	75	1.231	1.760	2.098	2.757	3.521
7	1.624	2.318	2.757	3.611	4.593	80	1.228	1.756	2.092	2.749	3.512
8	1.568	2.238	2.663	3.491	4.444	85	1.225	1.752	2.087	2.743	3.504
9	1.525	2.178	2.593	3.400	4.330	90	1.223	1.748	2.083	2.737	3.497
10	1.492	2.131	2.537	3.328	4.241	95	1.220	1.745	2.079	2.732	3.490
11	1.465	2.093	2.493	3.271	4.169	100	1.218	1.742	2.075	2.727	3.484
12	1.443	2.062	2.456	3.223	4.110	110	1.214	1.736	2.069	2.719	3.473
13	1.425	2.036	2.424	3.183	4.059	120	1.211	1.732	2.063	2.712	3.464
14	1.409	2.013	2.398	3.148	4.016	130	1.208	1.728	2.059	2.705	3.456
15	1.395	1.994	2.375	3.118	3.979	140	1.206	1.724	2.054	2.700	3.449
16	1.383	1.977	2.355	3.092	3.946	150	1.204	1.721	2.051	2.695	3.443
17	1.372	1.962	2.337	3.069	3.917	160	1.202	1.718	2.047	2.691	3.437
18	1.363	1.948	2.321	3.048	3.891	170	1.200	1.716	2.044	2.687	3.432
19	1.355	1.936	2.307	3.030	3.867	180	1.198	1.713	2.042	2.683	3.427
20	1.347	1.925	2.294	3.013	3.846	190	1.197	1.711	2.039	2.680	3.423
21	1.340	1.915	2.282	2.998	3.827	200	1.195	1.709	2.037	2.677	3.419
22	1.334	1.906	2.271	2.984	3.809	250	1.190	1.702	2.028	2.665	3.404
23	1.328	1.898	2.261	2.971	3.793	300	1.186	1.696	2.021	2.656	3.393
24	1.322	1.891	2.252	2.959	3.778	400	1.181	1.688	2.012	2.644	3.378
25	1.317	1.883	2.244	2.948	3.764	500	1.177	1.683	2.006	2.636	3.368
26	1.313	1.877	2.236	2.938	3.751	600	1.175	1.680	2.002	2.631	3.360
27	1.309	1.871	2.229	2.929	3.740	700	1.173	1.677	1.998	2.626	3.355
30	1.297	1.855	2.210	2.904	3.708	800	1.171	1.675	1.996	2.623	3.350
35	1.283	1.834	2.185	2.871	3.667	900	1.170	1.673	1.993	2.620	3.347
40	1.271	1.818	2.166	2.846	3.635	1000	1.169	1.671	1.992	2.617	3.344
45	1.262	1.805	2.150	2.826	3.609	∞	1.150	1.645	1.960	2.576	3.291
50	1.255	1.794	2.138	2.809	3.588						

TOLERANCE FACTORS FOR NORMAL DISTRIBUTIONS

λ = 0.90

N \ P	0.75	0.90	0.95	0.99	0.999	N \ P	0.75	0.90	0.95	0.99	0.999
2	11.407	15.978	18.800	24.167	30.227	55	1.329	1.901	2.265	2.976	3.801
3	4.132	5.847	6.919	8.974	11.309	60	1.320	1.887	2.248	2.955	3.774
4	2.932	4.166	4.943	6.440	8.149	65	1.312	1.875	2.235	2.937	3.751
5	2.454	3.494	4.152	5.423	6.879	70	1.304	1.865	2.222	2.920	3.730
6	2.196	3.131	3.723	4.870	6.188	75	1.298	1.856	2.211	2.906	3.712
7	2.034	2.902	3.452	4.521	5.750	80	1.292	1.848	2.202	2.894	3.696
8	1.921	2.743	3.264	4.278	5.446	85	1.287	1.841	2.193	2.882	3.682
9	1.839	2.626	3.125	4.098	5.220	90	1.283	1.834	2.185	2.872	3.669
10	1.775	2.535	3.018	3.950	5.046	95	1.278	1.828	2.178	2.863	3.657
11	1.724	2.463	2.933	3.849	4.906	100	1.275	1.822	2.172	2.854	3.646
12	1.683	2.404	2.863	3.758	4.792	110	1.268	1.813	2.160	2.839	3.626
13	1.648	2.355	2.805	3.682	4.697	120	1.262	1.804	2.150	2.826	3.610
14	1.619	2.314	2.756	3.618	4.615	130	1.257	1.797	2.141	2.814	3.595
15	1.594	2.278	2.713	3.562	4.545	140	1.252	1.791	2.134	2.804	3.582
16	1.572	2.246	2.676	3.514	4.484	150	1.248	1.785	2.127	2.795	3.571
17	1.552	2.219	2.643	3.471	4.430	160	1.245	1.780	2.121	2.787	3.561
18	1.535	2.194	2.614	3.433	4.382	170	1.242	1.775	2.116	2.780	3.552
19	1.520	2.172	2.588	3.399	4.339	180	1.239	1.771	2.111	2.774	3.543
20	1.506	2.152	2.564	3.368	4.300	190	1.236	1.767	2.106	2.768	3.536
21	1.493	2.135	2.543	3.340	4.264	200	1.234	1.764	2.102	2.762	3.429
22	1.482	2.118	2.524	3.315	4.232	250	1.224	1.750	2.085	2.740	3.501
23	1.471	2.103	2.506	3.292	4.203	300	1.217	1.740	2.073	2.725	3.481
24	1.462	2.089	2.489	3.270	4.176	400	1.207	1.726	2.057	2.703	3.453
25	1.453	2.077	2.474	3.251	4.151	500	1.201	1.717	2.046	2.689	3.434
26	1.444	2.065	2.460	3.232	4.127	600	1.196	1.710	2.038	2.678	3.421
27	1.437	2.054	2.447	3.215	4.106	700	1.192	1.705	2.032	2.670	3.411
30	1.417	2.025	2.413	3.170	4.049	800	1.189	1.701	2.027	2.663	3.402
35	1.390	1.988	2.368	3.112	3.974	900	1.187	1.697	2.023	2.658	3.396
40	1.370	1.959	2.334	3.066	3.917	1000	1.185	1.695	2.019	2.654	3.390
45	1.354	1.935	2.306	3.030	3.871	∞	1.150	1.645	1.960	2.576	3.291
50	1.340	1.916	2.284	3.001	3.833						

TOLERANCE FACTORS FOR NORMAL DISTRIBUTIONS

$\lambda = 0.95$

N \ P	0.75	0.90	0.95	0.99	0.999	N \ P	0.75	0.90	0.95	0.99	0.999
2	22.858	32.019	37.674	48.430	60.573	55	1.382	1.976	2.354	3.094	3.951
3	5.922	8.380	9.916	12.861	16.208	60	1.369	1.958	2.333	3.066	3.916
4	3.779	5.369	6.370	8.299	10.502	65	1.359	1.943	2.315	3.042	3.886
5	3.002	4.275	5.079	6.634	8.415	70	1.349	1.929	2.299	3.021	3.859
6	2.604	3.712	4.414	5.775	7.337	75	1.341	1.917	2.285	3.002	3.835
7	2.361	3.369	4.007	5.248	6.676	80	1.334	1.907	2.272	2.986	3.814
8	2.197	3.136	3.732	4.891	6.226	85	1.327	1.897	2.261	2.971	3.795
9	2.078	2.967	3.532	4.631	5.899	90	1.321	1.889	2.251	2.958	3.778
10	1.987	2.839	3.379	4.433	5.649	95	1.315	1.881	2.241	2.945	3.763
11	1.916	2.737	3.259	4.277	5.452	100	1.311	1.874	2.233	2.934	3.748
12	1.858	2.655	3.162	4.150	5.291	110	1.302	1.861	2.218	2.915	3.723
13	1.810	2.587	3.081	4.044	5.158	120	1.294	1.850	2.205	2.898	3.702
14	1.770	2.529	3.012	3.955	5.045	130	1.288	1.841	2.194	2.883	3.683
15	1.735	2.480	2.954	3.878	4.949	140	1.282	1.833	2.184	2.870	3.666
16	1.705	2.437	2.903	3.812	4.865	150	1.277	1.825	1.175	2.859	3.652
17	1.679	2.400	2.858	3.754	4.791	160	1.272	1.819	2.167	2.848	3.638
18	1.655	2.366	2.819	3.702	4.725	170	1.268	1.813	2.160	2.839	3.627
19	1.635	2.337	2.784	3.656	4.667	180	1.264	1.808	2.154	2.831	3.616
20	1.616	2.310	2.752	3.615	4.614	190	1.261	1.803	2.148	2.823	3.606
21	1.599	2.286	2.723	3.577	4.567	200	1.258	1.798	2.143	2.816	3.597
22	1.584	2.264	2.697	3.543	4.523	250	1.245	1.780	2.121	2.788	3.561
23	1.570	2.244	2.673	3.512	4.484	300	1.236	1.767	2.106	2.767	3.535
24	1.557	2.225	2.651	3.483	4.447	400	1.223	1.749	2.084	2.739	3.499
25	1.545	2.208	2.631	3.457	4.413	500	1.215	1.737	2.070	2.721	3.475
26	1.534	2.193	2.612	3.432	4.382	600	1.209	1.729	2.060	2.707	3.458
27	1.523	2.178	2.595	3.409	4.353	700	1.204	1.722	2.052	2.697	3.445
30	1.497	2.140	2.549	3.350	4.278	800	1.201	1.717	2.046	2.688	3.434
35	1.462	2.090	2.490	3.272	4.179	900	1.198	1.712	2.040	2.682	3.426
40	1.435	2.052	2.445	3.213	4.104	1000	1.195	1.709	2.036	2.676	3.418
45	1.414	2.021	2.408	3.165	4.042	∞	1.150	1.645	1.960	2.576	3.291
50	1.396	1.996	2.379	3.126	3.993						

TOLERANCE FACTORS FOR NORMAL DISTRIBUTIONS

$\lambda = 0.99$

N \ P	0.75	0.90	0.95	0.99	0.999	N \ P	0.75	0.90	0.95	0.99	0.999
2	114.363	160.193	188.491	242.300	303.054	55	1.490	2.130	2.538	3.335	4.260
3	13.378	18.930	22.401	29.055	36.616	60	1.471	2.103	2.506	3.293	4.206
4	6.614	9.398	11.150	14.527	18.383	65	1.455	2.080	2.478	3.257	4.160
5	4.643	6.612	7.855	10.260	13.015	70	1.440	2.060	2.454	3.225	4.120
6	3.743	5.337	6.345	8.301	10.548	75	1.428	2.042	2.433	3.197	4.084
7	3.233	4.613	5.488	7.187	9.142	80	1.417	2.026	2.414	3.173	4.053
8	2.905	4.147	4.936	6.468	8.234	85	1.407	2.012	2.397	3.150	4.024
9	2.677	3.822	4.550	5.966	7.600	90	1.398	1.999	2.382	3.130	3.999
10	2.508	3.582	4.265	5.594	7.129	95	1.390	1.987	2.368	3.112	3.976
11	2.378	3.397	4.045	5.308	6.766	100	1.383	1.977	2.355	3.096	3.954
12	2.274	3.250	3.870	5.079	6.477	110	1.369	1.958	2.333	3.066	3.917
13	2.190	3.130	3.727	4.893	6.240	120	1.358	1.942	2.314	3.041	3.885
14	2.120	3.029	3.608	4.737	6.043	130	1.349	1.928	2.298	3.019	3.857
15	2.060	2.945	3.507	4.605	5.876	140	1.340	1.916	2.283	3.000	3.833
16	2.009	2.872	3.421	4.492	5.732	150	1.332	1.905	2.270	2.983	3.811
17	1.965	2.808	3.345	4.393	5.607	160	1.326	1.896	2.259	2.968	3.792
18	1.926	2.753	3.270	4.307	5.497	170	1.320	1.887	2.248	2.955	3.774
19	1.891	2.703	3.221	4.230	5.399	180	1.314	1.879	2.239	2.942	3.759
20	1.860	2.659	3.168	4.161	5.312	190	1.309	1.872	2.230	2.931	3.744
21	1.833	2.620	3.121	4.100	5.234	200	1.304	1.865	2.222	2.921	3.731
22	1.808	2.584	3.078	4.044	5.163	250	1.286	1.839	2.191	2.880	3.678
23	1.785	2.551	3.040	3.993	5.098	300	1.273	1.820	2.169	2.850	3.641
24	1.764	2.522	3.004	3.947	5.039	400	1.255	1.794	2.138	2.809	3.589
25	1.745	2.494	2.972	3.904	4.985	500	1.243	1.777	2.117	2.783	3.555
26	1.727	2.469	2.941	3.865	4.935	600	1.234	1.764	2.102	2.763	3.530
27	1.711	2.446	2.914	3.828	4.888	700	1.227	1.755	2.091	2.748	3.511
30	1.668	2.385	2.841	3.733	4.768	800	1.222	1.747	2.082	2.736	3.495
35	1.613	2.306	2.748	3.611	4.611	900	1.218	1.741	2.075	2.726	3.483
40	1.571	2.247	2.677	3.518	4.493	1000	1.214	1.736	2.068	2.718	3.472
45	1.539	2.200	2.621	3.444	4.399	∞	1.150	1.645	1.960	2.576	3.291
50	1.512	2.162	2.576	3.385	4.323						

II.3 FACTORS FOR COMPUTING PROBABLE ERRORS

The probable error of a series of n measures $a_1, a_2, a_3 \cdots a_n$, the mean of which is m, is given by the expression,

$$e = \frac{0.6745}{\sqrt{n-1}} \sqrt{(m-a_1)^2 + (m-a_2)^2 + \cdots + (m-a_n)^2}\ .$$

The probable error of the mean is,

$$E = \frac{0.6745}{\sqrt{n(n-1)}} \sqrt{(m-a_1)^2 + (m-a_2)^2 + \cdots + (m-a_n)^2}$$

The following approximate equations are convenient forms for computation,

$$e = 0.8453 \frac{\Sigma d}{\sqrt{n(n-1)}}$$

$$E = 0.8453 \frac{\Sigma d}{n\sqrt{n-1}}\ .$$

The symbol Σd represents the arithmetical sum of the deviations.

For convenience in computing the probable error the value of several of the factors involved is given for values of n from 2 to 100.

FACTORS FOR COMPUTING PROBABLE ERRORS

n	$\frac{1}{\sqrt{n}}$	$\frac{1}{\sqrt{n(n-1)}}$	$\frac{.6745}{\sqrt{n-1}}$	$\frac{.6745}{\sqrt{n(n-1)}}$	$\frac{.8453}{n\sqrt{n-1}}$	$\frac{.8453}{\sqrt{n(n-1)}}$
2	.707107	.707107	.6745	.4769	.4227	.5978
3	.577350	.408248	.4769	.2754	.1993	.3451
4	.500000	.288675	.3894	.1947	.1220	.2440
5	.447214	.223607	.3372	.1508	.0845	.1890
6	.408248	.182574	.3016	.1231	.0630	.1543
7	.377964	.154303	.2754	.1041	.0493	.1304
8	.353553	.133631	.2549	.0901	.0399	.1130
9	.333333	.117851	.2385	.0795	.0332	.0996
10	.316228	.105409	.2248	.0711	.0282	.0891
11	.301511	.095346	.2133	.0643	.0243	.0806
12	.288675	.087039	.2034	.0587	.0212	.0736
13	.277350	.080064	.1947	.0540	.0188	.0677
14	.267261	.074125	.1871	.0500	.0167	.0627
15	.258199	.069007	.1803	.0465	.0151	.0583
16	.250000	.064550	.1742	.0435	.0136	.0546
17	.242536	.060634	.1686	.0409	.0124	.0513
18	.235702	.057166	.1636	.0386	.0114	.0483
19	.229416	.054074	.1590	.0365	.0105	.0457
20	.223607	.051299	.1547	.0346	.0097	.0434
21	.218218	.048795	.1508	.0329	.0090	.0412
22	.213201	.046524	.1472	.0314	.0084	.0393
23	.208514	.044455	.1438	.0300	.0078	.0376
24	.204124	.042563	.1406	.0287	.0073	.0360
25	.200000	.040825	.1377	.0275	.0069	.0345
26	.196116	.039223	.1349	.0265	.0065	.0332
27	.192450	.037743	.1323	.0255	.0061	.0319
28	.188982	.036370	.1298	.0245	.0058	.0307
29	.185695	.035093	.1275	.0237	.0055	.0297
30	.182574	.033903	.1252	.0229	.0052	.0287
31	.179605	.032791	.1231	.0221	.0050	.0277
32	.176777	.031750	.1211	.0214	.0047	.0268
33	.174078	.030773	.1192	.0208	.0045	.0260
34	.171499	.029854	.1174	.0201	.0043	.0252
35	.169031	.028989	.1157	.0196	.0041	.0245
36	.166667	.028172	.1140	.0190	.0040	.0238
37	.164399	.027400	.1124	.0185	.0038	.0232
38	.162221	.026669	.1109	.0180	.0037	.0225
39	.160128	.025976	.1094	.0175	.0035	.0220
40	.158114	.025318	.1080	.0171	.0034	.0214
41	.156174	.024693	.1066	.0167	.0033	.0209
42	.154303	.024098	.1053	.0163	.0031	.0204
43	.152499	.023531	.1041	.0159	.0030	.0199
44	.150756	.022990	.1029	.0155	.0029	.0194
45	.149071	.022473	.1017	.0152	.0028	.0190
46	.147442	.021979	.1005	.0148	.0027	.0186
47	.145865	.021507	.0994	.0145	.0027	.0182
48	.144338	.021054	.0984	.0142	.0026	.0178
49	.142857	.020620	.0974	.0139	.0025	.0174
50	.141421	.020203	.0964	.0136	.0024	.0171

FACTORS FOR COMPUTING PROBABLE ERRORS

n	$\frac{1}{\sqrt{n}}$	$\frac{1}{\sqrt{n(n-1)}}$	$\frac{.6745}{\sqrt{n-1}}$	$\frac{.6745}{\sqrt{n(n-1)}}$	$\frac{.8453}{n\sqrt{n-1}}$	$\frac{.8453}{\sqrt{n(n-1)}}$
50	.141421	.020203	.0964	.0136	.0024	.0171
51	.140028	.019803	.0954	.0134	.0023	.0167
52	.138675	.019418	.0945	.0131	.0023	.0164
53	.137361	.019048	.0935	.0129	.0022	.0161
54	.136083	.018692	.0927	.0126	.0022	.0158
55	.134840	.018349	.0918	.0124	.0021	.0155
56	.133631	.018019	.0910	.0122	.0020	.0152
57	.132453	.017700	.0901	.0119	.0020	.0150
58	.131306	.017392	.0893	.0117	.0019	.0147
59	.130189	.017095	.0886	.0115	.0019	.0145
60	.129099	.016807	.0878	.0113	.0018	.0142
61	.128037	.016529	.0871	.0112	.0018	.0140
62	.127000	.016261	.0864	.0110	.0018	.0138
63	.125988	.016001	.0857	.0108	.0017	.0135
64	.125000	.015749	.0850	.0106	.0017	.0133
65	.124035	.015504	.0843	.0105	.0016	.0131
66	.123091	.015268	.0837	.0103	.0016	.0129
67	.122169	.015038	.0830	.0101	.0016	.0127
68	.121268	.014815	.0824	.0100	.0015	.0125
69	.120386	.014599	.0818	.0099	.0015	.0123
70	.119523	.014389	.0812	.0097	.0015	.0122
71	.118678	.014185	.0806	.0096	.0014	.0120
72	.117851	.013986	.0801	.0094	.0014	.0118
73	.117041	.013793	.0795	.0093	.0014	.0117
74	.116248	.013606	.0789	.0092	.0013	.0115
75	.115470	.013423	.0784	.0091	.0013	.0113
76	.114708	.013245	.0779	.0089	.0013	.0112
77	.113961	.013072	.0773	.0088	.0013	.0111
78	.113228	.012904	.0769	.0087	.0012	.0109
79	.112509	.012739	.0764	.0086	.0012	.0108
80	.111803	.012579	.0759	.0085	.0012	.0106
81	.111111	.012423	.0754	.0084	.0012	.0105
82	.110432	.012270	.0749	.0083	.0012	.0104
83	.109764	.012121	.0745	.0082	.0011	.0103
84	.109109	.011976	.0740	.0081	.0011	.0101
85	.108465	.011835	.0736	.0080	.0011	.0100
86	.107833	.011696	.0732	.0079	.0011	.0099
87	.107211	.011561	.0727	.0078	.0011	.0098
88	.106600	.011429	.0723	.0077	.0010	.0097
89	.106000	.011300	.0719	.0076	.0010	.0096
90	.105409	.011173	.0715	.0075	.0010	.0094
91	.104828	.011050	.0711	.0075	.0010	.0093
92	.104257	.010929	.0707	.0074	.0010	.0092
93	.103695	.010811	.0703	.0073	.0010	.0091
94	.103142	.010695	.0699	.0072	.0009	.0090
95	.102598	.010582	.0696	.0071	.0009	.0089
96	.102062	.010471	.0692	.0071	.0009	.0089
97	.101535	.010363	.0688	.0070	.0009	.0088
98	.101015	.010257	.0685	.0069	.0009	.0087
99	.100504	.010152	.0681	.0069	.0009	.0086
100	.100000	.010050	.0678	.0068	.0008	.0085

II.4 PROBABILITY OF OCCURRENCE OF DEVIATIONS

The significance of deviations is indicated by this table. The probability of occurrence of deviations as great as or greater than any specific value is given for various ratios of deviation to probable error and also with respect to the standard deviation. The probability of occurrence is stated in per cent or chances in 100. The odds against occurrence are also stated. The probable error is 0.6745 × the standard deviation.

Ratio, dev. to P.E.	Probable occurrence %	Odds against, to 1	Ratio dev. to std. dev.	Probable occurrence %	Odds against, to 1
1.0	50.00	1.00	0.67449	50.00	1.00
1.1	45.81	1.18	0.7	48.39	1.07
1.2	41.83	1.39	0.8	42.37	1.36
1.3	38.00	1.63	0.9	36.81	1.72
1.4	34.50	1.90	1.0	31.73	2.15
1.5	31.17	2.21	1.1	27.13	2.69
1.6	28.05	2.57	1.2	23.01	3.35
1.7	25.15	2.98	1.3	19.36	4.17
1.8	22.47	3.45	1.4	16.15	5.19
1.9	20.00	4.00	1.5	13.36	6.48
2.0	17.73	4.64	1.6	10.96	8.12
2.1	15.67	5.38	1.7	8.91	10.22
2.2	13.78	6.25	1.8	7.19	12.92
2.3	12.08	7.28	1.9	5.74	16.41
2.4	10.55	8.48	2.0	4.55	20.98
2.5	9.18	9.90	2.1	3.57	26.99
2.6	7.95	11.58	2.2	2.78	34.96
2.7	6.86	13.58	2.3	2.14	45.62
2.8	5.89	15.96	2.4	1.64	59.99
2.9	5.05	18.82	2.5	1.24	79.52
3.0	4.30	22.24	2.6	.932	106.3
3.1	3.65	26.37	2.7	.693	143.2
3.2	3.09	31.36	2.8	.511	194.7
3.3	2.60	37.42	2.9	.373	267.0
3.4	2.18	44.80	3.0	.270	369.4
3.5	1.82	53.82	3.1	.194	515.7
3.6	1.52	64.89	3.2	.137	726.7
3.7	1.26	78.53	3.3	.0967	1033.
3.8	1.04	95.38	3.4	.0674	1483.
3.9	.853	116.3	3.5	.0465	2149.
4.0	.698	142.3	3.6	.0318	3142.
4.1	.569	174.9	3.7	.0216	4637.
4.2	.461	215.8	3.8	.0145	6915.
4.3	.373	267.2	3.9	.00962	10394.
4.4	.300	332.4	4.0	.00634	15772.
4.5	.240	415.0	5.0	5.73×10^{-5}	1.744×10^{6}
4.6	.192	520.4	6.0	2.0×10^{-7}	5.0×10^{8}
4.7	.152	655.3	7.0	2.6×10^{-10}	3.9×10^{11}
4.8	.121	828.3			
4.9	.0950	1052.			
5.0	.0745	1341.			
6.0	.0052	19300.			
7.0	.00023	4.27×10^{5}			
8.0	6.8×10^{-6}	1.47×10^{7}			
9.0	1.3×10^{-7}	7.30×10^{8}			
10.0	1.5×10^{-9}	6.5×10^{10}			

Valid for samples of size 30 or greater.

II.5 OPERATING CHARACTERISTIC (OC) CURVES FOR A TEST ON THE MEAN OF A NORMAL DISTRIBUTION WITH KNOWN STANDARD DEVIATION

The OC curves give the sample sizes needed for given values of $\alpha = P$ (Type I error) and $\beta = P$ (Type II error) for a test of the hypothesis Ho: $\mu = \mu_0$ where the standard deviation is known. The statistic used is $z = \frac{(\bar{x} - \mu_0)\sqrt{n}}{\sigma}$ which is distributed as the standard normal distribution. The required sample size is obtained by entering the appropriate set of curves for given α and β for various values of $\Delta = \frac{|\mu_1 - \mu_0|}{\sigma}$ for both one-sided and two-sided tests.

The OC curves can also be used to give the sample sizes for a test of the hypothesis H_0: $\mu_x = \mu_y$, where the standard deviations σ_x and σ_y are known. The statistic used is $z = \frac{\bar{x} - \bar{y}}{\sqrt{\frac{\sigma_x^2}{n_x} + \frac{\sigma_y^2}{n_y}}}$. The required sample size is obtained by entering the appropriate set of curves for given α and β for various values of $\Delta = \frac{|\mu_x - \mu_y|}{\sqrt{\sigma_x^2 + \sigma_y^2}}$ for both one-sided and two-sided tests.

OC CURVES FOR A TEST ON THE MEAN OF A NORMAL DISTRIBUTION WITH KNOWN STANDARD DEVIATION

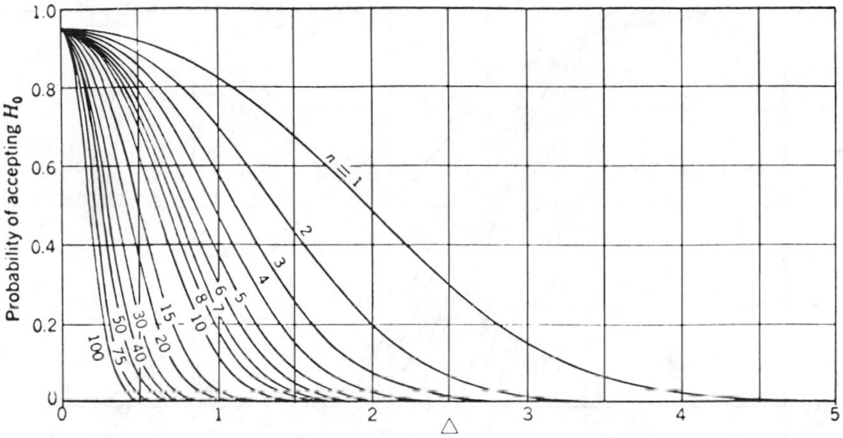

a) OC curves for different values of n for the two-sided normal test for a level of significance $\alpha = 0.05$.

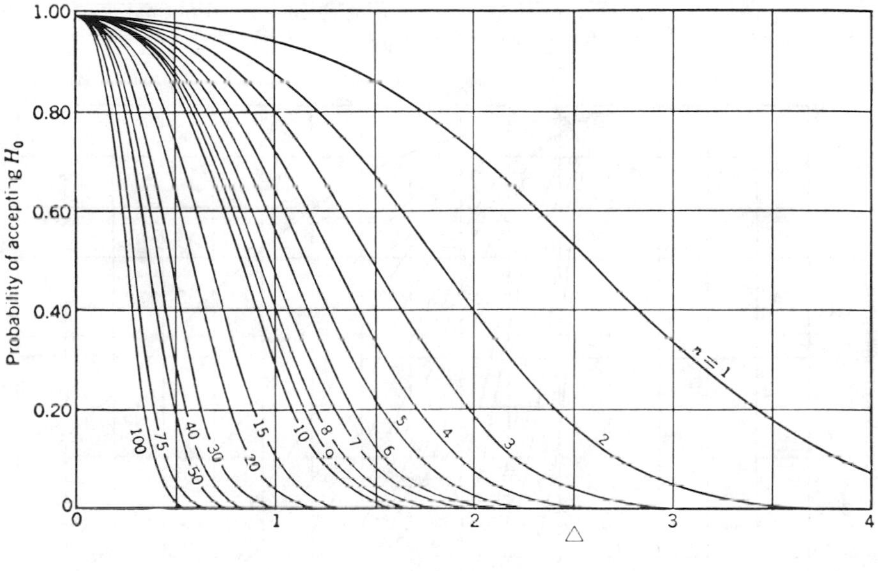

b) OC curves for different values of n for the two-sided normal test for a level of significance $\alpha = 0.01$.

OC CURVES FOR A TEST ON THE MEAN OF A NORMAL DISTRIBUTION WITH KNOWN STANDARD DEVIATION

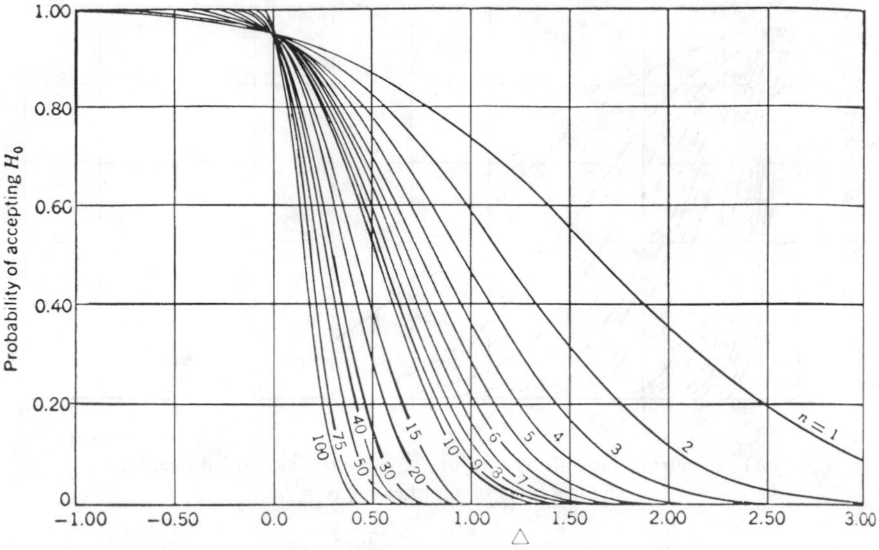

c) OC curves for different values of n for the one-sided normal test for a level of significance $\alpha = 0.05$.

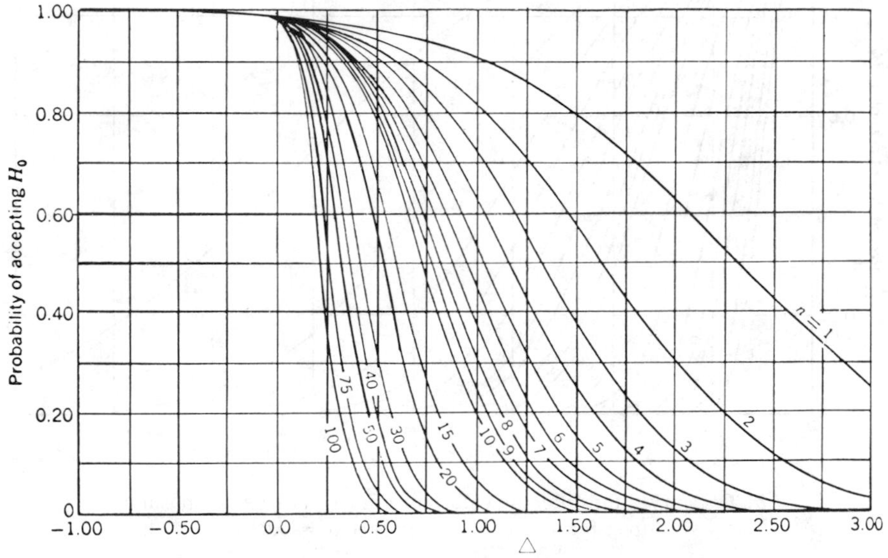

d) OC curves for different values of n for the one-sided normal test for a level of significance $\alpha = 0.01$.

II.6 BIVARIATE NORMAL PROBABILITIES

The joint probability density function of two random variables x and y, distributed as a bivariate normal distribution with zero means, unit variances, and correlation coefficient ρ, is given by

$$f(x,y;\rho) = \frac{1}{2\pi\sqrt{1-\rho^2}} \exp\left\{-\frac{1}{2(1-\rho^2)}(x^2 - 2\rho xy + y^2)\right\}.$$

The bivariate normal probability integral is then

$$Pr(x \geq h, y \geq k) = L(h,k;\rho) = \int_h^\infty dx \int_k^\infty f(x,y;\rho)\, dy.$$

$L(h,k;\rho)$ can be expressed as a function of $L(h,0;\rho)$ by use of

$$\begin{aligned} L(h,k;\rho) &= L\left(h, 0; \frac{(\rho h - k)(\operatorname{sgn} h)}{\sqrt{h^2 - 2\rho hk + k^2}}\right) \\ &\quad + L\left(k, 0; \frac{(\rho k - h)(\operatorname{sgn} k)}{\sqrt{h^2 - 2\rho hk + k^2}}\right) \\ &\quad - \begin{cases} 0 & \text{if } hk > 0 \quad \text{or} \quad hk = 0 \text{ and } h + k \geq 0 \\ \frac{1}{2} & \text{otherwise,} \end{cases} \end{aligned}$$

where sgn $h = 1$ if $h \geq 0$ and sgn $h = -1$ if $h < 0$. The graphs are plots of h versus ρ with constant contour lines such that $L(h,0;\rho) = 0.01$ (.01) .10 (.02) .50.

BIVARIATE NORMAL PROBABILITIES

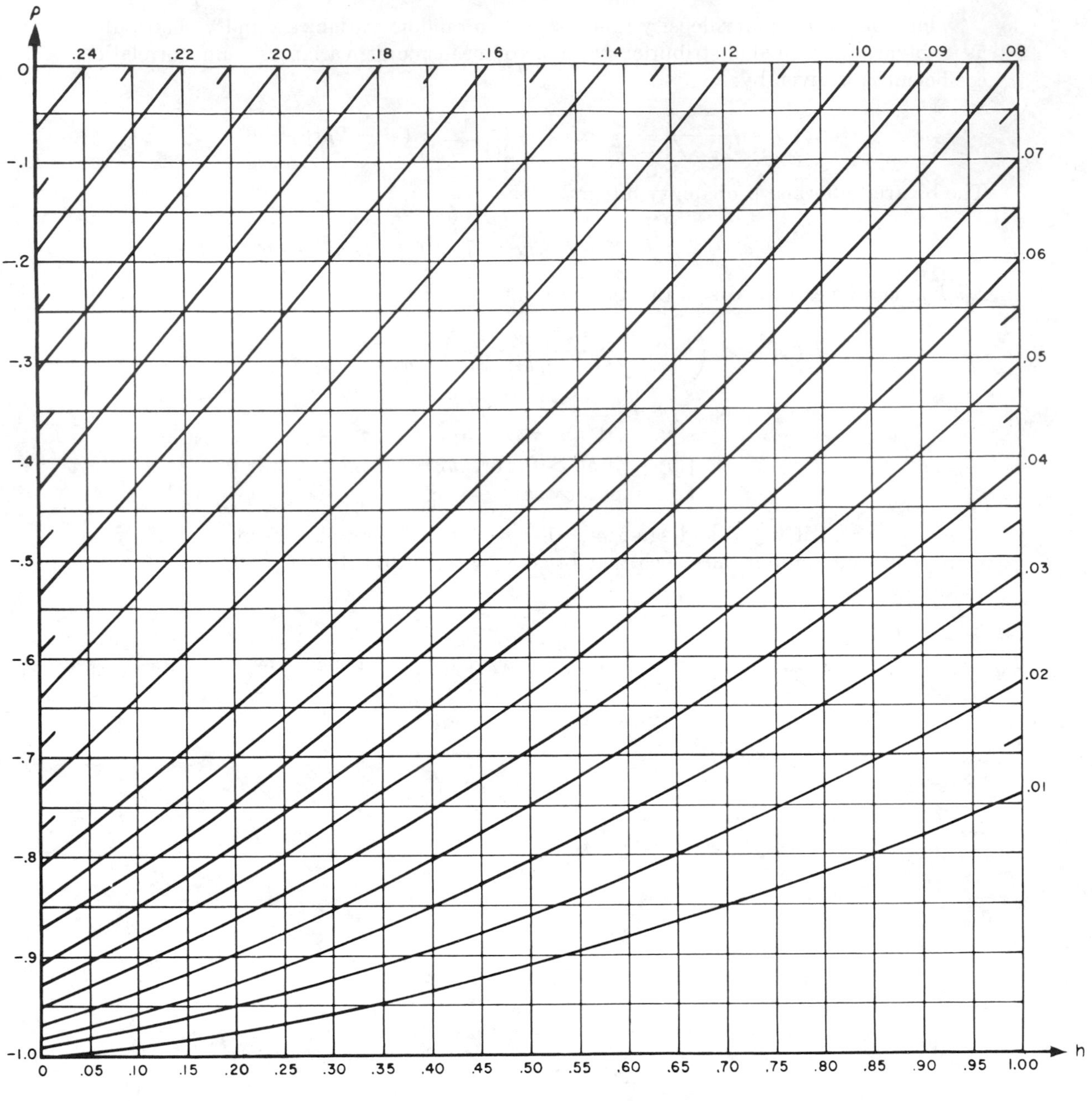

$L(h,0,\rho)$ *for* $0 \leq h \leq 1$ *and* $-1 \leq \rho \leq 0$.
Values for $h < 0$ can be obtained using $L(h,0,-\rho) = \frac{1}{2} - L(-h,0,\rho)$.

BIVARIATE NORMAL PROBABILITIES

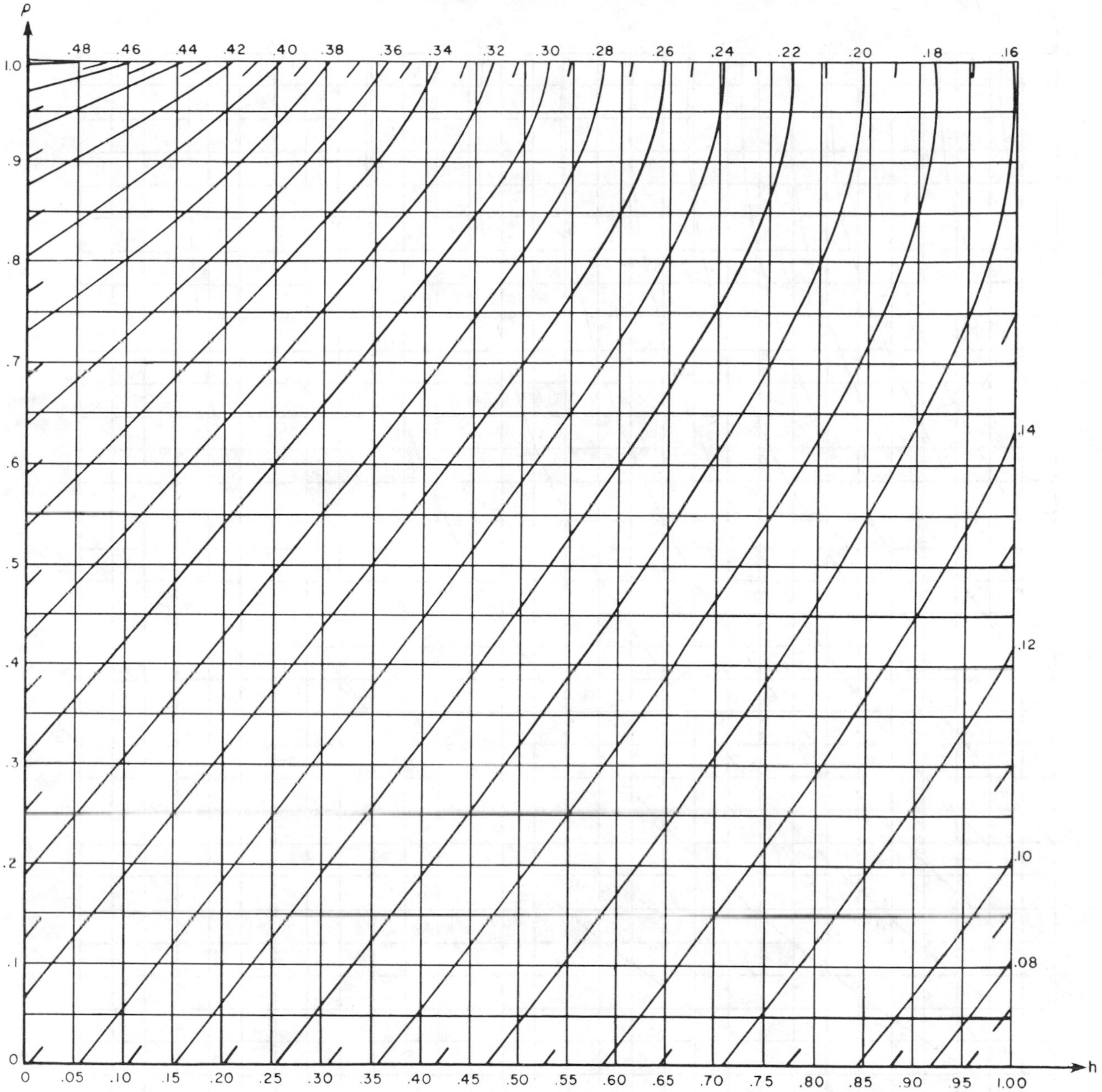

$L(h,0,\rho)$ *for* $0 \leq h \leq 1$ *and* $0 \leq \rho \leq 1$.

Values for $h < 0$ can be obtained using $L(h,0,-\rho) = \frac{1}{2} - L(-h,0,\rho)$.

BIVARIATE NORMAL PROBABILITIES

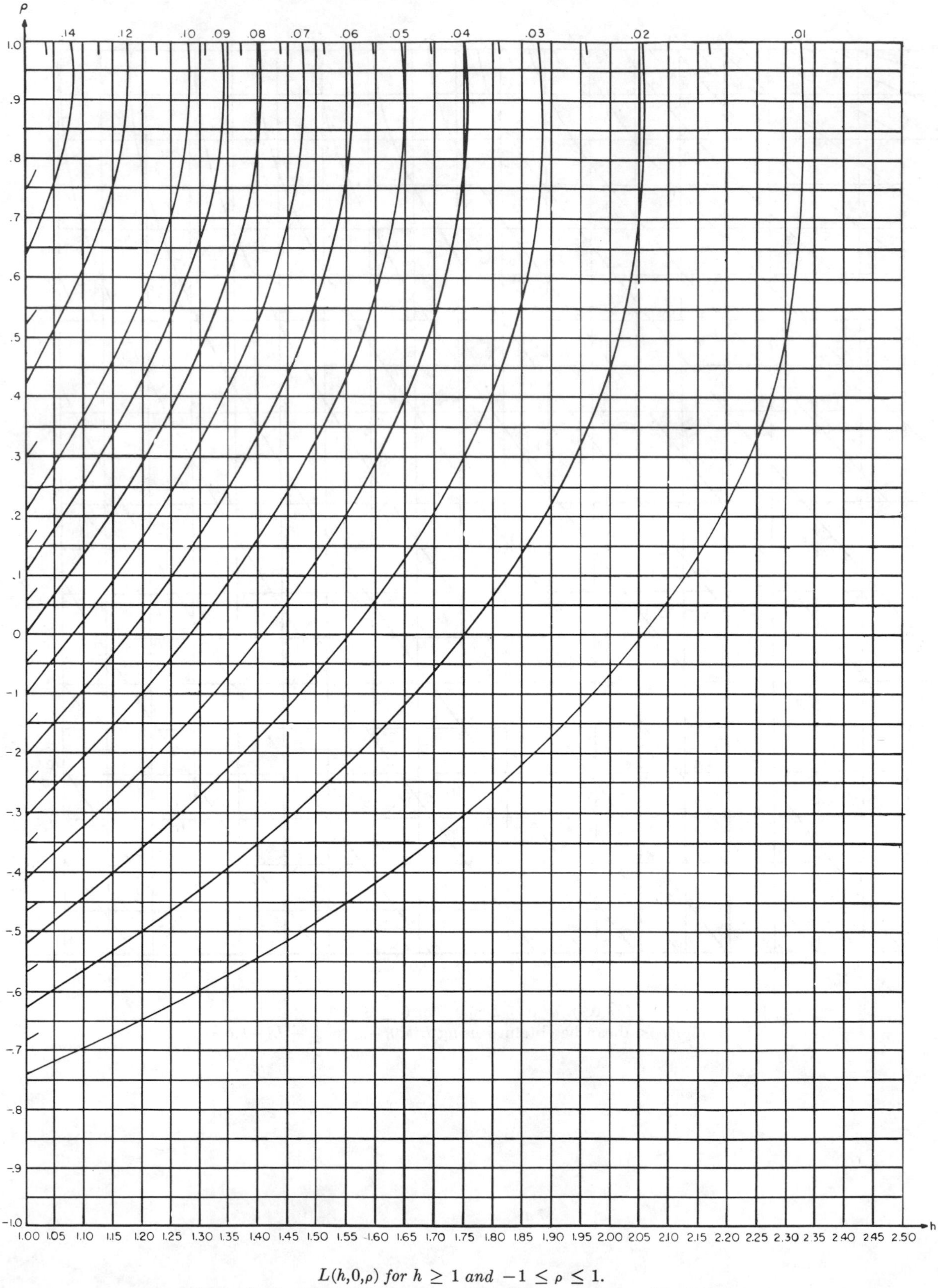

$L(h,0,\rho)$ *for* $h \geq 1$ *and* $-1 \leq \rho \leq 1$.
Values for $h < 0$ can be obtained using $L(h,0,-\rho) = \frac{1}{2} - L(-h,0,\rho.)$

II.7 CIRCULAR NORMAL PROBABILITIES

The joint probability density function of two random variables x and y, normally and independently distributed each with mean zero and standard deviation σ is given by

$$f(x,y) = \frac{1}{2\pi\sigma^2} \exp\left\{-\frac{1}{2\sigma^2}(x^2+y^2)\right\}.$$

The table gives values of

$$P\left(\frac{d}{\sigma}, \frac{R}{\sigma}\right) = \frac{1}{2\pi\sigma^2} \iint\limits_C \exp\left\{-\frac{1}{2\sigma^2}(x^2+y^2)\right\} dx\, dy$$

over a circle C of radius R with center at distance d from the origin.

CIRCULAR NORMAL PROBABILITIES

d/σ	R/σ									
	0.1	0.2	0.3	0.4	0.5	0.6	0.7	0.8	0.9	1.0
	P									
0.0	.0050	.020	.044	.077	.118	.165	.217	.274	.333	.393
0.1	.0050	.020	.044	.077	.117	.164	.216	.273	.332	.392
0.2	.0049	.019	.043	.075	.115	.162	.213	.269	.328	.387
0.3	.0048	.019	.042	.074	.113	.158	.209	.264	.321	.380
0.4	.0046	.018	.041	.071	.109	.153	.202	.256	.312	.370
0.5	.0044	.018	.039	.068	.104	.147	.195	.246	.301	.357
0.6	.0042	.017	.037	.065	.099	.140	.185	.235	.288	.342
0.7	.0039	.016	.035	.061	.093	.132	.175	.223	.273	.326
0.8	.0036	.014	.032	.057	.087	.123	.164	.209	.257	.307
0.9	.0033	.013	.030	.052	.080	.114	.152	.194	.240	.288
1.0	.0030	.012	.027	.048	.073	.104	.140	.179	.222	.267
1.1	.0027	.011	.024	.043	.067	.095	.127	.164	.203	.246
1.2	.0024	.010	.022	.038	.060	.085	.115	.148	.185	.225
1.3	.0022	.0086	.019	.034	.053	.076	.103	.133	.167	.204
1.4	.0019	.0075	.017	.030	.047	.067	.091	.119	.150	.184
1.5	.0016	.0065	.015	.026	.041	.059	.080	.105	.133	.164
1.6	.0014	.0056	.013	.022	.035	.051	.070	.092	.117	.145
1.7	.0012	.0047	.011	.019	.030	.044	.060	.080	.102	.127
1.8	.0010	.0040	.0090	.016	.026	.037	.052	.069	.088	.111
1.9	.0008	.0033	.0075	.014	.022	.032	.044	.059	.076	.096
2.0	.0007	.0027	.0062	.011	.018	.026	.037	.050	.064	.082
2.1	.0006	.0022	.0051	.0092	.015	.022	.031	.042	.054	.070
2.2	.0004	.0018	.0041	.0075	.012	.018	.025	.034	.045	.059
2.3	.0004	.0014	.0033	.0060	.0098	.015	.021	.028	.038	.049
2.4	.0003	.0011	.0026	.0048	.0078	.012	.017	.023	.031	.040
2.5	.0002	.0009	.0021	.0038	.0062	.0094	.014	.019	.025	.033
2.6	.0002	.0007	.0016	.0030	.0049	.0074	.011	.015	.020	.027
2.7	.0001	.0005	.0012	.0023	.0038	.0058	.0085	.012	.016	.022
2.8	.0001	.0004	.0010	.0018	.0029	.0045	.0066	.0094	.013	.017
2.9	.0001	.0003	.0007	.0014	.0022	.0035	.0051	.0073	.010	.014
3.0	.0001	.0002	.0005	.0010	.0017	.0026	.0039	.0057	.0079	.011
3.2		.0001	.0003	.0006	.0010	.0014	.0024	.0034	.0048	.0066
3.4		.0001	.0001	.0003	.0005	.0008	.0013	.0020	.0028	.0039
3.6				.0001	.0002	.0004	.0008	.0011	.0016	.0022
3.8					.0001	.0002	.0004	.0006	.0009	.0012
4.0					.0001	.0001	.0002	.0003	.0005	.0007
4.2						.0001	.0001	.0002	.0002	.0004
4.4							.0001	.0001	.0001	.0002
4.6									.0001	.0001
4.8										
5.0										
5.2										
5.4										
5.6										
5.8										
6.0										

CIRCULAR NORMAL PROBABILITIES

d/σ	R/σ 1.2	1.4	1.6	1.8	2.0	2.2	2.4	2.6	2.8	3.0
						P				
0.0	.513	.625	.722	.802	.865	.911	.944	.966	.980	.989
0.1	.512	.623	.720	.800	.863	.910	.943	.965	.980	.989
0.2	.506	.617	.715	.796	.859	.907	.941	.964	.979	.988
0.3	.498	.608	.706	.788	.852	.901	.937	.961	.977	.987
0.4	.486	.596	.694	.777	.843	.894	.931	.956	.974	.985
0.5	.471	.580	.678	.763	.831	.884	.923	.951	.970	.982
0.6	.454	.561	.660	.745	.816	.872	.914	.944	.965	.979
0.7	.434	.540	.639	.726	.799	.857	.902	.936	.959	.975
0.8	.412	.516	.615	.703	.778	.840	.889	.925	.952	.970
0.9	.388	.490	.588	.678	.756	.821	.873	.913	.943	.964
1.0	.364	.463	.560	.650	.731	.800	.856	.900	.933	.956
1.1	.338	.434	.530	.621	.704	.776	.836	.884	.921	.948
1.2	.312	.404	.498	.590	.674	.750	.814	.866	.907	.937
1.3	.285	.374	.466	.557	.643	.721	.789	.846	.891	.926
1.4	.259	.344	.433	.523	.610	.691	.763	.824	.873	.912
1.5	.234	.314	.400	.489	.576	.659	.734	.799	.853	.896
1.6	.210	.284	.367	.454	.541	.625	.703	.772	.831	.878
1.7	.186	.256	.334	.419	.505	.590	.671	.744	.806	.859
1.8	.164	.229	.303	.384	.469	.554	.637	.713	.780	.837
1.9	.144	.203	.272	.349	.433	.518	.601	.680	.751	.812
2.0	.125	.178	.243	.316	.396	.481	.565	.646	.720	.786
2.1	.107	.156	.215	.284	.361	.443	.528	.610	.687	.757
2.2	.092	.135	.189	.253	.327	.407	.490	.573	.653	.726
2.3	.078	.116	.165	.224	.294	.370	.452	.536	.617	.693
2.4	.065	.099	.143	.197	.262	.335	.415	.498	.580	.659
2.5	.054	.084	.123	.172	.232	.301	.378	.460	.542	.623
2.6	.045	.070	.105	.149	.204	.269	.342	.422	.504	.586
2.7	.037	.059	.089	.128	.178	.238	.308	.385	.466	.548
2.8	.030	.048	.074	.109	.154	.210	.275	.348	.428	.510
2.9	.024	.040	.062	.093	.133	.183	.244	.313	.390	.471
3.0	.019	.032	.051	.078	.113	.159	.215	.280	.353	.433
3.2	.012	.021	.034	.053	.080	.117	.163	.219	.284	.358
3.4	.007	.013	.022	.036	.055	.083	.119	.166	.222	.288
3.6	.004	.008	.014	.023	.037	.057	.085	.122	.169	.225
3.8	.002	.004	.008	.014	.024	.038	.059	.087	.124	.171
4.0	.0013	.0025	.0046	.0085	.015	.024	.039	.060	.088	.126
4.2	.0007	.0014	.0026	.0049	.0087	.015	.025	.040	.061	.090
4.4	.0004	.0007	.0014	.0027	.0051	.0090	.016	.026	.041	.062
4.6	.0002	.0004	.0008	.0015	.0028	.0052	.0093	.016	.026	.041
4.8	.0001	.0002	.0004	.0008	.0016	.0029	.0054	.0095	.016	.027
5.0			.0002	.0004	.0008	.0016	.0030	.0055	.0098	.017
5.2			.0001	.0002	.0004	.0008	.0016	.0030	.0056	.0100
5.4				.0001	.0002	.0004	.0009	.0016	.0031	.0058
5.6						.0002	.0005	.0009	.0017	.0033
5.8						.0001	.0002	.0005	.0009	.0017
6.0								.0002	.0005	.0009

II.8 CIRCULAR ERROR PROBABILITIES

The joint probability density function of two random variables x and y, normally and independently distributed each with mean zero and standard deviations σ_x and σ_y, respectively, is given by

$$f(x,y) = \frac{1}{2\pi\sigma_x\sigma_y} \exp\left\{-\frac{1}{2}\left[\left(\frac{x}{\sigma_x}\right)^2 + \left(\frac{y}{\sigma_y}\right)^2\right]\right\}.$$

The probability that a point (x,y), whose coordinates are chosen randomly and independently from this joint distribution, will lie within a circle with center at the origin and radius $K\sigma_x$ is given by

$$P(K,\sigma_x,\sigma_y) = \iint_R f(x,y)\, dx\, dy,$$

where R is the region $\sqrt{x^2 + y^2} < K\sigma_x$. For various values of $c = \frac{\sigma_y}{\sigma_x}$, where for convenience the components are labeled so that $\sigma_y \leq \sigma_x$, the table gives values of the probability P that the point of impact lies inside a circle with center at the target and radius $K\sigma_x$.

CIRCULAR ERROR PROBABILITIES

K \ c	0.0	0.1	0.2	0.3	0.4	0.5
0.1	.0796557	.0443987	.0242119	.0164176	.0123875	.0099377
0.2	.1585194	.1339783	.0884533	.0628396	.0482413	.0390193
0.3	.2358228	.2213804	.1739300	.1318281	.1039193	.0851535
0.4	.3108435	3010228	.2635181	.2139084	.1742045	.1451808
0.5	.3829249	.3755884	.3481790	.3003001	.2532953	.2152886
0.6	.4514938	.4457708	.4255605	.3846374	.3357384	.2914682
0.7	.5160727	.5115048	.4960683	.4633258	.4170862	.3699305
0.8	.5762892	.5725957	.5604457	.5349387	.4941882	.4474207
0.9	.6318797	.6288721	.6191354	.5993140	.5651564	.5213998
1.0	.6826895	.6802325	.6723586	.6568242	.6291249	.5900953
1.1	.7286679	.7266597	.7202682	.7079681	.6859367	.6524489
1.2	.7698607	.7682215	.7630305	.7532175	.7359558	.7079973
1.3	.8063990	.8050648	.8008554	.7929968	.7793550	.7567265
1.4	.8384867	.8374049	.8340018	.8277048	.8169851	.7989288
1.5	.8663856	.8655127	.8627728	.8577362	.8493071	.8350816
1.6	.8904014	.8897008	.8875060	.8834914	.8768644	.8657559
1.7	.9108691	.9103102	.9085619	.9053766	.9001746	.8915536
1.8	.9281394	.9276964	.9263125	.9237989	.9197275	.9130680
1.9	.9425669	.9422182	.9411299	.9391586	.9359855	.9308615
2.0	.9544997	.9542272	.9533775	.9518415	.9493815	.9454546
2.1	.9642712	.9640598	.9634011	.9622127	.9603170	.9573205
2.2	.9721931	.9720304	.9715237	.9706109	.9691597	.9668845
2.3	.9785518	.9784275	.9780408	.9773450	.9762419	.9745239
2.4	.9836049	.9835108	.9832180	.9826918	.9818594	.9805703
2.5	.9875807	.9875100	.9872900	.9868953	.9862720	.9853112
2.6	.9906776	.9906249	.9904612	.9901674	.9897045	.9889934
2.7	.9930661	.9930271	.9929062	.9926894	.9923483	.9918260
2.8	.9948897	.9948612	.9947727	.9946141	.9943649	.9939842
2.9	.9962684	.9962477	.9961834	.9960684	.9958878	.9956126
3.0	.9973002	.9972853	.9972391	.9971564	.9970266	.9968294
3.1	.9980648	.9980542	.9980212	.9979622	.9978699	.9977296
3.2	.9986257	.9986182	.9985949	.9985533	.9984880	.9983892
3.3	.9990332	.9990279	.9990116	.9989824	.9989368	.9988677
3.4	.9993261	.9993225	.9993112	.9992909	.9992593	.9992115
3.5	.9995347	.9995323	.9995245	.9995105	.9994888	.9994559
3.6	.9996818	.9996801	.9996748	.9996653	.9996505	.9996281
3.7	.9997844	.9997832	.9997797	.9997733	.9997633	.9997482
3.8	.9998553	.9998545	.9998522	.9998478	.9998412	.9998311
3.9	.9999038	.9999033	.9999018	.9998989	.9998945	.9998878
4.0	.9999367	.9999363	.9999353	.9999334	.9999305	.9999261
4.1	.9999587	.9999585	.9999578	.9999566	.9999547	.9999519
4.2	.9999733	.9999732	.9999727	.9999720	.9999707	.9999689
4.3	.9999829	.9999828	.9999826	.9999821	.9999813	.9999801
4.4	.9999892	.9999891	.9999889	.9999886	.9999881	.9999874
4.5	.9999932	.9999932	.9999931	.9999929	.9999925	.9999921
4.6	.9999958	.9999957	.9999957	.9999955	.9999954	.9999951
4.7	.9999974	.9999974	.9999973	.9999973	.9999971	.9999970
4.8	.9999984	.9999984	.9999984	.9999983	.9999983	.9999982
4.9	.9999990	.9999990	.9999990	.9999990	.9999990	.9999989
5.0	.9999994	.9999994	.9999994	.9999994	.9999994	.9999993
5.1	.9999997	.9999997	.9999997	.9999996	.9999996	.9999996
5.2	.9999998	.9999998	.9999998	.9999998	.9999998	.9999998
5.3	.9999999	.9999999	.9999999	.9999999	.9999999	.9999999
5.4	.9999999	.9999999	.9999999	.9999999	.9999999	.9999999
5.5	1.0000000	1.0000000	1.0000000	1.0000000	1.0000000	1.0000000

$P(K,c)$ = the probability that a point falls inside a circle whose center is at the origin and whose radius is K times the larger standard deviation, c being the ratio of the smaller standard deviation to the larger standard deviation.

CIRCULAR ERROR PROBABILITIES

K \ c	0.6	0.7	0.8	0.9	1.0
0.1	.0082940	.0071157	.0062299	.0055400	.0049875
0.2	.0327123	.0281415	.0246824	.0219757	.0198013
0.3	.0719102	.0621386	.0546598	.0487639	.0440025
0.4	.1237982	.1076237	.0950495	.0850326	.0768837
0.5	.1857448	.1626829	.1443941	.1296286	.1175031
0.6	.2548177	.2251114	.2009797	.1811783	.1647298
0.7	.3280302	.2925654	.2629373	.2381583	.2172955
0.8	.4025628	.3627122	.3283453	.2989700	.2738510
0.9	.4759375	.4333628	.3953279	.3620135	.3330232
1.0	.5461319	.5025790	.4621421	.4257553	.3934693
1.1	.6116316	.5687467	.5272462	.4887873	.4539256
1.2	.6714269	.6306168	.5893494	.5498736	.5132477
1.3	.7249673	.6873122	.6474394	.6079822	.5704426
1.4	.7720889	.7383089	.7007900	.6623035	.6246889
1.5	.8129287	.7833962	.7489500	.7122546	.6753475
1.6	.8478393	.8226246	.7917194	.7574708	.7219627
1.7	.8773116	.8562471	.8291137	.7977882	.7462539
1.8	.9019110	.8846624	.8613238	.8332175	.8021013
1.9	.9222277	.9083609	.8886731	.8639149	.8355255
2.0	.9388418	.9278799	.9115762	.8901495	.8646647
2.1	.9522999	.9437668	.9305013	.9122714	.8897495
2.2	.9631017	.9565522	.9459386	.9306821	.9110784
2.3	.9716934	.9667306	.9583739	.9458085	.9289946
2.4	.9784661	.9747495	.9682698	.9580804	.9438652
2.5	.9837569	.9810035	.9760522	.9679136	.9560631
2.6	.9878527	.9858331	.9821023	.9756969	.9659525
2.7	.9909944	.9895268	.9867530	.9817837	.9738786
2.8	.9933821	.9923249	.9902888	.9864876	.9801589
2.9	.9951798	.9944246	.9929482	.9900803	.9850792
3.0	.9965205	.9959854	.9949274	.9927925	.9888910
3.1	.9975109	.9971348	.9963851	.9948168	.9918113
3.2	.9982356	.9979733	.9974478	.9963105	.9940240
3.3	.9987607	.9985792	.9982147	.9974004	.9956822
3.4	.9991376	.9990129	.9987626	.9981868	.9969113
3.5	.9994053	.9993204	.9991502	.9987480	.9978125
3.6	.9995938	.9995364	.9994218	.9991442	.9984662
3.7	.9997251	.9996867	.9996102	.9994208	.9989352
3.8	.9998157	.9997902	.9997396	.9996119	.9992682
3.9	.9998776	.9998608	.9998276	.9997426	.9995020
4.0	.9999195	.9999085	.9998870	.9998309	.9996645
4.1	.9999475	.9999404	.9999266	.9998900	.9997763
4.2	.9999661	.9999616	.9999527	.9999292	.9998523
4.3	.9999783	.9999754	.9999698	.9999548	.9999034
4.4	.9999863	.9999845	.9999809	.9999715	.9999375
4.5	.9999914	.9999902	.9999881	.9999822	.9999599
4.6	.9999947	.9999939	.9999926	.9999889	.9999746
4.7	.9999967	.9999963	.9999955	.9999932	.9999840
4.8	.9999980	.9999977	.9999972	.9999959	.9999901
4.9	.9999988	.9999986	.9999983	.9999975	.9999939
5.0	.9999993	.9999992	.9999990	.9999985	.9999963
5.1	.9999996	.9999995	.9999994	.9999991	.9999978
5.2	.9999998	.9999997	.9999997	.9999995	.9999987
5.3	.9999999	.9999998	.9999998	.9999997	.9999992
5.4	.9999999	.9999999	.9999999	.9999998	.9999995
5.5	1.0000000	.9999999	.9999999	.9999999	.9999997
5.6		1.0000000	1.0000000	.9999999	.9999998
5.7				1.0000000	.9999999
5.8					1.0000000

$P(K,c)$ = the probability that a point falls inside a circle whose center is at the origin and whose radius is K times the larger standard deviation, c being the ratio of the smaller standard deviation to the larger standard deviation.

II.9 CHARTS OF THE UPPER 1%, 2.5%, AND 5% POINTS OF THE DISTRIBUTION OF THE LARGEST CHARACTERISTIC ROOT

Charts I–XII enable finding of $x_\alpha(s,m,n)$ such that

$$P[\theta_s \leq x_\alpha(s,m,n)] = 1 - \alpha,$$

where θ_s is the largest of s non-zero roots of the $(p \times p)$ matrix $S_{12}S_{22}^{-1}S_{12}'S_{11}^{-1}$, and where the covariance matrix from a $(p + q)$-variate normal population based on $N - 1$ degrees of freedom is

$$S = \begin{bmatrix} S_{11} & S_{12} \\ S_{12}' & S_{22} \end{bmatrix}.$$

The test of independence between the p-set of variates and the q-set is as follows: accept the null hypothesis at the α-level of significance if $c - \theta_s \leq x_\alpha$, and reject otherwise. If $2 \leq \min(p,q) \leq 5$, then x_α, for a given α, may be obtained by entering the charts with the following degrees of freedom:

$$s = \min(p,q), \qquad m = \frac{|p - q| - 1}{2}, \text{ and } n = \frac{N - p - q - 2}{2}.$$

If $\min(p,q) = 1$, the test is equivalent to the test for $\rho^2 = 0$ where ρ is the multiple correlation of the p set on the q set. These charts are also useful in testing the general linear hypothesis in multivariate analysis.

CHART I

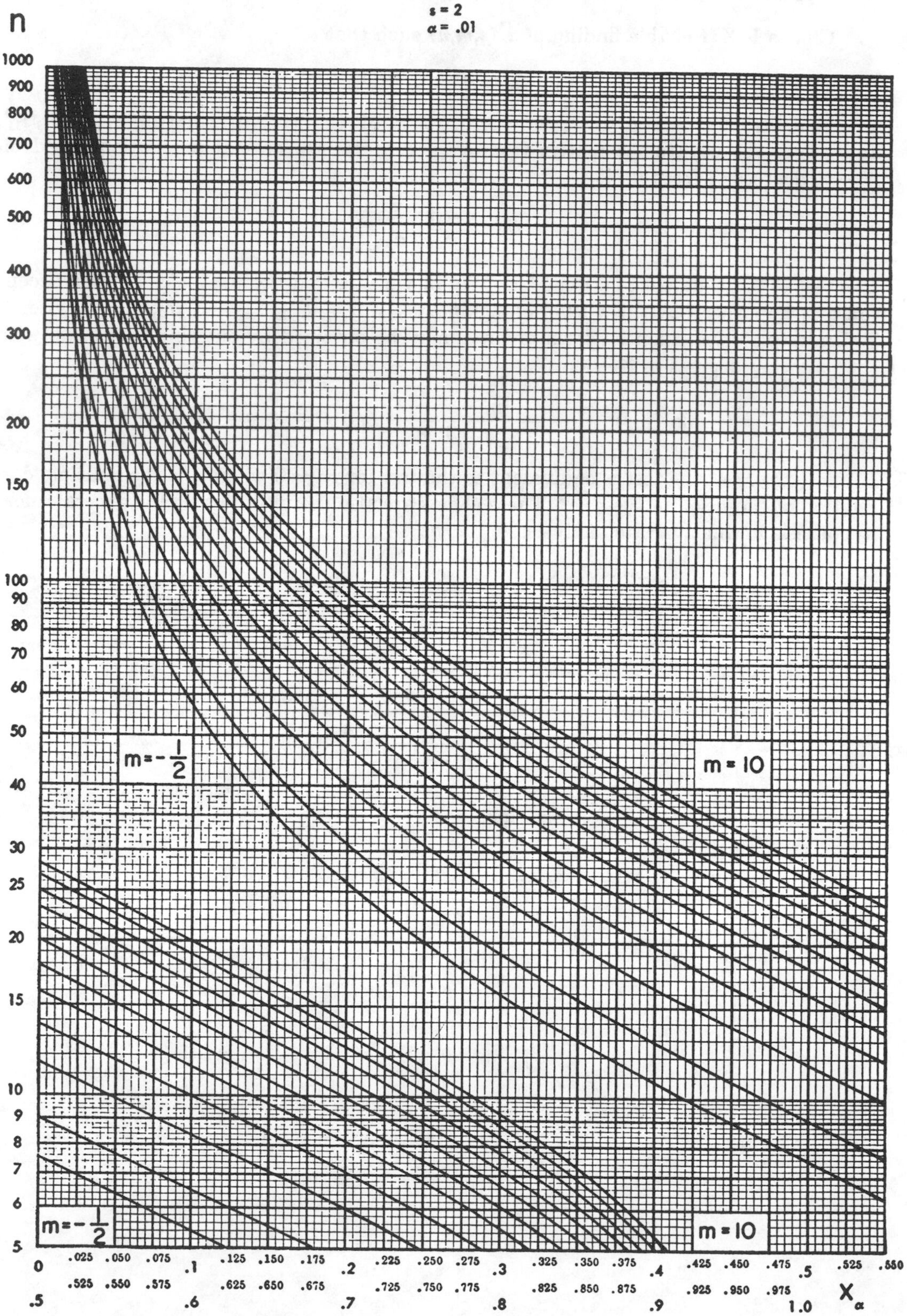
n
s = 2
α = .01
1000
900
800
700
600
500
400
300
200
150
100
90
80
70
60
50
40
30
25
20
15
10
9
8
7
6
5
m = - 1/2
m = 10
m = - 1/2
m = 10
0 .025 .050 .075 .1 .125 .150 .175 .2 .225 .250 .275 .3 .325 .350 .375 .4 .425 .450 .475 .5 .525 .550
.525 .550 .575 .625 .650 .675 .725 .750 .775 .825 .850 .875 .925 .950 .975
.5 .6 .7 .8 .9 1.0
X_α

CHART 11

s = 2
α = .025

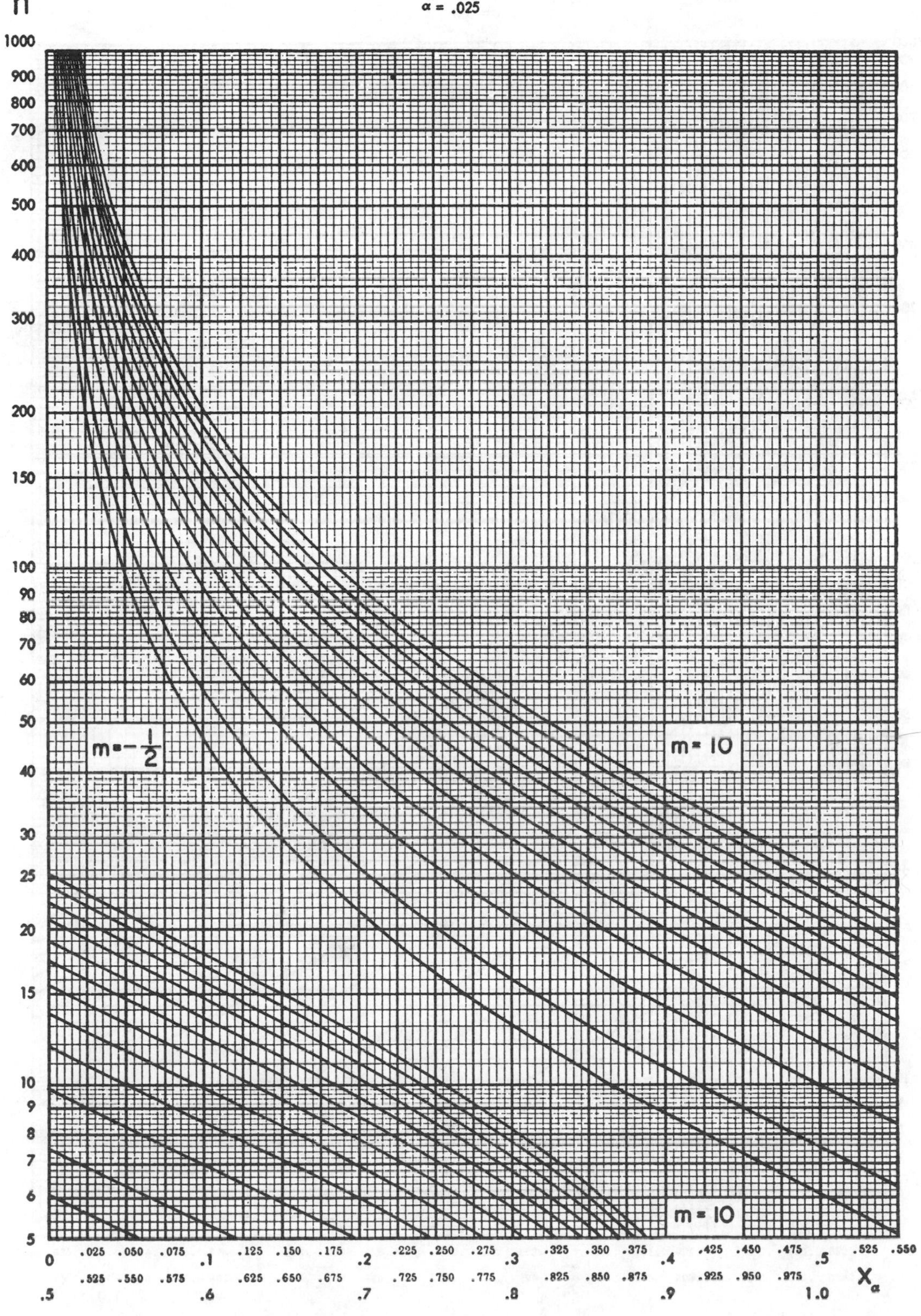

CHART III

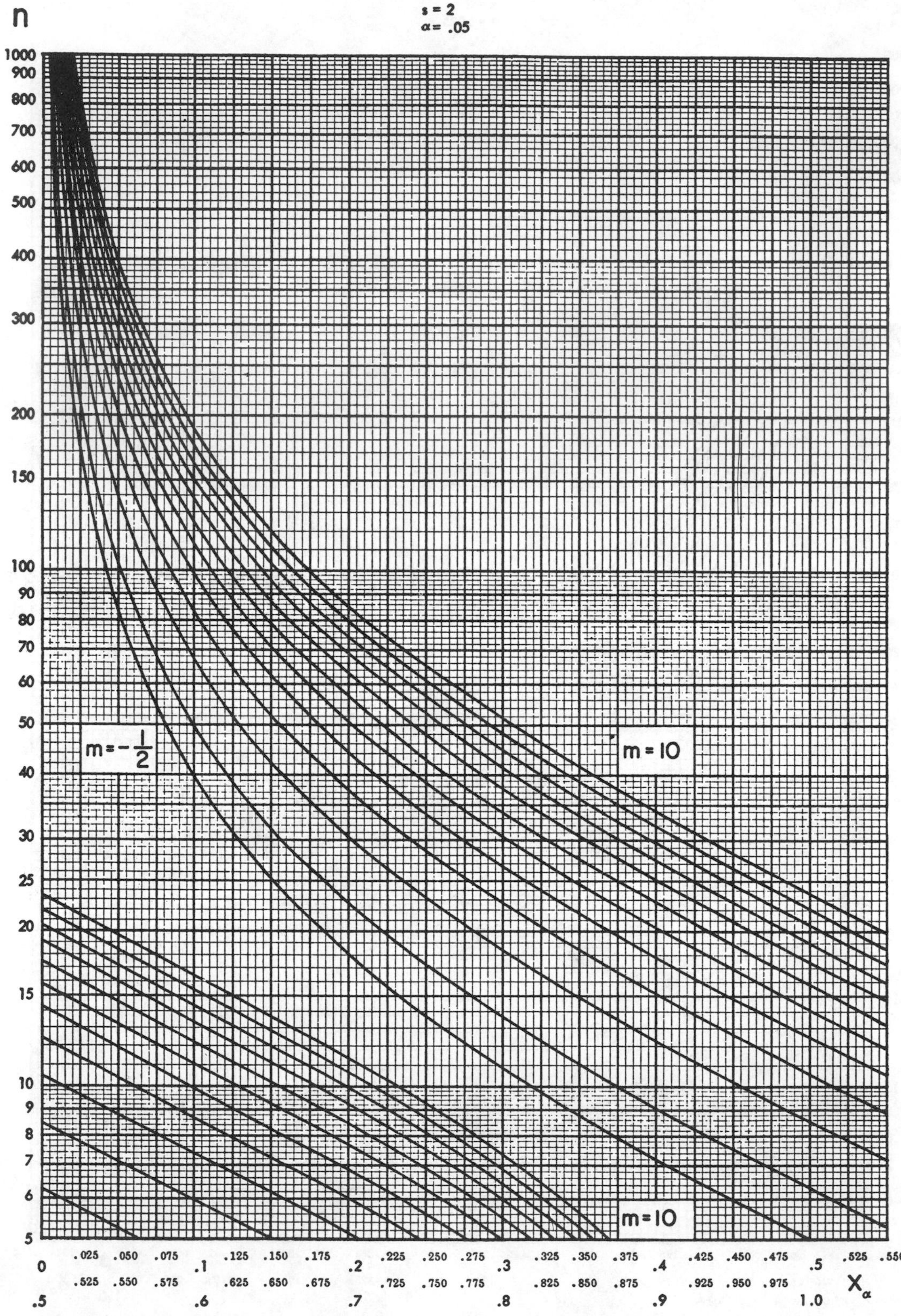
n
s = 2
α = .05
1000
900
800
700
600
500
400
300
200
150
100
90
80
70
60
50
40
30
25
20
15
10
9
8
7
6
5
m = − 1/2
m = 10
m = 10
0 .025 .050 .075 .1 .125 .150 .175 .2 .225 .250 .275 .3 .325 .350 .375 .4 .425 .450 .475 .5 .525 .550
.525 .550 .575 .625 .650 .675 .725 .750 .775 .825 .850 .875 .925 .950 .975
.5 .6 .7 .8 .9 1.0
X_α

CHART IV

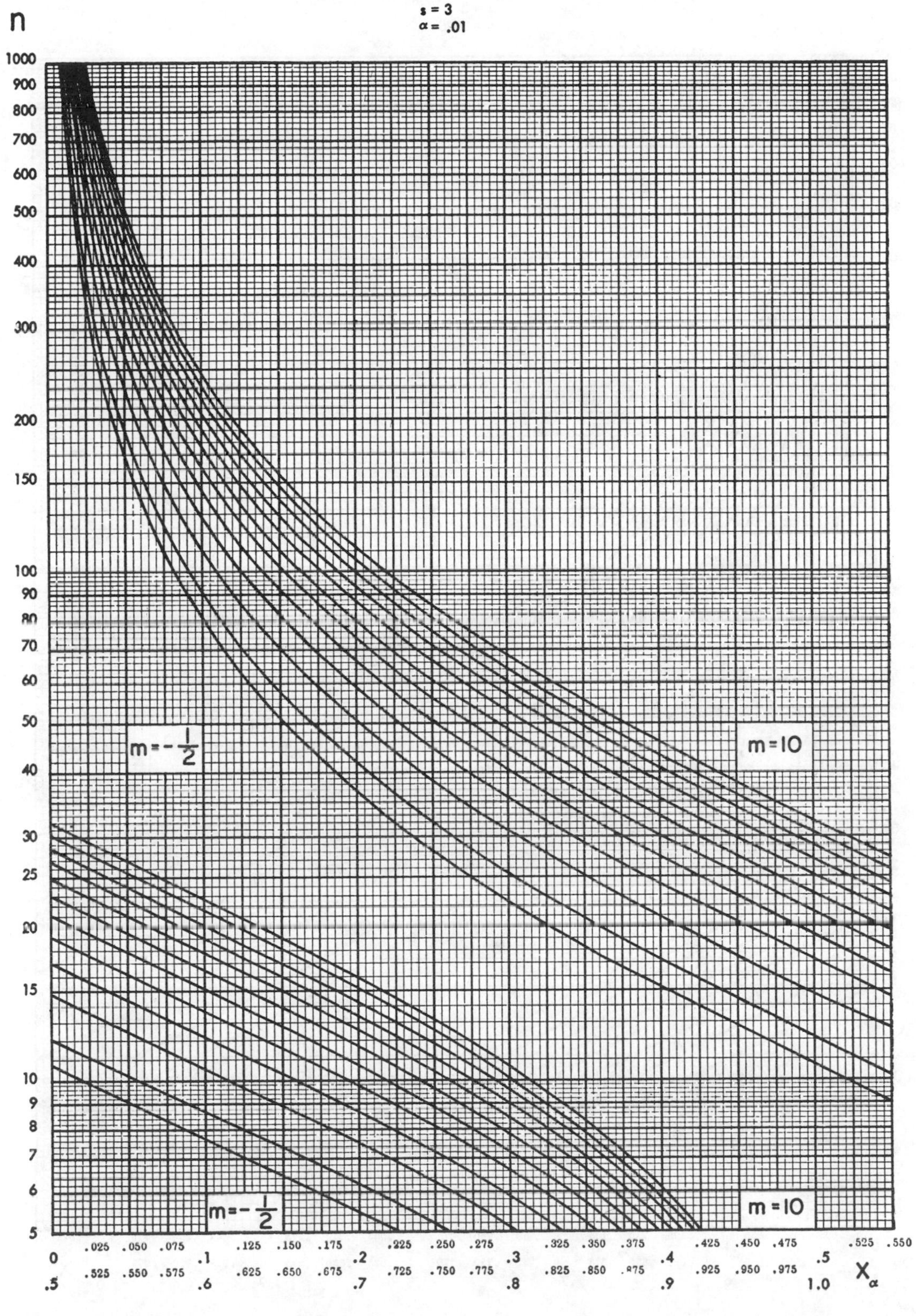
s = 3
α = .01
n
1000
900
800
700
600
500
400
300
200
150
100
90
80
70
60
50
40
30
25
20
15
10
9
8
7
6
5
m = - 1/2
m = 10
m = - 1/2
m = 10
0 .025 .050 .075 .1 .125 .150 .175 .2 .225 .250 .275 .3 .325 .350 .375 .4 .425 .450 .475 .5 .525 .550
.5 .525 .550 .575 .6 .625 .650 .675 .7 .725 .750 .775 .8 .825 .850 .875 .9 .925 .950 .975 1.0
X_α

CHART V

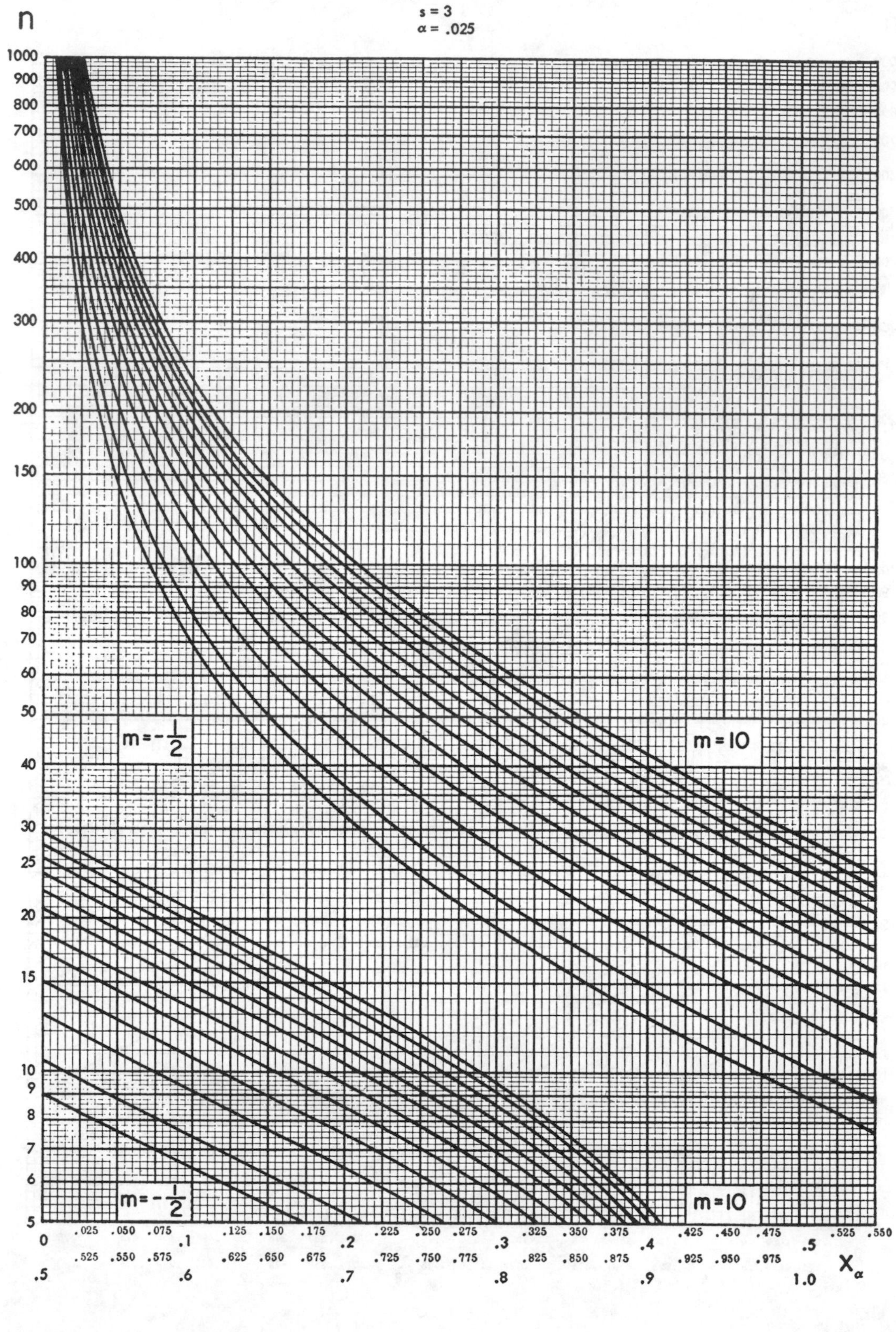
n
s = 3
α = .025
1000
900
800
700
600
500
400
300
200
150
100
90
80
70
60
50
40
30
25
20
15
10
9
8
7
6
5
m = −1/2
m = 10
m = −1/2
m = 10
0 .025 .050 .075 .1 .125 .150 .175 .2 .225 .250 .275 .3 .325 .350 .375 .4 .425 .450 .475 .5 .525 .550
.5 .525 .550 .575 .6 .625 .650 .675 .7 .725 .750 .775 .8 .825 .850 .875 .9 .925 .950 .975 1.0
X_α

CHART VI

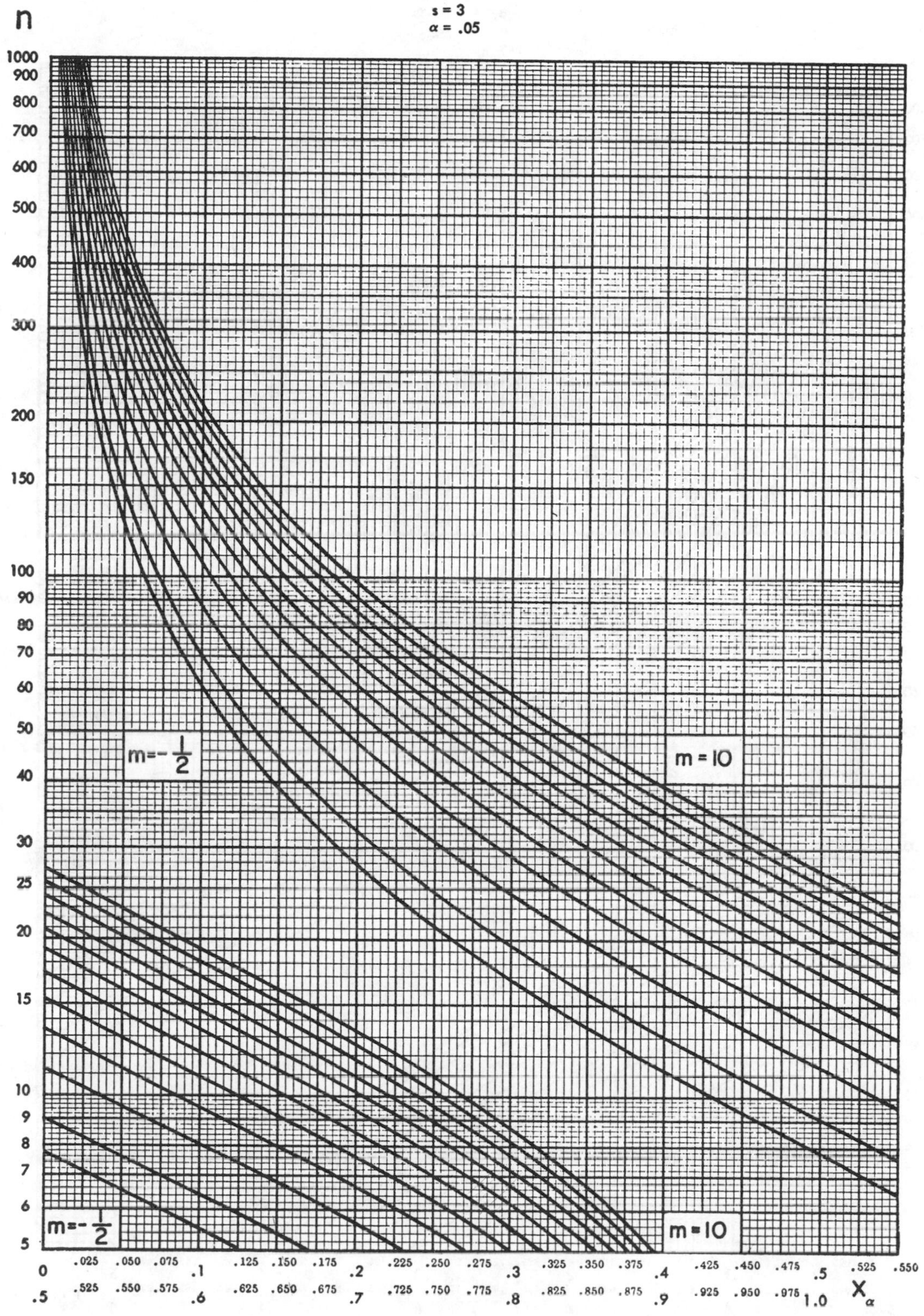
n
s = 3
α = .05
1000
900
800
700
600
500
400
300
200
150
100
90
80
70
60
50
40
30
25
20
15
10
9
8
7
6
5
m = −1/2
m = 10
m = −1/2
m = 10
0 .025 .050 .075 .1 .125 .150 .175 .2 .225 .250 .275 .3 .325 .350 .375 .4 .425 .450 .475 .5 .525 .550
.5 .525 .550 .575 .6 .625 .650 .675 .7 .725 .750 .775 .8 .825 .850 .875 .9 .925 .950 .975 1.0
X_α

CHART VII

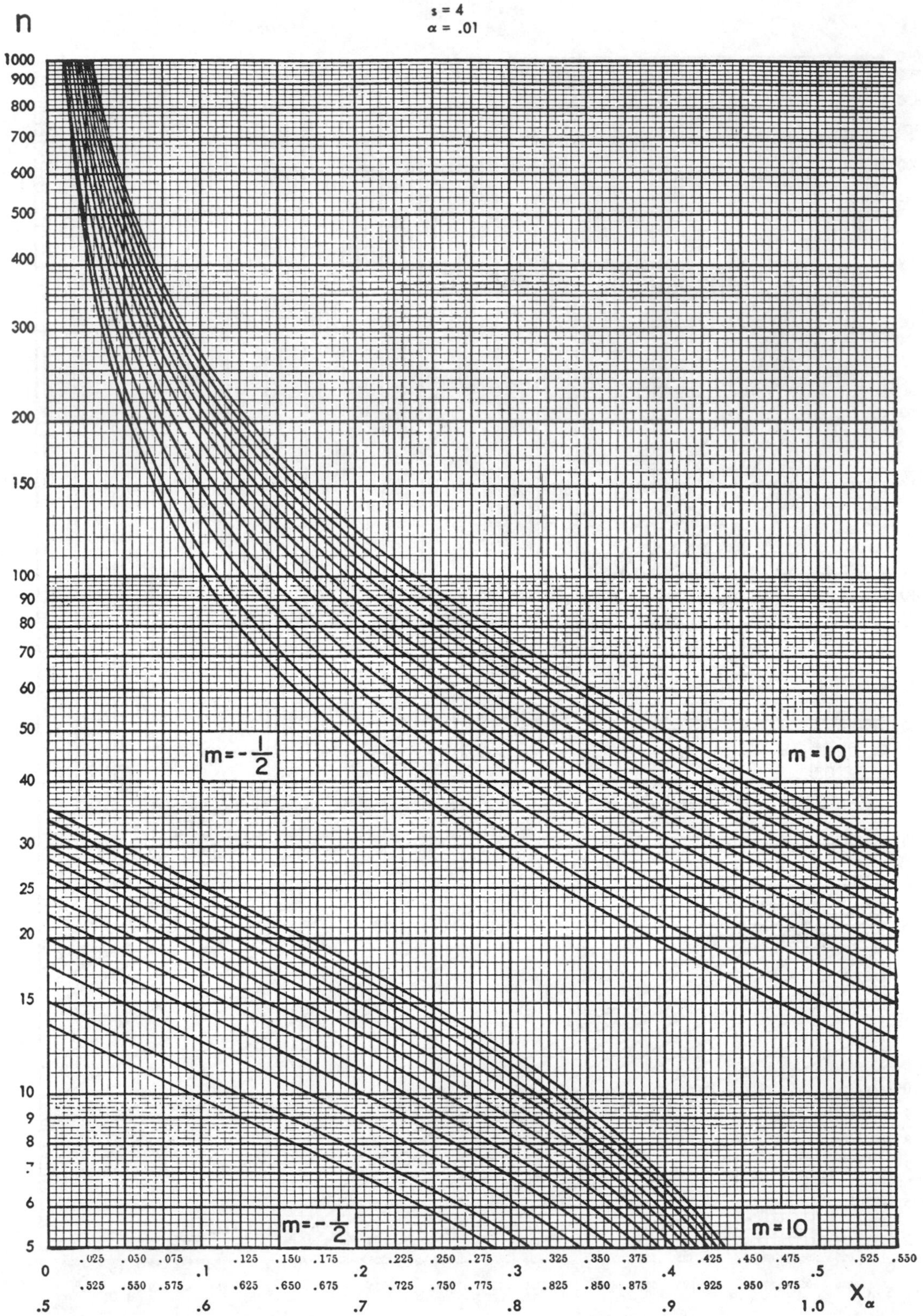
s = 4
α = .01
n
1000
900
800
700
600
500
400
300
200
150
100
90
80
70
60
50
40
30
25
20
15
10
9
8
7
6
5
m = - 1/2
m = 10
m = - 1/2
m = 10
0
.025
.050
.075
.1
.125
.150
.175
.2
.225
.250
.275
.3
.325
.350
.375
.4
.425
.450
.475
.5
.525
.550
.525
.550
.575
.625
.650
.675
.725
.750
.775
.825
.850
.875
.925
.950
.975
.5
.6
.7
.8
.9
1.0
X_α

CHART VIII

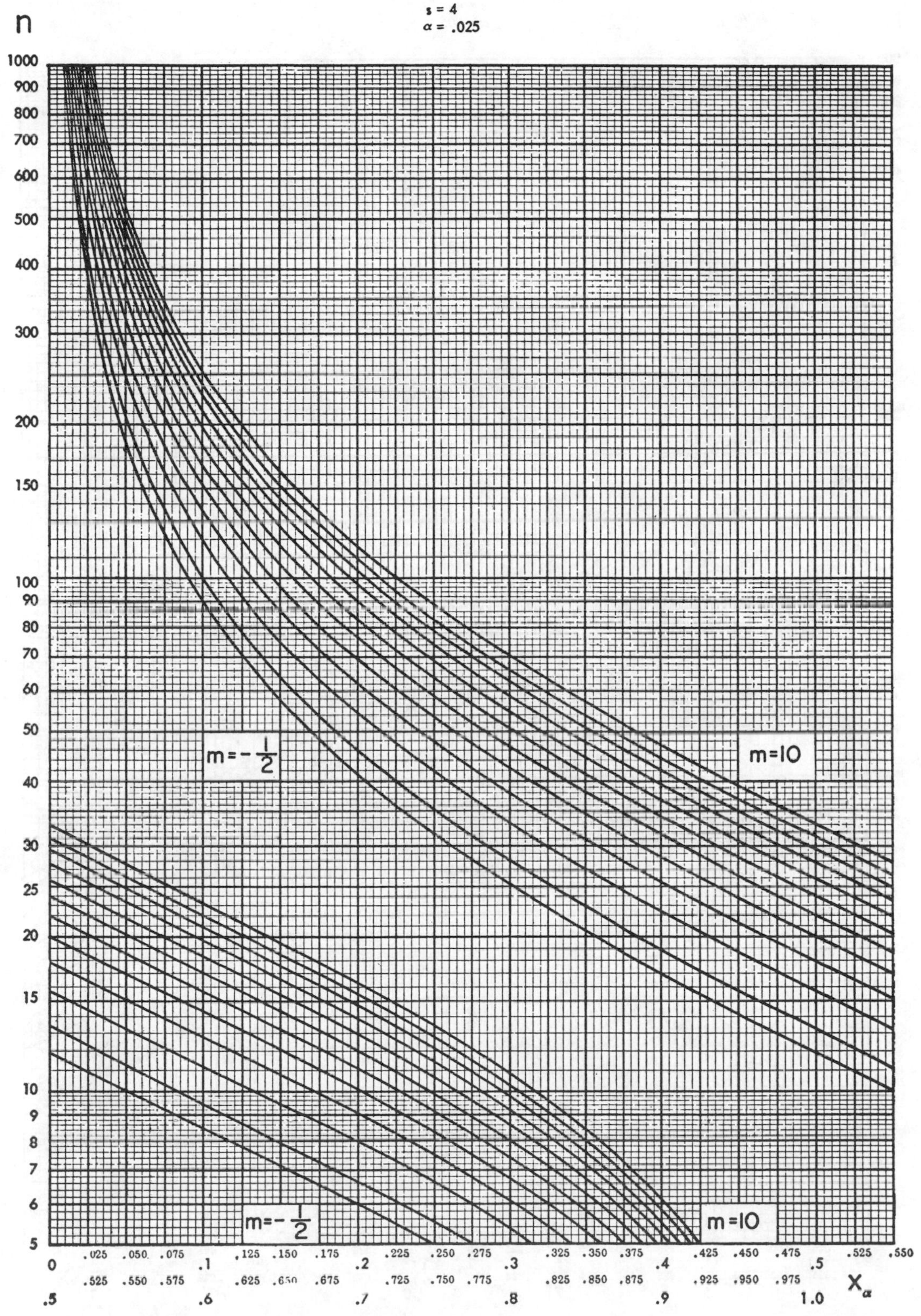
n
s = 4
α = .025
1000
900
800
700
600
500
400
300
200
150
100
90
80
70
60
50
40
30
25
20
15
10
9
8
7
6
5
m = − 1/2
m=10
m = − 1/2
m =10
0 .025 .050 .075 .1 .125 .150 .175 .2 .225 .250 .275 .3 .325 .350 .375 .4 .425 .450 .475 .5 .525 .550
.525 .550 .575 .625 .650 .675 .725 .750 .775 .825 .850 .875 .925 .950 .975
.5 .6 .7 .8 .9 1.0
X_α

CHART IX

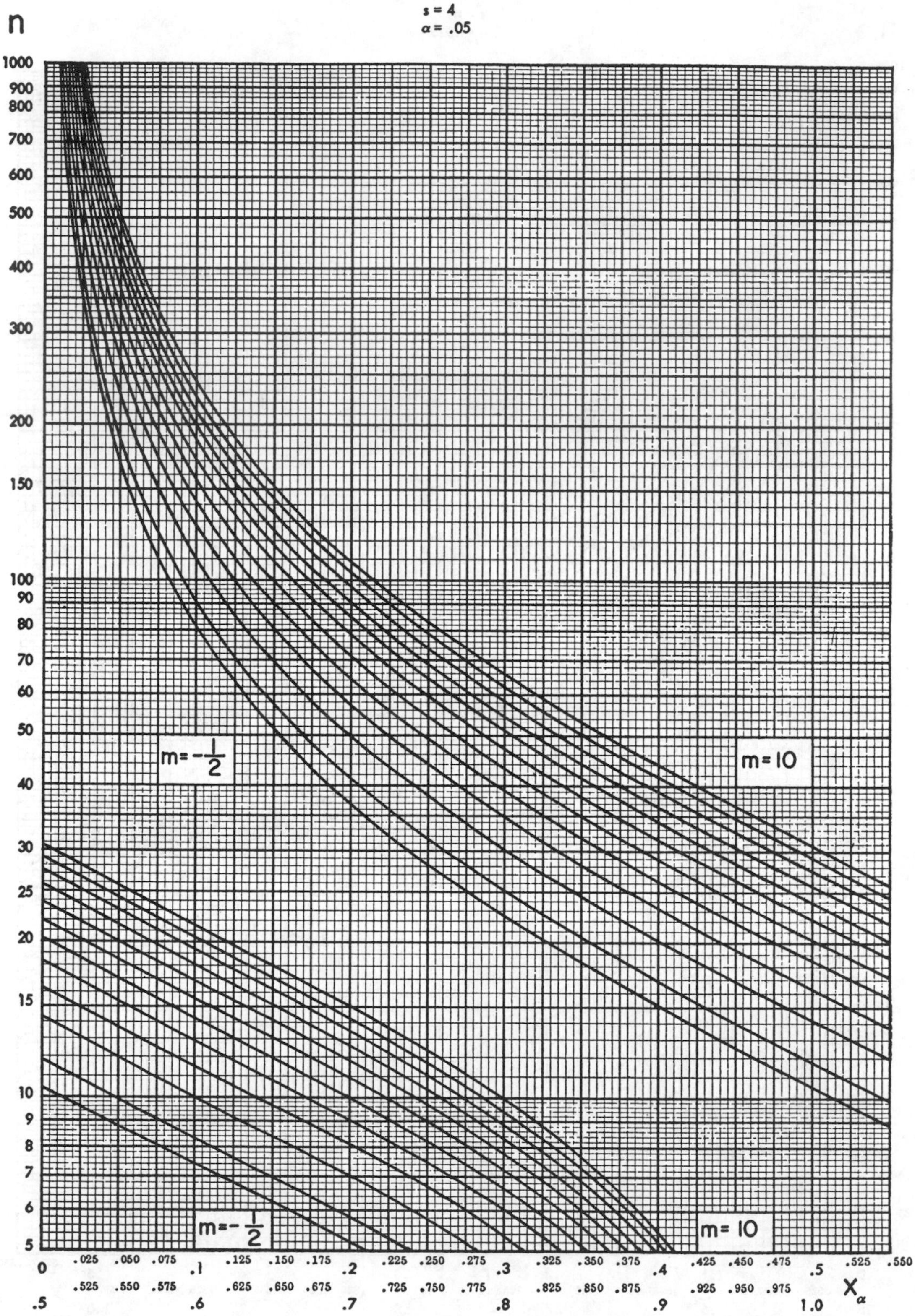
s = 4
α = .05
n
1000
900
800
700
600
500
400
300
200
150
100
90
80
70
60
50
40
30
25
20
15
10
9
8
7
6
5
m= −1/2
m= 10
m= −1/2
m= 10
0 .025 .050 .075 .1 .125 .150 .175 .2 .225 .250 .275 .3 .325 .350 .375 .4 .425 .450 .475 .5 .525 .550
.525 .550 .575 .625 .650 .675 .725 .750 .775 .825 .850 .875 .925 .950 .975
.5 .6 .7 .8 .9 1.0
X_α

CHART X

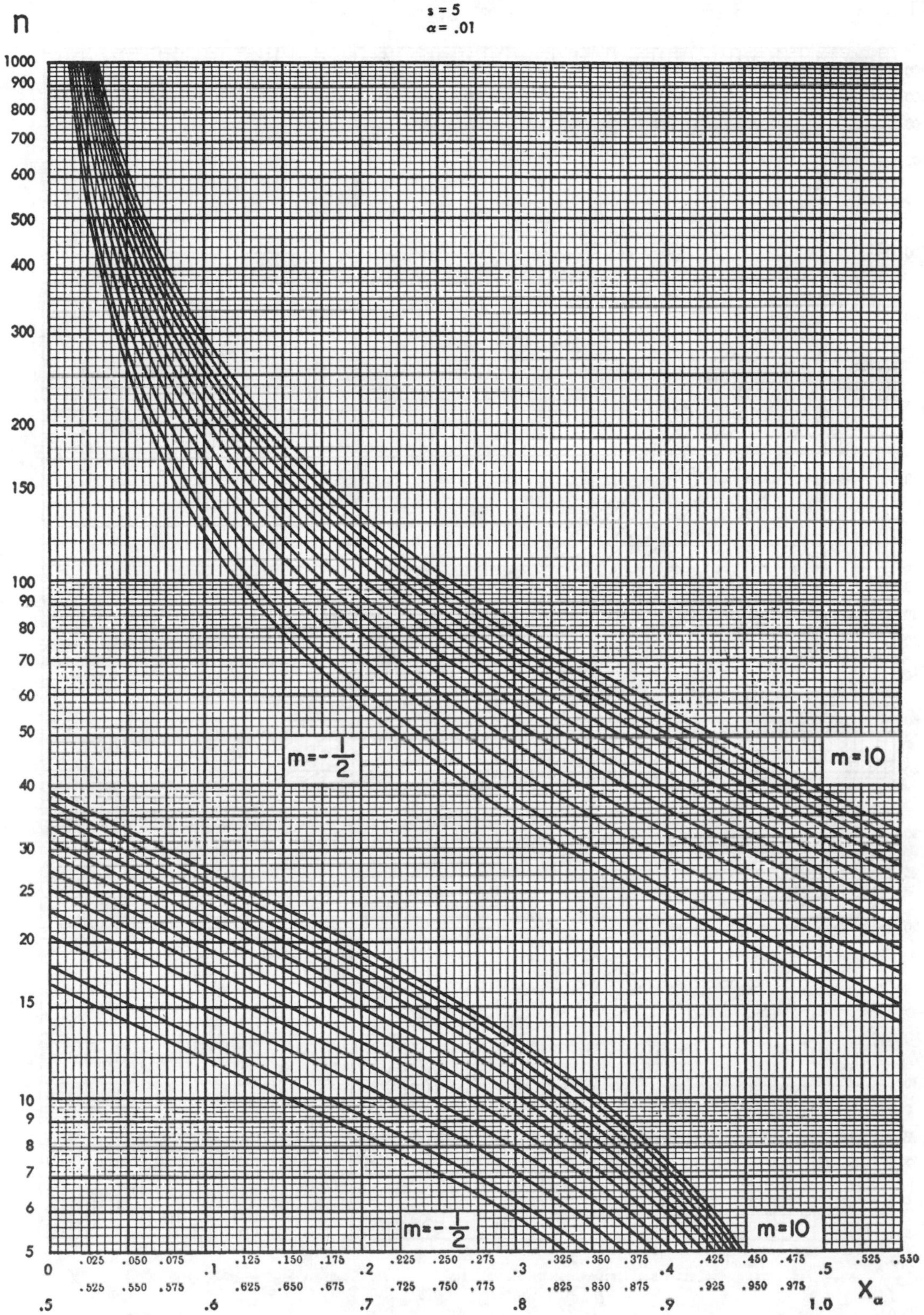

s = 5
α = .01
n
1000
900
800
700
600
500
400
300
200
150
100
90
80
70
60
50
40
30
25
20
15
10
9
8
7
6
5
m=-1/2
m=10
m=-1/2
m=10
0 .025 .050 .075 .1 .125 .150 .175 .2 .225 .250 .275 .3 .325 .350 .375 .4 .425 .450 .475 .5 .525 .550
.525 .550 .575 .625 .650 .675 .725 .750 .775 .825 .850 .875 .925 .950 .975
.5 .6 .7 .8 .9 1.0
X_α

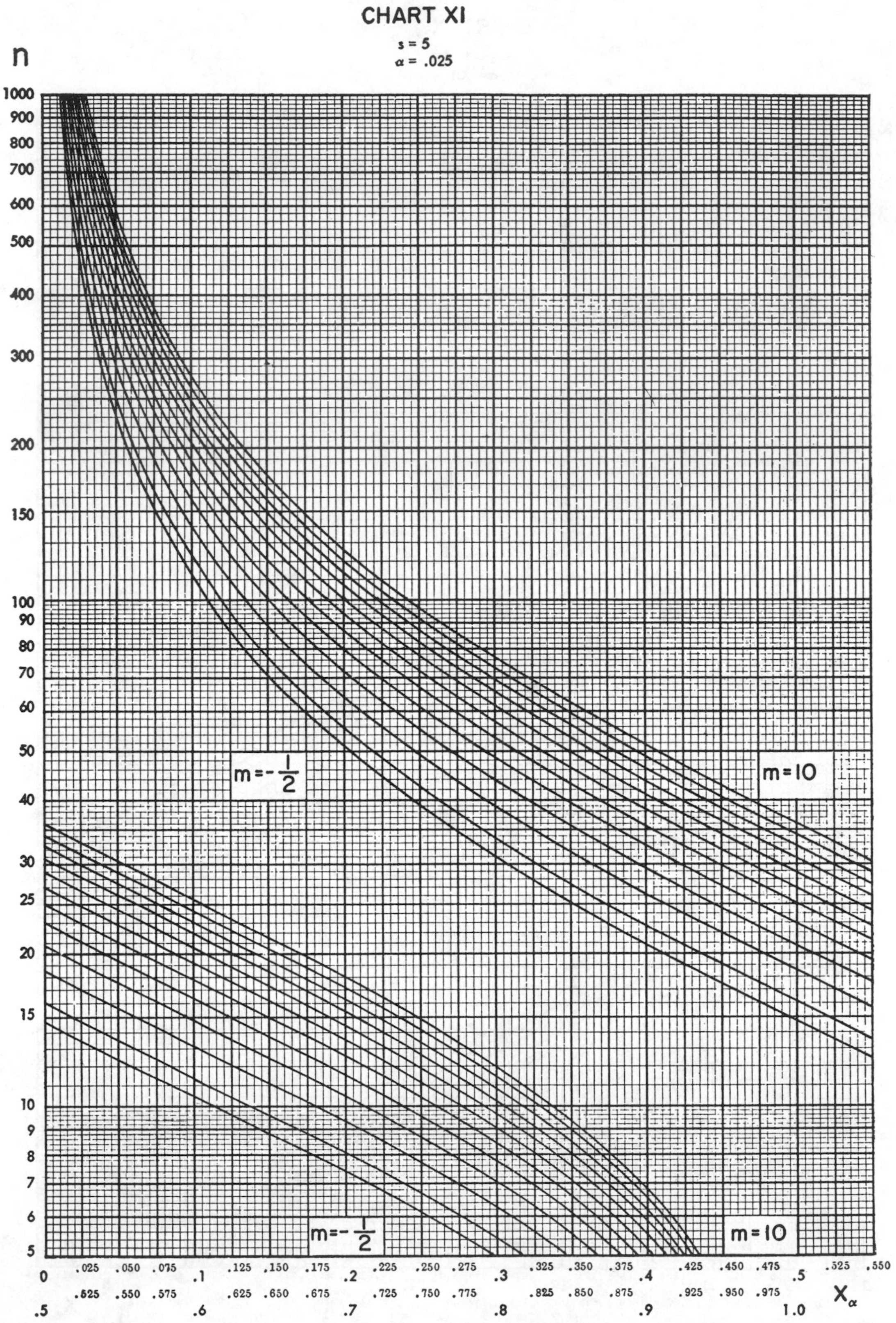
CHART XI
s = 5
α = .025
n
1000
900
800
700
600
500
400
300
200
150
100
90
80
70
60
50
40
30
25
20
15
10
9
8
7
6
5
m = -1/2
m = 10
m = -1/2
m = 10
0 .025 .050 .075 .1 .125 .150 .175 .2 .225 .250 .275 .3 .325 .350 .375 .4 .425 .450 .475 .5 .525 .550
.525 .550 .575 .625 .650 .675 .725 .750 .775 .825 .850 .875 .925 .950 .975
.5 .6 .7 .8 .9 1.0
Xα

CHART XII

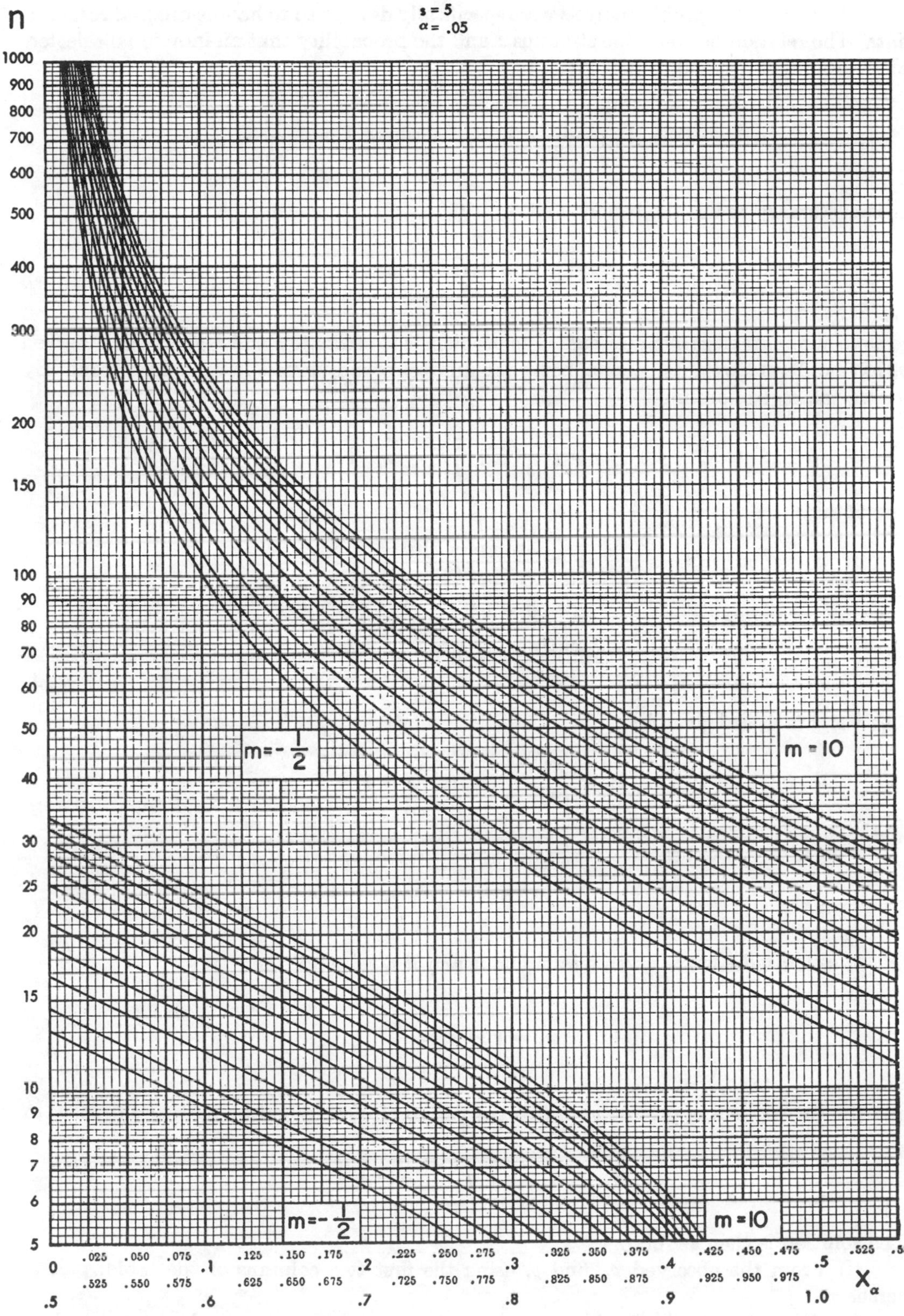
s = 5
α = .05
n
1000
900
800
700
600
500
400
300
200
150
100
90
80
70
60
50
40
30
25
20
15
10
9
8
7
6
5
m = - 1/2
m = 10
m = - 1/2
m = 10
0
.025
.050
.075
.1
.125
.150
.175
.2
.225
.250
.275
.3
.325
.350
.375
.4
.425
.450
.475
.5
.525
.550
.525
.550
.575
.625
.650
.675
.725
.750
.775
.825
.850
.875
.925
.950
.975
.5
.6
.7
.8
.9
1.0
X_α

II.10 PROBIT ANALYSIS

The methods of probit analysis were specifically developed to handle quantal response data. The relation between the stimulus x and the probability that an individual selected at random will respond to it is given by

$$P = \int_{-\infty}^{X} \frac{1}{\sqrt{2\pi}} e^{-\frac{1}{2}t^2}\, dt, \qquad \text{where } X = \frac{x-\mu}{\sigma}.$$

It is customary to use the probit

$$Y = \frac{x-\mu}{\sigma} + 5$$

so as to eliminate negative numbers. The problem is to estimate μ and σ where the observed y_i have different weights, $n_i w_i$, n_i being the number of individuals in each dose group. By fitting the regression line

$$y = \frac{5-\mu}{\sigma} + \frac{1}{\sigma}x = a + bx,$$

one obtains

$$b = \frac{\Sigma nw(x-\bar{x})(y-\bar{y})}{\Sigma nw(x-\bar{x})^2}$$

$$a = \bar{y} - b\bar{x},$$

where

$$\bar{x} = \frac{\Sigma nwx}{\Sigma nw} \quad \text{and} \quad \bar{y} = \frac{\Sigma nwy}{\Sigma nw}.$$

The weights w_i are given by

$$w_i = \frac{Z^2}{PQ}, \qquad \text{where } Q = 1 - P$$

and

$$Z = \frac{1}{\sqrt{2\pi}} e^{-\frac{1}{2}X^2}.$$

If n_i individuals are given a stimulus x_i and if r_i respond, then

$$p_i = 1 - q_i = \frac{r_i}{n_i}$$

and the corresponding probits y_i will be the values of Y obtained by inserting p_i for P in

$$P = \frac{1}{\sqrt{2\pi}} \int_{-\infty}^{Y-5} e^{-\frac{1}{2}t^2}\, dt.$$

The solution is then as follows:

(i) From the observed p_i, find y_i using the first two columns of the table; plot y_i versus x_i .

(ii) Fit a straight line to the points (x_i, y_i) by eye and obtain a set of expected probits Y_i' corresponding to x_i.

(iii) Obtain a set of working probits y_i' and their weighting coefficients w_i'. These working probits are obtained from either

$$y = Y + \frac{Q}{Z} - \frac{q}{Z}$$

or

$$y = Y - \frac{P}{Z} + \frac{p}{Z}.$$

A second approximation to the regression line is thus obtained. The following can be found by entering the table with the expected probits Y_i':

$$\text{range} = \frac{1}{Z}$$

$$\text{maximum working probit } Y_{\max} = Y + \frac{Q}{Z}$$

$$\text{minimum working probit } Y_{\min} = Y - \frac{P}{Z}.$$

(iv) By entering the table with Y_i', the appropriate weights $n_i w_i'$ are also found.

(v) These weights and the working probits y_i' are then used to compute a and b.

(vi) The values of the probits Y_i'' obtained from this second approximation may be used to repeat the above cycle. The iteration is continued until the line changes no further.

TABLE FOR PROBIT ANALYSIS

Proportion P	Expected probit Y	Maximum working probit $Y + Q/Z$	Minimum working probit $Y - P/Z$	Range $1/Z$	Weighting coefficient Z^2/PQ			
0.500	**5.00**	6.2533	3.7467	2.5066	0.6366	6.2533	3.7467	**5.00**
.504	**.01**	.2534	.7466	.5068	.6366	.2534	.7466	**4.99**
.508	**.02**	.2536	.7465	.5071	.6365	.2535	.7464	**.98**
.512	**.03**	.2539	.7461	.5078	.6364	.2539	.7461	**.97**
.516	**.04**	.2543	.7457	.5086	.6362	.2543	.7457	**.96**
0.520	**5.05**	6.2548	3.7450	2.5098	0.6360	6.2550	3.7452	**4.95**
.524	**.06**	.2555	.7444	.5111	.6358	.2556	.7445	**.94**
.528	**.07**	.2563	.7435	.5128	.6355	.2565	.7437	**.93**
.532	**.08**	.2572	.7425	.5147	.6351	.2575	.7428	**.92**
.536	**.09**	.2582	.7414	.5168	.6347	.2586	.7418	**.91**
0.540	**5.10**	6.2593	3.7401	2.5192	0.6343	6.2599	3.7407	**4.90**
.544	**.11**	.2605	.7387	.5218	.6338	.2613	.7395	**.89**
.548	**.12**	.2618	.7371	.5247	.6333	.2629	.7382	**.88**
.552	**.13**	.2632	.7353	.5279	.6327	.2647	.7368	**.87**
.556	**.14**	.2647	.7334	.5313	.6321	.2666	.7353	**.86**
0.560	**5.15**	6.2664	3.7314	2.5350	0.6314	6.2686	3.7336	**4.85**
.564	**.16**	.2681	.7292	.5389	.6307	.2708	.7319	**.84**
.567	**.17**	.2699	.7268	.5431	.6300	.2732	.7301	**.83**
.571	**.18**	.2718	.7242	.5476	.6292	.2758	.7282	**.82**
.575	**.19**	.2738	.7215	.5523	.6283	.2785	.7262	**.81**
0.579	**5.20**	6.2759	3.7186	2.5573	0.6274	6.2814	3.7241	**4.80**
.583	**.21**	.2781	.7156	.5625	.6265	.2844	.7219	**.79**
.587	**.22**	.2804	.7124	.5680	.6255	.2876	.7196	**.78**
.591	**.23**	.2828	.7090	.5738	.6245	.2910	.7172	**.77**
.595	**.24**	.2853	.7054	.5799	.6234	.2946	.7147	**.76**
0.599	**5.25**	6.2878	3.7016	2.5862	0.6223	6.2984	3.7122	**4.75**
.603	**.26**	.2905	.6977	.5928	.6211	.3023	.7095	**.74**
.606	**.27**	.2932	.6935	.5997	.6199	.3065	.7068	**.73**
.610	**.28**	.2960	.6892	.6068	.6187	.3108	.7040	**.72**
.614	**.29**	.2989	.6846	.6143	.6174	.3154	.7011	**.71**
0.618	**5.30**	6.3018	3.6798	2.6220	0.6161	6.3202	3.6982	**4.70**
.622	**.31**	.3049	.6749	.6300	.6147	.3251	.6951	**.69**
.626	**.32**	.3080	.6697	.6383	.6133	.3303	.6920	**.68**
.629	**.33**	.3112	.6643	.6469	.6119	.3357	.6888	**.67**
.633	**.34**	.3145	.6587	.6558	.6104	.3413	.6855	**.66**
0.637	**5.35**	6.3178	3.6528	2.6650	0.6088	6.3472	3.6822	**4.65**
.641	**.36**	.3213	.6469	.6744	.6072	.3531	.6787	**.64**
.644	**.37**	.3248	.6406	.6842	.6056	.3594	.6752	**.63**
.648	**.38**	.3283	.6340	.6943	.6040	.3660	.6717	**.62**
.652	**.39**	.3320	.6273	.7047	.6023	.3727	.6680	**.61**
0.655	**5.40**	6.3357	3.6203	2.7154	0.6005	6.3797	3.6643	**4.60**
$Z = e^{-\frac{1}{2}X^2}/\sqrt{(2\pi)}$ $Y = X + 5$ $P = 1 - Q = \int_{-\infty}^{X} Z(t)\,dt$				$1/Z$ Range	Z^2/PQ Weighting coefficient	$Y + Q/Z$ Maximum working probit	$Y - P/Z$ Minimum working probit	Y Expected probit

TABLE FOR PROBIT ANALYSIS

Proportion P	Expected probit Y	Maximum working probit $Y + Q/Z$	Minimum working probit $Y - P/Z$	Range $1/Z$	Weighting coefficient Z^2/PQ			
0.655	**5.40**	6.3357	3.6203	2.7154	0.6005	6.3797	3.6643	**4.60**
.659	**.41**	.3394	.6130	.7264	.5987	.3870	.6606	**.59**
.663	**.42**	.3433	.6055	.7378	.5969	.3945	.6567	**.58**
.666	**.43**	.3472	.5978	.7494	.5951	.4022	.6528	**.57**
.670	**.44**	.3512	.5898	.7614	.5932	.4102	.6488	**.56**
0.674	**5.45**	6.3552	3.5815	2.7737	0.5912	6.4185	3.6448	**4.55**
.677	**.46**	.3593	.5729	.7864	.5893	.4271	.6407	**.54**
.681	**.47**	.3635	.5641	.7994	.5872	.4359	.6365	**.53**
.684	**.48**	.3677	.5550	.8127	.5852	.4450	.6323	**.52**
.688	**.49**	.3720	.5456	.8264	.5831	.4544	.6280	**.51**
0.691	**5.50**	6.3764	3.5360	2.8404	0.5810	6.4640	3.6236	**4.50**
.695	**.51**	.3808	.5260	.8548	.5788	.4740	.6192	**.49**
.698	**.52**	.3852	.5157	.8695	.5766	.4843	.6148	**.48**
.702	**.53**	.3898	.5052	.8846	.5744	.4948	.6102	**.47**
.705	**.54**	.3944	.4943	.9001	.5722	.5057	.6056	**.46**
0.709	**5.55**	6.3990	3.4831	2.9159	0.5699	6.5169	3.6010	**4.45**
.712	**.56**	.4037	.4715	.9322	.5675	.5285	.5963	**.44**
.716	**.57**	.4085	.4597	.9488	.5652	.5403	.5915	**.43**
.719	**.58**	.4133	.4475	.9658	.5628	.5525	.5867	**.42**
.722	**.59**	.4181	.4349	.9832	.5603	.5651	.5819	**.41**
0.726	**5.60**	6.4230	3.4220	3.0010	0.5579	6.5780	3.5770	**4.40**
.729	**.61**	.4280	.4088	.0192	.5554	.5912	.5720	**.39**
.732	**.62**	.4330	.3952	.0378	.5529	.6048	.5670	**.38**
.736	**.63**	.4381	.3812	.0569	.5503	.6188	.5619	**.37**
.739	**.64**	.4432	.3669	.0763	.5477	.6331	.5568	**.36**
0.742	**5.65**	6.4484	3.3522	3.0962	0.5451	6.6478	3.5516	**4.35**
.745	**.66**	.4536	.3370	.1166	.5425	.6630	.5464	**.34**
.749	**.67**	.4588	.3214	.1374	.5398	.6786	.5412	**.33**
.752	**.68**	.4641	.3055	.1586	.5371	.6945	.5359	**.32**
.755	**.69**	.4695	.2892	.1803	.5343	.7108	.5305	**.31**
0.758	**5.70**	6.4749	3.2724	3.2025	0.5316	6.7276	3.5251	**4.30**
.761	**.71**	.4803	.2551	.2252	.5288	.7449	.5197	**.29**
.764	**.72**	.4858	.2375	.2483	.5260	.7625	.5142	**.28**
.767	**.73**	.4914	.2194	.2720	.5232	.7806	.5086	**.27**
.770	**.74**	.4969	.2008	.2961	.5203	.7992	.5031	**.26**
0.773	**5.75**	6.5026	3.1819	3.3207	0.5174	6.8181	3.4974	**4.25**
.776	**.76**	.5082	.1623	.3459	.5145	.8377	.4918	**.24**
.779	**.77**	.5139	.1423	.3716	.5116	.8577	.4861	**.23**
.782	**.78**	.5197	.1219	.3978	.5086	.8781	.4803	**.22**
.785	**.79**	.5255	.1009	.4246	.5056	.8991	.4745	**.21**
0.788	**5.80**	6.5313	3.0794	3.4519	0.5026	6.9206	3.4687	**4.20**
$Z = e^{-\frac{1}{2}X^2}/\sqrt{(2\pi)}$ $Y = X + 5$ $P = 1 - Q = \int_{-\infty}^{X} Z(t)\,dt$				$1/Z$ Range	Z^2/PQ Weighting coefficient	$Y + Q/Z$ Maximum working probit	$Y - P/Z$ Minimum working probit	Y Expected probit

TABLE FOR PROBIT ANALYSIS

Proportion P	Expected probit Y	Maximum working probit $Y + Q/Z$	Minimum working probit $Y - P/Z$	Range $1/Z$	Weighting coefficient Z^2/PQ			
0.788	**5.80**	6.5313	3.0794	3.4519	0.5026	6.9206	3.4687	**4.20**
.791	**.81**	.5372	.0574	.4798	.4996	.9426	.4628	**.19**
.794	**.82**	.5431	.0348	.5083	.4965	.9652	.4569	**.18**
.797	**.83**	.5490	.0116	.5374	.4935	.9884	.4510	**.17**
.800	**.84**	.5550	2.9880	.5670	.4904	7.0120	.4450	**.16**
0.802	**5.85**	6.5611	2.9638	3.5973	0.4873	7.0362	3.4389	**4.15**
.805	**.86**	.5671	.9389	.6282	.4841	.0611	.4329	**.14**
.808	**.87**	.5732	.9135	.6597	.4810	.0865	.4268	**.13**
.811	**.88**	.5794	.8875	.6919	.4778	.1125	.4206	**.12**
.813	**.89**	.5855	.8608	.7247	.4746	.1392	.4145	**.11**
0.816	**5.90**	6.5917	2.8335	3.7582	0.4714	7.1665	3.4083	**4.10**
.819	**.91**	.5980	.8056	.7924	.4682	.1944	.4020	**.09**
.821	**.92**	.6043	.7771	.8272	.4650	.2229	.3957	**.08**
.824	**.93**	.6106	.7478	.8628	.4617	.2522	.3894	**.07**
.826	**.94**	.6169	.7178	.8991	.4585	.2822	.3831	**.06**
0.829	**5.95**	6.6233	2.6872	3.9361	0.4552	7.3128	3.3767	**4.05**
.831	**.96**	.6297	.6558	.9739	.4519	.3442	.3703	**.04**
.834	**.97**	.6362	.6238	4.0124	.4486	.3762	.3638	**.03**
.836	**.98**	.6426	.5909	.0517	.4453	.4091	.3574	**.02**
.839	**.99**	.6491	.5573	.0918	.4420	.4427	.3509	**.01**
0.841	**6.00**	6.6557	2.5230	4.1327	0.4386	7.4770	3.3443	**4.00**
.844	**.01**	.6623	.4878	.1745	.4353	.5122	.3377	**3.99**
.846	**.02**	.6689	.4518	.2171	.4319	.5482	.3311	**.98**
.848	**.03**	.6755	.4150	.2605	.4285	.5850	.3245	**.97**
.851	**.04**	.6822	.3774	.3048	.4252	.6226	.3178	**.96**
0.853	**6.05**	6.6888	2.3387	4.3501	0.4218	7.6613	3.3112	**3.95**
.855	**.06**	.6956	.2994	.3962	.4184	.7006	.3044	**.94**
.858	**.07**	.7023	.2590	.4433	.4150	.7410	.2977	**.93**
.860	**.08**	.7091	.2178	.4913	.4116	.7822	.2909	**.92**
.862	**.09**	.7159	.1756	.5403	.4082	.8244	.2841	**.91**
0.864	**6.10**	6.7227	2.1324	4.5903	0.4047	7.8676	3.2773	**3.90**
.867	**.11**	.7296	.0883	.6413	.4013	.9117	.2704	**.89**
.869	**.12**	.7365	.0432	.6933	.3979	.9568	.2635	**.88**
.871	**.13**	.7434	1.9970	.7464	.3944	8.0030	.2566	**.87**
.873	**.14**	.7504	.9498	.8006	.3910	.0502	.2496	**.86**
0.875	**6.15**	6.7573	1.9014	4.8559	0.3876	8.0986	3.2427	**3.85**
.877	**.16**	.7643	.8520	.9123	.3841	.1480	.2357	**.84**
.879	**.17**	.7714	.8016	.9698	.3807	.1984	.2286	**.83**
.881	**.18**	.7784	.7498	5.0286	.3772	.2502	.2216	**.82**
.883	**.19**	.7855	.6970	.0885	.3738	.3030	.2145	**.81**
0.885	**6.20**	6.7926	1.6429	5.1497	0.3703	8.3571	3.2074	**3.80**
$Z = e^{-\frac{1}{2}X^2}/\sqrt{(2\pi)}$ $Y = X + 5$ $P = 1 - Q = \int_{-\infty}^{X} Z(t)\,dt$				$1/Z$ Range	Z^2/PQ Weighting coefficient	$Y + Q/Z$ Maximum working probit	$Y - P/Z$ Minimum working probit	Y Expected probit

TABLE FOR PROBIT ANALYSIS

Proportion P	Expected probit Y	Maximum working probit $Y + Q/Z$	Minimum working probit $Y - P/Z$	Range $1/Z$	Weighting coefficient Z^2/PQ			
0.885	**6.20**	6.7926	1.6429	5.1497	0.3703	8.3571	3.2074	**3.80**
.887	**.21**	.7997	.5876	.2121	.3669	.4124	.2003	**.79**
.889	**.22**	.8068	.5310	.2758	.3634	.4690	.1932	**.78**
.891	**.23**	.8140	.4731	.3409	.3600	.5269	.1860	**.77**
.893	**.24**	.8212	.4140	.4072	.3565	.5860	.1788	**.76**
0.894	**6.25**	6.8284	1.3534	5.4750	0.3531	8.6466	3.1716	**3.75**
.896	**.26**	.8357	.2916	.5441	.3496	.7084	.1643	**.74**
.898	**.27**	.8429	.2282	.6147	.3462	.7718	.1571	**.73**
.900	**.28**	.8502	.1635	.6867	.3428	.8365	.1498	**.72**
.901	**.29**	.8575	.0972	.7603	.3393	.9028	.1425	**.71**
0.903	**6.30**	6.8649	1.0295	5.8354	0.3359	8.9705	3.1351	**3.70**
.905	**.31**	.8722	0.9602	.9120	.3325	9.0398	.1278	**.69**
.907	**.32**	.8796	.8893	.9903	.3291	.1107	.1204	**.68**
.908	**.33**	.8870	.8168	6.0702	.3256	.1832	.1130	**.67**
.910	**.34**	.8944	.7426	.1518	.3222	.2574	.1056	**.66**
0.911	**6.35**	6.9019	0.6668	6.2351	0.3188	9.3332	3.0981	**3.65**
.913	**.36**	.9093	.5892	.3201	.3155	.4108	.0907	**.64**
.915	**.37**	.9168	.5098	.4070	.3121	.4902	.0832	**.63**
.916	**.38**	.9243	.4286	.4957	.3087	.5714	.0757	**.62**
.918	**.39**	.9318	.3455	.5863	.3053	.6545	.0682	**.61**
0.919	**6.40**	6.9394	0.2606	6.6788	0.3020	9.7394	3.0606	**3.60**
.921	**.41**	.9469	.1736	.7733	.2986	.8264	.0531	**.59**
.922	**.42**	.9545	.0847	.8698	.2953	.9153	.0455	**.58**
.924	**.43**	.9621		.9684	.2920		.0379	**.57**
.925	**.44**	.9697		7.0691	.2887		.0303	**.56**
0.926	**6.45**	6.9774		7.1720	0.2854		3.0226	**3.55**
.928	**.46**	.9850		.2771	.2821		.0150	**.54**
.929	**.47**	6.9927		.3845	.2788		.0073	**.53**
.931	**.48**	7.0004		.4943	.2756		2.9996	**.52**
.932	**.49**	.0081		.6064	.2723		.9919	**.51**
0.9332	**6.50**	7.0158		7.7210	0.2691		2.9842	**3.50**
345	**.51**	.0236		.8380	.2658		.9764	**.49**
357	**.52**	.0313		.9577	.2626		.9687	**.48**
370	**.53**	.0391		8.0800	.2594		.9609	**.47**
382	**.54**	.0469		.2050	.2563		.9531	**.46**
0.9394	**6.55**	7.0547		8.3327	0.2531		2.9453	**3.45**
406	**.56**	.0625		.4633	.2500		.9375	**.44**
418	**.57**	.0704		.5968	.2468		.9296	**.43**
429	**.58**	.0783		.7333	.2437		.9217	**.42**
441	**.59**	.0861		.8728	.2406		.9139	**.41**
0.9452	**6.60**	7.0940		9.0154	0.2375		2.9060	**3.40**
$Z = e^{-\frac{1}{2}X^2}/\sqrt{(2\pi)}$ $Y = X + 5$ $P = 1 - Q = \int_{-\infty}^{X} Z(t)\,dt$				$1/Z$ Range	Z^2/PQ Weighting coefficient	$Y + Q/Z$ Maximum working probit	$Y - P/Z$ Minimum working profit	Y Expected probit

TABLE FOR PROBIT ANALYSIS

Proportion P	Expected probit Y	Maximum working probit $Y + Q/Z$	Range $1/Z$	Weighting coefficient Z^2/PQ		
0.9452	**6.60**	7.0940	9.0154	0.2375	2.9060	**3.40**
463	**.61**	.1020	.1613	.2345	.8980	**.39**
474	**.62**	.1099	.3105	.2314	.8901	**.38**
484	**.63**	.1178	.4630	.2284	.8822	**.37**
495	**.64**	.1258	.6190	.2254	.8742	**.36**
0.9505	**6.65**	7.1338	9.7785	0.2224	2.8662	**3.35**
515	**.66**	.1417	.9417	.2194	.8583	**.34**
525	**.67**	.1498	10.1086	.2165	.8502	**.33**
535	**.68**	.1578	10.2794	.2135	.8422	**.32**
545	**.69**	.1658	10.4540	.2106	.8342	**.31**
0.9554	**6.70**	7.1739	10.6327	0.2077	2.8261	**3.30**
564	**.71**	.1819	10.8156	.2049	.8181	**.29**
573	**.72**	.1900	11.0027	.2020	.8100	**.28**
582	**.73**	.1981	11.1941	.1992	.8019	**.27**
591	**.74**	.2062	11.3900	.1964	.7938	**.26**
0.9599	**6.75**	7.2143	11.5905	0.1936	2.7857	**3.25**
608	**.76**	.2224	11.7957	.1908	.7776	**.24**
616	**.77**	.2306	12.0058	.1881	.7694	**.23**
625	**.78**	.2387	12.2208	.1853	.7613	**.22**
633	**.79**	.2469	12.4409	.1826	.7531	**.21**
0.9641	**6.80**	7.2551	12.6662	0.1799	2.7449	**3.20**
649	**.81**	.2633	12.8969	.1773	.7367	**.19**
656	**.82**	.2715	13.1331	.1746	.7285	**.18**
664	**.83**	.2797	13.3750	.1720	.7203	**.17**
671	**.84**	.2880	13.6227	.1694	.7120	**.16**
0.9678	**6.85**	7.2962	13.8764	0.1669	2.7038	**3.15**
686	**.86**	.3045	14.1362	.1643	.6955	**.14**
693	**.87**	.3128	14.4023	.1618	.6872	**.13**
699	**.88**	.3210	14.6749	.1593	.6790	**.12**
706	**.89**	.3293	14.9541	.1568	.6707	**.11**
0.9713	**6.90**	7.3376	15.2402	0.1544	2.6624	**3.10**
719	**.91**	.3460	15.5333	.1519	.6540	**.09**
726	**.92**	.3543	15.8337	.1495	.6457	**.08**
732	**.93**	.3626	16.1414	.1471	.6374	**.07**
738	**.94**	.3710	16.4568	.1448	.6290	**.06**
0.9744	**6.95**	7.3794	16.7800	0.1424	2.6206	**3.05**
750	**.96**	.3877	17.1113	.1401	.6123	**.04**
756	**.97**	.3961	17.4509	.1378	.6039	**.03**
761	**.98**	.4045	17.7989	.1356	.5955	**.02**
767	**.99**	.4129	18.1558	.1333	.5871	**.01**
0.9772	**7.00**	7.4214	18.5216	0.1311	2.5786	**3.00**
$Z = e^{-\frac{1}{2}X^2}/\sqrt{(2\pi)}$ $Y = X + 5$ $P = 1 - Q = \int_{-\infty}^{X} Z(t)\,dt$			$1/Z$ Range	Z^2/PQ Weighting coefficient	$Y - P/Z$ Minimum working probit	Y Expected probit

TABLE FOR PROBIT ANALYSIS

Proportion P	Expected probit Y	Maximum working probit $Y + Q/Z$	Range $1/Z$	Weighting coefficient Z^2/PQ		
0.9772	**7.00**	7.4214	18.5216	0.1311	2.5786	**3.00**
778	**.01**	.4298	18.8967	.1289	.5702	**2.99**
783	**.02**	.4382	19.2814	.1268	.5618	**.98**
788	**.03**	.4467	19.6758	.1246	.5533	**.97**
793	**.04**	.4552	20.0803	.1225	.5448	**.96**
0.9798	**7.05**	7.4636	20.4952	0.1204	2.5364	**2.95**
803	**.06**	.4721	20.9207	.1183	.5279	**.94**
808	**.07**	.4806	21.3572	.1163	.5194	**.93**
812	**.08**	.4891	21.8050	.1142	.5109	**.92**
817	**.09**	.4976	22.2644	.1122	.5024	**.91**
0.9821	**7.10**	7.5062	22.7357	0.1103	2.4938	**2.90**
826	**.11**	.5147	23.2194	.1083	.4853	**.89**
830	**.12**	.5232	23.7157	.1064	.4768	**.88**
834	**.13**	.5318	24.2251	.1045	.4682	**.87**
838	**.14**	.5404	24.7478	.1026	.4596	**.86**
0.9842	**7.15**	7.5489	25.2844	0.1007	2.4511	**2.85**
846	**.16**	.5575	25.8352	.0989	.4425	**.84**
850	**.17**	.5661	26.4006	.0971	.4339	**.83**
854	**.18**	.5747	26.9812	.0953	.4253	**.82**
857	**.19**	.5833	27.5772	.0935	.4167	**.81**
0.9861	**7.20**	7.5919	28.1892	0.0918	2.4081	**2.80**
864	**.21**	.6006	28.8177	.0901	.3994	**.79**
868	**.22**	.6092	29.4631	.0884	.3908	**.78**
871	**.23**	.6178	30.1260	.0867	.3822	**.77**
875	**.24**	.6265	30.8069	.0851	.3735	**.76**
0.9878	**7.25**	7.6351	31.5063	0.0834	2.3649	**2.75**
881	**.26**	.6438	32.2249	.0818	.3562	**.74**
884	**.27**	.6525	32.9631	.0802	.3475	**.73**
887	**.28**	.6612	33.7216	.0787	.3388	**.72**
890	**.29**	.6699	34.5010	.0771	.3301	**.71**
0.9893	**7.30**	7.6786	35.3020	0.0756	2.3214	**2.70**
896	**.31**	.6873	36.1251	.0741	.3127	**.69**
898	**.32**	.6960	36.9712	.0727	.3040	**.68**
901	**.33**	.7047	37.8408	.0712	.2953	**.67**
904	**.34**	.7135	38.7348	.0698	.2865	**.66**
0.9906	**7.35**	7.7222	39.6539	0.0684	2.2778	**2.65**
909	**.36**	.7310	40.5088	.0671	.2690	**.64**
911	**.37**	.7397	41.5704	.0656	.2603	**.63**
913	**.38**	.7485	42.5695	.0643	.2515	**.62**
916	**.39**	.7573	43.5970	.0630	.2427	**.61**
0.9918	**7.40**	7.7661	44.6538	0.0617	2.2339	**2.60**
$Z = e^{-\frac{1}{2}X^2}/\sqrt{(2\pi)}$; $Y = X + 5$; $P = 1 - Q = \int_{-\infty}^{X} Z(t)\,dt$			$1/Z$ Range	Z^2/PQ Weighting coefficient	$Y - P/Z$ Minimum working probit	Y Expected probit

TABLE FOR PROBIT ANALYSIS

Proportion P	Expected probit Y	Maximum working probit $Y + Q/Z$	Range $1/Z$	Weighting coefficient Z^2/PQ		
0.9918	**7.40**	7.7661	44.6538	0.0617	2.2339	**2.60**
920	**.41**	.7748	45.7407	.0604	.2252	**.59**
922	**.42**	.7836	46.8588	.0591	.2164	**.58**
925	**.43**	.7924	48.0090	.0579	.2076	**.57**
927	**.44**	.8013	49.1924	.0567	.1987	**.56**
0.9929	**7.45**	7.8101	50.4099	0.0555	2.1899	**2.55**
931	**.46**	.8189	51.6628	.0543	.1811	**.54**
932	**.47**	.8277	52.9521	.0532	.1723	**.53**
934	**.48**	.8366	54.2791	.0520	.1634	**.52**
936	**.49**	.8454	55.6448	.0509	.1546	**.51**
0.99379	**7.50**	7.8543	57.0506	0.0498	2.1457	**2.50**
396	**.51**	.8631	58.4978	.0487	.1369	**.49**
413	**.52**	.8720	59.9876	.0476	.1280	**.48**
430	**.53**	.8809	61.5216	.0466	.1191	**.47**
446	**.54**	.8897	63.1011	.0456	.1103	**.46**
0.99461	**7.55**	7.8986	64.7277	0.0446	2.1014	**2.45**
477	**.56**	.9075	66.4028	.0436	.0925	**.44**
492	**.57**	.9164	68.1280	.0426	.0836	**.43**
506	**.58**	.9253	69.9051	.0416	.0747	**.42**
520	**.59**	.9342	71.7357	.0407	.0658	**.41**
0.99534	**7.60**	7.9432	73.6216	0.0398	2.0568	**2.40**
547	**.61**	.9521	75.5646	.0389	.0479	**.39**
560	**.62**	.9610	77.5667	.0380	.0390	**.38**
573	**.63**	.9700	79.6298	.0371	.0300	**.37**
585	**.64**	.9789	81.7559	.0362	.0211	**.36**
0.99598	**7.65**	7.9879	83.9472	0.0354	2.0121	**2.35**
609	**.66**	.9968	86.2059	.0346	.0032	**.34**
621	**.67**	8.0058	88.5342	.0338	1.9942	**.33**
632	**.68**	.0147	90.9344	.0330	.9853	**.32**
643	**.69**	.0237	93.4091	.0322	.9763	**.31**
0.99653	**7.70**	8.0327	95.9607	0.0314	1.9673	**2.30**
664	**.71**	.0417	98.5918	.0307	.9583	**.29**
674	**.72**	.0507	101.3053	.0300	.9493	**.28**
683	**.73**	.0597	104.1038	.0292	.9403	**.27**
693	**.74**	.0687	106.9903	.0285	.9313	**.26**
0.99702	**7.75**	8.0777	109.9679	0.0278	1.9223	**2.25**
711	**.76**	.0867	113.0396	.0272	.9133	**.24**
720	**.77**	.0957	116.2088	.0265	.9043	**.23**
728	**.78**	.1047	119.4788	.0258	.8953	**.22**
736	**.79**	.1138	122.8530	.0252	.8862	**.21**
0.99744	**7.80**	8.1228	126.3352	0.0246	1.8772	**2.20**
$Z = e^{-\frac{1}{2}X^2}/\sqrt{(2\pi)}$ $Y = X + 5$ $P = 1 - Q = \int_{-\infty}^{X} Z(t)\,dt$			$1/Z$ Range	Z^2/PQ Weighting coefficient	$Y - P/Z$ Minimum working probit	Y Expected probit

TABLE FOR PROBIT ANALYSIS

Proportion P	Expected probit Y	Maximum working probit $Y + Q/Z$	Range $1/Z$	Weighting coefficient Z^2/PQ		
0.99744	**7.80**	8.1228	126.3352	0.0246	1.8772	**2.20**
752	**.81**	.1318	129.9290	.0240	.8682	**.19**
760	**.82**	.1409	133.6385	.0234	.8591	**.18**
767	**.83**	.1499	137.4676	.0228	.8501	**.17**
774	**.84**	.1590	141.4206	.0222	.8410	**.16**
0.99781	**7.85**	8.1681	145.5018	0.0217	1.8319	**2.15**
788	**.86**	.1771	149.7158	.0211	.8229	**.14**
795	**.87**	.1862	154.0671	.0206	.8138	**.13**
801	**.88**	.1953	158.5609	.0200	.8047	**.12**
807	**.89**	.2044	163.2020	.0195	.7956	**.11**
0.99813	**7.90**	8.2134	167.9957	0.0190	1.7866	**2.10**
819	**.91**	.2225	172.9476	.0185	.7775	**.09**
825	**.92**	.2316	178.0632	.0181	.7684	**.08**
831	**.93**	.2407	183.3485	.0176	.7593	**.07**
836	**.94**	.2498	188.8095	.0171	.7502	**.06**
0.99841	**7.95**	8.2590	194.4526	0.0167	1.7410	**2.05**
846	**.96**	.2681	200.2844	.0162	.7319	**.04**
851	**.97**	.2772	206.3118	.0158	.7228	**.03**
856	**.98**	.2863	212.5418	.0154	.7137	**.02**
861	**.99**	.2955	218.9818	.0150	.7045	**.01**
0.99865	**8.00**	8.3046	225.6395	0.0146	1.6954	**2.00**
869	**.01**	.3137	232.5229	.0142	.6863	**1.99**
874	**.02**	.3229	239.6402	.0138	.6771	**.98**
878	**.03**	.3320	247.0000	.0134	.6680	**.97**
882	**.04**	.3412	254.6114	.0131	.6588	**.96**
0.99886	**8.05**	8.3503	262.4836	0.0127	1.6497	**1.95**
889	**.06**	.3595	270.6262	.0124	.6405	**.94**
893	**.07**	.3687	279.0493	.0120	.6313	**.93**
896	**.08**	.3778	287.7634	.0117	.6222	**.92**
900	**.09**	.3870	296.7792	.0114	.6130	**.91**
0.99903	**8.10**	8.3962	306.1082	0.0110	1.6038	**1.90**
906	**.11**	.4054	315.7619	.0107	.5946	**.89**
910	**.12**	.4146	325.7527	.0104	.5854	**.88**
913	**.13**	.4238	336.0932	.0101	.5762	**.87**
916	**.14**	.4330	346.7966	.0099	.5670	**.86**
0.99918	**8.15**	8.4422	357.8732	0.0096	1.5578	**1.85**
921	**.16**	.4514	369.3477	.0093	.5486	**.84**
924	**.17**	.4606	381.2245	.0090	.5394	**.83**
926	**.18**	.4698	393.5226	.0088	.5302	**.82**
929	**.19**	.4790	406.2580	.0085	.5210	**.81**
0.99931	**8.20**	8.4882	419.4476	0.0083	1.5118	**1.80**
$Z = e^{-\frac{1}{2}X^2}/\sqrt{(2\pi)}$ $Y = X + 5$ $P = 1 - Q = \int_{-\infty}^{X} Z(t)\,dt$			$1/Z$ Range	Z^2/PQ Weighting coefficient	$Y - P/Z$ Minimum working probit	Y Expected probit

TABLE FOR PROBIT ANALYSIS

Proportion P	Expected probit Y	Maximum working probit $Y + Q/Z$	Range $1/Z$	Weighting coefficient Z^2/PQ		
0.99931	**8.20**	8.4882	419.4476	0.0083	1.5118	**1.80**
934	**.21**	.4974	433.1086	.0080	.5026	**.79**
936	**.22**	.5067	447.2593	.0078	.4933	**.78**
938	**.23**	.5159	461.9185	.0076	.4841	**.77**
940	**.24**	.5251	477.1059	.0074	.4749	**.76**
0.99942	**8.25**	8.5344	492.8419	0.0071	1.4656	**1.75**
944	**.26**	.5436	509.1479	.0069	.4564	**.74**
946	**.27**	.5529	526.0459	.0067	.4471	**.73**
948	**.28**	.5621	543.5592	.0065	.4379	**.72**
950	**.29**	.5714	561.7116	.0063	.4286	**.71**
0.99952	**8.30**	8.5806	580.5283	0.0061	1.4194	**1.70**
953	**.31**	.5899	600.0353	.0060	.4101	**.69**
955	**.32**	.5992	620.2599	.0058	.4008	**.68**
957	**.33**	.6084	641.2302	.0056	.3916	**.67**
958	**.34**	.6177	662.9758	.0054	.3823	**.66**
0.99960	**8.35**	8.6270	685.5274	0.0053	1.3730	**1.65**
961	**.36**	.6363	708.9171	.0051	.3637	**.64**
962	**.37**	.6456	733.1780	.0050	.3544	**.63**
964	**.38**	.6548	758.3451	.0048	.3452	**.62**
965	**.39**	.6641	784.4545	.0047	.3359	**.61**
0.99966	**8.40**	8.6734	811.5439	0.0045	1.3266	**1.60**
968	**.41**	.6827	839.6528	.0044	.3173	**.59**
969	**.42**	.6920	868.8222	.0042	.3080	**.58**
970	**.43**	.7013	899.0948	.0041	.2987	**.57**
971	**.44**	.7106	930.5153	.0040	.2894	**.56**
0.99972	**8.45**	8.7200	963.1301	0.0038	1.2800	**1.55**
973	**.46**	.7293	996.9878	.0037	.2707	**.54**
974	**.47**	.7386	1032.1389	.0036	.2614	**.53**
975	**.48**	.7479	1068.6362	.0035	.2521	**.52**
976	**.49**	.7572	1106.5347	.0034	.2428	**.51**
0.999767	**8.50**	8.7666	1145.8919	0.0033	1.2334	**1.50**
776	**.51**	.7759	1186.7675	.0032	.2241	**.49**
784	**.52**	.7852	1229.2242	.0031	.2148	**.48**
792	**.53**	.7946	1273.3271	.0030	.2054	**.47**
800	**.54**	.8039	1319.1443	.0029	.1961	**.46**
0.999807	**8.55**	8.8133	1366.7467	0.0028	1.1867	**1.45**
815	**.56**	.8226	1416.2085	.0027	.1774	**.44**
882	**.57**	.8320	1467.6071	.0026	.1680	**.43**
828	**.58**	.8413	1521.0232	.0025	.1587	**.42**
835	**.59**	.8507	1576.5411	.0024	.1493	**.41**
0.999841	**8.60**	8.8600	1634.2488	0.0024	1.1400	**1.40**
$Z = e^{-\frac{1}{2}X^2}/\sqrt{(2\pi)}$ $Y = X + 5$ $P = 1 - Q = \int_{-\infty}^{X} Z(t)\,dt$			$1/Z$ Range	Z^2/PQ Weighting coefficient	$Y - P/Z$ Minimum working probit	Y Expected probit

TABLE FOR PROBIT ANALYSIS

Proportion P	Expected probit Y	Maximum working probit $Y + Q/Z$	Range $1/Z$	Weighting coefficient Z^2/PQ		
0.999841	**8.60**	8.8600	1634.2488	0.0024	1.1400	**1.40**
847	**.61**	.8694	1694.2383	.0023	.1306	**.39**
853	**.62**	.8788	1756.6055	.0022	.1212	**.38**
858	**.63**	.8881	1821.4507	.0021	.1119	**.37**
864	**.64**	.8975	1888.8785	.0021	.1025	**.36**
0.999869	**8.65**	8.9069	1958.9983	0.0020	1.0931	**1.35**
874	**.66**	.9162	2031.9243	.0019	.0838	**.34**
879	**.67**	.9256	2107.7758	.0019	.0744	**.33**
883	**.68**	.9350	2186.6775	.0018	.0650	**.32**
888	**.69**	.9444	2268.7596	.0017	.0556	**.31**
0.999892	**8.70**	8.9538	2354.1583	0.0017	1.0462	**1.30**
896	**.71**	.9632	2443.0158	.0016	.0368	**.29**
900	**.72**	.9726	2535.4807	.0016	.0274	**.28**
904	**.73**	.9820	2631.7085	.0015	.0180	**.27**
908	**.74**	.9914	2731.8615	.0015	.0086	**.26**
0.999912	**8.75**	9.0008	2836.1096	0.0014	0.9992	**1.25**
915	**.76**	.0102	2944.6302	.0014	.9898	**.24**
918	**.77**	.0196	3057.6091	.0013	.9804	**.23**
922	**.78**	.0290	3175.2401	.0013	.9710	**.22**
925	**.79**	.0384	3297.7264	.0012	.9616	**.21**
0.999928	**8.80**	9.0478	3425.2801	0.0012	0.9522	**1.20**
931	**.81**	.0572	3558.1233	.0011	.9428	**.19**
933	**.82**	.0667	3696.4883	.0011	.9333	**.18**
936	**.83**	.0761	3840.6179	.0011	.9239	**.17**
938	**.84**	.0855	3990.7662	.0010	.9145	**.16**
0.999941	**8.85**	9.0949	4147.1994	0.0010	0.9051	**1.15**
943	**.86**	.1044	4310.1955	.0010	.8956	**.14**
946	**.87**	.1138	4480.0457	.0009	.8862	**.13**
948	**.88**	.1232	4657.0549	.0009	.8768	**.12**
950	**.89**	.1327	4841.5419	.0009	.8673	**.11**
0.999952	**8.90**	9.1421	5033.8407	0.0008	0.8579	**1.10**
954	**.91**	.1516	5234.3007	.0008	.8484	**.09**
956	**.92**	.1610	5443.2878	.0008	.0390	**.08**
958	**.93**	.1704	5661.1851	.0007	.8296	**.07**
959	**.94**	.1799	5888.3938	.0007	.8201	**.06**
0.999961	**8.95**	9.1894	6125.3338	0.0007	0.8106	**1.05**
963	**.96**	.1988	6372.4452	.0007	.8012	**.04**
964	**.97**	.2083	6630.1886	.0006	.7917	**.03**
966	**.98**	.2177	6899.0468	.0006	.7823	**.02**
967	**.99**	.2272	7179.5252	.0006	.7728	**.01**
0.999968	**9.00**	9.2367	7472.1536	0.0006	0.7633	**1.00**
$Z = e^{-\frac{1}{2}X^2}/\sqrt{(2\pi)}$ $Y = X + 5$ $P = 1 - Q = \int_{-\infty}^{X} Z(t)\,dt$			$1/Z$ Range	Z^2/PQ Weighting coefficient	$Y - P/Z$ Minimum working probit	Y Expected probit

III. Binomial, Poisson, Hypergeometric, and Negative Binomial Distributions

III.1 INDIVIDUAL TERMS, BINOMIAL DISTRIBUTION

The $(x + 1)^{st}$ term in the expansion of the binomial $[\theta + (1 - \theta)]^n$ is given by

$$f(x;n,\theta) = \binom{n}{x} \theta^x (1 - \theta)^{n-x}, \qquad x = 0, 1, 2, \ldots, n.$$

This is the probability of exactly x successes in n independent binomial trials with probability of success on a single trial equal to θ. This table contains the individual terms of $f(x;n,\theta)$ for specified choices of x, n, and θ.

For $\theta > 0.5$, the value of $\binom{n}{x} \theta^x (1 - \theta)^{n-x}$ is found by using the table entry for $\binom{n}{n-x} (1 - \theta)^{n-x} \theta^x$.

INDIVIDUAL TERMS, BINOMIAL DISTRIBUTION

						θ					
n	x	.05	.10	.15	.20	.25	.30	.35	.40	.45	.50
1	0	.9500	.9000	.8500	.8000	.7500	.7000	.6500	.6000	.5500	.5000
	1	.0500	.1000	.1500	.2000	.2500	.3000	.3500	.4000	.4500	.5000
2	0	.9025	.8100	.7225	.6400	.5625	.4900	.4225	.3600	.3025	.2500
	1	.0950	.1800	.2550	.3200	.3750	.4200	.4550	.4800	.4950	.5000
	2	.0025	.0100	.0225	.0400	.0625	.0900	.1225	.1600	.2025	.2500
3	0	.8574	.7290	.6141	.5120	.4219	.3430	.2746	.2160	.1664	.1250
	1	.1354	.2430	.3251	.3840	.4219	.4410	.4436	.4320	.4084	.3750
	2	.0071	.0270	.0574	.0960	.1406	.1890	.2389	.2880	.3341	.3750
	3	.0001	.0010	.0034	.0080	.0156	.0270	.0429	.0640	.0911	.1250
4	0	.8145	.0501	.5220	.4096	.3164	.2401	.1785	.1296	.0915	.0625
	1	.1715	.2916	.3685	.4096	.4219	.4116	.3845	.3456	.2995	.2500
	2	.0135	.0486	.0975	.1536	.2109	.2646	.3105	.3456	.3675	.3750
	3	.0005	.0036	.0115	.0256	.0469	.0756	.1115	.1536	.2005	.2500
	4	.0000	.0001	.0005	.0016	.0039	.0081	.0150	.0256	.0410	.0625
5	0	.7738	.5905	.4437	.3277	.2373	.1681	.1160	.0778	.0503	.0312
	1	.2036	.3280	.3915	.4096	.3955	.3602	.3124	.2592	.2059	.1562
	2	.0214	.0729	.1382	.2048	.2637	.3087	.3364	.3456	.3369	.3125
	3	.0011	.0081	.0244	.0512	.0879	.1323	.1811	.2304	.2757	.3125
	4	.0000	.0004	.0022	.0064	.0146	.0284	.0488	.0768	.1128	.1562
	5	.0000	.0000	.0001	.0003	.0010	.0024	.0053	.0102	.0185	.0312
6	0	.7351	.5314	.3771	.2621	.1780	.1176	.0754	.0467	.0277	.0156
	1	.2321	.3543	.3993	.3932	.3560	.3025	.2437	.1866	.1359	.0938
	2	.0305	.0984	.1762	.2458	.2966	.3241	.3280	.3110	.2780	.2344
	3	.0021	.0146	.0415	.0819	.1318	.1852	.2355	.2765	.3032	.3125
	4	.0001	.0012	.0055	.0154	.0330	.0595	.0951	.1382	.1861	.2344
	5	.0000	.0001	.0004	.0015	.0044	.0102	.0205	.0369	.0609	.0938
	6	.0000	.0000	.0000	.0001	.0002	.0007	.0018	.0041	.0083	.0156
7	0	.6983	.4783	.3206	.2097	.1335	.0824	.0490	.0280	.0152	.0078
	1	.2573	.3720	.3960	.3670	.3115	.2471	.1848	.1306	.0872	.0547
	2	.0406	.1240	.2097	.2753	.3115	.3177	.2985	.2613	.2140	.1641
	3	.0036	.0230	.0617	.1147	.1730	.2269	.2679	.2903	.2918	.2734
	4	.0002	.0026	.0109	.0287	.0577	.0972	.1442	.1935	.2388	.2734
	5	.0000	.0002	.0012	.0043	.0115	.0250	.0466	.0774	.1172	.1641
	6	.0000	.0000	.0001	.0004	.0013	.0036	.0084	.0172	.0320	.0547
	7	.0000	.0000	.0000	.0000	.0001	.0002	.0006	.0016	.0037	.0078
8	0	.6634	.4305	.2725	.1678	.1001	.0576	.0319	.0168	.0084	.0039
	1	.2793	.3826	.3847	.3355	.2670	.1977	.1373	.0896	.0548	.0312
	2	.0515	.1488	.2376	.2936	.3115	.2965	.2587	.2090	.1569	.1094
	3	.0054	.0331	.0839	.1468	.2076	.2541	.2786	.2787	.2568	.2188
	4	.0004	.0046	.0185	.0459	.0865	.1361	.1875	.2322	.2627	.2734
	5	.0000	.0004	.0026	.0092	.0231	.0467	.0808	.1239	.1719	.2188
	6	.0000	.0000	.0002	.0011	.0038	.0100	.0217	.0413	.0703	.1094
	7	.0000	.0000	.0000	.0001	.0004	.0012	.0033	.0079	.0164	.0312
	8	.0000	.0000	.0000	.0000	.0000	.0001	.0002	.0007	.0017	.0039

Linear interpolations with respect to θ will in general be accurate at most to two decimal places.

INDIVIDUAL TERMS, BINOMIAL DISTRIBUTION

		θ									
n	x	.05	.10	.15	.20	.25	.30	.35	.40	.45	.50
9	0	.6302	.3874	.2316	.1342	.0751	.0404	.0207	.0101	.0046	.0020
	1	.2985	.3874	.3679	.3020	.2253	.1556	.1004	.0605	.0339	.0176
	2	.0629	.1722	.2597	.3020	.3003	.2668	.2162	.1612	.1110	.0703
	3	.0077	.0446	.1069	.1762	.2336	.2668	.2716	.2508	.2119	.1641
	4	.0006	.0074	.0283	.0661	.1168	.1715	.2194	.2508	.2600	.2461
	5	.0000	.0008	.0050	.0165	.0389	.0735	.1181	.1672	.2128	.2461
	6	.0000	.0001	.0006	.0028	.0087	.0210	.0424	.0743	.1160	.1641
	7	.0000	.0000	.0000	.0003	.0012	.0039	.0098	.0212	.0407	.0703
	8	.0000	.0000	.0000	.0000	.0001	.0004	.0013	.0035	.0083	.0176
	9	.0000	.0000	.0000	.0000	.0000	.0000	.0001	.0003	.0008	.0020
10	0	.5987	.3487	.1969	.1074	.0563	.0282	.0135	.0060	.0025	.0010
	1	.3151	.3874	.3474	.2684	.1877	.1211	.0725	.0403	.0207	.0098
	2	.0746	.1937	.2759	.3020	.2816	.2335	.1757	.1209	.0763	.0439
	3	.0105	.0574	.1298	.2013	.2503	.2668	.2522	.2150	.1665	.1172
	4	.0010	.0112	.0401	.0881	.1460	.2001	.2377	.2508	.2384	.2051
	5	.0001	.0015	.0085	.0264	.0584	.1029	.1536	.2007	.2340	.2461
	6	.0000	.0001	.0012	.0055	.0162	.0368	.0689	.1115	.1596	.2051
	7	.0000	.0000	.0001	.0008	.0031	.0090	.0212	.0425	.0746	.1172
	8	.0000	.0000	.0000	.0001	.0004	.0014	.0043	.0106	.0229	.0439
	9	.0000	.0000	.0000	.0000	.0000	.0001	.0005	.0016	.0042	.0098
	10	.0000	.0000	.0000	.0000	.0000	.0000	.0000	.0001	.0003	.0010
11	0	.5688	.3138	.1673	.0859	.0422	.0198	.0088	.0036	.0014	.0004
	1	.3293	.3835	.3248	.2362	.1549	.0932	.0518	.0266	.0125	.0055
	2	.0867	.2131	.2866	.2953	.2581	.1998	.1395	.0887	.0513	.0269
	3	.0137	.0710	.1517	.2215	.2581	.2568	.2254	.1774	.1259	.0806
	4	.0014	.0158	.0536	.1107	.1721	.2201	.2428	.2365	.2060	.1611
	5	.0001	.0025	.0132	.0388	.0803	.1321	.1830	.2207	.2360	.2256
	6	.0000	.0003	.0023	.0097	.0268	.0566	.0985	.1471	.1931	.2256
	7	.0000	.0000	.0003	.0017	.0064	.0173	.0379	.0701	.1128	.1611
	8	.0000	.0000	.0000	.0002	.0011	.0037	.0102	.0234	.0462	.0806
	9	.0000	.0000	.0000	.0000	.0001	.0005	.0018	.0052	.0126	.0269
	10	.0000	.0000	.0000	.0000	.0000	.0000	.0002	.0007	.0021	.0054
	11	.0000	.0000	.0000	.0000	.0000	.0000	.0000	.0000	.0002	.0005
12	0	.5404	.2824	.1422	.0687	.0317	.0138	.0057	.0022	.0008	.0002
	1	.3413	.3766	.3012	.2062	.1267	.0712	.0368	.0174	.0075	.0029
	2	.0988	.2301	.2924	.2835	.2323	.1678	.1088	.0639	.0339	.0161
	3	.0173	.0852	.1720	.2362	.2581	.2397	.1954	.1419	.0923	.0537
	4	.0021	.0213	.0683	.1329	.1936	.2311	.2367	.2128	.1700	.1208
	5	.0002	.0038	.0193	.0532	.1032	.1585	.2039	.2270	.2225	.1934
	6	.0000	.0005	.0040	.0155	.0401	.0792	.1281	.1766	.2124	.2256
	7	.0000	.0000	.0006	.0033	.0115	.0291	.0591	.1009	.1489	.1934
	8	.0000	.0000	.0001	.0005	.0024	.0078	.0199	.0420	.0762	.1208
	9	.0000	.0000	.0000	.0001	.0004	.0015	.0048	.0125	.0277	.0537
	10	.0000	.0000	.0000	.0000	.0000	.0002	.0008	.0025	.0068	.0161
	11	.0000	.0000	.0000	.0000	.0000	.0000	.0001	.0003	.0010	.0029
	12	.0000	.0000	.0000	.0000	.0000	.0000	.0000	.0000	.0001	.0002

INDIVIDUAL TERMS, BINOMIAL DISTRIBUTION

		θ									
n	x	.05	.10	.15	.20	.25	.30	.35	.40	.45	.50
13	0	.5133	.2542	.1209	.0550	.0238	.0097	.0037	.0013	.0004	.0001
	1	.3512	.3672	.2774	.1787	.1029	.0540	.0259	.0113	.0045	.0016
	2	.1109	.2448	.2937	.2680	.2059	.1388	.0836	.0453	.0220	.0095
	3	.0214	.0997	.1900	.2457	.2517	.2181	.1651	.1107	.0660	.0349
	4	.0028	.0277	.0838	.1535	.2097	.2337	.2222	.1845	.1350	.0873
	5	.0003	.0055	.0266	.0691	.1258	.1803	.2154	.2214	.1989	.1571
	6	.0000	.0008	.0063	.0230	.0559	.1030	.1546	.1968	.2169	.2095
	7	.0000	.0001	.0011	.0058	.0186	.0442	.0833	.1312	.1775	.2095
	8	.0000	.0000	.0001	.0011	.0047	.0142	.0336	.0656	.1089	.1571
	9	.0000	.0000	.0000	.0001	.0009	.0034	.0101	.0243	.0495	.0873
	10	.0000	.0000	.0000	.0000	.0001	.0006	.0022	.0065	.0162	.0349
	11	.0000	.0000	.0000	.0000	.0000	.0001	.0003	.0012	.0036	.0095
	12	.0000	.0000	.0000	.0000	.0000	.0000	.0000	.0001	.0005	.0016
	13	.0000	.0000	.0000	.0000	.0000	.0000	.0000	.0000	.0000	.0001
14	0	.4877	.2288	.1028	.0440	.0178	.0068	.0024	.0008	.0002	.0001
	1	.3593	.3559	.2539	.1539	.0832	.0407	.0181	.0073	.0027	.0009
	2	.1229	.2570	.2912	.2501	.1802	.1134	.0634	.0317	.0141	.0056
	3	.0259	.1142	.2056	.2501	.2402	.1943	.1366	.0845	.0462	.0222
	4	.0037	.0349	.0998	.1720	.2202	.2290	.2022	.1549	.1040	.0611
	5	.0004	.0078	.0352	.0860	.1468	.1963	.2178	.2066	.1701	.1222
	6	.0000	.0013	.0093	.0322	.0734	.1262	.1759	.2066	.2088	.1833
	7	.0000	.0002	.0019	.0092	.0280	.0618	.1082	.1574	.1952	.2095
	8	.0000	.0000	.0003	.0020	.0082	.0232	.0510	.0918	.1398	.1833
	9	.0000	.0000	.0000	.0003	.0018	.0066	.0183	.0408	.0762	.1222
	10	.0000	.0000	.0000	.0000	.0003	.0014	.0049	.0136	.0312	.0611
	11	.0000	.0000	.0000	.0000	.0000	.0002	.0010	.0033	.0093	.0222
	12	.0000	.0000	.0000	.0000	.0000	.0000	.0001	.0005	.0019	.0056
	13	.0000	.0000	.0000	.0000	.0000	.0000	.0000	.0001	.0002	.0009
	14	.0000	.0000	.0000	.0000	.0000	.0000	.0000	.0000	.0000	.0001
15	0	.4633	.2059	.0874	.0352	.0134	.0047	.0016	.0005	.0001	.0000
	1	.3658	.3432	.2312	.1319	.0668	.0305	.0126	.0047	.0016	.0005
	2	.1348	.2669	.2856	.2309	.1559	.0916	.0476	.0219	.0090	.0032
	3	.0307	.1285	.2184	.2501	.2252	.1700	.1110	.0634	.0318	.0139
	4	.0049	.0428	.1156	.1876	.2252	.2186	.1792	.1268	.0780	.0417
	5	.0006	.0105	.0449	.1032	.1651	.2061	.2123	.1859	.1404	.0916
	6	.0000	.0019	.0132	.0430	.0917	.1472	.1906	.2066	.1914	.1527
	7	.0000	.0003	.0030	.0138	.0393	.0811	.1319	.1771	.2013	.1964
	8	.0000	.0000	.0005	.0035	.0131	.0348	.0710	.1181	.1647	.1964
	9	.0000	.0000	.0001	.0007	.0034	.0116	.0298	.0612	.1048	.1527
	10	.0000	.0000	.0000	.0001	.0007	.0030	.0096	.0245	.0515	.0916
	11	.0000	.0000	.0000	.0000	.0001	.0006	.0024	.0074	.0191	.0417
	12	.0000	.0000	.0000	.0000	.0000	.0001	.0004	.0016	.0052	.0139
	13	.0000	.0000	.0000	.0000	.0000	.0000	.0001	.0003	.0010	.0032
	14	.0000	.0000	.0000	.0000	.0000	.0000	.0000	.0000	.0001	.0005
	15	.0000	.0000	.0000	.0000	.0000	.0000	.0000	.0000	.0000	.0000

INDIVIDUAL TERMS, BINOMIAL DISTRIBUTION

						θ					
n	*x*	.05	.10	.15	.20	.25	.30	.35	.40	.45	.50
16	0	.4401	.1853	.0743	.0281	.0100	.0033	.0010	.0003	.0001	.0000
	1	.3706	.3294	.2097	.1126	.0535	.0228	.0087	.0030	.0009	.0002
	2	.1463	.2745	.2775	.2111	.1336	.0732	.0353	.0150	.0056	.0018
	3	.0359	.1423	.2285	.2463	.2079	.1465	.0888	.0468	.0215	.0085
	4	.0061	.0514	.1311	.2001	.2252	.2040	.1553	.1014	.0572	.0278
	5	.0008	.0137	.0555	.1201	.1802	.2099	.2008	.1623	.1123	.0667
	6	.0001	.0028	.0180	.0550	.1101	.1649	.1982	.1983	.1684	.1222
	7	.0000	.0004	.0045	.0197	.0524	.1010	.1524	.1889	.1969	.1746
	8	.0000	.0001	.0009	.0055	.0197	.0487	.0923	.1417	.1812	.1964
	9	.0000	.0000	.0001	.0012	.0058	.0185	.0442	.0840	.1318	.1746
	10	.0000	.0000	.0000	.0002	.0014	.0056	.0167	.0392	.0755	.1222
	11	.0000	.0000	.0000	.0000	.0002	.0013	.0049	.0142	.0337	.0667
	12	.0000	.0000	.0000	.0000	.0000	.0002	.0011	.0040	.0115	.0278
	13	.0000	.0000	.0000	.0000	.0000	.0000	.0002	.0008	.0029	.0085
	14	.0000	.0000	.0000	.0000	.0000	.0000	.0000	.0001	.0005	.0018
	15	.0000	.0000	.0000	.0000	.0000	.0000	.0000	.0000	.0001	.0002
	16	.0000	.0000	.0000	.0000	.0000	.0000	.0000	.0000	.0000	.0000
17	0	.4181	.1668	.0631	.0225	.0075	.0023	.0007	.0002	.0000	.0000
	1	.3741	.3150	.1893	.0957	.0426	.0169	.0060	.0019	.0005	.0001
	2	.1575	.2800	.2673	.1914	.1136	.0581	.0260	.0102	.0035	.0010
	3	.0415	.1556	.2359	.2393	.1893	.1245	.0701	.0341	.0144	.0052
	4	.9076	.0605	.1457	.2093	.2209	.1868	.1320	.0796	.0411	.0182
	5	.0010	.0175	.0668	.1361	.1914	.2081	.1849	.1379	.0875	.0472
	6	.0001	.0039	.0236	.0680	.1276	.1784	.1991	.1839	.1432	.0944
	7	.0000	.0007	.0065	.0267	.0668	.1201	.1685	.1927	.1841	.1484
	8	.0000	.0001	.0014	.0084	.0279	.0644	.1134	.1606	.1883	.1855
	9	.0000	.0000	.0003	.0021	.0093	.0276	.0611	.1070	.1540	.1855
	10	.0000	.0000	.0000	.0004	.0025	.0095	.0263	.0571	.1008	.1484
	11	.0000	.0000	.0000	.0001	.0005	.0026	.0090	.0242	.0525	.0944
	12	.0000	.0000	.0000	.0000	.0001	.0006	.0024	.0081	.0215	.0472
	13	.0000	.0000	.0000	.0000	.0000	.0001	.0005	.0021	.0068	.0182
	14	.0000	.0000	.0000	.0000	.0000	.0000	.0001	.0004	.0016	.0052
	15	.0000	.0000	.0000	.0000	.0000	.0000	.0000	.0001	.0003	.0010
	16	.0000	.0000	.0000	.0000	.0000	.0000	.0000	.0000	.0000	.0001
	17	.0000	.0000	.0000	.0000	.0000	.0000	.0000	.0000	.0000	.0000
18	0	.3972	.1501	.0536	.0180	.0056	.0016	.0004	.0001	.0000	.0000
	1	.3763	.3002	.1704	.0811	.0338	.0126	.0042	.0012	.0003	.0001
	2	.1683	.2835	.2556	.1723	.0958	.0458	.0190	.0069	.0022	.0006
	3	.0473	.1680	.2406	.2297	.1704	.1046	.0547	.0246	.0095	.0031
	4	.0093	.0700	.1592	.2153	.2130	.1681	.1104	.0614	.0291	.0117
	5	.0014	.0218	.0787	.1507	.1988	.2017	.1664	.1146	.0666	.0327
	6	.0002	.0052	.0301	.0816	.1436	.1873	.1941	.1655	.1181	.0708
	7	.0000	.0010	.0091	.0350	.0820	.1376	.1792	.1892	.1657	.1214
	8	.0000	.0002	.0022	.0120	.0376	.0811	.1327	.1734	.1864	.1669
	9	.0000	.0000	.0004	.0033	.0139	.0386	.0794	.1284	.1694	.1855
	10	.0000	.0000	.0001	.0008	.0042	.0149	.0385	.0771	.1248	.1669
	11	.0000	.0000	.0000	.0001	.0010	.0046	.0151	.0374	.0742	.1214

INDIVIDUAL TERMS, BINOMIAL DISTRIBUTION

		θ									
n	*x*	.05	.10	.15	.20	.25	.30	.35	.40	.45	.50
18	12	.0000	.0000	.0000	.0000	.0002	.0012	.0047	.0145	.0354	.0708
	13	.0000	.0000	.0000	.0000	.0000	.0002	.0012	.0045	.0134	.0327
	14	.0000	.0000	.0000	.0000	.0000	.0000	.0002	.0011	.0039	.0117
	15	.0000	.0000	.0000	.0000	.0000	.0000	.0000	.0002	.0009	.0031
	16	.0000	.0000	.0000	.0000	.0000	.0000	.0000	.0000	.0001	.0006
	17	.0000	.0000	.0000	.0000	.0000	.0000	.0000	.0000	.0000	.0001
	18	.0000	.0000	.0000	.0000	.0000	.0000	.0000	.0000	.0000	.0000
19	0	.3774	.1351	.0456	.0144	.0042	.0011	.0003	.0001	.0000	.0000
	1	.3774	.2852	.1529	.0685	.0268	.0093	.0029	.0008	.0002	.0000
	2	.1787	.2852	.2428	.1540	.0803	.0358	.0138	.0046	.0013	.0003
	3	.0533	.1796	.2428	.2182	.1517	.0869	.0422	.0175	.0062	.0018
	4	.0112	.0798	.1714	.2182	.2023	.1491	.0909	.0467	.0203	.0074
	5	.0018	.0266	.0907	.1636	.2023	.1916	.1468	.0933	.0497	.0222
	6	.0002	.0069	.0374	.0955	.1574	.1916	.1844	.1451	.0949	.0518
	7	.0000	.0014	.0122	.0443	.0974	.1525	.1844	.1797	.1443	.0961
	8	.0000	.0002	.0032	.0166	.0487	.0981	.1489	.1797	.1771	.1442
	9	.0000	.0000	.0007	.0051	.0198	.0514	.0980	.1464	.1771	.1762
	10	.0000	.0000	.0001	.0013	.0066	.0220	.0528	.0976	.1449	.1762
	11	.0000	.0000	.0000	.0003	.0018	.0077	.0233	.0532	.0970	.1442
	12	.0000	.0000	.0000	.0000	.0004	.0022	.0083	.0237	.0529	.0961
	13	.0000	.0000	.0000	.0000	.0001	.0005	.0024	.0085	.0233	.0518
	14	.0000	.0000	.0000	.0000	.0000	.0001	.0006	.0024	.0082	.0222
	15	.0000	.0000	.0000	.0000	.0000	.0000	.0001	.0005	.0022	.0074
	16	.0000	.0000	.0000	.0000	.0000	.0000	.0000	.0001	.0005	.0018
	17	.0000	.0000	.0000	.0000	.0000	.0000	.0000	.0000	.0001	.0003
	18	.0000	.0000	.0000	.0000	.0000	.0000	.0000	.0000	.0000	.0000
	19	.0000	.0000	.0000	.0000	.0000	.0000	.0000	.0000	.0000	.0000
20	0	.3585	.1216	.0388	.0115	.0032	.0008	.0002	.0000	.0000	.0000
	1	.3774	.2702	.1368	.0576	.0211	.0068	.0020	.0005	.0001	.0000
	2	.1887	.2852	.2293	.1369	.0669	.0278	.0100	.0031	.0008	.0002
	3	.0596	.1901	.2428	.2054	.1339	.0716	.0323	.0123	.0040	.0011
	4	.0133	.0898	.1821	.2182	.1897	.1304	.0738	.0350	.0139	.0046
	5	.0022	.0319	.1028	.1746	.2023	.1789	.1272	.0746	.0365	.0148
	6	.0003	.0089	.0454	.1091	.1686	.1916	.1712	.1244	.0746	.0370
	7	.0000	.0020	.0160	.0545	.1124	.1643	.1844	.1659	.1221	.0739
	8	.0000	.0004	.0046	.0222	.0609	.1144	.1614	.1797	.1623	.1201
	9	.0000	.0001	.0011	.0074	.0271	.0654	.1158	.1597	.1771	.1602
	10	.0000	.0000	.0002	.0020	.0099	.0308	.0686	.1171	.1593	.1762
	11	.0000	.0000	.0000	.0005	.0030	.0120	.0336	.0710	.1185	.1602
	12	.0000	.0000	.0000	.0001	.0008	.0039	.0136	.0355	.0727	.1201
	13	.0000	.0000	.0000	.0000	.0002	.0010	.0045	.0146	.0366	.0739
	14	.0000	.0000	.0000	.0000	.0000	.0002	.0012	.0049	.0150	.0370
	15	.0000	.0000	.0000	.0000	.0000	.0000	.0003	.0013	.0049	.0148
	16	.0000	.0000	.0000	.0000	.0000	.0000	.0000	.0003	.0013	.0046
	17	.0000	.0000	.0000	.0000	.0000	.0000	.0000	.0000	.0002	.0011
	18	.0000	.0000	.0000	.0000	.0000	.0000	.0000	.0000	.0000	.0002
	19	.0000	.0000	.0000	.0000	.0000	.0000	.0000	.0000	.0000	.0000
	20	.0000	.0000	.0000	.0000	.0000	.0000	.0000	.0000	.0000	.0000

INDIVIDUAL TERMS, BINOMIAL DISTRIBUTION

						θ					
n	x	.05	.10	.15	.20	.25	.30	.35	.40	.45	.50
21	0	.3406	.1094	.0329	.0092	.0024	.0006	.0001	.0000	.0000	.0000
	1	.3764	.2553	.1221	.0484	.0166	.0050	.0013	.0003	.0001	.0000
	2	.1981	.2837	.2155	.1211	.0555	.0215	.0072	.0020	.0005	.0001
	3	.0660	.1996	.2408	.1917	.1172	.0585	.0245	.0086	.0026	.0006
	4	.0156	.0998	.1912	.2156	.1757	.1128	.0593	.0259	.0095	.0029
	5	.0028	.0377	.1147	.1883	.1992	.1643	.1085	.0588	.0263	.0097
	6	.0004	.0112	.0540	.1222	.1770	.1878	.1558	.1045	.0574	.0259
	7	.0000	.0027	.0204	.0655	.1265	.1725	.1798	.1493	.1007	.0554
	8	.0000	.0005	.0063	.0286	.0738	.1294	.1694	.1742	.1442	.0970
	9	.0000	.0001	.0016	.0103	.0355	.0801	.1318	.1677	.1704	.1402
	10	.0000	.0000	.0003	.0031	.0142	.0412	.0851	.1342	.1673	.1682
	11	.0000	.0000	.0001	.0008	.0047	.0176	.0458	.0895	.1369	.1682
	12	.0000	.0000	.0000	.0002	.0013	.0063	.0206	.0500	.0933	.1402
	13	.0000	.0000	.0000	.0000	.0003	.0019	.0077	.0229	.0529	.0970
	14	.0000	.0000	.0000	.0000	.0001	.0005	.0024	.0087	.0247	.0554
	15	.0000	.0000	.0000	.0000	.0000	.0001	.0006	.0027	.0094	.0259
	16	.0000	.0000	.0000	.0000	.0000	.0000	.0001	.0007	.0029	.0097
	17	.0000	.0000	.0000	.0000	.0000	.0000	.0000	.0001	.0007	.0029
	18	.0000	.0000	.0000	.0000	.0000	.0000	.0000	.0000	.0001	.0006
	19	.0000	.0000	.0000	.0000	.0000	.0000	.0000	.0000	.0000	.0001
	20	.0000	.0000	.0000	.0000	.0000	.0000	.0000	.0000	.0000	.0000
	21	.0000	.0000	.0000	.0000	.0000	.0000	.0000	.0000	.0000	.0000
22	0	.3235	.0985	.0280	.0074	.0018	.0004	.0001	.0000	.0000	.0000
	1	.3746	.2407	.1087	.0406	.0131	.0037	.0009	.0001	.0000	.0000
	2	.2070	.2808	.2015	.1065	.0458	.0166	.0051	.0014	.0003	.0001
	3	.0726	.2080	.2370	.1775	.1017	.0474	.0184	.0060	.0016	.0004
	4	.0182	.1098	.1987	.2108	.1611	.0965	.0471	.0190	.0064	.0017
	5	.0034	.0439	.1262	.1897	.1933	.1489	.0913	.0456	.0187	.0063
	6	.0005	.0138	.0631	.1344	.1826	.1808	.1393	.0862	.0434	.0178
	7	.0001	.0035	.0255	.0768	.1391	.1771	.1714	.1314	.0812	.0407
	8	.0000	.0007	.0084	.0360	.0869	.1423	.1730	.1642	.1246	.0762
	9	.0000	.0001	.0023	.0140	.0451	.0949	.1449	.1703	.1586	.1186
	10	.0000	.0000	.0005	.0046	.0195	.0529	.1015	.1476	.1687	.1542
	11	.0000	.0000	.0001	.0012	.0071	.0247	.0596	.1073	.1506	.1682
	12	.0000	.0000	.0000	.0003	.0022	.0097	.0294	.0656	.1129	.1542
	13	.0000	.0000	.0000	.0001	.0006	.0032	.0121	.0336	.0711	.1186
	14	.0000	.0000	.0000	.0000	.0001	.0009	.0042	.0144	.0374	.0762
	15	.0000	.0000	.0000	.0000	.0000	.0002	.0012	.0051	.0163	.0407
	16	.0000	.0000	.0000	.0000	.0000	.0000	.0003	.0015	.0058	.0178
	17	.0000	.0000	.0000	.0000	.0000	.0000	.0001	.0004	.0017	.0063
	18	.0000	.0000	.0000	.0000	.0000	.0000	.0000	.0000	.0004	.0017
	19	.0000	.0000	.0000	.0000	.0000	.0000	.0000	.0000	.0001	.0004
	20	.0000	.0000	.0000	.0000	.0000	.0000	.0000	.0000	.0000	.0001
	21	.0000	.0000	.0000	.0000	.0000	.0000	.0000	.0000	.0000	.0000
	22	.0000	.0000	.0000	.0000	.0000	.0000	.0000	.0000	.0000	.0000
23	0	.3074	.0886	.0238	.0059	.0013	.0003	.0000	.0000	.0000	.0000
	1	.3721	.2265	.0966	.0339	.0103	.0027	.0006	.0001	.0000	.0000

INDIVIDUAL TERMS, BINOMIAL DISTRIBUTION

						θ					
n	x	.05	.10	.15	.20	.25	.30	.35	.40	.45	.50
23	2	.2154	.2768	.1875	.0933	.0376	.0127	.0037	.0009	.0002	.0000
	3	.0794	.2153	.2317	.1633	.0878	.0382	.0138	.0041	.0010	.0002
	4	.0209	.1196	.2044	.2042	.1463	.0818	.0371	.0138	.0042	.0011
	5	.0042	.0505	.1371	.1940	.1853	.1332	.0758	.0350	.0132	.0040
	6	.0007	.0168	.0726	.1455	.1853	.1712	.1225	.0700	.0323	.0120
	7	.0001	.0045	.0311	.0883	.1500	.1782	.1602	.1133	.0642	.0292
	8	.0000	.0010	.0110	.0442	.1000	.1527	.1725	.1511	.1051	.0585
	9	.0000	.0002	.0032	.0184	.0555	.1091	.1548	.1679	.1433	.0974
	10	.0000	.0000	.0008	.0064	.0259	.0655	.1167	.1567	.1642	.1364
	11	.0000	.0000	.0002	.0019	.0102	.0332	.0743	.1234	.1587	.1612
	12	.0000	.0000	.0000	.0005	.0034	.0142	.0400	.0823	.1299	.1612
	13	.0000	.0000	.0000	.0001	.0010	.0052	.0182	.0464	.0899	.1364
	14	.0000	.0000	.0000	.0000	.0002	.0016	.0070	.0221	.0525	.0974
	15	.0000	.0000	.0000	.0000	.0000	.0004	.0023	.0088	.0258	.0585
	16	.0000	.0000	.0000	.0000	.0000	.0001	.0006	.0029	.0106	.0292
	17	.0000	.0000	.0000	.0000	.0000	.0000	.0001	.0008	.0036	.0120
	18	.0000	.0000	.0000	.0000	.0000	.0000	.0000	.0002	.0010	.0040
	19	.0000	.0000	.0000	.0000	.0000	.0000	.0000	.0000	.0002	.0011
	20	.0000	.0000	.0000	.0000	.0000	.0000	.0000	.0000	.0000	.0002
	21	.0000	.0000	.0000	.0000	.0000	.0000	.0000	.0000	.0000	.0000
	22	.0000	.0000	.0000	.0000	.0000	.0000	.0000	.0000	.0000	.0000
	23	.0000	.0000	.0000	.0000	.0000	.0000	.0000	.0000	.0000	.0000
24	0	.2920	.0798	.0202	.0047	.0010	.0001	.0000	.0000	.0000	.0000
	1	.3688	.2127	.0857	.0283	.0080	.0020	.0004	.0001	.0000	.0000
	2	.2232	.2718	.1739	.0815	.0308	.0097	.0026	.0006	.0001	.0000
	3	.0862	.2215	.2251	.1493	.0752	.0305	.0102	.0028	.0007	.0001
	4	.0238	.1292	.2085	.1960	.1316	.0687	.0289	.0099	.0028	.0006
	5	.0050	.0574	.1472	.1960	.1755	.1177	.0622	.0265	.0091	.0025
	6	.0008	.0202	.0822	.1552	.1853	.1598	.1061	.0560	.0237	.0080
	7	.0001	.0058	.0373	.0998	.1588	.1761	.1470	.0960	.0499	.0206
	8	.0000	.0014	.0149	.0530	.1125	.1604	.1682	.1359	.0867	.0438
	9	.0000	.0003	.0044	.0236	.0667	.1222	.1610	.1612	.1261	.0779
	10	.0000	.0000	.0012	.0088	.0333	.0785	.1300	.1612	.1548	.1169
	11	.0000	.0000	.0003	.0028	.0141	.0428	.0891	.1367	.1612	.1488
	12	.0000	.0000	.0000	.0008	.0051	.0199	.0510	.0988	.1429	.1612
	13	.0000	.0000	.0000	.0002	.0016	.0079	.0258	.0608	.1079	.1488
	14	.0000	.0000	.0000	.0000	.0004	.0026	.0109	.0318	.0694	.1169
	15	.0000	.0000	.0000	.0000	.0001	.0008	.0039	.0141	.0378	.0779
	16	.0000	.0000	.0000	.0000	.0000	.0002	.0012	.0053	.0174	.0438
	17	.0000	.0000	.0000	.0000	.0000	.0000	.0003	.0017	.0067	.0206
	18	.0000	.0000	.0000	.0000	.0000	.0000	.0001	.0004	.0021	.0080
	19	.0000	.0000	.0000	.0000	.0000	.0000	.0000	.0001	.0006	.0025
	20	.0000	.0000	.0000	.0000	.0000	.0000	.0000	.0000	.0001	.0006
	21	.0000	.0000	.0000	.0000	.0000	.0000	.0000	.0000	.0000	.0001
	22	.0000	.0000	.0000	.0000	.0000	.0000	.0000	.0000	.0000	.0000
	23	.0000	.0000	.0000	.0000	.0000	.0000	.0000	.0000	.0000	.0000
	24	.0000	.0000	.0000	.0000	.0000	.0000	.0000	.0000	.0000	.0000

INDIVIDUAL TERMS, BINOMIAL DISTRIBUTION

						θ					
n	x	.05	.10	.15	.20	.25	.30	.35	.40	.45	.50
25	0	.2774	.0718	.0172	.0038	.0008	.0001	.0000	.0000	.0000	.0000
	1	.3650	.1994	.0759	.0236	.0063	.0014	.0003	.0000	.0000	.0000
	2	.2305	.2659	.1607	.0708	.0251	.0074	.0018	.0004	.0001	.0000
	3	.0930	.2265	.2174	.1358	.0641	.0243	.0076	.0019	.0004	.0001
	4	.0269	.1384	.2110	.1867	.1175	.0572	.0224	.0071	.0018	.0004
	5	.0060	.0646	.1564	.1960	.1645	.1030	.0506	.0199	.0063	.0016
	6	.0010	.0239	.0920	.1633	.1828	.1472	.0908	.0442	.0172	.0053
	7	.0001	.0072	.0441	.1108	.1654	.1712	.1327	.0800	.0381	.0143
	8	.0000	.0018	.0175	.0623	.1241	.1651	.1607	.1200	.0701	.0322
	9	.0000	.0004	.0058	.0294	.0781	.1336	.1635	.1511	.1084	.0609
	10	.0000	.0001	.0016	.0118	.0417	.0916	.1409	.1612	.1419	.0974
	11	.0000	.0000	.0004	.0040	.0189	.0536	.1034	.1465	.1583	.1328
	12	.0000	.0000	.0001	.0012	.0074	.0268	.0650	.1140	.1511	.1550
	13	.0000	.0000	.0000	.0003	.0025	.0115	.0350	.0760	.1236	.1550
	14	.0000	.0000	.0000	.0001	.0007	.0042	.0161	.0434	.0867	.1328
	15	.0000	.0000	.0000	.0000	.0002	.0013	.0064	.0212	.0520	.0974
	16	.0000	.0000	.0000	.0000	.0000	.0004	.0021	.0088	.0266	.0609
	17	.0000	.0000	.0000	.0000	.0000	.0001	.0006	.0031	.0115	.0322
	18	.0000	.0000	.0000	.0000	.0000	.0000	.0001	.0009	.0042	.0143
	19	.0000	.0000	.0000	.0000	.0000	.0000	.0000	.0002	.0013	.0053
	20	.0000	.0000	.0000	.0000	.0000	.0000	.0000	.0000	.0003	.0016
	21	.0000	.0000	.0000	.0000	.0000	.0000	.0000	.0000	.0001	.0004
	22	.0000	.0000	.0000	.0000	.0000	.0000	.0000	.0000	.0000	.0001
	23	.0000	.0000	.0000	.0000	.0000	.0000	.0000	.0000	.0000	.0000
	24	.0000	.0000	.0000	.0000	.0000	.0000	.0000	.0000	.0000	.0000
	25	.0000	.0000	.0000	.0000	.0000	.0000	.0000	.0000	.0000	.0000
30	0	.2146	.0424	.0076	.0012	.0002	.0000	.0000	.0000	.0000	.0000
	1	.3389	.1413	.0404	.0093	.0018	.0003	.0000	.0000	.0000	.0000
	2	.2586	.2277	.1034	.0337	.0086	.0018	.0003	.0000	.0000	.0000
	3	.1270	.2361	.1703	.0785	.0269	.0072	.0015	.0003	.0000	.0000
	4	.0451	.1771	.2028	.1325	.0604	.0208	.0056	.0012	.0002	.0000
	5	.0124	.1023	.1861	.1723	.1047	.0464	.0157	.0041	.0008	.0001
	6	.0027	.0474	.1368	.1795	.1455	.0829	.0353	.0115	.0029	.0006
	7	.0005	.0180	.0828	.1538	.1662	.1219	.0652	.0263	.0081	.0019
	8	.0001	.0058	.0420	.1106	.1593	.1501	.1009	.0505	.0191	.0055
	9	.0000	.0016	.0181	.0676	.1298	.1573	.1328	.0823	.0382	.0133
	10	.0000	.0004	.0067	.0355	.0909	.1416	.1502	.1152	.0656	.0280
	11	.0000	.0001	.0022	.0161	.0551	.1103	.1471	.1396	.0976	.0509
	12	.0000	.0000	.0006	.0064	.0291	.0749	.1254	.1474	.1265	.0806
	13	.0000	.0000	.0001	.0022	.0134	.0444	.0935	.1360	.1433	.1115
	14	.0000	.0000	.0000	.0007	.0054	.0231	.0611	.1101	.1424	.1354
	15	.0000	.0000	.0000	.0002	.0019	.0106	.0351	.0783	.1242	.1445
	16	.0000	.0000	.0000	.0000	.0006	.0042	.0177	.0489	.0953	.1354
	17	.0000	.0000	.0000	.0000	.0002	.0015	.0079	.0269	.0642	.1115
	18	.0000	.0000	.0000	.0000	.0000	.0005	.0031	.0129	.0379	.0806
	19	.0000	.0000	.0000	.0000	.0000	.0001	.0010	.0054	.0196	.0509
	20	.0000	.0000	.0000	.0000	.0000	.0000	.0003	.0020	.0088	.0280

INDIVIDUAL TERMS, BINOMIAL DISTRIBUTION

		θ									
n	x	.05	.10	.15	.20	.25	.30	.35	.40	.45	.50
30	21	.0000	.0000	.0000	.0000	.0000	.0000	.0001	.0006	.0034	.0133
	22	.0000	.0000	.0000	.0000	.0000	.0000	.0000	.0002	.0012	.0055
	23	.0000	.0000	.0000	.0000	.0000	.0000	.0000	.0000	.0003	.0019
	24	.0000	.0000	.0000	.0000	.0000	.0000	.0000	.0000	.0001	.0006
	25	.0000	.0000	.0000	.0000	.0000	.0000	.0000	.0000	.0000	.0001
	26	.0000	.0000	.0000	.0000	.0000	.0000	.0000	.0000	.0000	.0000
	27	.0000	.0000	.0000	.0000	.0000	.0000	.0000	.0000	.0000	.0000
	28	.0000	.0000	.0000	.0000	.0000	.0000	.0000	.0000	.0000	.0000
	29	.0000	.0000	.0000	.0000	.0000	.0000	.0000	.0000	.0000	.0000
	30	.0000	.0000	.0000	.0000	.0000	.0000	.0000	.0000	.0000	.0000
35	0	.1661	.0250	.0034	.0004	.0000	.0000	.0000	.0000	.0000	.0000
	1	.3059	.0973	.0209	.0035	.0005	.0001	.0000	.0000	.0000	.0000
	2	.2737	.1839	.0627	.0151	.0028	.0004	.0000	.0000	.0000	.0000
	3	.1585	.2247	.1218	.0415	.0103	.0020	.0003	.0000	.0000	.0000
	4	.0667	.1998	.1719	.0830	.0274	.0067	.0012	.0002	.0000	.0000
	5	.0218	.1376	.1881	.1286	.0566	.0178	.0042	.0007	.0001	.0000
	6	.0057	.0765	.1660	.1608	.0944	.0381	.0112	.0024	.0004	.0000
	7	.0012	.0352	.1213	.1665	.1303	.0676	.0250	.0068	.0013	.0002
	8	.0002	.0137	.0749	.1457	.1520	.1015	.0471	.0158	.0039	.0007
	9	.0000	.0046	.0397	.1093	.1520	.1305	.0761	.0316	.0095	.0021
	10	.0000	.0013	.0182	.0710	.1318	.1454	.1065	.0547	.0202	.0053
	11	.0000	.0003	.0073	.0404	.0998	.1416	.1303	.0829	.0375	.0121
	12	.0000	.0001	.0026	.0202	.0665	.1214	.1404	.1106	.0614	.0243
	13	.0000	.0000	.0008	.0089	.0392	.0920	.1337	.1304	.0889	.0430
	14	.0000	.0000	.0002	.0035	.0206	.0620	.1131	.1366	.1143	.0675
	15	.0000	.0000	.0001	.0012	.0096	.0372	.0853	.1275	.1309	.0945
	16	.0000	.0000	.0000	.0004	.0040	.0199	.0574	.1063	.1339	.1182
	17	.0000	.0000	.0000	.0001	.0015	.0095	.0345	.0792	.1225	.1321
	18	.0000	.0000	.0000	.0000	.0005	.0041	.0186	.0528	.1002	.1321
	19	.0000	.0000	.0000	.0000	.0001	.0016	.0090	.0315	.0733	.1182
	20	.0000	.0000	.0000	.0000	.0000	.0005	.0038	.0168	.0480	.0945
	21	.0000	.0000	.0000	.0000	.0000	.0002	.0015	.0080	.0281	.0675
	22	.0000	.0000	.0000	.0000	.0000	.0000	.0005	.0034	.0146	.0430
	23	.0000	.0000	.0000	.0000	.0000	.0000	.0002	.0013	.0068	.0243
	24	.0000	.0000	.0000	.0000	.0000	.0000	.0000	.0004	.0028	.0121
	25	.0000	.0000	.0000	.0000	.0000	.0000	.0000	.0001	.0010	.0053
	26	.0000	.0000	.0000	.0000	.0000	.0000	.0000	.0000	.0003	.0021
	27	.0000	.0000	.0000	.0000	.0000	.0000	.0000	.0000	.0001	.0007
	28	.0000	.0000	.0000	.0000	.0000	.0000	.0000	.0000	.0000	.0002
	29	.0000	.0000	.0000	.0000	.0000	.0000	.0000	.0000	.0000	.0000
	30	.0000	.0000	.0000	.0000	.0000	.0000	.0000	.0000	.0000	.0000
	31	.0000	.0000	.0000	.0000	.0000	.0000	.0000	.0000	.0000	.0000
	32	.0000	.0000	.0000	.0000	.0000	.0000	.0000	.0000	.0000	.0000
	33	.0000	.0000	.0000	.0000	.0000	.0000	.0000	.0000	.0000	.0000
	34	.0000	.0000	.0000	.0000	.0000	.0000	.0000	.0000	.0000	.0000
	35	.0000	.0000	.0000	.0000	.0000	.0000	.0000	.0000	.0000	.0000
40	0	.1285	.0148	.0015	.0001	.0000	.0000	.0000	.0000	.0000	.0000

INDIVIDUAL TERMS, BINOMIAL DISTRIBUTION

		θ									
n	x	.05	.10	.15	.20	.25	.30	.35	.40	.45	.50
40	1	.2706	.0657	.0106	.0013	.0001	.0000	.0000	.0000	.0000	.0000
	2	.2777	.1423	.0365	.0065	.0009	.0001	.0000	.0000	.0000	.0000
	3	.1851	.2003	.0816	.0205	.0037	.0005	.0001	.0000	.0000	.0000
	4	.0901	.2059	.1332	.0475	.0113	.0020	.0003	.0000	.0000	.0000
	5	.0342	.1647	.1692	.0854	.0272	.0061	.0010	.0001	.0000	.0000
	6	.0105	.1068	.1742	.1246	.0530	.0151	.0031	.0005	.0000	.0000
	7	.0027	.0576	.1493	.1513	.0857	.0315	.0080	.0015	.0002	.0000
	8	.0006	.0264	.1087	.1560	.1179	.0557	.0179	.0040	.0006	.0001
	9	.0001	.0104	.0682	.1387	.1397	.0849	.0342	.0095	.0018	.0002
	10	.0000	.0036	.0373	.1075	.1444	.1128	.0571	.0196	.0047	.0008
	11	.0000	.0011	.0180	.0733	.1312	.1319	.0837	.0357	.0105	.0021
	12	.0000	.0003	.0077	.0443	.1057	.1366	.1090	.0576	.0207	.0051
	13	.0000	.0001	.0029	.0238	.0759	.1261	.1265	.0827	.0365	.0109
	14	.0000	.0000	.0010	.0115	.0488	.1042	.1313	.1063	.0575	.0211
	15	.0000	.0000	.0003	.0050	.0281	.0774	.1226	.1228	.0816	.0366
	16	.0000	.0000	.0001	.0019	.0147	.0518	.1031	.1279	.1043	.0572
	17	.0000	.0000	.0000	.0007	.0069	.0314	.0784	.1204	.1205	.0807
	18	.0000	.0000	.0000	.0002	.0029	.0172	.0539	.1026	.1260	.1031
	19	.0000	.0000	.0000	.0001	.0011	.0085	.0336	.0792	.1194	.1194
	20	.0000	.0000	.0000	.0000	.0004	.0038	.0190	.0554	.1025	.1254
	21	.0000	.0000	.0000	.0000	.0001	.0016	.0097	.0352	.0799	.1194
	22	.0000	.0000	.0000	.0000	.0000	.0006	.0045	.0203	.0565	.1031
	23	.0000	.0000	.0000	.0000	.0000	.0002	.0019	.0106	.0362	.0807
	24	.0000	.0000	.0000	.0000	.0000	.0001	.0007	.0050	.0210	.0572
	25	.0000	.0000	.0000	.0000	.0000	.0000	.0003	.0021	.0110	.0366
	26	.0000	.0000	.0000	.0000	.0000	.0000	.0001	.0008	.0052	.0211
	27	.0000	.0000	.0000	.0000	.0000	.0000	.0001	.0003	.0022	.0109
	28	.0000	.0000	.0000	.0000	.0000	.0000	.0000	.0001	.0008	.0051
	29	.0000	.0000	.0000	.0000	.0000	.0000	.0000	.0000	.0003	.0021
	30	.0000	.0000	.0000	.0000	.0000	.0000	.0000	.0000	.0001	.0008
	31	.0000	.0000	.0000	.0000	.0000	.0000	.0000	.0000	.0000	.0002
	32	.0000	.0000	.0000	.0000	.0000	.0000	.0000	.0000	.0000	.0001
	33	.0000	.0000	.0000	.0000	.0000	.0000	.0000	.0000	.0000	.0000
	34	.0000	.0000	.0000	.0000	.0000	.0000	.0000	.0000	.0000	.0000
	35	.0000	.0000	.0000	.0000	.0000	.0000	.0000	.0000	.0000	.0000
	36	.0000	.0000	.0000	.0000	.0000	.0000	.0000	.0000	.0000	.0000
	37	.0000	.0000	.0000	.0000	.0000	.0000	.0000	.0000	.0000	.0000
	38	.0000	.0000	.0000	.0000	.0000	.0000	.0000	.0000	.0000	.0000
	39	.0000	.0000	.0000	.0000	.0000	.0000	.0000	.0000	.0000	.0000
	40	.0000	.0000	.0000	.0000	.0000	.0000	.0000	.0000	.0000	.0000
45	0	.0994	.0087	.0007	.0000	.0000	.0000	.0000	.0000	.0000	.0000
	1	.2355	.0436	.0053	.0005	.0000	.0000	.0000	.0000	.0000	.0000
	2	.2727	.1067	.0206	.0027	.0003	.0000	.0000	.0000	.0000	.0000
	3	.2057	.1699	.0520	.0097	.0013	.0001	.0000	.0000	.0000	.0000
	4	.1137	.1982	.0963	.0524	.0044	.0005	.0000	.0000	.0000	.0000
	5	.0491	.1806	.1394	.0520	.0120	.0019	.0002	.0000	.0000	.0000
	6	.0172	.1338	.1640	.0866	.0267	.0054	.0008	.0001	.0000	.0000
	7	.0050	.0828	.1612	.1206	.0495	.0129	.0022	.0003	.0000	.0000

INDIVIDUAL TERMS, BINOMIAL DISTRIBUTION

		θ									
n	x	.05	.10	.15	.20	.25	.30	.35	.40	.45	.50
45	8	.0013	.0437	.1351	.1433	.0784	.0263	.0058	.0009	.0001	.0000
	9	.0003	.0200	.0980	.1472	.1074	.0463	.0129	.0024	.0003	.0000
	10	.0001	.0080	.0623	.1325	.1289	.0714	.0249	.0058	.0009	.0001
	11	.0000	.0028	.0350	.1054	.1367	.0973	.0427	.0122	.0023	.0003
	12	.0000	.0009	.0175	.0747	.1291	.1182	.0651	.0230	.0054	.0008
	13	.0000	.0003	.0078	.0474	.1093	.1286	.0890	.0390	.0118	.0021
	14	.0000	.0001	.0032	.0271	.0833	.1259	.1096	.0594	.0208	.0047
	15	.0000	.0000	.0012	.0140	.0574	.1115	.1219	.0819	.0352	.0098
	16	.0000	.0000	.0004	.0066	.0358	.0896	.1231	.1023	.0540	.0184
	17	.0000	.0000	.0001	.0028	.0204	.0655	.1131	.1164	.0754	.0314
	18	.0000	.0000	.0000	.0011	.0106	.0437	.0947	.1207	.0960	.0488
	19	.0000	.0000	.0000	.0004	.0050	.0266	.0725	.1143	.1116	.0693
	20	.0000	.0000	.0000	.0001	.0021	.0148	.0507	.0991	.1187	.0901
	21	.0000	.0000	.0000	.0000	.0009	.0076	.0325	.0786	.1156	.1073
	22	.0000	.0000	.0000	.0000	.0003	.0035	.0191	.0572	.1032	.1170
	23	.0000	.0000	.0000	.0000	.0001	.0015	.0103	.0381	.0844	.1170
	24	.0000	.0000	.0000	.0000	.0000	.0006	.0051	.0233	.0633	.1073
	25	.0000	.0000	.0000	.0000	.0000	.0002	.0023	.0130	.0435	.0901
	26	.0000	.0000	.0000	.0000	.0000	.0001	.0010	.0067	.0274	.0693
	27	.0000	.0000	.0000	.0000	.0000	.0000	.0004	.0031	.0158	.0488
	28	.0000	.0000	.0000	.0000	.0000	.0000	.0001	.0013	.0083	.0314
	29	.0000	.0000	.0000	.0000	.0000	.0000	.0000	.0005	.0040	.0184
	30	.0000	.0000	.0000	.0000	.0000	.0000	.0000	.0002	.0017	.0098
	31	.0000	.0000	.0000	.0000	.0000	.0000	.0000	.0001	.0007	.0047
	32	.0000	.0000	.0000	.0000	.0000	.0000	.0000	.0000	.0002	.0021
	33	.0000	.0000	.0000	.0000	.0000	.0000	.0000	.0000	.0001	.0008
	34	.0000	.0000	.0000	.0000	.0000	.0000	.0000	.0000	.0000	.0003
	35	.0000	.0000	.0000	.0000	.0000	.0000	.0000	.0000	.0000	.0001
	36	.0000	.0000	.0000	.0000	.0000	.0000	.0000	.0000	.0000	.0000
	37	.0000	.0000	.0000	.0000	.0000	.0000	.0000	.0000	.0000	.0000
	38	.0000	.0000	.0000	.0000	.0000	.0000	.0000	.0000	.0000	.0000
	39	.0000	.0000	.0000	.0000	.0000	.0000	.0000	.0000	.0000	.0000
	40	.0000	.0000	.0000	.0000	.0000	.0000	.0000	.0000	.0000	.0000
	41	.0000	.0000	.0000	.0000	.0000	.0000	.0000	.0000	.0000	.0000
	42	.0000	.0000	.0000	.0000	.0000	.0000	.0000	.0000	.0000	.0000
	43	.0000	.0000	.0000	.0000	.0000	.0000	.0000	.0000	.0000	.0000
	44	.0000	.0000	.0000	.0000	.0000	.0000	.0000	.0000	.0000	.0000
	45	.0000	.0000	.0000	.0000	.0000	.0000	.0000	.0000	.0000	.0000

III.2 CUMULATIVE TERMS, BINOMIAL DISTRIBUTION

For the binomial probability function $f(x;n,\theta)$ the probability of observing x' or more successes is given by

$$\sum_{x=x'}^{n} \binom{n}{x} \theta^x (1-\theta)^{n-x},$$

This table contains the values of $\sum_{x=x'}^{n} \binom{n}{x} \theta^x (1-\theta)^{n-x}$ for specified values of n, x', and θ. If $\theta > 0.5$, the values for $\sum_{x=x'}^{n} \binom{n}{x} \theta^x (1-\theta)^{n-x}$ are obtained using the corresponding results obtained from

$$1 - \sum_{x=n-x'+1}^{n} \binom{n}{x} (1-\theta)^x \theta^{n-x}$$

The cumulative binomial distribution is related to the incomplete beta function as follows:

$$\sum_{x=x'}^{n} \binom{n}{x} \theta^x (1-\theta)^{n-x} = I_\theta(x', n - x' + 1),$$

$$\sum_{x=0}^{x'-1} \binom{n}{x} \theta^x (1-\theta)^{n-x} = 1 - I_\theta(x', n - x' + 1)$$

$$= 1 - \int_0^\theta u^{x'-1}(1-u)^{n-x'}\, du \Big/ \int_0^1 u^{x'-1}(1-u)^{n-x'}\, du\,.$$

The cumulative binomial distribution is related to the cumulative negative binomial distribution as follows:

$$1 - \sum_{x'=0}^{r-1} \binom{x+r}{x'} \theta^{x'}(1-\theta)^{x+r-x'} = \sum_{x'=0}^{x} \binom{x'+r-1}{r-1} \theta^r (1-\theta)^{x'}$$

or

$$\sum_{x'=r}^{x+r} \binom{x+r}{x'} \theta^{x'}(1-\theta)^{x+r-x'} = \sum_{x'=0}^{x} \binom{x'+r-1}{r-1} \theta^r (1-\theta)^{x'}\,.$$

CUMULATIVE TERMS, BINOMIAL DISTRIBUTION

						θ					
n	x'	.05	.10	.15	.20	.25	.30	.35	.40	.45	.50
2	1	.0975	.1900	.2775	.3600	.4375	.5100	.5775	.6400	.6975	.7500
	2	.0025	.0100	.0225	.0400	.0625	.0900	.1225	.1600	.2025	.2500
3	1	.1426	.2710	.3859	.4880	.5781	.6570	.7254	.7840	.8336	.8750
	2	.0072	.0280	.0608	.1040	.1562	.2160	.2818	.3520	.4252	.5000
	3	.0001	.0010	.0034	.0080	.0156	.0270	.0429	.0640	.0911	.1250
4	1	.1855	.3439	.4780	.5904	.6836	.7599	.8215	.8704	.9085	.9375
	2	.0140	.0523	.1095	.1808	.2617	.3483	.4370	.5248	.6090	.6875
	3	.0005	.0037	.0120	.0272	.0508	.0837	.1265	.1792	.2415	.3125
	4	.0000	.0001	.0005	.0016	.0039	.0081	.0150	.0256	.0410	.0625
5	1	.2262	.4095	.5563	.6723	.7627	.8319	.8840	.9222	.9497	.9688
	2	.0226	.0815	.1648	.2627	.3672	.4718	.5716	.6630	.7438	.8125
	3	.0012	.0086	.0266	.0579	.1035	.1631	.2352	.3174	.4069	.5000
	4	.0000	.0005	.0022	.0067	.0156	.0308	.0540	.0870	.1312	.1875
	5	.0000	.0000	.0001	.0003	.0010	.0024	.0053	.0102	.0185	.0312
6	1	.2649	.4686	.6229	.7379	.8220	.8824	.9246	.9533	.9723	.9844
	2	.0328	.1143	.2235	.3447	.4661	.5798	.6809	.7667	.8364	.8906
	3	.0022	.0158	.0473	.0989	.1694	.2557	.3529	.4557	.5585	.6562
	4	.0001	.0013	.0059	.0170	.0376	.0705	.1174	.1792	.2553	.3438
	5	.0000	.0001	.0004	.0016	.0046	.0109	.0223	.0410	.0692	.1094
	6	.0000	.0000	.0000	.0001	.0002	.0007	.0018	.0041	.0083	.0156
7	1	.3017	.5217	.6794	.7903	.8665	.9176	.9510	.9720	.9848	.9922
	2	.0444	.1497	.2834	.4233	.5551	.6706	.7662	.8414	.8976	.9375
	3	.0038	.0257	.0738	.1480	.2436	.3529	.4677	.5801	.6836	.7734
	4	.0002	.0027	.0121	.0333	.0706	.1260	.1998	.2898	.3917	.5000
	5	.0000	.0002	.0012	.0047	.0120	.0288	.0556	.0963	.1529	.2266
	6	.0000	.0000	.0001	.0004	.0013	.0038	.0090	.0188	.0357	.0625
	7	.0000	.0000	.0000	.0000	.0001	.0002	.0006	.0016	.0037	.0078
8	1	.3366	.5695	.7275	.8322	.8999	.9424	.9681	.9832	.9916	.9961
	2	.0572	.1869	.3428	.4967	.6329	.7447	.8309	.8936	.9368	.9648
	3	.0058	.0381	.1052	.2031	.3215	.4482	.5722	.6846	.7799	.8555
	4	.0004	.0050	.0214	.0563	.1138	.1941	.2936	.4059	.5230	.6367
	5	.0000	.0004	.0029	.0104	.0273	.0580	.1061	.1737	.2604	.3633
	6	.0000	.0000	.0002	.0012	.0042	.0113	.0253	.0498	.0885	.1445
	7	.0000	.0000	.0000	.0001	.0004	.0013	.0036	.0085	.0181	.0352
	8	.0000	.0000	.0000	.0000	.0000	.0001	.0002	.0007	.0017	.0039
9	1	.3698	.6126	.7684	.8658	.9249	.9596	.9793	.9899	.9954	.9980
	2	.0712	.2252	.4005	.5638	.6997	.8040	.8789	.9295	.9615	.9805
	3	.0084	.0530	.1409	.2618	.3993	.5372	.6627	.7682	.8505	.9102
	4	.0006	.0083	.0339	.0856	.1657	.2703	.3911	.5174	.6386	.7461
	5	.0000	.0009	.0056	.0196	.0489	.0988	.1717	.2666	.3786	.5000
	6	.0000	.0001	.0006	.0031	.0100	.0253	.0536	.0994	.1658	.2539
	7	.0000	.0000	.0000	.0003	.0013	.0043	.0112	.0250	.0498	.0898
	8	.0000	.0000	.0000	.0000	.0001	.0004	.0014	.0038	.0091	.0195
	9	.0000	.0000	.0000	.0000	.0000	.0000	.0001	.0003	.0008	.0020

Linear interpolation will be accurate at most to two decimal places.

CUMULATIVE TERMS, BINOMIAL DISTRIBUTION

n	x′	θ .05	.10	.15	.20	.25	.30	.35	.40	.45	.50
10	1	.4013	.6513	.8031	.8926	.9437	.9718	.9865	.9940	.9975	.9990
	2	.0861	.2639	.4557	.6242	.7560	.8507	.9140	.9536	.9767	.9893
	3	.0115	.0702	.1798	.3222	.4744	.6172	.7384	.8327	.9004	.9453
	4	.0010	.0128	.0500	.1209	.2241	.3504	.4862	.6177	.7340	.8281
	5	.0001	.0016	.0099	.0328	.0781	.1503	.2485	.3669	.4956	.6230
	6	.0000	.0001	.0014	.0064	.0197	.0473	.0949	.1662	.2616	.3770
	7	.0000	.0000	.0001	.0009	.0035	.0106	.0260	.0548	.1020	.1719
	8	.0000	.0000	.0000	.0001	.0004	.0016	.0048	.0123	.0274	.0547
	9	.0000	.0000	.0000	.0000	.0000	.0001	.0005	.0017	.0045	.0107
	10	.0000	.0000	.0000	.0000	.0000	.0000	.0000	.0001	.0003	.0010
11	1	.4312	.6862	.8327	.9141	.9578	.9802	.9912	.9964	.9986	.9995
	2	.1019	.3026	.5078	.6779	.8029	.8870	.9394	.9698	.9861	.9941
	3	.0152	.0896	.2212	.3826	.5448	.6873	.7999	.8811	.9348	.9673
	4	.0016	.0185	.0694	.1611	.2867	.4304	.5744	.7037	.8089	.8867
	5	.0001	.0028	.0159	.0504	.1146	.2103	.3317	.4672	.6029	.7256
	6	.0000	.0003	.0027	.0117	.0343	.0782	.1487	.2465	.3669	.5000
	7	.0000	.0000	.0003	.0020	.0076	.0216	.0501	.0994	.1738	.2744
	8	.0000	.0000	.0000	.0002	.0012	.0043	.0122	.0293	.0610	.1133
	9	.0000	.0000	.0000	.0000	.0001	.0006	.0020	.0059	.0148	.0327
	10	.0000	.0000	.0000	.0000	.0000	.0000	.0002	.0007	.0022	.0059
	11	.0000	.0000	.0000	.0000	.0000	.0000	.0000	.0000	.0002	.0005
12	1	.4596	.7176	.8578	.9313	.9683	.9862	.9943	.9978	.9992	.9998
	2	.1184	.3410	.5565	.7251	.8416	.9150	.9576	.9804	.9917	.9968
	3	.0196	.1109	.2642	.4417	.6093	.7472	.8487	.9166	.9579	.9807
	4	.0022	.0256	.0922	.2054	.3512	.5075	.6533	.7747	.8655	.9270
	5	.0002	.0043	.0239	.0726	.1576	.2763	.4167	.5618	.6956	.8062
	6	.0000	.0005	.0046	.0194	.0544	.1178	.2127	.3348	.4731	.6128
	7	.0000	.0001	.0007	.0039	.0143	.0386	.0846	.1582	.2607	.3872
	8	.0000	.0000	.0001	.0006	.0028	.0095	.0255	.0573	.1117	.1938
	9	.0000	.0000	.0000	.0001	.0004	.0017	.0056	.0153	.0356	.0730
	10	.0000	.0000	.0000	.0000	.0000	.0002	.0008	.0028	.0079	.0193
	11	.0000	.0000	.0000	.0000	.0000	.0000	.0001	.0003	.0011	.0032
	12	.0000	.0000	.0000	.0000	.0000	.0000	.0000	.0000	.0001	.0002
13	1	.4867	.7458	.8791	.9450	.9762	.9903	.9963	.9987	.9996	.9999
	2	.1354	.3787	.6017	.7664	.8733	.9363	.9704	.9874	.9951	.9983
	3	.0245	.1339	.2704	.4983	.6674	.7975	.8868	.9421	.9731	.9888
	4	.0031	.0342	.0967	.2527	.4157	.5794	.7217	.8314	.9071	.9539
	5	.0003	.0065	.0260	.0991	.2060	.3457	.4995	.6470	.7721	.8666
	6	.0000	.0009	.0053	.0300	.0802	.1654	.2841	.4256	.5732	.7095
	7	.0000	.0001	.0013	.0070	.0243	.0624	.1295	.2288	.3563	.5000
	8	.0000	.0000	.0002	.0012	.0056	.0182	.0462	.0977	.1788	.2905
	9	.0000	.0000	.0000	.0002	.0010	.0040	.0126	.0321	.0698	.1334
	10	.0000	.0000	.0000	.0000	.0001	.0007	.0025	.0078	.0203	.0461
	11	.0000	.0000	.0000	.0000	.0000	.0001	.0003	.0013	.0041	.0112
	12	.0000	.0000	.0000	.0000	.0000	.0000	.0000	.0001	.0005	.0017
	13	.0000	.0000	.0000	.0000	.0000	.0000	.0000	.0000	.0000	.0001

CUMULATIVE TERMS, BINOMIAL DISTRIBUTION

		θ									
n	*x'*	.05	.10	.15	.20	.25	.30	.35	.40	.45	.50
14	1	.5123	.7712	.8972	.9560	.9822	.9932	.9976	.9992	.9998	.9999
	2	.1530	.4154	.6433	.8021	.8990	.9525	.9795	.9919	.9971	.9991
	3	.0301	.1584	.3521	.5519	.7189	.8392	.9161	.9602	.9830	.9935
	4	.0042	.0441	.1465	.3018	.4787	.6448	.7795	.8757	.9368	.9713
	5	.0004	.0092	.0467	.1298	.2585	.4158	.5773	.7207	.8328	.9102
	6	.0000	.0015	.0115	.0439	.1117	.2195	.3595	.5141	.6627	.7880
	7	.0000	.0002	.0022	.0116	.0383	.0933	.1836	.3075	.4539	.6047
	8	.0000	.0000	.0003	.0024	.0103	.0315	.0753	.1501	.2586	.3953
	9	.0000	.0000	.0000	.0004	.0022	.0083	.0243	.0583	.1189	.2120
	10	.0000	.0000	.0000	.0000	.0003	.0017	.0060	.0175	.0426	.0898
	11	.0000	.0000	.0000	.0000	.0000	.0002	.0011	.0039	.0114	.0287
	12	.0000	.0000	.0000	.0000	.0000	.0000	.0001	.0006	.0022	.0065
	13	.0000	.0000	.0000	.0000	.0000	.0000	.0000	.0001	.0003	.0009
	14	.0000	.0000	.0000	.0000	.0000	.0000	.0000	.0000	.0000	.0001
15	1	.5367	.7941	.9126	.9648	.9866	.9953	.9984	.9995	.9999	1.0000
	2	.1710	.4510	.6814	.8329	.9198	.9647	.9858	.9948	.9983	.9995
	3	.0362	.1841	.3958	.6020	.7639	.8732	.9383	.9729	.9893	.9963
	4	.0055	.0556	.1773	.3518	.5387	.7031	.8273	.9095	.9576	.9824
	5	.0006	.0127	.0617	.1642	.3135	.4845	.6481	.7827	.8796	.9408
	6	.0001	.0022	.0168	.0611	.1484	.2784	.4357	.5968	.7392	.8491
	7	.0000	.0003	.0036	.0181	.0566	.1311	.2452	.3902	.5478	.6964
	8	.0000	.0000	.0006	.0042	.0173	.0500	.1132	.2131	.3465	.5000
	9	.0000	.0000	.0001	.0008	.0042	.0152	.0422	.0950	.1818	.3036
	10	.0000	.0000	.0000	.0001	.0008	.0037	.0124	.0338	.0769	.1509
	11	.0000	.0000	.0000	.0000	.0001	.0007	.0028	.0093	.0255	.0592
	12	.0000	.0000	.0000	.0000	.0000	.0001	.0005	.0010	.0063	.0176
	13	.0000	.0000	.0000	.0000	.0000	.0000	.0001	.0003	.0011	.0037
	14	.0000	.0000	.0000	.0000	.0000	.0000	.0000	.0000	.0001	.0005
	15	.0000	.0000	.0000	.0000	.0000	.0000	.0000	.0000	.0000	.0000
16	1	.5599	.8147	.9257	.9719	.9900	.9967	.9990	.9997	.9999	1.0000
	2	.1892	.4853	.7161	.8593	.9365	.9739	.9902	.9967	.9990	.9997
	3	.0429	.2108	.4386	.6482	.8029	.9006	.9549	.9817	.9934	.9979
	4	.0070	0684	.2101	.4019	.5950	.7541	.8661	.0340	.0710	.0804
	5	.0009	.0170	.0791	.2018	.3698	.5501	.7108	.8334	.9147	.9616
	6	.0001	.0033	.0235	.0817	.1897	.3402	.5100	.6712	.8024	.8949
	7	.0000	.0005	.0056	.0267	.0796	.1753	.3119	.4728	.6340	.7228
	8	.0000	.0001	.0011	.0070	.0271	.0744	.1594	.2839	.4371	.5982
	9	.0000	.0000	.0002	.0015	.0075	.0257	.0671	.1423	.2559	.4018
	10	.0000	.0000	.0000	.0002	.0016	.0071	.0229	.0583	.1241	.2272
	11	.0000	.0000	.0000	.0000	.0003	.0016	.0062	.0191	.0486	.1051
	12	.0000	.0000	.0000	.0000	.0000	.0003	.0013	.0049	.0149	.0384
	13	.0000	.0000	.0000	.0000	.0000	.0000	.0002	.0009	.0035	.0106
	14	.0000	.0000	.0000	.0000	.0000	.0000	.0000	.0001	.0006	.0021
	15	.0000	.0000	.0000	.0000	.0000	.0000	.0000	.0000	.0001	.0003
	16	.0000	.0000	.0000	.0000	.0000	.0000	.0000	.0000	.0000	.0000

CUMULATIVE TERMS, BINOMIAL DISTRIBUTION

n	x′	θ .05	.10	.15	.20	.25	.30	.35	.40	.45	.50
17	1	.5819	.8332	.9369	.9775	.9925	.9977	.9993	.9998	1.0000	1.0000
	2	.2078	.5182	.7475	.8818	.9499	.9807	.9933	.9979	.9994	.9999
	3	.0503	.2382	.4802	.6904	.8363	.9226	.9673	.9877	.9959	.9988
	4	.0088	.0826	.2444	.4511	.6470	.7981	.8972	.9536	.9816	.9936
	5	.0012	.0221	.0987	.2418	.4261	.6113	.7652	.8740	.9404	.9755
	6	.0001	.0047	.0319	.1057	.2347	.4032	.5803	.7361	.8529	.9283
	7	.0000	.0008	.0083	.0377	.1071	.2248	.3812	.5522	.7098	.8338
	8	.0000	.0001	.0017	.0109	.0402	.1046	.2128	.3595	.5257	.6855
	9	.0000	.0000	.0003	.0026	.0124	.0403	.0994	.1989	.3374	.5000
	10	.0000	.0000	.0000	.0005	.0031	.0127	.0383	.0919	.1834	.3145
	11	.0000	.0000	.0000	.0001	.0006	.0032	.0120	.0348	.0826	.1662
	12	.0000	.0000	.0000	.0000	.0001	.0007	.0030	.0106	.0301	.0717
	13	.0000	.0000	.0000	.0000	.0000	.0001	.0006	.0025	.0086	.0245
	14	.0000	.0000	.0000	.0000	.0000	.0000	.0000	.0005	.0019	.0064
	15	.0000	.0000	.0000	.0000	.0000	.0000	.0000	.0001	.0003	.0012
	16	.0000	.0000	.0000	.0000	.0000	.0000	.0000	.0000	.0000	.0001
	17	.0000	.0000	.0000	.0000	.0000	.0000	.0000	.0000	.0000	.0000
18	1	.6028	.8499	.9464	.9820	.9944	.9984	.9996	.9999	1.0000	1.0000
	2	.2265	.5497	.7759	.9009	.9605	.9858	.9954	.9987	.9997	.9999
	3	.0581	.2662	.5203	.7287	.8647	.9400	.9764	.9918	.9975	.9993
	4	.0109	.0982	.2798	.4990	.6943	.8354	.9217	.9672	.9880	.9962
	5	.0015	.0282	.1206	.2836	.4813	.6673	.8114	.9058	.9589	.9846
	6	.0002	.0064	.0419	.1329	.2825	.4656	.6450	.7912	.8923	.9519
	7	.0000	.0012	.0118	.0513	.1390	.2783	.4509	.6257	.7742	.8811
	8	.0000	.0002	.0027	.0163	.0569	.1407	.2717	.4366	.6085	.7597
	9	.0000	.0000	.0005	.0043	.0193	.0596	.1391	.2632	.4222	.5927
	10	.0000	.0000	.0001	.0009	.0054	.0210	.0597	.1347	.2527	.4073
	11	.0000	.0000	.0000	.0002	.0012	.0061	.0212	.0576	.1280	.2403
	12	.0000	.0000	.0000	.0000	.0002	.0014	.0062	.0203	.0537	.1189
	13	.0000	.0000	.0000	.0000	.0000	.0003	.0014	.0058	.0183	.0481
	14	.0000	.0000	.0000	.0000	.0000	.0000	.0003	.0013	.0049	.0154
	15	.0000	.0000	.0000	.0000	.0000	.0000	.0000	.0002	.0010	.0038
	16	.0000	.0000	.0000	.0000	.0000	.0000	.0000	.0000	.0001	.0007
	17	.0000	.0000	.0000	.0000	.0000	.0000	.0000	.0000	.0000	.0001
	18	.0000	.0000	.0000	.0000	.0000	.0000	.0000	.0000	.0000	.0000
19	1	.6226	.8649	.9544	.9856	.9958	.9989	.9997	.9999	1.0000	1.0000
	2	.2453	.5797	.8015	.9171	.9690	.9896	.9969	.9992	.9998	1.0000
	3	.0665	.2946	.5587	.7631	.8887	.9538	.9830	.9945	.9985	.9996
	4	.0132	.1150	.3159	.5449	.7369	.8668	.9409	.9770	.9923	.9978
	5	.0020	.0352	.1444	.3267	.5346	.7178	.8500	.9304	.9720	.9904
	6	.0002	.0086	.0537	.1631	.3322	.5261	.7032	.8371	.9223	.9682
	7	.0000	.0017	.0163	.0676	.1749	.3345	.5188	.6919	.8273	.9165
	8	.0000	.0003	.0041	.0233	.0775	.1820	.3344	.5122	.6831	.8204
	9	.0000	.0000	.0008	.0067	.0287	.0839	.1855	.3325	.5060	.6762
	10	.0000	.0000	.0001	.0016	.0089	.0326	.0875	.1861	.3290	.5000

CUMULATIVE TERMS, BINOMIAL DISTRIBUTION

		θ									
n	*x'*	.05	.10	.15	.20	.25	.30	.35	.40	.45	.50
19	11	.0000	.0000	.0000	.0003	.0023	.0105	.0347	.0885	.1841	.3238
	12	.0000	.0000	.0000	.0000	.0005	.0028	.0114	.0352	.0871	.1796
	13	.0000	.0000	.0000	.0000	.0001	.0006	.0031	.0116	.0342	.0835
	14	.0000	.0000	.0000	.0000	.0000	.0001	.0007	.0031	.0109	.0318
	15	.0000	.0000	.0000	.0000	.0000	.0000	.0001	.0006	.0028	.0096
	16	.0000	.0000	.0000	.0000	.0000	.0000	.0000	.0001	.0005	.0022
	17	.0000	.0000	.0000	.0000	.0000	.0000	.0000	.0000	.0001	.0004
	18	.0000	.0000	.0000	.0000	.0000	.0000	.0000	.0000	.0000	.0000
	19	.0000	.0000	.0000	.0000	.0000	.0000	.0000	.0000	.0000	.0000
20	1	.6415	.8784	.9612	.9885	.9968	.9992	.9998	1.0000	1.0000	1.0000
	2	.2642	.6083	.8244	.9308	.9757	.9924	.9979	.9995	.9999	1.0000
	3	.0755	.3231	.5951	.7939	.9087	.9645	.9879	.9964	.9991	.9998
	4	.0159	.1330	.3523	.5886	.7748	.8929	.9556	.9840	.9951	.9987
	5	.0026	.0432	.1702	.3704	.5852	.7625	.8818	.9490	.9811	.9941
	6	.0003	.0113	.0673	.1958	.3828	.5836	.7546	.8744	.9447	.9793
	7	.0000	.0024	.0219	.0867	.2142	.3920	.5834	.7500	.8701	.9423
	8	.0000	.0004	.0059	.0321	.1018	.2277	.3990	.5841	.7480	.8684
	9	.0000	.0001	.0013	.0100	.0409	.1133	.2376	.4044	.5857	.7483
	10	.0000	.0000	.0002	.0026	.0139	.0480	.1218	.2447	.4086	.5881
	11	.0000	.0000	.0000	.0006	.0039	.0171	.0532	.1275	.2493	.4119
	12	.0000	.0000	.0000	.0001	.0009	.0051	.0196	.0565	.1308	.2517
	13	.0000	.0000	.0000	.0000	.0002	.0013	.0060	.0210	.0580	.1316
	14	.0000	.0000	.0000	.0000	.0000	.0003	.0015	.0065	.0214	.0577
	15	.0000	.0000	.0000	.0000	.0000	.0000	.0003	.0016	.0064	.0207
	16	.0000	.0000	.0000	.0000	.0000	.0000	.0000	.0003	.0015	.0059
	17	.0000	.0000	.0000	.0000	.0000	.0000	.0000	.0000	.0003	.0013
	18	.0000	.0000	.0000	.0000	.0000	.0000	.0000	.0000	.0000	.0002
	19	.0000	.0000	.0000	.0000	.0000	.0000	.0000	.0000	.0000	.0000
	20	.0000	.0000	.0000	.0000	.0000	.0000	.0000	.0000	.0000	.0000
21	1	.6594	.8906	.9671	.9908	.9976	.9994	.9999	1.0000	1.0000	1.0000
	2	.2830	.6353	.8450	.9424	.9810	.9944	.9996	.9997	.9999	1.0000
	3	.0849	.3516	.6295	.8213	.9255	.9729	.9914	.9976	.9994	.9999
	4	.0189	.1520	.3887	.6296	.8083	.9144	.9669	.9890	.9969	.9993
	5	.0032	.0522	.1975	.4140	.6326	.8016	.9076	.9630	.9874	.9967
	6	.0004	.0144	.0827	.2307	.4334	.6373	.7991	.9043	.9611	.9867
	7	.0000	.0033	.0287	.1085	.2564	.4495	.6433	.7998	.9036	.9608
	8	.0000	.0006	.0083	.0431	.1299	.2770	.4635	.6505	.8029	.9054
	9	.0000	.0001	.0020	.0144	.0561	.1477	.2941	.4763	.6587	.8083
	10	.0000	.0000	.0004	.0041	.0206	.0676	.1632	.3086	.4883	.6682
	11	.0000	.0000	.0001	.0010	.0064	.0264	.0772	.1744	.3210	.5000
	12	.0000	.0000	.0000	.0002	.0017	.0087	.0313	.0849	.1841	.3318
	13	.0000	.0000	.0000	.0000	.0004	.0024	.0108	.0352	.0908	.1917
	14	.0000	.0000	.0000	.0000	.0001	.0006	.0031	.0123	.0379	.0946
	15	.0000	.0000	.0000	.0000	.0000	.0001	.0007	.0036	.0132	.0392
	16	.0000	.0000	.0000	.0000	.0000	.0000	.0001	.0008	.0037	.0133
	17	.0000	.0000	.0000	.0000	.0000	.0000	.0000	.0002	.0008	.0036
	18	.0000	.0000	.0000	.0000	.0000	.0000	.0000	.0000	.0001	.0007
	19	.0000	.0000	.0000	.0000	.0000	.0000	.0000	.0000	.0000	.0001

CUMULATIVE TERMS, BINOMIAL DISTRIBUTION

		θ									
n	x′	.05	.10	.15	.20	.25	.30	.35	.40	.45	.50
21	20	.0000	.0000	.0000	.0000	.0000	.0000	.0000	.0000	.0000	.0000
	21	.0000	.0000	.0000	.0000	.0000	.0000	.0000	.0000	.0000	.0000
22	1	.6765	.9015	.9720	.9926	.9982	.9966	.9999	1.0000	1.0000	1.0000
	2	.3018	.6608	.8633	.9520	.9851	.9959	.9990	.9998	1.0000	1.0000
	3	.0948	.3800	.6618	.8455	.9394	.9793	.9399	.9984	.9997	.9999
	4	.0222	.1719	.4248	.6680	.8376	.9319	.9755	.9924	.9980	.9996
	5	.0040	.0621	.2262	.4571	.6765	.8355	.9284	.9734	.9917	.9978
	6	.0006	.0182	.0999	.2674	.4832	.6866	.8371	.9278	.9729	.9915
	7	.0001	.0044	.0368	.1330	.3006	.5058	.6978	.8416	.9295	.9738
	8	.0000	.0009	.0114	.0561	.1615	.3287	.5264	.7102	.8482	.9331
	9	.0000	.0001	.0030	.0201	.0746	.1865	.3534	.5460	.7236	.8569
	10	.0000	.0000	.0007	.0061	.0295	.0916	.2084	.3756	.5650	.7383
	11	.0000	.0000	.0001	.0016	.0100	.0387	.1070	.2281	.3963	.5841
	12	.0000	.0000	.0000	.0003	.0029	.0140	.0474	.1207	.2457	.4159
	13	.0000	.0000	.0000	.0001	.0007	.0043	.0180	.0551	.1328	.2617
	14	.0000	.0000	.0000	.0000	.0001	.0011	.0058	.0215	.0617	.1431
	15	.0000	.0000	.0000	.0000	.0000	.0002	.0015	.0070	.0243	.0669
	16	.0000	.0000	.0000	.0000	.0000	.0000	.0003	.0019	.0080	.0262
	17	.0000	.0000	.0000	.0000	.0000	.0000	.0001	.0004	.0021	.0085
	18	.0000	.0000	.0000	.0000	.0000	.0000	.0000	.0001	.0005	.0022
	19	.0000	.0000	.0000	.0000	.0000	.0000	.0000	.0000	.0001	.0004
	20	.0000	.0000	.0000	.0000	.0000	.0000	.0000	.0000	.0000	.0001
	21	.0000	.0000	.0000	.0000	.0000	.0000	.0000	.0000	.0000	.0000
	22	.0000	.0000	.0000	.0000	.0000	.0000	.0000	.0000	.0000	.0000
23	1	.6926	.9114	.9762	.9941	.9987	.9997	1.0000	1.0000	1.0000	1.0000
	2	.3206	.6849	.8796	.9602	.9884	.9970	.9993	.9999	1.0000	1.0000
	3	.1052	.4080	.6920	.8668	.9508	.9843	.9957	.9990	1.0000	1.0000
	4	.0258	.1927	.4604	.7035	.8630	.9462	.9819	.9948	.9988	.9998
	5	.0049	.0731	.2560	.4993	.7168	.8644	.9449	.9810	.9945	.9987
	6	.0008	.0226	.1189	.3053	.5315	.7312	.8691	.9460	.9814	.9947
	7	.0001	.0058	.0463	.1598	.3463	.5601	.7466	.8760	.9490	.9827
	8	.0000	.0012	.0152	.0715	.1963	.3819	.5864	.7627	.8848	.9534
	9	.0000	.0002	.0042	.0273	.0963	.2291	.4140	.6116	.7797	.8950
	10	.0000	.0000	.0010	.0089	.0408	.1201	.2592	.4438	.6364	.7976
	11	.0000	.0000	.0002	.0025	.0149	.0546	.1425	.2871	.4722	.6612
	12	.0000	.0000	.0000	.0006	.0046	.0214	.0682	.1636	.3135	.5000
	13	.0000	.0000	.0000	.0001	.0012	.0072	.0283	.0813	.1836	.3388
	14	.0000	.0000	.0000	.0000	.0003	.0021	.0100	.0349	.0937	.2024
	15	.0000	.0000	.0000	.0000	.0001	.0005	.0030	.0128	.0411	.1050
	16	.0000	.0000	.0000	.0000	.0000	.0001	.0008	.0040	.0153	.0466
	17	.0000	.0000	.0000	.0000	.0000	.0000	.0002	.0010	.0048	.0173
	18	.0000	.0000	.0000	.0000	.0000	.0000	.0000	.0002	.0012	.0053
	19	.0000	.0000	.0000	.0000	.0000	.0000	.0000	.0000	.0002	.0013
	20	.0000	.0000	.0000	.0000	.0000	.0000	.0000	.0000	.0000	.0002
	21	.0000	.0000	.0000	.0000	.0000	.0000	.0000	.0000	.0000	.0000
	22	.0000	.0000	.0000	.0000	.0000	.0000	.0000	.0000	.0000	.0000
	23	.0000	.0000	.0000	.0000	.0000	.0000	.0000	.0000	.0000	.0000

CUMULATIVE TERMS, BINOMIAL DISTRIBUTION

					θ						
n	*x′*	.05	.10	.15	.20	.25	.30	.35	.40	.45	.50
24	1	.7080	.9202	.9798	.9953	.9990	.9998	1.0000	1.0000	1.0000	1.0000
	2	.3391	.7075	.8941	.9669	.9910	.9978	.9995	.9999	1.0000	1.0000
	3	.1159	.4357	.7202	.8855	.9602	.9881	.9970	.9993	.9999	1.0000
	4	.0298	.2143	.4951	.7361	.8850	.9576	.9867	.9965	.9992	.9999
	5	.0060	.0851	.2866	.5401	.7534	.8889	.9578	.9866	.9964	.9992
	6	.0010	.0277	.1394	.3441	.5778	.7712	.8956	.9600	.9873	.9967
	7	.0001	.0075	.0572	.1889	.3926	.6114	.7894	.9040	.9636	.9887
	8	.0000	.0017	.0199	.0892	.2338	.4353	.6425	.8081	.9137	.9680
	9	.0000	.0003	.0059	.0362	.1213	.2750	.4743	.6721	.8270	.9242
	10	.0000	.0001	.0015	.0126	.0547	.1528	.3134	.5109	.7009	.8463
	11	.0000	.0000	.0003	.0038	.0213	.0742	.1833	.3498	.5461	.7294
	12	.0000	.0000	.0001	.0010	.0072	.0314	.0942	.2130	.3849	.5806
	13	.0000	.0000	.0000	.0002	.0021	.0115	.0423	.1143	.2420	.4194
	14	.0000	.0000	.0000	.0000	.0005	.0036	.0164	.0535	.1341	.2706
	15	.0000	.0000	.0000	.0000	.0001	.0010	.0055	.0217	.0648	.1537
	16	.0000	.0000	.0000	.0000	.0000	.0002	.0016	.0075	.0269	.0758
	17	.0000	.0000	.0000	.0000	.0000	.0000	.0004	.0022	.0095	.0320
	18	.0000	.0000	.0000	.0000	.0000	.0000	.0001	.0005	.0028	.0113
	19	.0000	.0000	.0000	.0000	.0000	.0000	.0000	.0001	.0007	.0033
	20	.0000	.0000	.0000	.0000	.0000	.0000	.0000	.0000	.0001	.0008
	21	.0000	.0000	.0000	.0000	.0000	.0000	.0000	.0000	.0000	.0001
	22	.0000	.0000	.0000	.0000	.0000	.0000	.0000	.0000	.0000	.0000
	23	.0000	.0000	.0000	.0000	.0000	.0000	.0000	.0000	.0000	.0000
	24	.0000	.0000	.0000	.0000	.0000	.0000	.0000	.0000	.0000	.0000
25	1	.7226	.9282	.9828	.9962	.9992	.9999	1.0000	1.0000	1.0000	1.0000
	2	.3576	.7288	.9069	.9726	.9930	.9984	.9997	.9999	1.0000	1.0000
	3	.1271	.4629	.7463	.9018	.9679	.9910	.9979	.9996	.9999	1.0000
	4	.0341	.2364	.5289	.7660	.9038	.9668	.9903	.9976	.9995	.9999
	5	.0072	.0980	.3179	.5793	.7863	.9095	.9680	.9905	.9977	.9995
	6	.0012	.0334	.1615	.3833	.6217	.8065	.9174	.9706	.9914	.9980
	7	.0002	.0095	.0695	.2200	.4389	.6593	.8266	.9264	.9742	.9927
	8	.0000	.0023	.0255	.1091	.2735	.4882	.6939	.8464	.9361	.9784
	9	.0000	.0005	.0080	.0468	.1494	.3231	.5332	.7265	.8660	.9461
	10	.0000	.0001	.0021	.0173	.0713	.1894	.3697	.5754	.7576	.8852
	11	.0000	.0000	.0005	.0056	.0297	.0978	.2288	.4142	.6157	.7878
	12	.0000	.0000	.0001	.0015	.0107	.0442	.1254	.2677	.4574	.6550
	13	.0000	.0000	.0000	.0004	.0034	.0175	.0604	.1538	.3063	.5000
	14	.0000	.0000	.0000	.0001	.0009	.0060	.0255	.0778	.1827	.3450
	15	.0000	.0000	.0000	.0000	.0002	.0018	.0093	.0344	.0960	.2122
	16	.0000	.0000	.0000	.0000	.0000	.0005	.0029	.0132	.0440	.1148
	17	.0000	.0000	.0000	.0000	.0000	.0001	.0008	.0043	.0174	.0539
	18	.0000	.0000	.0000	.0000	.0000	.0000	.0002	.0012	.0058	.0216
	19	.0000	.0000	.0000	.0000	.0000	.0000	.0000	.0003	.0016	.0073
	20	.0000	.0000	.0000	.0000	.0000	.0000	.0000	.0001	.0004	.0020
	21	.0000	.0000	.0000	.0000	.0000	.0000	.0000	.0000	.0001	.0005
	22	.0000	.0000	.0000	.0000	.0000	.0000	.0000	.0000	.0000	.0001
	23	.0000	.0000	.0000	.0000	.0000	.0000	.0000	.0000	.0000	.0000
	24	.0000	.0000	.0000	.0000	.0000	.0000	.0000	.0000	.0000	.0000

CUMULATIVE TERMS, BINOMIAL DISTRIBUTION

n	x′	θ .05	.10	.15	.20	.25	.30	.35	.40	.45	.50
25	25	.0000	.0000	.0000	.0000	.0000	.0000	.0000	.0000	.0000	.0000
30	1	.7854	.9576	.9924	.9988	.9998	1.0000	1.0000	1.0000	1.0000	1.0000
	2	.4465	.8163	.9520	.9895	.9980	.9997	1.0000	1.0000	1.0000	1.0000
	3	.1878	.5886	.8486	.9558	.9894	.9979	.9997	1.0000	1.0000	1.0000
	4	.0608	.3526	.6783	.8773	.9626	.9907	.9981	.9997	1.0000	1.0000
	5	.0156	.1755	.4755	.7448	.9021	.9698	.9925	.9985	.9998	1.0000
	6	.0033	.0732	.2894	.5725	.7974	.9234	.9767	.9943	.9989	.9998
	7	.0006	.0258	.1526	.3930	.6519	.8405	.9414	.9828	.9960	.9993
	8	.0001	.0078	.0698	.2392	.4857	.7186	.8762	.9565	.9879	.9974
	9	.0000	.0020	.0278	.1287	.3264	.5685	.7753	.9060	.9688	.9919
	10	.0000	.0005	.0097	.0611	.1966	.4112	.6425	.8237	.9306	.9786
	11	.0000	.0001	.0029	.0256	.1057	.2696	.4922	.7085	.8650	.9506
	12	.0000	.0000	.0008	.0095	.0507	.1593	.3452	.5689	.7673	.8998
	13	.0000	.0000	.0002	.0031	.0216	.0845	.2198	.4215	.6408	.8192
	14	.0000	.0000	.0000	.0009	.0082	.0401	.1263	.2855	.4975	.7077
	15	.0000	.0000	.0000	.0002	.0027	.0169	.0652	.1754	.3552	.5722
	16	.0000	.0000	.0000	.0001	.0008	.0064	.0301	.0971	.2309	.4278
	17	.0000	.0000	.0000	.0000	.0002	.0021	.0124	.0481	.1356	.2923
	18	.0000	.0000	.0000	.0000	.0001	.0006	.0045	.0212	.0714	.1808
	19	.0000	.0000	.0000	.0000	.0000	.0002	.0014	.0083	.0334	.1002
	20	.0000	.0000	.0000	.0000	.0000	.0000	.0004	.0029	.0138	.0494
	21	.0000	.0000	.0000	.0000	.0000	.0000	.0001	.0009	.0050	.0214
	22	.0000	.0000	.0000	.0000	.0000	.0000	.0000	.0002	.0016	.0081
	23	.0000	.0000	.0000	.0000	.0000	.0000	.0000	.0000	.0004	.0026
	24	.0000	.0000	.0000	.0000	.0000	.0000	.0000	.0000	.0001	.0007
	25	.0000	.0000	.0000	.0000	.0000	.0000	.0000	.0000	.0000	.0002
	26	.0000	.0000	.0000	.0000	.0000	.0000	.0000	.0000	.0000	.0000
	27	.0000	.0000	.0000	.0000	.0000	.0000	.0000	.0000	.0000	.0000
	28	.0000	.0000	.0000	.0000	.0000	.0000	.0000	.0000	.0000	.0000
	29	.0000	.0000	.0000	.0000	.0000	.0000	.0000	.0000	.0000	.0000
	30	.0000	.0000	.0000	.0000	.0000	.0000	.0000	.0000	.0000	.0000
35	1	.8339	.9750	.9966	.9996	1.0000	1.0000	1.0000	1.0000	1.0000	1.0000
	2	.5280	.8776	.9757	.9960	.9995	.9999	1.0000	1.0000	1.0000	1.0000
	3	.2542	.6937	.9130	.9810	.9967	.9995	.9999	1.0000	1.0000	1.0000
	4	.0958	.4690	.7912	.9395	.9864	.9976	.9997	1.0000	1.0000	1.0000
	5	.0290	.2693	.6193	.8565	.9590	.9909	.9984	.9998	1.0000	1.0000
	6	.0073	.1316	.4311	.7279	.9024	.9731	.9942	.9990	.9999	1.0000
	7	.0015	.0552	.2652	.5672	.8080	.9350	.9830	.9966	.9995	.9999
	8	.0003	.0200	.1438	.4007	.6777	.8674	.9581	.9898	.9981	.9997
	9	.0000	.0063	.0689	.2550	.5257	.7659	.9110	.9740	.9943	.9991
	10	.0000	.0017	.0292	.1457	.3737	.6354	.8349	.9425	.9848	.9970
	11	.0000	.0004	.0110	.0747	.2419	.4900	.7284	.8877	.9646	.9917
	12	.0000	.0001	.0037	.0344	.1421	.3484	.5981	.8048	.9271	.9795
	13	.0000	.0000	.0011	.0142	.0756	.2271	.4577	.6943	.8656	.9552
	14	.0000	.0000	.0003	.0053	.0363	.1350	.3240	.5639	.7767	.9123
	15	.0000	.0000	.0001	.0018	.0158	.0731	.2109	.4272	.6624	.8447
	16	.0000	.0000	.0000	.0005	.0062	.0359	.1256	.2997	.5315	.7502

CUMULATIVE TERMS, BINOMIAL DISTRIBUTION

n	x′	.05	.10	.15	.20	θ .25	.30	.35	.40	.45	.50
35	17	.0000	.0000	.0000	.0001	.0022	.0160	.0682	.1935	.3976	.6321
	18	.0000	.0000	.0000	.0000	.0007	.0064	.0336	.1143	.2751	.5000
	19	.0000	.0000	.0000	.0000	.0002	.0023	.0150	.0615	.1749	.3679
	20	.0000	.0000	.0000	.0000	.0001	.0008	.0061	.0300	.1016	.2498
	21	.0000	.0000	.0000	.0000	.0000	.0002	.0022	.0133	.0536	.1553
	22	.0000	.0000	.0000	.0000	.0000	.0001	.0007	.0053	.0255	.0877
	23	.0000	.0000	.0000	.0000	.0000	.0000	.0002	.0019	.0109	.0448
	24	.0000	.0000	.0000	.0000	.0000	.0000	.0001	.0006	.0042	.0205
	25	.0000	.0000	.0000	.0000	.0000	.0000	.0000	.0002	.0014	.0083
	26	.0000	.0000	.0000	.0000	.0000	.0000	.0000	.0000	.0004	.0030
	27	.0000	.0000	.0000	.0000	.0000	.0000	.0000	.0000	.0001	.0009
	28	.0000	.0000	.0000	.0000	.0000	.0000	.0000	.0000	.0000	.0003
	29	.0000	.0000	.0000	.0000	.0000	.0000	.0000	.0000	.0000	.0001
	30	.0000	.0000	.0000	.0000	.0000	.0000	.0000	.0000	.0000	.0000
	31	.0000	.0000	.0000	.0000	.0000	.0000	.0000	.0000	.0000	.0000
	32	.0000	.0000	.0000	.0000	.0000	.0000	.0000	.0000	.0000	.0000
	33	.0000	.0000	.0000	.0000	.0000	.0000	.0000	.0000	.0000	.0000
	34	.0000	.0000	.0000	.0000	.0000	.0000	.0000	.0000	.0000	.0000
	35	.0000	.0000	.0000	.0000	.0000	.0000	.0000	.0000	.0000	.0000
40	1	.8715	.9852	.9985	.9999	1.0000	1.0000	1.0000	1.0000	1.0000	1.0000
	2	.6009	.9195	.9879	.9985	.9999	1.0000	1.0000	1.0000	1.0000	1.0000
	3	.3233	.7772	.9514	.9921	.9990	.9999	1.0000	1.0000	1.0000	1.0000
	4	.1381	.5769	.8698	.9715	.9953	.9994	.9999	1.0000	1.0000	1.0000
	5	.0480	.3710	.7367	.9241	.9840	.9974	.9997	1.0000	1.0000	1.0000
	6	.0139	.2063	.5675	.8387	.9567	.9914	.9987	.9999	1.0000	1.0000
	7	.0034	.0995	.3933	.7141	.9038	.9762	.9956	.9994	.9999	1.0000
	8	.0007	.0419	.2441	.5629	.8180	.9447	.9876	.9979	.9998	1.0000
	9	.0001	.0155	.1354	.4069	.7002	.8890	.9697	.9939	.9991	.9999
	10	.0000	.0051	.0672	.2682	.5605	.8041	.9356	.9844	.9973	.9997
	11	.0000	.0015	.0299	.1608	.4161	.6913	.8785	.9648	.9926	.9989
	12	.0000	.0004	.0120	.0875	.2849	.5594	.7947	.9291	.9821	.9968
	13	.0000	.0001	.0043	.0432	.1791	.4228	.6857	.8715	.9614	.9917
	14	.0000	.0000	.0014	.0194	.1032	.2968	.5592	.7888	.9249	.9808
	15	.0000	.0000	.0004	.0079	.0544	.1926	.4279	.6826	.8674	.9597
	16	.0000	.0000	.0001	.0029	.0262	.1151	.3054	.5598	.7858	.9231
	17	.0000	.0000	.0000	.0010	.0116	.0633	.2022	.4319	.6815	.8659
	18	.0000	.0000	.0000	.0003	.0047	.0320	.1239	.3115	.5609	.7852
	19	.0000	.0000	.0000	.0001	.0017	.0148	.0699	.2089	.4349	.6821
	20	.0000	.0000	.0000	.0000	.0006	.0063	.0363	.1298	.3156	.5627
	21	.0000	.0000	.0000	.0000	.0002	.0024	.0173	.0744	.2130	.4373
	22	.0000	.0000	.0000	.0000	.0000	.0009	.0075	.0392	.1331	.3179
	23	.0000	.0000	.0000	.0000	.0000	.0003	.0030	.0189	.0767	.2148
	24	.0000	.0000	.0000	.0000	.0000	.0001	.0011	.0083	.0405	.1341
	25	.0000	.0000	.0000	.0000	.0000	.0000	.0004	.0034	.0196	.0769
	26	.0000	.0000	.0000	.0000	.0000	.0000	.0001	.0012	.0086	.0403
	27	.0000	.0000	.0000	.0000	.0000	.0000	.0000	.0004	.0034	.0192
	28	.0000	.0000	.0000	.0000	.0000	.0000	.0000	.0001	.0012	.0083
	29	.0000	.0000	.0000	.0000	.0000	.0000	.0000	.0000	.0004	.0032

CUMULATIVE TERMS, BINOMIAL DISTRIBUTION

		θ									
n	x'	.05	.10	.15	.20	.25	.30	.35	.40	.45	.50
40	30	.0000	.0000	.0000	.0000	.0000	.0000	.0000	.0000	.0001	.0011
	31	.0000	.0000	.0000	.0000	.0000	.0000	.0000	.0000	.0000	.0003
	32	.0000	.0000	.0000	.0000	.0000	.0000	.0000	.0000	.0000	.0001
	33	.0000	.0000	.0000	.0000	.0000	.0000	.0000	.0000	.0000	.0000
	34	.0000	.0000	.0000	.0000	.0000	.0000	.0000	.0000	.0000	.0000
	35	.0000	.0000	.0000	.0000	.0000	.0000	.0000	.0000	.0000	.0000
	36	.0000	.0000	.0000	.0000	.0000	.0000	.0000	.0000	.0000	.0000
	37	.0000	.0000	.0000	.0000	.0000	.0000	.0000	.0000	.0000	.0000
	38	.0000	.0000	.0000	.0000	.0000	.0000	.0000	.0000	.0000	.0000
	39	.0000	.0000	.0000	.0000	.0000	.0000	.0000	.0000	.0000	.0000
	40	.0000	.0000	.0000	.0000	.0000	.0000	.0000	.0000	.0000	.0000
45	1	.9006	.9913	.9993	1.0000	1.0000	1.0000	1.0000	1.0000	1.0000	1.0000
	2	.6650	.9476	.9940	.9995	1.0000	1.0000	1.0000	1.0000	1.0000	1.0000
	3	.3923	.8410	.9735	.9968	.9997	1.0000	1.0000	1.0000	1.0000	1.0000
	4	.1866	.6711	.9215	.9871	.9984	.9999	1.0000	1.0000	1.0000	1.0000
	5	.0729	.4729	.8252	.9618	.9941	.9993	.9999	1.0000	1.0000	1.0000
	6	.0239	.2923	.6858	.9098	.9821	.9974	.9997	1.0000	1.0000	1.0000
	7	.0066	.1585	.5218	.8232	.9554	.9920	.9990	.9999	1.0000	1.0000
	8	.0016	.0757	.3606	.7025	.9059	.9791	.9967	.9996	1.0000	1.0000
	9	.0003	.0320	.2255	.5593	.8275	.9529	.9909	.9988	.9999	1.0000
	10	.0001	.0120	.1274	.4120	.7200	.9066	.9780	.9964	.9996	1.0000
	11	.0000	.0040	.0651	.2795	.5911	.8353	.9531	.9906	.9987	.9999
	12	.0000	.0012	.0302	.1741	.4543	.7380	.9104	.9784	.9964	.9996
	13	.0000	.0003	.0127	.0995	.3252	.6198	.8453	.9554	.9910	.9988
	14	.0000	.0001	.0048	.0521	.2159	.4912	.7563	.9164	.9799	.9967
	15	.0000	.0000	.0017	.0250	.1327	.3653	.6467	.8570	.9591	.9920
	16	.0000	.0000	.0005	.0110	.0753	.2538	.5248	.7751	.9238	.9822
	17	.0000	.0000	.0002	.0044	.0395	.1642	.4017	.6728	.8698	.9638
	18	.0000	.0000	.0000	.0017	.0191	.0986	.2887	.5564	.7944	.9324
	19	.0000	.0000	.0000	.0006	.0085	.0549	.1940	.4357	.6985	.8837
	20	.0000	.0000	.0000	.0002	.0035	.0283	.1215	.3214	.5869	.8144
	21	.0000	.0000	.0000	.0001	.0013	.0135	.0708	.2223	.4682	.7243
	22	.0000	.0000	.0000	.0000	.0005	.0060	.0382	.1436	.3526	.6170
	23	.0000	.0000	.0000	.0000	.0001	.0024	.0191	.0865	.2494	.5000
	24	.0000	.0000	.0000	.0000	.0000	.0009	.0089	.0483	.1650	.3830
	25	.0000	.0000	.0000	.0000	.0000	.0003	.0038	.0250	.1017	.2757
	26	.0000	.0000	.0000	.0000	.0000	.0001	.0015	.0120	.0582	.1856
	27	.0000	.0000	.0000	.0000	.0000	.0000	.0005	.0053	.0308	.1163
	28	.0000	.0000	.0000	.0000	.0000	.0000	.0002	.0021	.0150	.0676
	29	.0000	.0000	.0000	.0000	.0000	.0000	.0001	.0008	.0068	.0362
	30	.0000	.0000	.0000	.0000	.0000	.0000	.0000	.0003	.0028	.0178
	31	.0000	.0000	.0000	.0000	.0000	.0000	.0000	.0001	.0010	.0080
	32	.0000	.0000	.0000	.0000	.0000	.0000	.0000	.0000	.0004	.0033
	33	.0000	.0000	.0000	.0000	.0000	.0000	.0000	.0000	.0001	.0012
	34	.0000	.0000	.0000	.0000	.0000	.0000	.0000	.0000	.0000	.0004
	35	.0000	.0000	.0000	.0000	.0000	.0000	.0000	.0000	.0000	.0001
	36	.0000	.0000	.0000	.0000	.0000	.0000	.0000	.0000	.0000	.0000

CUMULATIVE TERMS, BINOMIAL DISTRIBUTION

						θ					
n	x'	.05	.10	.15	.20	.25	.30	.35	.40	.45	.50
45	37	.0000	.0000	.0000	.0000	.0000	.0000	.0000	.0000	.0000	.0000
	38	.0000	.0000	.0000	.0000	.0000	.0000	.0000	.0000	.0000	.0000
	39	.0000	.0000	.0000	.0000	.0000	.0000	.0000	.0000	.0000	.0000
	40	.0000	.0000	.0000	.0000	.0000	.0000	.0000	.0000	.0000	.0000
	41	.0000	.0000	.0000	.0000	.0000	.0000	.0000	.0000	.0000	.0000
	42	.0000	.0000	.0000	.0000	.0000	.0000	.0000	.0000	.0000	.0000
	43	.0000	.0000	.0000	.0000	.0000	.0000	.0000	.0000	.0000	.0000
	44	.0000	.0000	.0000	.0000	.0000	.0000	.0000	.0000	.0000	.0000
	45	.0000	.0000	.0000	.0000	.0000	.0000	.0000	.0000	.0000	.0000

III.3 INDIVIDUAL TERMS, POISSON DISTRIBUTION

The Poisson probability function is given by

$$f(x;\lambda) = \frac{\lambda^x e^{-\lambda}}{x!}, \qquad \lambda > 0,\ x = 0, 1, 2, \ldots .$$

This table contains the individual terms of $f(x;\lambda)$ for specified values of x and λ.

INDIVIDUAL TERMS, POISSON DISTRIBUTION

	λ									
x	0.1	0.2	0.3	0.4	0.5	0.6	0.7	0.8	0.9	1.0
0	.9048	.8187	.7408	.6703	.6065	.5488	.4966	.4493	.4066	.3679
1	.0905	.1637	.2222	.2681	.3033	.3293	.3476	.3595	.3659	.3679
2	.0045	.0164	.0333	.0536	.0758	.0988	.1217	.1438	.1647	.1839
3	.0002	.0011	.0033	.0072	.0126	.0198	.0284	.0383	.0494	.0613
4	.0000	.0001	.0003	.0007	.0016	.0030	.0050	.0077	.0111	.0153
5	.0000	.0000	.0000	.0001	.0002	.0004	.0007	.0012	.0020	.0031
6	.0000	.0000	.0000	.0000	.0000	.0000	.0001	.0002	.0003	.0005
7	.0000	.0000	.0000	.0000	.0000	.0000	.0000	.0000	.0000	.0001

	λ									
x	1.1	1.2	1.3	1.4	1.5	1.6	1.7	1.8	1.9	2.0
0	.3329	.3012	.2725	.2466	.2231	.2019	.1827	.1653	.1496	.1353
1	.3662	.3614	.3543	.3452	.3347	.3230	.3106	.2975	.2842	.2707
2	.2014	.2169	.2303	.2417	.2510	.2584	.2640	.2678	.2700	.2707
3	.0738	.0867	.0998	.1128	.1255	.1378	.1496	.1607	.1710	.1804
4	.0203	.0260	.0324	.0395	.0471	.0551	.0636	.0723	.0812	.0902
5	.0045	.0062	.0084	.0111	.0141	.0176	.0216	.0260	.0309	.0361
6	.0008	.0012	.0018	.0026	.0035	.0047	.0061	.0078	.0098	.0120
7	.0001	.0002	.0003	.0005	.0008	.0011	.0015	.0020	.0027	.0034
8	.0000	.0000	.0001	.0001	.0001	.0002	.0003	.0005	.0006	.0009
9	.0000	.0000	.0000	.0000	.0000	.0000	.0001	.0001	.0001	.0002

	λ									
x	2.1	2.2	2.3	2.4	2.5	2.6	2.7	2.8	2.9	3.0
0	.1225	.1108	.1003	.0907	.0821	.0743	.0672	.0608	.0550	.0498
1	.2572	.2438	.2306	.2177	.2052	.1931	.1815	.1703	.1596	.1494
2	.2700	.2681	.2652	.2613	.2565	.2510	.2450	.2384	.2314	.2240
3	.1890	.1966	.2033	.2090	.2138	.2176	.2205	.2225	.2237	.2240
4	.0992	.1082	.1169	.1254	.1336	.1414	.1488	.1557	.1622	.1680
5	.0417	.0476	.0538	.0602	.0668	.0735	.0804	.0872	.0940	.1008
6	.0146	.0174	.0206	.0241	.0278	.0319	.0362	.0407	.0455	.0504
7	.0044	.0055	.0068	.0083	.0099	.0118	.0139	.0163	.0188	.0216
8	.0011	.0015	.0019	.0025	.0031	.0038	.0047	.0057	.0068	.0081
9	.0003	.0004	.0005	.0007	.0009	.0011	.0014	.0018	.0022	.0027
10	.0001	.0001	.0001	.0002	.0002	.0003	.0004	.0005	.0006	.0008
11	.0000	.0000	.0000	.0000	.0000	.0001	.0001	.0001	.0002	.0002
12	.0000	.0000	.0000	.0000	.0000	.0000	.0000	.0000	.0000	.0001

	λ									
x	3.1	3.2	3.3	3.4	3.5	3.6	3.7	3.8	3.9	4.0
0	.0450	.0408	.0369	.0334	.0302	.0273	.0247	.0224	.0202	.0183
1	.1397	.1304	.1217	.1135	.1057	.0984	.0915	.0850	.0789	.0733
2	.2165	.2087	.2008	.1929	.1850	.1771	.1692	.1615	.1539	.1465
3	.2237	.2226	.2209	.2186	.2158	.2125	.2087	.2046	.2001	.1954
4	.1734	.1781	.1823	.1858	.1888	.1912	.1931	.1944	.1951	.1954
5	.1075	.1140	.1203	.1264	.1322	.1377	.1429	.1477	.1522	.1563
6	.0555	.0608	.0662	.0716	.0771	.0826	.0881	.0936	.0989	.1042
7	.0246	.0278	.0312	.0348	.0385	.0425	.0466	.0508	.0551	.0595
8	.0095	.0111	.0129	.0148	.0169	.0191	.0215	.0241	.0269	.0298
9	.0033	.0040	.0047	.0056	.0066	.0076	.0089	.0102	.0116	.0132

INDIVIDUAL TERMS, POISSON DISTRIBUTION

x	λ = 3.1	3.2	3.3	3.4	3.5	3.6	3.7	3.8	3.9	4.0
10	.0010	.0013	.0016	.0019	.0023	.0028	.0033	.0039	.0045	.0053
11	.0003	.0004	.0005	.0006	.0007	.0009	.0011	.0013	.0016	.0019
12	.0001	.0001	.0001	.0002	.0002	.0003	.0003	.0004	.0005	.0006
13	.0000	.0000	.0000	.0000	.0001	.0001	.0001	.0001	.0002	.0002
14	.0000	.0000	.0000	.0000	.0000	.0000	.0000	.0000	.0000	.0001

x	λ = 4.1	4.2	4.3	4.4	4.5	4.6	4.7	4.8	4.9	5.0
0	.0166	.0150	.0136	.0123	.0111	.0101	.0091	.0082	.0074	.0067
1	.0679	.0630	.0583	.0540	.0500	.0462	.0427	.0395	.0365	.0337
2	.1393	.1323	.1254	.1188	.1125	.1063	.1005	.0948	.0894	.0842
3	.1904	.1852	.1798	.1743	.1687	.1631	.1574	.1517	.1460	.1404
4	.1951	.1944	.1933	.1917	.1898	.1875	.1849	.1820	.1789	.1755
5	.1600	.1633	.1662	.1687	.1708	.1725	.1738	.1747	.1753	.1755
6	.1093	.1143	.1191	.1237	.1281	.1323	.1362	.1398	.1432	.1462
7	.0640	.0686	.0732	.0778	.0824	.0869	.0914	.0959	.1002	.1044
8	.0328	.0360	.0393	.0428	.0463	.0500	.0537	.0575	.0614	.0653
9	.0150	.0168	.0188	.0209	.0232	.0255	.0280	.0307	.0334	.0363
10	.0061	.0071	.0081	.0092	.0104	.0118	.0132	.0147	.0164	.0181
11	.0023	.0027	.0032	.0037	.0043	.0049	.0056	.0064	.0073	.0082
12	.0008	.0009	.0011	.0014	.0016	.0019	.0022	.0026	.0030	.0034
13	.0002	.0003	.0004	.0005	.0006	.0007	.0008	.0009	.0011	.0013
14	.0001	.0001	.0001	.0001	.0002	.0002	.0003	.0003	.0004	.0005
15	.0000	.0000	.0000	.0000	.0001	.0001	.0001	.0001	.0001	.0002

x	λ = 5.1	5.2	5.3	5.4	5.5	5.6	5.7	5.8	5.9	6.0
0	.0061	.0055	.0050	.0045	.0041	.0037	.0033	.0030	.0027	.0025
1	.0311	.0287	.0265	.0244	.0225	.0207	.0191	.0176	.0162	.0149
2	.0793	.0746	.0701	.0659	.0618	.0580	.0544	.0509	.0477	.0446
3	.1348	.1293	.1239	.1185	.1133	.1082	.1033	.0985	.0938	.0892
4	.1719	.1681	.1641	.1600	.1558	.1515	.1472	.1428	.1383	.1339
5	.1753	.1748	.1740	.1728	.1714	.1697	.1678	.1656	.1632	.1606
6	.1490	.1515	.1537	.1555	.1571	.1584	.1594	.1601	.1605	.1606
7	.1086	.1125	.1163	.1200	.1234	.1267	.1298	.1326	.1353	.1377
8	.0692	.0731	.0771	.0810	.0849	.0887	.0925	.0962	.0998	.1033
9	.0392	.0423	.0454	.0486	.0519	.0552	.0586	.0620	.0654	.0688
10	.0200	.0220	.0241	.0262	.0285	.0309	.0334	.0359	.0386	.0413
11	.0093	.0104	.0116	.0129	.0143	.0157	.0173	.0190	.0207	.0225
12	.0039	.0045	.0051	.0058	.0065	.0073	.0082	.0092	.0102	.0113
13	.0015	.0018	.0021	.0024	.0028	.0032	.0036	.0041	.0046	.0052
14	.0006	.0007	.0008	.0009	.0011	.0013	.0015	.0017	.0019	.0022
15	.0002	.0002	.0003	.0003	.0004	.0005	.0006	.0007	.0008	.0009
16	.0001	.0001	.0001	.0001	.0001	.0002	.0002	.0002	.0003	.0003
17	.0000	.0000	.0000	.0000	.0000	.0000	.0001	.0001	.0001	.0001

INDIVIDUAL TERMS, POISSON DISTRIBUTION

	λ									
x	6.1	6.2	6.3	6.4	6.5	6.6	6.7	6.8	6.9	7.0
0	.0022	.0020	.0018	.0017	.0015	.0014	.0012	.0011	.0010	.0009
1	.0137	.0126	.0116	.0106	.0098	.0090	.0082	.0076	.0070	.0064
2	.0417	.0390	.0364	.0340	.0318	.0296	.0276	.0258	.0240	.0223
3	.0848	.0806	.0765	.0726	.0688	.0652	.0617	.0584	.0552	.0521
4	.1294	.1249	.1205	.1162	.1118	.1076	.1034	.0992	.0952	.0912
5	.1579	.1549	.1519	.1487	.1454	.1420	.1385	.1349	.1314	.1277
6	.1605	.1601	.1595	.1586	.1575	.1562	.1546	.1529	.1511	.1490
7	.1399	.1418	.1435	.1450	.1462	.1472	.1480	.1486	.1489	.1490
8	.1066	.1099	.1130	.1160	.1188	.1215	.1240	.1263	.1284	.1304
9	.0723	.0757	.0791	.0825	.0858	.0891	.0923	.0954	.0985	.1014
10	.0441	.0469	.0498	.0528	.0558	.0588	.0618	.0649	.0679	.0710
11	.0245	.0265	.0285	.0307	.0330	.0353	.0377	.0401	.0426	.0452
12	.0124	.0137	.0150	.0164	.0179	.0194	.0210	.0227	.0245	.0264
13	.0058	.0065	.0073	.0081	.0089	.0098	.0108	.0119	.0130	.0142
14	.0025	.0029	.0033	.0037	.0041	.0046	.0052	.0058	.0064	.0071
15	.0010	.0012	.0014	.0016	.0018	.0020	.0023	.0026	.0029	.0033
16	.0004	.0005	.0005	.0006	.0007	.0008	.0010	.0011	.0013	.0014
17	.0001	.0002	.0002	.0002	.0003	.0003	.0004	.0004	.0005	.0006
18	.0000	.0001	.0001	.0001	.0001	.0001	.0001	.0002	.0002	.0002
19	.0000	.0000	.0000	.0000	.0000	.0000	.0000	.0001	.0001	.0001

	λ									
x	7.1	7.2	7.3	7.4	7.5	7.6	7.7	7.8	7.9	8.0
0	.0008	.0007	.0007	.0006	.0006	.0005	.0005	.0004	.0004	.0003
1	.0059	.0054	.0049	.0045	.0041	.0038	.0035	.0032	.0029	.0027
2	.0208	.0194	.0180	.0167	.0156	.0145	.0134	.0125	.0116	.0107
3	.0492	.0464	.0438	.0413	.0389	.0366	.0345	.0324	.0305	.0286
4	.0874	.0836	.0799	.0764	.0729	.0696	.0663	.0632	.0602	.0573
5	.1241	.1204	.1167	.1130	.1094	.1057	.1021	.0986	.0951	.0916
6	.1468	.1445	.1420	.1394	.1367	.1339	.1311	.1282	.1252	.1221
7	.1489	.1486	.1481	.1474	.1465	.1454	.1442	.1428	.1413	.1396
8	.1321	.1337	.1351	.1363	.1373	.1382	.1388	.1392	.1395	.1396
9	.1042	.1070	.1096	.1121	.1144	.1167	.1187	.1207	.1224	.1241
10	.0740	.0770	.0800	.0829	.0858	.0887	.0914	.0941	.0967	.0993
11	.0478	.0504	.0531	.0558	.0585	.0613	.0640	.0667	.0695	.0722
12	.0283	.0303	.0323	.0344	.0366	.0388	.0411	.0434	.0457	.0481
13	.0154	.0168	.0181	.0196	.0211	.0227	.0243	.0260	.0278	.0296
14	.0078	.0086	.0095	.0104	.0113	.0123	.0134	.0145	.0157	.0169
15	.0037	.0041	.0046	.0051	.0057	0062	.0069	.0075	.0083	.0090
16	.0016	.0019	.0021	.0024	.0026	.0030	.0033	.0037	.0041	.0045
17	.0007	.0008	.0009	.0010	.0012	.0013	.0015	.0017	.0019	.0021
18	.0003	.0003	.0004	.0004	.0005	.0006	.0006	.0007	.0008	.0009
19	.0001	.0001	.0001	.0002	.0002	.0002	.0003	.0003	.0003	.0004
20	.0000	.0000	.0001	.0001	.0001	.0001	.0001	.0001	.0001	.0002
21	.0000	.0000	.0000	.0000	.0000	.0000	.0000	.0000	.0001	.0001

INDIVIDUAL TERMS, POISSON DISTRIBUTION

	λ									
x	8.1	8.2	8.3	8.4	8.5	8.6	8.7	8.8	8.9	9.0
0	.0003	.0003	.0002	.0002	.0002	.0002	.0002	.0002	.0001	.0001
1	.0025	.0023	.0021	.0019	.0017	.0016	.0014	.0013	.0012	.0011
2	.0100	.0092	.0086	.0079	.0074	.0068	.0063	.0058	.0054	.0050
3	.0269	.0252	.0237	.0222	.0208	.0195	.0183	.0171	.0160	.0150
4	.0544	.0517	.0491	.0466	.0443	.0420	.0398	.0377	.0357	.0337
5	.0882	.0849	.0816	.0784	.0752	.0722	.0692	.0663	.0635	.0607
6	.1191	.1160	.1128	.1097	.1066	.1034	.1003	.0972	.0941	.0911
7	.1378	.1358	.1338	.1317	.1294	.1271	.1247	.1222	.1197	.1171
8	.1395	.1392	.1388	.1382	.1375	.1366	.1356	.1344	.1332	.1318
9	.1256	.1269	.1280	.1290	.1299	.1306	.1311	.1315	.1317	.1318
10	.1017	.1040	.1063	.1084	.1104	.1123	.1140	.1157	.1172	.1186
11	.0749	.0776	.0802	.0828	.0853	.0878	.0902	.0925	.0948	.0970
12	.0505	.0530	.0555	.0579	.0604	.0629	.0654	.0679	.0703	.0728
13	.0315	.0334	.0354	.0374	.0395	.0416	.0438	.0459	.0481	.0504
14	.0182	.0196	.0210	.0225	.0240	.0256	.0272	.0289	.0306	.0324
15	.0098	.0107	.0116	.0126	.0136	.0147	.0158	.0169	.0182	.0194
16	.0050	.0055	.0060	.0066	.0072	.0079	.0086	.0093	.0101	.0109
17	.0024	.0026	.0029	.0033	.0036	.0040	.0044	.0048	.0053	.0058
18	.0011	.0012	.0014	.0015	.0017	.0019	.0021	.0024	.0026	.0029
19	.0005	.0005	.0006	.0007	.0008	.0009	.0010	.0011	.0012	.0014
20	.0002	.0002	.0002	.0003	.0003	.0004	.0004	.0005	.0005	.0006
21	.0001	.0001	.0001	.0001	.0001	.0002	.0002	.0002	.0002	.0003
22	.0000	.0000	.0000	.0000	.0001	.0001	.0001	.0001	.0001	.0001

	λ									
x	9.1	9.2	9.3	9.4	9.5	9.6	9.7	9.8	9.9	10
0	.0001	.0001	.0001	.0001	.0001	.0001	.0001	.0001	.0001	.0000
1	.0010	.0009	.0009	.0008	.0007	.0007	.0006	.0005	.0005	.0005
2	.0046	.0043	.0040	.0037	.0034	.0031	.0029	.0027	.0025	.0023
3	.0140	.0131	.0123	.0115	.0107	.0100	.0093	.0087	.0081	.0076
4	.0319	.0302	.0285	.0269	.0254	.0240	.0226	.0213	.0201	.0189
5	.0581	.0555	.0530	.0506	.0483	.0460	.0439	.0418	.0398	.0378
6	.0881	.0851	.0822	.0793	.0764	.0736	.0709	.0682	.0656	.0631
7	.1145	.1118	.1091	.1064	.1037	.1010	.0982	.0955	.0928	.0901
8	.1302	.1286	.1269	.1251	.1232	.1212	.1191	.1170	.1148	.1126
9	.1317	.1315	.1311	.1306	.1300	.1293	.1284	.1274	.1263	.1251
10	.1198	.1210	.1219	.1228	.1235	.1241	.1245	.1249	.1250	.1251
11	.0991	.1012	.1031	.1049	.1067	.1083	.1098	.1112	.1125	.1137
12	.0752	.0776	.0799	.0822	.0844	.0866	.0888	.0908	.0928	.0948
13	.0526	.0549	.0572	.0594	.0617	.0640	.0662	.0685	.0707	.0729
14	.0342	.0361	.0380	.0399	.0419	.0439	.0459	.0479	.0500	.0521
15	.0208	.0221	.0235	.0250	.0265	.0281	.0297	.0313	.0330	.0347
16	.0118	.0127	.0137	.0147	.0157	.0168	.0180	.0192	.0204	.0217
17	.0063	.0069	.0075	.0081	.0088	.0095	.0103	.0111	.0119	.0128
18	.0032	.0035	.0039	.0042	.0046	.0051	.0055	.0060	.0065	.0071
19	.0015	.0017	.0019	.0021	.0023	.0026	.0028	.0031	.0034	.0037

INDIVIDUAL TERMS, POISSON DISTRIBUTION

	λ									
x	9.1	9.2	9.3	9.4	9.5	9.6	9.7	9.8	9.9	10
20	.0007	.0008	.0009	.0010	.0011	.0012	.0014	.0015	.0017	.0019
21	.0003	.0003	.0004	0004	.0005	.0006	.0006	.0007	.0008	.0009
22	.0001	.0001	.0002	.0002	.0002	.0002	.0003	.0003	.0004	.0004
23	.0000	.0001	.0001	.0001	.0001	.0001	.0001	.0001	.0002	.0002
24	.0000	.0000	.0000	.0000	.0000	.0000	.0000	.0001	.0001	.0001

	λ									
x	11	12	13	14	15	16	17	18	19	20
0	.0000	.0000	.0000	.0000	.0000	.0000	.0000	.0000	.0000	.0000
1	.0002	.0001	.0000	.0000	.0000	.0000	.0000	.0000	.0000	.0000
2	.0010	.0004	.0002	.0001	.0000	.0000	.0000	.0000	.0000	.0000
3	.0037	.0018	.0008	.0004	.0002	.0001	.0000	.0000	.0000	.0000
4	.0102	.0053	.0027	.0013	.0006	.0003	.0001	.0001	.0000	.0000
5	.0224	.0127	.0070	.0037	.0019	.0010	.0005	.0002	.0001	.0001
6	.0411	.0255	.0152	.0087	.0048	.0026	.0014	.0007	.0004	.0002
7	.0646	.0437	.0281	.0174	.0104	.0060	.0034	.0018	.0010	.0005
8	.0888	.0655	.0457	.0304	.0194	.0120	.0072	.0042	.0024	.0013
9	.1085	.0874	.0661	.0473	.0324	.0213	.0135	.0083	.0050	.0029
10	.1194	.1048	.0859	.0663	.0486	.0341	.0230	.0150	.0095	.0058
11	.1194	.1144	.1015	.0844	.0663	.0496	.0355	.0245	.0164	.0106
12	.1094	.1144	.1099	.0984	.0829	.0661	.0504	.0368	.0259	.0176
13	.0926	.1056	.1099	.1060	.0956	.0814	.0658	.0509	.0378	.0271
14	.0728	.0905	.1021	.1060	.1024	.0930	.0800	.0655	.0514	.0387
15	.0534	.0724	.0885	.0989	.1024	.0992	.0906	.0786	.0650	.0516
16	.0367	.0543	.0719	.0866	.0960	.0992	.0963	.0884	.0772	.0646
17	.0237	.0383	.0550	.0713	.0847	.0934	.0963	.0936	.0863	.0760
18	.0145	.0256	.0397	.0554	.0706	.0830	.0909	.0936	.0911	.0844
19	.0084	.0161	.0272	.0409	.0557	.0699	.0814	.0887	.0911	.0888
20	.0046	.0097	.0177	.0286	.0418	.0559	.0692	.0798	.0866	.0888
21	.0024	.0055	.0109	.0191	.0299	.0426	.0560	.0684	.0783	.0846
22	.0012	.0030	.0065	.0121	.0204	.0310	.0433	.0560	.0676	.0769
23	.0006	.0016	.0037	.0074	.0133	.0216	.0320	.0438	.0559	.0669
24	.0003	.0008	.0020	.0043	.0083	.0144	.0226	.0328	.0442	.0557
25	.0001	.0004	.0010	.0024	.0050	.0092	.0154	.0237	.0336	.0446
26	.0000	.0002	.0005	.0013	.0029	.0057	.0101	.0164	.0246	.0343
27	.0000	.0001	.0002	.0007	.0016	.0034	.0063	.0109	.0173	.0254
28	.0000	.0000	.0001	.0003	.0009	.0019	.0038	.0070	.0117	.0181
29	.0000	.0000	.0001	.0002	.0004	.0011	.0023	.0044	.0077	.0125
30	.0000	.0000	.0000	.0001	.0002	.0006	.0013	.0026	.0049	.0083
31	.0000	.0000	.0000	.0000	.0001	.0003	.0007	.0015	.0030	.0054
32	.0000	.0000	.0000	.0000	.0001	.0001	.0004	.0009	.0018	.0034
33	.0000	.0000	.0000	.0000	.0000	.0001	.0002	.0005	.0010	.0020
34	.0000	.0000	.0000	.0000	.0000	.0000	.0001	.0002	.0006	.0012
35	.0000	.0000	.0000	.0000	.0000	.0000	.0000	.0001	.0003	.0007
36	.0000	.0000	.0000	.0000	.0000	.0000	.0000	.0001	.0002	.0004
37	.0000	.0000	.0000	.0000	.0000	.0000	.0000	.0000	.0001	.0002
38	.0000	.0000	.0000	.0000	.0000	.0000	.0000	.0000	.0000	.0001
39	.0000	.0000	.0000	.0000	.0000	.0000	.0000	.0000	.0000	.0001

III.4 CUMULATIVE TERMS, POISSON DISTRIBUTION

This table contains the values of

$$\sum_{x=x'}^{\infty} \frac{e^{-\lambda}\lambda^x}{x!}$$

for specified values of x' and λ. The cumulative Poisson distribution and the cumulative chi-square (χ^2) distribution are related as follows:

$$\sum_{x=0}^{x'-1} \frac{e^{-\lambda}\lambda^x}{x!} = 1 - F(\chi^2)$$

$$= \frac{1}{2^{\frac{n}{2}}\Gamma\left(\frac{n}{2}\right)} \int_{\chi^2}^{\infty} x^{\frac{n}{2}-1} e^{-\frac{x}{2}}\, dx$$

where $\lambda = \frac{1}{2}\chi^2$ and $x' = \frac{1}{2}n$.

CUMULATIVE TERMS, POISSON DISTRIBUTION

	λ									
x'	0.1	0.2	0.3	0.4	0.5	0.6	0.7	0.8	0.9	1.0
0	1.0000	1.0000	1.0000	1.0000	1.0000	1.0000	1.0000	1.0000	1.0000	1.0000
1	.0952	.1813	.2592	.3297	.3935	.4512	.5034	.5507	.5934	.6321
2	.0047	.0175	.0369	.0616	.0902	.1219	.1558	.1912	.2275	.2642
3	.0002	.0011	.0036	.0079	.0144	.0231	.0341	.0474	.0629	.0803
4	.0000	.0001	.0003	.0008	.0018	.0034	.0058	.0091	.0135	.0190
5	.0000	.0000	.0000	.0001	.0002	.0004	.0008	.0014	.0023	.0037
6	.0000	.0000	.0000	.0000	.0000	.0000	.0001	.0002	.0003	.0006
7	.0000	.0000	.0000	.0000	.0000	.0000	.0000	.0000	.0000	.0001

	λ									
x'	1.1	1.2	1.3	1.4	1.5	1.6	1.7	1.8	1.9	2.0
0	1.0000	1.0000	1.0000	1.0000	1.0000	1.0000	1.0000	1.0000	1.0000	1.0000
1	.6671	.6988	.7275	.7534	.7769	.7981	.8173	.8347	.8504	.8647
2	.3010	.3374	.3732	.4082	.4422	.4751	.5068	.5372	.5663	.5940
3	.0996	.1205	.1429	.1665	.1912	.2166	.2428	.2694	.2963	.3233
4	.0257	.0338	.0431	.0537	.0656	.0788	.0932	.1087	.1253	.1429
5	.0054	.0077	.0107	.0143	.0186	.0237	.0296	.0364	.0441	.0527
6	.0010	.0015	.0022	.0032	.0045	.0060	.0080	.0104	.0132	.0166
7	.0001	.0003	.0004	.0006	.0009	.0013	.0019	.0026	.0034	.0045
8	.0000	.0000	.0001	.0001	.0002	.0003	.0004	.0006	.0008	.0011
9	.0000	.0000	.0000	.0000	.0000	.0000	.0001	.0001	.0002	.0002

	λ									
x'	2.1	2.2	2.3	2.4	2.5	2.6	2.7	2.8	2.9	3.0
0	1.0000	1.0000	1.0000	1.0000	1.0000	1.0000	1.0000	1.0000	1.0000	1.0000
1	.8775	.8892	.8997	.9093	.9179	.9257	.9328	.9392	.9450	.9502
2	.6204	.6454	.6691	.6916	.7127	.7326	.7513	.7689	.7854	.8009
3	.3504	.3773	.4040	.4303	.4562	.4816	.5064	.5305	.5540	.5768
4	.1614	.1806	.2007	.2213	.2424	.2640	.2859	.3081	.3304	.3528
5	.0621	.0725	.0838	.0959	.1088	.1226	.1371	.1523	.1682	.1847
6	.0204	.0249	.0300	.0357	.0420	.0490	.0567	.0651	.0742	.0839
7	.0059	.0075	.0094	.0116	.0142	.0172	.0206	.0244	.0287	.0335
8	.0015	.0020	.0026	.0033	.0042	.0053	.0066	.0081	.0099	.0119
9	.0003	.0005	.0006	.0009	.0011	.0015	.0019	.0024	.0031	.0038
10	.0001	.0001	.0001	.0002	.0003	.0004	.0005	.0007	.0009	.0011
11	.0000	.0000	.0000	.0000	.0001	.0001	.0001	.0002	.0002	.0003
12	.0000	.0000	.0000	.0000	.0000	.0000	.0000	.0000	.0001	.0001

	λ									
x'	3.1	3.2	3.3	3.4	3.5	3.6	3.7	3.8	3.9	4.0
0	1.0000	1.0000	1.0000	1.0000	1.0000	1.0000	1.0000	1.0000	1.0000	1.0000
1	.9550	.9592	.9631	.9666	.9698	.9727	.9753	.9776	.9798	.9817
2	.8153	.8288	.8414	.8532	.8641	.8743	.8838	.8926	.9008	.9084
3	.5988	.6201	.6406	.6603	.6792	.6973	.7146	.7311	.7469	.7619
4	.3752	.3975	.4197	.4416	.4634	.4848	.5058	.5265	.5468	.5665

CUMULATIVE TERMS, POISSON DISTRIBUTION

λ

x'	3.1	3.2	3.3	3.4	3.5	3.6	3.7	3.8	3.9	4.0
5	.2018	.2194	.2374	.2558	.2746	.2936	.3128	.3322	.3516	.3712
6	.0943	.1054	.1171	.1295	.1424	.1559	.1699	.1844	.1994	.2149
7	.0388	.0446	.0510	.0579	.0653	.0733	.0818	.0909	.1005	.1107
8	.0142	.0168	.0198	.0231	.0267	.0308	.0352	.0401	.0454	.0511
9	.0047	.0057	.0069	.0083	.0099	.0117	.0137	.0160	.0185	.0214
10	.0014	.0018	.0022	.0027	.0033	.0040	.0048	.0058	.0069	.0081
11	.0004	.0005	.0006	.0008	.0010	.0013	.0016	.0019	.0023	.0028
12	.0001	.0001	.0002	.0002	.0003	.0004	.0005	.0006	.0007	.0009
13	.0000	.0000	.0000	.0001	.0001	.0001	.0001	.0002	.0002	.0003
14	.0000	.0000	.0000	.0000	.0000	.0000	.0000	.0000	.0001	.0001

λ

x'	4.1	4.2	4.3	4.4	4.5	4.6	4.7	4.8	4.9	5.0
0	1.0000	1.0000	1.0000	1.0000	1.0000	1.0000	1.0000	1.0000	1.0000	1.0000
1	.9834	.9850	.9864	.9877	.9889	.9899	.9909	.9918	.9926	.9933
2	.9155	.9220	.9281	.9337	.9389	.9437	.9482	.9523	.9561	.9596
3	.7762	.7898	.8026	.8149	.8264	.8374	.8477	.8575	.8667	.8753
4	.5858	.6046	.6228	.6406	.6577	.6743	.6903	.7058	.7207	.7350
5	.3907	.4102	.4296	.4488	.4679	.4868	.5054	.5237	.5418	.5595
6	.2307	.2469	.2633	.2801	.2971	.3142	.3316	.3490	.3665	.3840
7	.1214	.1325	.1442	.1564	.1689	.1820	.1954	.2092	.2233	.2378
8	.0573	.0639	.0710	.0786	.0866	.0951	.1040	.1133	.1231	.1334
9	.0245	.0279	.0317	.0358	.0403	.0451	.0503	.0558	.0618	.0681
10	.0095	.0111	.0129	.0149	.0171	.0195	.0222	.0251	.0283	.0318
11	.0034	.0041	.0048	.0057	.0067	.0078	.0090	.0104	.0120	.0137
12	.0011	.0014	.0017	.0020	.0024	.0029	.0034	.0040	.0047	.0055
13	.0003	.0004	.0005	.0007	.0008	.0010	.0012	.0014	.0017	.0020
14	.0001	.0001	.0002	.0002	.0003	.0003	.0004	.0005	.0006	.0007
15	.0000	.0000	.0000	.0001	.0001	.0001	.0001	.0001	.0002	.0002
16	.0000	.0000	.0000	.0000	.0000	.0000	.0000	.0000	.0001	.0001

λ

x'	5.1	5.2	5.3	5.4	5.5	5.6	5.7	5.8	5.9	6.0
0	1.0000	1.0000	1.0000	1.0000	1.0000	1.0000	1.0000	1.0000	1.0000	1.0000
1	.9939	.9945	.9950	.9955	.9959	.9963	.9967	.9970	.9973	.9975
2	.9628	.9658	.9686	.9711	.9734	.9756	.9776	.9794	.9811	.9826
3	.8835	.8912	.8984	.9052	.9116	.9176	.9232	.9285	.9334	.9380
4	.7487	.7619	.7746	.7867	.7983	.8094	.8200	.8300	.8396	.8488
5	.5769	.5939	.6105	.6267	.6425	.6579	.6728	.6873	.7013	.7149
6	.4016	.4191	.4365	.4539	.4711	.4881	.5050	.5217	.5381	.5543
7	.2526	.2676	.2829	.2983	.3140	.3297	.3456	.3616	.3776	.3937
8	.1440	.1551	.1665	.1783	.1905	.2030	.2159	.2290	.2424	.2560
9	.0748	.0819	.0894	.0974	.1056	.1143	.1234	.1328	.1426	.1528

CUMULATIVE TERMS, POISSON DISTRIBUTION

x \ λ	5.1	5.2	5.3	5.4	5.5	5.6	5.7	5.8	5.9	6.0
10	.0356	.0397	.0441	.0488	.0538	.0591	.0648	.0708	.0772	.0839
11	.0156	.0177	.0200	.0225	.0253	.0282	.0314	.0349	.0386	.0426
12	.0063	.0073	.0084	.0096	.0110	.0125	.0141	.0160	.0179	.0201
13	.0024	.0028	.0033	.0038	.0045	.0051	.0059	.0068	.0078	.0088
14	.0008	.0010	.0012	.0014	.0017	.0020	.0023	.0027	.0031	.0036
15	.0003	.0003	.0004	.0005	.0006	.0007	.0009	.0010	.0012	.0014
16	.0001	.0001	.0001	.0002	.0002	.0002	.0003	.0004	.0004	.0005
17	.0000	.0000	.0000	.0001	.0001	.0001	.0001	.0001	.0001	.0002
18	.0000	.0000	.0000	.0000	.0000	.0000	.0000	.0000	.0000	.0001

x' \ λ	6.1	6.2	6.3	6.4	6.5	6.6	6.7	6.8	6.9	7.0
0	1.0000	1.0000	1.0000	1.0000	1.0000	1.0000	1.0000	1.0000	1.0000	1.0000
1	.9978	.9980	.9982	.9983	.9985	.9986	.9988	.9989	.9990	.9991
2	.9841	.9854	.9866	.9877	.9887	.9897	.9905	.9913	.9920	.9927
3	.9423	.9464	.9502	.9537	.9570	.9600	.9629	.9656	.9680	.9704
4	.8575	.8658	.8736	.8811	.8882	.8948	.9012	.9072	.9129	.9182
5	.7281	.7408	.7531	.7649	.7763	.7873	.7978	.8080	.8177	.8270
6	.5702	.5859	.6012	.6163	.6310	.6453	.6594	.6730	.6863	.6993
7	.4098	.4258	.4418	.4577	.4735	.4892	.5047	.5201	.5353	.5503
8	.2699	.2840	.2983	.3127	.3272	.3419	.3567	.3715	.3864	.4013
9	.1633	.1741	.1852	.1967	.2084	.2204	.2327	.2452	.2580	.2709
10	.0910	.0984	.1061	.1142	.1226	.1314	.1404	.1498	.1505	.1695
11	.0469	.0514	.0563	.0614	.0668	.0726	.0786	.0849	.0916	.0985
12	.0224	.0250	.0277	.0307	.0339	.0373	.0409	.0448	.0490	.0534
13	.0100	.0113	.0127	.0143	.0160	.0179	.0199	.0221	.0245	.0270
14	.0042	.0048	.0055	.0063	.0071	.0080	.0091	.0102	.0115	.0128
15	.0016	.0019	.0022	.0026	.0030	.0034	.0039	.0044	.0050	.0057
16	.0006	.0007	.0008	.0010	.0012	.0014	.0016	.0018	.0021	.0024
17	.0002	.0003	.0003	.0004	.0004	.0005	.0006	.0007	.0008	.0010
18	.0001	.0001	.0001	.0001	.0002	.0002	.0002	.0003	.0003	.0004
19	.0000	.0000	.0000	.0000	.0001	.0001	.0001	.0001	.0001	.0001

x' \ λ	7.1	7.2	7.3	7.4	7.5	7.6	7.7	7.8	7.9	8.0
0	1.0000	1.0000	1.0000	1.0000	1.0000	1.0000	1.0000	1.0000	1.0000	1.0000
1	.9992	.9993	.9993	.9994	.9994	.9995	.9995	.9996	.9996	.9997
2	.9933	.9939	.9944	.9949	.9953	.9957	.9961	.9964	.9967	.9970
3	.9725	.9745	.9764	.0781	.9797	.9812	.9826	.9839	.9851	.9862
4	.9233	.9281	.9326	.9368	.9409	.9446	.9482	.9515	.9547	.9576
5	.8359	.8445	.8527	.8605	.8679	.8751	.8819	.8883	.8945	.9004
6	.7119	.7241	.7360	.7474	.7586	.7693	.7797	.7897	.7994	.8088
7	.5651	.5796	.5940	.6080	.6218	.6354	.6486	.6616	.6743	.6866
8	.4162	.4311	.4459	.4607	.4754	.4900	.5044	.5188	.5330	.5470
9	.2840	.2973	.3108	.3243	.3380	.3518	.3657	.3796	.3935	.4075
10	.1798	.1904	.2012	.2123	.2236	.2351	.2469	.2589	.2710	.2834
11	.1058	.1133	.1212	.1293	.1378	.1465	.1555	.1648	.1743	.1841
12	.0580	.0629	.0681	.0735	.0792	.0852	.0915	.0980	.1048	.1119
13	.0297	.0327	.0358	.0391	.0427	.0464	.0504	.0546	.0591	.0638
14	.0143	.0159	.0176	.0195	.0216	.0238	.0261	.0286	.0313	.0342

CUMULATIVE TERMS, POISSON DISTRIBUTION

x'	λ 7.1	7.2	7.3	7.4	7.5	7.6	7.7	7.8	7.9	8.0
15	.0065	.0073	.0082	.0092	.0103	.0114	.0127	.0141	.0156	.0173
16	.0028	.0031	.0036	.0041	.0046	.0052	.0059	.0066	.0074	.0082
17	.0011	.0013	.0015	.0017	.0020	.0022	.0026	.0029	.0033	.0037
18	.0004	.0005	.0006	.0007	.0008	.0009	.0011	.0012	.0014	.0016
19	.0002	.0002	.0002	.0003	.0003	.0004	.0004	.0005	.0006	.0006
20	.0001	.0001	.0001	.0001	.0001	.0001	.0002	.0002	.0002	.0003
21	.0000	.0000	.0000	.0000	.0000	.0000	.0001	.0001	.0001	.0001

x'	λ 8.1	8.2	8.3	8.4	8.5	8.6	8.7	8.8	8.9	9.0
0	1.0000	1.0000	1.0000	1.0000	1.0000	1.0000	1.0000	1.0000	1.0000	1.0000
1	.9997	.9997	.9998	.9998	.9998	.9998	.9998	.9998	.9999	.9999
2	.9972	.9975	.9977	.9979	.9981	.9982	.9984	.9985	.9987	.9988
3	.9873	.9882	.9891	.9900	.9907	.9914	.9921	.9927	.9932	.9938
4	.9604	.9630	.9654	.9677	.9699	.9719	.9738	.9756	.9772	.9788
5	.9060	.9113	.9163	.9211	.9256	.9299	.9340	.9379	.9416	.9450
6	.8178	.8264	.8347	.8427	.8504	.8578	.8648	.8716	.8781	.8843
7	.6987	.7104	.7219	.7330	.7438	.7543	.7645	.7744	.7840	.7932
8	.5609	.5746	.5881	.6013	.6144	.6272	.6398	.6522	.6643	.6761
9	.4214	.4353	.4493	.4631	.4769	.4906	.5042	.5177	.5311	.5443
10	.2959	.3085	.3212	.3341	.3470	.3600	.3731	.3863	.3994	.4126
11	.1942	.2045	.2150	.2257	.2366	.2478	.2591	.2706	.2822	.2940
12	.1193	.1269	.1348	.1429	.1513	.1600	.1689	.1780	.1874	.1970
13	.0687	.0739	.0793	.0850	.0909	.0971	.1035	.1102	.1171	.1242
14	.0372	.0405	.0439	.0476	.0514	.0555	.0597	.0642	.0689	.0739
15	.0190	.0209	.0229	.0251	.0274	.0299	.0325	.0353	.0383	.0415
16	.0092	.0102	.0113	.0125	.0138	.0152	.0168	.0184	.0202	.0220
17	.0042	.0047	.0053	.0059	.0066	.0074	.0082	.0091	.0101	.0111
18	.0018	.0021	.0023	.0027	.0030	.0034	.0038	.0043	.0048	.0053
19	.0008	.0009	.0010	.0011	.0013	.0015	.0017	.0019	.0022	.0024
20	.0003	.0003	.0004	.0005	.0005	.0006	.0007	.0008	.0009	.0011
21	.0001	.0001	.0002	.0002	.0002	.0002	.0003	.0003	.0004	.0004
22	.0000	.0000	.0001	.0001	.0001	.0001	.0001	.0001	.0002	.0002
23	.0000	.0000	.0000	.0000	.0000	.0000	0000	.0000	.0001	.0001

x'	λ 9.1	9.2	9.3	9.4	9.5	9.6	9.7	9.8	9.9	10
0	1.0000	1.0000	1.0000	1.0000	1.0000	1.0000	1.0000	1.0000	1.0000	1.0000
1	.9999	.9999	.9999	.9999	.9999	.9999	.9999	.9999	1.0000	1.0000
2	.9989	.9990	.9991	.9991	.9992	.9993	.9993	.9994	.9995	.9995
3	.9942	.9947	.9951	.9955	.9958	.9962	.9965	.9967	.9970	.9972
4	.9802	.9816	.9828	.9840	.9851	.9862	.9871	.9880	.9889	.9897
5	.9483	.9514	.9544	.9571	.9597	.9622	.9645	.9667	.9688	.9707
6	.8902	.8959	.9014	.9065	.9115	.9162	.9207	.9250	.9290	.9329
7	.8022	.8108	.8192	.8273	.8351	.8426	.8498	.8567	.8634	.8699
8	.6877	.6990	.7101	.7208	.7313	.7416	.7515	.7612	.7706	.7798
9	.5574	.5704	.5832	.5958	.6082	.6204	.6324	.6442	.6558	.6672

CUMULATIVE TERMS, POISSON DISTRIBUTION

x'	λ = 9.1	9.2	9.3	9.4	9.5	9.6	9.7	9.8	9.9	10
10	.4258	.4389	.4521	.4651	.4782	.4911	.5040	.5168	.5295	.5421
11	.3059	.3180	.3301	.3424	.3547	.3671	.3795	.3920	.4045	.4170
12	.2068	.2168	.2270	.2374	.2480	.2588	.2697	.2807	.2919	.3032
13	.1316	.1393	.1471	.1552	.1636	.1721	.1809	.1899	.1991	.2084
14	.0790	.0844	.0900	.0958	.1019	.1081	.1147	.1214	.1284	.1355
15	.0448	.0483	.0520	.0559	.0600	.0643	.0688	.0735	.0784	.0835
16	.0240	.0262	.0285	.0309	.0335	.0362	.0391	.0421	.0454	.0487
17	.0122	.0135	.0148	.0162	.0177	.0194	.0211	.0230	.0249	.0270
18	.0059	.0066	.0073	.0081	.0089	.0098	.0108	.0119	.0130	.0143
19	.0027	.0031	.0034	.0038	.0043	.0048	.0053	.0059	.0065	.0072
20	.0012	.0014	.0015	.0017	.0020	.0022	.0025	.0028	.0031	.0035
21	.0005	.0006	.0007	.0008	.0009	.0010	.0011	.0013	.0014	.0016
22	.0002	.0002	.0003	.0003	.0004	.0004	.0005	.0005	.0006	.0007
23	.0001	.0001	.0001	.0001	.0001	.0002	.0002	.0002	.0003	.0003
24	.0000	.0000	.0000	.0000	.0001	.0001	.0001	.0001	.0001	.0001

x'	λ = 11	12	13	14	15	16	17	18	19	20
0	1.0000	1.0000	1.0000	1.0000	1.0000	1.0000	1.0000	1.0000	1.0000	1.0000
1	1.0000	1.0000	1.0000	1.0000	1.0000	1.0000	1.0000	1.0000	1.0000	1.0000
2	.9998	.9999	1.0000	1.0000	1.0000	1.0000	1.0000	1.0000	1.0000	1.0000
3	.0088	.0005	.0008	.9999	1.0000	1.0000	1.0000	1.0000	1.0000	1.0000
4	.9951	.9977	.9990	.9995	.9998	.9999	1.0000	1.0000	1.0000	1.0000
5	.9849	.9924	.9963	.9982	.9991	.9996	.9998	.9999	1.0000	1.0000
6	.9625	.9797	.9893	.9945	.9972	.9986	.9993	.9997	.9998	.9999
7	.9214	.9542	.9741	.9858	.9924	.9960	.9979	.9990	.9995	.9997
8	.8568	.9105	.9460	.9684	.9820	.9900	.9946	.9971	.9985	.9992
9	.7680	.8450	.9002	.9379	.9626	.9780	.9874	.9929	.9961	.9979
10	.6595	.7576	.8342	.8906	.9301	.9567	.9739	.9846	.9911	.9950
11	.5401	.6528	.7483	.8243	.8815	.9226	.9509	.9696	.9817	.9892
12	.4207	.5384	.6468	.7400	.8152	.8730	.9153	.9451	.9653	.9786
13	.3113	.4240	.5369	.6415	.7324	.8069	.8650	.9083	.9394	.9610
14	.2187	.3185	.4270	.5356	.6368	.7255	.7991	.8574	.9016	.9339
15	.1460	.2280	.3249	.4296	.5343	.6325	.7192	.7919	.8503	.8951
16	.0926	.1556	.2364	.3306	.4319	.5333	.6285	.7133	.7852	.8435
17	.0559	.1013	.1645	.2441	.3359	.4340	.5323	.6250	.7080	.7789
18	.0322	.0630	.1095	.1728	.2511	.3407	.4360	.5314	.6216	.7030
19	.0177	.0374	.0698	.1174	.1805	.2577	.3450	.4378	.5305	.6186
20	.0093	.0213	.0427	.0765	.1248	.1878	.2637	.3491	.4394	.5297
21	.0047	.0116	.0250	.0479	.0830	.1318	.1945	.2693	.3528	.4409
22	.0023	.0061	.0141	.0288	.0531	.0892	.1385	.2009	.2745	.3563
23	.0010	.0030	.0076	.0167	.0327	.0582	.0953	.1449	.2069	.2794
24	.0005	.0015	.0040	.0093	.0195	.0367	.0633	.1011	.1510	.2125
25	.0002	.0007	.0020	.0050	.0112	.0223	.0406	.0683	.1067	.1568
26	.0001	.0003	.0010	.0026	.0062	.0131	.0252	.0446	.0731	.1122
27	.0000	.0001	.0005	.0013	.0033	.0075	.0152	.0282	.0486	.0779
28	.0000	.0001	.0002	.0006	.0017	.0041	.0088	.0173	.0313	.0525
29	.0000	.0000	.0001	.0003	.0009	.0022	.0050	.0103	.0195	.0343

CUMULATIVE TERMS, POISSON DISTRIBUTION

	λ									
x′	**11**	**12**	**13**	**14**	**15**	**16**	**17**	**18**	**19**	**20**
30	.0000	.0000	.0000	.0001	.0004	.0011	.0027	.0059	.0118	.0218
31	.0000	.0000	.0000	.0001	.0002	.0006	.0014	.0033	.0070	.0135
32	.0000	.0000	.0000	.0000	.0001	.0003	.0007	.0018	.0040	.0081
33	.0000	.0000	.0000	.0000	.0000	.0001	.0004	.0010	.0022	.0047
34	.0000	.0000	.0000	.0000	.0000	.0001	.0002	.0005	.0012	.0027
35	.0000	.0000	.0000	.0000	.0000	.0000	.0001	.0002	.0006	.0015
36	.0000	.0000	.0000	.0000	.0000	.0000	.0000	.0001	.0003	.0008
37	.0000	.0000	.0000	.0000	.0000	.0000	.0000	.0001	.0002	.0004
38	.0000	.0000	.0000	.0000	.0000	.0000	.0000	.0000	.0001	.0002
39	.0000	.0000	.0000	.0000	.0000	.0000	.0000	.0000	.0000	.0001
40	.0000	.0000	.0000	.0000	.0000	.0000	.0000	.0000	.0000	.0001

III.5 CONFIDENCE LIMITS FOR PROPORTIONS

The general term of the binomial expansion is given by

$$f(x;n,\theta) = \binom{n}{x}\theta^x(1-\theta)^{n-x}, \qquad x = 0, 1, 2, \ldots, n.$$

For known n, and for a given value of x', the values of the confidence limits θ_a and θ_b, $(\theta_a < \theta_b)$ are defined by

$$\sum_{x=x'}^{n} f(x;n,\theta_a) = \alpha \qquad \text{and} \qquad \sum_{x=0}^{x'} f(x;n,\theta_b) = \alpha,$$

where the cumulative sums may be evaluated conveniently from the cumulative binomial distribution tables.

The charts show confidence limits for θ for

$$1 - 2\alpha = .95, \text{ and } .99$$

or

$$\alpha = .025, \text{ and } .005$$

and for $n = 8, 10, 12, 16, 20, 24, 30, 40, 60, 100, 200, 400, 1000$.

The tables show confidence limits for θ for

$$1 - 2\alpha = .95, \text{ and } .99$$

or

$$\alpha = .025, \text{ and } .005.$$

Example: Observed relative frequency $8/30 = 0.267$. The 95 per cent confidence limits for θ are 0.123 and 0.459.

Example: Observed relative frequency $8/30 = 0.267$. The 99 per cent confidence limits for θ are 0.093 and 0.516.

CONFIDENCE LIMITS FOR PROPORTIONS (CONFIDENCE COEFFICIENT 0.95)

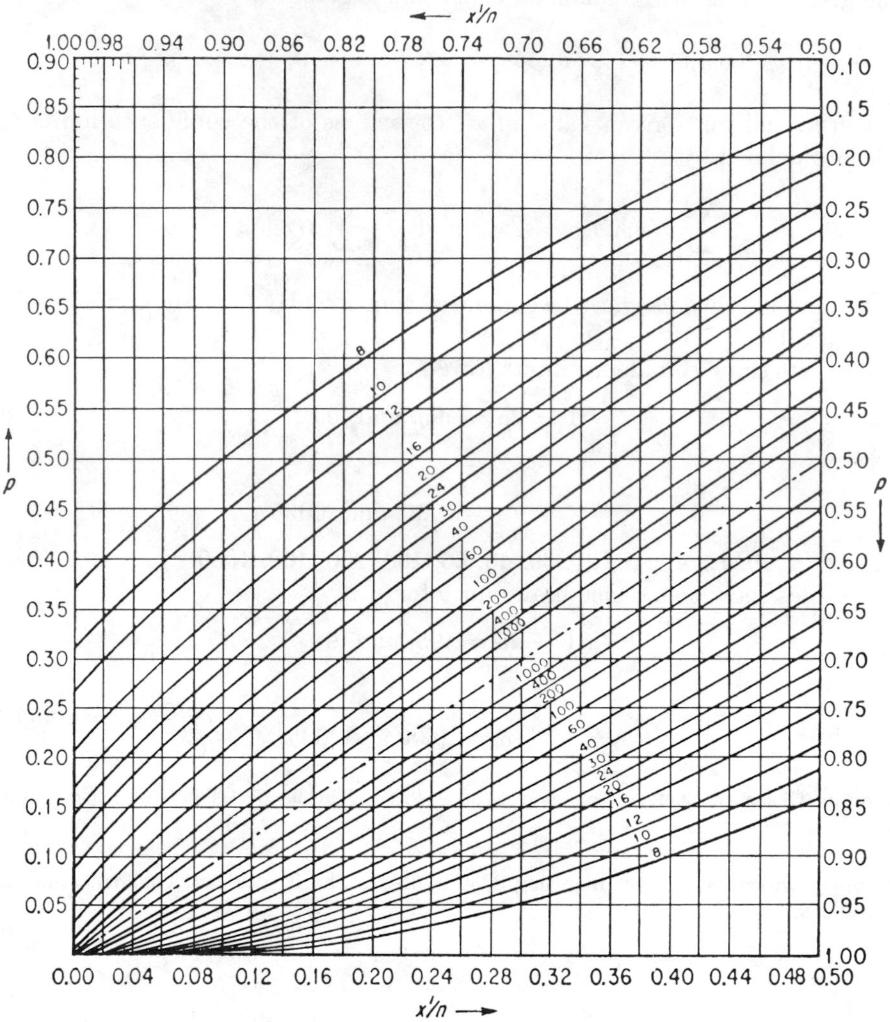

CONFIDENCE LIMITS FOR PROPORTIONS
(CONFIDENCE COEFFICIENT 0.99)

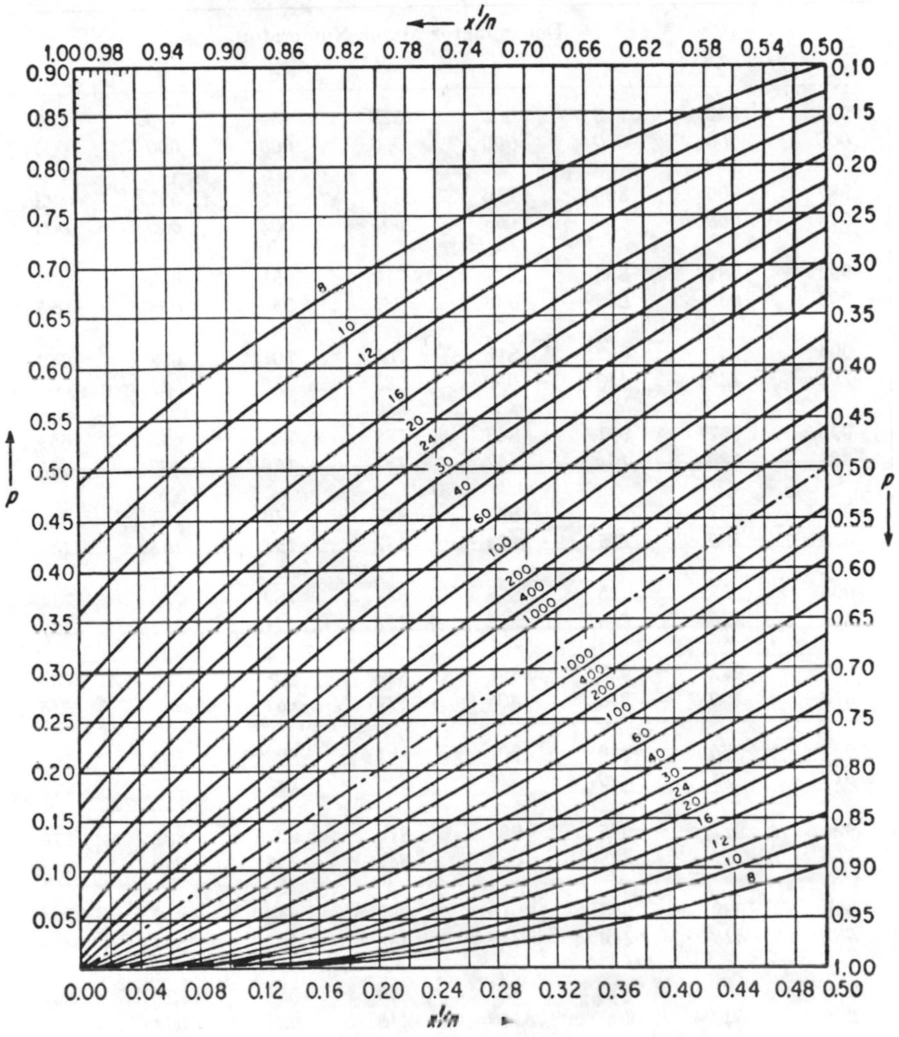

CONFIDENCE LIMITS FOR PROPORTIONS (CONFIDENCE COEFFICIENT .95)

x Denotes the Numerator and n the Denominator of the Relative Frequency

x (Numerator of the Relative Frequency) \ $n-x$ (Denominator Minus Numerator)	1	2	3	4	5	6	7	8	9
0	975	842	708	602	522	459	410	369	336
	000	*000*	*000*	*000*	*000*	*000*	*000*	*000*	*000*
1	987	906	806	716	641	579	527	483	445
	013	*008*	*006*	*005*	*004*	*004*	*003*	*003*	*003*
2	992	932	853	777	710	651	600	556	518
	094	*068*	*053*	*043*	*037*	*032*	*028*	*025*	*023*
3	994	947	882	816	755	701	652	610	572
	194	*147*	*118*	*099*	*085*	*075*	*067*	*060*	*055*
4	995	957	901	843	788	738	692	651	614
	284	*223*	*184*	*157*	*137*	*122*	*109*	*099*	*091*
5	996	963	915	863	813	766	723	684	649
	359	*290*	*245*	*212*	*187*	*167*	*151*	*139*	*128*
6	996	968	925	878	833	789	749	711	677
	421	*349*	*299*	*262*	*234*	*211*	*192*	*177*	*163*
7	997	972	933	891	849	808	770	734	701
	473	*400*	*348*	*308*	*277*	*251*	*230*	*213*	*198*
8	997	975	940	901	861	823	787	753	722
	517	*444*	*390*	*349*	*316*	*289*	*266*	*247*	*230*
9	997	977	945	909	872	837	802	770	740
	555	*482*	*428*	*386*	*351*	*323*	*299*	*278*	*260*
10	998	979	950	916	882	848	816	785	756
	587	*516*	*462*	*419*	*384*	*354*	*329*	*308*	*289*
11	998	981	953	922	890	858	827	797	769
	615	*546*	*492*	*449*	*413*	*383*	*357*	*335*	*315*
12	998	982	957	927	897	867	837	809	782
	640	*572*	*519*	*476*	*440*	*410*	*384*	*361*	*340*
13	998	983	960	932	903	874	846	819	793
	661	*595*	*544*	*501*	*465*	*435*	*408*	*384*	*364*
14	998	984	962	936	909	881	854	828	803
	681	*617*	*566*	*524*	*488*	*457*	*430*	*407*	*385*
15	998	985	964	939	913	887	861	836	812
	698	*636*	*586*	*544*	*509*	*478*	*451*	*427*	*406*
16	999	986	966	943	918	893	868	844	820
	713	*653*	*604*	*563*	*529*	*498*	*471*	*447*	*425*
17	999	987	968	946	922	898	874	851	828
	727	*669*	*621*	*581*	*547*	*516*	*488*	*465*	*443*

CONFIDENCE LIMITS FOR PROPORTIONS (CONFIDENCE COEFFICIENT .95)

x DENOTES THE NUMERATOR AND n THE DENOMINATOR OF THE RELATIVE FREQUENCY

Numerator of the Relative Frequency x \ $n-x$ Denominator minus Numerator	1	2	3	4	5	6	7	8	9
18	999 *740*	988 *683*	970 *637*	948 *597*	925 *564*	902 *533*	879 *506*	857 *482*	835 *460*
19	999 *751*	988 *696*	971 *651*	950 *612*	929 *579*	906 *549*	884 *522*	862 *498*	841 *476*
20	999 *762*	989 *708*	972 *664*	953 *626*	932 *593*	910 *564*	889 *537*	868 *513*	847 *492*
22	999 *781*	990 *730*	975 *688*	956 *651*	937 *619*	917 *590*	897 *565*	877 *541*	858 *519*
24	999 *797*	991 *749*	976 *708*	960 *673*	942 *642*	923 *614*	904 *589*	885 *566*	867 *545*
26	999 *810*	991 *765*	978 *726*	962 *693*	945 *663*	928 *636*	910 *611*	893 *588*	875 *567*
28	999 *822*	992 *779*	980 *743*	965 *710*	949 *681*	932 *655*	916 *631*	899 *609*	882 *588*
30	999 *833*	992 *792*	981 *757*	967 *725*	952 *697*	936 *672*	920 *649*	904 *627*	889 *607*
35	999 *855*	993 *818*	983 *786*	971 *758*	958 *732*	944 *708*	930 *686*	916 *666*	902 *647*
40	999 *871*	994 *838*	985 *809*	975 *783*	963 *759*	951 *737*	938 *717*	925 *698*	912 *679*
45	999 *885*	995 *855*	987 *828*	977 *804*	967 *782*	956 *761*	944 *742*	933 *724*	921 *707*
50	1000 *896*	995 *868*	988 *843*	979 *821*	970 *800*	960 *781*	949 *763*	939 *746*	928 *730*
60	1000 *912*	996 *888*	990 *867*	983 *848*	975 *830*	966 *813*	957 *797*	948 *782*	939 *767*
80	1000 *933*	997 *915*	992 *898*	987 *882*	981 *868*	974 *855*	967 *842*	960 *829*	953 *816*
100	1000 *946*	998 *931*	994 *917*	989 *904*	984 *892*	979 *881*	973 *870*	967 *859*	962 *849*
200	1000 *973*	999 *965*	997 *957*	995 *951*	992 *944*	989 *938*	986 *932*	983 *926*	980 *920*
500	1000 *989*	1000 *986*	999 *983*	998 *980*	997 *977*	996 *974*	995 *972*	993 *969*	992 *967*
∞	1000 *1000*	1000 *1000*	1000 *1000*	1000 *1000*	1000 *1000*	1000 *1000*	1000 *1000*	1000 *1000*	1000 *1000*

CONFIDENCE LIMITS FOR PROPORTIONS (CONFIDENCE COEFFICIENT .95)

x Denotes the Numerator and n the Denominator of the Relative Frequency

Numerator of the Relative Frequency (x) / Denominator minus Numerator ($n-x$)

x \ $n-x$	10	11	12	13	14	15	16	17	18
0	308	285	265	247	232	218	206	195	185
	000	*000*	*000*	*000*	*000*	*000*	*000*	*000*	*000*
1	413	385	360	339	319	302	287	273	260
	002	*002*	*002*	*002*	*002*	*002*	*001*	*001*	*001*
2	484	454	428	405	383	364	347	331	317
	021	*019*	*018*	*017*	*016*	*015*	*014*	*013*	*012*
3	538	508	481	456	434	414	396	379	363
	050	*047*	*043*	*040*	*038*	*036*	*034*	*032*	*030*
4	581	551	524	499	476	456	437	419	403
	084	*078*	*073*	*068*	*064*	*061*	*057*	*054*	*052*
5	616	587	560	535	512	491	471	453	436
	118	*110*	*103*	*097*	*091*	*087*	*082*	*078*	*075*
6	646	617	590	565	543	522	502	484	467
	152	*142*	*133*	*126*	*119*	*113*	*107*	*102*	*098*
7	671	643	616	592	570	549	529	512	494
	184	*173*	*163*	*154*	*146*	*139*	*132*	*126*	*121*
8	692	665	639	616	593	573	553	535	518
	215	*203*	*191*	*181*	*172*	*164*	*156*	*149*	*143*
9	711	685	660	636	615	594	575	557	540
	244	*231*	*218*	*207*	*197*	*188*	*180*	*172*	*165*
10	728	702	678	655	634	614	595	577	560
	272	*257*	*244*	*232*	*221*	*211*	*202*	*194*	*186*
11	743	718	694	672	651	631	612	594	578
	298	*282*	*268*	*256*	*244*	*234*	*224*	*215*	*207*
12	756	732	709	687	666	647	628	611	594
	322	*306*	*291*	*278*	*266*	*255*	*245*	*235*	*227*
13	768	744	722	701	680	661	643	626	609
	345	*328*	*313*	*299*	*287*	*275*	*264*	*255*	*245*
14	779	756	734	713	694	675	657	640	624
	366	*349*	*334*	*320*	*306*	*295*	*283*	*273*	*264*
15	789	766	745	725	705	687	669	653	637
	386	*369*	*353*	*339*	*325*	*313*	*302*	*291*	*281*
16	798	776	755	736	717	698	681	665	649
	405	*388*	*372*	*357*	*343*	*331*	*319*	*308*	*298*
17	806	785	765	745	727	709	692	676	660
	423	*406*	*389*	*374*	*360*	*347*	*335*	*324*	*314*

CONFIDENCE LIMITS FOR PROPORTIONS (CONFIDENCE COEFFICIENT .95)

x Denotes the Numerator and n the Denominator of the Relative Frequency

x (Numerator of the Relative Frequency) \ $n-x$ (Denominator minus Numerator)	10	11	12	13	14	15	16	17	18
18	814 *440*	793 *422*	773 *406*	755 *391*	736 *376*	719 *363*	702 *351*	686 *340*	671 *329*
19	821 *456*	801 *439*	782 *422*	763 *406*	745 *392*	728 *379*	712 *366*	696 *355*	681 *344*
20	827 *472*	808 *454*	789 *437*	771 *421*	753 *407*	737 *393*	720 *381*	705 *369*	690 *358*
22	839 *500*	820 *481*	803 *465*	785 *449*	768 *434*	752 *421*	737 *408*	722 *396*	707 *385*
24	849 *525*	831 *507*	814 *490*	798 *475*	782 *460*	766 *446*	751 *433*	737 *421*	723 *410*
26	858 *548*	841 *530*	825 *513*	809 *497*	794 *483*	779 *469*	764 *456*	750 *444*	736 *432*
28	866 *569*	850 *551*	834 *535*	819 *519*	804 *504*	790 *491*	776 *478*	762 *465*	749 *453*
30	873 *588*	858 *571*	843 *554*	828 *539*	814 *524*	800 *510*	786 *498*	773 *485*	760 *473*
35	888 *628*	874 *612*	860 *596*	847 *581*	834 *567*	821 *554*	809 *541*	797 *529*	785 *517*
40	900 *662*	887 *646*	875 *631*	862 *616*	850 *602*	838 *590*	827 *578*	815 *566*	804 *555*
45	909 *690*	898 *675*	886 *661*	875 *647*	864 *633*	853 *621*	842 *609*	831 *598*	821 *587*
50	917 *714*	906 *700*	896 *686*	885 *673*	875 *660*	865 *648*	854 *636*	844 *625*	835 *614*
60	929 *752*	920 *740*	911 *727*	902 *715*	893 *703*	884 *692*	874 *681*	866 *670*	857 *660*
80	945 *804*	938 *793*	931 *783*	923 *773*	916 *763*	909 *753*	901 *744*	894 *734*	887 *726*
100	955 *838*	949 *829*	943 *820*	937 *811*	931 *802*	925 *794*	919 *786*	913 *778*	907 *770*
200	977 *914*	974 *909*	970 *903*	967 *898*	964 *893*	961 *888*	957 *883*	954 *878*	950 *873*
500	991 *964*	989 *962*	988 *960*	986 *957*	985 *955*	984 *953*	982 *950*	981 *948*	979 *946*
∞	1000 *1000*	1000 *1000*	1000 *1000*	1000 *1000*	1000 *1000*	1000 *1000*	1000 *1000*	1000 *1000*	1000 *1000*

CONFIDENCE LIMITS FOR PROPORTIONS (CONFIDENCE COEFFICIENT .95)

x Denotes the Numerator and n the Denominator of the Relative Frequency

Numerator of the Relative Frequency (x); Denominator minus Numerator ($n-x$)

x \ $n-x$	19	20	22	24	26	28	30	35	40
0	176 *000*	168 *000*	154 *000*	142 *000*	132 *000*	123 *000*	116 *000*	100 *000*	088 *000*
1	249 *001*	238 *001*	219 *001*	203 *001*	190 *001*	178 *001*	167 *001*	145 *001*	129 *001*
2	304 *012*	292 *011*	270 *010*	251 *009*	235 *009*	221 *008*	208 *008*	182 *007*	162 *006*
3	349 *029*	336 *028*	312 *025*	292 *024*	274 *022*	257 *020*	243 *019*	214 *017*	191 *015*
4	388 *050*	374 *047*	349 *044*	327 *040*	307 *038*	290 *035*	275 *033*	242 *029*	217 *025*
5	421 *071*	407 *068*	381 *063*	358 *058*	337 *055*	319 *051*	303 *048*	268 *042*	241 *037*
6	451 *094*	436 *090*	410 *083*	386 *077*	364 *072*	345 *068*	328 *064*	292 *056*	263 *049*
7	478 *116*	463 *111*	435 *103*	411 *096*	389 *090*	369 *084*	351 *080*	314 *070*	283 *062*
8	502 *138*	487 *132*	459 *123*	434 *115*	412 *107*	391 *101*	373 *096*	334 *084*	302 *075*
9	524 *159*	508 *153*	481 *142*	455 *133*	433 *125*	412 *118*	393 *111*	353 *098*	321 *088*
10	544 *179*	528 *173*	500 *161*	475 *151*	452 *142*	431 *134*	412 *127*	372 *112*	338 *100*
11	561 *199*	546 *192*	519 *180*	493 *169*	470 *159*	449 *150*	429 *142*	388 *126*	354 *113*
12	578 *218*	563 *211*	535 *197*	510 *186*	487 *175*	465 *166*	446 *157*	404 *140*	369 *125*
13	594 *237*	579 *229*	551 *215*	525 *202*	503 *191*	481 *181*	461 *172*	419 *153*	384 *138*
14	608 *255*	593 *247*	566 *232*	540 *218*	517 *206*	496 *196*	476 *186*	433 *166*	398 *150*
15	621 *272*	607 *263*	579 *248*	554 *234*	531 *221*	509 *210*	490 *200*	446 *179*	410 *162*
16	634 *288*	619 *280*	592 *263*	567 *249*	544 *236*	522 *224*	502 *214*	459 *191*	422 *173*
17	645 *304*	631 *295*	604 *278*	579 *263*	556 *250*	535 *238*	515 *227*	471 *203*	434 *185*

CONFIDENCE LIMITS FOR PROPORTIONS (CONFIDENCE COEFFICIENT .95)

x Denotes the Numerator and n the Denominator of the Relative Frequency

x (Numerator of the Relative Frequency) \ $n-x$ (Denominator minus Numerator)	19	20	22	24	26	28	30	35	40
18	656	642	615	590	568	547	527	483	445
	319	*310*	*293*	*277*	*264*	*251*	*240*	*215*	*196*
19	666	652	626	601	578	557	538	494	456
	334	*324*	*307*	*291*	*277*	*264*	*252*	*227*	*207*
20	676	662	636	612	589	568	548	504	467
	348	*338*	*320*	*304*	*289*	*276*	*264*	*238*	*217*
22	693	680	654	631	614	588	568	524	487
	374	*364*	*346*	*329*	*314*	*300*	*287*	*260*	*237*
24	709	696	671	648	626	605	586	543	505
	399	*388*	*369*	*352*	*337*	*322*	*309*	*281*	*257*
26	723	711	686	663	642	622	603	559	522
	422	*411*	*386*	*374*	*358*	*343*	*330*	*300*	*276*
28	736	724	700	678	657	637	618	575	538
	443	*432*	*412*	*395*	*378*	*363*	*349*	*319*	*294*
30	748	736	713	691	670	651	632	590	552
	462	*452*	*432*	*414*	*397*	*382*	*368*	*337*	*311*
35	773	762	740	719	700	681	663	622	586
	506	*496*	*476*	*457*	*441*	*425*	*410*	*378*	*351*
40	793	783	763	743	724	706	689	649	614
	544	*533*	*513*	*495*	*478*	*462*	*448*	*414*	*386*
45	811	801	781	763	745	728	711	673	639
	576	*566*	*546*	*528*	*511*	*495*	*480*	*447*	*419*
50	825	816	797	780	763	746	731	694	660
	604	*594*	*575*	*557*	*540*	*525*	*510*	*476*	*447*
60	848	840	823	807	792	777	763	728	697
	650	*641*	*622*	*605*	*589*	*574*	*559*	*526*	*497*
80	880	874	860	846	833	820	808	778	750
	717	*708*	*692*	*676*	*662*	*647*	*634*	*603*	*575*
100	901	895	883	872	860	847	838	812	787
	762	*755*	*740*	*726*	*713*	*700*	*687*	*658*	*632*
200	947	943	937	930	923	917	910	894	878
	868	*863*	*854*	*845*	*836*	*828*	*819*	*799*	*780*
500	978	976	973	970	967	964	961	954	947
	944	*941*	*937*	*933*	*928*	*924*	*920*	*910*	*901*
∞	1000	1000	1000	1000	1000	1000	1000	1000	1000
	1000	*1000*	*1000*	*1000*	*1000*	*1000*	*1000*	*1000*	*1000*

CONFIDENCE LIMITS FOR PROPORTIONS (CONFIDENCE COEFFICIENT .95)

x Denotes the Numerator and n the Denominator of the Relative Frequency

x \ $n-x$	Denominator minus Numerator							
	45	50	60	80	100	200	500	∞
0	079	071	060	045	036	018	007	000
	000	*000*	*000*	*000*	*000*	*000*	*000*	*000*
1	115	104	088	067	054	027	011	000
	001	*001*	*000*	*000*	*000*	*000*	*000*	*000*
2	145	132	112	085	069	035	014	000
	005	*005*	*004*	*003*	*002*	*001*	*000*	*000*
3	172	157	133	102	083	043	017	000
	013	*012*	*010*	*008*	*006*	*003*	*001*	*000*
4	196	179	152	118	096	049	020	000
	023	*021*	*017*	*013*	*011*	*005*	*002*	*000*
5	218	200	170	132	108	056	023	000
	033	*030*	*025*	*019*	*016*	*008*	*003*	*000*
6	239	219	187	145	119	062	026	000
	044	*040*	*034*	*026*	*021*	*011*	*004*	*000*
7	258	237	203	158	130	068	028	000
	056	*051*	*043*	*033*	*027*	*014*	*005*	*000*
8	276	254	218	171	141	074	031	000
	067	*061*	*052*	*040*	*033*	*017*	*007*	*000*
9	293	270	233	184	151	080	033	000
	079	*072*	*061*	*047*	*038*	*020*	*008*	*000*
10	310	286	248	196	162	086	036	000
	091	*083*	*071*	*055*	*045*	*023*	*009*	*000*
11	325	300	260	207	171	091	038	000
	102	*094*	*080*	*062*	*051*	*026*	*011*	*000*
12	339	314	273	217	180	097	040	000
	114	*104*	*089*	*069*	*057*	*030*	*012*	*000*
13	353	327	285	227	189	102	043	000
	125	*115*	*098*	*077*	*063*	*033*	*014*	*000*
14	367	340	297	237	198	107	045	000
	136	*125*	*107*	*084*	*069*	*036*	*015*	*000*
15	379	352	308	247	206	112	047	000
	147	*135*	*116*	*091*	*075*	*039*	*016*	*000*
16	391	364	319	256	214	117	050	000
	158	*146*	*126*	*099*	*081*	*043*	*018*	*000*
17	402	375	330	266	222	122	052	000
	169	*156*	*134*	*106*	*087*	*046*	*019*	*000*

Numerator of the Relative Frequency

CONFIDENCE LIMITS FOR PROPORTIONS (CONFIDENCE COEFFICIENT .95)

x DENOTES THE NUMERATOR AND n THE DENOMINATOR OF THE RELATIVE FREQUENCY

x (Numerator of the Relative Frequency) \ $n-x$ (Denominator minus Numerator)	45	50	60	80	100	200	500	∞
18	413	386	340	274	230	127	054	000
	179	*165*	*143*	*113*	*093*	*050*	*021*	*000*
19	424	396	350	283	238	132	056	000
	189	*175*	*152*	*120*	*099*	*053*	*022*	*000*
20	434	406	359	292	245	137	059	000
	199	*184*	*160*	*126*	*105*	*057*	*024*	*000*
22	454	425	378	308	260	146	063	000
	219	*203*	*177*	*140*	*117*	*063*	*027*	*000*
24	472	443	395	324	274	155	067	000
	237	*220*	*193*	*154*	*128*	*070*	*030*	*000*
26	489	460	411	338	287	164	072	000
	255	*237*	*208*	*167*	*140*	*077*	*033*	*000*
28	505	475	426	353	300	172	076	000
	272	*254*	*223*	*180*	*153*	*083*	*036*	*000*
30	520	490	441	366	313	181	080	000
	289	*269*	*237*	*192*	*162*	*090*	*039*	*000*
35	553	524	474	397	342	201	090	000
	327	*306*	*272*	*222*	*188*	*106*	*046*	*000*
40	581	553	503	425	368	220	099	000
	361	*340*	*303*	*250*	*213*	*122*	*053*	*000*
45	607	579	529	451	392	238	109	000
	393	*370*	*332*	*276*	*236*	*137*	*061*	*000*
50	630	602	552	474	415	255	118	000
	421	*398*	*359*	*301*	*259*	*152*	*068*	*000*
60	668	641	593	515	455	287	136	000
	471	*448*	*407*	*345*	*300*	*181*	*083*	*000*
80	724	699	655	580	520	342	169	000
	549	*526*	*485*	*420*	*370*	*234*	*111*	*000*
100	764	741	700	630	571	395	199	000
	608	*585*	*545*	*480*	*429*	*280*	*138*	*000*
200	863	848	819	766	720	550	319	000
	762	*745*	*713*	*658*	*605*	*450*	*253*	*000*
500	939	932	917	889	862	747	531	000
	891	*882*	*864*	*831*	*801*	*681*	*469*	*000*
∞	1000	1000	1000	1000	1000	1000	1000	—
	1000	*1000*	*1000*	*1000*	*1000*	*1000*	*1000*	—

CONFIDENCE LIMITS FOR PROPORTIONS (CONFIDENCE COEFFICIENT .99)

x Denotes the Numerator and n the Denominator of the Relative Frequency

x \ $n-x$ (Numerator of the Relative Frequency / Denominator minus Numerator)	1	2	3	4	5	6	7	8	9
0	995	929	829	734	653	586	531	484	445
	000	*000*	*000*	*000*	*000*	*000*	*000*	*000*	*000*
1	997	959	889	815	746	685	632	585	544
	003	*002*	*001*	*001*	*001*	*001*	*001*	*001*	*001*
2	998	971	917	856	797	742	693	648	608
	041	*029*	*023*	*019*	*016*	*014*	*012*	*011*	*010*
3	999	977	934	882	830	781	735	693	655
	111	*083*	*066*	*055*	*047*	*042*	*037*	*033*	*030*
4	999	981	945	900	854	809	767	728	691
	185	*144*	*118*	*100*	*087*	*077*	*069*	*062*	*057*
5	999	984	953	913	872	831	791	755	720
	254	*203*	*170*	*146*	*128*	*114*	*103*	*094*	*087*
6	999	986	958	923	886	848	811	777	744
	315	*258*	*219*	*191*	*169*	*152*	*138*	*127*	*117*
7	999	988	963	931	897	862	828	795	764
	368	*307*	*265*	*233*	*209*	*189*	*172*	*159*	*147*
8	999	989	967	938	906	873	841	811	781
	415	*352*	*307*	*272*	*245*	*223*	*205*	*189*	*176*
9	999	990	970	943	913	883	853	824	795
	456	*392*	*345*	*309*	*280*	*256*	*236*	*219*	*205*
10	1000	991	972	947	920	891	863	835	808
	491	*427*	*379*	*342*	*312*	*286*	*265*	*247*	*232*
11	1000	992	974	951	925	899	872	845	819
	523	*459*	*411*	*373*	*342*	*315*	*293*	*274*	*257*
12	1000	992	976	955	930	905	879	854	829
	551	*488*	*439*	*401*	*369*	*342*	*319*	*299*	*282*
13	1000	993	978	957	935	910	886	862	838
	576	*514*	*466*	*427*	*395*	*367*	*343*	*323*	*305*
14	1000	993	979	960	938	915	892	869	846
	598	*537*	*490*	*451*	*418*	*390*	*366*	*345*	*326*
15	1000	994	980	962	942	920	898	875	854
	619	*559*	*512*	*473*	*440*	*412*	*388*	*366*	*347*
16	1000	994	981	964	945	924	903	881	860
	637	*578*	*532*	*493*	*461*	*433*	*408*	*386*	*366*
17	1000	994	982	966	947	927	907	887	866
	654	*596*	*551*	*512*	*480*	*452*	*427*	*405*	*385*

CONFIDENCE LIMITS FOR PROPORTIONS (CONFIDENCE COEFFICIENT .99)

x DENOTES THE NUMERATOR AND n THE DENOMINATOR OF THE RELATIVE FREQUENCY

x (Numerator of the Relative Frequency) \ $n-x$	Denominator minus Numerator								
	1	2	3	4	5	6	7	8	9
18	1000	995	983	968	950	931	911	891	872
	669	*613*	*568*	*530*	*498*	*469*	*445*	*422*	*402*
19	1000	995	984	969	952	934	915	896	877
	683	*628*	*584*	*547*	*515*	*486*	*462*	*439*	*419*
20	1000	995	985	971	954	936	918	900	881
	696	*642*	*599*	*562*	*530*	*502*	*478*	*455*	*435*
22	1000	996	986	973	958	941	924	907	890
	719	*668*	*626*	*590*	*559*	*531*	*507*	*484*	*464*
24	1000	996	987	975	961	946	930	913	897
	738	*690*	*649*	*615*	*584*	*557*	*533*	*511*	*490*
26	1000	996	988	977	963	949	934	919	903
	755	*709*	*670*	*637*	*607*	*580*	*557*	*535*	*515*
28	1000	996	989	978	966	952	938	924	909
	770	*726*	*689*	*656*	*627*	*602*	*578*	*557*	*537*
30	1000	997	989	980	968	955	942	928	914
	784	*741*	*705*	*674*	*646*	*621*	*598*	*577*	*557*
35	1000	997	991	982	972	961	949	937	924
	811	*773*	*740*	*711*	*685*	*661*	*639*	*619*	*600*
40	1000	998	992	984	975	965	955	944	933
	832	*797*	*767*	*740*	*716*	*694*	*673*	*654*	*636*
45	1000	998	993	986	978	969	959	949	939
	849	*817*	*790*	*765*	*742*	*721*	*701*	*683*	*666*
50	1000	998	994	987	980	972	963	954	945
	863	*834*	*808*	*785*	*763*	*743*	*725*	*708*	*691*
60	1000	998	995	989	983	976	969	961	953
	884	*859*	*830*	*810*	*797*	*780*	*763*	*748*	*733*
80	1000	999	996	992	987	982	976	970	964
	912	*892*	*874*	*857*	*842*	*827*	*814*	*801*	*788*
100	1000	999	997	993	990	985	981	976	971
	929	*912*	*897*	*884*	*871*	*858*	*847*	*836*	*825*
200	1000	999	998	997	995	992	990	988	985
	964	*955*	*947*	*939*	*932*	*925*	*919*	*913*	*907*
500	1000	1000	999	999	998	997	996	995	994
	985	*982*	*978*	*975*	*972*	*969*	*967*	*964*	*961*
∞	1000	1000	1000	1000	1000	1000	1000	1000	1000
	1000	*1000*	*1000*	*1000*	*1000*	*1000*	*1000*	*1000*	*1000*

CONFIDENCE LIMITS FOR PROPORTIONS (CONFIDENCE COEFFICIENT .99)

x Denotes the Numerator and n the Denominator of the Relative Frequency

x (Numerator of the Relative Frequency) \ $n-x$ (Denominator minus Numerator)	10	11	12	13	14	15	16	17	18
0	411	382	357	335	315	298	282	268	255
	000	*000*	*000*	*000*	*000*	*000*	*000*	*000*	*000*
1	509	477	449	424	402	381	363	346	331
	000	*000*	*000*	*000*	*000*	*000*	*000*	*000*	*000*
2	573	541	512	486	463	441	422	404	387
	009	*008*	*008*	*007*	*007*	*006*	*006*	*006*	*005*
3	621	589	561	534	510	488	468	449	432
	028	*026*	*024*	*022*	*021*	*020*	*019*	*018*	*017*
4	658	627	599	573	549	527	507	488	470
	053	*049*	*045*	*043*	*040*	*038*	*036*	*034*	*032*
5	688	658	631	605	582	560	539	520	502
	080	*075*	*070*	*065*	*062*	*058*	*055*	*053*	*050*
6	714	685	658	633	610	588	567	548	531
	109	*101*	*095*	*090*	*085*	*080*	*076*	*073*	*069*
7	735	707	681	657	634	612	592	573	555
	137	*128*	*121*	*114*	*108*	*102*	*097*	*093*	*089*
8	753	726	701	677	655	634	614	595	578
	165	*155*	*146*	*138*	*131*	*125*	*119*	*113*	*109*
9	768	743	718	695	674	653	634	615	598
	192	*181*	*171*	*162*	*154*	*146*	*140*	*134*	*128*
10	782	758	734	712	690	670	651	633	616
	218	*205*	*195*	*185*	*176*	*168*	*161*	*154*	*148*
11	795	771	748	726	705	686	667	649	632
	242	*229*	*218*	*207*	*197*	*189*	*181*	*173*	*167*
12	805	782	760	739	719	700	682	664	647
	266	*252*	*240*	*228*	*218*	*209*	*200*	*192*	*185*
13	815	793	772	751	731	713	695	678	661
	288	*274*	*261*	*249*	*238*	*228*	*219*	*211*	*203*
14	824	803	782	762	743	724	707	691	674
	310	*295*	*281*	*269*	*257*	*247*	*237*	*228*	*220*
15	832	811	791	772	753	735	718	702	685
	330	*314*	*300*	*287*	*276*	*265*	*255*	*246*	*237*
16	839	819	800	781	763	745	728	712	696
	349	*333*	*318*	*305*	*293*	*282*	*272*	*262*	*253*
17	846	827	808	789	772	754	738	722	706
	367	*351*	*336*	*322*	*309*	*298*	*288*	*278*	*269*

CONFIDENCE LIMITS FOR PROPORTIONS (CONFIDENCE COEFFICIENT .99)

x DENOTES THE NUMERATOR AND n THE DENOMINATOR OF THE RELATIVE FREQUENCY

Numerator of the Relative Frequency (x); Denominator minus Numerator ($n-x$)

x \ $n-x$	10	11	12	13	14	15	16	17	18
18	852	833	815	797	780	763	747	731	716
	384	*368*	*353*	*339*	*326*	*315*	*304*	*294*	*284*
19	858	840	822	804	787	771	755	740	725
	401	*384*	*369*	*355*	*342*	*330*	*319*	*308*	*299*
20	863	845	828	811	794	778	763	748	733
	417	*400*	*384*	*370*	*357*	*345*	*334*	*323*	*313*
22	873	856	839	823	807	792	777	762	748
	445	*429*	*413*	*398*	*385*	*372*	*361*	*350*	*339*
24	881	865	849	834	819	804	789	775	762
	471	*455*	*439*	*424*	*410*	*398*	*386*	*375*	*364*
26	888	873	858	843	829	814	800	787	774
	496	*479*	*463*	*448*	*434*	*422*	*410*	*398*	*388*
28	894	880	866	852	838	824	811	798	785
	518	*501*	*485*	*471*	*457*	*444*	*432*	*420*	*409*
30	900	886	873	859	846	833	820	807	795
	539	*522*	*506*	*492*	*478*	*464*	*452*	*441*	*430*
35	912	900	887	875	863	851	839	827	816
	582	*566*	*550*	*535*	*522*	*510*	*498*	*486*	*475*
40	921	910	899	888	876	865	854	844	833
	619	*603*	*588*	*574*	*560*	*548*	*536*	*525*	*514*
45	929	919	908	898	888	877	867	857	847
	649	*634*	*620*	*606*	*593*	*582*	*570*	*558*	*547*
50	935	926	916	906	897	888	878	869	859
	676	*661*	*648*	*634*	*621*	*610*	*599*	*588*	*577*
60	945	937	928	920	912	904	895	887	878
	719	*705*	*693*	*680*	*668*	*657*	*646*	*636*	*626*
80	957	951	944	938	931	924	918	911	904
	776	*765*	*754*	*743*	*733*	*724*	*715*	*705*	*696*
100	965	960	955	949	943	938	932	927	921
	815	*805*	*795*	*786*	*777*	*769*	*761*	*753*	*745*
200	982	979	976	973	970	967	964	961	958
	901	*896*	*890*	*884*	*878*	*873*	*868*	*863*	*858*
500	993	992	990	989	988	987	985	984	982
	959	*956*	*953*	*951*	*949*	*946*	*944*	*941*	*939*
∞	1000	1000	1000	1000	1000	1000	1000	1000	1000
	1000	*1000*	*1000*	*1000*	*1000*	*1000*	*1000*	*1000*	*1000*

CONFIDENCE LIMITS FOR PROPORTIONS (CONFIDENCE COEFFICIENT .99)

x Denotes the Numerator and n the Denominator of the Relative Frequency

Numerator of the Relative Frequency (x) / Denominator minus Numerator ($n-x$)

x \ $n-x$	19	20	22	24	26	28	30	35	40
0	243 *000*	233 *000*	214 *000*	198 *000*	184 *000*	172 *000*	162 *000*	140 *000*	124 *000*
1	317 *000*	304 *000*	281 *000*	262 *000*	245 *000*	230 *000*	216 *000*	189 *000*	168 *000*
2	372 *005*	358 *005*	332 *004*	310 *004*	291 *004*	274 *004*	259 *003*	227 *003*	203 *002*
3	416 *016*	401 *015*	374 *014*	351 *013*	330 *012*	311 *011*	295 *011*	260 *009*	233 *008*
4	453 *031*	438 *029*	410 *027*	385 *025*	363 *023*	344 *022*	326 *020*	289 *018*	260 *016*
5	485 *048*	470 *046*	441 *042*	416 *039*	393 *037*	373 *034*	354 *032*	315 *028*	284 *025*
6	514 *066*	498 *064*	469 *059*	443 *054*	420 *051*	398 *048*	379 *045*	339 *039*	306 *035*
7	538 *085*	522 *082*	493 *076*	467 *070*	443 *066*	422 *062*	402 *058*	361 *051*	327 *045*
8	561 *104*	545 *100*	516 *093*	489 *087*	465 *081*	443 *076*	423 *072*	381 *063*	346 *056*
9	581 *123*	565 *119*	536 *110*	510 *103*	485 *097*	463 *091*	443 *086*	400 *076*	364 *067*
10	599 *142*	583 *137*	555 *127*	529 *119*	504 *112*	482 *106*	461 *100*	418 *088*	381 *079*
11	616 *160*	600 *155*	571 *144*	545 *135*	521 *127*	499 *120*	478 *114*	434 *100*	397 *090*
12	631 *178*	616 *172*	587 *161*	561 *151*	537 *142*	515 *134*	494 *127*	450 *113*	412 *101*
13	645 *196*	630 *189*	602 *177*	576 *166*	552 *157*	529 *148*	508 *141*	465 *125*	426 *112*
14	658 *213*	643 *206*	615 *193*	590 *181*	566 *171*	543 *162*	522 *154*	478 *137*	440 *124*
15	670 *229*	655 *222*	628 *208*	602 *196*	578 *186*	556 *176*	536 *167*	490 *149*	452 *135*
16	681 *245*	666 *237*	639 *223*	614 *211*	590 *200*	568 *189*	548 *180*	502 *161*	464 *146*
17	692 *260*	677 *252*	650 *238*	625 *225*	602 *213*	580 *202*	559 *193*	514 *173*	475 *156*

CONFIDENCE LIMITS FOR PROPORTIONS (CONFIDENCE COEFFICIENT .99)

x Denotes the Numerator and n the Denominator of the Relative Frequency

x (Numerator of the Relative Frequency) \ $n-x$ (Denominator minus Numerator)	19	20	22	24	26	28	30	35	40
18	701	687	661	636	612	591	570	525	486
	275	*267*	*252*	*238*	*226*	*215*	*205*	*184*	*167*
19	711	697	670	646	623	601	581	536	497
	289	*281*	*265*	*251*	*239*	*228*	*217*	*195*	*177*
20	719	705	679	655	632	611	591	546	507
	303	*295*	*279*	*264*	*251*	*239*	*229*	*206*	*187*
22	735	721	696	673	650	629	609	565	526
	330	*321*	*304*	*289*	*274*	*263*	*251*	*227*	*207*
24	749	736	711	688	666	646	626	582	543
	354	*345*	*327*	*312*	*298*	*285*	*273*	*247*	*226*
26	761	749	726	702	681	661	642	598	560
	377	*368*	*350*	*334*	*319*	*306*	*293*	*267*	*244*
28	772	761	737	715	694	675	656	613	575
	399	*389*	*371*	*354*	*339*	*325*	*312*	*285*	*262*
30	783	771	749	727	707	688	669	626	589
	419	*409*	*391*	*374*	*358*	*344*	*331*	*303*	*278*
35	805	794	773	753	733	715	697	657	620
	464	*454*	*435*	*418*	*402*	*387*	*374*	*343*	*318*
40	823	813	793	774	756	738	722	682	646
	503	*493*	*474*	*457*	*440*	*425*	*411*	*380*	*354*
45	838	828	810	792	775	758	742	704	670
	537	*527*	*508*	*491*	*474*	*459*	*445*	*413*	*386*
50	850	842	824	807	791	775	759	723	690
	567	*557*	*538*	*521*	*505*	*490*	*475*	*443*	*415*
60	870	863	847	832	817	802	788	755	724
	616	*606*	*589*	*572*	*556*	*541*	*527*	*495*	*466*
80	898	891	878	866	853	841	829	800	773
	687	*679*	*663*	*647*	*632*	*618*	*605*	*574*	*547*
100	916	910	899	888	878	867	857	831	807
	737	*729*	*714*	*700*	*687*	*674*	*661*	*632*	*606*
200	955	952	946	939	933	927	921	905	890
	853	*848*	*838*	*829*	*820*	*811*	*803*	*782*	*763*
500	981	980	977	974	971	969	966	959	952
	937	*934*	*930*	*925*	*921*	*917*	*912*	*902*	*892*
∞	1000	1000	1000	1000	1000	1000	1000	1000	1000
	1000	*1000*	*1000*	*1000*	*1000*	*1000*	*1000*	*1000*	*1000*

CONFIDENCE LIMITS FOR PROPORTIONS (CONFIDENCE COEFFICIENT .99)

x Denotes the Numerator and n the Denominator of the Relative Frequency

x (Numerator of the Relative Frequency) \ $n-x$ (Denominator minus Numerator)	45	50	60	80	100	200	500	∞
0	111	101	085	064	052	026	011	000
	000	*000*	*000*	*000*	*000*	*000*	*000*	*000*
1	151	137	116	088	071	036	015	000
	000	*000*	*000*	*000*	*000*	*000*	*000*	*000*
2	183	166	141	108	088	045	018	000
	002	*002*	*002*	*001*	*001*	*001*	*000*	*000*
3	210	192	164	126	103	053	022	000
	007	*006*	*005*	*004*	*003*	*002*	*001*	*000*
4	235	215	184	143	116	061	025	000
	014	*013*	*011*	*008*	*007*	*003*	*001*	*000*
5	258	237	203	158	129	068	028	000
	022	*020*	*017*	*013*	*010*	*005*	*002*	*000*
6	279	257	220	173	142	075	031	000
	031	*028*	*024*	*018*	*015*	*008*	*003*	*000*
7	299	275	237	186	153	081	033	000
	041	*037*	*031*	*024*	*019*	*010*	*004*	*000*
8	317	292	252	199	164	087	036	000
	051	*046*	*039*	*030*	*024*	*012*	*005*	*000*
9	334	309	267	212	175	093	039	000
	061	*055*	*047*	*036*	*029*	*015*	*006*	*000*
10	351	324	281	224	185	099	041	000
	071	*065*	*055*	*043*	*035*	*018*	*007*	*000*
11	366	339	295	235	195	104	044	000
	081	*074*	*063*	*049*	*040*	*021*	*008*	*000*
12	380	352	307	246	205	110	047	000
	092	*084*	*072*	*056*	*045*	*024*	*010*	*000*
13	394	366	320	257	214	116	049	000
	102	*094*	*080*	*062*	*051*	*027*	*011*	*000*
14	407	379	332	267	223	122	051	000
	112	*103*	*088*	*069*	*057*	*030*	*012*	*000*
15	418	390	343	276	231	127	054	000
	123	*112*	*096*	*076*	*062*	*033*	*013*	*000*
16	430	401	354	285	239	132	056	000
	133	*122*	*105*	*082*	*068*	*036*	*015*	*000*
17	442	412	364	295	247	137	059	000
	143	*131*	*113*	*089*	*073*	*039*	*016*	*000*

CONFIDENCE LIMITS FOR PROPORTIONS (CONFIDENCE COEFFICIENT .99)

x Denotes the Numerator and n the Denominator of the Relative Frequency

x \ $n-x$ (Numerator of the Relative Frequency \ Denominator minus Numerator)	45	50	60	80	100	200	500	∞
18	453 *153*	423 *141*	374 *122*	304 *096*	255 *079*	142 *042*	061 *018*	000 *000*
19	463 *162*	433 *150*	384 *130*	313 *102*	263 *084*	147 *045*	063 *019*	000 *000*
20	473 *172*	443 *158*	394 *137*	321 *109*	271 *090*	152 *048*	066 *020*	000 *000*
22	492 *190*	462 *176*	411 *153*	337 *122*	286 *101*	162 *054*	070 *023*	000 *000*
24	509 *208*	479 *193*	428 *168*	353 *134*	300 *112*	171 *061*	075 *026*	000 *000*
26	526 *225*	495 *209*	444 *183*	368 *147*	313 *122*	180 *067*	079 *029*	000 *000*
28	541 *242*	510 *225*	459 *198*	382 *159*	326 *133*	189 *073*	083 *031*	000 *000*
30	555 *258*	525 *241*	473 *212*	395 *171*	339 *143*	197 *079*	088 *034*	000 *000*
35	587 *296*	557 *277*	505 *245*	426 *200*	368 *169*	218 *095*	098 *041*	000 *000*
40	614 *330*	585 *310*	534 *276*	453 *227*	394 *193*	237 *110*	108 *048*	000 *000*
45	638 *362*	609 *341*	559 *305*	478 *253*	418 *216*	255 *125*	118 *055*	000 *000*
50	659 *391*	631 *369*	581 *332*	501 *277*	440 *238*	273 *139*	127 *062*	000 *000*
60	695 *441*	668 *419*	620 *380*	541 *301*	479 *278*	305 *167*	145 *076*	000 *000*
80	747 *522*	723 *499*	679 *459*	604 *396*	543 *349*	360 *219*	179 *103*	000 *000*
100	784 *582*	762 *560*	722 *521*	651 *457*	593 *407*	407 *265*	209 *129*	000 *000*
200	875 *745*	861 *727*	833 *695*	781 *640*	735 *593*	565 *435*	332 *243*	000 *000*
500	945 *882*	938 *873*	924 *855*	897 *821*	871 *791*	757 *668*	541 *459*	000 *000*
∞	1000 *1000*	1000 *1000*	1000 *1000*	1000 *1000*	1000 *1000*	1000 *1000*	1000 *1000*	— —

III.6 CONFIDENCE LIMITS FOR THE EXPECTED VALUE OF A POISSON DISTRIBUTION

The general term of a Poisson distributed variable is given by

$$f(x;\lambda) = \frac{e^{-\lambda}\lambda^x}{x!}, \qquad x = 0, 1, 2, \ldots .$$

For any given value x' and $\alpha < 0.5$, lower and upper limits of λ may be determined, say λ_a and λ_b, such that $\lambda_a < \lambda_b$ and

$$\sum_{x=x'}^{\infty} \frac{e^{-\lambda_a}\lambda_a^x}{x!} = \alpha \qquad \text{and} \qquad \sum_{x=0}^{x'} \frac{e^{-\lambda_b}\lambda_b^x}{x!} = \alpha.$$

Within the range of tabulation, λ_a and λ_b may be determined from the cumulative Poisson distribution tables, or from a table of percentage points of the χ^2 distribution, since

$$1 - P(\chi^2;n) = \sum_{x=0}^{x'-1} \frac{e^{-\lambda}\lambda^x}{x!}.$$

This table gives values of λ_a and λ_b for values of x' and for $2\alpha = 0.01$ and 0.05. Beyond $x' = 50$, λ_a and λ_b may be computed from

$$\lambda_b = \tfrac{1}{2}\chi_1^2 \qquad \text{where } 1 - P(\chi^2;n) = \alpha,\ n = 2(x'+1)$$
$$\lambda_a = \tfrac{1}{2}\chi_2^2 \qquad \text{where } P(\chi^2;n) = \alpha,\ n = 2x' .$$

CONFIDENCE LIMITS FOR THE EXPECTED VALUE OF A POISSON DISTRIBUTION

Total observed count $x' = \Sigma x_i$	Significance level				Total observed count $x' = \Sigma x_i$	Significance level			
	$2\alpha = 0.01$		$2\alpha = 0.05$			$2\alpha = 0.01$		$2\alpha = 0.05$	
	Lower Limit	*Upper Limit*	*Lower Limit*	*Upper Limit*		*Lower Limit*	*Upper Limit*	*Lower Limit*	*Upper Limit*
0	0.0	5.3	0.0	3.7					
1	0.0	7.4	0.1	5.6	26	14.7	42.2	17.0	38.0
2	0.1	9.3	0.2	7.2	27	15.4	43.5	17.8	39.2
3	0.3	11.0	0.6	8.8	28	16.2	44.8	18.6	40.4
4	0.6	12.6	1.0	10.2	29	17.0	46.0	19.4	41.6
5	1.0	14.1	1.6	11.7	30	17.7	47.2	20.2	42.8
6	1.5	15.6	2.2	13.1	31	18.5	48.4	21.0	44.0
7	2.0	17.1	2.8	14.4	32	19.3	49.6	21.8	45.1
8	2.5	18.5	3.4	15.8	33	20.0	50.8	22.7	46.3
9	3.1	20.0	4.0	17.1	34	20.8	52.1	23.5	47.5
10	3.7	21.3	4.7	18.4	35	21.6	53.3	24.3	48.7
11	4.3	22.6	5.4	19.7	36	22.4	54.5	25.1	49.8
12	4.9	24.0	6.2	21.0	37	23.2	55.7	26.0	51.0
13	5.5	25.4	6.9	22.3	38	24.0	56.9	26.8	52.2
14	6.2	26.7	7.7	23.5	39	24.8	58.1	27.7	53.3
15	6.8	28.1	8.4	24.8	40	25.6	59.3	28.6	54.5
16	7.5	29.4	9.4	26.0	41	26.4	60.5	29.4	55.6
17	8.2	30.7	9.9	27.2	42	27.2	61.7	30.3	56.8
18	8.9	32.0	10.7	28.4	43	28.0	62.9	31.1	57.9
19	9.6	33.3	11.5	29.6	44	28.8	64.1	32.0	59.0
20	10.3	34.6	12.2	30.8	45	29.6	65.3	32.8	60.2
21	11.0	35.9	13.0	32.0	46	30.4	66.5	33.6	61.3
22	11.8	37.2	13.8	33.2	47	31.2	67.7	34.5	62.5
23	12.5	38.4	14.6	34.4	48	32.0	68.9	35.3	63.6
24	13.2	39.7	15.4	35.6	49	32.8	70.1	36.1	64.8
25	14.0	41.0	16.2	36.8	50	33.6	71.3	37.0	65.9

III.7 VARIOUS FUNCTIONS OF p AND q = 1 − p

The columns of this table give values of the various functions

$$pq,\ \sqrt{pq},\ 1 - p^2,\ \sqrt{1 - p^2},\ \frac{1}{\sqrt{1 - p^2}},\ p^2 + q^2,\ 1 - q^2,\ \Gamma(1 + p),\ \log_{10} \Gamma(1 + p),$$
$$2 \text{ arc sin } \sqrt{p},\ 2 \text{ arc sin } \sqrt{q}.$$

The transformed variable, $y = 2 \text{ arc sin } \sqrt{p}$, is approximately normally distributed with mean $2 \text{ arc sin } \sqrt{\theta}$ and variance $\frac{1}{n}$ for $n\theta(1 - \theta) > 9$. Here p is the probability of success in a sample of n drawn from an infinite population where the probability of success is θ.

VARIOUS FUNCTIONS OF p AND $q = 1 - p$

p	$q = 1 - p$	pq	$\sqrt{(pq)}$	$1 - p^2$	$\sqrt{(1 - p^2)}$	$\frac{1}{\sqrt{(1 - p^2)}}$
0.00	**1.00**	0.0000	0.00000	1.0000	1.00000	1.00000
0.01	**0.99**	0.0099	0.09950	0.9999	0.99995	1.00005
0.02	**0.98**	0.0196	0.14000	0.9996	0.99980	1.00020
0.03	**0.97**	0.0291	0.17059	0.9991	0.99955	1.00045
0.04	**0.96**	0.0384	0.19596	0.9984	0.99920	1.00080
0.05	**0.95**	0.0475	0.21794	0.9975	0.99875	1.00125
0.06	**0.94**	0.0564	0.23749	0.9964	0.99820	1.00180
0.07	**0.93**	0.0651	0.25515	0.9951	0.99755	1.00246
0.08	**0.92**	0.0736	0.27129	0.9936	0.99679	1.00322
0.09	**0.91**	0.0819	0.28618	0.9919	0.99594	1.00407
0.10	**0.90**	0.0900	0.30000	0.9900	0.99499	1.00504
0.11	**0.89**	0.0979	0.31289	0.9879	0.99393	1.00611
0.12	**0.88**	0.1056	0.32496	0.9856	0.99277	1.00728
0.13	**0.87**	0.1131	0.33630	0.9831	0.99151	1.00856
0.14	**0.86**	0.1204	0.34699	0.9804	0.99015	1.00995
0.15	**0.85**	0.1275	0.35707	0.9775	0.98869	1.01144
0.16	**0.84**	0.1344	0.36661	0.9744	0.98712	1.01305
0.17	**0.83**	0.1411	0.37563	0.9711	0.98544	1.01477
0.18	**0.82**	0.1476	0.38419	0.9676	0.98367	1.01660
0.19	**0.81**	0.1539	0.39230	0.9639	0.98178	1.01855
0.20	**0.80**	0.1600	0.40000	0.9600	0.97980	1.02062
0.21	**0.79**	0.1659	0.40731	0.9559	0.97770	1.02281
0.22	**0.78**	0.1716	0.41425	0.9516	0.97550	1.02512
0.23	**0.77**	0.1771	0.42083	0.9471	0.97319	1.02755
0.24	**0.76**	0.1824	0.42708	0.9424	0.97077	1.03011
0.25	**0.75**	0.1875	0.43301	0.9375	0.96825	1.03280
0.26	**0.74**	0.1924	0.43863	0.9324	0.96561	1.03562
0.27	**0.73**	0.1971	0.44396	0.9271	0.96286	1.03857
0.28	**0.72**	0.2016	0.44900	0.9216	0.96000	1.04167
0.29	**0.71**	0.2059	0.45376	0.9159	0.95703	1.04490
0.30	**0.70**	0.2100	0.45826	0.9100	0.95394	1.04828
0.31	**0.69**	0.2139	0.46249	0.9039	0.95074	1.05182
0.32	**0.68**	0.2176	0.46648	0.8976	0.94742	1.05550
0.33	**0.67**	0.2211	0.47021	0.8911	0.94398	1.05934
0.34	**0.66**	0.2244	0.47371	0.8844	0.94043	1.06335
0.35	**0.65**	0.2275	0.47697	0.8775	0.93675	1.06752
0.36	**0.64**	0.2304	0.48000	0.8704	0.93295	1.07187
0.37	**0.63**	0.2331	0.48280	0.8631	0.92903	1.07639
0.38	**0.62**	0.2356	0.48539	0.8556	0.92499	1.08110
0.39	**0.61**	0.2379	0.48775	0.8479	0.92081	1.08599
0.40	**0.60**	0.2400	0.48990	0.8400	0.91652	1.09109
0.41	**0.59**	0.2419	0.49183	0.8319	0.91209	1.09639
0.42	**0.58**	0.2436	0.49356	0.8236	0.90752	1.10190
0.43	**0.57**	0.2451	0.49508	0.8151	0.90283	1.10763
0.44	**0.56**	0.2464	0.49639	0.8064	0.89800	1.11359
0.45	**0.55**	0.2475	0.49749	0.7975	0.89303	1.11979
0.46	**0.54**	0.2484	0.49840	0.7884	0.88792	1.12623
0.47	**0.53**	0.2491	0.49910	0.7791	0.88267	1.13293
0.48	**0.52**	0.2496	0.49960	0.7696	0.87727	1.13990
0.49	**0.51**	0.2499	0.49990	0.7599	0.87172	1.14715
0.50	**0.50**	0.2500	0.50000	0.7500	0.86603	1.15470

VARIOUS FUNCTIONS OF p AND $q = 1 - p$

p	$q = 1 - p$	$p^2 + q^2$	$1 - q^2$	$\Gamma(1 + p)$	$\log_{10} \Gamma(1 + p)$	$2 \arcsin \sqrt{p}$	$2 \arcsin \sqrt{q}$
0.00	**1.00**	1.0000	0.0000	1.0000 000	0.0000 000	0.0000	3.1416
0.01	**0.99**	0.9802	0.0199	0.9943 259	$\bar{1}$.9975 287	0.2003	2.9413
0.02	**0.98**	0.9608	0.0396	0.9888 442	$\bar{1}$.9951 279	0.2838	2.8578
0.03	**0.97**	0.9418	0.0591	0.9835 500	$\bar{1}$.9927 964	0.3482	2.7934
0.04	**0.96**	0.9232	0.0784	0.9784 382	$\bar{1}$.9905 334	0.4027	2.7389
0.05	**0.95**	0.9050	0.0975	0.9735 043	$\bar{1}$.9883 379	0.4510	2.6906
0.06	**0.94**	0.8872	0.1164	0.9687 436	$\bar{1}$.9862 089	0.4949	2.6467
0.07	**0.93**	0.8698	0.1351	0.9641 520	$\bar{1}$.9841 455	0.5355	2.6061
0.08	**0.92**	0.8528	0.1536	0.9597 253	$\bar{1}$.9821 469	0.5735	2.5681
0.09	**0.91**	0.8362	0.1719	0.9554 595	$\bar{1}$.9802 123	0.6094	2.5322
0.10	**0.90**	0.8200	0.1900	0.9513 508	$\bar{1}$.9783 407	0.6435	2.4981
0.11	**0.89**	0.8042	0.2079	0.9473 955	$\bar{1}$.9765 313	0.6761	2.4655
0.12	**0.88**	0.7888	0.2256	0.9435 902	$\bar{1}$.9747 834	0.7075	2.4341
0.13	**0.87**	0.7738	0.2431	0.9399 314	$\bar{1}$.9730 962	0.7377	2.4039
0.14	**0.86**	0.7592	0.2604	0.9364 161	$\bar{1}$.9714 689	0.7670	2.3746
0.15	**0.85**	0.7450	0.2775	0.9330 409	$\bar{1}$.9699 007	0.7954	2.3462
0.16	**0.84**	0.7312	0.2944	0.9298 031	$\bar{1}$.9683 910	0.8230	2.3186
0.17	**0.83**	0.7178	0.3111	0.9266 996	$\bar{1}$.9669 390	0.8500	2.2916
0.18	**0.82**	0.7048	0.3276	0.9237 278	$\bar{1}$.9655 440	0.8763	2.2653
0.19	**0.81**	0.6922	0.3439	0.9208 850	$\bar{1}$.9642 054	0.9021	2.2395
0.20	**0.80**	0.6800	0.3600	0.9181 687	$\bar{1}$.9629 225	0.9273	2.2143
0.21	**0.79**	0.6682	0.3759	0.9155 765	$\bar{1}$.9616 946	0.9521	2.1895
0.22	**0.78**	0.6568	0.3916	0.9131 059	$\bar{1}$.9605 212	0.9764	2.1652
0.23	**0.77**	0.6458	0.4071	0.9107 549	$\bar{1}$.9594 015	1.0004	2.1412
0.24	**0.76**	0.6352	0.4224	0.9085 211	$\bar{1}$.9583 350	1.0239	2.1176
0.25	**0.75**	0.6250	0.4375	0.9064 025	$\bar{1}$.9573 211	1.0472	2.0944
0.26	**0.74**	0.6152	0.4524	0.9043 971	$\bar{1}$.9563 592	1.0701	2.0715
0.27	**0.73**	0.6058	0.4671	0.9025 031	$\bar{1}$.9554 487	1.0928	2.0488
0.28	**0.72**	0.5968	0.4816	0.9007 185	$\bar{1}$.9545 891	1.1152	2.0264
0.29	**0.71**	0.5882	0.4959	0.8990 416	$\bar{1}$.9537 798	1.1374	2.0042
0.30	**0.70**	0.5800	0.5100	0.8974 707	$\bar{1}$.9530 203	1.1593	1.9823
0.31	**0.69**	0.5722	0.5239	0.8960 042	$\bar{1}$.9523 100	1.1810	1.9606
0.32	**0.68**	0.5648	0.5376	0.8946 405	$\bar{1}$.9516 485	1.2025	1.9391
0.33	**0.67**	0.5578	0.5511	0.8933 781	$\bar{1}$.9510 353	1.2239	1.9177
0.34	**0.66**	0.5512	0.5644	0.8922 155	$\bar{1}$.9504 698	1.2451	1.8965
0.35	**0.65**	0.5450	0.5775	0.8911 514	$\bar{1}$.9499 515	1.2661	1.8755
0.36	**0.64**	0.5392	0.5904	0.8901 845	$\bar{1}$.9494 800	1.2870	1.8546
0.37	**0.63**	0.5338	0.6031	0.8893 135	$\bar{1}$.9490 549	1.3078	1.8338
0.38	**0.62**	0.5288	0.6156	0.8885 371	$\bar{1}$.9486 756	1.3284	1.8132
0.39	**0.61**	0.5242	0.6279	0.8878 543	$\bar{1}$.9483 417	1.3490	1.7926
0.40	**0.60**	0.5200	0.6400	0.8872 638	$\bar{1}$.9480 528	1.3694	1.7722
0.41	**0.59**	0.5162	0.6519	0.8867 647	$\bar{1}$.9478 084	1.3898	1.7518
0.42	**0.58**	0.5128	0.6636	0.8863 558	$\bar{1}$.9476 081	1.4101	1.7315
0.43	**0.57**	0.5098	0.6751	0.8860 362	$\bar{1}$.9474 515	1.4303	1.7113
0.44	**0.56**	0.5072	0.6864	0.8858 051	$\bar{1}$.9473 382	1.4505	1.6911
0.45	**0.55**	0.5050	0.6975	0.8856 614	$\bar{1}$.9472 677	1.4706	1.6710
0.46	**0.54**	0.5032	0.7084	0.8856 043	$\bar{1}$.9472 397	1.4907	1.6509
0.47	**0.53**	0.5018	0.7191	0.8856 331	$\bar{1}$.9472 539	1.5108	1.6308
0.48	**0.52**	0.5008	0.7296	0.8857 470	$\bar{1}$.9473 097	1.5308	1.6108
0.49	**0.51**	0.5002	0.7399	0.8859 451	$\bar{1}$.9474 068	1.5508	1.5908
0.50	**0.50**	0.5000	0.7500	0.8862 269	$\bar{1}$.9475 449	1.5708	1.5708

VARIOUS FUNCTIONS OF p AND $q = 1 - p$

p	$q = 1 - p$	pq	$\sqrt{(pq)}$	$1 - p^2$	$\sqrt{(1 - p^2)}$	$\frac{1}{\sqrt{(1 - p^2)}}$
0.50	**0.50**	0.2500	0.50000	0.7500	0.86603	1.15470
0.51	**0.49**	0.2499	0.49990	0.7399	0.86017	1.16255
0.52	**0.48**	0.2496	0.49960	0.7296	0.85417	1.17073
0.53	**0.47**	0.2491	0.49910	0.7191	0.84800	1.17925
0.54	**0.46**	0.2484	0.49840	0.7084	0.84167	1.18812
0.55	**0.45**	0.2475	0.49749	0.6975	0.83516	1.19737
0.56	**0.44**	0.2464	0.49639	0.6864	0.82849	1.20701
0.57	**0.43**	0.2451	0.49508	0.6751	0.82164	1.21707
0.58	**0.42**	0.2436	0.49356	0.6636	0.81462	1.22757
0.59	**0.41**	0.2419	0.49183	0.6519	0.80740	1.23854
0.60	**0.40**	0.2400	0.48990	0.6400	0.80000	1.25000
0.61	**0.39**	0.2379	0.48775	0.6279	0.79240	1.26199
0.62	**0.38**	0.2356	0.48539	0.6156	0.78460	1.27453
0.63	**0.37**	0.2331	0.48280	0.6031	0.77660	1.28767
0.64	**0.36**	0.2304	0.48000	0.5904	0.76837	1.30145
0.65	**0.35**	0.2275	0.47697	0.5775	0.75993	1.31590
0.66	**0.34**	0.2244	0.47371	0.5644	0.75127	1.33109
0.67	**0.33**	0.2211	0.47021	0.5511	0.74236	1.34705
0.68	**0.32**	0.2176	0.46648	0.5376	0.73321	1.36386
0.69	**0.31**	0.2139	0.46249	0.5239	0.72381	1.38158
0.70	**0.30**	0.2100	0.45826	0.5100	0.71414	1.40028
0.71	**0.29**	0.2059	0.45376	0.4959	0.70420	1.42005
0.72	**0.28**	0.2016	0.44900	0.4816	0.69397	1.44098
0.73	**0.27**	0.1971	0.44396	0.4671	0.68345	1.46317
0.74	**0.26**	0.1924	0.43863	0.4524	0.67261	1.48675
0.75	**0.25**	0.1875	0.43301	0.4375	0.66144	1.51186
0.76	**0.24**	0.1824	0.42708	0.4224	0.64992	1.53864
0.77	**0.23**	0.1771	0.42083	0.4071	0.63804	1.56729
0.78	**0.22**	0.1716	0.41425	0.3916	0.62578	1.59801
0.79	**0.21**	0.1659	0.40731	0.3759	0.61311	1.63104
0.80	**0.20**	0.1600	0.40000	0.3600	0.60000	1.66667
0.81	**0.19**	0.1539	0.39230	0.3439	0.58643	1.70523
0.82	**0.18**	0.1476	0.38419	0.3276	0.57236	1.74714
0.83	**0.17**	0.1411	0.37563	0.3111	0.55776	1.79287
0.84	**0.16**	0.1344	0.36661	0.2944	0.54259	1.84302
0.85	**0.15**	0.1275	0.35707	0.2775	0.52678	1.89832
0.86	**0.14**	0.1204	0.34699	0.2604	0.51029	1.95965
0.87	**0.13**	0.1131	0.33630	0.2431	0.49305	2.02818
0.88	**0.12**	0.1056	0.32496	0.2256	0.47497	2.10538
0.89	**0.11**	0.0979	0.31289	0.2079	0.45596	2.19317
0.90	**0.10**	0.0900	0.30000	0.1900	0.43589	2.29416
0.91	**0.09**	0.0819	0.28618	0.1719	0.41461	2.41192
0.92	**0.08**	0.0736	0.27129	0.1536	0.39192	2.55155
0.93	**0.07**	0.0651	0.25515	0.1351	0.36756	2.72065
0.94	**0.06**	0.0564	0.23749	0.1164	0.34117	2.93105
0.95	**0.05**	0.0475	0.21794	0.0975	0.31225	3.20256
0.96	**0.04**	0.0384	0.19596	0.0784	0.28000	3.57143
0.97	**0.03**	0.0291	0.17059	0.0591	0.24310	4.11345
0.98	**0.02**	0.0196	0.14000	0.0396	0.19900	5.02519
0.99	**0.01**	0.0099	0.09950	0.0199	0.14107	7.08881
1.00	**0.00**	0.0000	0.00000	0.0000	0.00000	∞

VARIOUS FUNCTIONS OF p AND $q = 1 - p$

p	$q = 1 - p$	$p^2 + q^2$	$1 - q^2$	$\Gamma(1 + p)$	$\log_{10} \Gamma(1 + p)$	$2 \text{ arc sin } \sqrt{p}$	$2 \text{ arc sin } \sqrt{q}$
0.50	**0.50**	0.5000	0.7500	0.8862 269	$\bar{1}$.9475 449	1.5708	1.5708
0.51	**0.49**	0.5002	0.7599	0.8865 917	$\bar{1}$.9477 237	1.5908	1.5508
0.52	**0.48**	0.5008	0.7696	0.8870 388	$\bar{1}$.9479 426	1.6108	1.5308
0.53	**0.47**	0.5018	0.7791	0.8875 676	$\bar{1}$.9482 015	1.6308	1.5108
0.54	**0.46**	0.5032	0.7884	0.8881 777	$\bar{1}$.9484 998	1.6509	1.4907
0.55	**0.45**	0.5050	0.7975	0.8888 683	$\bar{1}$.9488 374	1.6710	1.4706
0.56	**0.44**	0.5072	0.8064	0.8896 392	$\bar{1}$.9492 139	1.6911	1.4505
0.57	**0.43**	0.5098	0.8151	0.8904 897	$\bar{1}$.9496 289	1.7113	1.4303
0.58	**0.42**	0.5128	0.8236	0.8914 196	$\bar{1}$.9500 822	1.7315	1.4101
0.59	**0.41**	0.5162	0.8319	0.8924 282	$\bar{1}$.9505 733	7.7518	1.3898
0.60	**0.40**	0.5200	0.8400	0.8935 153	$\bar{1}$.9511 020	1.7722	1.3694
0.61	**0.39**	0.5242	0.8479	0.8946 806	$\bar{1}$.9516 680	1.7926	1.3490
0.62	**0.38**	0.5288	0.8556	0.8959 237	$\bar{1}$.9522 710	1.8132	1.3284
0.63	**0.37**	0.5338	0.8631	0.8972 442	$\bar{1}$.9529 107	1.8338	1.3078
0.64	**0.36**	0.5392	0.8704	0.8986 420	$\bar{1}$.9535 867	1.8546	1.2870
0.65	**0.35**	0.5450	0.8775	0.9001 168	$\bar{1}$.9542 989	1.8755	1.2661
0.66	**0.34**	0.5512	0.8844	0.9016 684	$\bar{1}$.9550 468	1.8965	1.2451
0.67	**0.33**	0.5578	0.8911	0.9032 965	$\bar{1}$.9558 303	1.9177	1.2239
0.68	**0.32**	0.5648	0.8976	0.9050 010	$\bar{1}$.9566 491	1.9391	1.2025
0.69	**0.31**	0.5722	0.9039	0.9067 818	$\bar{1}$.9575 028	1.9606	1.1810
0.70	**0.30**	0.5800	0.9100	0.9086 387	$\bar{1}$.9583 912	1.9823	1.1593
0.71	**0.29**	0.5882	0.9159	0.9105 717	$\bar{1}$.9593 141	2.0042	1.1374
0.72	**0.28**	0.5968	0.9216	0.9125 806	$\bar{1}$.9602 712	2.0264	1.1152
0.73	**0.27**	0.6058	0.9271	0.9146 654	$\bar{1}$.9612 622	2.0488	1.0928
0.74	**0.26**	0.6152	0.9324	0.9168 260	$\bar{1}$.9622 869	2.0715	1.0701
0.75	**0.25**	0.6250	0.9375	0.9190 625	$\bar{1}$.9633 451	2.0944	1.0472
0.76	**0.24**	0.6352	0.9424	0.9213 749	$\bar{1}$.9644 364	2.1176	1.0239
0.77	**0.23**	0.6458	0.9471	0.9237 631	$\bar{1}$.9655 606	2.1412	1.0004
0.78	**0.22**	0.6568	0.9516	0.9262 273	$\bar{1}$.9667 176	2.1652	0.9764
0.79	**0.21**	0.6682	0.9559	0.9287 675	$\bar{1}$.9679 070	2.1895	0.9521
0.80	**0.20**	0.6800	0.9600	0.9313 838	$\bar{1}$.9691 287	2.2143	0.9273
0.81	**0.19**	0.6922	0.9639	0.9340 763	$\bar{1}$.9703 823	2.2395	0.9021
0.82	**0.18**	0.7048	0.9676	0.9368 451	$\bar{1}$.9716 678	2.2653	0.8763
0.83	**0.17**	0.7178	0.9711	0.9396 904	$\bar{1}$.9729 848	2.2916	0.8500
0.84	**0.16**	0.7312	0.9744	0.9426 124	$\bar{1}$.9743 331	2.3186	0.8230
0.85	**0.15**	0.7450	0.9775	0.9456 112	$\bar{1}$.9757 126	2.3462	0.7954
0.86	**0.14**	0.7592	0.9804	0.9486 870	$\bar{1}$.9771 230	2.3746	0.7670
0.87	**0.13**	0.7738	0.9831	0.9518 402	$\bar{1}$.9785 640	2.4039	0.7377
0.88	**0.12**	0.7888	0.9856	0.9550 709	$\bar{1}$.9800 356	2.4341	0.7075
0.89	**0.11**	0.8042	0.9879	0.9583 793	$\bar{1}$.9815 374	2.4655	0.6761
0.90	**0.10**	0.8200	0.9900	0.9617 658	$\bar{1}$.9830 693	2.4981	0.6435
0.91	**0.09**	0.8362	0.9919	0.9652 307	$\bar{1}$.9846 311	2.5322	0.6094
0.92	**0.08**	0.8528	0.9936	0.9687 743	$\bar{1}$.9862 226	2.5681	0.5735
0.93	**0.07**	0.8698	0.9951	0.9723 969	$\bar{1}$.9878 436	2.6061	0.5355
0.94	**0.06**	0.8872	0.9964	0.9760 989	$\bar{1}$.9894 938	2.6467	0.4949
0.95	**0.05**	0.9050	0.9975	0.9798 807	$\bar{1}$.9911 732	2.6906	0.4510
0.96	**0.04**	0.9232	0.9984	0.9837 425	$\bar{1}$.9928 815	2.7389	0.4027
0.97	**0.03**	0.9418	0.9991	0.9876 850	$\bar{1}$.9946 185	2.7934	0.3482
0.98	**0.02**	0.9608	0.9996	0.9917 084	$\bar{1}$.9963 840	2.8578	0.2838
0.99	**0.01**	0.9802	0.9999	0.9958 133	$\bar{1}$.9981 779	2.9413	0.2003
1.00	**0.00**	1.0000	1.0000	1.0000 000	0.0000 000	3.1416	0.0000

III.8 HYPERGEOMETRIC DISTRIBUTION

The hypergeometric probability function is given by

$$f(x;N,n,k) = \frac{\binom{k}{x}\binom{N-k}{n-x}}{\binom{N}{n}} = \frac{\dfrac{k!}{x!(k-x)!}\,\dfrac{(N-k)!}{(n-x)!(N-k-n+x)!}}{\dfrac{N!}{n!(N-n)!}}$$

$$= \frac{k!n!}{x!(k-x)!(n-x)!}\,\frac{(N-k)!(N-n)!}{N!(N-k-n+x)!},$$

where N = number of items in a finite population consisting of A successes and B failures $(A + B = N)$
n = number of items drawn in sample without replacement, from the N items
k = number of failures in finite population $= B$
x = number of failures in sample .

$f(x;N,n,k)$ gives the probability of exactly x failures and $n - x$ successes in the sample of n items.

$$F(x;N,n,k) = \sum_{r=0}^{x} \frac{\binom{k}{r}\binom{N-k}{n-r}}{\binom{N}{n}}.$$

$F(x;N,n,k)$ gives the probability of x or fewer failures in the sample of n items.

HYPERGEOMETRIC PROBABILITY AND DISTRIBUTION FUNCTIONS

$$f(x;N,n,k) = \frac{\binom{k}{x}\binom{N-k}{n-x}}{\binom{N}{n}}, \qquad F(x;N,n,k) = \sum_{r=0}^{x} \frac{\binom{k}{r}\binom{N-k}{n-r}}{\binom{N}{n}}$$

N	n	k	x	$F(x)$	$f(x)$	N	n	k	x	$F(x)$	$f(x)$
2	1	1	0	0.500000	0.500000	6	2	2	2	1.000000	0.066667
2	1	1	1	1.000000	0.500000	6	3	1	0	0.500000	0.500000
3	1	1	0	0.666667	0.666667	6	3	1	1	1.000000	0.500000
3	1	1	1	1.000000	0.333333	6	3	2	0	0.200000	0.200000
3	2	1	0	0.333333	0.333333	6	3	2	1	0.800000	0.600000
3	2	1	1	1.000000	0.666667	6	3	2	2	1.000000	0.200000
3	2	2	1	0.666667	0.666667	6	3	3	0	0.050000	0.050000
3	2	2	2	1.000000	0.333333	6	3	3	1	0.500000	0.450000
4	1	1	0	0.750000	0.750000	6	3	3	2	0.950000	0.450000
4	1	1	1	1.000000	0.250000	6	3	3	3	1.000000	0.050000
4	2	1	0	0.500000	0.500000	6	4	1	0	0.333333	0.333333
4	2	1	1	1.000000	0.500000	6	4	1	1	1.000000	0.666667
4	2	2	0	0.166667	0.166667	6	4	2	0	0.066667	0.066667
4	2	2	1	0.833333	0.666667	6	4	2	1	0.600000	0.533333
4	2	2	2	1.000000	0.166667	6	4	2	2	1.000000	0.400000
4	3	1	0	0.250000	0.250000	6	4	3	1	0.200000	0.200000
4	3	1	1	1.000000	0.750000	6	4	3	2	0.800000	0.600000
4	3	2	1	0.500000	0.500000	6	4	3	3	1.000000	0.200000
4	3	2	2	1.000000	0.500000	6	4	4	2	0.400000	0.400000
4	3	3	2	0.750000	0.750000	6	4	4	3	0.933333	0.533333
4	3	3	3	1.000000	0.250000	6	4	4	4	1.000000	0.066667
5	1	1	0	0.800000	0.800000	6	5	1	0	0.166667	0.166667
5	1	1	1	1.000000	0.200000	6	5	1	1	1.000000	0.833333
5	2	1	0	0.600000	0.600000	6	5	2	1	0.333333	0.333333
5	2	1	1	1.000000	0.400000	6	5	2	2	1.000000	0.666667
5	2	2	0	0.300000	0.300000	6	5	3	2	0.500000	0.500000
5	2	2	1	0.900000	0.600000	6	5	3	3	1.000000	0.500000
5	2	2	2	1.000000	0.100000	6	5	4	3	0.666667	0.666667
5	3	1	0	0.400000	0.400000	6	5	4	4	1.000000	0.333333
5	3	1	1	1.000000	0.600000	6	5	5	4	0.833333	0.833333
5	3	2	0	0.100000	0.100000	6	5	5	5	1.000000	0.166667
5	3	2	1	0.700000	0.600000	7	1	1	0	0.857143	0.857143
5	3	2	2	1.000000	0.300000	7	1	1	1	1.000000	0.142857
5	3	3	1	0.300000	0.300000	7	2	1	0	0.714286	0.714286
5	3	3	2	0.900000	0.600000	7	2	1	1	1.000000	0.285714
5	3	3	3	1.000000	0.100000	7	2	2	0	0.476190	0.476190
5	4	1	0	0.200000	0.200000	7	2	2	1	0.952381	0.476190
5	4	1	1	1.000000	0.800000	7	2	2	2	1.000000	0.047619
5	4	2	1	0.400000	0.400000	7	3	1	0	0.571429	0.571429
5	4	2	2	0.000000	0.600000	7	3	1	1	1.000000	0.428571
5	4	3	2	0.600000	0.600000	7	3	2	0	0.285714	0.285714
5	4	3	3	1.000000	0.400000	7	3	2	1	0.857143	0.571429
5	4	4	3	0.800000	0.800000	7	3	2	2	1.000000	0.142857
5	4	4	4	1.000000	0.200000	7	3	3	0	0.114286	0.114286
6	1	1	0	0.833333	0.833333	7	3	3	1	0.628571	0.514286
6	1	1	1	1.000000	0.166667	7	3	3	2	0.971428	0.342857
6	2	1	0	0.666667	0.666667	7	3	3	3	1.000000	0.028571
6	2	1	1	1.000000	0.333333	7	4	1	0	0.428571	0.428571
6	2	2	0	0.400000	0.400000	7	4	1	1	1.000000	0.571429
6	2	2	1	0.933333	0.533333	7	4	2	0	0.142857	0.142857

HYPERGEOMETRIC PROBABILITY AND DISTRIBUTION FUNCTIONS

N	n	k	x	$F(x)$	$f(x)$	N	n	k	x	$F(x)$	$f(x)$
7	4	2	1	0.714286	0.571429	8	3	3	2	0.982143	0.267857
7	4	2	2	1.000000	0.285714	8	3	3	3	1.000000	0.017857
7	4	3	0	0.028571	0.028571	8	4	1	0	0.500000	0.500000
7	4	3	1	0.371429	0.342857	8	4	1	1	1.000000	0.500000
7	4	3	2	0.885714	0.514286	8	4	2	0	0.214286	0.214286
7	4	3	3	1.000000	0.114286	8	4	2	1	0.785714	0.571429
7	4	4	1	0.114286	0.114286	8	4	2	2	1.000000	0.214286
7	4	4	2	0.628571	0.514286	8	4	3	0	0.071429	0.071429
7	4	4	3	0.971428	0.342857	8	4	3	1	0.500000	0.428571
7	4	4	4	1.000000	0.028571	8	4	3	2	0.928571	0.428571
7	5	1	0	0.285714	0.285714	8	4	3	3	1.000000	0.071429
7	5	1	1	1.000000	0.714286	8	4	4	0	0.014286	0.014286
7	5	2	0	0.047619	0.047619	8	4	4	1	0.242857	0.228571
7	5	2	1	0.523809	0.476190	8	4	4	2	0.757143	0.514286
7	5	2	2	1.000000	0.476190	8	4	4	3	0.985714	0.228571
7	5	3	1	0.142857	0.142857	8	4	4	4	1.000000	0.014286
7	5	3	2	0.714286	0.571429	8	5	1	0	0.375000	0.375000
7	5	3	3	1.000000	0.285714	8	5	1	1	1.000000	0.625000
7	5	4	2	0.285714	0.285714	8	5	2	0	0.107143	0.107143
7	5	4	3	0.857143	0.571429	8	5	2	1	0.642857	0.535714
7	5	4	4	1.000000	0.142857	8	5	2	2	1.000000	0.357143
7	5	5	3	0.476190	0.476190	8	5	3	0	0.017857	0.017857
7	5	5	4	0.952381	0.476190	8	5	3	1	0.285714	0.267857
7	5	5	5	1.000000	0.047619	8	5	3	2	0.821429	0.535714
7	6	1	0	0.142857	0.142857	8	5	3	3	1.000000	0.178571
7	6	1	1	1.000000	0.857143	8	5	4	1	0.071429	0.071429
7	6	2	1	0.285714	0.285714	8	5	4	2	0.500000	0.428571
7	6	2	2	1.000000	0.714286	8	5	4	3	0.928571	0.428571
7	6	3	2	0.428571	0.428571	8	5	4	4	1.000000	0.071429
7	6	3	3	1.000000	0.571429	8	5	5	2	0.178571	0.178571
7	6	4	3	0.571429	0.571429	8	5	5	3	0.714286	0.535714
7	6	4	4	1.000000	0.428571	8	5	5	4	0.982143	0.267857
7	6	5	4	0.714286	0.714286	8	5	5	5	1.000000	0.017857
7	6	5	5	1.000000	0.285714	8	6	1	0	0.250000	0.250000
7	6	6	5	0.857143	0.857143	8	6	1	1	1.000000	0.750000
7	6	6	6	1.000000	0.142857	8	6	2	0	0.035714	0.035714
8	1	1	0	0.875000	0.875000	8	6	2	1	0.464286	0.428571
8	1	1	1	1.000000	0.125000	8	6	2	2	1.000000	0.535714
8	2	1	0	0.750000	0.750000	8	6	3	1	0.107143	0.107143
8	2	1	1	1.000000	0.250000	8	6	3	2	0.642857	0.535714
8	2	2	0	0.535714	0.535714	8	6	3	3	1.000000	0.357143
8	2	2	1	0.964286	0.428571	8	6	4	2	0.214286	0.214286
8	2	2	2	1.000000	0.035714	8	6	4	3	0.785714	0.571429
8	3	1	0	0.625000	0.625000	8	6	4	4	1.000000	0.214286
8	3	1	1	1.000000	0.375000	8	6	5	3	0.357143	0.357143
8	3	2	0	0.357143	0.357143	8	6	5	4	0.892857	0.535714
8	3	2	1	0.892857	0.535714	8	6	5	5	1.000000	0.107143
8	3	2	2	1.000000	0.107143	8	6	6	4	0.535714	0.535714
8	3	3	0	0.178571	0.178571	8	6	6	5	0.964286	0.428571
8	3	3	1	0.714286	0.535714	8	6	6	6	1.000000	0.035714

HYPERGEOMETRIC PROBABILITY AND DISTRIBUTION FUNCTIONS

N	n	k	x	F(x)	f(x)	N	n	k	x	F(x)	f(x)
8	7	1	0	0.125000	0.125000	9	5	3	1	0.404762	0.357143
8	7	1	1	1.000000	0.875000	9	5	3	2	0.880952	0.476190
8	7	2	1	0.250000	0.250000	9	5	3	3	1.000000	0.119048
8	7	2	2	1.000000	0.750000	9	5	4	0	0.007936	0.007936
8	7	3	2	0.375000	0.375000	9	5	4	1	0.166667	0.158730
8	7	3	3	1.000000	0.625000	9	5	4	2	0.642857	0.476190
8	7	4	3	0.500000	0.500000	9	5	4	3	0.960317	0.317460
8	7	4	4	1.000000	0.500000	9	5	4	4	1.000000	0.039683
8	7	5	4	0.625000	0.625000	9	5	5	1	0.039683	0.039683
8	7	5	5	1.000000	0.375000	9	5	5	2	0.357143	0.317460
8	7	6	5	0.750000	0.750000	9	5	5	3	0.833333	0.476190
8	7	6	6	1.000000	0.250000	9	5	5	4	0.992063	0.158730
8	7	7	6	0.875000	0.875000	9	5	5	5	1.000000	0.007936
8	7	7	7	1.000000	0.125000	9	6	1	0	0.333333	0.333333
9	1	1	0	0.888889	0.888889	9	6	1	1	1.000000	0.666667
9	1	1	1	1.000000	0.111111	9	6	2	0	0.083333	0.083333
9	2	1	0	0.777778	0.777778	9	6	2	1	0.583333	0.500000
9	2	1	1	1.000000	0.222222	9	6	2	2	1.000000	0.416667
9	2	2	0	0.583333	0.583333	9	6	3	0	0.011905	0.011905
9	2	2	1	0.972222	0.388889	9	6	3	1	0.226190	0.214286
9	2	2	2	1.000000	0.027778	9	6	3	2	0.761905	0.535714
9	3	1	0	0.666667	0.666667	9	6	3	3	1.000000	0.238095
9	3	1	1	1.000000	0.333333	9	6	4	1	0.047619	0.047619
9	3	2	0	0.416667	0.416667	9	6	4	2	0.404762	0.357143
9	3	2	1	0.916667	0.500000	9	6	4	3	0.880952	0.476190
9	3	2	2	1.000000	0.083333	9	6	4	4	1.000000	0.119048
9	3	3	0	0.238095	0.238095	9	6	5	2	0.119048	0.119048
9	3	3	1	0.773809	0.535714	9	6	5	3	0.595238	0.476190
9	3	3	2	0.988095	0.214286	9	6	5	4	0.952381	0.357143
9	3	3	3	1.000000	0.011905	9	6	5	5	1.000000	0.047619
9	4	1	0	0.555556	0.555556	9	6	6	3	0.238095	0.238095
9	4	1	1	1.000000	0.444444	9	6	6	4	0.773809	0.535714
9	4	2	0	0.277778	0.277778	9	6	6	5	0.988095	0.214286
9	4	2	1	0.833333	0.555556	9	6	6	6	1.000000	0.011905
9	4	2	2	1.000000	0.166667	9	7	1	0	0.222222	0.222222
9	4	3	0	0.119048	0.119048	9	7	1	1	1.000000	0.777778
9	4	3	1	0.595238	0.476190	9	7	2	0	0.027778	0.027778
9	4	3	2	0.952381	0.357143	9	7	2	1	0.416667	0.388889
9	4	3	3	1.000000	0.047619	9	7	2	2	1.000000	0.583333
9	4	4	0	0.039683	0.039683	9	7	3	1	0.083333	0.083333
9	4	4	1	0.357143	0.317460	9	7	3	2	0.583333	0.500000
9	4	4	2	0.833333	0.476190	9	7	3	3	1.000000	0.416667
9	4	4	3	0.992063	0.158730	9	7	4	2	0.166667	0.166667
9	4	4	4	1.000000	0.007936	9	7	4	3	0.722222	0.555556
9	5	1	0	0.444444	0.444444	9	7	4	4	1.000000	0.277778
9	5	1	1	1.000000	0.555556	9	7	5	3	0.277778	0.277778
9	5	2	0	0.166667	0.166667	9	7	5	4	0.833333	0.555556
9	5	2	1	0.722222	0.555556	9	7	5	5	1.000000	0.166667
9	5	2	2	1.000000	0.277778	9	7	6	4	0.416667	0.416667
9	5	3	0	0.047619	0.047619	9	7	6	5	0.916667	0.500000

HYPERGEOMETRIC PROBABILITY AND DISTRIBUTION FUNCTIONS

N	n	k	x	$F(x)$	$f(x)$	N	n	k	x	$F(x)$	$f(x)$
9	7	6	6	1.000000	0.083333	10	5	1	0	0.500000	0.500000
9	7	7	5	0.583333	0.583333	10	5	1	1	1.000000	0.500000
9	7	7	6	0.972222	0.388889	10	5	2	0	0.222222	0.222222
9	7	7	7	1.000000	0.027778	10	5	2	1	0.777778	0.555556
9	8	1	0	0.111111	0.111111	10	5	2	2	1.000000	0.222222
9	8	1	1	1.000000	0.888889	10	5	3	0	0.083333	0.083333
9	8	2	1	0.222222	0.222222	10	5	3	1	0.500000	0.416667
9	8	2	2	1.000000	0.777778	10	5	3	2	0.916667	0.416667
9	8	3	2	0.333333	0.333333	10	5	3	3	1.000000	0.083333
9	8	3	3	1.000000	0.666667	10	5	4	0	0.023810	0.023810
9	8	4	3	0.444444	0.444444	10	5	4	1	0.261905	0.238095
9	8	4	4	1.000000	0.555556	10	5	4	2	0.738095	0.476190
9	8	5	4	0.555556	0.555556	10	5	4	3	0.976190	0.238095
9	8	5	5	1.000000	0.444444	10	5	4	4	1.000000	0.023810
9	8	6	5	0.666667	0.666667	10	5	5	0	0.003968	0.003968
9	8	6	6	1.000000	0.333333	10	5	5	1	0.103175	0.099206
9	8	7	6	0.777778	0.777778	10	5	5	2	0.500000	0.396825
9	8	7	7	1.000000	0.222222	10	5	5	3	0.896825	0.396825
9	8	8	7	0.888889	0.888889	10	5	5	4	0.996032	0.099206
9	8	8	8	1.000000	0.111111	10	5	5	5	1.000000	0.003968
10	1	1	0	0.900000	0.900000	10	6	1	0	0.400000	0.400000
10	1	1	1	1.000000	0.100000	10	6	1	1	1.000000	0.600000
10	2	1	0	0.800000	0.800000	10	6	2	0	0.133333	0.133333
10	2	1	1	1.000000	0.200000	10	6	2	1	0.666667	0.533333
10	2	2	0	0.622222	0.622222	10	6	2	2	1.000000	0.333333
10	2	2	1	0.977778	0.355556	10	6	3	0	0.033333	0.033333
10	2	2	2	1.000000	0.022222	10	6	3	1	0.333333	0.300000
10	3	1	0	0.700000	0.700000	10	6	3	2	0.833333	0.500000
10	3	1	1	1.000000	0.300000	10	6	3	3	1.000000	0.166667
10	3	2	0	0.466667	0.466667	10	6	4	0	0.004762	0.004762
10	3	2	1	0.933333	0.466667	10	6	4	1	0.119048	0.114286
10	3	2	2	1.000000	0.066667	10	6	4	2	0.547619	0.428571
10	3	3	0	0.291667	0.291667	10	6	4	3	0.928571	0.380952
10	3	3	1	0.816667	0.525000	10	6	4	4	1.000000	0.071429
10	3	3	2	0.991667	0.175000	10	6	5	1	0.023810	0.023810
10	3	3	3	1.000000	0.008333	10	6	5	2	0.261905	0.238095
10	4	1	0	0.600000	0.600000	10	6	5	3	0.738095	0.476190
10	4	1	1	1.000000	0.400000	10	6	5	4	0.976190	0.238095
10	4	2	0	0.333333	0.333333	10	6	5	5	1.000000	0.023810
10	4	2	1	0.866667	0.533333	10	6	6	2	0.071429	0.071429
10	4	2	2	1.000000	0.133333	10	6	6	3	0.452381	0.380952
10	4	3	0	0.166667	0.166667	10	6	6	4	0.880952	0.428571
10	4	3	1	0.666667	0.500000	10	6	6	5	0.995238	0.114286
10	4	3	2	0.966667	0.300000	10	6	6	6	1.000000	0.004762
10	4	3	3	1.000000	0.033333	10	7	1	0	0.300000	0.300000
10	4	4	0	0.071429	0.071429	10	7	1	1	1.000000	0.700000
10	4	4	1	0.452381	0.380952	10	7	2	0	0.066667	0.066667
10	4	4	2	0.880952	0.428571	10	7	2	1	0.533333	0.466667
10	4	4	3	0.995238	0.114286	10	7	2	2	1.000000	0.466667
10	4	4	4	1.000000	0.004762	10	7	3	0	0.008333	0.008333

III.9 NEGATIVE BINOMIAL DISTRIBUTION

The negative binomial probability function is given by

$$f(x;r,\theta) = \binom{x+r-1}{r-1} \theta^r (1-\theta)^x, \qquad x = 0, 1, 2, \ldots ;$$

where θ is the probability of success and $1 - \theta$ the probability of failure of a given event.

$f(x)$ is the probability that exactly $x + r$ trials will be required to produce r successes.

The cumulative distribution is given by

$$F(x;r,\theta) = \sum_{x'=0}^{x} \binom{x'+r-1}{r-1} \theta^r (1-\theta)^{x'} .$$

The cumulative negative binomial distribution is related to the cumulative binomial distribution as follows:

$$\sum_{x'=0}^{x} \binom{x'+r-1}{r-1} \theta^r (1-\theta)^{x'} = \sum_{x'=r}^{x+r} \binom{x+r}{x'} \theta^{x'} (1-\theta)^{x+r-x'} .$$

NEGATIVE BINOMIAL PROBABILITY AND DISTRIBUTION FUNCTIONS

$$f(x;r,\theta) = \binom{x+r-1}{r-1} \theta^r (1-\theta)^x, \qquad F(x;r,\theta) = \sum_{x'=0}^{x} \binom{x'+r-1}{r-1} \theta^r (1-\theta)^{x'}$$

$\theta = 0.900,\ r = 1$		
$x + r$	$f(x)$	$F(x)$
1	0.90000	0.9000
2	0.09000	0.9900

$\theta = 0.900,\ r = 2$		
$x + r$	$f(x)$	$F(x)$
2	0.81000	0.8100
3	0.16200	0.9720
4	0.02430	0.9963

$\theta = 0.900,\ r = 3$		
$x + r$	$f(x)$	$F(x)$
3	0.72900	0.7290
4	0.21870	0.9477
5	0.04374	0.9914

$\theta = 0.900,\ r = 4$		
$x + r$	$f(x)$	$F(x)$
4	0.65610	0.6561
5	0.26244	0.9185
6	0.06561	0.9841
7	0.01312	0.9973

$\theta = 0.900,\ r = 5$		
$x + r$	$f(x)$	$F(x)$
5	0.59049	0.5905
6	0.29524	0.8857
7	0.08857	0.9743
8	0.02067	0.9950

$\theta = 0.900,\ r = 6$		
$x + r$	$f(x)$	$F(x)$
6	0.53144	0.5314
7	0.31886	0.8503
8	0.11160	0.9619
9	0.02976	0.9917

III.10 PERCENTAGE POINTS OF THE BETA DISTRIBUTION

The incomplete beta function is defined as

$$I_x(a,b) = \frac{B_x(a,b)}{B(a,b)}$$
$$= \frac{\Gamma(a+b)}{\Gamma(a)\Gamma(b)} \int_0^x u^{a-1}(1-u)^{b-1}\,du.$$

This table gives lower percentage points of the distribution of x, i.e. the roots of $I_x(a,b) = P$ for various values of P. The corresponding upper percentage points can be obtained from

$$I_x(a,b) = 1 - I_{1-x}(b,a).$$

The incomplete beta function is related to the cumulative binomial distribution as follows:

$$I_\theta(x', n - x' + 1) = \sum_{x=x'}^{n} \binom{n}{x} \theta^x (1-\theta)^{n-x}.$$

PERCENTAGE POINTS OF THE BETA DISTRIBUTION

50% points for x

$\nu_1 = 2b,\ \nu_2 = 2a$

$\nu_2 \backslash \nu_1$	1	2	3	4	5	6	7	8	9
1	0.50000	0.25000	0.16319	0.12061	0.095526	0.079033	0.067378	0.058711	0.052015
2	.75000	.50000	.37004	.29289	.24214	.20630	.17966	.15910	.14276
3	.83681	.62996	.50000	.41363	.35245	.30695	.27181	.24386	.22112
4	.87939	.70711	.58637	.50000	.43556	.38573	.34609	.31381	.28703
5	0.90447	0.75786	0.64755	0.56444	0.50000	0.44867	0.40684	0.37213	0.34286
6	.92097	.79370	.69305	.61427	.55133	.50000	.45737	.42141	.39068
7	.93262	.82034	.72819	.65391	.59316	.54263	.50000	.46355	.43205
8	.94129	.84090	.75614	.68619	.62787	.57859	.53645	.50000	.46818
9	.94799	.85724	.77888	.71297	.65714	.60932	.56795	.53182	.50000
10	0.95331	0.87055	0.79775	0.73555	0.68214	0.63588	0.59546	0.55984	0.52824
11	.95765	.88159	.81366	.75484	.70376	.65907	.61968	.58471	.55346
12	.96125	.89090	.82725	.77151	.72262	.67948	.64116	.60692	.57613
13	.96429	.89885	.83899	.78606	.73923	.69759	.66035	.62687	.59661
14	.96689	.90572	.84924	.79887	.75396	.71376	.67760	.64490	.61520
15	0.96913	0.91172	0.85827	0.81023	0.76712	0.72830	0.69318	0.66127	0.63216
16	.97109	.91700	.86627	.82038	.77894	.74143	.70732	.67620	.64768
17	.97282	.92169	.87342	.82950	.78963	.75334	.72022	.68986	.66195
18	.97435	.92587	.87985	.83774	.79932	.76421	.73203	.70242	.67511
19	.97572	.92964	.88565	.84522	.80817	.77417	.74288	.71401	.68728
20	0.97695	0.93303	0.89092	0.85204	0.81626	0.78331	0.75289	0.72472	0.69858
21	.97806	.93612	.89573	.85828	.82370	.79175	.76215	.73467	.70909
22	.97907	.93893	.90013	.86402	.83057	.79955	.77074	.74392	.71889
23	.97999	.94151	.90417	.86931	.83692	.80679	.77873	.75254	.72805
24	.98083	.94387	.90790	.87421	.84281	.81353	.78618	.76061	.73663
25	0.98161	0.94606	0.91135	0.87875	0.84828	0.81981	0.79315	0.76816	0.74469
26	.98232	.94808	.91455	.88298	.85340	.82568	.79968	.77526	.75227
27	.98298	.94995	.91753	.88692	.85817	.83118	.80581	.78193	.75941
28	.98360	.95170	.92031	.89060	.86265	.83635	.81157	.78821	.76615
29	.98417	.95332	.92290	.89406	.86685	.84120	.81701	.79415	.77253
30	0.98470	0.95484	0.92534	0.89730	0.87080	0.84578	0.82214	0.79976	0.77856
40	.98855	.96594	.94324	.92136	.90038	.88030	.86107	.84266	.82501
60	.99238	.97716	.96164	.94645	.93166	.91731	.90338	.88985	.87672
120	.99620	.98851	.98056	.97264	.96482	.95710	.94951	.94202	.93465
∞	1.00000	1.00000	1.00000	1.00000	1.00000	1.00000	1.00000	1.00000	1.00000

This table gives the values of x for which

$$I_x(a, b) = \int_0^x u^{a-1}(1-u)^{b-1}\,du \Big/ \int_0^1 u^{a-1}(1-u)^{b-1}\,du = 0.50,$$

where $a = \frac{1}{2}\nu_2$, $b = \frac{1}{2}\nu_1$.

PERCENTAGE POINTS OF THE BETA DISTRIBUTION

50% points for x

$\nu_1 = 2b,\ \nu_2 = 2a$

ν_2 \ ν_1	10	12	15	20	24	30	40	60	120
1	0.046687	0.038746	0.030867	0.023052	0.019168	0.015301	0.011450	0.0076165	0.0037997
2	.12945	.10910	.088278	.066967	.056126	.045158	.034064	.022840	.011486
3	.20225	.17275	.14173	.10908	.092099	.074664	.056756	.038355	.019443
4	.26445	.22849	.18977	.14796	.12579	.10270	.078644	.053552	.027361
5	0.31786	0.27738	0.23288	0.18374	0.15719	0.12920	0.099622	0.068335	0.035184
6	.36412	.32052	.27170	.21669	.18647	.15422	.11970	.082690	.042896
7	.40454	.35884	.30682	.24711	.21382	.17786	.13893	.096624	.050494
8	.44016	.39308	.33873	.27528	.23939	.20024	.15734	.11015	.057977
9	.47176	.42387	.36784	.30142	.26337	.22144	.17499	.12328	.065345
10	0.50000	0.45169	0.39451	0.32575	0.28589	0.24154	0.19192	0.13603	0.072602
11	.52538	.47696	.41902	.34845	.30707	.26064	.20818	.14842	.079747
12	.54831	.50000	.44162	.36967	.32704	.27880	.22379	.16046	.086785
13	.56912	.52110	.46254	.38956	.34589	.29610	.23880	.17217	.093716
14	.58811	.54049	.48194	.40823	.36371	.31258	.25325	.18355	.10054
15	0.60549	0.55838	0.50000	0.42579	0.38059	0.32832	0.26715	0.19463	0.10727
16	.62147	.57492	.51684	.44234	.39660	.34335	.28055	.20541	.11390
17	.03021	.59027	.53258	.45797	.41181	.35772	.29347	.21591	.12043
18	.64984	.60456	.54733	.47274	.42626	.37147	.30593	.22613	.12686
19	.66248	.61788	.56118	.48673	.44002	.38465	.31796	.23609	.13320
20	0.67425	0.63033	0.57421	0.50000	0.45314	0.39729	0.32958	0.24580	0.13945
21	.68522	.64200	.58649	.51260	.46566	.40942	.34082	.25527	.14561
22	.69548	.65295	.59807	.52458	.47762	.42108	.35168	.26450	.15168
23	.70509	.66325	.60903	.53599	.48905	.43228	.36219	.27350	.15767
24	.71411	67296	.61941	.54686	.50000	.44305	.37237	.28229	.16357
25	0.72260	0.68213	0.62924	0.55723	0.51049	0.45343	0.38222	0.29086	0.16939
26	.73060	.69079	.63859	.56714	.52054	.46342	.39177	.29924	.17513
27	.73815	.69900	.64747	.57662	.53019	.47306	.40103	.30741	.18079
28	.74529	.70678	.65593	.58569	.53946	.48236	.41001	.31540	.18638
29	.75205	.71417	.66399	.59437	.54837	.49133	.41873	.32321	.19189
30	0.75846	0.72120	0.67168	0.60271	0.55695	0.50000	0.42720	0.33084	0.19732
40	.80808	.77621	.73285	.67042	.62763	.57280	.50000	.39866	.24791
60	.86397	.83954	.80537	.75420	.71771	.66916	.60134	.50000	.33209
120	.92740	.91321	.89273	.86055	.83643	.80268	.75209	.66791	.50000
∞	1.00000	1.00000	1.00000	1.00000	1.00000	1.00000	1.00000	1.00000	1.00000

For $\nu_1 = \infty,\ x = 0$

PERCENTAGE POINTS OF THE BETA DISTRIBUTION

Lower 25% points for x

$\nu_1 = 2b,\ \nu_2 = 2a$

ν_2 \ ν_1	1	2	3	4	5	6	7	8	9
1	0.14645	0.062500	0.039063	0.028309	0.022173	0.018215	0.015453	0.013416	0.011853
2	.43750	.25000	.17452	.13397	.10870	.091440	.078908	.069395	.061929
3	.59715	.39685	.29801	.23885	.19937	.17113	.14991	.13339	.12015
4	.68878	.50000	.39448	.32635	.27852	.24302	.21560	.19376	.17596
5	0.74711	0.57435	0.46936	0.39775	0.34546	0.30550	0.27390	0.24828	0.22707
6	.78726	.62996	.52848	.45632	.40198	.35944	.32516	.29692	.27323
7	.81650	.67295	.57609	.50494	.45001	.40614	.37021	.34022	.31478
8	.83872	.70711	.61516	.54582	.49117	.44680	.40996	.37885	.35219
9	.85616	.73487	.64773	.58060	.52678	.48245	.44521	.41343	.38597
10	0.87021	0.75786	0.67529	0.61052	0.55783	0.51390	0.47662	0.44451	0.41655
11	.88177	.77720	.69888	.63651	.58513	.54184	.50475	.47257	.44435
12	.89144	.79370	.71931	.65929	.60930	.56679	.53009	.49801	.46970
13	.89966	.80793	.73716	.67941	.63085	.58921	.55300	.52116	.49289
14	.90672	.82034	.75288	.69730	.65017	.60946	.57382	.54230	.51419
15	0.91285	0.83124	0.76684	0.71332	0.66758	0.62782	0.59282	0.56169	0.53380
16	.91823	.84090	.77932	.72773	.68336	.64456	.61021	.57953	.55192
17	.92298	.84951	.79053	.74077	.69772	.65986	.62619	.59599	.56870
18	.92721	.85724	.80066	.75263	.71084	.67391	.64093	.61122	.58428
19	.93100	.86422	.80986	.76345	.72287	.68686	.65456	.62536	.59879
20	0.93442	0.87055	0.81825	0.77337	0.73395	0.69882	0.66720	0.63852	0.61234
21	.93751	.87632	.82593	.78250	.74418	.70991	.67895	.65079	.62500
22	.94033	.88159	.83299	.79092	.75366	.72021	.68991	.66226	.63688
23	.94290	.88644	.83950	.79871	.76246	.72981	.70015	.67300	.64803
24	.94526	.89090	.84553	.80595	.77066	.73878	.70973	.68309	.65852
25	0.94744	0.89503	0.85112	0.81268	0.77831	0.74717	0.71873	0.69258	0.66840
26	.94944	.89885	.85632	.81896	.78547	.75505	.72719	.70151	.67774
27	.95130	.90241	.86116	.82484	.79218	.76244	.73515	.70995	.68657
28	.95303	.90572	.86570	.83035	.79848	.76941	.74267	.71793	.69492
29	.95464	.90882	.86994	.83552	.80442	.77598	.74977	.72548	.70285
30	0.95614	0.91172	0.87393	0.84039	0.81002	0.78219	0.75649	0.73263	0.71038
40	.96706	.93303	.90351	.87685	.85230	.82947	.80809	.78797	.76896
60	.97801	.95484	.93434	.91548	.89782	.88113	.86525	.85009	.83557
120	.98899	.97716	.96648	.95647	.94692	.93774	.92887	.92025	.91187
∞	1.00000	1.00000	1.00000	1.00000	1.00000	1.00000	1.00000	1.00000	1.00000

This table gives the values of x for which

$$I_x(a, b) = \int_0^x u^{a-1}(1-u)^{b-1}\,du \Big/ \int_0^1 u^{a-1}(1-u)^{b-1}\,du = 0.25,$$

where $a = \frac{1}{2}\nu_2$, $b = \frac{1}{2}\nu_1$.

PERCENTAGE POINTS OF THE BETA DISTRIBUTION

Lower 25% points for x

$\nu_1 = 2b,\ \nu_2 = 2a$

ν_2 \ ν_1	10	12	15	20	24	30	40	60	120
1	0.010616	0.0087814	0.0069734	0.0051914	0.0043101	0.0034353	0.0025669	0.0017049	$0.0^3 84926$
2	.055913	.046816	.037631	.028358	.023689	.018996	.014281	.0095436	.0047832
3	.10930	.092592	.075324	.057467	.048307	.038986	.029500	.019844	.010012
4	.16116	.13797	.11350	.087610	.074095	.060174	.045827	.031031	.015764
5	0.20922	0.18082	0.15026	0.11726	0.099749	0.081498	0.062458	0.042571	0.021774
6	.25307	.22058	.18500	.14585	.12475	.10251	.079043	.054222	.027923
7	.29291	.25724	.21758	.17316	.14888	.12301	.095405	.065857	.034143
8	.32908	.29099	.24802	.19913	.17203	.14289	.11145	.077403	.040396
9	.36198	.32205	.27644	.22376	.19420	.16211	.12712	.088814	.046656
10	0.39196	0.35068	0.30297	0.24710	0.21538	0.18064	0.14240	0.10006	0.052904
11	.41938	.37712	.32776	.26921	.23562	.19850	.15726	.11113	.059127
12	.44451	.40158	.35094	.29017	.25493	.21570	.17171	.12200	.065317
13	.46762	.42426	.37265	.31004	.27338	.23226	.18575	.13267	.071466
14	.48893	.44534	.39302	.32889	.29100	.24819	.19938	.14314	.077570
15	0.50863	0.46497	0.41215	0.34679	0.30785	0.26353	0.21261	0.15341	0.083624
16	.52691	.48330	.43016	.36380	.32395	.27831	.22546	.16347	.089625
17	.54389	.50043	.44712	.38008	.33936	.29251	.23703	.17332	.095571
18	.55972	.51649	.46312	.39539	.35411	.30625	.25004	.18298	.10146
19	.57449	.53156	.47825	.41008	.36824	.31946	.26179	.19244	.10729
20	0.58832	0.54574	0.49256	0.42409	0.38179	0.33221	0.27321	0.20170	0.11307
21	.60129	.55909	.50613	.43746	.39478	.34450	.28430	.21078	.11878
22	.61348	.57169	.51900	.45025	.40726	.35637	.29507	.21966	.12443
23	.62495	.58360	.53122	.46247	.41925	.36783	.30554	.22837	.13003
24	.63576	.59487	.54285	.47418	.43078	.37891	.31572	.23690	.13556
25	0.64597	0.60556	0.55392	0.48539	0.44186	0.38961	0.32561	0.24525	0.14103
26	.65563	.61570	.56447	.49615	.45253	.39996	.33524	.25343	.14645
27	.66478	.62533	.57455	.50647	.46281	.40997	.34460	.26145	.15180
28	.67346	.63450	.58417	.51639	.47272	.41967	.35371	.26931	.15710
29	.68170	.64323	.59337	.52591	.48228	.42906	.36259	.27701	.16234
30	0.68954	0.65156	0.60217	0.53508	0.49150	0.43815	0.37122	0.28455	0.16752
40	.75095	.71758	.67308	.61054	.56853	.51555	.44650	.35245	.21626
60	.82163	.79529	.75915	.70620	.66914	.62056	.55390	.45636	.29913
120	.90370	.88794	.86554	.83103	.80557	.77041	.71852	.63381	.46918
∞	1.00000	1.00000	1.00000	1.00000	1.00000	1.00000	1.00000	1.00000	1.00000

For $\nu_1 = \infty,\ x = 0$

PERCENTAGE POINTS OF THE BETA DISTRIBUTION

Lower 10% points for x

$\nu_1 = 2b,\ \nu_2 = 2a$

ν_2 \ ν_1	1	2	3	4	5	6	7	8	9
1	0.024472	0.010000	0.0061812	0.0044577	0.0034818	0.0028553	0.0024193	0.0020986	0.0018528
2	.19000	.10000	.067830	.051317	.041268	.034511	.029654	.025996	.023141
3	.35136	.21544	.15648	.12310	.10154	.086434	.075257	.066647	.059809
4	.46812	.31623	.24136	.19580	.16493	.14256	.12558	.11224	.10147
5	0.55185	0.39811	0.31529	0.26204	0.22457	0.19664	0.17498	0.15766	0.14349
6	.61375	.46416	.37816	.32046	.27858	.24664	.22139	.20091	.18394
7	.66104	.51795	.43151	.37151	.32685	.29210	.26421	.24127	.22207
8	.69821	.56234	.47700	.41611	.36982	.33319	.30339	.27860	.25764
9	.72814	.59948	.51610	.45522	.40811	.37029	.33915	.31299	.29067
10	0.75273	0.63096	0.54996	0.48968	0.44232	0.40382	0.37178	0.34462	0.32128
11	.77328	.65793	.57954	.52022	.47300	.43419	.40159	.37374	.34963
12	.79069	.68129	.60555	.54744	.50062	.46178	.42889	.40058	.37592
13	.80564	.70170	.62860	.57181	.52560	.48693	.45393	.42535	.40032
14	.81861	.71969	.64915	.59375	.54827	.50992	.47697	.44827	.42299
15	0.82996	0.73564	0.66758	0.61360	0.56893	0.53100	0.49822	0.46951	0.44410
16	.83998	.74989	.68419	.63164	.58783	.55040	.51787	.48924	.46380
17	.84889	.76270	.69923	.64809	.60517	.56829	.53608	.50760	.48219
18	.85686	.77426	.71293	.66315	.62114	.58484	.55300	.52473	.49942
19	.86403	.78476	.72544	.67699	.63588	.60020	.56876	.54074	.51557
20	0.87052	0.79433	0.73691	0.68976	0.64954	0.61448	0.58347	0.55574	0.53073
21	.87643	.80309	.74747	.70156	.66222	.62779	.59722	.56980	.54500
22	.88181	.81113	.75722	.71250	.67403	.64022	.61011	.58302	.55845
23	.88675	.81855	.76625	.72268	.68504	.65187	.62222	.59547	.57115
24	.89129	.82540	.77464	.73216	.69535	.66279	.63361	.60721	.58314
25	0.89549	0.83176	0.78245	0.74103	0.70500	0.67305	0.64434	0.61829	0.59450
26	.89937	.83768	.78973	.74933	.71407	.68271	.65446	.62878	.60526
27	.90297	.84319	.79655	.75711	.72260	.69183	.66403	.63871	.61548
28	.90633	.84834	.80294	.76443	.73064	.70044	.67309	.64813	.62518
29	.90946	.85317	.80894	.77132	.73823	.70858	.68168	.65708	.63442
30	0.91239	0.85770	0.81459	0.77783	0.74541	0.71630	0.68984	0.66559	0.64322
40	.93381	.89125	.85693	.82706	.80025	.77578	.75319	.73219	.71255
60	.95555	.92612	.90182	.88023	.86048	.84212	.82490	.80864	.79321
120	.97761	.96235	.94944	.93773	.92679	.91643	.90653	.89702	.88785
∞	1.00000	1.00000	1.00000	1.00000	1.00000	1.00000	1.00000	1.00000	1.00000

This table gives the values of x for which

$$I_x(a, b) = \int_0^x u^{a-1}(1-u)^{b-1}\,du \Big/ \int_0^1 u^{a-1}(1-u)^{b-1}\,du = 0.10,$$

where $a = \frac{1}{2}\nu_2,\ b = \frac{1}{2}\nu_1$.

PERCENTAGE POINTS OF THE BETA DISTRIBUTION

Lower 10% points for x

$\nu_1 = 2b,\ \nu_2 = 2a$

ν_2 \ ν_1	10	12	15	20	24	30	40	60	120
1	0.0016585	0.0013709	0.0010878	$0.0^{3}80919$	$0.0^{3}67157$	$0.0^{3}53506$	$0.0^{3}39965$	$0.0^{3}26535$	$0.0^{3}13213$
2	.020852	.017407	.013950	.010481	.0087416	.0069994	.0052542	.0035059	.0017545
3	.054245	.045740	.037035	.028119	.023579	.018982	.014327	.0096132	.0048379
4	.092595	.078823	.064482	.049452	.041691	.033749	.025617	.017288	.0087521
5	0.13167	0.11307	0.093336	0.072324	0.061295	0.049889	0.038083	0.025851	0.013167
6	.16964	.14685	.12228	.095653	.081477	.066668	.051174	.034941	.017906
7	.20573	.17941	.15059	.11886	.10173	.083668	.064573	.044345	.022866
8	.23966	.21040	.17792	.14161	.12177	.10064	.078083	.053928	.027978
9	.27139	.23970	.20411	.16374	.14141	.11743	.091577	.063600	.033196
10	0.30097	0.26732	0.22908	0.18513	0.16056	0.13394	0.10497	0.073298	0.038489
11	.32853	.29330	.25284	.20576	.17915	.15010	.11820	.082977	.043832
12	.35422	.31772	.27540	.22559	.19716	.16587	.13123	.092604	.049206
13	.37817	.34068	.29682	.24464	.21457	.18124	.14403	.10215	.054597
14	.40053	.36228	.31715	.26292	.23139	.19619	.15659	.11161	.059993
15	0.42143	0.38261	0.33645	0.28045	0.24762	0.21072	0.16889	0.12096	0.065386
16	.44100	.40176	.35478	.29726	.26327	.22483	.18093	.13019	.070768
17	.45934	.41983	.37219	.31338	.27837	.23853	.19270	.13930	.076134
18	.47657	.43689	.38875	.32885	.29293	.25182	.20420	.14828	.081478
19	.49277	.45302	.40451	.34369	.30697	.26471	.21544	.15712	.086796
20	0.50803	0.46829	0.41952	0.35793	0.32051	0.27721	0.22642	0.16583	0.092085
21	.52243	.48276	.43382	.37161	.33358	.28934	.23713	.17440	.097342
22	.53603	.49649	.44746	.38475	.34619	.30111	.24759	.18283	.10257
23	.54889	.50953	.46049	.39738	.35836	.31253	.25781	.19112	.10775
24	.56108	.52193	.47294	.40954	.37012	.32361	.26778	.19928	.11290
25	0.57263	0.53373	0.48485	0.42123	0.38147	0.33437	0.27751	0.20730	0.11801
26	.58361	.54498	.49624	.43248	.39245	.34481	.28701	.21518	.12308
27	.59405	.55571	.50716	.44333	.40306	.35495	.29629	.22293	.12811
28	.60398	.56595	.51763	.45378	.41332	.36479	.30534	.23054	.13310
29	.61344	.57574	.52767	.46386	.42325	.37436	.31419	.23803	.13804
30	0.62247	.058511	0.53731	0.47359	0.43286	0.38366	0.32283	0.24539	0.14295
40	.69412	.66034	.61599	.55476	.51428	.46386	.39910	.31243	.18960
60	.77851	.75104	.71386	.66029	.62333	.57545	.51067	.41750	.27063
120	.87897	.86198	.83814	.80192	.77553	.73946	.68688	.60235	.44158
∞	1.00000	1.00000	1.00000	1.00000	1.00000	1.00000	1.00000	1.00000	1.00000

For $\nu_1 = \infty,\ x = 0$

PERCENTAGE POINTS OF THE BETA DISTRIBUTION

Lower 5% points for x

$\nu_1 = 2b,\ \nu_2 = 2a$

ν_2 \ ν_1	1	2	3	4	5	6	7	8	9
1	0.0061558	0.0025000	0.0015429	0.0011119	$0.0^3 86820$	$0.0^3 71179$	$0.0^3 60300$	$0.0^3 52300$	$0.0^3 46170$
2	.097500	.050000	.033617	.025321	.020308	.016952	.014548	.012741	.011334
3	.22852	.13572	.097308	.076010	.062412	.052962	.046007	.040671	.036447
4	.34163	.22361	.16825	.13535	.11338	.097611	.085728	.076440	.068979
5	0.43074	0.30171	0.23553	0.19403	0.16528	0.14408	0.12778	0.11482	0.10427
6	.50053	.36840	.29599	.24860	.21477	.18926	.16927	.15316	.13989
7	.55593	.42489	.34929	.29811	.26063	.23182	.20890	.19019	.17461
8	.60071	.47287	.39607	.34259	.30260	.27134	.24613	.22532	.20783
9	.63751	.51390	.43716	.38245	.34080	.30777	.28082	.25835	.23930
10	0.66824	0.54928	0.47338	0.41820	0.37553	0.34126	0.31301	0.28924	0.26894
11	.69425	.58003	.50546	.45033	.40712	.37203	.34283	.31807	.29677
12	.71654	.60696	.53402	.47930	.43590	.40031	.37044	.34494	.32286
13	.73583	.63073	.55958	.50551	.46219	.42635	.39604	.37000	.34732
14	.75268	.65184	.58256	.52932	.48626	.45036	.41980	.39338	.37025
15	0.76754	0.67070	0.60333	0.55102	0.50836	0.47255	0.44187	0.41521	0.39176
16	.78072	.68766	.62217	.57086	.52872	.49310	.46242	.43563	.41196
17	.79249	.70297	.63933	.58907	.54750	.51217	.48158	.45474	.43094
18	.80307	.71687	.65503	.60584	.56490	.52991	.49949	.47267	.44880
19	.81263	.72954	.66944	.62131	.58103	.54645	.51624	.48951	.46564
20	0.82131	0.74113	0.68271	0.63564	0.59605	0.56189	0.53194	0.50535	0.48152
21	.82923	.75178	.69496	.64894	.61004	.57635	.54669	.52027	.49652
22	.83647	.76160	.70632	.66132	.62312	.58990	.56056	.53434	.51071
23	.84313	.77067	.71687	.67287	.63536	.60263	.57363	.54764	.52415
24	.84927	.77908	.72669	.68366	.64684	.61461	.58596	.56022	.53689
25	0.85494	0.78690	0.73586	0.69377	0.65764	0.62590	0.59761	0.57213	0.54898
26	.86021	.79418	.74444	.70327	.66780	.63656	.60864	.58343	.56048
27	.86511	.80099	.75249	.71219	.67738	.64663	.61909	.59416	.57141
28	.86967	.80736	.76004	.72060	.68643	.65617	.62900	.60436	.58183
29	.87394	.81334	.76715	.72854	.69499	.66522	.63842	.61407	.59177
30	0.87794	0.81896	0.77386	0.73604	0.70311	0.67381	0.64738	0.62332	0.60125
40	.90734	.86089	.82447	.79327	.76559	.74053	.71758	.69636	.67663
60	.93748	.90497	.87881	.85591	.83517	.81606	.79824	.78150	.76569
120	.96837	.95130	.93720	.92458	.91290	.90192	.89148	.88150	.87191
∞	1.00000	1.00000	1.00000	1.00000	1.00000	1.00000	1.00000	1.00000	1.00000

This table gives the values of x for which

$$I_x(a, b) = \int_0^x u^{a-1}(1-u)^{b-1}\,du \Big/ \int_0^1 u^{a-1}(1-u)^{b-1}\,du = 0.05,$$

where $a = \frac{1}{2}\nu_2$, $b = \frac{1}{2}\nu_1$.

PERCENTAGE POINTS OF THE BETA DISTRIBUTION

Lower 5% points for x

$\nu_1 = 2b,\ \nu_2 = 2a$

ν_2 \ ν_1	10	12	15	20	24	30	40	60	120
1	$0.0^3 41325$	$0.0^3 34155$	$0.0^3 27098$	$0.0^3 20156$	$0.0^3 16727$	$0.0^3 13326$	$0.0^4 99535$	$0.0^4 66082$	$0.0^4 32904$
2	.010206	.0085124	.0068158	.0051162	.0042653	.0034137	.0025614	.0017083	$.0^3 85452$
3	.033020	.027794	.022465	.017026	.014264	.011472	.0086511	.0057991	.0029157
4	.062850	.053375	.043541	.033319	.028053	.022679	.017191	.011585	.0058567
5	0.095510	0.081790	0.067312	0.051995	0.043994	0.035747	0.027240	0.018458	0.0093841
6	.12876	.11111	.092207	.071870	.061103	.049898	.038224	.026043	.013317
7	.16142	.14029	.11733	.092238	.078783	.064651	.049781	.034103	.017540
8	.19290	.16875	.14216	.11267	.096658	.079695	.061675	.042481	.021976
9	.22292	.19618	.16638	.13288	.11449	.094827	.073748	.051068	.026572
10	0.25137	0.22244	0.18984	0.15272	0.13211	0.10991	0.085885	0.059785	0.031288
11	.27823	.24746	.21244	.17207	.14943	.12484	.098008	.068575	.036094
12	.30354	.27125	.23413	.19086	.16636	.13955	.11006	.077394	.040967
13	.32737	.29383	.25492	.20908	.18288	.15401	.12199	.086209	.045889
14	.34981	.31524	.27481	.22669	.19895	.16818	.13377	.094994	.050847
15	0.37095	0.33554	0.29382	0.24370	0.21457	0.18203	0.14539	0.10373	0.055827
16	.39086	.35480	.31199	.26011	.22972	.19556	.15682	.11240	.060821
17	.40965	.37307	.32936	.27594	.24441	.20877	.16805	.12099	.065820
18	.42738	.39041	.34596	.29120	.25865	.22164	.17908	.12950	.070818
19	.44414	.40689	.36183	.30591	.27244	.23418	.18989	.13791	.075809
20	0.45999	0.42256	0.37701	0.32009	0.28580	0.24639	0.20050	0.14622	0.080789
21	.47501	.43746	.39154	.33375	.29874	.25828	.21088	.15442	.085753
22	.48925	.45165	.40544	.34693	.31126	.26985	.22106	.16252	.090698
23	.50276	.46518	.41877	.35964	.32340	.28112	.23102	.17051	.095621
24	.51560	.47808	.43154	.37190	.33515	.29208	.24078	.17838	.10052
25	0.52782	0.49040	0.44379	0.38373	0.34653	0.30275	0.25032	0.18615	0.10539
26	.53945	.50217	.45554	.39516	.35756	.31314	.25966	.19379	.11024
27	.55054	.51343	.46683	.40619	.36826	.32325	.26880	.20133	.11505
28	.56112	.52420	.47768	.41685	.37862	.33309	.27775	.20875	.11983
29	.57122	.53452	.48812	.42715	.38867	.34267	.28650	.21606	.12458
30	0.58088	0.54442	0.49816	0.43711	0.39842	0.35200	0.29507	0.22326	0.12930
40	.65819	.62460	.58083	.52099	.48175	.43321	.37136	.28936	.17453
60	.75070	.72282	.68535	.63185	.59522	.54807	.48477	.39458	.25416
120	.86266	.84504	.82047	.78342	.75661	.72016	.66738	.58326	.42519
∞	1.00000	1.00000	1.00000	1.00000	1.00000	1.00000	1.00000	1.00000	1.00000

For $\nu_1 = \infty$, $x = 0$

PERCENTAGE POINTS OF THE BETA DISTRIBUTION

Lower 2.5% points for x

$\nu_1 = 2b,\ \nu_2 = 2a$

ν_2 \ ν_1	1	2	3	4	5	6	7	8	9
1	0.0015413	$0.0^3 62500$	$0.0^3 38558$	$0.0^3 27783$	$0.0^3 21691$	$0.0^3 17782$	$0.0^3 15064$	$0.0^3 13065$	$0.0^3 11533$
2	.049375	.025000	.016737	.012579	.010076	.0084038	.0072076	.0063095	.0056104
3	.14675	.085499	.060830	.047316	.038748	.032820	.028471	.025143	.022513
4	.24664	.15811	.11786	.094299	.078706	.067586	.059243	.052745	.047539
5	0.33318	0.22865	0.17674	0.14471	0.12275	0.10669	0.094390	0.084663	0.076770
6	.40505	.29240	.23259	.19412	.16695	.14663	.13081	.11812	.10770
7	.46442	.34855	.28375	.24063	.20942	.18562	.16681	.15153	.13886
8	.51378	.39764	.32993	.28358	.24933	.22278	.20151	.18405	.16944
9	.55524	.44054	.37137	.32290	.28642	.25774	.23450	.21523	.19897
10	0.59043	0.47818	0.40855	0.35877	0.32071	0.29042	0.26561	0.24486	0.22722
11	.62062	.51135	.44194	.39146	.35234	.32085	.29482	.27288	.25409
12	.64677	.54074	.47202	.42128	.38149	.34914	.32219	.29930	.27957
13	.66961	.56693	.49920	.44853	.40838	.37545	.34779	.32416	.30368
14	.68973	.59038	.52385	.47349	.43321	.39991	.37175	.34755	.32646
15	0.70756	0.61149	0.54628	0.49641	0.45618	0.42268	0.39418	0.36955	0.34799
16	.72349	.63058	.56676	.51750	.47746	.44390	.41520	.39026	.36833
17	.73778	.64792	.58553	.53697	.49723	.46372	.43490	.40976	.38756
18	.75069	.66373	.60278	.55498	.51561	.48224	.45341	.42814	.40575
19	.76239	.67821	.61869	.57169	.53276	.49959	.47081	.44549	.42297
20	0.77305	0.69150	0.63339	0.58722	0.54877	0.51586	0.48719	0.46187	0.43928
21	.78280	.70376	.64702	.60169	.56375	.53115	.50263	.47736	.45475
22	.79176	.71509	.65970	.61520	.57780	.54553	.51720	.49202	.46943
23	.80001	.72559	.67150	.62785	.59100	.55908	.53098	.50592	.48338
24	.80763	.73535	.68253	.63970	.60341	.57187	.54401	.51911	.49664
25	0.81469	0.74445	0.69285	0.65084	0.61511	0.58396	0.55636	0.53163	0.50927
26	.82126	.75295	.70253	.66132	.62615	.59540	.56808	.54354	.52130
27	.82738	.76090	.71162	.67119	.63658	.60624	.57922	.55488	.53278
28	.83310	.76836	.72018	.68052	.64646	.61652	.58980	.56568	.54373
29	.83845	.77538	.72825	.68933	.65582	.62630	.59988	.57599	.55420
30	0.84347	0.78198	0.73587	0.69768	0.66471	0.63559	0.60948	0.58582	0.56421
40	.88059	.83157	.79381	.76184	.73369	.70839	.68532	.66411	.64446
60	.91904	.88430	.85681	.83298	.81156	.79193	.77372	.75668	.74065
120	.95883	.94037	.92535	.91201	.89975	.88828	.87743	.86708	.85717
∞	1.00000	1.00000	1.00000	1.00000	1.00000	1.00000	1.00000	1.00000	1.00000

This table gives the values of x for which

$$I_x(a, b) = \int_0^x u^{a-1}(1-u)^{b-1}\,du \Big/ \int_0^1 u^{a-1}(1-u)^{b-1}\,du = 0.025,$$

where $a = \frac{1}{2}\nu_2$, $b = \frac{1}{2}\nu_1$.

PERCENTAGE POINTS OF THE BETA DISTRIBUTION

Lower 2.5% points for x

$\nu_1 = 2b,\ \nu_2 = 2a$

ν_2 \ ν_1	10	12	15	20	24	30	40	60	120
1	$0.0^{3}10323$	$0.0^{4}85313$	$0.0^{4}67686$	$0.0^{4}50345$	$0.0^{4}41780$	$0.0^{4}33285$	$0.0^{4}24860$	$0.0^{4}16505$	$0.0^{5}82180$
2	.0050508	.0042107	.0033700	.0025286	.0021076	.0016864	.0012651	$.0^{3}84357$	$.0^{3}42187$
3	.020382	.017139	.013838	.010477	.0087725	.0070519	.0053148	.0035607	.0017893
4	.043272	.036693	.029885	.022831	.019207	.015514	.011749	.0079110	.0039956
5	0.070233	0.060028	0.049302	0.038002	0.032119	0.026068	0.019841	0.013428	0.0068184
6	.098988	.085233	.070563	.054861	.046579	0.37985	.029056	.019767	.010092
7	.12818	.11113	.092695	.072663	.061969	.050772	.039029	.026691	.013702
8	.15701	.13700	.11508	.090920	.077871	0.64092	0.49508	0.34033	0.17569
9	.18504	.16240	.13732	.10931	.094004	.077712	.060314	.041675	.021634
10	0.21201	0.18709	0.15917	0.12760	0.11017	0.091466	0.071319	0.049528	0.025854
11	.23780	.21091	.18048	.14565	.12623	.10523	.082426	.057528	.030196
12	.26238	.23379	.20115	.16336	.14210	.11893	.093564	.065622	.034634
13	.28573	.25571	.22112	.18067	.15770	.13249	.10468	.073771	.039147
14	.30790	.27667	.24039	.19753	.17299	.14588	.11573	.081944	.043718
15	0.32893	0.29668	0.25893	0.21392	0.18793	0.15905	0.12669	0.090115	0.048335
16	.34888	.31578	.27676	.22983	.20252	.17198	.13753	.098266	.052985
17	.30779	.33400	.29389	.24525	.21674	.18466	.14823	.10638	.057659
18	.38574	.35138	.31034	.26019	.23058	.19708	.15878	.11444	.062348
19	.40278	.36797	.32614	.27465	.24404	.20922	.16916	.12244	.067047
20	0.41896	0.38380	0.34132	0.28864	0.25713	0.22110	0.17938	0.13038	0.071749
21	.43435	.39893	.35589	.30218	.26985	.23270	.18943	.13823	.076450
22	.44900	.41338	.36990	.31528	.28221	.24402	.19930	.14601	.081144
23	.46294	.42720	.38335	.32795	.29422	.25508	.20899	.15370	.085828
24	.47623	.44042	.39629	.34021	.30588	.26587	.21850	.16130	.090500
25	0.48801	0.45307	0.40874	0.35207	0.31721	0.27640	0.22783	0.16881	0.095156
26	.50101	.46520	.42071	.36355	.32821	.28667	.23698	.17622	.099794
27	.51257	.47682	.43223	.37466	.33890	.29669	.24596	.18354	.10441
28	.52363	.48797	.44334	.38542	.34928	.30647	.25476	.19076	.10901
29	.53421	.49867	.45403	.39584	.35937	.31601	.26339	.19789	.11358
30	0.54435	0.50895	0.46434	0.40594	0.36918	0.32532	0.27185	0.20492	0.11812
40	.62616	.59296	.54999	.49168	.45370	.40697	.34780	.26997	.16201
60	.72550	.69743	.65992	.60674	.57056	.52422	.46239	.37498	.24027
120	.84764	.82954	.80442	.76678	.73968	.70299	.65017	.56658	.41107
∞	1.00000	1.00000	1.00000	1.00000	1.00000	1.00000	1.00000	1.00000	1.00000

For $\nu_1 = \infty,\ x = 0$

PERCENTAGE POINTS OF THE BETA DISTRIBUTION

Lower 1% points for x

$\nu_1 = 2b,\ \nu_2 = 2a$

$\nu_2 \backslash \nu_1$	1	2	3	4	5	6	7	8	9
1	$0.0^{3}24672$	$0.0^{3}10000$	$0.0^{4}61686$	$0.0^{4}44446$	$0.0^{4}34699$	$0.0^{4}28446$	$0.0^{4}24097$	$0.0^{4}20897$	$0.0^{4}18449$
2	.019900	.010000	.0066778	.0050126	.0040121	.0033445	.0028674	.0025094	.0022309
3	.080827	.046416	.032834	.025458	.020807	.017599	.015252	.013458	.012043
4	.15875	.10000	.073960	.058903	.049014	.041999	.036754	.032682	.029426
5	0.23520	0.15849	0.12142	0.098877	0.083563	0.072429	0.063948	0.057264	0.051857
6	.30387	.21544	.16979	.14087	.12065	.10564	.094014	.084730	.077136
7	.36370	.26827	.21636	.18236	.15801	.13959	.12511	.11341	.10375
8	.41540	.31623	.25997	.22207	.19437	.17307	.15612	.14227	.13073
9	.46009	.35938	.30024	.25945	.22910	.20543	.18637	.17066	.15745
10	0.49889	0.39811	0.33719	0.29431	0.26191	0.23632	0.21551	0.19820	0.18355
11	.53279	.43288	.37099	.32667	.29271	.26560	.24335	.22469	.20879
12	.56258	.46416	.40191	.35664	.32153	.29323	.26981	.25003	.23307
13	.58893	.49239	.43020	.38437	.34845	.31924	.29487	.27417	.25631
14	.61238	.51795	.45615	.41006	.37358	.34369	.31858	.29712	.27851
15	0.63336	0.54117	0.47999	0.43387	0.39706	0.36666	0.34098	0.31891	0.29968
16	.65224	.56234	.50194	.45597	.41899	.38826	.36214	.33958	.31985
17	.66930	.58171	.52219	.47651	.43951	.40857	.38213	.35920	.33905
18	.68479	.59948	.54094	.49565	.45872	.42768	.40103	.37781	.35733
19	.69892	.61585	.55832	.51350	.47674	.44568	.41890	.39547	.37474
20	0.71185	0.63096	0.57447	0.53018	0.49366	0.46266	0.43581	0.41224	0.39131
21	.72372	.64495	.58952	.54581	.50958	.47868	.45184	.42818	.40711
22	.73467	.65793	.60357	.56046	.52456	.49383	.46703	.44333	.42217
23	.74479	.67002	.61671	.57422	.53869	.50816	.48144	.45775	.43653
24	.75417	.68129	.62903	.58717	.55204	.52174	.49514	.47149	.45025
25	0.76290	0.69183	0.64059	0.59938	0.56466	0.53461	0.50816	0.48458	0.46335
26	.77103	.70170	.65147	.61090	.57660	.54683	.52055	.49706	.47587
27	.77862	.71097	.66172	.62180	.58793	.55845	.53236	.50899	.48785
28	.78573	.71969	.67139	.63211	.59868	.56951	.54362	.52038	.49932
29	.79240	.72790	.68054	.64188	.60890	.58004	.55437	.53127	.51031
30	0.79867	0.73564	0.68919	0.65116	0.61862	0.59008	0.56464	0.54170	0.52085
40	.84541	.79433	.75561	.72316	.69482	.66950	.64656	.62555	.60617
60	.89449	.85770	.82898	.80433	.78233	.76227	.74376	.72651	.71034
120	.94599	.92612	.91014	.89607	.88321	.87124	.85995	.84924	.83900
∞	1.00000	1.00000	1.00000	1.00000	1.00000	1.00000	1.00000	1.00000	1.00000

This table gives the values of x for which

$$I_x(a, b) = \int_0^x u^{a-1}(1-u)^{b-1}\,du \Big/ \int_0^1 u^{a-1}(1-u)^{b-1}\,du = 0.01,$$

where $a = \frac{1}{2}\nu_2$, $b = \frac{1}{2}\nu_1$.

PERCENTAGE POINTS OF THE BETA DISTRIBUTION

Lower 1% points for x

$\nu_1 = 2b,\ \nu_2 = 2a$

ν_2 \ ν_1	10	12	15	20	24	30	40	60	120
1	$0.0^{4}16513$	$0.0^{4}13647$	$0.0^{4}10827$	$0.0^{5}80531$	$0.0^{5}66831$	$0.0^{5}53242$	$0.0^{5}39766$	$0.0^{5}26400$	$0.0^{5}13145$
2	.0020080	.0016737	.0013391	.0010045	$.0^{3}83718$	$.0^{3}66980$	$.0^{3}50239$	$.0^{3}33496$	$.0^{3}16749$
3	.010898	.0091569	.0073877	.0055887	.0046777	.0037588	.0028317	.0018964	$.0^{3}95252$
4	.026763	.022665	.018435	.014065	.011824	.0095436	.0072226	.0048595	.0024525
5	0.047389	0.040434	0.033149	0.025503	0.021534	0.017459	0.013275	0.0089747	0.0045520
6	.070804	.060840	.050258	.038982	.033057	.026923	.020567	.013973	.0071235
7	.095627	.082714	.068820	.053801	.045816	.037481	.028767	.019640	.010065
8	.12095	.10526	.088177	.069456	.059390	.048797	.037625	.025815	.013300
9	.14619	.12796	.10787	.085584	.073472	.060623	.046956	.032376	.016768
10	0.17097	0.15044	0.12760	0.10193	0.087838	0.072776	0.056621	0.039229	0.020426
11	.19506	.17250	.14713	.11830	.10232	.085117	.066512	.046303	.024237
12	.21834	.19398	.16633	.13458	.11681	.097542	.076547	.053541	.028173
13	.24073	.21479	.18511	.15065	.13120	.10997	.086660	.060897	.032212
14	.26220	.23489	.20338	.16646	.14544	.12235	.096802	.068334	.036335
15	0.28276	0.25426	0.22113	0.18196	0.15948	0.13462	0.10693	0.075824	0.040526
16	.30240	.27289	.23833	.19711	.17327	.14676	.11702	.083341	.044772
17	.32117	.29079	.25497	.21189	.18681	.15873	.12704	.090866	.049062
18	.33910	.30797	.27105	.22630	.20005	.17053	.13697	.098383	.053386
19	.35622	.32446	.28658	.24032	.21301	.18212	.14680	.10588	.057738
20	0.37257	0.34029	0.30157	0.25395	0.22567	0.19351	0.15651	0.11334	0.062109
21	.38818	.35548	.31603	.26721	.23803	.20468	.16609	.12076	.066494
22	.40311	.37005	.32999	.28008	.25008	.21563	.17554	.12812	.070888
23	.41738	.38405	.34345	.29258	.26184	.22636	.18486	.13543	.075285
24	.43103	.39749	.35645	.30472	.27329	.23687	.19403	.14268	.079683
25	0.44410	0.41040	0.36899	0.31651	0.28446	0.24716	0.20305	0.14986	0.084077
26	.45661	.42280	.38109	.32795	.29534	.25722	.21193	.15697	.088465
27	.46861	.43473	.39278	.33906	.30594	.26707	.22066	.16401	.092843
28	.48011	.44621	.40407	.34985	.31626	.27670	.22925	.17096	.097210
29	.49115	.45726	.41497	.36032	.32632	.28612	.23768	.17785	.10156
30	0.50175	0.46789	0.42552	0.37049	0.33612	0.29534	0.24597	0.18465	0.10590
40	.58819	.55573	.51398	.45778	.42144	.37700	.32111	.24819	.14811
60	.69511	.66701	.62969	.57717	.54167	.49647	.43655	.35258	.22459
120	.82918	.81062	.78497	.74677	.71942	.68259	.62988	.54709	.39479
∞	1.00000	1.00000	1.00000	1.00000	1.00000	1.00000	1.00000	1.00000	1.00000

For $\nu_1 = \infty,\ x = 0$

PERCENTAGE POINTS OF THE BETA DISTRIBUTION

Lower 0.5% points for x

$\nu_1 = 2b,\ \nu = 2a$

ν_2 \ ν_1	1	2	3	4	5	6	7	8	9
1	$0.0^{4}61684$	$0.0^{4}25000$	$0.0^{4}15421$	$0.0^{4}11111$	$0.0^{5}86745$	$0.0^{5}71112$	$0.0^{5}60240$	$0.0^{5}52245$	$0.0^{5}46121$
2	0099750	0050000	0033361	.0025031	.0020030	.0016695	.0014311	.0012524	.0011133
3	.051237	.029240	.020632	.015976	.013046	.011028	.0095530	.0084269	.0075388
4	.11321	.070711	.052099	.041400	.034399	.029445	.025748	.022881	.020592
5	0.17996	0.12011	0.091593	0.074378	0.062737	0.054301	0.047891	0.042849	0.038776
6	.24356	.17100	.13408	.11088	.094759	.082829	.073619	.066279	.060287
7	.30126	.22007	.17656	.14830	.12818	.11303	.10116	.091593	.083707
8	.35261	.26591	.21745	.18510	.16159	.14360	.12933	.11770	.10804
9	.39799	.30808	.25604	.22046	.19415	.17373	.15736	.14389	.13261
10	0.43809	0.34657	0.29204	0.25399	0.22542	0.20297	0.18478	0.16970	0.15697
11	.47360	.38162	.32543	.28554	.25517	.23105	.21132	.19484	.18083
12	.50517	.41352	.35632	.31509	.28332	.25783	.23682	.21914	.20402
13	.53337	.44258	.38487	.34270	.30986	.28328	.26120	.24250	.22642
14	.55865	.46912	.41127	.36848	.33484	.30739	.28444	.26489	.24798
15	0.58144	0.49340	0.43569	0.39255	0.35833	0.33022	0.30656	0.28629	0.26869
16	.60206	.51567	.45832	.41503	.38042	.35180	.32757	.30672	.28852
17	.62080	.53616	.47932	.43605	.40120	.37221	.34754	.32620	.30752
18	.63789	.55505	.49885	.45571	.42076	.39151	.36650	.34478	.32568
19	.65354	.57251	.51703	.47414	.43917	.40976	.38451	.36248	.34305
20	0.66792	0.58870	0.53400	0.49144	0.45654	0.42705	0.40162	0.37936	0.35966
21	.68117	.60375	.54986	.50768	.47293	.44343	.41789	.39546	.37554
22	.69341	.61775	.56472	.52297	.48841	.45896	.43336	.41082	.39073
23	.70477	.63083	.57866	.53738	.50306	.47369	.44810	.42547	.40527
24	.71532	.64305	.59176	.55098	.51692	.48769	.46213	.43947	.41918
25	0.72516	0.65451	0.60409	0.56382	0.53007	0.50100	0.47551	0.45285	0.43251
26	.73434	.66527	.61571	.57597	.54255	.51367	.48827	.46564	.44528
27	.74294	.67539	.62669	.58749	.55441	.52574	.50046	.47788	.45752
28	.75100	.68492	.63707	.59841	.56568	.53724	.51210	.48960	.46927
29	.75857	.69392	.64690	.60878	.57642	.54822	.52324	.50083	.48054
30	0.76570	0.70242	0.65622	0.61864	0.58665	0.55871	0.53389	0.51159	0.49137
40	.81920	.76727	.72823	.69571	.66744	.64229	.61956	.59882	.57973
60	.87598	.83811	.80877	.78370	.76142	.74119	.72256	.70526	.68907
120	.93619	.91548	.89893	.88442	.87120	.85892	.84739	.83645	.82602
∞	1.00000	1.00000	1.00000	1.00000	1.00000	1.00000	1.00000	1.00000	1.00000

This table gives the values of x for which

$$I_x(a, b) = \int_0^x u^{a-1}(1-u)^{b-1}\,du \Big/ \int_0^1 u^{a-1}(1-u)^{b-1}\,du = 0.005,$$

where $a = \frac{1}{2}\nu_2$, $b = \frac{1}{2}\nu_1$.

PERCENTAGE POINTS OF THE BETA DISTRIBUTION

Lower 0.5% points for x

$\nu_1 = 2b,\ \nu_2 = 2a$

ν_2 \ ν_1	11	12	15	20	24	30	40	60	120
1	$0.0^{5}41280$	$0.0^{5}34116$	$0.0^{5}27067$	$0.0^{5}20132$	$0.0^{5}16707$	$0.0^{5}13310$	$0.0^{6}99411$	$0.0^{6}65998$	$0.0^{6}32862$
2	.0010020	$.0^{3}83507$	$.0^{3}66812$	$.0^{3}50113$	$.0^{3}41762$	$.0^{3}33411$	$.0^{3}25060$	$.0^{3}16707$	$.0^{4}83539$
3	.0068204	.0057290	.0046206	.0034943	.0029242	.0023493	.0017696	.0011848	$.0^{3}59503$
4	.018721	.015844	.012879	.0098197	.0082522	.0066584	.0050373	.0033880	.0017093
5	0.035415	0.030191	0.024729	0.019006	0.016040	0.012998	0.0098777	0.0066743	0.0033833
6	.055299	.047464	.039162	.030337	.025709	.020924	.015973	.010844	.0055240
7	.077090	.066593	.055329	.043189	.036749	.030038	.023034	.015712	.0080441
8	.099867	.086787	.072586	.057076	.048760	.040023	.030828	.021129	.010873
9	.12300	.10749	.090464	.071635	.061433	.050635	.039174	.026976	.013953
10	0.14606	0.12831	0.10862	0.086595	0.074540	0.061684	0.047930	0.033162	0.017241
11	.16876	.14898	.12683	.10175	.087903	.073027	.056985	.039611	.020700
12	.19092	.16931	.14489	.11696	.10139	.084550	.066252	.046265	.024302
13	.21242	.18919	.16270	.13210	.11490	.096167	.075662	.053076	.028022
14	.23320	.20853	.18017	.14710	.12835	.10781	.085158	.060005	.031841
15	0.25323	0.22728	0.19725	0.16190	0.14170	0.11942	0.094697	0.067019	0.035743
16	.27248	.24543	.21388	.17644	.15488	.13097	.10424	.074093	.039714
17	.29098	.26295	.23000	.19070	.16787	.14241	.11377	.081204	.043741
18	.30872	.27986	.24576	.20465	.18065	.15373	.12324	.088334	.047815
19	.32574	.29615	.26099	.21829	.19319	.16489	.13265	.095467	.051928
20	0.34200	0.31184	0.27575	0.23160	0.20549	0.17590	0.14198	0.10259	0.056070
21	.35770	.32696	.29004	.24458	.21753	.18673	.15122	.10969	.060237
22	.37269	.34151	.30387	.25723	.22932	.19738	.16036	.11676	.064421
23	.38707	.35552	.31725	.26954	.24084	.20784	.16938	.12380	.068619
24	.40087	.36901	.33020	.28153	.25210	.21811	.17829	.13078	.072825
25	0.41411	0.38200	0.34272	0.29320	0.26309	0.22818	0.18707	0.13772	0.077036
26	.42682	.39452	.35484	.30456	.27383	.23806	.19573	.14461	.081248
27	.43903	.40658	.36657	.31560	.28432	.24775	.20426	.15143	.085459
28	.45076	.41821	.37792	.32635	.29455	.25724	.21266	.15819	.089665
29	.46204	.42942	.38891	.33681	.30454	.26654	.22093	.16489	.093863
30	0.47289	0.44024	0.39954	0.34698	0.31429	0.27565	0.22907	0.17152	0.098050
40	.56205	.53024	.48950	.43493	.39980	.35700	.30341	.23388	.13907
60	.67384	.64584	.60879	.55688	.52194	.47762	.41913	.33759	.21421
120	.81604	.79720	.77125	.73277	.70531	.66845	.61590	.53378	.38380
∞	1.00000	1.00000	1.00000	1.00000	1.00000	1.00000	1.00000	1.00000	1.00000

For $\nu_1 = \infty,\ x = 0$

III.11 TESTS OF SIGNIFICANCE IN 2 × 2 CONTINGENCY TABLES

Suppose that N elements are categorized as 1 or 2 and simultaneously as I or II. The 2 × 2 contingency table in standard form is represented by

	I	II	Totals
1	a	$A - a$	A
2	b	$B - b$	B
Totals	r	$N - r$	N

The probability of a given configuration, given fixed marginal totals is

$$f(a|r,A,B) = \frac{A!B!r!(N-r)!}{a!b!(A-a)!(B-b)!N!}\,.$$

This table is designed to provide a significance test for the discrepancy of observed from expected frequencies. The table shows, in bold type, for given a, A, and B, the highest value of $b(<a)$ which is just significant at the significance levels .05, .025, .01, .005.

Rules to follow in using the table:

(i) Category 1 in the sense of the 2 × 2 table is that for which $A \geq B$.

(ii) $\frac{a}{A} \geq \frac{b}{B}$ (or $aB \geq bA$)

(iii) If b is less than or equal to the integer in bold type, $\frac{a}{A}$ is significantly greater than $\frac{b}{B}$ (single-tail test) at the probability level indicated by the column heading. For a double-tail test, if b is less than or equal to the integer in bold type, $\frac{a}{A}$ is significantly different from $\frac{b}{B}$ at a probability level equal to twice that indicated by the column heading.

(iv) A dash for some combination of A, B, and a indicates that no 2 × 2 table in that class can show a significant effect at that level.

(v) The true probability that, for given r, b will be less than or equal to the integer in bold type, is shown in small type following an entry.

TESTS OF SIGNIFICANCE IN A 2 × 2 CONTINGENCY TABLE

	a	Probability			
		0.05	0.025	0.01	0.005
$A = 3$ $B = 3$	3	0.050	—	—	—
$A = 4$ $B = 4$	4	0.014	0.014	—	—
3	4	0.029	—	—	—
$A = 5$ $B = 5$	5	1.024	1.024	0.004	0.004
	4	0.024	0.024	—	—
4	5	1.048	0.008	0.008	—
	4	0.040	—	—	—
3	5	0.018	0.018	—	—
2	5	0.048	—	—	—
$A = 6$ $B = 6$	6	2.030	1.008	1.008	0.001
	5	1.040	0.008	0.008	—
	4	0.030	—	—	—
5	6	1.015+	0.015+	0.002	0.002
	5	0.013	0.013	—	—
	4	0.045+	—	—	—
4	6	1.033	0.005−	0.005−	0.005−
	5	0.024	0.024	—	—
3	6	0.012	0.012	—	—
	5	0.048	—	—	—
2	6	0.036	—	—	—
$A = 7$ $B = 7$	7	3.035−	2.010+	1.002	1.002
	6	1.015−	1.015−	0.002	0.002
	5	0.010+	0.010+	—	—
	4	0.035−	—	—	—
6	7	2.021	2.021	1.005−	1.005−
	6	1.025+	0.004	0.004	0.004
	5	0.016	0.016	—	—
	4	0.049	—	—	—
5	7	2.045+	1.010+	0.001	0.001
	6	1.045+	0.008	0.008	—
	5	0.027	—	—	—
4	7	1.024	1.024	0.003	0.003
	6	0.015+	0.015+	—	—
	5	0.045+	—	—	—
3	7	0.008	0.008	0.008	—
	6	0.033	—	—	—
2	7	0.028	—	—	—
$A = 8$ $B = 8$	8	4.038	3.013	2.003	2.003
	7	2.020	2.020	1.005+	0.001
	6	1.020	1.020	0.003	0.003
	5	0.013	0.013	—	—
	4	0.038	—	—	—
7	8	3.026	2.007	2.007	1.001
	7	2.035−	1.009	1.009	0.001
	6	1.032	0.006	0.006	—
	5	0.019	0.019	—	—
6	8	2.015−	2.015−	1.003	1.003
	7	1.016	1.016	0.002	0.002
	6	0.009	0.009	0.009	—
	5	0.028	—	—	—
5	8	2.035−	1.007	1.007	0.001
	7	1.032	0.005−	0.005−	0.005−
$A = 8$ $B = 5$	6	0.016	0.016	—	—
	5	0.044	—	—	—
4	8	1.018	1.018	0.002	0.002
	7	0.010+	0.010+	—	—
	6	0.030	—	—	—
3	8	0.006	0.006	0.006	—
	7	0.024	0.024	—	—
2	8	0.022	0.022	—	—
$A = 9$ $B = 9$	9	5.041	4.015−	3.005−	3.005−
	8	3.025−	3.025−	2.008	1.002
	7	2.028	1.008	1.008	0.001
	6	1.025−	1.025−	0.005−	0.005−
	5	0.015−	0.015−	—	—
	4	0.041	—	—	—
8	9	4.029	3.009	3.009	2.002
	8	3.043	2.013	1.003	1.003
	7	2.044	1.012	0.002	0.002
	6	1.036	0.007	0.007	—
	5	0.020	0.020	—	—
7	9	3.019	3.019	2.005−	2.005−
	8	2.024	2.024	1.006	0.001
	7	1.020	1.020	0.003	0.003
	6	0.010+	0.010+	—	—
	5	0.029	—	—	—
6	9	3.044	2.011	1.002	1.002
	8	2.047	1.011	0.001	0.001
	7	1.035−	0.006	0.006	—
	6	0.017	0.017	—	—
	5	0.042	—	—	—
5	9	2.027	1.005−	1.005−	1.005−
	8	1.023	1.023	0.003	0.003
	7	0.010+	0.010+	—	—
	6	0.028	—	—	—
4	9	1.014	1.014	0.001	0.001
	8	0.007	0.007	0.007	—
	7	0.021	0.021	—	—
	6	0.040	—	—	—
3	9	1.045+	0.005−	0.005−	0.005−
	8	0.018	0.018	—	—
	7	0.045+	—	—	—
2	9	0.018	0.018	—	—
$A = 10$ $B = 10$	10	6.043	5.016	4.005+	3.002
	9	4.029	3.010−	3.010−	2.003
	8	3.035−	2.012	1.003	1.003
	7	2.035−	1.010−	1.010−	0.002
	6	1.029	0.005+	0.005+	—
	5	0.016	0.016	—	—
	4	0.043	—	—	—
9	10	5.033	4.011	3.003	3.003
	9	4.050−	3.017	2.005−	2.005−
	8	2.019	2.019	1.004	1.004
	7	1.015−	1.015−	0.002	0.002
	6	1.040	0.008	0.008	—
	5	0.022	0.022	—	—

TESTS OF SIGNIFICANCE IN A 2 × 2 CONTINGENCY TABLE

	a	Probability			
		0.05	0.025	0.01	0.005
$A = 10$ $B = 8$	10	4.023	4.023	3.007	2.002
	9	3.032	2.009	2.009	1.002
	8	2.031	1.008	1.008	0.001
	7	1.023	1.023	0.004	0.004
	6	0.011	0.011	—	—
	5	0.029	—	—	—
7	10	3.015−	3.015−	2.003	2.003
	9	2.018	2.018	1.004	1.004
	8	1.013	1.013	0.002	0.002
	7	1.036	0.006	0.006	—
	6	0.017	0.017	—	—
	5	0.041	—	—	—
6	10	3.036	2.008	2.008	1.001
	9	2.036	1.008	1.008	0.001
	8	1.024	1.024	0.003	0.003
	7	0.010+	0.010+	—	—
	6	0.026	—	—	—
5	10	2.022	2.022	1.004	1.004
	9	1.017	1.017	0.002	0.002
	8	1.047	0.007	0.007	—
	7	0.019	0.019	—	—
	6	0.042	—	—	—
4	10	1.011	1.011	0.001	0.001
	9	1.041	0.005−	0.005−	0.005−
	8	0.015−	0.015−	—	—
	7	0.035−	—	—	—
3	10	1.038	0.003	0.003	0.003
	9	0.014	0.014	—	—
	8	0.035−	—	—	—
2	10	0.015+	0.015+	—	—
	9	0.045+	—	—	—

	a	Probability			
		0.05	0.025	0.01	0.005
$A = 11$ $B = 11$	11	7.045+	6.018	5.006	4.002
	10	5.032	4.012	3.004	3.004
	9	4.040	3.015−	2.004	2.004
	8	3.043	2.015−	1.004	1.004
	7	2.040	1.012	0.002	0.002
	6	1.032	0.006	0.006	—
	5	0.018	0.018	—	—
	4	0.045+	—	—	—
10	11	6.035+	5.012	4.004	4.004
	10	4.021	4.021	3.007	2.002
	9	3.024	3.024	2.007	1.002
	8	2.023	2.023	1.006	0.001
	7	1.017	1.017	0.003	0.003
	6	1.043	0.009	0.009	—
	5	0.023	0.023	—	—
9	11	5.026	4.008	4.008	3.002
	10	4.038	3.012	2.003	2.003
	9	3.040	2.012	1.003	1.003
	8	2.035−	1.009	1.009	0.001
	7	1.025−	1.025−	0.004	0.004
	6	0.012	0.012	—	—
	5	0.030	—	—	—
8	11	4.018	4.018	3.005−	3.005−
	10	3.024	3.024	2.006	1.001

	a	Probability			
		0.05	0.025	0.01	0.005
$A = 11$ $B = 8$	9	2.022	2.022	1.005−	1.005−
	8	1.015−	1.015−	0.002	0.002
	7	1.037	0.007	0.007	—
	6	0.017	0.017	—	—
	5	0.040	—	—	—
7	11	4.043	3.011	2.002	2.002
	10	3.047	2.013	1.002	1.002
	9	2.039	1.009	1.009	0.001
	8	1.025−	1.025−	0.004	0.004
	7	0.010+	0.010+	—	—
	6	0.025−	0.025−	—	—
6	11	3.029	2.006	2.006	1.001
	10	2.028	1.005+	1.005+	0.001
	9	1.018	1.018	0.002	0.002
	8	1.043	0.007	0.007	—
	7	0.017	0.017	—	—
	6	0.037	—	—	—
5	11	2.018	2.018	1.003	1.003
	10	1.013	1.013	0.001	0.001
	9	1.036	0.005−	0.005−	0.005−
	8	0.013	0.013	—	—
	7	0.029	—	—	—
4	11	1.009	1.009	1.009	0.001
	10	1.033	0.004	0.004	0.004
	9	0.011	0.011	—	—
	8	0.026	—	—	—
3	11	1.033	0.003	0.003	0.003
	10	0.011	0.011	—	—
	9	0.027	—	—	—
2	11	0.013	0.013	—	—
	10	0.038	—	—	—

	a	Probability			
		0.05	0.025	0.01	0.005
$A = 12$ $B = 12$	12	8.047	7.019	6.007	5.002
	11	6.034	5.014	4.005−	4.005−
	10	5.045−	4.018	3.006	2.002
	9	4.050−	3.020	2.006	1.001
	8	3.050−	2.018	1.005−	1.005−
	7	2.045−	1.014	0.002	0.002
	6	1.034	0.007	0.007	—
	5	0.019	0.019	—	—
	4	0.047	—	—	—
11	12	7.037	6.014	5.005−	5.005−
	11	5.024	5.024	4.008	3.002
	10	4.029	3.010+	2.003	2.003
	9	3.030	2.009	2.009	1.002
	8	2.026	1.007	1.007	0.001
	7	1.019	1.019	0.003	0.003
	6	1.045−	0.009	0.009	—
	5	0.024	0.024	—	—
10	12	6.029	5.010−	5.010−	4.003
	11	5.043	4.015+	3.005−	3.005−
	10	4.048	3.017	2.005−	2.005−
	9	3.046	2.015−	1.004	1.004
	8	2.038	1.010+	0.002	0.002
	7	1.026	0.005−	0.005−	0.005−
	6	0.012	0.012	—	—

TESTS OF SIGNIFICANCE IN A 2 × 2 CONTINGENCY TABLE

	a	Probability 0.05	0.025	0.01	0.005
A = 12 *B* = 10	5	0.030	—	—	—
9	12	5.021	5.021	4.006	3.002
	11	4.029	3.009	3.009	2.002
	10	3.029	2.008	2.008	1.002
	9	2.024	2.024	1.006	0.001
	8	1.016	1.016	0.002	0.002
	7	1.037	0.007	0.007	—
	6	0.017	0.017	—	—
	5	0.039	—	—	—
8	12	5.049	4.014	3.004	3.004
	11	3.018	3.018	2.004	2.004
	10	2.015+	2.015+	1.003	1.003
	9	2.040	1.010−	1.010−	0.001
	8	1.025−	1.025−	0.004	0.004
	7	0.010+	0.010+	—	—
	6	0.024	0.024	—	—
7	12	4.030	3.009	3.009	2.002
	11	3.038	2.010−	2.010−	1.002
	10	2.029	1.006	1.006	0.001
	9	1.017	1.017	0.002	0.002
	8	1.040	0.007	0.007	—
	7	0.016	0.016	—	—
	6	0.034	—	—	—
6	12	3.025−	3.025−	2.005−	2.005−
	11	2.022	2.022	1.004	1.004
	10	1.013	1.013	0.002	0.002
	9	1.032	0.005−	0.005−	0.005−
	8	0.011	0.011	—	—
	7	0.025−	0.025−	—	—
	6	0.050−	—	—	—
5	12	2.015−	2.015−	1.002	1.002
	11	1.010−	1.010−	1.010−	0.001
	10	1.028	0.003	0.003	0.003
	9	0.009	0.009	0.009	—
	8	0.020	0.020	—	—
	7	0.041	—	—	—
4	12	2.050	1.007	1.007	0.001
	11	1.027	0.003	0.003	0.003
	10	0.008	0.008	0.008	—
	9	0.019	0.019	—	—
	8	0.038	—	—	—
3	12	1.029	0.002	0.002	0.002
	11	0.009	0.009	0.009	—
	10	0.022	0.022	—	—
	9	0.044	—	—	—
2	12	0.011	0.011	—	—
	11	0.033	—	—	—
A = 13 *B* = 13	13	9.048	8.020	7.007	6.003
	12	7.037	6.015+	5.006	4.002
	11	6.048	5.021	4.008	3.002
	10	4.024	4.024	3.008	2.002
	9	3.024	3.024	2.008	1.002
	8	2.021	2.021	1.006	0.001
	7	2.048	1.015+	0.003	0.003
	6	1.037	0.007	0.007	—
A = 13 *B* = 13	5	0.020	0.020	—	—
	4	0.048	—	—	—
12	13	8.039	7.015−	6.005+	5.002
	12	6.027	5.010−	5.010−	4.003
	11	5.033	4.013	3.004	3.004
	10	4.036	3.013	2.004	2.004
	9	3.034	2.011	1.003	1.003
	8	2.029	1.008	1.008	0.001
	7	1.020	1.020	0.004	0.004
	6	1.046	0.010−	0.010−	—
	5	0.024	0.024		—
11	13	7.031	6.011	5.003	5.003
	12	6.048	5.018	4.006	3.002
	11	4.021	4.021	3.007	2.002
	10	3.021	3.021	2.006	1.001
	9	3.050−	2.017	1.004	1.004
	8	2.040	1.011	0.002	0.002
	7	1.027	0.005−	0.005−	0.005−
	6	0.013	0.013	—	—
	5	0.030	—	—	—
10	13	6.024	6.024	5.007	4.002
	12	5.035−	4.012	3.003	3.003
	11	4.037	3.012	2.003	2.003
	10	3.033	2.010+	1.002	1.002
	9	2.026	1.006	1.006	0.001
	8	1.017	1.017	0.003	0.003
	7	1.038	0.007	0.007	—
	6	0.017	0.017	—	—
	5	0.038	—	—	—
9	13	5.017	5.017	4.005−	4.005−
	12	4.023	4.023	3.007	2.001
	11	3.022	3.022	2.006	1.001
	10	2.017	2.017	1.004	1.004
	9	2.040	1.010+	0.001	0.001
	8	1.025−	1.025−	0.004	0.004
	7	0.010+	0.010+	—	—
	6	0.023	0.023	—	—
	5	0.049	—	—	—
8	13	5.042	4.012	3.003	3.003
	12	4.047	3.014	2.003	2.003
	11	3.041	2.011	1.002	1.002
	10	2.029	1.007	1.007	0.001
	9	1.017	1.017	0.002	0.002
	8	1.037	0.006	0.006	—
	7	0.015−	0.015−	—	—
	6	0.032	—	—	—
7	13	4.031	3.007	3.007	2.001
	12	3.031	2.007	2.007	1.001
	11	2.022	2.022	1.004	1.004
	10	1.012	1.012	0.002	0.002
	9	1.029	0.004	0.004	0.004
	8	0.010+	0.010+	—	—
	7	0.022	0.022	—	—
	6	0.044	—	—	—
6	13	3.021	3.021	2.004	2.004

TESTS OF SIGNIFICANCE IN A 2 × 2 CONTINGENCY TABLE

	a	Probability 0.05	0.025	0.01	0.005
A = 13 B = 6	12	2.017	2.017	1.003	1.003
	11	2.046	1.010−	1.010−	0.001
	10	1.024	1.024	0.003	0.003
	9	1.050−	0.008	0.008	—
	8	0.017	0.017	—	—
	7	0.034	—	—	—
5	13	2.012	2.012	1.002	1.002
	12	2.044	1.008	1.008	0.001
	11	1.022	1.022	0.002	0.002
	10	1.047	0.007	0.007	—
	9	0.015−	0.015−	—	—
	8	0.029	—	—	—
4	13	2.044	1.006	1.006	0.000
	12	1.022	1.022	0.002	0.002
	11	0.006	0.006	0.006	—
	10	0.015−	0.015−	—	—
	9	0.029	—	—	—
3	13	1.025	1.025	0.002	0.002
	12	0.007	0.007	0.007	—
	11	0.018	0.018	—	—
	10	0.036	—	—	—
2	13	0.010−	0.010−	0.010−	—
	12	0.029	—	—	—
A = 14 B = 14	14	10.049	9.020	8.008	7.003
	13	8.038	7.016	6.006	5.002
	12	6.023	6.023	5.009	4.003
	11	5.027	4.011	3.004	3.004
	10	4.028	3.011	2.003	2.003
	9	3.027	2.009	2.009	1.002
	8	2.023	2.023	1.006	0.001
	7	1.016	1.016	0.003	0.003
	6	1.038	0.008	0.008	—
	5	0.020	0.020	—	—
	4	0.049	—	—	—
13	14	9.041	8.016	7.006	6.002
	13	7.029	6.011	5.004	5.004
	12	6.037	5.015+	4.005+	3.002
	11	5.041	4.017	3.006	2.001
	10	4.041	3.016	2.005−	2.005−
	9	3.038	2.013	1.003	1.003
	8	2.031	1.009	1.009	0.001
	7	1.021	1.021	0.004	0.004
	6	1.048	0.010+	—	—
	5	0.025−	0.025−	—	—
12	14	8.033	7.012	6.004	6.004
	13	6.021	6.021	5.007	4.002
	12	5.025+	4.009	4.009	3.003
	11	4.026	3.009	3.009	2.002
	10	3.024	3.024	2.007	1.002
	9	2.019	2.019	1.005−	1.005−
	8	2.042	1.012	0.002	0.002
	7	1.028	0.005+	0.005+	—
	6	0.013	0.013	—	—
	5	0.030	—	—	—
11	14	7.026	6.009	6.009	5.003
A = 14 B = 11	13	6.039	5.014	4.004	4.004
	12	5.043	4.016	3.005−	3.005−
	11	4.042	3.015−	2.004	2.004
	10	3.036	2.011	1.003	1.003
	9	2.027	1.007	1.007	0.001
	8	1.017	1.017	0.003	0.003
	7	1.038	0.007	0.007	—
	6	0.017	0.017	—	—
	5	0.038	—	—	—
10	14	6.020	6.020	5.006	4.002
	13	5.028	4.009	4.009	3.002
	12	4.028	3.009	3.009	2.002
	11	3.024	3.024	2.007	1.001
	10	2.018	2.018	1.004	1.004
	9	2.040	1.011	0.002	0.002
	8	1.024	1.024	0.004	0.004
	7	0.010−	0.010−	0.010−	—
	6	0.022	0.022	—	—
	5	0.047	—	—	—
9	14	6.047	5.014	4.004	4.004
	13	4.018	4.018	3.005−	3.005−
	12	3.017	3.017	2.004	2.004
	11	3.042	2.012	1.002	1.002
	10	2.029	1.007	1.007	0.001
	9	1.017	1.017	0.002	0.002
	8	1.036	0.006	0.006	—
	7	0.014	0.014	—	—
	6	0.030	—	—	—
8	14	5.036	4.010−	4.010−	3.002
	13	4.039	3.011	2.002	2.002
	12	3.032	2.008	2.008	1.001
	11	2.022	2.022	1.005−	1.005−
	10	2.048	1.012	0.002	0.002
	9	1.026	0.004	0.004	0.004
	8	0.009	0.009	0.009	—
	7	0.020	0.020	—	—
	6	0.040	—	—	—
7	14	4.026	3.006	3.006	2.001
	13	3.025	2.006	2.006	1.001
	12	2.017	2.017	1.003	1.003
	11	2.041	1.009	1.009	0.001
	10	1.021	1.021	0.003	0.003
	9	1.043	0.007	0.007	—
	8	0.015−	0.015−	—	—
	7	0.030	—	—	—
6	14	3.018	3.018	2.003	2.003
	13	2.014	2.014	1.002	1.002
	12	2.037	1.007	1.007	0.001
	11	1.018	1.018	0.002	0.002
	10	1.038	0.005+	0.005+	—
	9	0.012	0.012	—	—
	8	0.024	0.024	—	—
	7	0.044	—	—	—
5	14	2.010+	2.010+	1.001	1.001
	13	2.037	1.006	1.006	0.001

TESTS OF SIGNIFICANCE IN A 2 × 2 CONTINGENCY TABLE

	a	Probability 0.05	0.025	0.01	0.005
$A = 14$ $B = 5$	12	1.017	1.017	0.002	0.002
	11	1.038	0.005−	0.005−	0.005−
	10	0.011	0.011	—	—
	9	0.022	0.022	—	—
	8	0.040	—	—	—
4	14	2.039	1.005−	1.005−	1.005−
	13	1.019	1.019	0.002	0.002
	12	1.044	0.005−	0.005−	0.005−
	11	0.011	0.011	—	—
	10	0.023	0.023	—	—
	9	0.041	—	—	—
3	14	1.022	1.022	0.001	0.001
	13	0.006	0.006	0.006	—
	12	0.015−	0.015−	—	—
	11	0.029	—	—	—
2	14	0.008	0.008	0.008	—
	13	0.025	0.025	—	—
	12	0.050	—	—	—
$A = 15$ $B = 15$	15	11.050−	10.021	9.008	8.003
	14	9.040	8.018	7.007	6.003
	13	7.025+	6.010+	5.004	5.004
	12	6.030	5.013	4.005−	4.005−
	11	5.033	4.013	3.005−	3.005−
	10	4.033	3.013	2.001	2.001
	9	3.030	2.010+	1.003	1.003
	8	2.025+	1.007	1.007	0.001
	7	1.018	1.018	0.003	0.003
	6	1.040	0.008	0.008	—
	5	0.021	0.021	—	—
	4	0.050−	—	—	—
14	15	10.042	9.017	8.006	7.002
	14	8.031	7.013	6.005−	6.005−
	13	7.041	6.017	5.007	4.002
	12	6.046	5.020	4.007	3.002
	11	5.048	4.020	3.007	2.002
	10	4.046	3.018	2.006	1.001
	9	3.041	2.014	1.004	1.004
	8	2.033	1.009	1.009	0.001
	7	1.022	1.022	0.004	0.004
	6	1.049	0.011	—	—
	5	0.025+	—	—	—
13	15	9.035−	8.013	7.005−	7.005−
	14	7.023	7.023	6.009	5.003
	13	6.029	5.011	4.004	4.004
	12	5.031	4.012	3.004	3.004
	11	4.030	3.011	2.003	2.003
	10	3.026	2.008	2.008	1.002
	9	2.020	2.020	1.005+	0.001
	8	2.043	1.013	0.002	0.002
	7	1.029	0.005+	0.005+	—
	6	0.013	0.013	—	—
	5	0.031	—	—	—
12	15	8.028	7.010−	7.010−	6.003
	14	7.043	6.016	5.006	4.002
	13	6.049	5.019	4.007	3.002

	a	Probability 0.05	0.025	0.01	0.005
$A = 15$ $B = 12$	12	5.049	4.019	3.006	2.002
	11	4.045+	3.017	2.005−	2.005−
	10	3.038	2.012	1.003	1.003
	9	2.028	1.007	1.007	0.001
	8	1.018	1.018	0.003	0.003
	7	1.038	0.007	0.007	—
	6	0.017	0.017	—	—
	5	0.037	—	—	—
11	15	7.022	7.022	6.007	5.002
	14	6.032	5.011	4.003	4.003
	13	5.034	4.012	3.003	3.003
	12	4.032	3.010+	2.003	2.003
	11	3.026	2.008	2.008	1.002
	10	2.019	2.019	1.004	1.004
	9	2.040	1.011	0.002	0.002
	8	1.024	1.024	0.004	0.004
	7	1.040	0.010−	0.010−	—
	6	0.022	0.022	—	—
	5	0.046	—	—	—
10	15	6.017	6.017	5.005−	5.005−
	14	5.023	5.023	4.007	3.002
	13	4.022	4.022	3.007	2.001
	12	3.018	3.018	2.005−	2.005−
	11	3.042	2.013	1.003	1.003
	10	2.029	1.007	1.007	0.001
	9	1.016	1.016	0.002	0.002
	8	1.034	0.006	0.006	—
	7	0.013	0.013	—	—
	6	0.028	—	—	—
9	15	6.042	5.012	4.003	4.003
	14	5.047	4.015−	3.004	3.004
	13	4.042	3.013	2.003	2.003
	12	3.032	2.009	2.009	1.002
	11	2.021	2.021	1.005−	1.005−
	10	2.045−	1.011	0.002	0.002
	9	1.024	1.024	0.004	0.004
	8	1.048	0.009	0.009	—
	7	0.019	0.019	—	—
	6	0.037	—	—	—
8	15	5.032	4.008	4.008	3.002
	14	4.033	3.009	3.009	2.002
	13	3.026	2.006	2.006	1.001
	12	2.017	2.017	1.003	1.003
	11	2.037	1.008	1.008	0.001
	10	1.019	1.019	0.003	0.003
	9	1.038	0.006	0.006	—
	8	0.013	0.013	—	—
	7	0.026	—	—	—
	6	0.050−	—	—	—
7	15	4.023	4.023	3.005−	3.005−
	14	3.021	3.021	2.004	2.004
	13	2.014	2.014	1.002	1.002
	12	2.032	1.007	1.007	0.001
	11	1.015+	1.015+	0.002	0.002
	10	1.032	0.005−	0.005−	0.005−

TESTS OF SIGNIFICANCE IN A 2 × 2 CONTINGENCY TABLE

	a	Probability 0.05	0.025	0.01	0.005
A = 15 *B* = 7	9	0.010+	0.010+	—	—
	8	0.020	0.020	—	—
	7	0.038	—	—	—
6	15	3.015+	3.015+	2.003	2.003
	14	2.011	2.011	1.002	1.002
	13	2.031	1.006	1.006	0.001
	12	1.014	1.014	0.002	0.002
	11	1.029	0.004	0.004	0.004
	10	0.009	0.009	0.009	—
	9	0.017	0.017	—	—
	8	0.032	—	—	—
5	15	2.009	2.009	2.009	1.001
	14	2.032	1.005−	1.005−	1.005−
	13	1.014	1.014	0.001	0.001
	12	1.031	0.004	0.004	0.004
	11	0.008	0.008	0.008	—
	10	0.016	0.016	—	—
	9	0.030	—	—	—
4	15	2.035+	1.004	1.004	1.004
	14	1.016	1.016	0.001	0.001
	13	1.037	0.004	0.004	0.004
	12	0.009	0.009	0.009	—
	11	0.018	0.018	—	—
	10	0.033	—	—	—
3	15	1.020	1.020	0.001	0.001
	14	0.005−	0.005−	0.005−	0.005−
	13	0.012	0.012	—	—
	12	0.025−	0.025−	—	—
	11	0.043	—	—	—
2	15	0.007	0.007	0.007	—
	14	0.022	0.022	—	—
	13	10.044	—	—	—
A = 16 *B* = 16	16	11.022	11.022	10.009	9.003
	15	10.041	9.019	8.008	7.003
	14	8.027	7.012	6.005−	6.005−
	13	7.033	6.015−	5.006	4.002
	12	6.037	5.016	4.006	3.002
	11	5.038	4.016	3.006	2.002
	10	4.037	3.015−	2.005−	2.005−
	9	3.033	2.012	1.003	1.003
	8	2.027	1.008	1.008	0.001
	7	1.019	1.019	0.003	0.003
	6	1.041	0.009	0.009	—
	5	0.022	0.022	—	—
15	16	11.043	10.018	9.007	8.002
	15	9.033	8.014	7.005+	6.002
	14	8.044	7.019	6.008	5.003
	13	6.023	6.023	5.009	4.003
	12	5.024	5.024	4.009	3.003
	11	4.023	4.023	3.008	2.002
	10	4.049	3.020	2.006	1.001
	9	3.043	2.016	1.004	1.004
	8	2.035−	1.010+	0.002	0.002
	7	1.023	1.023	0.004	0.004
	6	0.011	0.011	—	—
A = 16 *B* = 15	5	0.026	—	—	—
14	16	10.037	9.014	8.005+	7.002
	15	8.025+	7.010−	7.010−	6.003
	14	7.032	6.013	5.005−	5.005−
	13	6.035+	5.014	4.005+	3.001
	12	5.035+	4.014	3.005−	3.005−
	11	4.033	3.012	2.004	2.004
	10	3.028	2.009	2.009	1.002
	9	2.021	2.021	1.006	0.001
	8	2.015−	1.013	0.002	0.002
	7	1.030	0.006	0.006	—
	6	0.013	0.013	—	—
	5	0.031	—	—	—
13	16	9.030	8.011	7.004	7.004
	15	8.037	7.019	6.007	5.002
	14	6.023	6.023	5.008	4.003
	13	5.023	5.023	4.008	3.003
	12	4.022	4.022	3.007	2.002
	11	4.078	3.018	2.005+	1.001
	10	3.039	2.013	1.003	1.003
	9	2.029	1.008	1.008	0.001
	8	1.018	1.018	0.003	0.003
	7	1.038	0.007	0.007	—
	6	0.017	0.017	—	—
	5	0.033	—	—	—
12	16	8.024	8.024	7.008	6.002
	15	7.036	6.013	5.004	5.004
	14	6.040	5.015−	4.005−	4.005−
	13	5.039	4.014	3.004	3.004
	12	4.034	3.012	2.003	2.003
	11	3.027	2.008	2.008	1.002
	10	2.019	2.019	1.005−	1.005−
	9	2.040	1.011	0.002	0.002
	8	1.024	1.024	0.004	0.004
	7	1.048	0.010−	0.010−	—
	6	0.021	0.021	—	—
	5	0.044	—	—	—
11	16	7.019	7.019	6.005	5.002
	15	6.027	5.009	5.009	4.002
	14	5.027	4.009	4.009	3.002
	13	4.024	4.024	3.008	2.002
	12	3.019	3.019	2.005+	1.001
	11	3.041	2.013	1.003	1.003
	10	2.028	1.007	1.007	0.001
	9	1.016	1.016	0.002	0.002
	8	1.033	0.006	0.066	—
	7	0.013	0.013	—	—
	6	0.027	—	—	—
10	16	7.046	6.014	5.004	5.004
	15	5.018	5.018	4.005+	3.001
	14	4.017	4.017	3.005−	3.005−
	13	4.042	3.014	2.003	2.003
	12	3.032	2.009	2.009	1.002
	11	2.021	2.021	1.005−	1.005−
	10	2.042	1.011	0.002	0.002

TESTS OF SIGNIFICANCE IN A 2 × 2 CONTINGENCY TABLE

	a	Probability 0.05	0.025	0.01	0.005
$A = 16$ $B = 10$	9	1.023	1.023	0.004	0.004
	8	1.045−	0.008	0.008	—
	7	0.017	0.017	—	—
	6	0.035−	—	—	—
9	16	6.037	5.010−	5.010−	4.002
	15	5.040	4.012	3.003	3.003
	14	4.034	3.010−	3.010−	2.002
	13	3.025+	2.007	2.007	1.001
	12	2.016	2.016	1.003	1.003
	11	2.033	1.008	1.008	0.001
	10	1.017	1.017	0.002	0.002
	9	1.034	0.006	0.006	—
	8	0.012	0.012	—	—
	7	0.024	0.024	—	—
	6	0.045+	—	—	—
8	16	5.028	4.007	4.007	3.001
	15	4.028	3.007	3.007	2.001
	14	3.021	3.021	2.005−	2.005−
	13	3.047	2.013	1.002	1.002
	12	2.028	1.006	1.006	0.001
	11	1.014	1.014	0.002	0.002
	10	1.027	0.004	0.004	0.004
	9	0.009	0.009	0.009	—
	8	0.017	0.017	—	—
	7	0.033	—	—	—
7	16	4.020	4.020	3.004	3.004
	15	3.017	3.017	2.003	2.003
	14	3.045+	2.011	1.002	1.002
	13	2.026	1.005−	1.005−	1.005−
	12	1.012	1.012	0.001	0.001
	11	1.024	1.024	0.003	0.003
	10	1.045−	0.007	0.007	—
	9	0.014	0.014	—	—
	8	0.026	—	—	—
	7	0.047	—	—	—
6	16	3.013	3.013	2.002	2.002
	15	3.046	2.009	2.009	1.001
	14	2.025+	1.004	1.004	1.004
	13	1.011	1.011	0.001	0.001
	12	1.023	1.023	0.003	0.003
	11	1.043	0.006	0.006	—
	10	0.012	0.012	—	—
	9	0.023	0.023	—	—
	8	0.040	—	—	—
5	16	3.048	2.008	2.008	1.001
	15	2.028	1.004	1.004	1.004
	14	1.011	1.011	0.001	0.001
	13	1.025+	0.003	0.003	0.003
	12	1.047	0.006	0.006	—
	11	0.012	0.012	—	—
	10	0.023	0.023	—	—
	9	0.039	—	—	—
4	16	2.032	1.004	1.004	1.004
	15	1.013	1.013	0.001	0.001
	14	1.032	0.003	0.003	0.003
$A = 16$ $B = 4$	13	0.007	0.007	0.007	—
	12	0.014	0.014	—	—
	11	0.026	—	—	—
	10	0.043	—	—	—
3	16	1.018	1.018	0.001	0.001
	15	0.004	0.004	0.004	0.004
	14	0.010+	0.010+	—	—
	13	0.021	0.021	—	—
	12	0.036	—	—	—
2	16	0.007	0.007	0.007	—
	15	0.020	0.020	—	—
	14	0.039	—	—	—
$A = 17$ $B = 17$	17	12.022	12.022	11.009	10.004
	16	11.043	10.020	9.008	8.003
	15	9.029	8.013	7.005+	6.002
	14	8.035+	7.016	6.007	5.002
	13	7.040	6.018	5.007	4.003
	12	6.042	5.019	4.007	3.002
	11	5.042	4.018	3.007	2.002
	10	4.040	3.016	2.005+	1.001
	9	3.035+	2.013	1.003	1.003
	8	2.029	1.008	1.008	0.001
	7	1.020	1.020	0.004	0.004
	6	1.043	0.009	0.009	—
	5	0.022	0.022	—	—
16	17	12.044	11.018	10.007	9.003
	16	10.035−	9.015−	8.006	7.002
	15	9.046	8.021	7.009	6.003
	14	7.025+	6.011	5.004	5.004
	13	6.027	5.011	4.001	4.001
	12	5.027	4.011	3.004	3.004
	11	4.025+	3.009	3.009	2.003
	10	3.022	3.022	2.007	1.002
	9	3.046	2.017	1.004	1.004
	8	2.036	1.011	0.002	0.002
	7	1.024	1.024	0.005−	0.005−
	6	0.011	0.011	—	—
	5	0.026	—	—	—
15	17	11.038	10.015−	9.006	8.002
	16	9.027	8.011	7.004	7.004
	15	8.035+	7.015−	6.006	5.002
	14	7.040	6.017	5.006	4.002
	13	6.041	5.017	4.006	3.002
	12	5.039	4.016	3.005+	2.001
	11	4.035+	3.013	2.004	2.004
	10	3.029	2.010−	2.010−	1.002
	9	2.022	2.022	1.006	0.001
	8	2.046	1.014	0.002	0.002
	7	1.030	0.006	0.006	—
	6	0.014	0.014	—	—
	5	0.031	—	—	—
14	17	10.032	9.012	8.004	8.004
	16	8.021	8.021	7.008	6.003
	15	7.026	6.010−	6.010−	5.003
	14	6.028	5.011	4.004	4.004

TESTS OF SIGNIFICANCE IN A 2 × 2 CONTINGENCY TABLE

	a	Probability 0.05	0.025	0.01	0.005
$A = 17$ $B = 14$	13	5.027	4.010−	4.010−	3.003
	12	4.024	4.024	3.008	2.002
	11	4.049	3.019	2.006	1.001
	10	3.040	2.014	1.003	1.003
	9	2.029	1.008	1.008	0.001
	8	1.018	1.018	0.003	0.003
	7	1.038	0.007	0.007	—
	6	0.017	0.017	—	—
	5	0.036	—	—	—
13	17	9.026	8.009	8.009	7.003
	16	8.040	7.015+	6.005+	5.002
	15	7.045+	6.018	5.006	4.002
	14	6.045+	5.018	4.006	3.002
	13	5.042	4.016	3.005+	2.001
	12	4.035+	3.013	2.004	2.004
	11	3.028	2.009	2.009	1.002
	10	2.019	2.019	1.005−	1.005−
	9	2.040	1.011	0.002	0.002
	8	1.024	1.024	0.004	0.004
	7	1.047	0.010−	0.010−	—
	6	0.021	0.021	—	—
	5	0.043	—	—	—
12	17	8.021	8.021	7.007	6.002
	16	7.030	6.011	5.003	5.003
	15	6.033	5.012	4.004	4.004
	14	5.030	4.011	3.003	3.003
	13	4.026	3.008	3.008	2.002
	12	3.020	3.020	2.006	1.001
	11	3.041	2.013	1.003	1.003
	10	2.028	1.007	1.007	0.001
	9	1.016	1.016	0.002	0.002
	8	1.032	0.006	0.006	—
	7	0.012	0.012	—	—
	6	0.026	—	—	—
11	17	7.016	7.016	6.005−	6.005−
	16	6.022	6.022	5.007	4.002
	15	5.022	5.022	4.007	3.002
	14	4.019	4.019	3.006	2.001
	13	4.042	3.014	2.004	2.004
	12	3.031	2.009	2.009	1.002
	11	2.020	2.020	1.005−	1.005−
	10	2.040	1.011	0.001	0.001
	9	1.022	1.022	0.004	0.004
	8	1.042	0.008	0.008	—
	7	0.016	0.016	—	—
	6	0.033	—	—	—
10	17	7.041	6.012	5.003	5.003
	16	6.047	5.015+	4.004	4.004
	15	5.043	4.014	3.004	3.004
	14	4.034	3.010+	2.002	2.002
	13	3.024	3.024	2.007	1.001
	12	3.049	2.015+	1.003	1.003
	11	2.031	1.007	1.007	0.001
	10	1.016	1.016	0.002	0.002
	9	1.031	0.005+	0.005+	—
$A = 17$ $B = 10$	8	0.011	0.011	—	—
	7	0.022	0.022	—	—
	6	0.042	—	—	—
9	17	6.032	5.008	5.008	4.002
	16	5.034	4.010−	4.010−	3.002
	15	4.028	3.008	3.008	2.002
	14	3.020	3.020	2.005−	2.005−
	13	3.042	2.012	1.002	1.002
	12	2.025+	1.006	1.006	0.001
	11	2.048	1.012	0.002	0.002
	10	1.024	1.024	0.004	0.004
	9	1.045−	0.008	0.008	—
	8	0.016	0.016	—	—
	7	0.030	—	—	—
8	17	5.024	5.024	4.006	3.001
	16	4.023	4.023	3.006	2.001
	15	3.017	3.017	2.004	2.004
	14	3.039	2.010−	2.010−	1.002
	13	2.022	2.022	1.004	1.004
	12	2.043	1.010−	1.010−	0.001
	11	1.020	1.020	0.003	0.003
	10	1.038	0.006	0.006	—
	9	0.012	0.012	—	—
	8	0.022	0.022	—	—
	7	0.040	—	—	—
7	17	4.017	4.017	3.003	3.003
	16	3.014	3.014	2.003	2.003
	15	3.038	2.009	2.009	1.001
	14	2.021	2.021	1.004	1.004
	13	2.042	1.009	1.009	0.001
	12	1.018	1.018	0.002	0.002
	11	1.034	0.005−	0.005−	0.005−
	10	0.010−	0.010−	0.010−	—
	9	0.019	0.019	—	—
	8	0.033	—	—	—
6	17	3.011	3.011	2.002	2.002
	16	3.040	2.008	2.008	1.001
	15	2.021	2.021	1.003	1.003
	14	2.045+	1.009	1.009	0.001
	13	1.018	1.018	0.002	0.002
	12	1.035−	0.005−	0.005−	0.005−
	11	0.009	0.009	0.009	—
	10	0.017	0.017	—	—
	9	0.030	—	—	—
	8	0.050−	—	—	—
5	17	3.043	2.006	2.006	1.001
	16	2.024	2.024	1.003	1.003
	15	1.009	1.009	1.009	0.001
	14	1.021	1.021	0.002	0.002
	13	1.039	0.005−	0.005−	0.005−
	12	0.010−	0.010−	0.010−	—
	11	0.018	0.018	—	—
	10	0.030	—	—	—
	9	0.049	—	—	—
4	17	2.029	1.003	1.003	1.003

TESTS OF SIGNIFICANCE IN A 2 × 2 CONTINGENCY TABLE

	a	Probability 0.05	0.025	0.01	0.005
$A = 17$ $B = 4$	16	1.012	1.012	0.001	0.001
	15	1.028	0.003	0.003	0.003
	14	0.006	0.006	0.006	—
	13	0.012	0.012	—	—
	12	0.021	0.021	—	—
	11	0.035+	—	—	—
3	17	1.016	1.016	0.001	0.001
	16	1.046	0.004	0.004	0.004
	15	0.009	0.009	0.009	—
	14	0.018	0.018	—	—
	13	0.031	—	—	—
	12	0.049	—	—	—
2	17	0.006	0.006	0.006	—
	16	0.018	0.018	—	—
	15	0.035+	—	—	—
$A = 18$ $B = 18$	18	13.023	13.023	12.010−	11.004
	17	12.044	11.020	10.009	9.004
	16	10.030	9.014	8.006	7.002
	15	9.038	8.018	7.008	6.003
	14	8.043	7.020	6.009	5.003
	13	7.046	6.022	5.009	4.003
	12	6.047	5.022	4.009	3.003
	11	5.046	4.020	3.008	2.002
	10	4.043	3.018	2.006	1.001
	9	3.038	2.014	1.004	1.004
	8	2.030	1.009	1.009	0.001
	7	1.020	1.020	0.004	0.004
	6	1.044	0.010−	0.010−	—
	5	0.023	0.023	—	—
17	10	10.040+	12.019	11.008	10.003
	17	11.036	10.016	9.007	8.002
	16	10.049	9.023	8.010−	7.004
	15	8.028	7.012	6.005−	6.005−
	14	7.030	6.013	5.005+	4.002
	13	6.031	5.013	4.005−	4.005−
	12	5.030	4.012	3.004	3.004
	11	4.028	3.010+	2.003	2.003
	10	3.023	3.023	2.008	1.002
	9	3.047	2.018	1.005−	1.005−
	8	2.037	1.011	0.002	0.002
	7	1.025−	1.025−	0.005−	0.005−
	6	0.011	0.011	—	—
	5	0.026	—	—	—
16	18	12.039	11.016	10.006	9.002
	17	10.029	9.012	8.005−	8.005−
	16	9.038	8.017	7.007	6.002
	15	8.043	7.019	6.008	5.003
	14	7.046	6.020	5.008	4.003
	13	6.045+	5.020	4.007	3.002
	12	5.042	4.018	3.006	2.002
	11	4.037	3.015−	2.004	2.004
	10	3.031	2.011	1.003	1.003
	9	2.023	2.023	1.006	0.001
	8	2.046	1.014	0.002	0.002
	7	1.030	0.006	0.006	—
$A = 18$ $B = 16$	6	0.014	0.014	—	—
	5	0.031	—	—	—
15	18	11.033	10.013	9.005−	9.005−
	17	9.023	9.023	8.009	7.003
	16	8.029	7.012	6.004	6.004
	15	7.031	6.013	5.005−	5.005−
	14	6.031	5.013	4.004	4.004
	13	5.029	4.011	3.004	3.004
	12	4.025+	3.009	3.009	2.003
	11	3.020	3.020	2.006	1.001
	10	3.041	2.014	1.004	1.004
	9	2.030	1.008	1.008	0.001
	8	1.018	1.018	0.003	0.003
	7	1.038	0.007	0.007	—
	6	0.017	0.017	—	—
	5	0.036	—	—	—
14	18	10.028	9.010−	9.010−	8.003
	17	9.043	8.017	7.006	6.002
	16	8.050−	7.021	6.008	5.003
	15	6.022	6.022	5.008	4.003
	14	6.049	5.020	4.007	3.002
	13	5.044	4.017	3.006	2.001
	12	4.037	3.013	2.004	2.004
	11	3.028	2.009	2.009	1.002
	10	2.020	2.020	1.005−	1.005−
	9	2.039	1.011	0.002	0.002
	8	1.024	1.024	0.004	0.004
	7	1.047	0.009	0.009	—
	6	0.020	0.020	—	—
	5	0.043	—	—	—
13	18	9.023	9.023	8.008	7.002
	17	8.034	7.012	6.004	6.004
	16	7.037	6.014	5.005−	5.005−
	15	6.036	5.014	4.004	4.004
	14	5.032	4.012	3.004	3.004
	13	4.027	3.009	3.009	2.002
	12	3.020	3.020	2.006	1.001
	11	3.040	2.013	1.003	1.003
	10	2.027	1.007	1.007	0.001
	9	1.015+	1.015+	0.002	0.002
	8	1.031	0.006	0.006	—
	7	0.012	0.012	—	—
	6	0.025+	—	—	—
12	18	8.018	8.018	7.006	6.002
	17	7.026	6.009	6.009	5.003
	16	6.027	5.009	5.009	4.003
	15	5.024	5.024	4.008	3.002
	14	4.020	4.020	3.006	2.001
	13	4.042	3.014	2.004	2.004
	12	3.030	2.009	2.009	1.002
	11	2.019	2.019	1.005−	1.005−
	10	2.038	1.010+	0.001	0.001
	9	1.021	1.021	0.003	0.003
	8	1.040	0.007	0.007	—
	7	0.016	0.016	—	—

TESTS OF SIGNIFICANCE IN A 2 × 2 CONTINGENCY TABLE

	a	Probability 0.05	0.025	0.01	0.005
$A = 18$ $B = 12$	6	0.031	—	—	—
11	18	8.045+	7.014	6.004	6.004
	17	6.018	6.018	5.006	4.001
	16	5.018	5.018	4.005+	3.001
	15	5.043	4.015−	3.004	3.004
	14	4.033	3.011	2.003	2.003
	13	3.023	3.023	2.007	1.001
	12	3.046	2.014	1.003	1.003
	11	2.029	1.007	1.007	0.001
	10	1.015−	1.015−	0.002	0.002
	9	1.029	0.005−	0.005−	0.005−
	8	0.010+	0.010+	—	—
	7	0.020	0.020	—	—
	6	0.039	—	—	—
10	18	7.037	6.010+	5.003	5.003
	17	6.041	5.013	4.003	4.003
	16	5.036	4.011	3.003	3.003
	15	4.028	3.008	3.008	2.002
	14	3.019	3.019	2.005−	2.005−
	13	3.039	2.011	1.002	1.002
	12	2.023	2.023	1.005+	0.001
	11	2.043	1.011	0.001	0.001
	10	1.022	1.022	0.003	0.003
	9	1.040	0.007	0.007	—
	8	0.014	0.014	—	—
	7	0.027	—	—	—
	6	0.049	—	—	—
9	18	6.029	5.007	5.007	4.002
	17	5.030	4.008	4.008	3.002
	16	4.023	4.023	3.006	2.001
	15	3.016	3.016	2.004	2.004
	14	3.034	2.009	2.009	1.002
	13	2.019	2.019	1.004	1.004
	12	2.037	1.009	1.009	0.001
	11	1.018	1.018	0.002	0.002
	10	1.033	0.005+	0.005+	—
	9	0.010+	0.010+	—	—
	8	0.020	0.020	—	—
	7	0.036	—	—	—
8	18	5.022	5.022	4.005−	4.005−
	17	4.020	4.020	3.004	3.004
	16	3.014	3.014	2.003	2.003
	15	3.032	2.008	2.008	1.001
	14	2.017	2.017	1.003	1.003
	13	2.034	1.007	1.007	0.001
	12	1.015+	1.015+	0.002	0.002
	11	1.023	0.004	0.004	0.004
	10	1.049	0.008	0.008	—
	9	0.016	0.016	—	—
	8	0.028	—	—	—
	7	0.048	—	—	—
7	18	4.015+	4.015+	3.003	3.003
	17	3.012	3.012	2.002	2.002
	16	3.032	2.007	2.007	1.001
	15	2.017	2.017	1.003	1.003

	a	Probability 0.05	0.025	0.01	0.005
$A = 18$ $B = 7$	14	2.034	1.007	1.007	0.001
	13	1.014	1.014	0.002	0.002
	12	1.027	0.004	0.004	0.004
	11	1.046	0.007	0.007	—
	10	0.013	0.013	—	—
	9	0.024	0.024	—	—
	8	0.040	—	—	—
6	18	3.010−	3.010−	3.010−	2.001
	17	3.035+	2.006	2.006	1.001
	16	2.018	2.018	1.003	1.003
	15	2.038	1.007	1.007	0.001
	14	1.015−	1.015−	0.002	0.002
	13	1.028	0.003	0.003	0.003
	12	1.048	0.007	0.007	—
	11	0.013	0.013	—	—
	10	0.022	0.022	—	—
	9	0.037	—	—	—
5	18	3.040	2.006	2.006	1.001
	17	2.021	2.021	1.003	1.003
	16	2.048	1.008	1.008	0.001
	15	1.017	1.017	0.002	0.002
	14	1.033	0.004	0.004	0.004
	13	0.007	0.007	0.007	—
	12	0.014	0.014	—	—
	11	0.024	0.024	—	—
	10	0.038	—	—	—
4	18	2.026	1.003	1.003	1.033
	17	1.010−	1.010−	1.010−	0.001
	16	1.024	1.024	0.002	0.002
	15	1.046	0.005−	0.005−	0.005−
	14	0.010−	0.010−	0.010−	—
	13	0.017	0.017	—	—
	12	0.029	—	—	—
	11	0.045+	—	—	—
3	18	1.014	1.014	0.001	0.001
	17	1.041	0.003	0.003	0.003
	16	0.008	0.008	0.008	—
	15	0.015+	0.015+	—	—
	14	0.026	—	—	—
	13	0.042	—	—	—
2	18	0.005+	0.005+	0.005+	—
	17	0.016	0.016	—	—
	16	0.032	—	—	—
$A = 19$ $B = 19$	19	14.023	14.023	13.010−	12.004
	18	13.045−	12.021	11.009	10.004
	17	11.031	10.015−	9.006	8.003
	16	10.039	9.019	8.009	7.003
	15	9.046	8.022	6.004	6.004
	14	8.050−	7.024	5.004	5.004
	13	6.025+	5.011	4.004	4.004
	12	5.024	5.024	3.003	3.003
	11	5.050−	4.022	3.009	2.003
	10	4.046	3.019	2.006	1.002
	9	3.039	2.015−	1.004	1.004
	8	2.031	1.009	1.009	0.002

TESTS OF SIGNIFICANCE IN A 2 × 2 CONTINGENCY TABLE

		a	Probability 0.05	0.025	0.01	0.005
$A = 19$	$B = 19$	7	1.021	1.021	0.004	0.004
		6	1.045−	0.010−	0.010−	—
		5	0.023	0.023	—	—
	18	19	14.046	13.020	12.008	11.003
		18	12.037	11.017	10.007	9.003
		17	10.024	10.024	8.004	8.004
		16	9.030	8.014	7.006	6.002
		15	8.033	7.015+	6.006	5.002
		14	7.035+	6.016	5.006	4.002
		13	6.035−	5.015+	4.006	3.002
		12	5.033	4.014	3.005−	3.005−
		11	4.030	3.011	2.004	2.004
		10	3.025−	3.025−	2.008	1.002
		9	3.049	2.019	1.005+	0.001
		8	2.038	1.012	0.002	0.002
		7	1.025+	0.005−	0.005−	0.005−
		7	0.012	0.012	—	—
		5	0.027	—	—	—
	17	19	13.040	12.016	11.006	10.002
		18	11.030	10.013	9.005+	8.002
		17	10.040	9.018	8.008	7.003
		16	9.047	8.022	7.009	6.003
		15	8.050−	7.023	6.010−	5.004
		14	6.023	6.023	5.010−	4.003
		13	6.049	5.022	4.008	3.003
		12	5.045−	4.019	3.007	2.002
		11	4.039	3.015+	2.005−	2.005−
		10	3.032	2.011	1.003	1.003
		9	2.024	2.024	1.007	0.001
		8	2.047	1.015−	0.002	0.002
		7	1.031	0.006	0.006	—
		6	0.014	0.014	—	—
		5	0.031	—	—	—
	16	19	12.035−	11.013	10.005−	10.005−
		18	10.024	10.024	9.010−	8.004
		17	9.031	8.013	7.005+	6.002
		16	8.035−	7.015+	6.006	5.002
		15	7.036	6.015+	5.006	4.002
		14	6.034	5.014	4.005+	3.002
		13	5.031	4.012	3.004	3.004
		12	4.027	3.010−	3.010−	2.003
		11	3.021	3.021	2.007	1.002
		10	3.042	2.015−	1.004	1.004
		9	2.030	1.009	1.009	0.001
		8	1.018	1.018	0.003	0.003
		7	1.037	0.007	0.007	—
		6	0.017	0.017	—	—
		5	0.036	—	—	—
	15	19	11.029	10.011	9.004	9.004
		18	10.046	9.019	8.007	7.002
		17	8.023	8.023	7.009	6.003
		16	7.025−	7.025−	6.010−	5.003
		15	6.024	6.024	5.009	4.003
		14	5.022	5.022	4.008	3.002
		13	5.045+	4.018	3.006	2.002
$A = 19$	$B = 15$	12	4.037	3.014	2.004	2.004
		11	3.029	2.009	2.009	1.002
		10	2.020	2.020	1.005+	0.001
		9	2.039	1.011	0.002	0.002
		8	1.023	1.023	0.004	0.004
		7	1.046	0.009	0.009	—
		6	0.020	0.020	—	—
		5	0.042	—	—	—
	14	19	10.024	10.024	9.008	8.003
		18	9.037	8.014	7.005−	7.005−
		17	8.042	7.017	6.006	5.002
		16	7.042	6.017	5.006	4.002
		15	6.039	5.015+	4.005+	3.001
		14	5.034	4.013	3.004	3.004
		13	4.027	3.009	3.009	2.003
		12	3.020	3.020	2.006	1.001
		11	3.040	2.013	1.003	1.003
		10	2.027	1.007	1.007	0.001
		9	1.015−	1.015−	0.002	0.002
		8	1.030	0.005+	0.005+	—
		7	0.012	0.012	—	—
		6	0.024	0.024	—	—
		5	0.049	—	—	—
	13	19	9.020	9.020	8.006	7.002
		18	8.029	7.010+	6.003	6.003
		17	7.031	6.011	5.004	5.004
		16	6.029	5.011	4.003	4.003
		15	5.025+	4.009	4.009	3.003
		14	4.020	4.020	3.006	2.002
		13	4.041	3.015−	2.004	2.004
		12	3.029	2.009	2.009	1.002
		11	2.019	2.019	1.005−	1.005−
		10	2.036	1.010−	1.010−	0.001
		9	1.020	1.020	0.003	0.003
		8	1.038	0.007	0.007	—
		7	0.015−	0.015−	—	—
		6	0.030	—	—	—
	12	19	9.049	8.016	7.005−	7.005−
		18	7.022	7.022	6.007	5.002
		17	6.022	6.022	5.007	4.002
		16	5.019	5.019	4.006	3.002
		15	5.042	4.015+	3.004	3.004
		14	4.032	3.011	2.003	2.003
		13	3.023	3.023	2.006	1.001
		12	3.043	2.014	1.003	1.003
		11	2.027	1.007	1.007	0.001
		10	2.050−	1.014	0.002	0.002
		9	1.027	0.005−	0.005−	0.005−
		8	1.050−	0.010−	0.010−	—
		7	0.019	0.019	—	—
		6	0.037	—	—	—
	11	19	8.041	7.012	6.003	6.003
		18	7.047	6.016	5.004	5.004
		17	6.043	5.015−	4.004	4.004
		16	5.035+	4.012	3.003	3.003

TESTS OF SIGNIFICANCE IN A 2 × 2 CONTINGENCY TABLE

	a	Probability 0.05	0.025	0.01	0.005
A = 19 B = 11	15	4.027	3.008	3.008	2.002
	14	3.018	3.018	2.005−	2.005−
	13	3.035+	2.010+	1.002	1.002
	12	2.021	2.021	1.005−	1.005−
	11	2.040	1.010+	0.001	0.001
	10	1.020	1.020	0.003	0.003
	9	1.037	0.006	0.006	—
	8	0.013	0.013	—	—
	7	0.025−	0.025−	—	—
	6	0.046	—	—	—
10	19	7.033	6.009	6.009	5.002
	18	6.036	5.011	4.003	4.003
	17	5.030	4.009	4.009	3.002
	16	4.022	4.022	3.006	2.001
	15	4.047	3.015−	2.004	2.004
	14	3.030	2.008	2.008	1.002
	13	2.017	2.017	1.004	1.004
	12	2.033	1.008	1.008	0.001
	11	1.016	1.016	0.002	0.002
	10	1.029	0.005−	0.005−	0.005−
	9	0.009	0.009	0.009	—
	8	0.018	0.018	—	—
	7	0.032	—	—	—
9	19	6.026	5.006	5.006	4.001
	18	5.026	4.007	4.007	3.001
	17	4.020	4.020	3.005−	3.005−
	16	4.044	3.013	2.003	2.003
	15	3.028	2.007	2.007	1.001
	14	2.015−	2.015−	1.003	1.003
	13	2.029	1.006	1.006	0.001
	12	1.013	1.013	0.002	0.002
	11	1.024	1.024	0.004	0.004
	10	1.042	0.007	0.007	—
	9	0.013	0.013	—	—
	8	0.024	0.024	—	—
	7	0.043	—	—	—
8	19	5.019	5.019	4.004	4.004
	18	4.017	4.017	3.004	3.004
	17	4.044	3.011	2.002	2.002
	16	3.027	2.006	2.006	1.001
	15	2.014	2.014	1.002	1.002
	14	2.027	1.006	1.006	0.001
	13	2.049	1.011	0.001	0.001
	12	1.021	1.021	0.003	0.003
	11	1.038	0.006	0.006	—
	10	0.011	0.011	—	—
	9	0.020	0.020	—	—
	8	0.034	—	—	—
7	19	4.013	4.013	3.002	3.002
	18	4.047	3.010+	2.002	2.002
	17	3.028	2.006	2.006	1.001
	16	2.014	2.014	1.002	1.002
	15	2.028	1.005+	1.005+	0.001
	14	1.011	1.011	0.001	0.001
	13	1.021	1.021	0.003	0.003

	a	Probability 0.05	0.025	0.01	0.005
A = 19 B = 7	12	1.037	0.005+	0.005+	—
	11	0.010−	0.010−	0.010−	—
	10	0.017	0.017	—	—
	9	0.030	—	—	—
	8	0.048	—	—	—
6	19	4.050	3.009	3.009	2.001
	18	3.031	2.005+	2.005+	1.001
	17	2.015+	2.015+	1.002	1.002
	16	2.032	1.006	1.006	0.000
	15	1.012	1.012	0.001	0.001
	14	1.023	1.023	0.003	0.003
	13	1.039	0.005+	0.005+	—
	12	0.010−	0.010−	0.010−	—
	11	0.017	0.017	—	—
	10	0.028	—	—	—
	9	0.045+	—	—	—
5	19	3.036	2.005−	2.005−	2.005−
	18	2.018	2.018	1.002	1.002
	17	2.042	1.006	1.006	0.000
	16	1.014	1.014	0.001	0.001
	15	1.028	0.003	0.003	0.003
	14	1.047	0.006	0.006	—
	13	0.011	0.011	—	—
	12	0.019	0.019	—	—
	11	0.030	—	—	—
	10	0.047	—	—	—
4	19	2.024	2.024	1.002	1.002
	18	1.009	1.009	1.009	0.001
	17	1.021	1.021	0.002	0.002
	16	1.040	0.004	0.004	0.004
	15	0.008	0.008	0.008	—
	14	0.014	0.014	—	—
	13	0.024	0.024	—	—
	12	0.037	—	—	—
3	19	1.013	1.013	0.001	0.001
	19	1.038	0.003	0.003	0.003
	17	0.006	0.006	0.006	—
	16	0.013	0.013	—	—
	15	0.023	0.023	—	—
	14	0.036	—	—	—
2	19	0.005−	0.005−	0.005−	0.005−
	18	0.014	0.014	—	—
	17	0.029	—	—	—
	16	0.048	—	—	—
A = 20 B = 20	20	15.024	15.024	13.004	13.004
	19	14.046	13.022	12.010−	11.004
	18	12.032	11.015+	10.007	9.003
	17	11.041	10.020	9.009	8.004
	16	10.048	9.024	7.005−	7.005−
	15	8.027	7.012	6.005+	5.002
	14	7.028	6.013	5.005+	4.002
	13	6.028	5.012	4.005−	4.005−
	12	5.027	4.011	3.004	3.004
	11	4.024	4.024	3.009	2.003
	10	4.048	3.020	2.007	1.002

TESTS OF SIGNIFICANCE IN A 2 × 2 CONTINGENCY TABLE

	a	Probability 0.05	0.025	0.01	0.005
$A = 20$ $B = 20$	9	3.041	2.015+	1.004	1.004
	8	2.032	1.010−	1.010−	0.002
	7	1.022	1.022	0.004	0.004
	6	1.046	0.010+	—	—
	5	0.024	0.024	—	—
19	20	15.047	14.020	13.008	12.003
	19	13.039	12.018	11.008	10.003
	18	11.026	10.012	9.005−	9.005−
	17	10.032	9.015−	8.006	7.002
	16	9.036	8.017	7.007	6.003
	15	8.038	7.018	6.008	5.003
	14	7.039	6.018	5.007	4.003
	13	6.038	5.017	4.007	3.002
	12	5.035+	4.015+	3.005+	2.002
	11	4.031	3.012	2.004	2.004
	10	3.026	2.009	2.009	1.002
	9	2.019	2.019	1.005+	0.001
	8	2.039	1.012	0.002	0.002
	7	1.026	0.005+	0.005+	—
	6	0.012	0.012	—	—
	5	0.027	—	—	—
18	20	14.041	13.017	12.007	11.003
	19	12.032	11.014	10.006	9.002
	18	11.043	10.020	9.008	8.003
	17	10.050−	9.024	7.004	7.004
	16	8.026	7.011	6.005−	6.005−
	15	7.027	6.012	5.004	5.004
	14	6.026	5.011	4.004	4.004
	13	5.024	5.024	4.009	3.003
	12	5.047	4.020	3.007	2.002
	11	4.041	3.016	2.005+	1.001
	10	3.033	2.012	1.003	1.003
	9	2.024	2.024	1.007	0.001
	8	2.048	1.015−	0.003	0.003
	7	1.031	0.006	0.006	—
	6	0.014	0.014	—	—
	5	0.031	—	—	—
17	20	13.036	12.014	11.005+	10.002
	19	11.026	10.011	9.004	9.004
	18	10.034	9.015−	8.006	7.002
	17	9.038	8.017	7.007	6.003
	16	8.040	7.018	6.007	5.003
	15	7.039	6.017	5.007	4.002
	14	6.037	5.016	4.006	3.002
	13	5.033	4.013	3.005−	3.005−
	12	4.028	3.010+	2.003	2.003
	11	3.022	3.022	2.007	1.002
	10	3.042	2.015+	1.004	1.004
	9	2.031	1.009	1.009	0.001
	8	1.019	1.019	0.003	0.003
	7	1.037	0.008	0.008	—
	6	0.017	0.017	—	—
	5	0.036	—	—	—
16	20	12.031	11.012	10.004	10.004
	19	11.049	10.021	9.008	8.003
$A = 20$ $B = 16$	18	9.026	8.011	7.004	7.004
	17	8.028	7.012	6.004	6.004
	16	7.028	6.012	5.004	5.004
	15	6.026	5.011	4.004	4.004
	14	5.023	5.023	4.009	3.003
	13	5.046	4.019	3.007	2.002
	12	4.038	3.014	2.004	2.004
	11	3.029	2.010−	2.010−	1.002
	10	2.020	2.020	1.005+	0.001
	9	2.039	1.011	0.002	0.002
	8	1.023	1.023	0.004	0.004
	7	1.045+	0.009	0.009	—
	6	0.020	0.020	—	—
	5	0.041	—	—	—
15	20	11.026	10.009	10.009	9.003
	19	10.040	9.016	8.006	7.002
	18	9.046	8.019	7.007	6.002
	17	8.047	7.020	6.008	5.003
	16	7.045−	6.019	5.007	4.002
	15	6.040	5.017	4.006	3.002
	14	5.034	4.013	3.004	3.004
	13	4.028	3.010−	3.010−	2.003
	12	3.020	3.020	2.006	1.001
	11	3.039	2.013	1.003	1.003
	10	2.026	1.007	1.007	0.001
	9	2.049	1.015−	0.002	0.002
	8	1.029	0.005+	0.005+	—
	7	0.012	0.012	—	—
	6	0.024	0.024	—	—
	5	0.048	—	—	—
14	20	10.022	10.022	9.007	8.002
	19	9.032	8.012	7.004	7.004
	18	8.035+	7.014	6.005−	6.005−
	17	7.035−	6.013	5.005−	5.005
	16	6.031	5.012	4.004	4.004
	15	5.026	4.009	4.009	3.003
	14	4.020	4.020	3.007	2.002
	13	4.040	3.015−	2.004	2.004
	12	3.029	2.009	2.009	1.002
	11	2.018	2.018	1.005−	1.005−
	10	2.035+	1.010−	1.010−	0.001
	9	1.019	1.019	0.003	0.003
	8	1.037	0.007	0.007	—
	7	0.014	0.014	—	—
	6	0.029	—	—	—
13	20	9.017	9.017	8.005	7.002
	19	8.025−	8.025−	7.008	6.003
	18	7.026	6.009	6.009	5.003
	17	6.024	6.024	5.008	4.002
	16	5.020	5.020	4.007	3.002
	15	5.041	4.015+	3.005	3.005
	14	4.031	3.011	2.003	2.003
	13	3.022	3.022	2.006	1.001
	12	3.041	2.013	1.003	1.003
	11	2.026	1.007	1.007	0.001

TESTS OF SIGNIFICANCE IN A 2 × 2 CONTINGENCY TABLE

	a	Probability			
		0.05	0.025	0.01	0.005
$A = 20$ $B = 13$	10	2.047	1.013	0.002	0.002
	9	1.026	0.004	0.004	0.004
	8	1.047	0.009	0.009	—
	7	0.018	0.018	—	—
	6	0.035−	—	—	—
12	20	9.044	8.014	7.004	7.004
	19	7.018	7.018	6.006	5.002
	18	6.018	6.018	5.006	4.002
	17	6.043	5.016	4.005−	4.005−
	16	5.034	4.012	3.003	3.003
	15	4.025+	3.008	3.008	2.002
	14	4.049	3.017	2.005−	2.005−
	13	3.033	2.010−	2.010−	1.002
	12	2.020	2.020	1.005−	1.005−
	11	2.036	1.009	1.009	0.001
	10	1.018	1.018	0.003	0.003
	9	1.034	0.006	0.006	—
	8	0.012	0.012	—	—
	7	0.023	0.023	—	—
	6	0.043	—	—	—
11	20	8.037	7.010+	6.003	6.003
	19	7.042	6.013	5.004	5.004
	18	6.037	5.012	4.003	4.003
	17	5.029	4.009	4.009	3.002
	16	4.021	4.021	3.006	2.001
	15	4.042	3.003	2.003	2.003
	14	3.028	2.008	2.008	1.001
	13	2.016	2.016	1.003	1.003
	12	2.029	1.007	1.007	0.001
	11	1.014	1.014	0.002	0.002
	10	1.026	0.004	0.004	0.004
	9	1.046	0.008	0.008	—
	8	0.016	0.016	—	—
	7	0.029	—	—	—
10	20	7.030	6.008	6.008	5.002
	19	6.031	5.009	5.009	4.002
	18	5.026	4.007	4.007	3.002
	17	4.018	4.018	3.005−	3.005−
	16	4.039	3.012	2.003	2.003
	15	3.024	3.024	2.006	1.001
	14	3.045+	2.013	1.003	1.003
	13	2.025+	1.006	1.006	0.001
	12	2.045−	1.011	0.001	0.001
	11	1.021	1.021	0.003	0.003
	10	1.037	0.006	0.006	—
	9	0.012	0.012	—	—
	8	0.022	0.022	—	—
	7	0.038	—	—	—
9	20	6.023	6.023	5.005+	4.001
	19	5.022	5.022	4.005+	3.001
	18	4.016	4.016	3.004	3.004
	17	4.037	3.010+	2.002	2.002
	16	3.022	3.022	2.005+	1.001
	15	3.043	2.012	1.002	1.002
	14	2.023	2.023	1.005−	1.005−
$A = 20$ $B = 9$	13	2.041	1.009	1.009	0.001
	12	1.018	1.018	0.002	0.002
	11	1.032	0.005−	0.005−	0.005−
	10	0.009	0.009	0.009	—
	9	0.017	0.017	—	—
	8	0.029	—	—	—
	7	0.050−	—	—	—
8	20	5.017	5.017	4.003	4.003
	19	4.015−	4.015−	3.003	3.003
	18	4.038	3.009	3.009	2.002
	17	3.022	3.022	2.005−	2.005−
	16	3.044	2.011	1.002	1.002
	15	0.022	2.022	1.004	1.004
	14	2.040	1.009	1.009	0.001
	13	1.016	1.016	0.002	0.002
	12	1.029	0.004	0.004	0.004
	11	1.048	0.008	0.008	—
	10	0.014	0.014	—	—
	9	0.024	0.024	—	—
	8	0.041	—	—	—
7	20	4.012	4.012	3.002	3.002
	19	4.042	3.009	3.009	2.001
	18	3.024	3.024	2.005−	2.005−
	17	3.050−	2.011	1.002	1.002
	16	2.023	2.023	1.004	1.004
	15	2.043	1.009	1.009	0.001
	14	1.016	1.016	0.002	0.002
	13	1.029	0.004	0.004	0.004
	12	1.048	0.007	0.007	—
	11	0.013	0.013	—	—
	10	0.022	0.022	—	—
	9	0.036	—	—	—
6	20	4.046	3.008	3.008	2.001
	19	3.028	2.005−	2.005−	2.005−
	18	2.013	2.013	1.002	1.002
	17	2.028	1.004	1.004	1.004
	16	1.010−	1.010−	1.010−	0.001
	15	1.018	1.018	0.002	0.002
	14	1.032	0.004	0.004	0.004
	13	0.007	0.007	0.007	—
	12	0.013	0.013	—	—
	11	0.022	0.022	—	—
	10	0.035−	—	—	—
5	20	3.033	2.004	2.004	2.004
	19	2.016	2.016	1.002	1.002
	18	2.038	1.005+	1.005+	0.000
	17	1.012	1.012	0.001	0.001
	16	1.023	1.023	0.002	0.002
	15	1.040	0.005−	0.005−	0.005−
	14	0.009	0.009	0.009	—
	13	0.015−	0.015−	—	—
	12	0.024	0.024	—	—
	11	0.038	—	—	—
4	20	2.022	2.022	1.002	1.002
	19	1.008	1.008	1.008	0.000

TESTS OF SIGNIFICANCE IN A 2 × 2 CONTINGENCY TABLE

	a	Probability					a	Probability			
		0.05	0.025	0.01	0.005			0.05	0.025	0.01	0.005
$A = 20$ $B = 4$	18	**1**.018	**1**.018	**0**.001	**0**.001	$A = 20$ $B = 3$	17	**0**.011	**0**.011	—	—
	17	**1**.035+	**0**.003	**0**.003	**0**.003		16	**0**.020	**0**.020	—	—
	16	**0**.007	**0**.007	**0**.007	—		15	**0**.032	—	—	—
	15	**0**.012	**0**.012	—	—		14	**0**.047	—	—	—
	14	**0**.020	**0**.020	—	—	2	20	**0**.004	**0**.004	**0**.004	**0**.004
	13	**0**.031	—	—	—		19	**0**.013	**0**.013	—	—
	12	**0**.047	—	—	—		18	**0**.026	—	—	—
3	20	**1**.012	**1**.012	**0**.001	**0**.001		17	**0**.043	—	—	—
	19	**1**.034	**0**.002	**0**.002	**0**.002	1	20	**0**.048	—	—	—
	18	**0**.000	**0**.000	**0**.000	—						

IV. Student's *t*-Distribution

IV.1 PERCENTAGE POINTS, STUDENT'S *t*-DISTRIBUTION

This table gives values of t such that

$$F(t) = \int_{-\infty}^{t} \frac{\Gamma\left(\frac{n+1}{2}\right)}{\sqrt{n\pi}\,\Gamma\left(\frac{n}{2}\right)} \left(1 + \frac{x^2}{n}\right)^{-\frac{n+1}{2}} dx$$

for n, the number of degrees of freedom, equal to 1, 2, . . . , 30, 40, 60, 120, ∞; and for $F(t) = 0.60, 0.75, 0.90, 0.95, 0.975, 0.99, 0.995$, and 0.9995. The t-distribution is symmetrical, so that $F(-t) = 1 - F(t)$.

PERCENTAGE POINTS, STUDENTS *t*-DISTRIBUTION

$$F(t) = \int_{-\infty}^{t} \frac{\Gamma\left(\frac{n+1}{2}\right)}{\sqrt{n\pi}\,\Gamma\left(\frac{n}{2}\right)} \left(1 + \frac{x^2}{n}\right)^{-\frac{n+1}{2}} dx$$

n \ F	.60	.75	.90	.95	.975	.99	.995	.9995
1	.325	1.000	3.078	6.314	12.706	31.821	63.657	636.619
2	.289	.816	1.886	2.920	4.303	6.965	9.925	31.598
3	.277	.765	1.638	2.353	3.182	4.541	5.841	12.924
4	.271	.741	1.533	2.132	2.776	3.747	4.604	8.610
5	.267	.727	1.476	2.015	2.571	3.365	4.032	6.869
6	.265	.718	1.440	1.943	2.447	3.143	3.707	5.959
7	.263	.711	1.415	1.895	2.365	2.998	3.499	5.408
8	.262	.706	1.397	1.860	2.306	2.896	3.355	5.041
9	.261	.703	1.383	1.833	2.262	2.821	3.250	4.781
10	.260	.700	1.372	1.812	2.228	2.764	3.169	4.587
11	.260	.697	1.363	1.796	2.201	2.718	3.106	4.437
12	.259	.695	1.356	1.782	2.179	2.681	3.055	4.318
13	.259	.694	1.350	1.771	2.160	2.650	3.012	4.221
14	.258	.692	1.345	1.761	2.145	2.624	2.977	4.140
15	.258	.691	1.341	1.753	2.131	2.602	2.947	4.073
16	.258	.690	1.337	1.746	2.120	2.583	2.921	4.015
17	.257	.689	1.333	1.740	2.110	2.567	2.898	3.965
18	.257	.688	1.330	1.734	2.101	2.552	2.878	3.922
19	.257	.688	1.328	1.729	2.093	2.539	2.861	3.883
20	.257	.687	1.325	1.725	2.086	2.528	2.845	3.850
21	.257	.686	1.323	1.721	2.080	2.518	2.831	3.819
22	.256	.686	1.321	1.717	2.074	2.508	2.819	3.792
23	.256	.685	1.319	1.714	2.069	2.500	2.807	3.767
24	.256	.685	1.318	1.711	2.064	2.492	2.797	3.745
25	.256	.684	1.316	1.708	2.060	2.485	2.787	3.725
26	.256	.684	1.315	1.706	2.056	2.479	2.779	3.707
27	.256	.684	1.314	1.703	2.052	2.473	2.771	3.690
28	.256	.683	1.313	1.701	2.048	2.467	2.763	3.674
29	.256	.683	1.311	1.699	2.045	2.462	2.756	3.659
30	.256	.683	1.310	1.697	2.042	2.457	2.750	3.646
40	.255	.681	1.303	1.684	2.021	2.423	2.704	3.551
60	.254	.679	1.296	1.671	2.000	2.390	2.660	3.460
120	.254	.677	1.289	1.658	1.980	2.358	2.617	3.373
∞	.253	.674	1.282	1.645	1.960	2.326	2.576	3.291

IV.2 POWER FUNCTION OF THE t-TEST

Any statistic of the form

$$t' = \frac{z + \delta}{s_z} = \frac{z'}{s_z},$$

where z is normally distributed with expectation zero and standard deviation σ_z, s_z^2 is an independent estimate of σ_z^2 based on ν degrees of freedom, and δ is the noncentrality parameter, is distributed as the non-central t-distribution, denoted by $f(t')$.

The power function of the t-test is the value of the following integrals considered as a function of $\frac{\delta}{\sigma_z}$

(a) $$\int_{-\infty}^{-t_{\alpha/2}} f(t')\,dt' + \int_{t_{\alpha/2}}^{\infty} f(t')\,dt' \qquad \text{for the double-tail } t\text{-test}$$

(b) $$\int_{t_\alpha}^{\infty} f(t')\,dt' \qquad \text{for the single-tail } t\text{-test } (\delta \geq 0)\ ,$$

where t_α denotes the α-level significance point for t.

The graph in this table shows the integral (a) for $\alpha = 0.05$ and 0.01, and for various values of ν, the degrees of freedom associated with s_z. The horizontal scale is in terms of $\phi = \frac{\delta}{\sigma_z\sqrt{2}}$. The graph can also be used to give the integral (b) for significance levels $\alpha = 0.025$ and 0.005.

POWER FUNCTION OF THE *t*-TEST

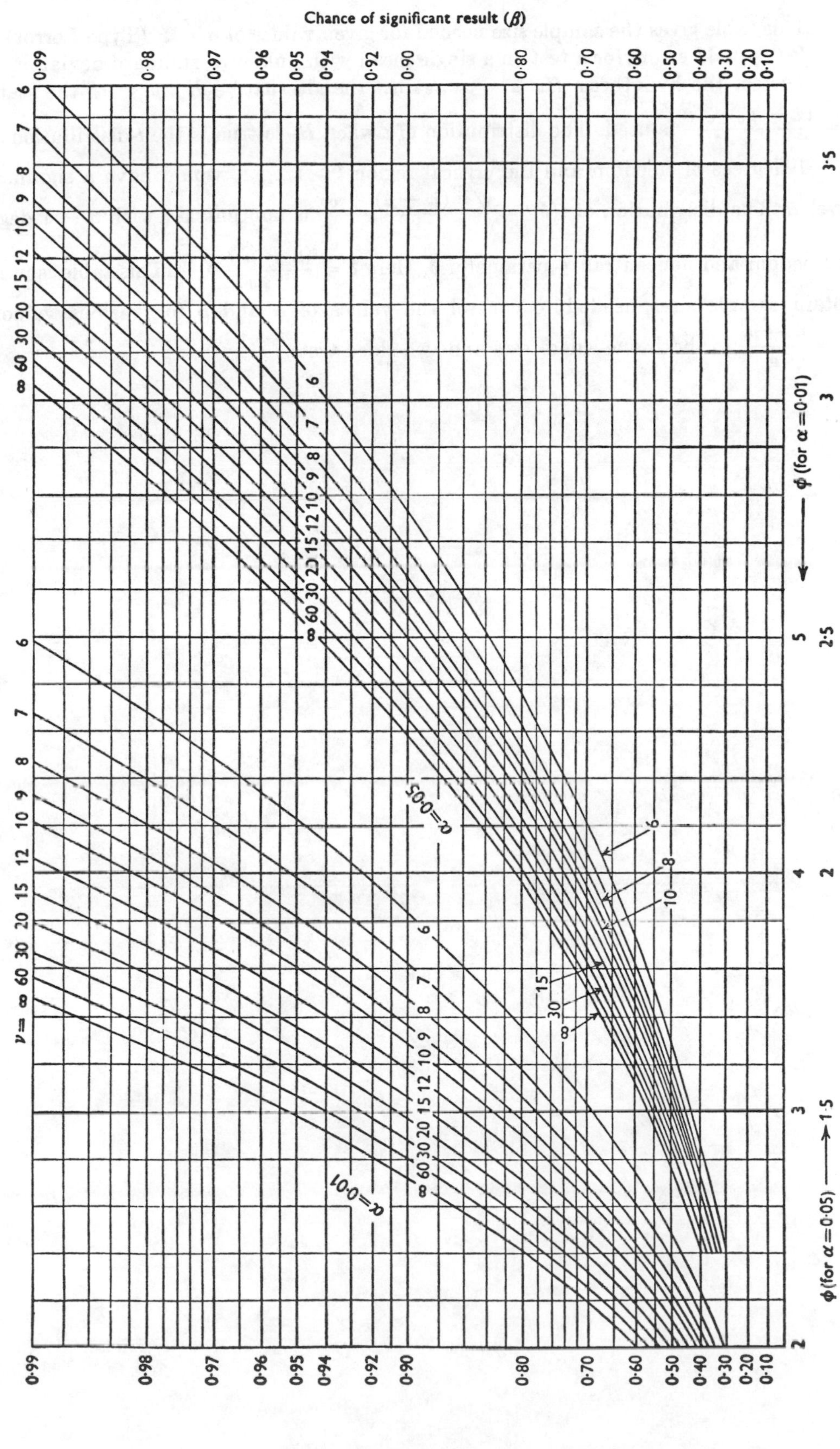

IV.3 NUMBER OF OBSERVATIONS FOR t-TEST OF MEAN

This table gives the sample size needed for given values of $\alpha = P$ (Type I error) and $\beta = P$ (Type II error) for a test on a single mean with unknown standard deviation.

To test the hypothesis H_0: $\mu = \mu_0$ against the alternative H_a: $\mu < \mu_0$, the statistic $t = \frac{(\bar{x} - \mu_0)\sqrt{n}}{s}$ is used. The distribution of t when H_0 is true is the t-distribution with $n - 1$ degrees of freedom and the critical region $t > t_{n-1,1-\alpha}$ would have a significance level α. The distribution of $t(\delta) = \frac{\sqrt{n}(\bar{x} - \mu) + \delta\sigma}{s}$ is noncentral t with $n - 1$ degrees of freedom and noncentrality parameter δ. Here $\delta = \frac{(\mu - \mu_0)\sqrt{n}}{\sigma}$. This table is used to obtain sample sizes needed to control the values of α and β for various values of $\Delta = \frac{\mu - \mu_0}{\sigma}$ for both one-sided tests and two-sided tests.

NUMBER OF OBSERVATIONS FOR *t*-TEST OF MEAN

Value of $\Delta = \frac{\mu - \mu_0}{\sigma}$	Level of *t*-test																				
Single-sided test	$\alpha = 0.005$					$\alpha = 0.01$					$\alpha = 0.025$					$\alpha = 0.05$					
Double-sided test	$\alpha = 0.01$					$\alpha = 0.02$					$\alpha = 0.05$					$\alpha = 0.1$					
$\beta =$	0.01	0.05	0.1	0.2	0.5	0.01	0.05	0.1	0.2	0.5	0.01	0.05	0.1	0.2	0.5	0.01	0.05	0.1	0.2	0.5	
0.05																					0.05
0.10																					0.10
0.15																				122	0.15
0.20										139					99					70	0.20
0.25					110					90				128	64			139	101	45	0.25
0.30				134	78				115	63			119	90	45		122	97	71	32	0.30
0.35			125	99	58			109	85	47		109	88	67	34		90	72	52	24	0.35
0.40		115	97	77	45		101	85	66	37	117	84	68	51	26	101	70	55	40	19	0.40
0.45		92	77	62	37	110	81	68	53	30	93	67	54	41	21	80	55	44	33	15	0.45
0.50	100	75	63	51	30	90	66	55	43	25	76	54	44	34	18	65	45	36	27	13	0.50
0.55	83	63	53	42	26	75	55	46	36	21	63	45	37	28	15	54	38	30	22	11	0.55
0.60	71	53	45	36	22	63	47	39	31	18	53	38	32	24	13	46	32	26	19	9	0.60
0.65	61	46	39	31	20	55	41	34	27	16	46	33	27	21	12	39	28	22	17	8	0.65
0.70	53	40	34	28	17	47	35	30	24	14	40	29	24	19	10	34	24	19	15	8	0.70
0.75	47	30	30	25	16	42	31	27	21	13	35	26	21	16	9	30	21	17	13	7	0.75
0.80	41	32	27	22	14	37	28	24	19	12	31	22	19	15	9	27	19	15	12	6	0.80
0.85	37	29	24	20	13	33	25	21	17	11	28	21	17	13	8	24	17	14	11	6	0.85
0.90	34	26	22	18	12	29	23	19	16	10	25	19	16	12	7	21	15	13	10	5	0.90
0.95	31	24	20	17	11	27	21	18	14	9	23	17	14	11	7	19	14	11	9	5	0.95
1.00	28	22	19	16	10	25	19	16	13	9	21	16	13	10	6	18	13	11	8	5	1.00
1.1	24	19	16	14	9	21	16	14	12	8	18	13	11	9	6	15	11	9	7		1.1
1.2	21	16	14	12	8	18	14	12	10	7	15	12	10	8	5	13	10	8	6		1.2
1.3	18	15	13	11	8	16	13	11	9	6	14	10	9	7		11	8	7	6		1.3
1.4	16	13	12	10	7	14	11	10	9	6	12	9	8	7		10	8	7	5		1.4
1.5	15	12	11	9	7	13	10	9	8	6	11	8	7	6		9	7	6			1.5
1.6	13	11	10	8	6	12	10	9	7	5	10	8	7	6		8	6	6			1.6
1.7	12	10	9	8	6	11	9	8	7		9	7	6	5		8	6	5			1.7
1.8	12	10	9	8	6	10	8	7	7		8	7	6			7	6				1.8
1.9	11	9	8	7	6	10	8	7	6		8	6	6			7	5				1.9
2.0	10	8	8	7	5	9	7	7	6		7	6	5			6					2.0
2.1	10	8	7	7		8	7	6	6		7	6				6					2.1
2.2	9	8	7	6		8	7	6	5		7	6				6					2.2
2.3	9	7	7	6		8	6	6			6	5				5					2.3
2.4	8	7	7	6		7	6	6			6										2.4
2.5	8	7	6	6		7	6	6			6										2.5
3.0	7	6	6	5		6	5	5			5										3.0
3.5	6	5	5			5															3.5
4.0	6																				4.0

IV.4 NUMBER OF OBSERVATIONS FOR *t*-TEST OF DIFFERENCE BETWEEN TWO MEANS

This table gives the sample size needed for given values of $\alpha = P$ (Type I error) and $\beta = P$ (Type II error) for a test of the hypothesis of the equality of two means H_0: $\mu_x = \mu_y$, where there is a common but unknown variance. The statistic used is

$$t = \frac{\bar{x} - \bar{y}}{s\sqrt{\dfrac{1}{n_x} + \dfrac{1}{n_y}}}$$

which is distributed as Students *t*-distribution with $n_x + n_y - 2$ degrees of freedom. Here

$$s = \left[\frac{(n_x - 1)s_x^2 + (n_y - 1)s_y^2}{n_x + n_y - 2}\right]^{\frac{1}{2}}.$$

The noncentrality parameter in this case is

$$\sigma = \frac{\mu_x - \mu_y}{\sigma\sqrt{\dfrac{1}{n_x} + \dfrac{1}{n_y}}}.$$

This table is used to obtain sample sizes needed to control the values of α and β for various values of $\Delta = \dfrac{\mu_x - \mu_y}{\sigma}$ for both one-sided and two-sided tests, where it is assumed $n_x = n_y = n$.

NUMBER OF OBSERVATIONS FOR *t*-TEST OF DIFFERENCE BETWEEN TWO MEANS

	Level of *t*-test																				
Single-sided test	$\alpha = 0.005$					$\alpha = 0.01$					$\alpha = 0.025$					$\alpha = 0.05$					
Double-sided test	$\alpha = 0.01$					$\alpha = 0.02$					$\alpha = 0.05$					$\alpha = 0.1$					
$\beta =$	0.01	0.05	0.1	0.2	0.5	0.01	0.05	0.1	0.2	0.5	0.01	0.05	0.1	0.2	0.5	0.01	0.05	0.1	0.2	0.5	
0.05																					0.05
0.10																					0.10
0.15																					0.15
0.20																				137	0.20
0.25															124					88	0.25
0.30										123					87					61	0.30
0.35					110					90					64				102	45	0.35
0.40					85					70				100	50			108	78	35	0.40
0.45				118	68				101	55			105	79	39		108	86	62	28	0.45
0.50				96	55			106	82	45		106	86	64	32		88	70	51	23	0.50
0.55			101	79	46		106	88	68	38		87	71	53	27	112	73	58	42	19	0.55
0.60		101	85	67	39		90	74	58	32	104	74	60	45	23	89	61	49	36	16	0.60
0.65		87	73	57	34	104	77	64	49	27	88	63	51	39	20	76	52	42	30	14	0.65
0.70	100	75	63	50	29	90	66	55	43	24	76	55	44	34	17	66	45	36	26	12	0.70
0.75	88	66	55	44	26	79	58	48	38	21	67	48	30	20	15	57	40	32	23	11	0.75
0.80	77	58	49	39	23	70	51	43	33	19	59	42	34	26	14	50	35	28	21	10	0.80
0.85	69	51	43	35	21	62	46	38	30	17	52	37	31	23	12	45	31	25	18	9	0.85
0.90	62	46	39	31	19	55	41	34	27	15	47	34	27	21	11	40	28	22	16	8	0.90
Value of 0.95	55	42	35	28	17	50	37	31	24	14	42	30	25	19	10	36	25	20	15	7	0.95
$\Delta = \frac{\mu_x - \mu}{\sigma}$ 1.00	50	38	32	26	15	45	33	28	22	13	38	27	23	17	9	33	23	18	14	7	1.00
1.1	42	32	27	22	13	38	28	23	19	11	32	23	19	14	8	27	19	15	12	6	1.1
1.2	36	27	23	18	11	32	24	20	16	9	27	20	16	12	7	23	16	13	10	5	1.2
1.3	31	23	20	16	10	28	21	17	14	8	23	17	14	11	6	20	14	11	9	5	1.3
1.4	27	20	17	14	9	24	18	15	12	8	20	15	12	10	6	17	12	10	8	4	1.4
1.5	24	18	15	13	8	21	16	14	11	7	18	13	11	9	5	15	11	9	7	4	1.5
1.6	21	16	14	11	7	19	14	12	10	6	16	12	10	8	5	14	10	8	6	4	1.6
1.7	19	15	13	10	7	17	13	11	9	6	14	11	9	7	4	12	9	7	6	3	1.7
1.8	17	13	11	10	6	15	12	10	8	5	13	10	8	6	4	11	8	7	5		1.8
1.9	16	12	11	9	6	14	11	9	8	5	12	9	7	6	4	10	7	6	5		1.9
2.0	14	11	10	8	6	13	10	9	7	5	11	8	7	6	4	9	7	6	4		2.0
2.1	13	10	9	8	5	12	9	8	7	5	10	8	6	5	3	8	6	5	4		2.1
2.2	12	10	8	7	5	11	9	7	6	4	9	7	6	5		8	6	5	4		2.2
2.3	11	9	8	7	5	10	8	7	6	4	9	7	6	5		7	5	5	4		2.3
2.4	11	9	8	6	5	10	8	7	6	4	8	6	5	4		7	5	4	4		2.4
2.5	10	8	7	6	4	9	7	6	5	4	8	6	5	4		6	5	4	3		2.5
3.0	8	6	6	5	4	7	6	5	4	3	6	5	4	4		5	4	3			3.0
3.5	6	5	5	4	3	6	5	4	4		5	4	4	3		4	3				3.5
4.0	6	5	4	4		5	4	4	3		4	4	3			4					4.0

IV.5 OPERATING CHARACTERISTIC (OC) CURVES FOR A TEST ON THE MEAN OF A NORMAL DISTRIBUTION WITH UNKNOWN STANDARD DEVIATION

The OC curves give the sample sizes needed for given values of $\alpha = P$ (Type I error) and $\beta = P$ (Type II error) for a test of the hypothesis H_0: $\mu = \mu_0$, where the standard deviation is unknown. The statistic used is $t = \dfrac{(\bar{x} - \mu_0)\sqrt{n}}{s}$ which is distributed as Student's t-distribution with $n - 1$ degrees of freedom. The required sample size is obtained by entering the appropriate set of curves for given α and β for various values of $\Delta = \dfrac{|\mu_1 - \mu_0|}{\sigma}$ for both one-sided and two-sided tests.

The OC curves can also be used to give the sample sizes for a test of the hypothesis Ho: $\mu_x = \mu_y$ where the standard deviations σ_x and σ_y are unknown. If $\sigma_x = \sigma_y = \sigma$, then the statistic used is

$$t = \frac{\bar{x} - \bar{y}}{\sqrt{\dfrac{(n_x - 1)s_x^2 + (n_y - 1)s_y^2}{n_x + n_y - 2}}\sqrt{\dfrac{1}{n_x} + \dfrac{1}{n_y}}}$$

which is distributed as Student's t-distribution with $(n_x + n_y - 2)$ degrees of freedom. The required sample size is obtained by entering the appropriate set of curves for given α and β for various values of $\Delta = \dfrac{|\mu_x - \mu_y|}{2\sigma}$ for both one-sided and two-sided tests, where it is assumed that $n_x = n_y = n$. If the value read from the OC curve is denoted by n', the required sample size is given by $n = \dfrac{n' + 1}{2}$.

OC CURVES FOR A TEST ON THE MEAN OF A NORMAL DISTRIBUTION WITH UNKNOWN STANDARD DEVIATION

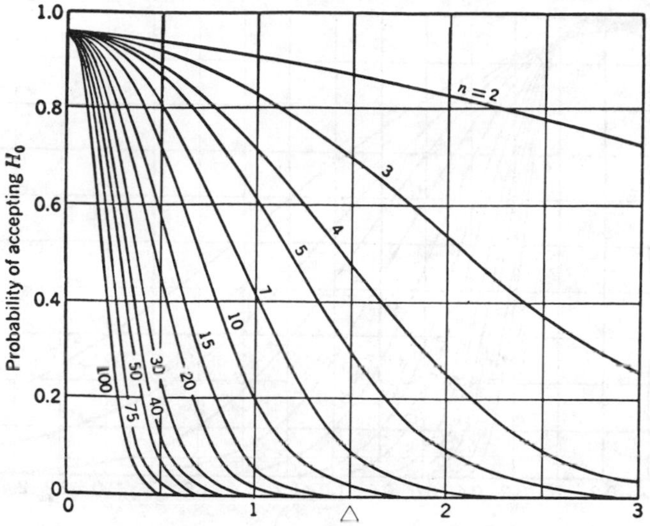

a) OC curves for different values of n for the two-sided t test for a level of significance $\alpha = 0.05$.

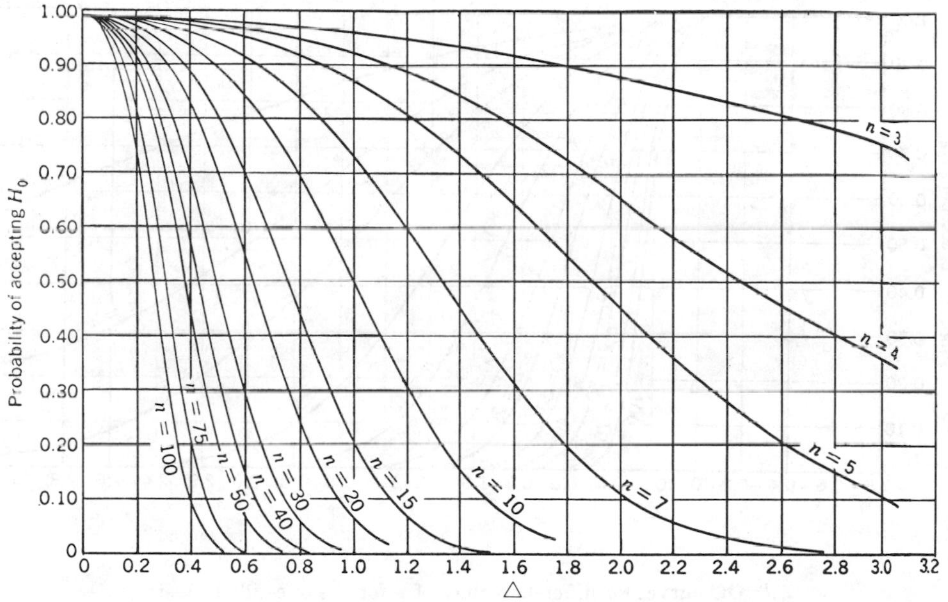

b) OC curves for different values of n for the two-sided t test for a level of significance $\alpha = 0.01$.

OC CURVES FOR A TEST ON THE MEAN OF A NORMAL DISTRIBUTION WITH UNKNOWN STANDARD DEVIATION

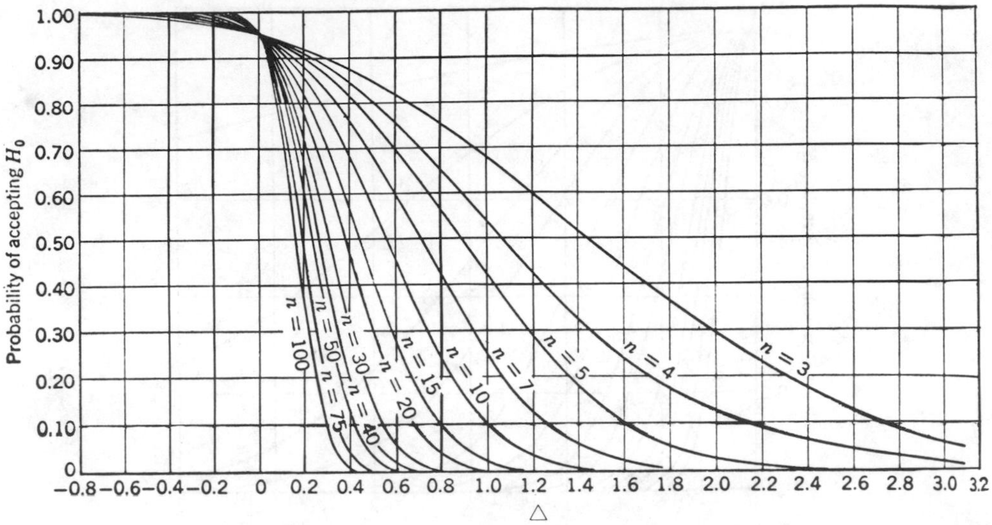

c) OC curves for different values of n for the one-sided t test for a level of significance $\alpha = 0.05$.

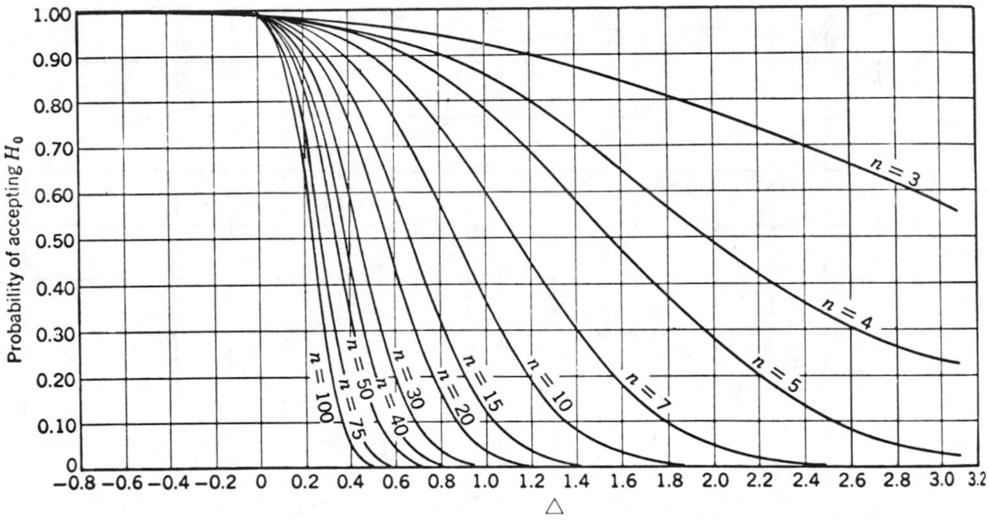

d) OC curves for different values of n for the one-sided t test for a level of significance $\alpha = 0.01$.

V. Chi-Square Distribution

V.1 PERCENTAGE POINTS, CHI-SQUARE DISTRIBUTION

This table gives values of χ^2 such that

$$F(\chi^2) = \int_0^{\chi^2} \frac{1}{2^{\frac{n}{2}}\,\Gamma\left(\frac{n}{2}\right)} x^{\frac{n-2}{2}} e^{-\frac{x}{2}}\,dx$$

for n, the number of degrees of freedom, equal to 1, 2, . . . , 30. For $n > 30$, a normal approximation is quite accurate. The expression $\sqrt{2\chi^2} - \sqrt{2n-1}$ is approximately normally distributed as the standard normal distribution. Thus χ^2_α, the α-point of the distribution, may be computed by the formula

$$\chi^2_\alpha = \tfrac{1}{2}[x_\alpha + \sqrt{2n-1}]^2,$$

where x_α is the α-point of the cumulative normal distribution. For even values of n, $F(\chi^2)$ can be written as

$$1 - F(\chi^2) = \sum_{x=0}^{x'-1} \frac{e^{-\lambda}\lambda^x}{x!}$$

with $\lambda = \frac{1}{2}\chi^2$ and $x' = \frac{1}{2}n$. Thus the cumulative Chi-Square distribution is related to the cumulative Poisson distribution.

PERCENTAGE POINTS, CHI-SQUARE DISTRIBUTION

$$F(\chi^2) = \int_0^{\chi^2} \frac{1}{2^{\frac{n}{2}}\,\Gamma\left(\frac{n}{2}\right)} x^{\frac{n-2}{2}} e^{-\frac{x}{2}}\,dx$$

n \ F	.005	.010	.025	.050	.100	.250	.500	.750	.900	.950	.975	.990	.995
1	.0000393	.000157	.000982	.00393	.0158	.102	.455	1.32	2.71	3.84	5.02	6.63	7.88
2	.0100	.0201	.0506	.103	.211	.575	1.39	2.77	4.61	5.99	7.38	9.21	10.6
3	.0717	.115	.216	.352	.584	1.21	2.37	4.11	6.25	7.81	9.35	11.3	12.8
4	.207	.297	.484	.711	1.06	1.92	3.36	5.39	7.78	9.49	11.1	13.3	14.9
5	.412	.554	.831	1.15	1.61	2.67	4.35	6.63	9.24	11.1	12.8	15.1	16.7
6	.676	.872	1.24	1.64	2.20	3.45	5.35	7.84	10.6	12.6	14.4	16.8	18.5
7	.989	1.24	1.69	2.17	2.83	4.25	6.35	9.04	12.0	14.1	16.0	18.5	20.3
8	1.34	1.65	2.18	2.73	3.49	5.07	7.34	10.2	13.4	15.5	17.5	20.1	22.0
9	1.73	2.09	2.70	3.33	4.17	5.90	8.34	11.4	14.7	16.9	19.0	21.7	23.6
10	2.16	2.56	3.25	3.94	4.87	6.74	9.34	12.5	16.0	18.3	20.5	23.2	25.2
11	2.60	3.05	3.82	4.57	5.58	7.58	10.3	13.7	17.3	19.7	21.9	24.7	26.8
12	3.07	3.57	4.40	5.23	6.30	8.44	11.3	14.8	18.5	21.0	23.3	26.2	28.3
13	3.57	4.11	5.01	5.89	7.04	9.30	12.3	16.0	19.8	22.4	24.7	27.7	29.8
14	4.07	4.66	5.63	6.57	7.79	10.2	13.3	17.1	21.1	23.7	26.1	29.1	31.3
15	4.60	5.23	6.26	7.26	8.55	11.0	14.3	18.2	22.3	25.0	27.5	30.6	32.8
16	5.14	5.81	6.91	7.96	9.31	11.9	15.3	19.4	23.5	26.3	28.8	32.0	34.3
17	5.70	6.41	7.56	8.67	10.1	12.8	16.3	20.5	24.8	27.6	30.2	33.4	35.7
18	6.26	7.01	8.23	9.39	10.9	13.7	17.3	21.6	26.0	28.9	31.5	34.8	37.2
19	6.84	7.63	8.91	10.1	11.7	14.6	18.3	22.7	27.2	30.1	32.9	36.2	38.6
20	7.43	8.26	9.59	10.9	12.4	15.5	19.3	23.8	28.4	31.4	34.2	37.6	40.0
21	8.03	8.90	10.3	11.6	13.2	16.3	20.3	24.9	29.6	32.7	35.5	38.9	41.4
22	8.64	9.54	11.0	12.3	14.0	17.2	21.3	26.0	30.8	33.9	36.8	40.3	42.8
23	9.26	10.2	11.7	13.1	14.8	18.1	22.3	27.1	32.0	35.2	38.1	41.6	44.2
24	9.89	10.9	12.4	13.8	15.7	19.0	23.3	28.2	33.2	36.4	39.4	43.0	45.6
25	10.5	11.5	13.1	14.6	16.5	19.9	24.3	29.3	34.4	37.7	40.6	44.3	46.9
26	11.2	12.2	13.8	15.4	17.3	20.8	25.3	30.4	35.6	38.9	41.9	45.6	48.3
27	11.8	12.9	14.6	16.2	18.1	21.7	26.3	31.5	36.7	40.1	43.2	47.0	49.6
28	12.5	13.6	15.3	16.9	18.9	22.7	27.3	32.6	37.9	41.3	44.5	48.3	51.0
29	13.1	14.3	16.0	17.7	19.8	23.6	28.3	33.7	39.1	42.6	45.7	49.6	52.3
30	13.8	15.0	16.8	18.5	20.6	24.5	29.3	34.8	40.3	43.8	47.0	50.9	53.7

V.2 PERCENTAGE POINTS, CHI-SQUARE OVER DEGREES OF FREEDOM DISTRIBUTION

This table gives the percentage points of the sampling distribution of $\frac{s^2}{\sigma^2}$, referred to as the percentage points of the $\frac{\chi^2}{\text{d.f.}}$ distribution (read "chi-square over degrees of freedom"). The percentage points are different for different sample sizes.

PERCENTAGE POINTS, CHI-SQUARE OVER DEGREES OF FREEDOM DISTRIBUTION

F / n	Probability in per cent						Probability in per cent					
	0.05	0.1	0.5	1.0	2.5	5.0	95.0	97.5	99.0	99.5	99.9	99.95
1	.0000	.0000	.0000	.0002	.0010	.0039	3.8410	5.0240	6.6350	7.8790	10.8280	12.1160
2	.0005	.0010	.0050	.0100	.0253	.0515	2.9955	3.6890	4.6050	5.2985	6.9080	7.6010
3	.0051	.0081	.0239	.0383	.0720	.1173	2.6050	3.1160	3.7817	4.2793	5.4220	5.9100
4	.0160	.0227	.0518	.0742	.1210	.1778	2.3720	2.7858	3.3192	3.7150	4.6168	4.9995
5	.0316	.0420	.0824	.1108	.1662	.2290	2.2140	2.5664	3.0172	3.3500	4.1030	4.4210
6	.0499	.0635	.1127	.1453	.2062	.2725	2.0987	2.4082	2.8020	3.0913	3.7430	4.0172
7	.0693	.0854	.1413	.1770	.2414	.3096	2.0096	2.2876	2.6393	2.8969	3.4746	3.7169
8	.0888	.1071	.1680	.2058	.2725	.3416	1.9384	2.1919	2.5112	2.7444	3.2656	3.4835
9	.1080	.1281	.1928	.2320	.3000	.3694	1.8799	2.1137	2.4073	2.6210	3.0974	3.2962
10	.1265	.1479	.2156	.2558	.3247	.3940	1.8307	2.0483	2.3209	2.5188	2.9588	3.1419
11	.1443	.1667	.2366	.2775	.3469	.4159	1.7886	1.9927	2.2477	2.4325	2.8422	3.0124
12	.1612	.1845	.2562	.2976	.3670	.4355	1.7522	1.9447	2.1848	2.3583	2.7424	2.9018
13	.1773	.2013	.2742	.3159	.3853	.4532	1.7202	1.9028	2.1298	2.2938	2.6560	2.8060
14	.1926	.2172	.2911	.3329	.4021	.4694	1.6918	1.8656	2.0815	2.2371	2.5802	2.7221
15	.2072	.2322	.3067	.3486	.4175	.4841	1.6664	1.8325	2.0385	2.1867	2.5131	2.6479
16	.2210	.2464	.3214	.3632	.4318	.4976	1.6435	1.8028	2.0000	2.1417	2.4532	2.5818
17	.2341	.2598	.3351	.3769	.4449	.5101	1.6228	1.7759	1.9652	2.1011	2.3994	2.5223
18	.2466	.2725	.3481	.3897	.4573	.5217	1.6038	1.7514	1.9336	2.0642	2.3507	2.4686
19	.2585	.2846	.3602	.4017	.4688	.5325	1.5865	1.7291	1.9048	2.0306	2.3063	2.4196
20	.2699	.2961	.3717	.4130	.4796	.5426	1.5705	1.7085	1.8783	1.9998	2.2658	2.3749
21	.2808	.3070	.3826	.4237	.4897	.5520	1.5558	1.6895	1.8539	1.9715	2.2284	2.3338
22	.2911	.3174	.3929	.4337	.4992	.5608	1.5420	1.6719	1.8313	1.9453	2.1940	2.2960
23	.3010	.3273	.4026	.4433	.5082	.5692	1.5292	1.6555	1.8103	1.9209	2.1621	2.2609
24	.3105	.3369	.4119	.4523	.5167	.5770	1.5173	1.6402	1.7908	1.8982	2.1325	2.2283
25	.3196	.3460	.4208	.4610	.5248	.5844	1.5061	1.6258	1.7726	1.8771	2.1048	2.1979
26	.3284	.3547	.4292	.4692	.5325	.5915	1.4956	1.6124	1.7555	1.8573	2.0789	2.1695
27	.3368	.3631	.4373	.4770	.5397	.5982	1.4857	1.5998	1.7394	1.8387	2.0547	2.1429
28	.3449	.3711	.4450	.4845	.5467	.6046	1.4763	1.5879	1.7242	1.8212	2.0319	2.1179
29	.3527	.3788	.4524	.4916	.5533	.6106	1.4675	1.5766	1.7099	1.8047	2.0104	2.0943
30	.3601	.3863	.4596	.4984	.5597	.6164	1.4591	1.5660	1.6964	1.7891	1.9901	2.0720
31	.3674	.3934	.4664	.5050	.5658	.6220	1.4511	1.5559	1.6836	1.7743	1.9709	2.0510
32	.3743	.4003	.4729	.5113	.5716	.6272	1.4436	1.5462	1.6714	1.7602	1.9527	2.0311
33	.3811	.4070	.4792	.5174	.5772	.6323	1.4364	1.5371	1.6599	1.7469	1.9355	2.0122
34	.3876	.4134	.4853	.5232	.5825	.6372	1.4295	1.5284	1.6489	1.7342	1.9190	1.9942
35	.3939	.4197	.4912	.5288	.5877	.6419	1.4229	1.5201	1.6383	1.7221	1.9034	1.9771
36	.4000	.4257	.4969	.5342	.5927	.6464	1.4166	1.5121	1.6283	1.7106	1.8885	1.9608
37	.4059	.4315	.5023	.5395	.5975	.6507	1.4106	1.5045	1.6187	1.6995	1.8742	1.9452
38	.4117	.4371	.5076	.5445	.6021	.6548	1.4048	1.4972	1.6095	1.6890	1.8606	1.9303
39	.4173	.4426	.5127	.5494	.6065	.6588	1.3993	1.4903	1.6007	1.6789	1.8476	1.9160
40	.4226	.4479	.5177	.5541	.6108	.6627	1.3940	1.4836	1.5923	1.6692	1.8350	1.9024
41	.4279	.4530	.5225	.5587	.6150	.6665	1.3888	1.4771	1.5841	1.6598	1.8230	1.8892
42	.4330	.4580	.5271	.5631	.6190	.6701	1.3839	1.4709	1.5763	1.6509	1.8115	1.8767
43	.4380	.4629	.5316	.5674	.6229	.6736	1.3792	1.4649	1.5688	1.6422	1.8004	1.8646
44	.4428	.4676	.5360	.5715	.6267	.6770	1.3746	1.4591	1.5616	1.6339	1.7898	1.8529
45	.4475	.4722	.5402	.5756	.6304	.6803	1.3701	1.4536	1.5546	1.6259	1.7795	1.8417
46	.4520	.4767	.5444	.5795	.6339	.6835	1.3659	1.4482	1.5478	1.6182	1.7696	1.8309
47	.4565	.4811	.5484	.5833	.6374	.6866	1.3617	1.4430	1.5413	1.6107	1.7600	1.8204
48	.4609	.4853	.5523	.5870	.6407	.6895	1.3577	1.4380	1.5351	1.6035	1.7508	1.8104
49	.4651	.4894	.5561	.5906	.6440	.6924	1.3539	1.4331	1.5290	1.5966	1.7418	1.8006
50	.4692	.4935	.5598	.5941	.6471	.6953	1.3501	1.4284	1.5231	1.5898	1.7332	1.7912

PERCENTAGE POINTS, CHI-SQUARE OVER DEGREES OF FREEDOM DISTRIBUTION

F / n	Probability in per cent						Probability in per cent					
	0.05	0.1	0.5	1.0	2.5	5.0	95.0	97.5	99.0	99.5	99.9	99.95
51	.4733	.4974	.5634	.5975	.6502	.6980	1.3465	1.4238	1.5174	1.5833	1.7249	1.7821
52	.4772	.5012	.5669	.6009	.6532	.7007	1.3429	1.4194	1.5118	1.5769	1.7168	1.7733
53	.4810	.5050	.5704	.6041	.6562	.7033	1.3395	1.4151	1.5065	1.5708	1.7089	1.7648
54	.4848	.5087	.5737	.6073	.6590	.7059	1.3362	1.4110	1.5013	1.5649	1.7013	1.7565
55	.4885	.5122	.5770	.6104	.6618	.7083	1.3329	1.4069	1.4962	1.5591	1.6939	1.7484
56	.4921	.5157	.5802	.6134	.6645	.7107	1.3298	1.4030	1.4913	1.5535	1.6868	1.7406
57	.4956	.5191	.5833	.6163	.6671	.7131	1.3267	1.3992	1.4865	1.5480	1.6798	1.7331
58	.4990	.5225	.5863	.6192	.6697	.7154	1.3238	1.3954	1.4819	1.5427	1.6731	1.7257
59	.5024	.5258	.5893	.6220	.6722	.7176	1.3209	1.3918	1.4774	1.5375	1.6665	1.7185
60	.5057	.5290	.5922	.6248	.6747	.7198	1.3180	1.3883	1.4730	1.5325	1.6601	1.7116
61	.5089	.5321	.5951	.6274	.6771	.7219	1.3153	1.3849	1.4687	1.5276	1.6539	1.7048
62	.5121	.5352	.5979	.6300	.6795	.7240	1.3126	1.3815	1.4645	1.5229	1.6478	1.6982
63	.5152	.5382	.6006	.6326	.6817	.7260	1.3100	1.3783	1.4605	1.5182	1.6419	1.6918
64	.5182	.5411	.6033	.6351	.6840	.7280	1.3074	1.3751	1.4565	1.5137	1.6362	1.6855
65	.5212	.5440	.6059	.6376	.6862	.7300	1.3049	1.3720	1.4526	1.5093	1.6306	1.6794
66	.5241	.5469	.6085	.6400	.6883	.7319	1.3025	1.3689	1.4489	1.5050	1.6251	1.6735
67	.5270	.5496	.6110	.6424	.6905	.7338	1.3001	1.3660	1.4452	1.5008	1.6198	1.6677
68	.5298	.5524	.6134	.6447	.6925	.7356	1.2978	1.3631	1.4416	1.4967	1.6146	1.6620
69	.5325	.5550	.6159	.6469	.6946	.7374	1.2955	1.3602	1.4381	1.4927	1.6095	1.6565
70	.5352	.5577	.6182	.6492	.6965	.7391	1.2933	1.3575	1.4346	1.4888	1.6045	1.6511
71	.5379	.5602	.6205	.6514	.6985	.7408	1.2911	1.3548	1.4313	1.4850	1.5997	1.6458
72	.5405	.5628	.6228	.6535	.7004	.7425	1.2890	1.3521	1.4280	1.4812	1.5949	1.6407
73	.5431	.5653	.6251	.6556	.7023	.7442	1.2869	1.3495	1.4248	1.4776	1.5903	1.6356
74	.5456	.5677	.6273	.6576	.7041	.7458	1.2849	1.3470	1.4216	1.4740	1.5858	1.6307
75	.5481	.5701	.6294	.6597	.7059	.7474	1.2829	1.3445	1.4186	1.4705	1.5813	1.6259
76	.5505	.5724	.6316	.6617	.7077	.7489	1.2809	1.3421	1.4156	1.4670	1.5770	1.6212
77	.5529	.5748	.6336	.6636	.7094	.7505	1.2790	1.3397	1.4126	1.4637	1.5727	1.6166
78	.5553	.5771	.6357	.6655	.7111	.7520	1.2771	1.3374	1.4097	1.4604	1.5686	1.6120
79	.5576	.5793	.6377	.6674	.7128	.7534	1.2753	1.3351	1.4069	1.4572	1.5645	1.6076
80	.5599	.5815	.6396	.6692	.7144	.7549	1.2735	1.3329	1.4041	1.4540	1.5605	1.6033
81	.5621	.5837	.6416	.6711	.7160	.7563	1.2717	1.3307	1.4014	1.4509	1.5566	1.5990
82	.5643	.5858	.6435	.6729	.7176	.7577	1.2700	1.3285	1.3987	1.4479	1.5527	1.5948
83	.5665	.5879	.6454	.6746	.7192	.7591	1.2683	1.3264	1.3961	1.4449	1.5490	1.5908
84	.5687	.5900	.6472	.6763	.7207	.7604	1.2666	1.3243	1.3935	1.4420	1.5453	1.5868
85	.5708	.5920	.6491	.6780	.7222	.7618	1.2650	1.3223	1.3910	1.4391	1.5417	1.5828
86	.5728	.5940	.6508	.6797	.7237	.7631	1.2633	1.3203	1.3885	1.4363	1.5381	1.5790
87	.5749	.5960	.6526	.6814	.7252	.7643	1.2618	1.3183	1.3861	1.4335	1.5346	1.5752
88	.5769	.5979	.6543	.6830	.7266	.7656	1.2602	1.3164	1.3837	1.4308	1.5312	1.5715
89	.5789	.5998	.6561	.6846	.7280	.7668	1.2587	1.3145	1.3814	1.4282	1.5278	1.5678
90	.5808	.6017	.6577	.6862	.7294	.7681	1.2572	1.3126	1.3791	1.4255	1.5245	1.5643
91	.5828	.6036	.6594	.6877	.7308	.7693	1.2557	1.3108	1.3768	1.4230	1.5213	1.5607
92	.5847	.6054	.6610	.6892	.7321	.7705	1.2542	1.3090	1.3746	1.4204	1.5181	1.5573
93	.5865	.6072	.6626	.6907	.7335	.7716	1.2528	1.3072	1.3724	1.4180	1.5150	1.5539
94	.5884	.6090	.6642	.6922	.7348	.7728	1.2514	1.3055	1.3702	1.4155	1.5119	1.5505
95	.5902	.6108	.6658	.6937	.7361	.7739	1.2500	1.3038	1.3681	1.4131	1.5089	1.5473
96	.5920	.6125	.6673	.6951	.7373	.7750	1.2487	1.3021	1.3661	1.4108	1.5059	1.5440
97	.5938	.6142	.6688	.6965	.7386	.7761	1.2473	1.3004	1.3640	1.4084	1.5030	1.5409
98	.5955	.6159	.6703	.6979	.7398	.7772	1.2460	1.2988	1.3620	1.4062	1.5001	1.5377
99	.5973	.6175	.6718	.6993	.7410	.7782	1.2447	1.2972	1.3600	1.4039	1.4973	1.5347
100	.5990	.6192	.6733	.7007	.7422	.7793	1.2434	1.2956	1.3581	1.4017	1.4945	1.5317

PERCENTAGE POINTS, CHI-SQUARE OVER DEGREES OF FREEDOM DISTRIBUTION

n \ *F*	Probability in per cent						Probability in per cent					
	0.05	0.1	0.5	1.0	2.5	5.0	95.0	97.5	99.0	99.5	99.9	99.95
100	.5990	.6192	.6733	.7007	.7422	.7793	1.2434	1.2956	1.3581	1.4017	1.4945	1.5317
105	.6072	.6271	.6802	.7071	.7480	.7843	1.2373	1.2881	1.3488	1.3911	1.4812	1.5173
110	.6148	.6344	.6868	.7132	.7534	.7890	1.2316	1.2811	1.3401	1.3813	1.4689	1.5040
115	.6221	.6414	.6930	.7190	.7584	.7934	1.2263	1.2746	1.3321	1.3722	1.4575	1.4916
120	.6289	.6480	.6988	.7243	.7632	.7975	1.2214	1.2685	1.3246	1.3637	1.4468	1.4801
125	.6353	.6542	.7042	.7294	.7676	.8014	1.2167	1.2627	1.3175	1.3557	1.4368	1.4692
130	.6414	.6600	.7094	.7342	.7718	.8051	1.2124	1.2574	1.3109	1.3484	1.4275	1.4592
135	.6473	.6656	.7143	.7388	.7757	.8085	1.2083	1.2523	1.3047	1.3413	1.4187	1.4496
140	.6528	.6709	.7190	.7431	.7795	.8119	1.2043	1.2475	1.2988	1.3346	1.4104	1.4406
145	.6581	.6760	.7234	.7472	.7831	.8150	1.2007	1.2430	1.2933	1.3284	1.4026	1.4321
150	.6631	.6808	.7276	.7511	.7865	.8180	1.1972	1.2387	1.2880	1.3224	1.3951	1.4241
155	.6679	.6854	.7316	.7549	.7898	.8208	1.1939	1.2346	1.2830	1.3168	1.3881	1.4166
160	.6725	.6898	.7355	.7584	.7930	.8235	1.1907	1.2308	1.2783	1.3114	1.3813	1.4093
165	.6769	.6939	.7392	.7618	.7959	.8260	1.1877	1.2270	1.2737	1.3063	1.3751	1.4024
170	.6811	.6980	.7427	.7651	.7987	.8285	1.1848	1.2235	1.2694	1.3014	1.3690	1.3958
175	.6852	.7019	.7461	.7682	.8015	.8309	1.1821	1.2201	1.2653	1.2968	1.3632	1.3896
180	.6891	.7056	.7494	.7712	.8041	.8332	1.1795	1.2170	1.2614	1.2924	1.3577	1.3836
185	.6929	.7092	.7525	.7741	.8066	.8353	1.1769	1.2138	1.2576	1.2881	1.3523	1.3779
190	.6964	.7127	.7555	.7768	.8090	.8374	1.1745	1.2109	1.2541	1.2840	1.3472	1.3725
195	.6999	.7160	.7584	.7795	.8114	.8394	1.1722	1.2081	1.2506	1.2801	1.3424	1.3672
200	.7033	.7192	.7612	.7821	.8136	.8414	1.1700	1.2053	1.2473	1.2763	1.3377	1.3622
210	.7097	.7254	.7665	.7870	.8179	.8451	1.1657	1.2001	1.2409	1.2692	1.3288	1.3526
220	.7157	.7311	.7715	.7916	.8219	.8485	1.1618	1.1953	1.2351	1.2626	1.3207	1.3438
230	.7213	.7365	.7762	.7959	.8256	.8517	1.1582	1.1908	1.2297	1.2564	1.3131	1.3356
240	.7266	.7415	.7805	.7999	.8291	.8547	1.1547	1.1867	1.2246	1.2507	1.3060	1.3279
250	.7317	.7463	.7847	.8037	.8324	.8576	1.1515	1.1828	1.2198	1.2453	1.2994	1.3207
260	.7364	.7507	.7886	.8073	.8355	.8602	1.1485	1.1791	1.2153	1.2403	1.2931	1.3140
270	.7408	.7550	.7923	.8107	.8384	.8628	1.1457	1.1756	1.2111	1.2356	1.2872	1.3077
280	.7450	.7590	.7958	.8139	.8412	.8652	1.1430	1.1723	1.2071	1.2312	1.2817	1.3017
290	.7491	.7629	.7991	.8170	.8438	.8674	1.1404	1.1692	1.2033	1.2269	1.2764	1.2961
300	.7529	.7665	.8023	.8199	.8463	.8696	1.1380	1.1663	1.1997	1.2229	1.2714	1.2907
350	.7698	.7826	.8160	.8326	.8573	.8790	1.1275	1.1535	1.1843	1.2055	1.2500	1.2676
400	.7836	.7957	.8272	.8429	.8662	.8866	1.1191	1.1433	1.1718	1.1915	1.2378	1.2491
450	.7951	.8066	.8366	.8515	.8736	.8929	1.1121	1.1349	1.1616	1.1801	1.2187	1.2340
500	.8050	.8160	.8446	.8588	.8799	.8983	1.1063	1.1277	1.1530	1.1704	1.2070	1.2214
550	.8135	.8239	.8515	.8651	.8853	.9029	1.1012	1.1216	1.1456	1.1622	1.1968	1.2105
600	.8208	.8310	.8575	.8706	.8900	.9070	1.0968	1.1163	1.1392	1.1550	1.1880	1.2010
650	.8275	.8373	.8629	.8755	.8942	.9106	1.0929	1.1116	1.1335	1.1487	1.1803	1.1927
700	.8334	.8429	.8677	.8799	.8980	.9137	1.0895	1.1074	1.1285	1.1430	1.1734	1.1853
750	.8387	.8480	.8720	.8838	.9013	.9166	1.0864	1.1037	1.1240	1.1380	1.1672	1.1787
800	.8436	.8526	.8759	.8874	.9044	.9192	1.0836	1.1004	1.1200	1.1335	1.1617	1.1728
850	.8480	.8568	.8795	.8906	.9072	.9216	1.0811	1.0973	1.1163	1.1294	1.1567	1.1674
900	.8521	.8606	.8827	.8936	.9097	.9237	1.0788	1.0945	1.1129	1.1256	1.1520	1.1624
950	.8559	.8642	.8858	.8964	.9121	.9257	1.0767	1.0919	1.1098	1.1221	1.1478	1.1579
1000	.8594	.8675	.8886	.8989	.9143	.9276	1.0747	1.0895	1.1070	1.1190	1.1440	1.1538
2000	.8992	.9051	.9204	.9279	.9390	.9486	1.0526	1.0629	1.0750	1.0833	1.1006	1.1074
3000	.9172	.9221	.9348	.9409	.9500	.9579	1.0429	1.0513	1.0611	1.0678	1.0817	1.0872
4000	.9280	.9323	.9433	.9487	.9566	.9635	1.0370	1.0443	1.0527	1.0585	1.0705	1.0752
5000	.9355	.9393	.9493	.9541	.9612	.9673	1.0331	1.0396	1.0471	1.0523	1.0630	1.0671
10000	.9541	.9569	.9640	.9674	.9725	.9769	1.0234	1.0279	1.0332	1.0368	1.0443	1.0472

V.3 NUMBER OF OBSERVATIONS REQUIRED FOR THE COMPARISON OF A POPULATION VARIANCE WITH A STANDARD VALUE USING THE CHI-SQUARE TEST

The tabular entries show the value of the ratio R of the population variance σ_1^2 to a standard variance σ_0^2 which is undetected with probability β in a χ^2 test at significance level α of an estimate s_1^2 of σ_1^2 based on n degrees of freedom.

NUMBER OF OBSERVATIONS REQUIRED FOR THE COMPARISON OF A POPULATION VARIANCE WITH A STANDARD VALUE USING THE CHI-SQUARE TEST

n	$\alpha = 0.01$				$\alpha = 0.05$			
	$\beta = 0.01$	$\beta = 0.05$	$\beta = 0.1$	$\beta = 0.5$	$\beta = 0.01$	$\beta = 0.05$	$\beta = 0.1$	$\beta = 0.5$
1	42,240	1,687	420.2	14.58	25,450	977.0	243.3	8.444
2	458.2	89.78	43.71	6.644	298.1	58.40	28.43	4.322
3	98.79	32.24	19.41	4.795	68.05	22.21	13.37	3.303
4	44.69	18.68	12.48	3.955	31.93	13.35	8.920	2.826
5	27.22	13.17	9.369	3.467	19.97	9.665	6.875	2.544
6	19.28	10.28	7.628	3.144	14.44	7.699	5.713	2.354
7	14.91	8.524	6.521	2.911	11.35	6.491	4.965	2.217
8	12.20	7.352	5.757	2.736	9.418	5.675	4.444	2.112
9	10.38	6.510	5.198	2.597	8.103	5.088	4.059	2.028
10	9.072	5.890	4.770	2.484	7.156	4.646	3.763	1.960
12	7.343	5.017	4.159	2.312	5.889	4.023	3.335	1.854
15	5.847	4.211	3.578	2.132	4.780	3.442	2.925	1.743
20	4.548	3.462	3.019	1.943	3.802	2.895	2.524	1.624
24	3.959	3.104	2.745	1.842	3.354	2.630	2.326	1.560
30	3.403	2.752	2.471	1.735	2.927	2.367	2.125	1.492
40	2.874	2.403	2.192	1.619	2.516	2.103	1.919	1.418
60	2.358	2.046	1.902	1.490	2.110	1.831	1.702	1.333
120	1.829	1.661	1.580	1.332	1.686	1.532	1.457	1.228
∞	1.000	1.000	1.000	1.000	1.000	1.000	1.000	1.000

Examples

Testing for an increase in variance. Let $\alpha = 0.05$, $\beta = 0.01$, and $R = 4$. Entering the table with these values it is found that the value 4 occurs between the rows corresponding to $n = 15$ and $n = 20$. Using rough interpolation it is indicated that the estimate of variance should be based on 19 degrees of freedom.

Testing for a decrease in variance. Let $\alpha = 0.05$, $\beta = 0.01$, and $R = 0.33$. The table is entered with $\alpha' = \beta = 0.01$, $\beta' = \alpha = 0.05$, and $R' = 1/R = 3$. It is found that the value 3 occurs between the rows corresponding to $n = 24$ and $n = 30$. Using rough interpolation it is indicated that the estimate of variance should be based on 26 degrees of freedom.

V.4 OPERATING CHARACTERISTIC (OC) CURVES FOR A TEST ON THE STANDARD DEVIATION OF A NORMAL DISTRIBUTION

The OC curves give the sample sizes needed for given values of $\alpha = P$ (Type I error) and $\beta = P$ (Type II error) for a test of the hypothesis $H_0\colon \sigma = \sigma_0$. The statistic used is $\chi^2 = \dfrac{(n-1)s^2}{{\sigma_0}^2}$, which is distributed as the Chi-square distribution with $n - 1$ degrees of freedom. The required sample size is obtained by entering the appropriate set of curves for given α and β for various values of $\lambda = \dfrac{\sigma_1}{\sigma_0}$ for both one-sided and two-sided tests.

OC CURVES FOR A TEST ON THE STANDARD DEVIATION OF A NORMAL DISTRIBUTION

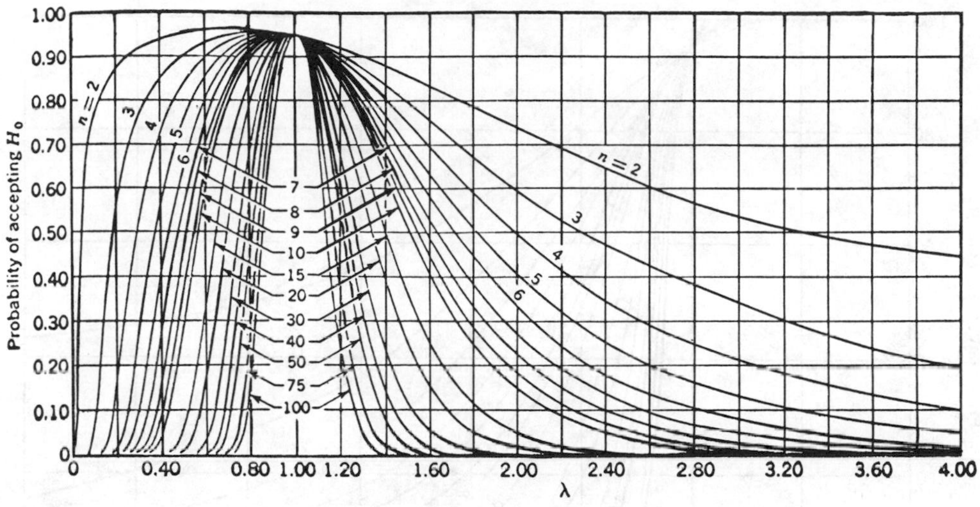

a) OC curves for different values of *n* for the two-sided chi-square test for a level of significance $\alpha = 0.05$.

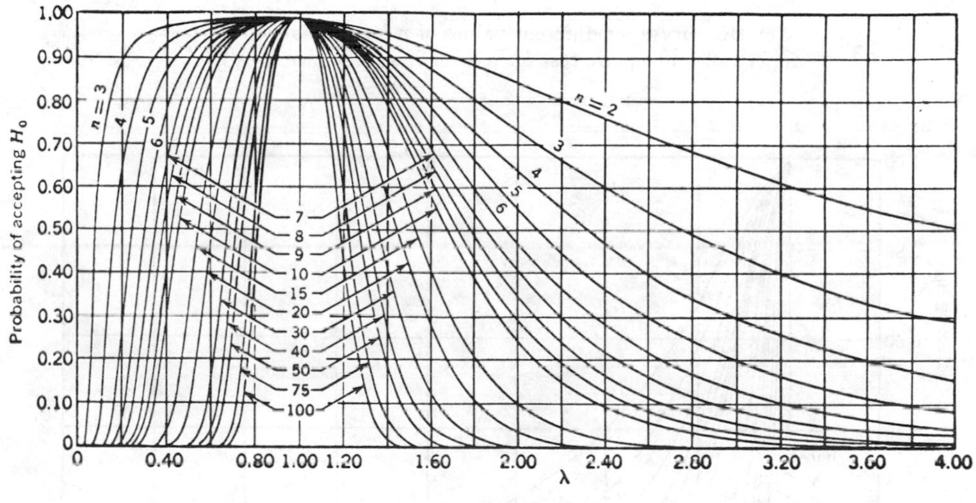

b) OC curves for different values of *n* for the two-sided chi-square test for a level of significance $\alpha = 0.01$.

OC CURVES FOR A TEST ON THE STANDARD DEVIATION OF A NORMAL DISTRIBUTION

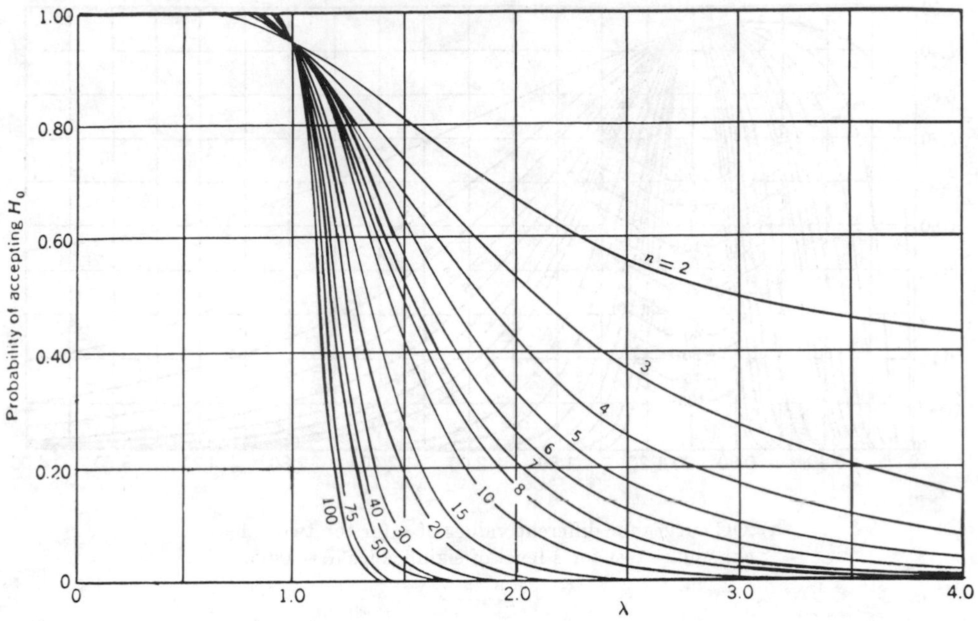

c) OC curves for different values of n for the one-sided (upper tail) chi-square test for a level of significance $\alpha = 0.05$.

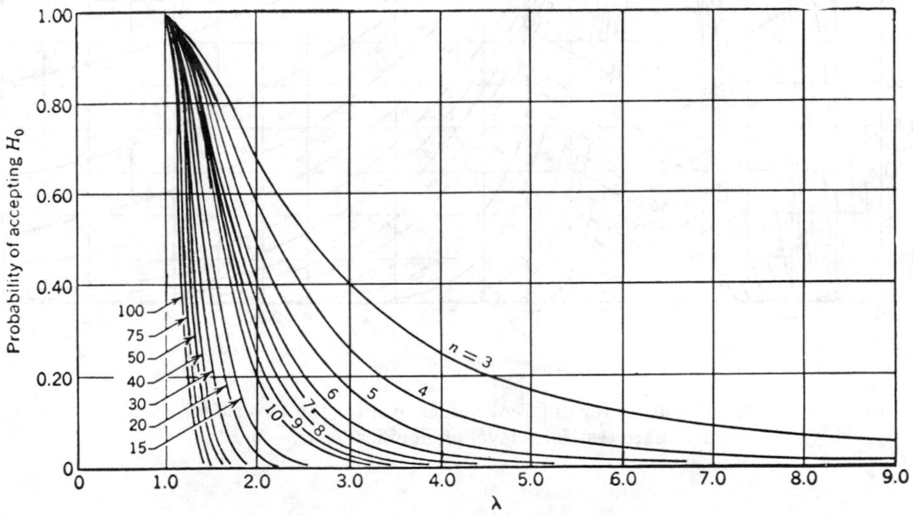

d) OC curves for different values of n for the one-sided (upper tail) chi-square test for a level of significance $\alpha = 0.01$.

OC CURVES FOR A TEST ON THE STANDARD DEVIATION OF A NORMAL DISTRIBUTION

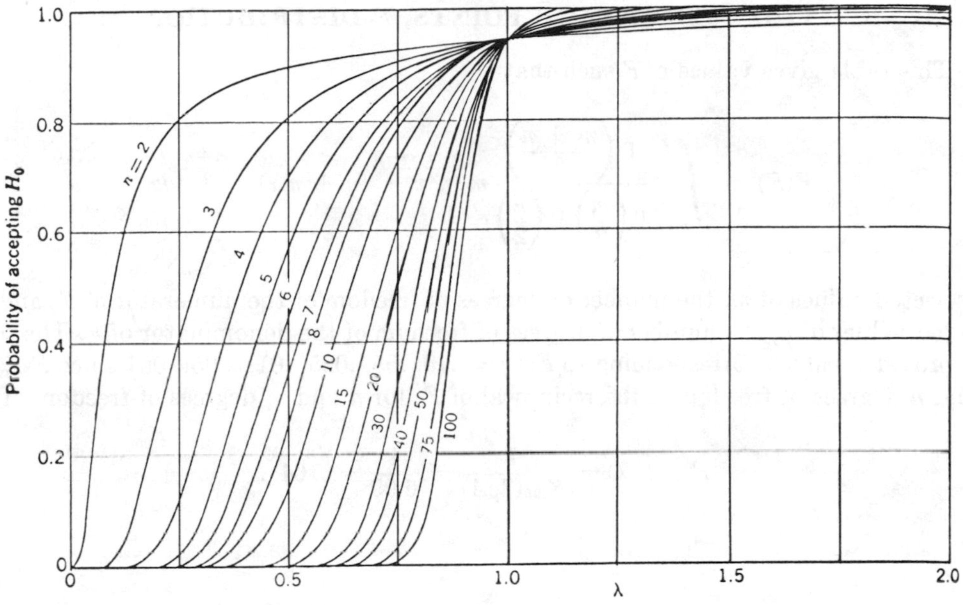

e) OC curves for different values of *n* for the one-sided (lower tail) chi-square test for a level of significance $\alpha = 0.05$.

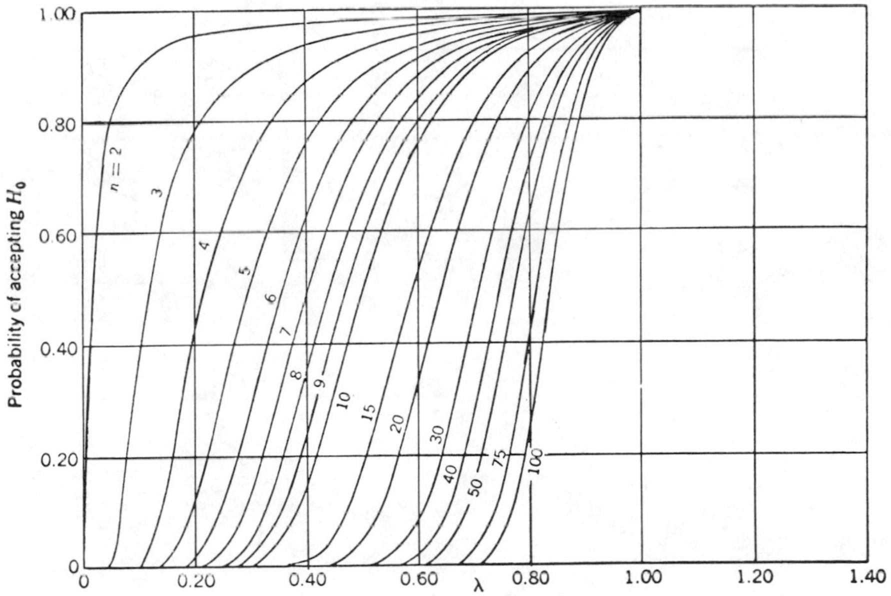

f) OC curves for different values of *n* for the one-sided (lower tail) chi-square test for a level of significance $\alpha = 0.01$.

VI. *F*-Distribution

VI.1 PERCENTAGE POINTS, *F*-DISTRIBUTION

This table gives values of F such that

$$F(F) = \int_0^F \frac{\Gamma\left(\frac{m+n}{2}\right)}{\Gamma\left(\frac{m}{2}\right)\Gamma\left(\frac{n}{2}\right)} m^{\frac{m}{2}} n^{\frac{n}{2}} x^{\frac{m-2}{2}} (n + mx)^{-\frac{m+n}{2}} dx$$

for selected values of m, the number of degrees of freedom of the numerator of F; and for selected values of n, the number of degrees of freedom of the denominator of F. The table also provides values corresponding to $F(F) = .10, .05, .025, .01, .005, .001$ since $F_{1-\alpha}$ for m and n degrees of freedom is the reciprocal of F_α for n and m degrees of freedom. Thus

$$F_{.05}(4, 7) = \frac{1}{F_{.95}(7, 4)} = \frac{1}{6.09} = .164 \ .$$

PERCENTAGE POINTS, F-DISTRIBUTION

$$F(F) = \int_0^F \frac{\Gamma\left(\frac{m+n}{2}\right)}{\Gamma\left(\frac{m}{2}\right)\Gamma\left(\frac{n}{2}\right)} m^{\frac{m}{2}} n^{\frac{n}{2}} x^{\frac{m}{2}-1} (n+mx)^{-\frac{m+n}{2}} dx = .90$$

n \ m	1	2	3	4	5	6	7	8	9	10	12	15	20	24	30	40	60	120	∞
1	39.86	49.50	53.59	55.83	57.24	58.20	58.91	59.44	59.86	60.19	60.71	61.22	61.74	62.00	62.26	62.53	62.79	63.06	63.33
2	8.53	9.00	9.16	9.24	9.29	9.33	9.35	9.37	9.38	9.39	9.41	9.42	9.44	9.45	9.46	9.47	9.47	9.48	9.49
3	5.54	5,46	5.39	5.34	5.31	5.28	5.27	5.25	5.24	5.23	5.22	5.20	5.18	5.18	5.17	5.16	5.15	5.14	5.13
4	4.54	4.32	4.19	4.11	4.05	4.01	3.98	3.95	3.94	3.92	3.90	3.87	3.84	3.83	3.82	3.80	3.79	3.78	3.76
5	4.06	3.78	3.62	3.52	3.45	3.40	3.37	3.34	3.32	3.30	3.27	3.24	3.21	3.19	3.17	3.16	3.14	3.12	3.10
6	3.78	3.46	3.29	3.18	3.11	3.05	3.01	2.98	2.96	2.94	2.90	2.87	2.84	2.82	2.80	2.78	2.76	2.74	2.72
7	3.59	3.26	3.07	2.96	2.88	2.83	2.78	2.75	2.72	2.70	2.67	2.63	2.59	2.58	2.56	2.54	2.51	2.49	2.47
8	3.46	3.11	2.92	2.81	2.73	2.67	2.62	2.59	2.56	2.54	2.50	2.46	2.42	2.40	2.38	2.36	2.34	2.32	2.29
9	3.36	3.01	2.81	2.69	2.61	2.55	2.51	2.47	2.44	2.42	2.38	2.34	2.30	2.28	2.25	2.23	2.21	2.18	2.16
10	3.29	2.92	2.73	2.61	2.52	2.46	2.41	2.38	2.35	2.32	2.28	2.24	2.20	2.18	2.16	2.13	2.11	2.08	2.06
11	3.23	2.86	2.66	2.54	2.45	2.39	2.34	2.30	2.27	2.25	2.21	2.17	2.12	2.10	2.08	2.05	2.03	2.00	1.97
12	3.18	2.81	2.61	2.48	2.39	2.33	2.28	2.24	2.21	2.19	2.15	2.10	2.06	2.04	2.01	1.99	1.96	1.93	1.90
13	3.14	2.76	2.56	2.43	2.35	2.28	2.23	2.20	2.16	2.14	2.10	2.05	2.01	1.98	1.96	1.93	1.90	1.88	1.85
14	3.10	2.73	2.52	2.39	2.31	2.24	2.19	2.15	2.12	2.10	2.05	2.01	1.96	1.94	1.91	1.89	1.86	1.83	1.80
15	3.07	2.70	2.49	2.36	2.27	2.21	2.16	2.12	2.09	2.06	2.02	1.97	1.92	1.90	1.87	1.85	1.82	1.79	1.76
16	3.05	2.67	2.46	2.33	2.24	2.18	2.13	2.09	2.06	2.03	1.99	1.94	1.89	1.87	1.84	1.81	1.78	1.75	1.72
17	3.03	2.64	2.44	2.31	2.22	2.15	2.10	2.06	2.03	2.00	1.96	1.91	1.86	1.84	1.81	1.78	1.75	1.72	1.69
18	3.01	2.62	2.42	2.29	2.20	2.13	2.08	2.04	2.00	1.98	1.93	1.89	1.84	1.81	1.78	1.75	1.72	1.69	1.66
19	2.99	2.61	2.40	2.27	2.18	2.11	2.06	2.02	1.98	1.96	1.91	1.86	1.81	1.79	1.76	1.73	1.70	1.67	1.63
20	2.97	2.59	2.38	2.25	2.16	2.09	2.04	2.00	1.96	1.94	1.89	1.84	1.79	1.77	1.74	1.71	1.68	1.64	1.61
21	2.96	2.57	2.36	2.23	2.14	2.08	2.02	1.98	1.95	1.92	1.87	1.83	1.78	1.75	1.72	1.69	1.66	1.62	1.59
22	2.95	2.56	2.35	2.22	2.13	2.06	2.01	1.97	1.93	1.90	1.86	1.81	1.76	1.73	1.70	1.67	1.64	1.60	1.57
23	2.94	2.55	2.34	2.21	2.11	2.05	1.99	1.95	1.92	1.89	1.84	1.80	1.74	1.72	1.69	1.66	1.62	1.59	1.55
24	2.93	2.54	2.33	2.19	2.10	2.04	1.98	1.94	1.91	1.88	1.83	1.78	1.73	1.70	1.67	1.64	1.61	1.57	1.53
25	2.92	2.53	2.32	2.18	2.09	2.02	1.97	1.93	1.89	1.87	1.82	1.77	1.72	1.69	1.66	1.63	1.59	1.56	1.52
26	2.91	2.52	2.31	2.17	2.08	2.01	1.96	1.92	1.88	1.86	1.81	1.76	1.71	1.68	1.65	1.61	1.58	1.54	1.50
27	2.90	2.51	2.30	2.17	2.07	2.00	1.95	1.91	1.87	1.85	1.80	1.75	1.70	1.67	1.64	1.60	1.57	1.53	1.49
28	2.89	2.50	2.29	2.16	2.06	2.00	1.94	1.90	1.87	1.84	1.79	1.74	1.69	1.66	1.63	1.59	1.56	1.52	1.48
29	2.89	2.50	2.28	2.15	2.06	1.99	1.93	1.89	1.86	1.83	1.78	1.73	1.68	1.65	1.62	1.58	1.55	1.51	1.47
30	2.88	2.49	2.28	2.14	2.05	1.98	1.93	1.88	1.85	1.82	1.77	1.72	1.67	1.64	1.61	1.57	1.54	1.50	1.46
40	2.84	2.44	2.23	2.09	2.00	1.93	1.87	1.83	1.79	1.76	1.71	1.66	1.61	1.57	1.54	1.51	1.47	1.42	1.38
60	2.79	2.39	2.18	2.04	1.95	1.87	1.82	1.77	1.74	1.71	1.66	1.60	1.54	1.51	1.48	1.44	1.40	1.35	1.29
120	2.75	2.35	2.13	1.99	1.90	1.82	1.77	1.72	1.68	1.65	1.60	1.55	1.48	1.45	1.41	1.37	1.32	1.26	1.19
∞	2.71	2.30	2.08	1.94	1.85	1.77	1.72	1.67	1.63	1.60	1.55	1.49	1.42	1.38	1.34	1.30	1.24	1.17	1.00

$F = \frac{s_1^2}{s_2^2} = \frac{S_1}{m} \Big/ \frac{S_2}{n}$, where $s_1^2 = S_1/m$ and $s_2^2 = S_2/n$ are independent mean squares estimating a common variance σ^2 and based on m and n degrees of freedom, respectively.

PERCENTAGE POINTS, F-DISTRIBUTION

$$F(F) = \int_0^F \frac{\Gamma\left(\frac{m+n}{2}\right)}{\Gamma\left(\frac{m}{2}\right)\Gamma\left(\frac{n}{2}\right)} m^{\frac{m}{2}} n^{\frac{n}{2}} x^{\frac{m}{2}-1} (n+mx)^{-\frac{m+n}{2}} dx = .95$$

n \ m	1	2	3	4	5	6	7	8	9	10	12	15	20	24	30	40	60	120	∞
1	161.4	199.5	215.7	224.6	230.2	234.0	236.8	238.9	240.5	241.9	243.9	245.9	248.0	249.1	250.1	251.1	252.2	253.3	254.3
2	18.51	19.00	19.16	19.25	19.30	19.33	19.35	19.37	19.38	19.40	19.41	19.43	19.45	19.45	19.46	19.47	19.48	19.49	19.50
3	10.13	9.55	9.28	9.12	9.01	8.94	8.89	8.85	8.81	8.79	8.74	8.70	8.66	8.64	8.62	8.59	8.57	8.55	8.53
4	7.71	6.94	6.59	6.39	6.26	6.16	6.09	6.04	6.00	5.96	5.91	5.86	5.80	5.77	5.75	5.72	5.69	5.66	5.63
5	6.61	5.79	5.41	5.19	5.05	4.95	4.88	4.82	4.77	4.74	4.68	4.62	4.56	4.53	4.50	4.46	4.43	4.40	4.36
6	5.99	5.14	4.76	4.53	4.39	4.28	4.21	4.15	4.10	4.06	4.00	3.94	3.87	3.84	3.81	3.77	3.74	3.70	3.67
7	5.59	4.74	4.35	4.12	3.97	3.87	3.79	3.73	3.68	3.64	3.57	3.51	3.44	3.41	3.38	3.34	3.30	3.27	3.23
8	5.32	4.46	4.07	3.84	3.69	3.58	3.50	3.44	3.39	3.35	3.28	3.22	3.15	3.12	3.08	3.04	3.01	2.97	2.93
9	5.12	4.26	3.86	3.63	3.48	3.37	3.29	3.23	3.18	3.14	3.07	3.01	2.94	2.90	2.86	2.83	2.79	2.75	2.71
10	4.96	4.10	3.71	3.48	3.33	3.22	3.14	3.07	3.02	2.98	2.91	2.85	2.77	2.74	2.70	2.66	2.62	2.58	2.54
11	4.84	3.98	3.59	3.36	3.20	3.09	3.01	2.95	2.90	2.85	2.79	2.72	2.65	2.61	2.57	2.53	2.49	2.45	2.40
12	4.75	3.89	3.49	3.26	3.11	3.00	2.91	2.85	2.80	2.75	2.69	2.62	2.54	2.51	2.47	2.43	2.38	2.34	2.30
13	4.67	3.81	3.41	3.18	3.03	2.92	2.83	2.77	2.71	2.67	2.60	2.53	2.46	2.42	2.38	2.34	2.30	2.25	2.21
14	4.60	3.74	3.34	3.11	2.96	2.85	2.76	2.70	2.65	2.60	2.53	2.46	2.39	2.35	2.31	2.27	2.22	2.18	2.13
15	4.54	3.68	3.29	3.06	2.90	2.79	2.71	2.64	2.59	2.54	2.48	2.40	2.33	2.29	2.25	2.20	2.16	2.11	2.07
16	4.49	3.63	3.24	3.01	2.85	2.74	2.66	2.59	2.54	2.49	2.42	2.35	2.28	2.24	2.19	2.15	2.11	2.06	2.01
17	4.45	3.59	3.20	2.96	2.81	2.70	2.61	2.55	2.49	2.45	2.38	2.31	2.23	2.19	2.15	2.10	2.06	2.01	1.96
18	4.41	3.55	3.16	2.93	2.77	2.66	2.58	2.51	2.46	2.41	2.34	2.27	2.19	2.15	2.11	2.06	2.02	1.97	1.92
19	4.38	3.52	3.13	2.90	2.74	2.63	2.54	2.48	2.42	2.38	2.31	2.23	2.16	2.11	2.07	2.03	1.98	1.93	1.88
20	4.35	3.49	3.10	2.87	2.71	2.60	2.51	2.45	2.39	2.35	2.28	2.20	2.12	2.08	2.04	1.99	1.95	1.90	1.84
21	4.32	3.47	3.07	2.84	2.68	2.57	2.49	2.42	2.37	2.32	2.25	2.18	2.10	2.05	2.01	1.96	1.92	1.87	1.81
22	4.30	3.44	3.05	2.82	2.66	2.55	2.46	2.40	2.34	2.30	2.23	2.15	2.07	2.03	1.98	1.94	1.89	1.84	1.78
23	4.28	3.42	3.03	2.80	2.64	2.53	2.44	2.37	2.32	2.27	2.20	2.13	2.05	2.01	1.96	1.91	1.86	1.81	1.76
24	4.26	3.40	3.01	2.78	2.62	2.51	2.42	2.36	2.30	2.25	2.18	2.11	2.03	1.98	1.94	1.89	1.84	1.79	1.73
25	4.24	3.39	2.99	2.76	2.60	2.49	2.40	2.34	2.28	2.24	2.16	2.09	2.01	1.96	1.92	1.87	1.82	1.77	1.71
26	4.23	3.37	2.98	2.74	2.59	2.47	2.39	2.32	2.27	2.22	2.15	2.07	1.99	1.95	1.90	1.85	1.80	1.75	1.69
27	4.21	3.35	2.96	2.73	2.57	2.46	2.37	2.31	2.25	2.20	2.13	2.06	1.97	1.93	1.88	1.84	1.79	1.73	1.67
28	4.20	3.34	2.95	2.71	2.56	2.45	2.36	2.29	2.24	2.19	2.12	2.04	1.96	1.91	1.87	1.82	1.77	1.71	1.65
29	4.18	3.33	2.93	2.70	2.55	2.43	2.35	2.28	2.22	2.18	2.10	2.03	1.94	1.90	1.85	1.81	1.75	1.70	1.64
30	4.17	3.32	2.92	2.69	2.53	2.42	2.33	2.27	2.21	2.16	2.09	2.01	1.93	1.89	1.84	1.79	1.74	1.68	1.62
40	4.08	3.23	2.84	2.61	2.45	2.34	2.25	2.18	2.12	2.08	2.00	1.92	1.84	1.79	1.74	1.69	1.64	1.58	1.51
60	4.00	3.15	2.76	2.53	2.37	2.25	2.17	2.10	2.04	1.99	1.92	1.84	1.75	1.70	1.65	1.59	1.53	1.47	1.39
120	3.92	3.07	2.68	2.45	2.29	2.17	2.09	2.02	1.96	1.91	1.83	1.75	1.66	1.61	1.55	1.50	1.43	1.35	1.25
∞	3.84	3.00	2.60	2.37	2.21	2.10	2.01	1.94	1.88	1.83	1.75	1.67	1.57	1.52	1.46	1.39	1.32	1.22	1.00

$F = \frac{s_1^2}{s_2^2} = \frac{S_1}{m} \Big/ \frac{S_2}{n}$, where $s_1^2 = S_1/m$ and $s_2^2 = S_2/n$ are independent mean squares estimating a common variance σ^2 and based on m and n degrees of freedom, respectively.

PERCENTAGE POINTS, *F*-DISTRIBUTION

$$F(F) = \int_0^F \frac{\Gamma\left(\frac{m+n}{2}\right)}{\Gamma\left(\frac{m}{2}\right)\Gamma\left(\frac{n}{2}\right)} m^{\frac{m}{2}} n^{\frac{n}{2}} x^{\frac{m}{2}-1} (n+mx)^{-\frac{m+n}{2}} dx = .975$$

n \ m	1	2	3	4	5	6	7	8	9	10	12	15	20	24	30	40	60	120	∞
1	647.8	799.5	864.2	899.6	921.8	937.1	948.2	956.7	963.3	968.6	976.7	984.9	993.1	997.2	1001	1006	1010	1014	1018
2	38.51	39.00	39.17	39.25	39.30	39.33	39.36	39.37	39.39	39.40	39.41	39.43	39.45	39.46	39.46	39.47	39.48	39.49	39.50
3	17.44	16.04	15.44	15.10	14.88	14.73	14.62	14.54	14.47	14.42	14.34	14.25	14.17	14.12	14.08	14.04	13.99	13.95	13.90
4	12.22	10.65	9.98	9.60	9.36	9.20	9.07	8.98	8.90	8.84	8.75	8.66	8.56	8.51	8.46	8.41	8.36	8.31	8.26
5	10.01	8.43	7.76	7.39	7.15	6.98	6.85	6.76	6.68	6.62	6.52	6.43	6.33	6.28	6.23	6.18	6.12	6.07	6.02
6	8.81	7.26	6.60	6.23	5.99	5.82	5.70	5.60	5.52	5.46	5.37	5.27	5.17	5.12	5.07	5.01	4.96	4.90	4.85
7	8.07	6.54	5.89	5.52	5.29	5.12	4.99	4.90	4.82	4.76	4.67	4.57	4.47	4.42	4.36	4.31	4.25	4.20	4.14
8	7.57	6.06	5.42	5.05	4.82	4.65	4.53	4.43	4.36	4.30	4.20	4.10	4.00	3.95	3.89	3.84	3.78	3.73	3.67
9	7.21	5.71	5.08	4.72	4.48	4.32	4.20	4.10	4.03	3.96	3.87	3.77	3.67	3.61	3.56	3.51	3.45	3.39	3.33
10	6.94	5.46	4.83	4.47	4.24	4.07	3.95	3.85	3.78	3.72	3.62	3.52	3.42	3.37	3.31	3.26	3.20	3.14	3.08
11	6.72	5.26	4.63	4.28	4.04	3.88	3.76	3.66	3.59	3.53	3.43	3.33	3.23	3.17	3.12	3.06	3.00	2.94	2.88
12	6.55	5.10	4.47	4.12	3.89	3.73	3.61	3.51	3.44	3.37	3.28	3.18	3.07	3.02	2.96	2.91	2.85	2.79	2.72
13	6.41	4.97	4.35	4.00	3.77	3.60	3.48	3.39	3.31	3.25	3.15	3.05	2.95	2.89	2.84	2.78	2.72	2.66	2.60
14	6.30	4.86	4.24	3.89	3.66	3.50	3.38	3.29	3.21	3.15	3.05	2.95	2.84	2.79	2.73	2.67	2.61	2.55	2.49
15	6.20	4.77	4.15	3.80	3.58	3.41	3.29	3.20	3.12	3.06	2.96	2.86	2.76	2.70	2.64	2.59	2.52	2.46	2.40
16	6.12	4.69	4.08	3.73	3.50	3.34	3.22	3.12	3.05	2.99	2.89	2.79	2.68	2.63	2.57	2.51	2.45	2.38	2.32
17	6.04	4.62	4.01	3.66	3.44	3.28	3.16	3.06	2.98	2.92	2.82	2.72	2.62	2.56	2.50	2.44	2.38	2.32	2.25
18	5.98	4.56	3.95	3.61	3.38	3.22	3.10	3.01	2.93	2.87	2.77	2.67	2.56	2.50	2.44	2.38	2.32	2.26	2.19
19	5.92	4.51	3.90	3.56	3.33	3.17	3.05	2.96	2.88	2.82	2.72	2.62	2.51	2.45	2.39	2.33	2.27	2.20	2.13
20	5.87	4.46	3.86	3.51	3.29	3.13	3.01	2.91	2.84	2.77	2.68	2.57	2.46	2.41	2.35	2.29	2.22	2.16	2.09
21	5.83	4.42	3.82	3.48	3.25	3.09	2.97	2.87	2.80	2.73	2.64	2.53	2.42	2.37	2.31	2.25	2.18	2.11	2.04
22	5.79	4.38	3.78	3.44	3.22	3.05	2.93	2.84	2.76	2.70	2.60	2.50	2.39	2.33	2.27	2.21	2.14	2.08	2.00
23	5.75	4.35	3.75	3.41	3.18	3.02	2.90	2.81	2.73	2.67	2.57	2.47	2.36	2.30	2.24	2.18	2.11	2.04	1.97
24	5.72	4.32	3.72	3.38	3.15	2.99	2.87	2.78	2.70	2.64	2.54	2.44	2.33	2.27	2.21	2.15	2.08	2.01	1.94
25	5.69	4.29	3.69	3.35	3.13	2.97	2.85	2.75	2.68	2.61	2.51	2.41	2.30	2.24	2.18	2.12	2.05	1.98	1.91
26	5.66	4.27	3.67	3.33	3.10	2.94	2.82	2.73	2.65	2.59	2.49	2.39	2.28	2.22	2.16	2.09	2.03	1.95	1.88
27	5.63	4.24	3.65	3.31	3.08	2.92	2.80	2.71	2.63	2.57	2.47	2.36	2.25	2.19	2.13	2.07	2.00	1.93	1.85
28	5.61	4.22	3.63	3.29	3.06	2.90	2.78	2.69	2.61	2.55	2.45	2.34	2.23	2.17	2.11	2.05	1.98	1.91	1.83
29	5.59	4.20	3.61	3.27	3.04	2.88	2.76	2.67	2.59	2.53	2.43	2.32	2.21	2.15	2.09	2.03	1.96	1.89	1.81
30	5.57	4.18	3.59	3.25	3.03	2.87	2.75	2.65	2.57	2.51	2.41	2.31	2.20	2.14	2.07	2.01	1.94	1.87	1.79
40	5.42	4.05	3.46	3.13	2.90	2.74	2.62	2.53	2.45	2.39	2.29	2.18	2.07	2.01	1.94	1.88	1.80	1.72	1.64
60	5.29	3.93	3.34	3.01	2.79	2.63	2.51	2.41	2.33	2.27	2.17	2.06	1.94	1.88	1.82	1.74	1.67	1.58	1.48
120	5.15	3.80	3.23	2.89	2.67	2.52	2.39	2.30	2.22	2.16	2.05	1.94	1.82	1.76	1.69	1.61	1.53	1.43	1.31
∞	5.02	3.69	3.12	2.79	2.57	2.41	2.29	2.19	2.11	2.05	1.94	1.83	1.71	1.64	1.57	1.48	1.39	1.27	1.00

$F = \frac{s_1^2}{s_2^2} = \frac{S_1}{m} \Big/ \frac{S_2}{n}$, where $s_1^2 = S_1/m$ and $s_2^2 = S_2/n$ are independent mean squares estimating a common variance σ^2 and based on m and n degrees of freedom, respectively.

PERCENTAGE POINTS, *F*-DISTRIBUTION

$$F(F) = \int_0^F \frac{\Gamma\left(\frac{m+n}{2}\right)}{\Gamma\left(\frac{m}{2}\right)\Gamma\left(\frac{n}{2}\right)} m^{\frac{m}{2}} n^{\frac{n}{2}} x^{\frac{m}{2}-1} (n+mx)^{-\frac{m+n}{2}}\, dx = .99$$

n \ m	1	2	3	4	5	6	7	8	9	10	12	15	20	24	30	40	60	120	∞
1	4052	4999.5	5403	5625	5764	5859	5928	5982	6022	6056	6106	6157	6209	6235	6261	6287	6313	6339	6366
2	98.50	99.00	99.17	99.25	99.30	99.33	99.36	99.37	99.39	99.40	99.42	99.43	99.45	99.46	99.47	99.47	99.48	99.49	99.50
3	34.12	30.82	29.46	28.71	28.24	27.91	27.67	27.49	27.35	27.23	27.05	26.87	26.69	26.60	26.50	26.41	26.32	26.22	26.13
4	21.20	18.00	16.69	15.98	15.52	15.21	14.98	14.80	14.66	14.55	14.37	14.20	14.02	13.93	13.84	13.75	13.65	13.56	13.46
5	16.26	13.27	12.06	11.39	10.97	10.67	10.46	10.29	10.16	10.05	9.89	9.72	9.55	9.47	9.38	9.29	9.20	9.11	9.02
6	13.75	10.92	9.78	9.15	8.75	8.47	8.26	8.10	7.98	7.87	7.72	7.56	7.40	7.31	7.23	7.14	7.06	6.97	6.88
7	12.25	9.55	8.45	7.85	7.46	7.19	6.99	6.84	6.72	6.62	6.47	6.31	6.16	6.07	5.99	5.91	5.82	5.74	5.65
8	11.26	8.65	7.59	7.01	6.63	6.37	6.18	6.03	5.91	5.81	5.67	5.52	5.36	5.28	5.20	5.12	5.03	4.95	4.86
9	10.56	8.02	6.99	6.42	6.06	5.80	5.61	5.47	5.35	5.26	5.11	4.96	4.81	4.73	4.65	4.57	4.48	4.40	4.31
10	10.04	7.56	6.55	5.99	5.64	5.39	5.20	5.06	4.94	4.85	4.71	4.56	4.41	4.33	4.25	4.17	4.08	4.00	3.91
11	9.65	7.21	6.22	5.67	5.32	5.07	4.89	4.74	4.63	4.54	4.40	4.25	4.10	4.02	3.94	3.86	3.78	3.69	3.60
12	9.33	6.93	5.95	5.41	5.06	4.82	4.64	4.50	4.39	4.30	4.16	4.01	3.86	3.78	3.70	3.62	3.54	3.45	3.36
13	9.07	6.70	5.74	5.21	4.86	4.62	4.44	4.30	4.19	4.10	3.96	3.82	3.66	3.59	3.51	3.43	3.34	3.25	3.17
14	8.86	6.51	5.56	5.04	4.69	4.46	4.28	4.14	4.03	3.94	3.80	3.66	3.51	3.43	3.35	3.27	3.18	3.09	3.00
15	8.68	6.36	5.42	4.89	4.56	4.32	4.14	4.00	3.89	3.80	3.67	3.52	3.37	3.29	3.21	3.13	3.05	2.96	2.87
16	8.53	6.23	5.29	4.77	4.44	4.20	4.03	3.89	3.78	3.69	3.55	3.41	3.26	3.18	3.10	3.02	2.93	2.84	2.75
17	8.40	6.11	5.18	4.67	4.34	4.10	3.93	3.79	3.68	3.59	3.46	3.31	3.16	3.08	3.00	2.92	2.83	2.75	2.65
18	8.29	6.01	5.09	4.58	4.25	4.01	3.84	3.71	3.60	3.51	3.37	3.23	3.08	3.00	2.92	2.84	2.75	2.66	2.57
19	8.18	5.93	5.01	4.50	4.17	3.94	3.77	3.63	3.52	3.43	3.30	3.15	3.00	2.92	2.84	2.76	2.67	2.58	2.49
20	8.10	5.85	4.94	4.43	4.10	3.87	3.70	3.56	3.46	3.37	3.23	3.09	2.94	2.86	2.78	2.69	2.61	2.52	2.42
21	8.02	5.78	4.87	4.37	4.04	3.81	3.64	3.51	3.40	3.31	3.17	3.03	2.88	2.80	2.72	2.64	2.55	2.46	2.36
22	7.95	5.72	4.82	4.31	3.99	3.76	3.59	3.45	3.35	3.26	3.12	2.98	2.83	2.75	2.67	2.58	2.50	2.40	2.31
23	7.88	5.66	4.76	4.26	3.94	3.71	3.54	3.41	3.30	3.21	3.07	2.93	2.78	2.70	2.62	2.54	2.45	2.35	2.26
24	7.82	5.61	4.72	4.22	3.90	3.67	3.50	3.36	3.26	3.17	3.03	2.89	2.74	2.66	2.58	2.49	2.40	2.31	2.21
25	7.77	5.57	4.68	4.18	3.85	3.63	3.46	3.32	3.22	3.13	2.99	2.85	2.70	2.62	2.54	2.45	2.36	2.27	2.17
26	7.72	5.53	4.64	4.14	3.82	3.59	3.42	3.29	3.18	3.09	2.96	2.81	2.66	2.58	2.50	2.42	2.33	2.23	2.13
27	7.68	5.49	4.60	4.11	3.78	3.56	3.39	3.26	3.15	3.06	2.93	2.78	2.63	2.55	2.47	2.38	2.29	2.20	2.10
28	7.64	5.45	4.57	4.07	3.75	3.53	3.36	3.23	3.12	3.03	2.90	2.75	2.60	2.52	2.44	2.35	2.26	2.17	2 06
29	7.60	5.42	4.54	4.04	3.73	3.50	3.33	3.20	3.09	3.00	2.87	2.73	2.57	2.49	2.41	2.33	2.23	2 14	2.03
30	7.56	5.39	4.51	4.02	3.70	3.47	3.30	3.17	3.07	2.98	2.84	2.70	2.55	2.47	2.39	2.30	2.21	2.11	2.01
40	7.31	5.18	4.31	3.83	3.51	3.29	3.12	2.99	2.89	2.80	2.66	2.52	2.37	2.29	2.20	2.11	2.02	1.92	1.80
60	7.08	4.98	4.13	3.65	3.34	3.12	2.95	2.82	2.72	2.63	2.50	2.35	2.20	2.12	2.03	1.94	1.84	1.73	1.60
120	6.85	4.79	3.95	3.48	3.17	2.96	2.79	2.66	2.56	2.47	2.34	2.19	2.03	1.95	1.86	1.76	1.66	1.53	1.38
∞	6.63	4.61	3.78	3.32	3.02	2.80	2.64	2.51	2.41	2.32	2.18	2.04	1.88	1.79	1.70	1.59	1.47	1.32	1.00

$F = \frac{s_1^2}{s_2^2} = \frac{S_1}{m} \Big/ \frac{S_2}{n}$, where $s_1^2 = S_1/m$ and $s_2^2 = S_2/n$ are independent mean squares estimating a common variance σ^2 and based on m and n degrees of freedom, respectively.

PERCENTAGE POINTS, F-DISTRIBUTION

$$F(F) = \int_0^F \frac{\Gamma\left(\frac{m+n}{2}\right)}{\Gamma\left(\frac{m}{2}\right)\Gamma\left(\frac{n}{2}\right)} m^{\frac{m}{2}} n^{\frac{n}{2}} x^{\frac{m}{2}-1} (n+mx)^{-\frac{m+n}{2}} dx = .995$$

n \ m	1	2	3	4	5	6	7	8	9	10	12	15	20	24	30	40	60	120	∞
1	16211	20000	21615	22500	23056	23437	23715	23925	24091	24224	24426	24630	24836	24940	25044	25148	25253	25359	25465
2	198.5	199.0	199.2	199.2	199.3	199.3	199.4	199.4	199.4	199.4	199.4	199.4	199.4	199.5	199.5	199.5	199.5	199.5	199.5
3	55.55	49.80	47.47	46.19	45.39	44.84	44.43	44.13	43.88	43.69	43.39	43.08	42.78	42.62	42.47	42.31	42.15	41.99	41.83
4	31.33	26.28	24.26	23.15	22.46	21.97	21.62	21.35	21.14	20.97	20.70	20.44	20.17	20.03	19.89	19.75	19.61	19.47	19.32
5	22.78	18.31	16.53	15.56	14.94	14.51	14.20	13.96	13.77	13.62	13.38	13.15	12.90	12.78	12.66	12.53	12.40	12.27	12.14
6	18.63	14.54	12.92	12.03	11.46	11.07	10.79	10.57	10.39	10.25	10.03	9.81	9.59	9.47	9.36	9.24	9.12	9.00	8.88
7	16.24	12.40	10.88	10.05	9.52	9.16	8.89	8.68	8.51	8.38	8.18	7.97	7.75	7.65	7.53	7.42	7.31	7.19	7.08
8	14.69	11.04	9.60	8.81	8.30	7.95	7.69	7.50	7.34	7.21	7.01	6.81	6.61	6.50	6.40	6.29	6.18	6.06	5.95
9	13.61	10.11	8.72	7.96	7.47	7.13	6.88	6.69	6.54	6.42	6.23	6.03	5.83	5.73	5.62	5.52	5.41	5.30	5.19
10	12.83	9.43	8.08	7.34	6.87	6.54	6.30	6.12	5.97	5.85	5.66	5.47	5.27	5.17	5.07	4.97	4.86	4.75	4.64
11	12.23	8.91	7.60	6.88	6.42	6.10	5.86	5.68	5.54	5.42	5.24	5.05	4.86	4.76	4.65	4.55	4.44	4.34	4.23
12	11.75	8.51	7.23	6.52	6.07	5.76	5.52	5.35	5.20	5.09	4.91	4.72	4.53	4.43	4.33	4.23	4.12	4.01	3.90
13	11.37	8.19	6.93	6.23	5.79	5.48	5.25	5.08	4.94	4.82	4.64	4.46	4.27	4.17	4.07	3.97	3.87	3.76	3.65
14	11.06	7.92	6.68	6.00	5.56	5.26	5.03	4.86	4.72	4.60	4.43	4.25	4.06	3.96	3.86	3.76	3.66	3.55	3.44
15	10.80	7.70	6.48	5.80	5.37	5.07	4.85	4.67	4.54	4.42	4.25	4.07	3.88	3.79	3.69	3.58	3.48	3.37	3.26
16	10.58	7.51	6.30	5.64	5.21	4.91	4.69	4.52	4.38	4.27	4.10	3.92	3.73	3.64	3.54	3.44	3.33	3.22	3.11
17	10.38	7.35	6.16	5.50	5.07	4.78	4.56	4.39	4.25	4.14	3.97	3.79	3.61	3.51	3.41	3.31	3.21	3.10	2.98
18	10.22	7.21	6.03	5.37	4.96	4.66	4.44	4.28	4.14	4.03	3.86	3.68	3.50	3.40	3.30	3.20	3.10	2.99	2.87
19	10.07	7.09	5.92	5.27	4.85	4.56	4.34	4.18	4.04	3.93	3.76	3.59	3.40	3.31	3.21	3.11	3.00	2.89	2.78
20	9.94	6.99	5.82	5.17	4.76	4.47	4.26	4.09	3.96	3.85	3.68	3.50	3.32	3.22	3.12	3.02	2.92	2.81	2.69
21	9.83	6.89	5.73	5.09	4.68	4.39	4.18	4.01	3.88	3.77	3.60	3.43	3.24	3.15	3.05	2.95	2.84	2.73	2.61
22	9.73	6.81	5.65	5.02	4.61	4.32	4.11	3.94	3.81	3.70	3.54	3.36	3.18	3.08	2.98	2.88	2.77	2.66	2.55
23	9.63	6.73	5.58	4.95	4.54	4.26	4.05	3.88	3.75	3.64	3.47	3.30	3.12	3.02	2.92	2.82	2.71	2.60	2.48
24	9.55	6.66	5.52	4.89	4.49	4.20	3.99	3.83	3.69	3.59	3.42	3.25	3.06	2.97	2.87	2.77	2.66	2.55	2.43
25	9.48	6.60	5.46	4.84	4.43	4.15	3.94	3.78	3.64	3.54	3.37	3.20	3.01	2.92	2.82	2.72	2.61	2.50	2.38
26	9.41	6.54	5.41	4.79	4.38	4.10	3.89	3.73	3.60	3.49	3.33	3.15	2.97	2.87	2.77	2.67	2.56	2.45	2.33
27	9.34	6.49	5.36	4.74	4.34	4.06	3.85	3.69	3.56	3.45	3.28	3.11	2.93	2.83	2.73	2.63	2.52	2.41	2.25
28	9.28	6.44	5.32	4.70	4.30	4.02	3.81	3.65	3.52	3.41	3.25	3.07	2.89	2.79	2.69	2.59	2.48	2.37	2.29
29	9.23	6.40	5.28	4.66	4.26	3.98	3.77	3.61	3.48	3.38	3.21	3.04	2.86	2.76	2.66	2.56	2.45	2.33	2.24
30	9.18	6.35	5.24	4.62	4.23	3.95	3.74	3.58	3.45	3.34	3.18	3.01	2.82	2.73	2.63	2.52	2.42	2.30	2.18
40	8.83	6.07	4.98	4.37	3.99	3.71	3.51	3.35	3.22	3.12	2.95	2.78	2.60	2.50	2.40	2.30	2.18	2.06	1.93
60	8.49	5.79	4.73	4.14	3.76	3.49	3.29	3.13	3.01	2.90	2.74	2.57	2.39	2.29	2.19	2.08	1.96	1.83	1.69
120	8.18	5.54	4.50	3.92	3.55	3.28	3.09	2.93	2.81	2.71	2.54	2.37	2.19	2.09	1.98	1.87	1.75	1.61	1.43
∞	7.88	5.30	4.28	3.72	3.35	3.09	2.90	2.74	2.62	2.52	2.36	2.19	2.00	1.90	1.79	1.67	1.53	1.36	1.00

$F = \frac{s_1^2}{s_2^2} = \frac{S_1}{m} \Big/ \frac{S_2}{n}$, where $s_1^2 = S_1/m$ and $s_2^2 = S_2/n$ are independent mean squares estimating a common variance σ^2 and based on m and n degrees of freedom, respectively.

PERCENTAGE POINTS, F-DISTRIBUTION

$$F(F) = \int_0^F \frac{\Gamma\left(\frac{m+n}{2}\right)}{\Gamma\left(\frac{m}{2}\right)\Gamma\left(\frac{n}{2}\right)} m^{\frac{m}{2}} n^{\frac{n}{2}} x^{\frac{m}{2}-1} (n+mx)^{-\frac{m+n}{2}} dx = .999$$

n \ m	1	2	3	4	5	6	7	8	9	10	12	15	20	24	30	40	60	120	∞
1	4053*	5000*	5404*	5625*	5764*	5859*	5929*	5981*	6023*	6056*	6107*	6158*	6209*	6235*	6261*	6287*	6313*	6340*	6366*
2	998.5	999.0	999.2	999.2	999.3	999.3	999.4	999.4	999.4	999.4	999.4	999.4	999.4	999.5	999.5	999.5	999.5	999.5	999.5
3	167.0	148.5	141.1	137.1	134.6	132.8	131.6	130.6	129.9	129.2	128.3	127.4	126.4	125.9	125.4	125.0	124.5	124.0	123.5
4	74.14	61.25	56.18	53.44	51.71	50.53	49.66	49.00	48.47	48.05	47.41	46.76	46.10	45.77	45.43	45.09	44.75	44.40	44.05
5	47.18	37.12	33.20	31.09	29.75	28.84	28.16	27.64	27.24	26.92	26.42	25.91	25.39	25.14	24.87	24.60	24.33	24.06	23.79
6	35.51	27.00	23.70	21.92	20.81	20.03	19.46	19.03	18.69	18.41	17.99	17.56	17.12	16.89	16.67	16.44	16.21	15.99	15.75
7	29.25	21.69	18.77	17.19	16.21	15.52	15.02	14.63	14.33	14.08	13.71	13.32	12.93	12.73	12.53	12.33	12.12	11.91	11.70
8	25.42	18.49	15.83	14.39	13.49	12.86	12.40	12.04	11.77	11.54	11.19	10.84	10.48	10.30	10.11	9.92	9.73	9.53	9.33
9	22.86	16.39	13.90	12.56	11.71	11.13	10.70	10.37	10.11	9.89	9.57	9.24	8.90	8.72	8.55	8.37	8.19	8.00	7.81
10	21.04	14.91	12.55	11.28	10.48	9.92	9.52	9.20	8.96	8.75	8.45	8.13	7.80	7.64	7.47	7.30	7.12	6.94	6.76
11	19.69	13.81	11.56	10.35	9.58	9.05	8.66	8.35	8.12	7.92	7.63	7.32	7.01	6.85	6.68	6.52	6.35	6.17	6.00
12	18.64	12.97	10.80	9.63	8.89	8.38	8.00	7.71	7.48	7.29	7.00	6.71	6.40	6.25	6.09	5.93	5.76	5.59	5.42
13	17.81	12.31	10.21	9.07	8.35	7.86	7.49	7.21	6.98	6.80	6.52	6.23	5.93	5.78	5.63	5.47	5.30	5.14	4.97
14	17.14	11.78	9.73	8.62	7.92	7.43	7.08	6.80	6.58	6.40	6.13	5.85	5.56	5.41	5.25	5.10	4.94	4.77	4.60
15	16.59	11.34	9.34	8.25	7.57	7.09	6.74	6.47	6.26	6.08	5.81	5.54	5.25	5.10	4.95	4.80	4.64	4.47	4.31
16	16.12	10.97	9.00	7.94	7.27	6.81	6.46	6.19	5.98	5.81	5.55	5.27	4.99	4.85	4.70	4.54	4.39	4.23	4.06
17	15.72	10.66	8.73	7.68	7.02	6.56	6.22	5.96	5.75	5.58	5.32	5.05	4.78	4.63	4.48	4.33	4.18	4.02	3.85
18	15.38	10.39	8.49	7.46	6.81	6.35	6.02	5.76	5.56	5.39	5.13	4.87	4.59	4.45	4.30	4.15	4.00	3.84	3.67
19	15.08	10.16	8.28	7.26	6.62	6.18	5.85	5.59	5.39	5.22	4.97	4.70	4.43	4.29	4.14	3.99	3.84	3.68	3.51
20	14.82	9.95	8.10	7.10	6.46	6.02	5.69	5.44	5.24	5.08	4.82	4.56	4.29	4.15	4.00	3.86	3.70	3.54	3.38
21	14.59	9.77	7.94	6.95	6.32	5.88	5.56	5.31	5.11	4.95	4.70	4.44	4.17	4.03	3.88	3.74	3.58	3.42	3.26
22	14.38	9.61	7.80	6.81	6.19	5.76	5.44	5.19	4.99	4.83	4.58	4.33	4.06	3.92	3.78	3.63	3.48	3.32	3.15
23	14.19	9.47	7.67	6.69	6.08	5.65	5.33	5.09	4.89	4.73	4.48	4.23	3.96	3.82	3.68	3.53	3.38	3.22	3.05
24	14.03	9.34	7.55	6.59	5.98	5.55	5.23	4.99	4.80	4.64	4.39	4.14	3.87	3.74	3.59	3.45	3.29	3.14	2.97
25	13.88	9.22	7.45	6.49	5.88	5.46	5.15	4.91	4.71	4.56	4.31	4.06	3.79	3.66	3.52	3.37	3.22	3.06	2.89
26	13.74	9.12	7.36	6.41	5.80	5.38	5.07	4.83	4.64	4.48	4.24	3.99	3.72	3.59	3.44	3.30	3.15	2.99	2.82
27	13.61	9.02	7.27	6.33	5.73	5.31	5.00	4.76	4.57	4.41	4.17	3.92	3.66	3.52	3.38	3.23	3.08	2.92	2.75
28	13.50	8.93	7.19	6.25	5.66	5.24	4.93	4.69	4.50	4.35	4.11	3.86	3.60	3.46	3.32	3.18	3.02	2.86	2.69
29	13.39	8.85	7.12	6.19	5.59	5.18	4.87	4.64	4.45	4.29	4.05	3.80	3.54	3.41	3.27	3.12	2.97	2.81	2.64
30	13.29	8.77	7.05	6.12	5.53	5.12	4.82	4.58	4.39	4.24	4.00	3.75	3.49	3.36	3.22	3.07	2.92	2.76	2.59
40	12.61	8.25	6.60	5.70	5.13	4.73	4.44	4.21	4.02	3.87	3.64	3.40	3.15	3.01	2.87	2.73	2.57	2.41	2.23
60	11.97	7.76	6.17	5.31	4.76	4.37	4.09	3.87	3.69	3.54	3.31	3.08	2.83	2.69	2.55	2.41	2.25	2.08	1.89
120	11.38	7.32	5.79	4.95	4.42	4.04	3.77	3.55	3.38	3.24	3.02	2.78	2.53	2.40	2.26	2.11	1.95	1.76	1.54
∞	10.83	6.91	5.42	4.62	4.10	3.74	3.47	3.27	3.10	2.96	2.74	2.51	2.27	2.13	1.99	1.84	1.66	1.45	1.00

* Multiply these entries by 100.

VI.2 POWER FUNCTIONS OF THE ANALYSIS-OF-VARIANCE TESTS

The noncentral F-distribution, $f(F')$, arises in the ratio of a non-central chi-square with m degrees of freedom and noncentrality parameter λ to an independent chi-square with n degrees of freedom.

P. C. Tang has compiled tables of

$$\int_0^{F_\alpha} f(F')\, dF'$$

for certain values of F_α. These tables are given in terms of E^2, where

$$E^2 = \frac{mF'}{mF' + n} \cdot$$

If the frequency function of E^2 is denoted by $g(E^2;m,n,\lambda)$, $g(E^2)$ is a beta distribution if $\lambda = 0$ and a noncentral beta distribution if $\lambda \neq 0$.

The integral

$$\int_0^{E_\alpha^2} g(E^2;m,n,\lambda)\, dE^2$$

equals $1 - \beta(\lambda)$, or unity minus the power of the test, which is the probability of a type II error. Here E_α^2 is obtained from the integral

$$\int_{E_\alpha^2}^1 g(E^2;m,n,\ \lambda = 0)\, dE^2 = \lambda.$$

P. C. Tang evaluated the integral

$$P(\text{II}) = 1 - \beta(\phi) = \int_0^{E_\alpha^2} g(E^2;f_1,f_2,\phi)\, dE^2$$

for various values of f_1, f_2, ϕ, and E_α^2 for $\alpha = 0.05$ and 0.01, where

$$\phi = \sqrt{\frac{2\lambda}{f_1 + 1}}$$

and where f_1 is the degrees of freedom in the numerator of the F statistic.

In this table, graphs are shown with $1 - \beta$ on the vertical scale corresponding to ϕ on the horizontal. The graphs are for two levels of significance, $\alpha = 0.01$ and 0.05, for eight values of ν_1, the number of degrees of freedom for the numerator, and several values of ν_2, the number of degrees of freedom for the denominator of the F ratio. There is a different curve for each set of values α, ν_1, and ν_2.

POWER OF THE ANALYSIS-OF-VARIANCE TEST

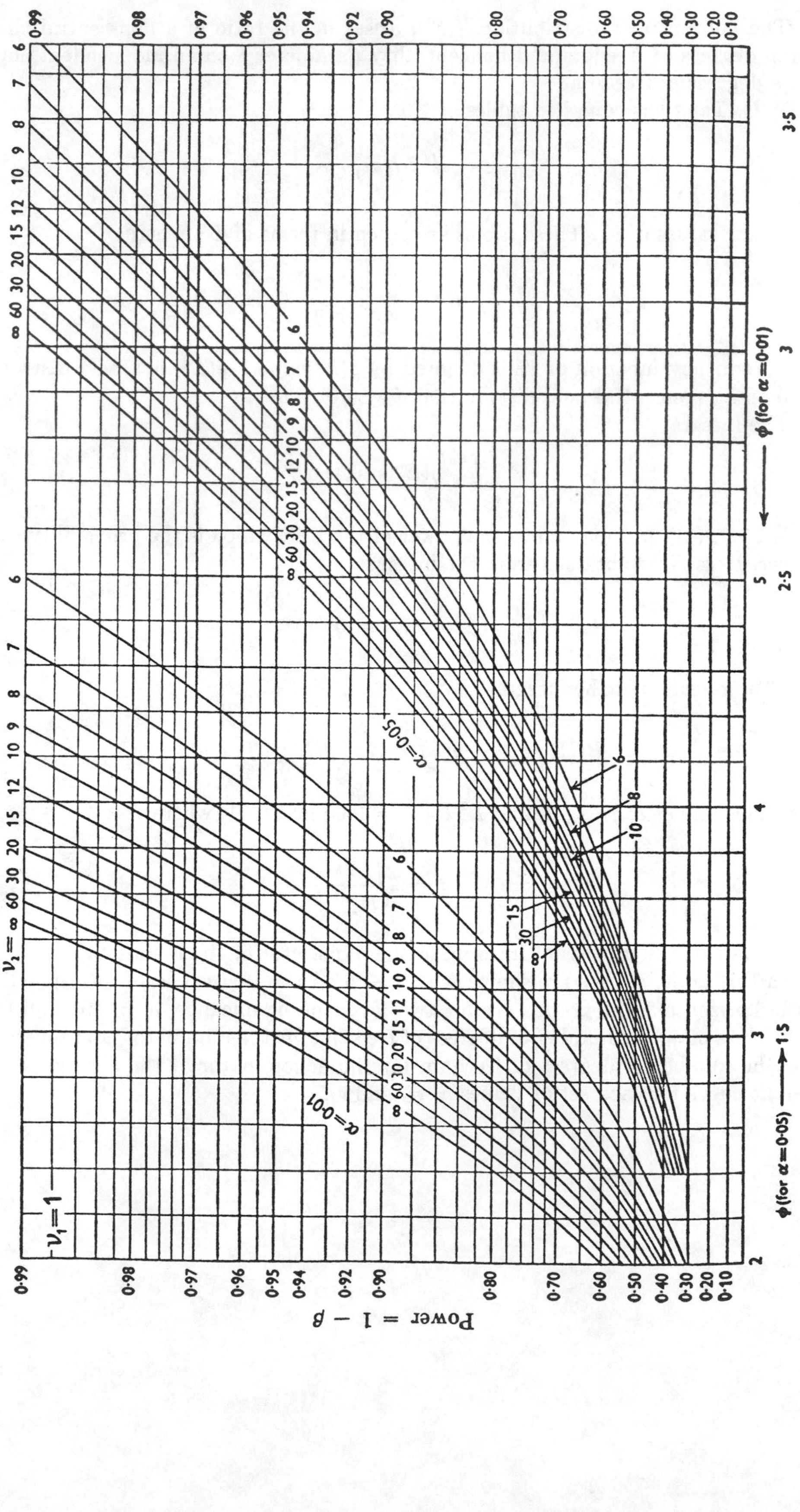

POWER OF THE ANALYSIS-OF-VARIANCE TEST

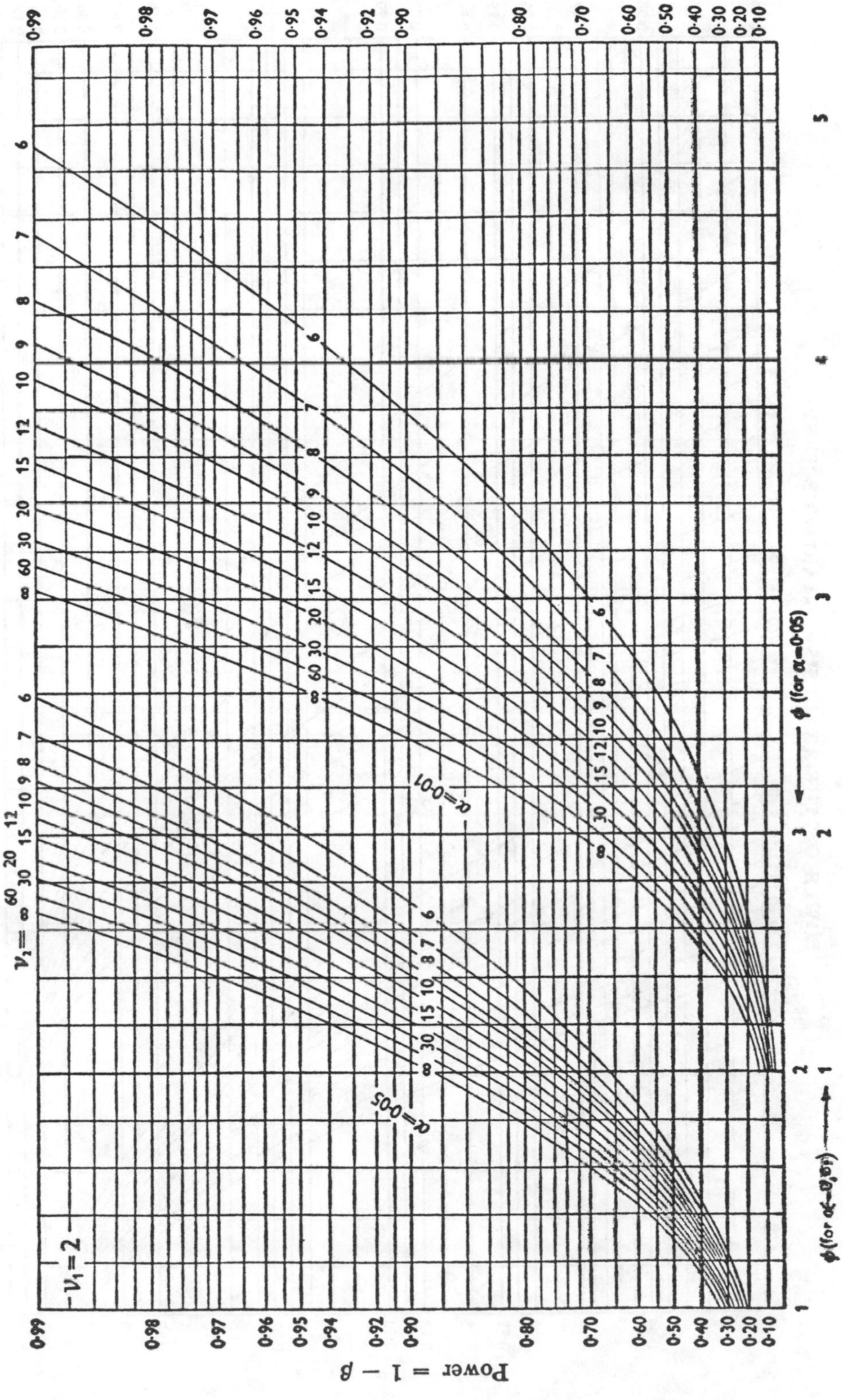

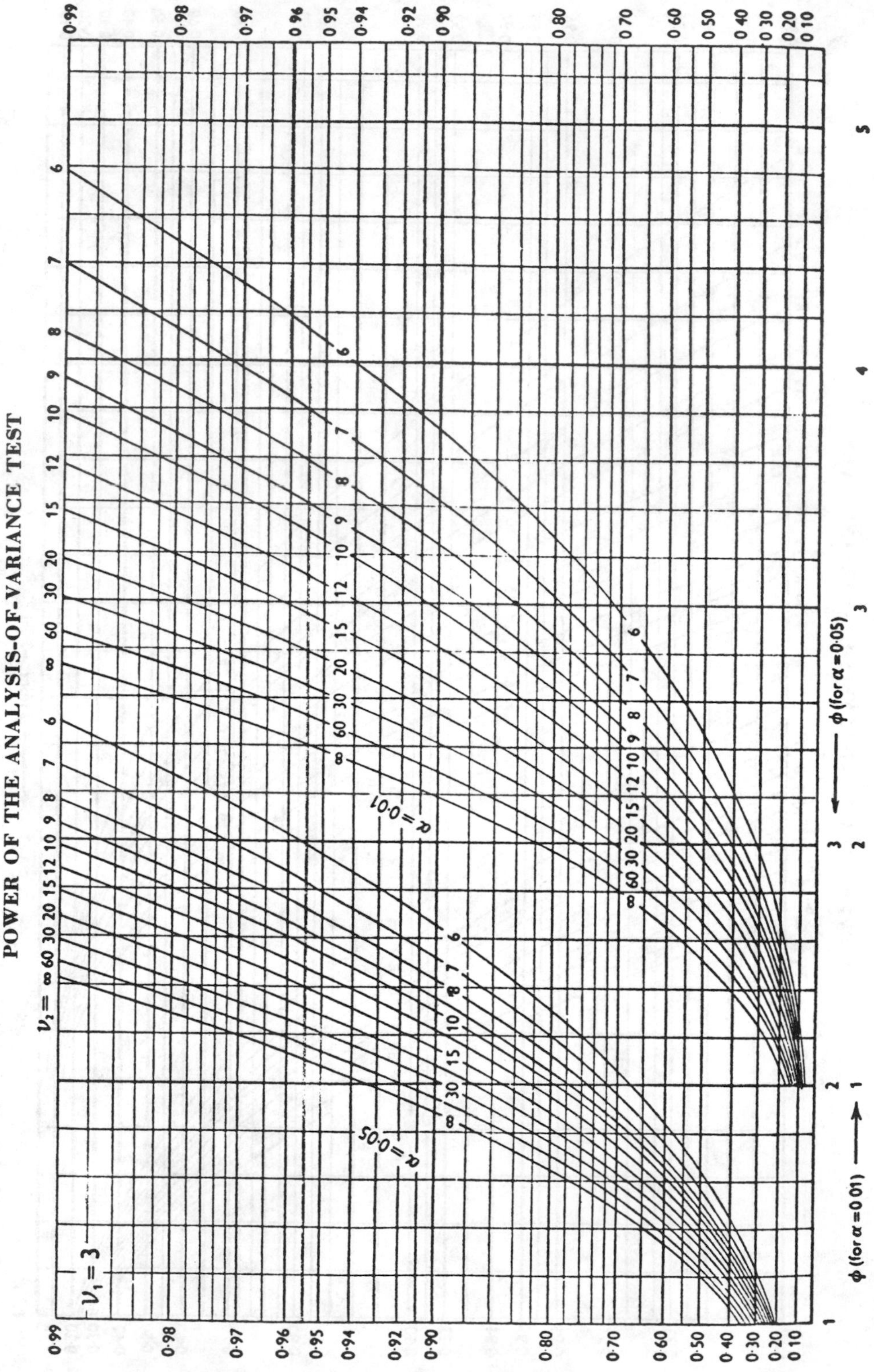
POWER OF THE ANALYSIS-OF-VARIANCE TEST
ν1 = 3
ν2 = ∞ 60 30 20 15 12 10 9 8 7 6 ∞ 60 30 20 15 12 10 9 8 7 6
α = 0·05
α = 0·01
Power = 1 − β
0·99 0·98 0·97 0·96 0·95 0·94 0·92 0·90 0·80 0·70 0·60 0·50 0·40 0·30 0·20 0·10
φ (for α = 0·01) ⟶ 1 2 3
⟵ φ (for α = 0·05) 1 2 3 4 5

POWER OF THE ANALYSIS-OF-VARIANCE TEST

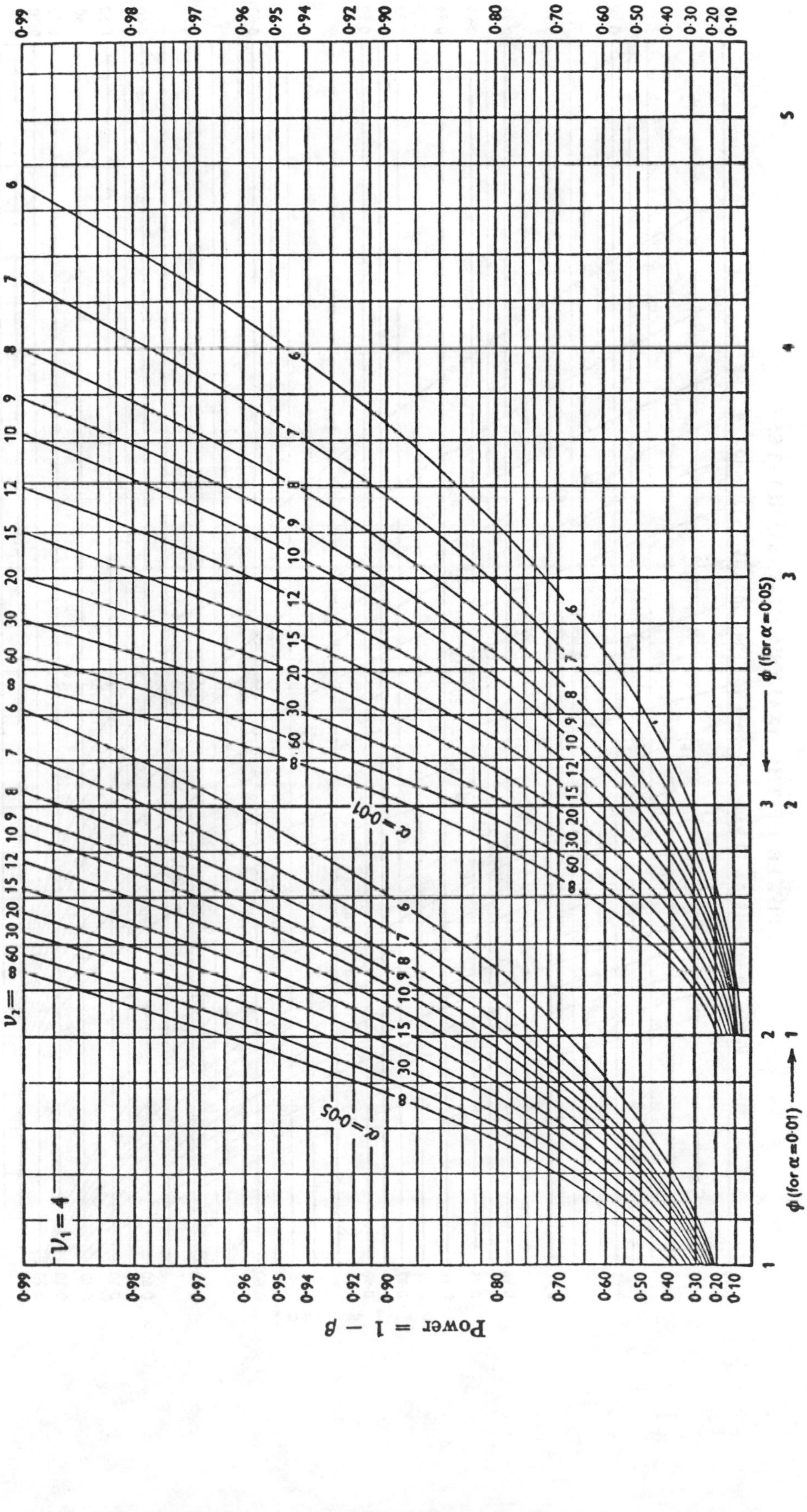

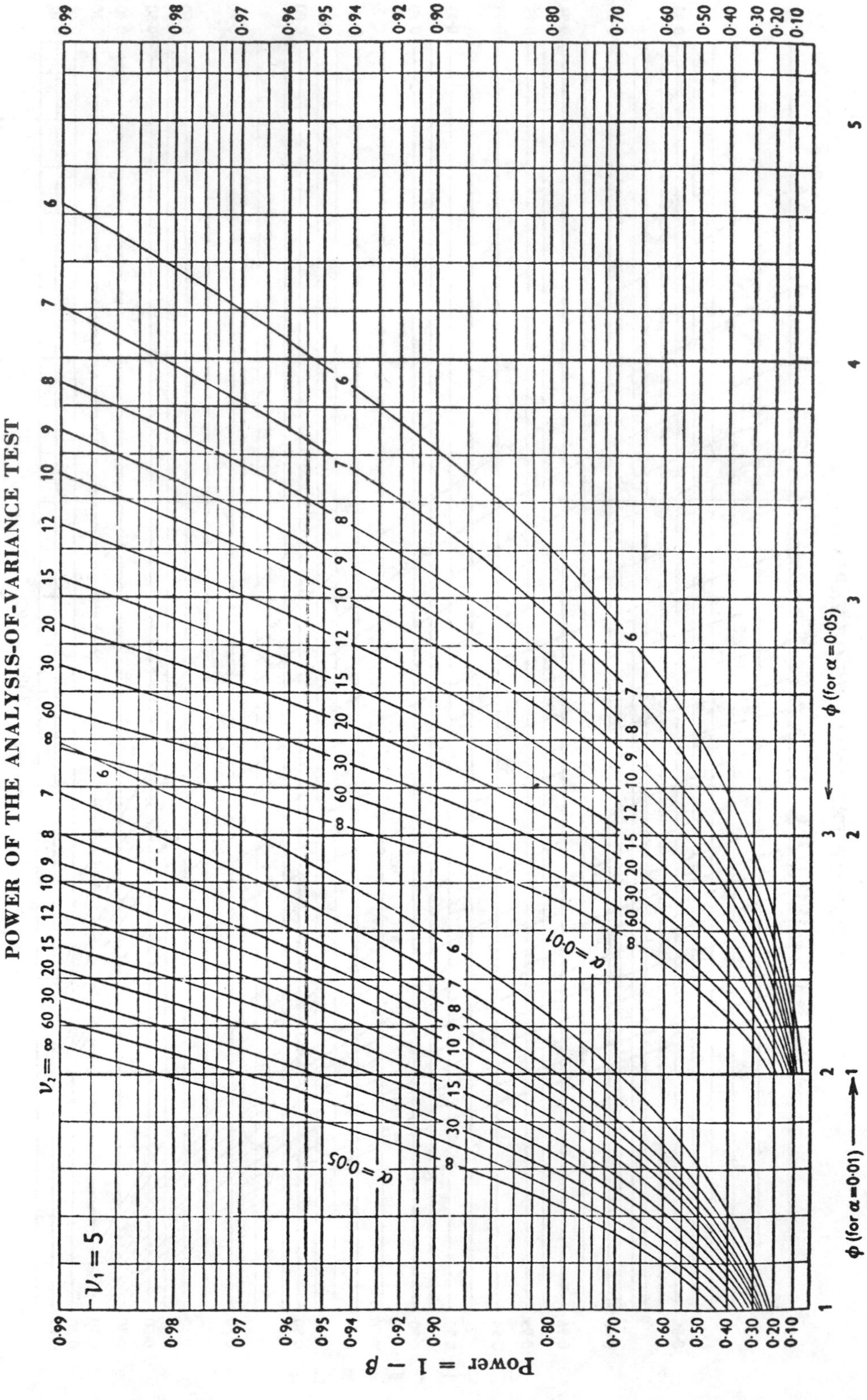
POWER OF THE ANALYSIS-OF-VARIANCE TEST
$\nu_1 = 5$
$\nu_2 = \infty$ 60 30 20 15 12 10 9 8 7 6
∞ 60 30 20 15 12 10 9 8 7 6
α = 0·05
α = 0·01
Power = 1 − β
0·99 0·98 0·97 0·96 0·95 0·94 0·92 0·90 0·80 0·70 0·60 0·50 0·40 0·30 0·20 0·10
φ (for α = 0·01) ⟶ 1 2 3
φ (for α = 0·05) ⟵ 1 2 3 4 5

POWER OF THE ANALYSIS-OF-VARIANCE TEST

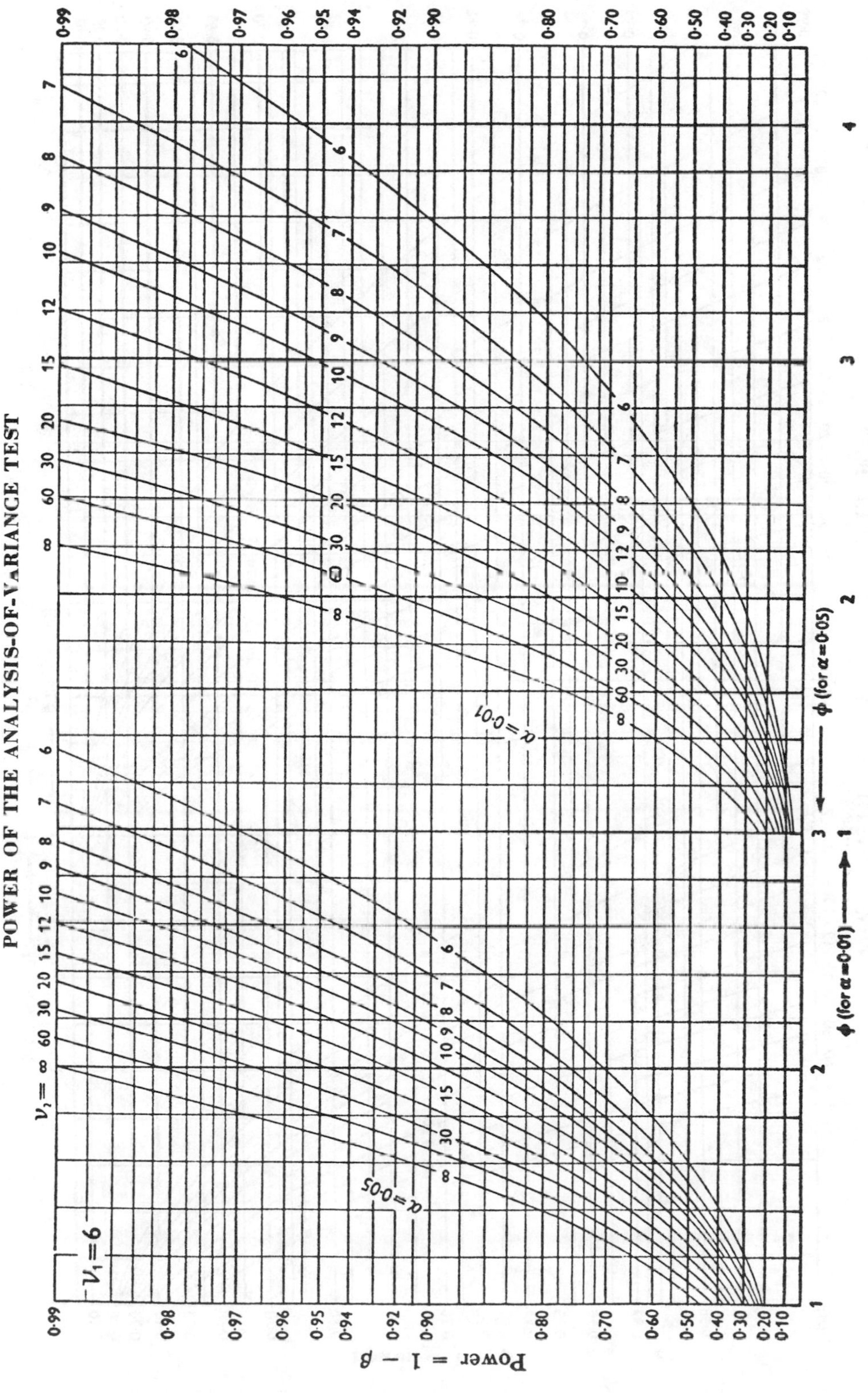

POWER OF THE ANALYSIS-OF-VARIANCE TEST

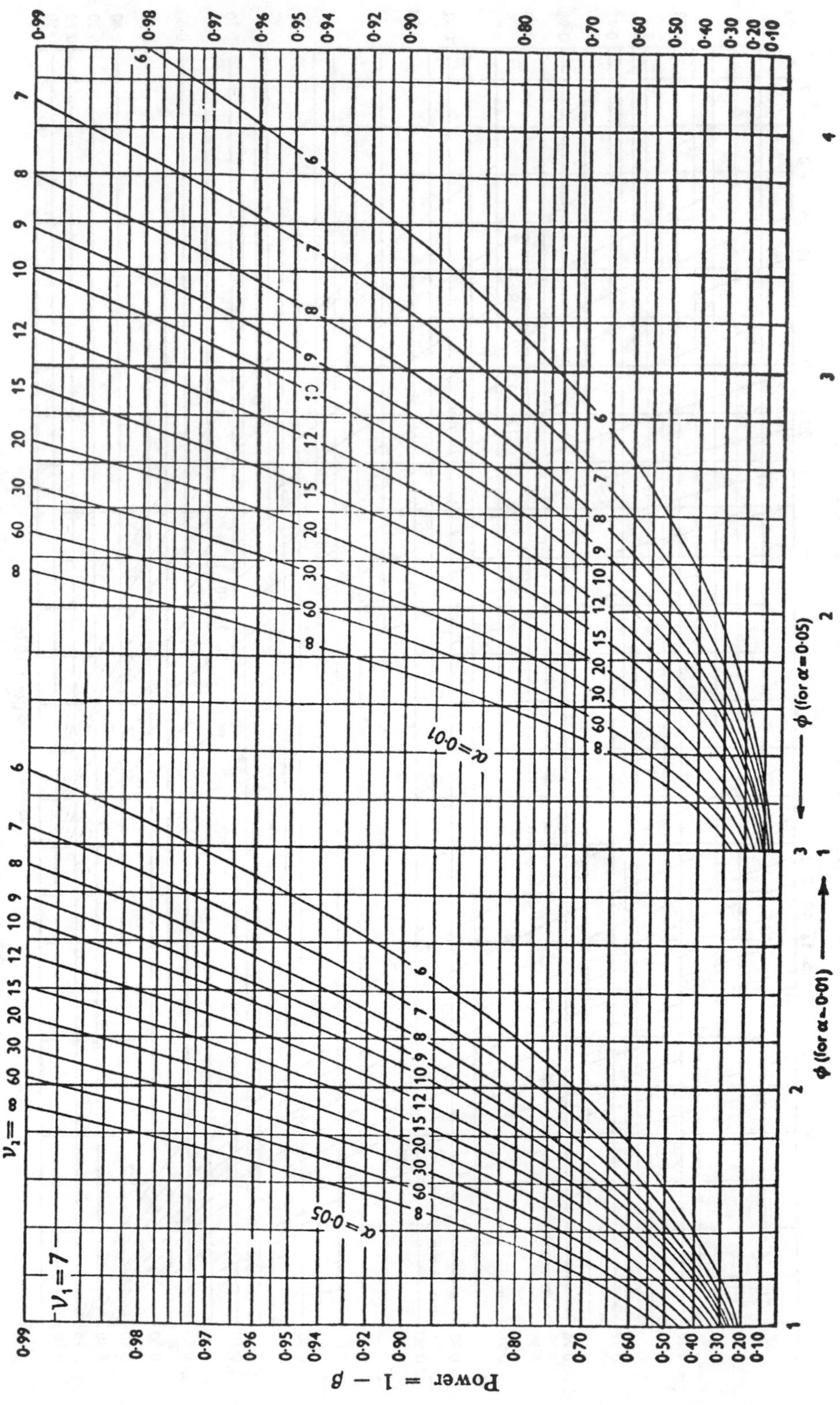

POWER OF THE ANALYSIS-OF-VARIANCE TEST

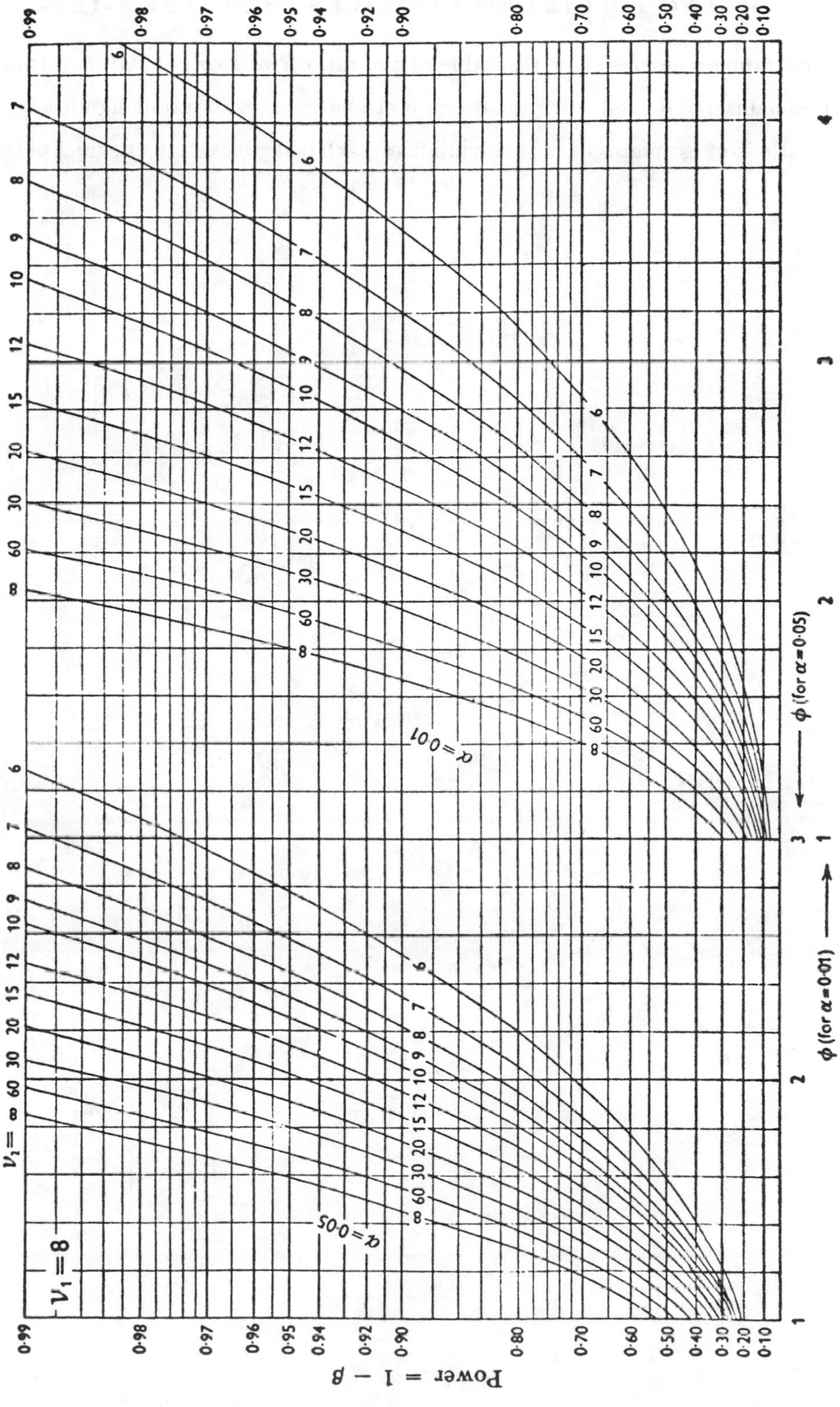

VI.3 NUMBER OF OBSERVATIONS REQUIRED FOR THE COMPARISON OF TWO POPULATION VARIANCES USING THE *F*-TEST

The tabular entries show the value of the ratio R of two population variances $\frac{\sigma_2^2}{\sigma_1^2}$, which remains undetected with probability β in a variance ratio test at significance level α of the ratio $\frac{s_2^2}{s_1^2}$ of estimates of the two variances, each being based on n degrees of freedom.

NUMBER OF OBSERVATIONS REQUIRED FOR THE COMPARISON OF TWO POPULATION VARIANCES USING THE *F*-TEST

	$\alpha = 0.01$				$\alpha = 0.05$				$\alpha = 0.5$			
η	$\beta = 0.01$	$\beta = 0.05$	$\beta = 0.1$	$\beta = 0.5$	$\beta = 0.01$	$\beta = 0.05$	$\beta = 0.1$	$\beta = 0.5$	$\beta = 0.01$	$\beta = 0.05$	$\beta = 0.1$	$\beta = 0.5$
1	16,420,000	654,200	161,500	4052	654,200	26,070	6,436	161.5	4,052	161.5	39.85	1.000
2	9,000	1,881	891.0	99.00	1,881	361.0	171.0	19.00	99.00	19.00	9.000	1.000
3	867.7	273.3	158.8	29.46	273.3	86.06	50.01	9.277	29.46	9.277	5.391	1.000
4	255.3	102.1	65.62	15.98	102.1	40.81	26.24	6.388	15.98	6.388	4.108	1.000
5	120.3	55.39	37.87	10.97	55.39	25.51	17.44	5.050	10.97	5.050	3.453	1.000
6	71.67	36.27	25.86	8.466	36.27	18.35	13.09	4.284	8.466	4.284	3.056	1.000
7	48.90	26.48	19.47	6.993	26.48	14.34	10.55	3.787	6.993	3.787	2.786	1.000
8	36.35	20.73	15.61	6.029	20.73	11.82	8.902	3.438	6.029	3.438	2.589	1.000
9	28.63	17.01	13.06	5.351	17.01	10.11	7.757	3.179	5.351	3.179	2.440	1.000
10	23.51	14.44	11.26	4.849	14.44	8.870	6.917	2.978	4.849	2.978	2.323	1.000
12	17.27	11.16	8.923	4.155	11.16	7.218	5.769	2.687	4.155	2.687	2.147	1.000
15	12.41	8.466	6.946	3.522	8.466	5.777	4.740	2.404	3.522	2.404	1.972	1.000
20	8.630	6.240	5.270	2.938	6.240	4.512	3.810	2.124	2.938	2.124	1.794	1.000
24	7.071	5.275	4.526	2.659	5.275	3.935	3.376	1.984	2.659	1.984	1.702	1.000
30	5.693	4.392	3.833	2.386	4.392	3.389	2.957	1.841	2.386	1.841	1.606	1.000
40	4.470	3.579	3.183	2.114	3.579	2.866	2.549	1.693	2.114	1.693	1.506	1.000
60	3.372	2.817	2.562	1.836	2.817	2.354	2.141	1.534	1.836	1.534	1.396	1.000
120	2.350	2.072	1.939	1.533	2.072	1.828	1.710	1.352	1.533	1.352	1.265	1.000
∞	1.000	1.000	1.000	1.000	1.000	1.000	1.000	1.000	1.000	1.000	1.000	1.000

VI.4 OPERATING CHARACTERISTIC (OC) CURVES FOR A TEST ON THE STANDARD DEVIATIONS OF TWO NORMAL DISTRIBUTIONS

The OC curves give the sample sizes needed for given values of $\alpha = P$ (Type I error) and $\beta = P$ (Type II error) for a test of the hypothesis $H_0: \sigma_x = \sigma_y$. The test statistic used is $F = \frac{s_x^2}{s_y^2}$ which is distributed as the F-distribution with $n_x - 1$ and $n_y - 1$ degrees of freedom. The required sample size is obtained by entering the appropriate set of curves for given α and β and for various values of $\lambda = \frac{\sigma_x}{\sigma_y}$ for both one-sided and two-sided tests for the case $n_x = n_y = n$.

OC CURVES FOR A TEST ON THE STANDARD DEVIATIONS OF TWO NORMAL DISTRIBUTIONS

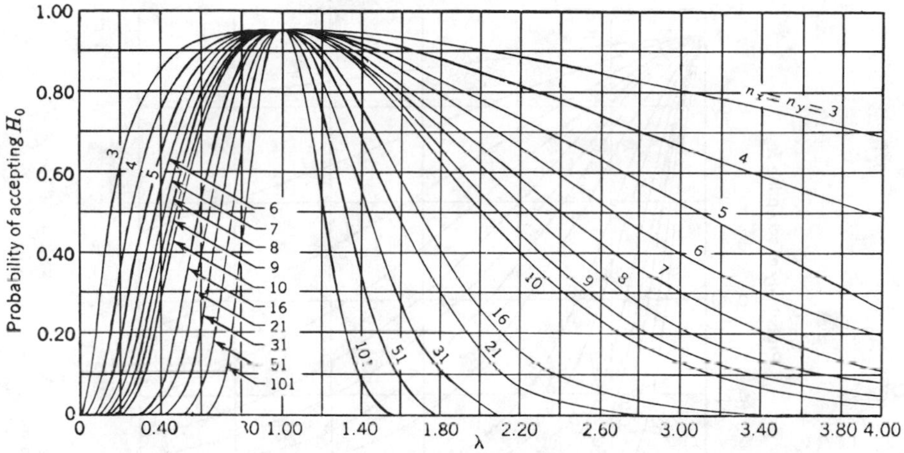

a) OC curves for different values of n for the two-sided F test for a level of significance $\alpha = 0.05$.

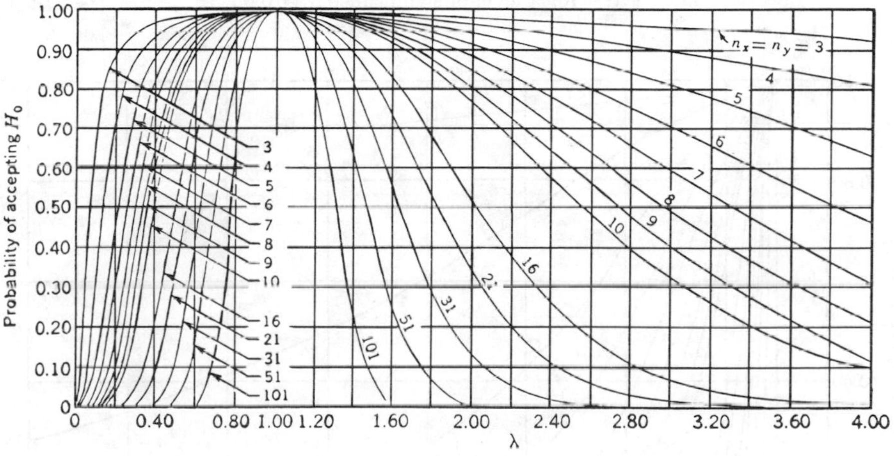

b) OC curves for different values of n for the two-sided F test for a level of significance $\alpha = 0.01$.

OC CURVES FOR A TEST ON THE STANDARD DEVIATIONS OF TWO NORMAL DISTRIBUTIONS

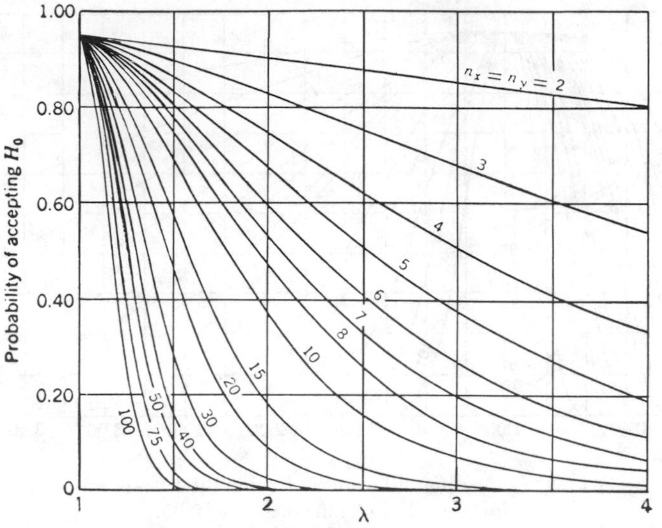

c) OC curves for different values of n for the one-sided F test for a level of significance $\alpha = 0.05$.

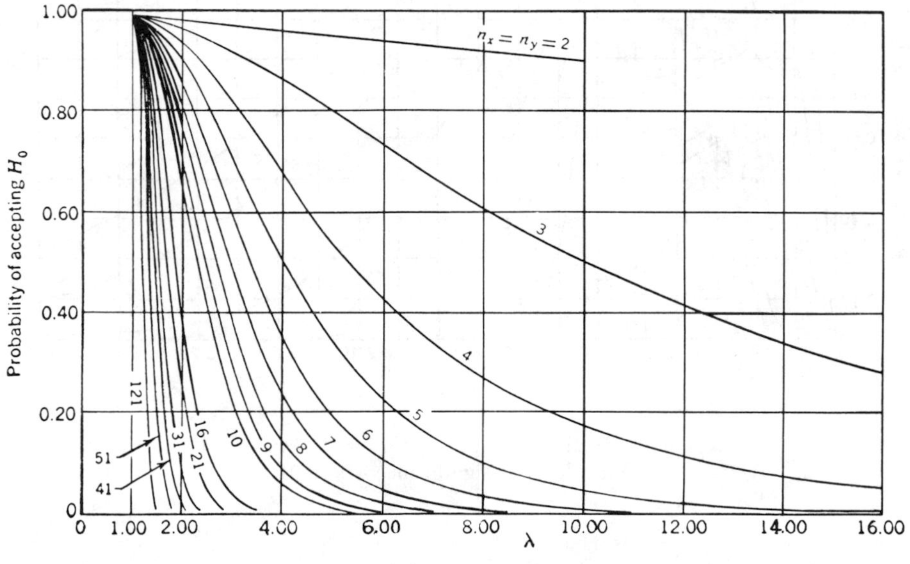

d) OC curves for different values of n for the one sided F test for a level of significance $\alpha = 0.01$.

VI.5 COCHRAN'S TEST FOR THE HOMOGENEITY OF VARIANCES

Let s_i^2, $i = 1, 2, \ldots, k$ denote a set of mean squares which are independent estimates of σ_i^2, respectively, each based upon n independent normally distributed random variables. Let

$$g = \frac{\max s_i^2}{\sum_{i=1}^{k} s_i^2}$$

be the ratio of the largest s^2 to their total. The hypothesis that $\sigma_1^2 = \sigma_2^2 = \cdots = \sigma_k^2$ is accepted if

$$g \leq g_\alpha$$

where g_α is given in the table for levels of significance α, equal to 0.05 and 0.01. The table is entered with n, the number of observations within each group, and k, the number of variances being considered.

UPPER 1 PERCENTAGE POINTS OF THE RATIO OF THE LARGEST TO THE SUM OF k INDEPENDENT ESTIMATES OF VARIANCE, EACH OF WHICH IS BASED ON n OBSERVATIONS

k \ n	2	3	4	5	6	7	8	9	10	11	17	37	145	∞
2	0.9999	0.9950	0.9794	0.9586	0.9373	0.9172	0.8988	0.8823	0.8674	0.8539	0.7949	0.7067	0.6062	0.5000
3	0.9933	0.9423	0.8831	0.8335	0.7933	0.7606	0.7335	0.7107	0.6912	0.6743	0.6059	0.5153	0.4230	0.3333
4	0.9676	0.8643	0.7814	0.7212	0.6761	0.6410	0.6129	0.5897	0.5702	0.5536	0.4884	0.4057	0.3251	0.2500
5	0.9279	0.7885	0.6957	0.6329	0.5875	0.5531	0.5259	0.5037	0.4854	0.4697	0.4094	0.3351	0.2644	0.2000
6	0.8828	0.7218	0.6258	0.5635	0.5195	0.4866	0.4608	0.4401	0.4229	0.4084	0.3529	0.2858	0.2229	0.1667
7	0.8376	0.6644	0.5685	0.5080	0.4659	0.4347	0.4105	0.3911	0.3751	0.3616	0.3105	0.2494	0.1929	0.1429
8	0.7945	0.6152	0.5209	0.4627	0.4226	0.3932	0.3704	0.3522	0.3373	0.3248	0.2779	0.2214	0.1700	0.1250
9	0.7544	0.5727	0.4810	0.4251	0.3870	0.3592	0.3378	0.3207	0.3067	0.2950	0.2514	0.1992	0.1521	0.1111
10	0.7175	0.5358	0.4469	0.3934	0.3572	0.3308	0.3106	0.2945	0.2813	0.2704	0.2297	0.1811	0.1376	0.1000
12	0.6528	0.4751	0.3919	0.3428	0.3099	0.2861	0.2680	0.2535	0.2419	0.2320	0.1961	0.1535	0.1157	0.0833
15	0.5747	0.4069	0.3317	0.2882	0.2593	0.2386	0.2228	0.2104	0.2002	0.1918	0.1612	0.1251	0.0934	0.0667
20	0.4799	0.3297	0.2654	0.2288	0.2048	0.1877	0.1748	0.1646	0.1567	0.1501	0.1248	0.0960	0.0709	0.0500
24	0.4247	0.2871	0.2295	0.1970	0.1759	0.1608	0.1495	0.1406	0.1338	0.1283	0.1060	0.0810	0.0595	0.0417
30	0.3632	0.2412	0.1913	0.1635	0.1454	0.1327	0.1232	0.1157	0.1100	0.1054	0.0867	0.0658	0.0480	0.0333
40	0.2940	0.1915	0.1508	0.1281	0.1135	0.1033	0.0957	0.0898	0.0853	0.0816	0.0668	0.0503	0.0363	0.0250
60	0.2151	0.1371	0.1069	0.0902	0.0796	0.0722	0.0668	0.0625	0.0594	0.0567	0.0461	0.0344	0.0245	0.0167
120	0.1225	0.0759	0.0585	0.0489	0.0429	0.0387	0.0357	0.0334	0.0316	0.0302	0.0242	0.0178	0.0125	0.0083
∞	0	0	0	0	0	0	0	0	0	0	0	0	0	0

UPPER 5 PERCENTAGE POINTS OF THE RATIO OF THE LARGEST TO THE SUM OF k INDEPENDENT ESTIMATES OF VARIANCE, EACH OF WHICH IS BASED ON n OBSERVATIONS

k \ n	2	3	4	5	6	7	8	9	10	11	17	37	145	∞
2	0.9985	0.9750	0.9392	0.9057	0.8772	0.8534	0.8332	0.8159	0.8010	0.7880	0.7341	0.6602	0.5813	0.5000
3	0.9669	0.8709	0.7977	0.7457	0.7071	0.6771	0.6530	0.6333	0.6167	0.6025	0.5466	0.4748	0.4031	0.3333
4	0.9065	0.7679	0.6841	0.6287	0.5895	0.5598	0.5365	0.5175	0.5017	0.4884	0.4366	0.3720	0.3093	0.2500
5	0.8412	0.6838	0.5981	0.5441	0.5065	0.4783	0.4564	0.4387	0.4241	0.4118	0.3645	0.3066	0.2513	0.2000
6	0.7808	0.6161	0.5321	0.4803	0.4447	0.4184	0.3980	0.3817	0.3682	0.3568	0.3135	0.2612	0.2119	0.1667
7	0.7271	0.5612	0.4800	0.4307	0.3974	0.3726	0.3535	0.3384	0.3259	0.3154	0.2756	0.2278	0.1833	0.1429
8	0.6798	0.5157	0.4377	0.3910	0.3595	0.3362	0.3185	0.3043	0.2926	0.2829	0.2462	0.2022	0.1616	0.1250
9	0.6385	0.4775	0.4027	0.3584	0.3286	0.3067	0.2901	0.2768	0.2659	0.2568	0.2226	0.1820	0.1446	0.1111
10	0.6020	0.4450	0.3733	0.3311	0.3029	0.2823	0.2666	0.2541	0.2439	0.2353	0.2032	0.1655	0.1308	0.1000
12	0.5410	0.3924	0.3264	0.2880	0.2624	0.2439	0.2299	0.2187	0.2098	0.2020	0.1737	0.1403	0.1100	0.0833
15	0.4709	0.3346	0.2758	0.2419	0.2195	0.2034	0.1911	0.1815	0.1736	0.1671	0.1429	0.1144	0.0889	0.0667
20	0.3894	0.2705	0.2205	0.1921	0.1735	0.1602	0.1501	0.1422	0.1357	0.1303	0.1108	0.0879	0.0675	0.0500
24	0.3434	0.2354	0.1907	0.1656	0.1493	0.1374	0.1286	0.1216	0.1160	0.1113	0.0942	0.0743	0.0567	0.0417
30	0.2929	0.1980	0.1593	0.1377	0.1237	0.1137	0.1061	0.1002	0.0958	0.0921	0.0771	0.0604	0.0457	0.0333
40	0.2370	0.1576	0.1259	0.1082	0.0968	0.0887	0.0827	0.0780	0.0745	0.0713	0.0595	0.0462	0.0347	0.0250
60	0.1737	0.1131	0.0895	0.0765	0.0682	0.0623	0.0583	0.0552	0.0520	0.0497	0.0411	0.0316	0.0234	0.0167
120	0.0998	0.0632	0.0495	0.0419	0.0371	0.0337	0.0312	0.0292	0.0279	0.0266	0.0218	0.0165	0.0120	0.0083
∞	0	0	0	0	0	0	0	0	0	0	0	0	0	0

VI.6 PERCENTAGE POINTS OF THE MAXIMUM F-RATIO

The maximum F-ratio $s^2_{\max}/s^2_{\min}$ can be used as a short-cut test for the heterogeneity of variance. Let s_i^2, $i = 1, 2, \ldots, k$ denote a set of mean squares, each based on ν degrees of freedom and arranged in ascending order of magnitude. Then

$$\begin{aligned} \log_e (s^2_{\max}/s^2_{\min}) &= \log_e (s^2_{\max}) - \log_e (s^2_{\min}) \\ &= \text{range } (\log_e s_i^2). \end{aligned}$$

Since $(\log_e s_i^2)$ are approximately normally distributed with mean $\log_e \sigma^2$ and variance $\frac{2}{\nu - 1}$, approximate percentage points of $s^2_{\max}/s^2_{\min}$ can be computed from percentage points of the range in normal samples. This table gives 5% and 1% points of the maximum F-ratio.

PERCENTAGE POINTS OF THE MAXIMUM F-RATIO

Upper 5% points

ν \ k	2	3	4	5	6	7	8	9	10	11	12
2	39.0	87.5	142	202	266	333	403	475	550	626	704
3	15.4	27.8	39.2	50.7	62.0	72.9	83.5	93.9	104	114	124
4	9.60	15.5	20.6	25.2	29.5	33.6	37.5	41.1	44.6	48.0	51.4
5	7.15	10.8	13.7	16.3	18.7	20.8	22.9	24.7	26.5	28.2	29.9
6	5.82	8.38	10.4	12.1	13.7	15.0	16.3	17.5	18.6	19.7	20.7
7	4.99	6.94	8.44	9.70	10.8	11.8	12.7	13.5	14.3	15.1	15.8
8	4.43	6.00	7.18	8.12	9.03	9.78	10.5	11.1	11.7	12.2	12.7
9	4.03	5.34	6.31	7.11	7.80	8.41	8.95	9.45	9.91	10.3	10.7
10	3.72	4.85	5.67	6.34	6.92	7.42	7.87	8.28	8.66	9.01	9.34
12	3.28	4.16	4.79	5.30	5.72	6.09	6.42	6.72	7.00	7.25	7.48
15	2.86	3.54	4.01	4.37	4.68	4.95	5.19	5.40	5.59	5.77	5.93
20	2.46	2.95	3.29	3.54	3.76	3.94	4.10	4.24	4.37	4.49	4.59
30	2.07	2.40	2.61	2.78	2.91	3.02	3.12	3.21	3.29	3.36	3.39
60	1.67	1.85	1.96	2.04	2.11	2.17	2.22	2.26	2.30	2.33	2.36
∞	1.00	1.00	1.00	1.00	1.00	1.00	1.00	1.00	1.00	1.00	1.00

Upper 1% points

ν \ k	2	3	4	5	6	7	8	9	10	11	12
2	199	448	729	1036	1362	1705	2063	2432	2813	3204	3605
3	47.5	85	120	151	184	21(6)	24(9)	28(1)	31(0)	33(7)	36(1)
4	23.2	37	49	59	69	79	89	97	106	113	120
5	14.9	22	28	33	38	42	46	50	54	57	60
6	11.1	15.5	19.1	22	25	27	30	32	34	36	37
7	8.89	12.1	14.5	16.5	18.4	20	22	23	24	26	27
8	7.50	9.9	11.7	13.2	14.5	15.8	16.9	17.9	18.9	19.8	21
9	6.54	8.5	9.9	11.1	12.1	13.1	13.9	14.7	15.3	16.0	16.6
10	5.85	7.4	8.6	9.6	10.4	11.1	11.8	12.4	12.9	13.4	13.9
12	4.91	6.1	6.9	7.6	8.2	8.7	9.1	9.5	9.9	10.2	10.6
15	4.07	4.9	5.5	6.0	6.4	6.7	7.1	7.3	7.5	7.8	8.0
20	3.32	3.8	4.3	4.6	4.9	5.1	5.3	5.5	5.6	5.8	5.9
30	2.63	3.0	3.3	3.4	3.6	3.7	3.8	3.9	4.0	4.1	4.2
60	1.96	2.2	2.3	2.4	2.4	2.5	2.5	2.6	2.6	2.7	2.7
∞	1.00	1.0	1.0	1.0	1.0	1.0	1.0	1.0	1.0	1.0	1.0

s^2_{max} is the largest and s^2_{min} the smallest in a set of k independent mean squares, each based on ν degrees of freedom.

Values in the column $k = 2$ and in the rows $\nu = 2$ and ∞ are exact. Elsewhere the third digit may be in error by a few units for the 5% points and several units for the 1% points. The third digit figures in brackets for $\nu = 3$ are the most uncertain.

VII. Order Statistics

VII.1 EXPECTED VALUES OF ORDER STATISTICS FROM A STANDARD NORMAL POPULATION

If a sample of n observations $x_1, x_2, \ldots, x_n$ is drawn from a standard normal distribution, and the observations are arranged in ascending order of magnitude $x_{(1)}, \ldots, x_{(n)}$, the ith value of the set $\{x_{(i)}\}$ is called the ith normal order statistic and its expectation is given by

$$E[x_{(i)}] = \frac{n!}{(i-1)!(n-i)!} \int_{-\infty}^{\infty} x f(x) F^{i-1}(x)[1 - F(x)]^{n-i}\, dx \ ,$$

where $f(x) = \dfrac{1}{\sqrt{2\pi}} e^{-\frac{1}{2}x^2}$,

$$F(x) = \int_{-\infty}^{x} \frac{1}{\sqrt{2\pi}} e^{-t^2/2}\, dt.$$

This table gives value of $E[x_{(i)}]$ for various values of n. Missing values may be obtained by noting that

$$E[x_{(i)}] = -E[x_{(n-i+1)}].$$

Tabular values are the expected values of the ith largest normal order statistic from a sample of size n from $N(0,1)$; or when preceded by a minus sign, they are the expected values of the ith smallest normal order statistic.

EXPECTED VALUES OF NORMAL ORDER STATISTICS

i \ n	2	3	4	5	6	7	8	9
1	0.56419	0.84628	1.02938	1.16296	1.26721	1.35218	1.42360	1.48501
2	—	.00000	0.29701	0.49502	0.64176	0.75737	0.85222	0.93230
3	—	—	—	.00000	.20155	.35271	.47282	.57197
4	—	—	—	—	—	.00000	.15251	.27453
5	—	—	—	—	—	—	—	.00000

i \ n	10	11	12	13	14	15	16	17	18	19
1	1.53875	1.58644	1.62923	1.66799	1.70338	1.73591	1.76599	1.79394	1.82003	1.84448
2	1.00136	1.06192	1.11573	1.16408	1.20790	1.24794	1.28474	1.31878	1.35041	1.37994
3	0.65606	0.72884	0.79284	0.84983	0.90113	0.94769	0.99027	1.02946	1.06573	1.09945
4	.37576	.46198	.53684	.60285	.66176	.71488	.76317	0.80738	0.84812	0.88586
5	.12267	.22489	.31225	.38833	.45557	.51570	.57001	.61946	.66479	.70661
6	—	0.00000	0.10259	0.19052	0.26730	0.33530	0.39622	0.45133	0.50158	0.54771
7	—	—	—	.00000	0.08816	.16530	.23375	.29519	.35084	.40164
8	—	—	—	—	—	.00000	.07729	.14599	.20774	.26374
9	—	—	—	—	—	—	—	.00000	.06880	.13072
10	—	—	—	—	—	—	—	—	—	.00000

i \ n	20	21	22	23	24	25	26	27	28	29
1	1.86748	1.88917	1.90969	1.92916	1.94767	1.96531	1.98216	1.99827	2.01371	2.02852
2	1.40760	1.43362	1.45816	1.48137	1.50338	1.52430	1.54423	1.56326	1.58145	1.59888
3	1.13005	1.16047	1.18824	1.21445	1.23024	1.26275	1.28511	1.30641	1.32674	1.34610
4	0.92098	0.95380	0.98459	1.01356	1.04091	1.06679	1.09135	1.11471	1.13697	1.15822
5	.74538	.78150	.81527	0.84697	0.87682	0.90501	0.93171	0.95705	0.98115	1.00414
6	0.59030	0.62982	0.66667	0.70115	0.73354	0.76405	0.79289	0.82021	0.84615	0.87084
7	.44833	.49148	.53157	.56896	.60399	.63690	.66794	.69727	.72508	.75150
8	.31493	.36203	.40559	.44609	.48391	.51935	.55267	.58411	.61385	.64205
9	.18696	.23841	.28579	.32965	.37047	.40860	.44436	.47801	.50977	.53982
10	.06200	.11836	.16997	.21755	.26163	.30268	.34105	.37706	.41096	.44298
11	—	0.00000	0.05642	0.10813	0.15583	0.20006	0.24128	0.27983	0.31603	0.35013
12	—	—	—	.00000	.05176	.09953	.14387	.18520	.22380	.26023
13	—	—	—	—	—	.00000	.04781	.09220	.13361	.17240
14	—	—	—	—	—	—	—	.00000	.04442	.08588
15	—	—	—	—	—	—	—	—	—	.00000

i \ n	30	31	32	33	34	35	36	37	38	39
1	2.04276	2.05646	2.06967	2.08241	2.09471	2.10661	2.11812	2.12928	2.14009	2.15059
2	1.61560	1.63166	1.64712	1.66200	1.67636	1.69023	1.70362	1.71659	1.72914	1.74131
3	1.36481	1.38268	1.39985	1.41637	1.43228	1.44762	1.46244	1.47676	1.49061	1.50402
4	1.17855	1.19803	1.21672	1.23468	1.25196	1.26860	1.28466	1.30016	1.31514	1.32964
5	1.02609	1.04709	1.06721	1.08652	1.10509	1.12295	1.14016	1.15677	1.17280	1.18830
6	0.89439	0.91688	0.93841	0.95905	0.97886	0.99790	1.01624	1.03390	1.05095	1.06741
7	.77666	.80066	.82359	.84555	.86660	.88681	0.90625	0.92496	0.94300	0.96041
8	.66885	.69438	.71875	.74204	.76435	.78574	.80629	.82605	.84508	.86343
9	.56834	.59545	.62129	.64596	.66954	.69214	.71382	.73465	.75468	.77398
10	.47329	.50206	.52943	.55552	.58043	.60427	.62710	.64902	.67009	.69035
11	0.38235	0.41287	0.44185	0.46942	0.49572	0.52084	0.54488	0.56793	0.59005	0.61131
12	.29449	.32686	.35755	.38669	.41444	.44091	.46620	.49042	.51363	.53592
13	.20885	.24322	.27573	.30654	.33582	.36371	.39032	.41576	.44012	.46348
14	.12473	.16126	.19572	.22832	.25924	.28863	.31663	.34336	.36892	.39340
15	.04148	.08037	.11695	.15147	.18415	.21515	.24463	.27272	.29954	.32520
16	—	0.00000	0.03890	0.07552	0.11009	0.14282	0.17388	0.20342	0.23159	0.25849
17	—	—	—	.00000	.03663	.07123	.10399	.13509	.16469	.19292
18	—	—	—	—	—	.00000	.03461	.06739	.09853	.12817
19	—	—	—	—	—	—	—	.00000	.03280	.06395
20	—	—	—	—	—	—	—	—	—	.00000

VII.2 VARIANCES AND COVARIANCES OF ORDER STATISTICS

If a sample of n observations $x_1, x_2, \ldots, x_n$ is drawn from a standard normal distribution, and the observations are arranged in ascending order of magnitude $x_{(1)}, x_{(2)}, \ldots, x_{(n)}$, then the variances and covariances of these order statistics may be obtained from the following expressions for expected values and product moments:

$$E[x_{(i)}] = \frac{n!}{(i-1)!(n-i)!}\int_{-\infty}^{\infty} xf(x)[F(x)]^{i-1}[1-F(x)]^{n-i}\,dx,$$

$$E[x^2_{(i)}] = \frac{n!}{(i-1)!(n-i)!}\int_{-\infty}^{\infty} x^2f(x)[F(x)]^{i-1}[1-F(x)]^{n-i}\,dx,$$

$$E[x_{(i)}x_{(j)}] = \frac{n!}{(i-1)!(j-i-1)!(n-j)!}\int_{-\infty}^{\infty}\int_{-\infty}^{y} xyf(x)f(y)[F(x)]^{i-1}[1-F(y)]^{n-j}[F(y)-F(x)]^{j-i-1}\,dx\,dy\;,$$

where $f(x) = \dfrac{1}{\sqrt{2\pi}}e^{-\frac{1}{2}x^2}$,

$$F(x) = \int_{-\infty}^{x}\frac{1}{\sqrt{2\pi}}e^{-\frac{1}{2}t^2}\,dt.$$

This table gives the variances and covariances of order statistics in samples of sizes up to 20 from a standard normal distribution. Missing values may be supplied from $E[x_{(i)}] = -E[x_{(n-i+1)}]$; $E[x_{(i)}x_{(j)}] = E[x_{(j)}x_{(i)}] = E[x_{(n-i+1)}x_{(n-j+1)}]$.

VARIANCES AND COVARIANCES OF ORDER STATISTICS

n	*i*	*j*	Value	*n*	*i*	*j*	Value	*n*	*i*	*j*	Value
2	1	1	.6816901139	8				10	3		
		2	.3183098861		2	2	.2394010458			5	.1077445336
	2	2	.6816901139			3	.1631958727			6	.0892254012
3	1	1	.5594672038			4	.1232633317			7	.0749183943
		2	.2756644477			5	.0975647193			8	.0630332449
		3	.1648683485			6	.0787224662		4	4	.1579389144
	2	2	.4486711046			7	.0632466118			5	.1275089295
4	1	1	.4917152369		3	3	.2007687900			6	.1057858169
		2	.2455926930			4	.1523584312			7	.0889462026
		3	.1580080701			5	.1209637555		5	5	.1510539039
		4	.1046840000			6	.0978171355			6	.1255989678
	2	2	.3604553434		4	4	.1871862195	11	1	1	.3332474428
		3	.2359438935			5	.1491754908			2	.1653647712
5	1	1	.4475340691	9	1	1	.3573533264			3	.1123584351
		2	.2243309596			2	.1781434240			4	.0855170596
		3	.1481477252			3	.1207454442			5	.0688483064
		4	.1057719776			4	.0913071400			6	.0572007586
		5	.0742152685			5	.0727422354			7	.0483754063
	2	2	.3115189521			6	.0594831125			8	.0412423472
		3	.2084354440			7	.0490764061			9	.0351103357
		4	.1499426668			8	.0400936927			10	.0294198503
	3	3	.2868336616			9	.0310552188			11	.0233152868
6	1	1	.4159271090		2	2	.2256968778		2	2	.2051975798
		2	.2085030023			3	.1541163526			3	.1403096511
		3	.1394352565			4	.1170056918			4	.1071492595
		4	.1024293940			5	.0934477394			5	.0864430257
		5	.0773037839			6	.0765461431			6	.0719305024
		6	.0563414544			7	.0632354695			7	.0608869662
	2	2	.2795777392			8	.0517146091			8	.0519504506
		3	.1889859560		3	3	.1863826133			9	.0442549455
		4	.1396040004			4	.1420779776			10	.0371029977
		5	.1059054582			5	.1137680176		3	3	.1657242880
	3	3	.2462125354			6	.0933625386			4	.1269672925
		4	.1832727978			7	.0772351806			5	.1026407291
7	1	1	.3919177761		4	4	.1705588454			6	.0855178832
		2	.1961990246			5	.1369913669			7	.0724741050
		3	.1321155811			6	.1126671842			8	.0618873278
		4	.0984868607		5	5	.1661012814			9	.0527550069
		5	.0765598346	10	1	1	.3443438233		4	4	.1479546565
		6	.0599187124			2	.1712629030			5	.1198752861
		7	.0448022105			3	.1162590989			6	.1000346585
	2	2	.2567328862			4	.0882494247			7	.0848765182
		3	.1744833274			5	.0707413677			8	.0725451434
		4	.1307298656			6	.0583987134		5	5	.1396410804
		5	.1019550089			7	.0489206279			6	.1167449805
		6	.0799811748			8	.0410844589			7	.0991935960
	3	3	.2107215626			9	.0340406470		6	6	.1371024335
		4	.1655598429			10	.0266989351	12	1	1	.3236363870
		5	.1296048425		2	2	.2145241430			2	.1602373762
	4	4	.2104468615			3	.1466226180			3	.1089309641
8	1	1	.3728971434			4	.1117015961			4	.0830686767
		2	.1863073997			5	.0897428245			5	.0670884464
		3	.1259660300			6	.0741995414			6	.0559933694
		4	.0947230277			7	.0622278486			7	.0476620974
		5	.0747650242			8	.0523067222			8	.0410208554
		6	.0602075169			9	.0433711561			9	.0354439060
		7	.0482985508		3	3	.1750032834			10	.0305012591
		8	.0368353073			4	.1338022448			11	.0257945392

VARIANCES AND COVARIANCES OF ORDER STATISTICS

n	*i*	*j*	Value
12	1		
		12	.0206221233
	2	2	.1972646039
		3	.1349020328
		4	.1031959206
		5	.0835045822
		6	.0697859658
		7	.0594590652
		8	.0512113198
		9	.0442747124
		10	.0381191478
		11	.0322507340
	3	3	.1579786877
		4	.1212063211
		5	.0982605602
		6	.0822228461
		7	.0701213964
		8	.0604384621
		9	.0522825611
		10	.0450357615
	4	4	.1398109405
		5	.1135687821
		6	.0951645279
		7	.0812419810
		8	.0700795832
		9	.0606620874
	5	5	.1306137359
		6	.1096212247
		7	.0936951520
		8	.0808972960
	6	6	.1266377911
		7	.1083945831
13	1	1	.3152053842
		2	.1557272904
		3	.1058908842
		4	.0808649736
		5	.0654634499
		6	.0548221797
		7	.0468833088
		8	.0406132548
		9	.0354226462
		10	.0309322744
		11	.0268537250
		12	.0228858068
		13	.0184348220
	2	2	.1904130721
		3	.1302055829
		4	.0997262696
		5	.0808785938
		6	.0678145832
		7	.0580457285
		8	.0503167946
		9	.0439095087
		10	.0383601798
		11	.0333147765
		12	.0284018130
	3	3	.1513917013
		4	.1162698131
13	3		
		5	.0944566603
		6	.0792922993
		7	.0679282354
		8	.0589221432
		9	.0514460445
		10	.0449637542
		11	.0390643799
	4	4	.1330111820
		5	.1082512667
		6	.0909855605
		7	.0780173339
		8	.0677217143
		9	.0591628729
		10	.0517328050
	5	5	.1232503256
		6	.1037367701
		7	.0890434754
		8	.0773552864
		9	.0676230994
	6	6	.1183175325
		7	.1016824204
		8	.0884194610
	7	7	.1167989950
14	1	1	.3077301026
		2	.1517203662
		3	.1031719531
		4	.0788715916
		5	.0639657428
		6	.0537064714
		7	.0460899189
		8	.0401141688
		9	.0352141760
		10	.0310371163
		11	.0273362865
		12	.0239061001
		13	.0205080257
		14	.0166279801
	2	2	.1844200252
		3	.1260791989
		4	.0966524633
		5	.0785202981
		6	.0660028340
		7	.0566896715
		8	.0493708148
		9	.0433617156
		10	.0382337404
		11	.0336863221
		12	.0294681314
		13	.0252863928
	3	3	.1457045665
		4	.1119816877
		5	.0911181271
		6	.0766754957
		7	.0659084825
		8	.0574341188
		9	.0504677802
		10	.0445169192
14	3		
		11	.0392352316
		12	.0343322071
	4	4	.1272273070
		5	.1036931108
		6	.0873562483
		7	.0751519909
		8	.0655310936
		9	.0576120957
		10	.0508402240
		11	.0448243469
	5	5	.1171012461
		6	.0987747550
		7	.0850536546
		8	.0742181416
		9	.0652867776
		10	.0576401464
	6	6	.1115324579
		7	.0961405595
		8	.0839617110
		9	.0739069221
	7	7	.1090269480
		8	.0953087256
15	1	1	.3010415703
		2	.1481297708
		3	.1007223449
		4	.0770594060
		5	.0625845851
		6	.0526530129
		7	.0453078886
		8	.0395736673
		9	.0349035905
		10	.0309614122
		11	.0275211039
		12	.0244126313
		13	.0214819828
		14	.0185333263
		15	.0151137071
	2	2	.1791215291
		3	.1224176953
		4	.0939067144
		5	.0763912337
		6	.0643390895
		7	.0554074400
		8	.0484238833
		9	.0427294113
		10	.0379177516
		11	.0337151721
		12	.0299152347
		13	.0263303885
		14	.0227213594
	3	3	.1407322502
		4	.1082138452
		5	.0881605755
		6	.0743268436
		7	.0640558183
		8	.0560136122
		9	.0494485109

VARIANCES AND COVARIANCES OF ORDER STATISTICS

n	*i*	*j*	Value	*n*	*i*	*j*	Value	*n*	*i*	*j*	Value
15	3			16	2			17	1		
		10	.0438960670			14	.0237301562			14	.0199690651
		11	.0390426915			15	.0205785433			15	.0177476891
		12	.0346513382		3	3	.1363385612			16	.0154552071
		13	.0305060359			4	.1048706756			17	.0127264751
	4	4	.1222328270			5	.0855189036		2	2	.1701426762
		5	.0997323941			6	.0722075087			3	.1161866734
		6	.0841705696			7	.0623568515			4	.0891982557
		7	.0725946869			8	.0546749107			5	.0726970385
		8	.0635175907			9	.0484366096			6	.0613998459
		9	.0560990511			10	.0431979377			7	.0530761573
		10	.0498187836			11	.0386652995			8	.0466140918
		11	.0443247452			12	.0346277256			9	.0413928192
		12	.0393501820			13	.0309149135			10	.0370349110
	5	5	.1118698986			14	.0273595378			11	.0332940892
		6	.0945206004		4	4	.1178657554			12	.0299982825
		7	.0815891122			5	.0962513413			13	.0270170379
		8	.0714331681			6	.0813480448			14	.0242386812
		9	.0631224388			7	.0703000911			15	.0215459396
		10	.0560795065			8	.0616728990			16	.0187658306
		11	.0499127743			9	.0546595026		3	3	.1324207975
	6	6	.1058666366			10	.0487647746			4	.1018792434
		7	.0914683204			11	.0436607328			5	.0831421716
		8	.0801407559			12	.0391112669			6	.0702850403
		9	.0708582099			13	.0349253749			7	.0607964413
		10	.0629824402		5	5	.1073517089			8	.0534208202
	7	7	.1026916923			6	.0908232622			9	.0471555187
		8	.0900499964			7	.0785480532			10	.0424726884
		9	.0796738323			8	.0689488802			11	.0381925587
	8	8	.1016946521			9	.0611364182			12	.0344194567
16	1	1	.2950098090			10	.0545638941			13	.0310047771
		2	.1448881689			11	.0488684327			14	.0278210708
		3	.0985009764			12	.0437882959			15	.0247342095
		4	.0754040023		6	6	.1010461906		4	4	.1140068197
		5	.0613086724			7	.0874627156			5	.0931620339
		6	.0516624963			8	.0768239668			6	.0788266621
		7	.0445503705			9	.0681545540			7	.0682298909
		8	.0390194716			10	.0608534805			8	.0599826092
		9	.0345378158			11	.0545210724			9	.0533057575
		10	.0307810093		7	7	.0974026613			10	.0477239973
		11	.0275353612			8	.0856181916			11	.0429261816
		12	.0246479007			9	.0760015577			12	.0386942630
		13	.0219956755			10	.0678931922			13	.0348624030
		14	.0194585037		8	8	.0957213007			14	.0312881041
		15	.0168710289			9	.0850291218		5	5	.1034004377
		16	.0138287378	17	1	1	.2895330037			6	.0875729930
	2	2	.1743940788			2	.1419424629			7	.0758534534
		3	.1191409287			3	.0964748737			8	.0667204245
		4	.0914359918			4	.0738849615			9	.0593187706
		5	.0744591145			5	.0601272302			10	.0531257771
		6	.0628093909			6	.0507326948			11	.0477987292
		7	.0542033941			7	.0438236491			12	.0430970793
		8	.0475009769			8	.0384672834			13	.0388375657
		9	.0420638230			9	.0341441055		6	6	.0968824669
		10	.0375018250			10	.0305389548			7	.0839811738
		11	.0335574912			11	.0274465527			8	.0739130260
		12	.0300461298			12	.0247237144			9	.0657442736
		13	.0268189579			13	.0222620771			10	.0589030403

VARIANCES AND COVARIANCES OF ORDER STATISTICS

n	*i*	*j*	Value	*n*	*i*	*j*	Value	*n*	*i*	*j*	Value
17	6			18	3			19	1		
		11	.0530137275			15	.0252244786			14	.0204007370
		12	.0478122599			16	.0225161109			15	.0185431530
	7	7	.0929031780		4	4	.1105660331			16	.0167731147
		8	.0818194607			5	.0903973787			17	.0150223067
		9	.0728154074			6	.0765579277			18	.0131789994
		10	.0652667274			7	.0663522086			19	.0109382527
		11	.0587626219			8	.0584310521		2	2	.1627856651
	8	8	.0907361650			9	.0520394281			3	.1110590145
		9	.0808000267			10	.0467183404			4	.0852931053
		10	.0724599963			11	.0421694861			5	.0695970759
	9	9	.0900465814			12	.0381869632			6	.0588910196
18	1	1	.2845301297			13	.0346192645			7	.0510351093
		2	.1392501620			14	.0313452497			8	.0449652247
		3	.0946172637			15	.0282548286			9	.0400891754
		4	.0724851730		5	5	.0999084321			10	.0360490040
		5	.0590304274			6	.0846879168			11	.0326137544
		6	.0498600635			7	.0734460811			12	.0296258236
		7	.0431302310			8	.0647101858			13	.0269716592
		8	.0379260195			9	.0576543520			14	.0245641909
		9	.0337388141			10	.0517756675			15	.0223306885
		10	.0302610667			11	.0467468133			16	.0202017247
		11	.0272938041			12	.0423415563			17	.0180952193
		12	.0247002471			13	.0383932046			18	.0158767294
		13	.0223801573			14	.0347682770		3	3	.1257138904
		14	.0202537421		6	6	.0932407331			4	.0967367097
		15	.0182488619			7	.0809202644			5	.0790298792
		16	.0162850441			8	.0713338046			6	.0669273696
		17	.0142368875			9	.0635829688			7	.0580336124
		18	.0117719054			10	.0571197288			8	.0511541418
	2	2	.1662929294			11	.0515868552			9	.0456228816
		3	.1135058132			12	.0467370896			10	.0410365629
		4	.0871597604			13	.0423879846			11	.0371346427
		5	.0710825990		7	7	.0890167025			12	.0337391171
		6	.0600975754			8	.0785179677			13	.0307215918
		7	.0520217423			9	.0700199026			14	.0279835020
		8	.0457683625			10	.0629269074			15	.0254424108
		9	.0407317967			11	.0568501034			16	.0230195063
		10	.0365451034			12	.0515199092			17	.0206214645
		11	.0329704894		8	8	.0864960639		4	4	.1074740839
		12	.0298442464			9	.0771762286			5	.0879051965
		13	.0270462261			10	.0693891332			6	.0745033878
		14	.0244806359			11	.0627116906			7	.0646406188
		15	.0220607111		9	9	.0853127880			8	.0570032284
		16	.0196894667			10	.0767442321			9	.0508572608
		17	.0172154925	19	1	1	.2799358050			10	.0457576598
	3	3	.1288998943			2	.1367768168			11	.0414165091
		4	.0991828539			3	.0929061763			12	.0376368753
		5	.0809899792			4	.0711902425			13	.0342765540
		6	.0685324700			5	.0580094835			14	.0312262549
		7	.0593598602			6	.0490405678			15	.0283944527
		8	.0522488413			7	.0424705246			16	.0256935148
		9	.0465162123			8	.0374006329		5	5	.0967944745
		10	.0417473296			9	.0333319395			6	.0821055695
		11	.0376730987			10	.0299634144			7	.0712796742
		12	.0341080171			11	.0271011338			8	.0628870095
		13	.0309157650			12	.0246129452			9	.0561272025
		14	.0279875014			13	.0224037540			10	.0505141639

VARIANCES AND COVARIANCES OF ORDER STATISTICS

n	*i*	*j*	Value	*n*	*i*	*j*	Value	*n*	*i*	*j*	Value
19	5			20	1			20	4		
		11	.0457330144			18	.0139227072			14	.0310045146
		12	.0415681234			19	.0122530117			15	.0283650517
		13	.0378636088			20	.0102047204			16	.0258897454
		14	.0344995261		2	2	.1595731636			17	.0235070343
		15	.0313752928			3	.1088143707		5	5	.0939960007
	6	6	.0900218693			4	.0835758044			6	.0797773755
		7	.0782029063			5	.0682247554			7	.0693175756
		8	.0690294360			6	.0577699656			8	.0612251429
		9	.0616336896			7	.0501109523			9	.0547222526
		10	.0554877905			8	.0442041191			10	.0493374275
		11	.0502493169			9	.0394693443			11	.0447662310
		12	.0456834841			10	.0355565554			12	.0408014074
		13	.0416203596			11	.0322405467			13	.0372948400
		14	.0379290224			12	.0293684960			14	.0341351571
	7	7	.0856172981			13	.0268315105			15	.0312332040
		8	.0756153413			14	.0245479493			16	.0285109200
		9	.0675433161			15	.0224526609		6	6	.0871511254
		10	.0608297030			16	.0204888032			7	.0757703360
		11	.0551032224			17	.0185994024			8	.0669555789
		12	.0501089625			18	.0167136502			9	.0598659769
		13	.0456621835			19	.0147107671			10	.0539910639
	8	8	.0828330961		3	3	.1228134687			11	.0490008080
		9	.0740273546			4	.0945049010			12	.0446702771
		10	.0666958229			5	.0772355098			13	.0408385549
		11	.0604372723			6	.0654510179			14	.0373845194
		12	.0540752083			7	.0568056677			15	.0342111024
	9	9	.0812876330			8	.0501310269		7	7	.0826123955
		10	.0732703911			9	.0447763202			8	.0730383676
		11	.0664202898			10	.0403482354			9	.0653307665
	10	10	.0807909751			11	.0365934287			10	.0589387428
20	1	1	.2756966156			12	.0333397949			11	.0535056766
		2	.1344941714			13	.0304645792			12	.0487882257
		3	.0913234064			14	.0278756579			13	.0446121090
		4	.0699879991			15	.0254994381			14	.0408459989
		5	.0570566384			16	.0232716371		8	8	.0796309757
		6	.0482701093			17	.0211277373			9	.0712591607
		7	.0418437826			18	.0189874448			10	.0643103375
		8	.0368937058		4	4	.1046766243			11	.0583997310
		9	.0329296302			5	.0856442356			12	.0532644495
		10	.0296562523			6	.0726321560			13	.0487159834
		11	.0268838808			7	.0630731775		9	9	.0778118317
		12	.0244839567			8	.0556855081			10	.0702526464
		13	.0223649803			9	.0497539273			11	.0638176734
		14	.0204584277			10	.0448455403			12	.0582229133
		15	.0187096782			11	.0406811669		10	10	.0769474356
		16	.0170711408			12	.0370709493			11	.0699266198
		17	.0154951854			13	.0338793392				

VII.3 CONFIDENCE INTERVALS FOR MEDIANS

If the observations $x_1, x_2, \ldots, x_n$ are arranged in ascending order $x_{(1)}, x_{(2)}, \ldots, x_{(n)}$, a $100(1-\alpha)\%$ confidence interval on the median of the population can be found. This table gives values of k and α such that one can be $100(1-\alpha)\%$ confident that the population median is between $x_{(k)}$ and $x_{(n-k+1)}$.

CONFIDENCE INTERVALS FOR THE MEDIAN

n	Largest k	Actual $\alpha \le 0.05$	Largest k	Actual $\alpha \le 0.01$	N	Largest k	Actual $\alpha \le 0.05$	Largest k	Actual $\alpha \le 0.01$
6	1	0.031			36	12	0.029	10	0.004
7	1	0.016			37	13	0.047	11	0.008
8	1	0.008	1	0.008	38	13	0.034	11	0.005
9	2	0.039	1	0.004	39	13	0.024	12	0.009
10	2	0.021	1	0.002	40	14	0.038	12	0.006
11	2	0.012	1	0.001	41	14	0.028	12	0.004
12	3	0.039	2	0.006	42	15	0.044	13	0.008
13	3	0.022	2	0.003	43	15	0.032	13	0.005
14	3	0.013	2	0.002	44	16	0.049	14	0.010
15	4	0.035	3	0.007	45	16	0.036	14	0.007
16	4	0.021	3	0.004	46	16	0.026	14	0.005
17	5	0.049	3	0.002	47	17	0.040	15	0.008
18	5	0.031	4	0.008	48	17	0.029	15	0.006
19	5	0.019	4	0.004	49	18	0.044	16	0.009
20	6	0.041	4	0.003	50	18	0.033	16	0.007
21	6	0.027	5	0.007	51	19	0.049	16	0.005
22	6	0.017	5	0.004	52	19	0.036	17	0.008
23	7	0.035	5	0.003	53	19	0.027	17	0.005
24	7	0.023	6	0.007	54	20	0.040	18	0.009
25	8	0.043	6	0.004	55	20	0.030	18	0.006
26	8	0.029	7	0.009	56	21	0.044	18	0.005
27	8	0.019	7	0.006	57	21	0.033	19	0.008
28	9	0.036	7	0.004	58	22	0.048	19	0.005
29	9	0.024	8	0.008	59	22	0.036	20	0.009
30	10	0.043	8	0.005	60	22	0.027	20	0.006
31	10	0.029	8	0.003	61	23	0.040	21	0.010
32	10	0.020	9	0.007	62	23	0.030	21	0.007
33	11	0.035	9	0.005	63	24	0.043	21	0.005
34	11	0.024	10	0.009	64	24	0.033	22	0.008
35	12	0.041	10	0.006	65	25	0.046	22	0.006

VII.4 CRITICAL VALUES FOR TESTING OUTLIERS

Tests for outliers may be based on the largest deviation $\max_{i=1,2,\ldots,n} (x_i - \bar{x})$ of the observations from their mean or on the range w, where these statistics have to be divided by the standard deviation σ or by an estimate of σ, depending on whether σ is known or not. An alternate set of statistics is considered in this table.

The following ratios are suitable for detection of outliers.

a) For single outlier $x_{(1)}$:

$$r_{10} = \frac{x_{(2)} - x_{(1)}}{x_{(n)} - x_{(1)}}$$

$$\left(\text{or for } x_{(n)}\text{: } r_{10} = \frac{x_{(n)} - x_{(n-1)}}{x_{(n)} - x_{(1)}}\right)$$

b) For single outlier $x_{(1)}$ avoiding $x_{(n)}$:

$$r_{11} = \frac{x_{(2)} - x_{(1)}}{x_{(n-1)} - x_{(1)}}$$

$$\left(\text{or for } x_{(n)} \text{ avoiding } x_{(1)}\text{: } r_{11} = \frac{x_{(n)} - x_{(n-1)}}{x_{(n)} - x_{(2)}}\right)$$

c) For single outlier $x_{(1)}$, avoiding $x_{(n)}$, $x_{(n-1)}$:

$$r_{12} = \frac{x_{(2)} - x_{(1)}}{x_{(n-2)} - x_{(1)}}$$

$$\left(\text{or for } x_{(n)} \text{ avoiding } x_{(1)}, x_{(2)}\text{: } r_{12} = \frac{x_{(n)} - x_{(n-1)}}{x_{(n)} - x_{(3)}}\right)$$

d) For outlier $x_{(1)}$ avoiding $x_{(2)}$:

$$r_{20} = \frac{x_{(3)} - x_{(1)}}{x_{(n)} - x_{(1)}}$$

$$\left(\text{or for } x_{(n)} \text{ avoiding } x_{(n-1)}\text{: } r_{20} = \frac{x_{(n)} - x_{(n-2)}}{x_{(n)} - x_{(1)}}\right)$$

e) For outlier $x_{(1)}$ avoiding $x_{(2)}$ and $x_{(n)}$:

$$r_{21} = \frac{x_{(3)} - x_{(1)}}{x_{(n-1)} - x_{(1)}}$$

$$\left(\text{or for } x_{(n)} \text{ avoiding } x_{(n-1)}, x_{(1)}\text{: } r_{21} = \frac{x_{(n)} - x_{(n-2)}}{x_{(n)} - x_{(2)}}\right)$$

f) For outlier $x_{(1)}$ avoiding $x_{(2)}$ and $x_{(n)}$, $x_{(n-1)}$:

$$r_{22} = \frac{x_{(3)} - x_{(1)}}{x_{(n-2)} - x_{(1)}}$$

$$\left(\text{or for } x_{(n)} \text{ avoiding } x_{(n-1)}, x_{(1)}, x_{(2)}\text{: } r_{22} = \frac{x_{(n)} - x_{(n-2)}}{x_{(n)} - x_{(3)}}\right)$$

PERCENTAGE VALUES FOR r_{10}

$[\Pr (r_{10} > R) = \alpha]$

n \ α	.005	.01	.02	.05	.10	.20	.30	.40	.50	.60	.70	.80	.90	.95	α / n
3	.994	.988	.976	.941	.886	.781	.684	.591	.500	.409	.316	.219	.114	.059	3
4	.926	.889	.846	.765	.679	.560	.471	.394	.324	.257	.193	.130	.065	.033	4
5	.821	.780	.729	.642	.557	.451	.373	.308	.250	.196	.146	.097	.048	.023	5
6	.740	.698	.644	.560	.482	.386	.318	.261	.210	.164	.121	.079	.038	.018	6
7	.680	.637	.586	.507	.434	.344	.281	.230	.184	.143	.105	.068	.032	.016	7
8	.634	.590	.543	.468	.399	.314	.255	.208	.166	.128	.094	.060	.029	.014	8
9	.598	.555	.510	.437	.370	.290	.234	.191	.152	.118	.086	.055	.026	.013	9
10	.568	.527	.483	.412	.349	.273	.219	.178	.142	.110	.080	.051	.025	.012	10
11	.542	.502	.460	.392	.332	.259	.208	.168	.133	.103	.074	.048	.023	.011	11
12	.522	.482	.441	.376	.318	.247	.197	.160	.126	.097	.070	.045	.022	.011	12
13	.503	.465	.425	.361	.305	.237	.188	.153	.120	.092	.067	.043	.021	.010	13
14	.488	.450	.411	.349	.294	.228	.181	.147	.115	.088	.064	.041	.020	.010	14
15	.475	.438	.399	.338	.285	.220	.175	.141	.111	.085	.062	.040	.019	.010	15
16	.463	.426	.388	.329	.277	.213	.169	.136	.107	.082	.060	.039	.019	.009	16
17	.452	.416	.379	.320	.269	.207	.165	.132	.104	.080	.058	.038	.018	.009	17
18	.442	.407	.370	.313	.263	.202	.160	.128	.101	.078	.056	.036	.018	.009	18
19	.433	.398	.363	.306	.258	.197	.157	.125	.098	.076	.055	.036	.017	.008	19
20	.425	.391	.356	.300	.252	.193	.153	.122	.096	.074	.053	.035	.017	.008	20
21	.418	.384	.350	.295	.247	.189	.150	.119	.094	.072	.052	.034	.016	.008	21
22	.411	.378	.344	.290	.242	.185	.147	.117	.092	.071	.051	.033	.016	.008	22
23	.404	.372	.338	.285	.238	.182	.144	.115	.090	.069	.050	.033	.016	.008	23
24	.399	.367	.333	.281	.234	.179	.142	.113	.089	.068	.049	.032	.016	.008	24
25	.393	.362	.329	.277	.230	.176	.139	.111	.088	.067	.048	.032	.015	.008	25
26	.388	.357	.324	.273	.227	.173	.137	.109	.086	.066	.047	.031	.015	.007	26
27	.384	.353	.320	.269	.224	.171	.135	.108	.085	.065	.047	.031	.015	.007	27
28	.380	.349	.316	.266	.220	.168	.133	.106	.084	.064	.046	.030	.015	.007	28
29	.376	.345	.312	.263	.218	.166	.131	.105	.083	.063	.046	.030	.014	.007	29
30	.372	.341	.309	.260	.215	.164	.130	.103	.082	.062	.045	.029	.014	.007	30

PERCENTAGE VALUES FOR r_{11}

$[\Pr(r_{11} > R) = \alpha]$

n \ α	.005	.01	.02	.05	.10	.20	.30	.40	.50	.60	.70	.80	.90	.95	α / n
4	.995	.991	.981	.955	.910	.822	.737	.648	.554	.459	.362	.250	.131	.069	4
5	.937	.916	.876	.807	.728	.615	.524	.444	.369	.296	.224	.151	.078	.039	5
6	.839	.805	.763	.689	.609	.502	.420	.350	.288	.227	.169	.113	.056	.028	6
7	.782	.740	.689	.610	.530	.432	.359	.298	.241	.189	.140	.093	.045	.022	7
8	.725	.683	.631	.554	.479	.385	.318	.260	.210	.164	.121	.079	.037	.019	8
9	.677	.635	.587	.512	.441	.352	.288	.236	.189	.148	.107	.070	.033	.016	9
10	.639	.597	.551	.477	.409	.325	.265	.216	.173	.134	.098	.063	.030	.014	10
11	.606	.566	.521	.450	.385	.305	.248	.202	.161	.124	.090	.058	.028	.013	11
12	.580	.541	.498	.428	.367	.289	.234	.190	.150	.116	.084	.055	.026	.012	12
13	.558	.520	.477	.410	.350	.275	.222	.180	.142	.109	.079	.052	.025	.012	13
14	.539	.502	.460	.395	.336	.264	.212	.171	.135	.104	.075	.049	.024	.011	14
15	.522	.486	.445	.381	.323	.253	.203	.164	.129	.099	.072	.047	.023	.011	15
16	.508	.472	.432	.369	.313	.244	.196	.158	.124	.095	.069	.045	.022	.011	16
17	.495	.460	.420	.359	.303	.236	.190	.152	.119	.092	.067	.044	.021	.010	17
18	.484	.449	.410	.349	.295	.229	.184	.148	.116	.089	.065	.042	.020	.010	18
19	.473	.439	.400	.341	.288	.223	.179	.143	.112	.087	.063	.041	.020	.010	19
20	.464	.430	.392	.334	.282	.218	.174	.139	.110	.084	.061	.040	.019	.010	20
21	.455	.421	.384	.327	.276	.213	.170	.136	.107	.082	.059	.039	.019	.009	21
22	.446	.414	.377	.320	.270	.208	.166	.132	.104	.081	.058	.038	.018	.009	22
23	.439	.407	.371	.314	.265	.204	.163	.130	.102	.079	.056	.037	.018	.009	23
24	.432	.400	.365	.309	.260	.200	.160	.127	.100	.077	.055	.036	.018	.009	24
25	.426	.394	.359	.304	.255	.197	.156	.124	.098	.076	.054	.036	.017	.009	25
26	.420	.389	.354	.299	.250	.193	.154	.122	.096	.074	.053	.035	.017	.008	26
27	.414	.383	.349	.295	.246	.190	.151	.120	.095	.073	.052	.034	.017	.008	27
28	.409	.378	.344	.291	.243	.188	.149	.118	.093	.072	.051	.034	.016	.008	28
29	.404	.374	.340	.287	.239	.185	.146	.116	.092	.070	.051	.033	.016	.008	29
30	.399	.369	.336	.283	.236	.182	.144	.115	.090	.069	.050	.032	.016	.008	30

PERCENTAGE VALUES FOR r_{12}

$[\Pr(r_{12} > R) = \alpha]$

$n \backslash \alpha$	.005	.01	.02	.05	.10	.20	.30	.40	.50	.60	.70	.80	.90	.95	α / n
5	.996	.992	.984	.960	.919	.838	.755	.669	.579	.483	.381	.268	.143	.074	5
6	.951	.925	.891	.824	.745	.635	.545	.465	.390	.316	.240	.165	.088	.049	6
7	.875	.836	.791	.712	.636	.528	.445	.374	.307	.245	.183	.123	.064	.031	7
8	.797	.760	.708	.632	.557	.456	.382	.317	.258	.203	.152	.101	.056	.025	8
9	.739	.701	.656	.580	.504	.409	.339	.270	.227	.177	.130	.086	.044	.021	9
10	.694	.655	.610	.537	.454	.373	.308	.258	.204	.158	.116	.075	.038	.019	10
11	.658	.619	.575	.502	.431	.345	.283	.232	.187	.145	.106	.069	.035	.017	11
12	.629	.590	.546	.473	.406	.324	.265	.217	.174	.135	.098	.063	.032	.016	12
13	.612	.554	.521	.451	.387	.307	.250	.204	.163	.126	.092	.059	.030	.015	13
14	.580	.542	.501	.432	.369	.292	.237	.193	.153	.118	.086	.055	.028	.014	14
15	.560	.523	.482	.416	.354	.280	.226	.184	.146	.112	.082	.053	.026	.013	15
16	.544	.508	.467	.401	.341	.269	.217	.177	.139	.107	.078	.050	.025	.013	16
17	.529	.493	.453	.388	.330	.259	.209	.170	.134	.103	.075	.048	.024	.012	17
18	.516	.480	.440	.377	.320	.251	.202	.163	.129	.099	.072	.047	.023	.012	18
19	.504	.469	.429	.367	.311	.243	.196	.157	.125	.096	.069	.045	.022	.011	19
20	.493	.458	.419	.358	.303	.237	.191	.153	.121	.093	.067	.044	.022	.011	20
21	.483	.449	.410	.349	.296	.231	.186	.148	.118	.090	.065	.042	.021	.010	21
22	.474	.440	.402	.342	.290	.225	.181	.145	.114	.088	.063	.041	.020	.010	22
23	.465	.432	.394	.336	.284	.220	.176	.141	.112	.086	.062	.040	.020	.010	23
24	.457	.423	.387	.330	.278	.216	.173	.138	.109	.084	.060	.039	.019	.010	24
25	.450	.417	.381	.324	.273	.212	.169	.135	.107	.082	.059	.038	.019	.009	25
26	.443	.411	.375	.319	.268	.208	.166	.132	.105	.080	.058	.037	.019	.009	26
27	.437	.405	.370	.314	.263	.204	.163	.130	.103	.079	.057	.037	.018	.009	27
28	.431	.399	.365	.309	.259	.201	.160	.128	.101	.077	.056	.036	.018	.009	28
29	.426	.394	.360	.305	.255	.197	.157	.126	.099	.076	.055	.035	.017	.009	29
30	.420	.389	.355	.301	.251	.194	.154	.124	.098	.075	.054	.035	.017	.009	30

PERCENTAGE VALUES FOR r_{20}

$[\Pr(r_{20} > R) = \alpha]$

n \ α	.005	.01	.02	.05	.10	.20	.30	.40	.50	.60	.70	.80	.90	.95	α / n
4	.996	.992	.987	.967	.935	.871	.807	.743	.676	.606	.529	.440	.321	.235	4
5	.950	.929	.901	.845	.782	.694	.623	.560	.500	.440	.377	.306	.218	.155	5
6	.865	.836	.800	.736	.670	.585	.520	.463	.411	.358	.305	.245	.172	.126	6
7	.814	.778	.732	.661	.596	.516	.454	.402	.355	.306	.261	.208	.144	.099	7
8	.746	.710	.670	.607	.545	.468	.410	.361	.317	.274	.230	.184	.125	.085	8
9	.700	.667	.627	.565	.505	.432	.378	.331	.288	.250	.208	.166	.114	.077	9
10	.664	.632	.592	.531	.474	.404	.354	.307	.268	.231	.192	.153	.104	.070	10
11	.627	.603	.564	.504	.449	.381	.334	.290	.253	.217	.181	.143	.097	.065	11
12	.612	.579	.540	.481	.429	.362	.316	.274	.239	.205	.172	.136	.091	.060	12
13	.590	.557	.520	.461	.411	.345	.301	.261	.227	.195	.164	.129	.086	.057	13
14	.571	.538	.502	.445	.395	.332	.288	.250	.217	.187	.157	.123	.082	.054	14
15	.554	.522	.486	.430	.382	.320	.277	.241	.209	.179	.150	.118	.079	.052	15
16	.539	.508	.472	.418	.370	.310	.268	.233	.202	.173	.144	.113	.076	.050	16
17	.526	.495	.460	.406	.359	.301	.260	.226	.195	.167	.139	.109	.074	.049	17
18	.514	.484	.449	.397	.350	.293	.252	.219	.189	.162	.134	.105	.071	.048	18
19	.503	.473	.439	.379	.341	.286	.246	.213	.184	.157	.130	.101	.069	.047	19
20	.494	.464	.430	.372	.333	.279	.240	.208	.179	.152	.126	.098	.067	.046	20
21	.485	.455	.422	.365	.326	.273	.235	.203	.175	.148	.123	.096	.065	.045	21
22	.477	.447	.414	.358	.320	.267	.230	.199	.171	.145	.120	.094	.064	.044	22
23	.469	.440	.407	.352	.314	.262	.225	.195	.167	.142	.117	.092	.062	.043	23
24	.462	.434	.401	.347	.309	.258	.221	.192	.164	.139	.114	.090	.061	.042	24
25	.456	.428	.395	.343	.304	.254	.217	.189	.161	.136	.112	.089	.060	.041	25
26	.450	.422	.390	.338	.300	.250	.214	.186	.158	.134	.110	.087	.059	.041	26
27	.444	.417	.385	.334	.296	.246	.211	.183	.156	.132	.109	.086	.058	.040	27
28	.439	.412	.381	.330	.292	.243	.208	.180	.154	.130	.107	.085	.058	.040	28
29	.434	.407	.370	.320	.288	.239	.205	.177	.151	.128	.100	.083	.057	.039	29
30	.428	.402	.372	.322	.285	.236	.202	.175	.149	.126	.104	.082	.056	.039	30

PERCENTAGE VALUES FOR r_{21}

$[\Pr(r_{21} > R) = \alpha]$

n \ α	.005	.01	.02	.05	.10	.20	.30	.40	.50	.60	.70	.80	.90	.95	α / n
5	.998	.995	.990	.976	.952	.902	.850	.795	.735	.669	.594	.501	.374	.273	5
6	.970	.951	.924	.872	.821	.745	.680	.621	.563	.504	.439	.364	.268	.195	6
7	.919	.885	.842	.780	.725	.637	.575	.517	.462	.408	.350	.285	.198	.138	7
8	.868	.829	.780	.710	.650	.570	.509	.454	.402	.352	.298	.240	.166	.117	8
9	.816	.776	.725	.657	.594	.516	.458	.407	.360	.313	.265	.212	.146	.103	9
10	.760	.726	.678	.612	.551	.474	.420	.374	.329	.286	.240	.189	.130	.089	10
11	.713	.679	.638	.576	.517	.442	.391	.348	.305	.265	.221	.173	.118	.080	11
12	.675	.642	.605	.546	.490	.419	.370	.326	.285	.247	.206	.161	.110	.074	12
13	.649	.615	.578	.521	.467	.399	.351	.308	.269	.232	.194	.152	.104	.070	13
14	.627	.593	.556	.501	.448	.381	.334	.293	.256	.219	.184	.144	.099	.066	14
15	.607	.574	.537	.483	.431	.366	.319	.280	.245	.208	.175	.138	.094	.062	15
16	.589	.557	.521	.467	.416	.353	.307	.269	.235	.199	.167	.132	.090	.059	16
17	.573	.542	.507	.453	.403	.341	.296	.259	.225	.192	.161	.127	.086	.057	17
18	.559	.529	.494	.440	.391	.331	.287	.250	.218	.186	.155	.122	.082	.054	18
19	.547	.517	.482	.428	.380	.322	.279	.243	.211	.180	.150	.117	.078	.052	19
20	.536	.506	.472	.419	.371	.314	.271	.236	.205	.174	.145	.113	.075	.050	20
21	.526	.496	.462	.410	.363	.306	.264	.229	.199	.170	.141	.110	.073	.049	21
22	.517	.487	.453	.402	.356	.299	.258	.223	.194	.165	.137	.107	.071	.048	22
23	.509	.479	.445	.395	.349	.293	.252	.218	.189	.161	.133	.105	.069	.046	23
24	.501	.471	.438	.388	.343	.287	.247	.214	.185	.158	.130	.103	.068	.045	24
25	.493	.464	.431	.382	.337	.282	.242	.210	.181	.154	.127	.100	.067	.043	25
26	.486	.457	.424	.376	.331	.277	.238	.206	.178	.151	.125	.098	.066	.042	26
27	.479	.450	.418	.370	.325	.273	.234	.203	.175	.149	.123	.096	.064	.041	27
28	.472	.444	.412	.365	.320	.269	.230	.200	.172	.146	.121	.094	.063	.041	28
29	.466	.438	.406	.360	.316	.265	.227	.197	.170	.144	.119	.092	.062	.040	29
30	.460	.433	.401	.355	.312	.261	.224	.194	.167	.142	.117	.091	.061	.040	30

PERCENTAGE VALUES FOR r_{22}

$[\Pr(r_{22} > R) = \alpha]$

n \ α	.005	.01	.02	.05	.10	.20	.30	.40	.50	.60	.70	.80	.90	.95	α / n
6	.998	.995	.992	.983	.965	.930	.880	.830	.780	.720	.640	.540	.410	.300	6
7	.970	.945	.919	.881	.850	.780	.730	.670	.610	.540	.470	.390	.270	.200	7
8	.922	.890	.857	.803	.745	.664	.602	.546	.490	.434	.375	.309	.218	.156	8
9	.873	.840	.800	.737	.676	.592	.530	.478	.425	.373	.320	.261	.186	.128	9
10	.826	.791	.749	.682	.620	.543	.483	.433	.384	.335	.285	.231	.150	.111	10
11	.781	.745	.703	.637	.578	.503	.446	.397	.351	.305	.258	.208	.142	.099	11
12	.740	.704	.661	.600	.543	.470	.416	.370	.325	.282	.238	.190	.130	.090	12
13	.705	.670	.628	.570	.515	.443	.391	.347	.304	.263	.222	.177	.122	.084	13
14	.674	.641	.602	.546	.492	.421	.370	.328	.287	.247	.208	.166	.115	.079	14
15	.647	.616	.579	.525	.472	.402	.353	.312	.273	.234	.196	.156	.109	.075	15
16	.624	.595	.559	.507	.454	.386	.338	.298	.261	.223	.186	.148	.104	.071	16
17	.605	.577	.542	.490	.438	.373	.325	.286	.250	.214	.178	.142	.099	.067	17
18	.589	.561	.527	.475	.424	.361	.314	.276	.241	.206	.171	.135	.094	.063	18
19	.575	.547	.514	.462	.412	.350	.304	.268	.233	.199	.165	.130	.090	.060	19
20	.562	.535	.502	.450	.401	.340	.295	.260	.226	.193	.160	.125	.086	.057	20
21	.551	.524	.491	.440	.391	.331	.287	.252	.220	.187	.155	.120	.082	.054	21
22	.541	.514	.481	.430	.382	.323	.280	.245	.213	.182	.150	.116	.078	.051	22
23	.532	.505	.472	.421	.374	.316	.274	.239	.207	.177	.146	.113	.075	.049	23
24	.524	.497	.484	.413	.367	.310	.268	.232	.201	.172	.142	.111	.074	.047	24
25	.516	.489	.457	.406	.360	.304	.262	.227	.196	.168	.138	.108	.073	.045	25
26	.508	.486	.450	.399	.354	.298	.257	.222	.192	.164	.135	.106	.072	.044	26
27	.501	.475	.443	.393	.348	.292	.252	.218	.189	.161	.132	.104	.071	.043	27
28	.495	.469	.437	.387	.342	.287	.247	.215	.186	.158	.130	.102	.069	.042	28
29	.489	.463	.431	.381	.337	.282	.243	.211	.183	.155	.128	.100	.068	.041	29
30	.483	.457	.425	.376	.332	.278	.239	.208	.180	.153	.126	.098	.067	.041	30

VII.5 PERCENTILE ESTIMATES IN LARGE SAMPLES

A. Estimates of Population Mean

In sampling from a normal population with variance σ^2, the sampling distribution of the median has variance $\frac{1.57\sigma^2}{n}$ for large sample size n. For estimating the mean μ the efficiency of the median P_{50} is .637, i.e.

$$E_{P_{50}} = \frac{\sigma^2/n}{1.57\sigma^2/n} = .637 \ .$$

Higher efficiencies can be obtained from the mean of several percentile values. The efficiencies in this table are for the percentile estimates obtained from the mean of the indicated percentile.

B. Estimates of the Population Standard Deviation

This table gives the efficiencies for estimating the population standard deviation obtained from percentile estimates.

C. Estimates of Mean and Standard Deviation

This table gives percentile values for estimating both the mean and standard deviation and the efficiencies for the estimation of each. The values of K are the multipliers for the estimate of σ.

PERCENTILE ESTIMATES IN LARGE SAMPLES

A. Mean.

	Percentile estimate	Eff.
1	P_{50}	.64
2	$.5(P_{25} + P_{75})$	.81
3	$.3333(P_{17} + P_{50} + P_{83})$	.88
4	$.25(P_{12.5} + P_{37.5} + P_{62.5} + P_{87.5})$	.91
5	$.20(P_{10} + P_{30} + P_{50} + P_{70} + P_{90})$	.93
...	....	...
10	$.10(P_{05} + P_{15} + P_{25} + P_{35} + P_{45} + P_{55} + P_{65} + P_{75} + P_{85} + P_{95})$	.97

B. Standard deviation.

	Percentile estimate	Eff.
2	$.3388(P_{93} - P_{07})$	.65
4	$.1714(P_{97} + P_{85} - P_{15} - P_{03})$	.80
6	$.1180(P_{98} + P_{91} + P_{80} - P_{20} - P_{09} - P_{02})$	.87
8	$.0935(P_{98} + P_{93} + P_{86} + P_{77} - P_{23} - P_{14} - P_{07} - P_{02})$	.90
10	$.0739(P_{98.5} + P_{95} + P_{90} + P_{84} + P_{75} - P_{25} - P_{16} - P_{10} - P_{05} - P_{01.5})$	.92

C. Mean and standard deviation.

	Percentile	Efficiency		K
		Mean	Standard deviation	
2	15, 85	.73	.56	.4824
4	05, 30, 70, 95	.80	.74	.2305
6	05, 15, 40, 60, 85, 95	.89	.80	.1704
8	03, 10, 25, 45, 55, 75, 90, 97	.90	.86	.1262
10	03, 10, 20, 30, 50, 50, 70, 80, 90, 97	.94	.87	.1104

VII.6 SIMPLE ESTIMATES IN SMALL SAMPLES

The observations $x_1, x_2, \ldots, x_n$ are arranged in ascending order $x_{(1)}, x_{(2)}, \ldots, x_{(n)}$.

A. Estimates of the Population Mean

This tables gives variance and efficiency for several alternate estimates of the population mean. The midrange is defined as $(x_{(1)} + x_{(n)})/2$.

B. Estimates of the Population Standard Deviation

(i) The range is a biased estimate of σ. By multiplying the range by a factor, an unbiased estimate is obtained. This table gives values of this factor, along with variance and efficiency of the range.

(ii) The mean deviation can also be used to estimate σ. The mean deviation is given by

$$\text{M.D.} = \frac{1}{n} \sum_{i=1}^{n} |x_i - \bar{x}| \; .$$

It is easy to compute for small samples if the deviations are taken from the median. This table indicates the computation of the sum of these deviations. The multiplier to convert this sum to an unbiased estimate of σ and the efficiencies of this estimate are also included.

(iii) The efficiencies of the range and mean deviation are less than for estimates which are easier to compute than the mean deviation. This table indicates the values to use in computing an estimate of σ which will give the highest efficiency for an estimate of this type. The coefficient is such that this statistic will give an unbiased estimate of σ.

(iv) This table indicates the values to use in computing the best linear estimate of σ. The efficiency of each of these estimates is also given.

SIMPLE ESTIMATES IN SMALL SAMPLES

A. Several estimates of the mean. (Variance to be multiplied by σ^2.)

n	Median		Midrange		Av. of best two			$(x_2 + x_3 + \cdots + x_{n-1})/(n-2)$	
	Var.	Eff.	Var.	Eff.	Statistic	Var.	Eff.	Var.	Eff.
2	.500	1.000	.500	1.000	$\frac{1}{2}(x_1 + x_2)$	.500	1.000		
3	.449	.743	.362	.920	$\frac{1}{2}(x_1 + x_3)$	.362	.920	.449	.743
4	.298	.838	.298	.838	$\frac{1}{2}(x_2 + x_3)$	.298	.838	.298	.838
5	.287	.697	.261	.767	$\frac{1}{2}(x_2 + x_4)$	.231	.867	.227	.881
6	.215	.776	.236	.706	$\frac{1}{2}(x_2 + x_5)$	.193	.865	.184	.906
7	.210	.679	.218	.654	$\frac{1}{2}(x_2 + x_6)$	.168	.849	.155	.922
8	.168	.743	.205	.610	$\frac{1}{2}(x_3 + x_6)$	.149	.837	.134	.934
9	.166	.669	.194	.572	$\frac{1}{2}(x_3 + x_7)$	.132	.843	.118	.942
10	.138	.723	.186	.539	$\frac{1}{2}(x_3 + x_8)$	.119	.840	.105	.949
11	.137	.663	.178	.510	$\frac{1}{2}(x_3 + x_9)$	.109	.832	.0952	.955
12	.118	.709	.172	.484	$\frac{1}{2}(x_4 + x_9)$	.100	.831	.0869	.959
13	.117	.659	.167	.461	$\frac{1}{2}(x_4 + x_{10})$	.0924	.833	.0799	.963
14	.102	.699	.162	.440	$\frac{1}{2}(x_4 + x_{11})$	.0860	.830	.0739	.966
15	.102	.656	.158	.422	$\frac{1}{2}(x_4 + x_{12})$	.0808	.825	.0688	.969
16	.0904	.692	.154	.392	$\frac{1}{2}(x_5 + x_{12})$	.0756	.827	.0644	.971
17	.0901	.653	.151	.389	$\frac{1}{2}(x_5 + x_{13})$	.0711	.827	.0605	.973
18	.0810	.686	.148	.375	$\frac{1}{2}(x_5 + x_{14})$	.0673	.825	.0570	.975
19	.0808	.651	.145	.362	$\frac{1}{2}(x_6 + x_{14})$	.0040	.823	.0539	.976
20	.0734	.681	.143	.350	$\frac{1}{2}(x_6 + x_{15})$	.0607	.824	.0511	.978
∞	$\frac{1.57}{n}$	.637		.000	$\frac{1}{2}(P_{25} + P_{75})$	$\frac{1.24}{n}$	.808		1.000

B. Estimates of mean and dispersion in small samples.
(i) Unbiased estimate of σ using w. (Variance to be multiplied by σ^2.)

Sample size	Estimate	Variance	Eff.	Sample size	Estimate	Variance	Eff.
2	$.886w$	.571	1.000	11	$.315w$	.0616	.831
3	$.591w$	.275	.992	12	$.307w$	.0571	.814
4	$.486w$	.183	.975	13	$.300w$	.0533	.797
5	$.430w$	.138	.955	14	$.294w$	.0502	.781
6	$.395w$	.112	.933	15	$.288w$	.0474	.766
7	$.370w$	.0949	.911	16	$.283w$	.0451	.751
8	$.351w$	.0829	.890	17	$.279w$	.0430	.738
9	$.337w$	.0740	.869	18	$.275w$	.0412	.725
10	$.325w$	.0671	.850	19	$.271w$	.0395	.712
				20	$.268w$	.0381	.700

(ii) Mean deviation estimate of σ.

Sample size	Estimate	Eff.
2	$.8862(x_2 - x_1)$	1.00
3	$.5908(x_3 - x_1)$	.99
4	$.3770(x_4 + x_3 - x_2 - x_1)$	.91
5	$.3016(x_5 + x_4 - x_2 - x_1)$	.94
6	$.2369(x_6 + x_5 + x_4 - x_3 - x_2 - x_1)$	.90
7	$.2031(x_7 + x_6 + x_5 - x_3 - x_2 - x_1)$	.92
8	$.1723(x_8 + x_7 + x_6 + x_5 - x_4 - x_3 - x_2 - x_1)$	.90
9	$.1532(x_9 + x_8 + x_7 + x_6 - x_4 - x_3 - x_2 - x_1)$	.91
10	$.1353(x_{10} + x_9 + x_8 + x_7 + x_6 - x_5 - x_4 - x_3 - x_2 - x_1)$	.89

(iii) Modified linear estimate of σ. (Variance to be multiplied by σ^2.)

Sample size	Estimate	Variance	Eff.
2	$.8862(x_2 - x_1)$	.571	1.000
3	$.5908(x_3 - x_1)$	.275	.992
4	$.4857(x_4 - x_1)$	.183	.975
5	$.4299(x_5 - x_1)$	.138	.955
6	$.2619(x_6 + x_5 - x_2 - x_1)$	.109	.957
7	$.2370(x_7 + x_6 - x_2 - x_1)$	.0895	.967
8	$.2197(x_8 + x_7 - x_2 - x_1)$	.0761	.970
9	$.2068(x_9 + x_8 - x_2 - x_1)$	.0664	.968
10	$.1968(x_{10} + x_9 - x_2 - x_1)$	.0591	.964
11	$.1608(x_{11} + x_{10} + x_8 - x_4 - x_2 - x_1)$	.0529	.967
12	$.1524(x_{12} + x_{11} + x_9 - x_4 - x_2 - x_1)$	.0478	.972
13	$.1456(x_{13} + x_{12} + x_{10} - x_4 - x_2 - x_1)$	.0436	.975
14	$.1399(x_{14} + x_{13} + x_{11} - x_4 - x_2 - x_1)$	.0401	.977
15	$.1352(x_{15} + x_{14} + x_{12} - x_4 - x_2 - x_1)$	.0372	.977
16	$.1311(x_{16} + x_{15} + x_{13} - x_4 - x_2 - x_1)$	.0347	.975
17	$.1050(x_{17} + x_{16} + x_{15} + x_{13} - x_5 - x_3 - x_2 - x_1)$	.0325	.978
18	$.1020(x_{18} + x_{17} + x_{16} + x_{14} - x_5 - x_3 - x_2 - x_1)$	.0305	.978
19	$.09939(x_{19} + x_{18} + x_{17} + x_{15} - x_5 - x_3 - x_2 - x_1)$	.0288	.979
20	$.09706(x_{20} + x_{19} + x_{18} + x_{16} - x_5 - x_3 - x_2 - x_1)$	.0272	.978

(iv) Best linear estimate of σ.

Sample size	Estimate	Eff.
2	$.8862(x_2 - x_1)$	1.000
3	$.5908(x_3 - x_1)$	.992
4	$.4539(x_4 - x_1) + .1102(x_3 - x_2)$	.989
5	$.3724(x_5 - x_1) + .1352(x_4 - x_2)$	.988
6	$.3175(x_6 - x_1) + .1386(x_5 - x_2) + .0432(x_4 - x_3)$	.988
7	$.2778(x_7 - x_1) + .1351(x_6 - x_2) + .0625(x_5 - x_3)$	.989
8	$.2476(x_8 - x_1) + .1294(x_7 - x_2) + .0713(x_6 - x_3) + .0230(x_5 - x_4)$	.989
9	$.2237(x_9 - x_1) + .1233(x_8 - x_2) + .0751(x_7 - x_3) + .0360(x_6 - x_4)$	.989
10	$.2044(x_{10} - x_1) + .1172(x_9 - x_2) + .0763(x_8 - x_3) + .0436(x_7 - x_4)$ $+ .0142(x_6 - x_5)$	.990

VIII. Range and Studentized Range

VIII.1 PROBABILITY INTEGRAL OF THE RANGE

Let $x_1, x_2, \ldots, x_n$ denote a random sample of size n from a population with density function $f(x)$ and distribution function $F(x)$.

Let $x_{(1)}, x_{(2)}, \ldots, x_{(n)}$ denote the same values in ascending order of magnitude. Then the sample range w is defined by

$$w = x_{(n)} - x_{(1)} .$$

In standardized form

$$W = \frac{x_{(n)} - x_{(1)}}{\sigma} = X_{(n)} - X_{(1)} .$$

The probability integral for W for a sample of size n is given by

$$P(W;n) = n \int_{-\infty}^{\infty} [F(X + w) - F(X)]^{n-1} f(X)\, dX .$$

This table gives values of $P(W;n)$ for the normal density function $f(x) = \frac{1}{\sqrt{2\pi}} e^{-\frac{1}{2}x^2}$ and for various values of n and W.

PROBABILITY INTEGRAL OF THE RANGE

W \ n	2	3	4	5	6	7	8	9	10
0.00	0.0000	0.0000							
0.05	.0282	.0007	0.0000						
0.10	.0564	.0028	.0001						
0.15	.0845	.0062	.0004	0.0000					
0.20	.1125	.0110	.0010	.0001					
0.25	0.1403	0.0171	0.0020	0.0002					
0.30	.1680	.0245	.0034	.0004	0.0001				
0.35	.1955	.0332	.0053	.0008	.0001				
0.40	.2227	.0431	.0079	.0014	.0002	0.0000			
0.45	.2497	.0543	.0111	.0022	.0004	.0001			
0.50	0.2763	0.0666	0.0152	0.0033	0.0007	0.0002	0.0000		
0.55	.3027	.0800	.0200	.0048	.0011	.0003	.0001		
0.60	.3286	.0944	.0257	.0068	.0017	.0004	.0001	0.0000	
0.65	.3542	.1099	.0322	.0092	.0026	.0007	.0002	.0001	
0.70	.3794	.1263	.0398	.0121	.0036	.0011	.0003	.0001	
0.75	0.4041	0.1436	0.0483	0.0157	0.0050	0.0016	0.0005	0.0002	0.0000
0.80	.4284	.1616	.0578	.0200	.0068	.0023	.0008	.0002	.0001
0.85	.4522	.1805	.0682	.0250	.0090	.0032	.0011	.0004	.0001
0.90	.4755	.2000	.0797	.0308	.0117	.0044	.0016	.0006	.0002
0.95	.4983	.2201	.0922	.0375	.0150	.0059	.0023	.0009	.0003
1.00	0.5205	0.2407	0.1057	0.0450	0.0188	0.0078	0.0032	0.0013	0.0005
1.05	.5422	.2618	.1201	.0535	.0234	.0101	.0043	.0018	.0008
1.10	.5633	.2833	.1355	.0629	.0287	.0129	.0058	.0025	.0011
1.15	.5839	.3052	.1517	.0733	.0348	.0163	.0075	.0035	.0016
1.20	.6039	.3272	.1688	.0847	.0417	.0203	.0098	.0047	.0022
1.25	0.6232	0.3495	0.1867	0.0970	0.0495	0.0250	0.0125	0.0062	0.0030
1.30	.6420	.3719	.2054	.1104	.0583	.0304	.0157	.0080	.0041
1.35	.6602	.3943	.2248	.1247	.0680	.0366	.0195	.0103	.0054
1.40	.6778	.4168	.2448	.1400	.0787	.0437	.0240	.0131	.0071
1.45	.6948	.4392	.2654	.1562	.0904	0.516	.0292	.0164	.0092
1.50	0.7112	0.4614	0.2865	0.1733	0.1031	0.0606	0.0353	0.0204	0.0117
1.55	.7269	.4835	.3080	.1913	.1168	.0705	.0421	.0250	.0148
1.60	.7421	.5053	.3299	.2101	.1315	.0814	.0499	.0304	.0184
1.65	.7567	.5269	.3521	.2296	.1473	.0934	.0587	.0366	.0227
1.70	.7707	.5481	.3745	.2498	.1639	.1064	.0684	.0437	.0278
1.75	0.7841	0.5690	0.3970	0.2706	0.1815	0.1204	0.0792	0.0517	0.0336
1.80	.7969	.5894	.4197	.2920	.2000	.1355	.0910	.0607	.0403
1.85	.8092	.6094	.4423	.3138	.2193	.1516	.1039	.0707	.0479
1.90	.8209	.6290	.4649	.3361	.2394	.1686	.1178	.0818	.0565
1.95	.8321	.6480	.4874	.3587	.2602	.1867	.1329	.0939	.0661
2.00	0.8427	0.6665	0.5096	0.3816	0.2816	0.2056	0.1489	0.1072	0.0768
2.05	.8528	.6845	.5317	.4046	.3035	.2254	.1661	.1216	.0886
2.10	.8624	.7019	.5534	.4277	.3260	.2460	.1842	.1371	.1015
2.15	.8716	.7187	.5748	.4508	.3489	.2673	.2032	.1536	.1155
2.20	.8802	.7349	.5957	.4739	.3720	.2893	.2232	.1712	.1307
2.25	0.8884	0.7505	0.6163	0.4969	0.3955	0.3118	0.2440	0.1899	0.1470

PROBABILITY INTEGRAL OF THE RANGE

W \ n	11	12	13	14	15	16	17	18	19	20
0.85	0.0000									
0.90	.0001									
0.95	.0001	0.0000								
1.00	0.0002	0.0001	0.0000							
1.05	.0003	.0001	.0001	0.0000						
1.10	.0005	.0002	.0001	0.0001						
1.15	.0007	.0003	.0001	.0001	0.0000					
1.20	.0010	.0005	.0002	.0001	0.0001					
1.25	0.0015	0.0007	0.0004	0.0002	0.0001	0.0000				
1.30	.0021	.0010	.0005	.0003	.0001	.0001	0.0000	0.0000		
1.35	.0028	.0015	.0008	.0004	.0002	.0001	.0001	0.0001		
1.40	.0038	.0021	.0011	.0006	.0003	.0002	.0001	.0001		
1.45	.0051	.0028	.0016	.0009	.0005	.0003	.0001	.0001	0.0000	
1.50	0.0067	0.0038	0.0022	0.0012	0.0007	0.0004	0.0002	0.0001	0.0001	0.0000
1.55	.0087	.0051	.0030	.0017	.0010	.0006	.0003	.0002	.0001	.0001
1.60	.0111	.0067	.0040	.0024	.0014	.0008	.0005	.0003	.0002	.0001
1.65	.0140	.0086	.0053	.0032	.0020	.0012	.0007	.0004	.0003	.0002
1.70	.0176	.0111	.0070	.0044	.0027	.0017	.0011	.0007	.0004	.0003
1.75	0.0217	0.0140	0.0090	0.0058	0.0037	0.0023	0.0015	0.0010	0.0006	0.0004
1.80	.0266	.0175	.0115	.0075	.0049	.0032	.0021	.0014	.0009	.0006
1.85	.0323	.0217	.0145	.0097	.0065	.0043	.0029	.0019	.0013	.0008
1.90	.0388	.0266	.0182	.0124	.0084	.0057	.0039	.0026	.0018	.0012
1.95	.0463	.0323	.0070	.0044	.0108	.0075	.0052	.0036	.0024	.0017
2.00	0.0548	0.0389	0.0276	0.0195	0.0137	0.0097	0.0068	0.0048	0.0033	0.0023
2.05	.0643	.0465	.0335	.0241	.0173	.0124	.0088	.0063	.0045	.0032
2.10	.0748	.0550	.0403	.0295	.0215	.0156	.0114	.0082	.0060	.0043
2.15	.0866	.0646	.0481	.0357	.0265	.0196	.0144	.0106	.0078	.0058
2.20	.0994	.0753	.0569	.0429	.0323	.0242	.0182	.0136	.0102	.0076
2.25	0.1134	0.0872	0.0669	0.0511	0.0390	0.0297	0.0226	0.0172	0.0130	0.0099

PROBABILITY INTEGRAL OF THE RANGE

W \ n	2	3	4	5	6	7	8	9	10
2.25	0.8884	0.7505	0.6163	0.4969	0.3955	0.3118	0.2440	0.1899	0.1470
2.30	.8961	.7655	.6363	.5196	.4190	.3348	.2656	.2095	.1645
2.35	.9034	.7799	.6559	.5421	.4427	.3582	.2878	.2300	.1829
2.40	.9103	.7937	.6748	.5643	.4663	.3820	.3107	.2514	.2025
2.45	.9168	.8069	.6932	.5861	.4899	.4059	.3341	.2735	.2229
2.50	0.9229	0.8195	0.7110	0.6075	0.5132	0.4300	0.3579	0.2963	0.2443
2.55	.9286	.8315	.7282	.6283	.5364	.4541	.3820	.3198	.2665
2.60	.9340	.8429	.7448	.6487	.5592	.4782	.4064	.3437	.2894
2.65	.9390	.8537	.7607	.6685	.5816	.5022	.4310	.3680	.3130
2.70	.9438	.8640	.7759	.6877	.6036	.5259	.4555	.3927	.3372
2.75	0.9482	0.8737	0.7905	0.7063	0.6252	0.5494	0.4801	0.4175	0.3617
2.80	.9523	.8828	.8045	.7242	.6461	.5725	.5045	.4425	.3867
2.85	.9561	.8915	.8177	.7415	.6665	.5952	.5286	.4675	.4119
2.90	.9597	.8996	.8304	.7581	.6863	.6174	.5525	.4923	.4372
2.95	.9630	.9073	.8424	.7739	.7055	.6391	.5760	.5171	.4625
3.00	0.9661	0.9145	0.8537	0.7891	0.7239	0.6601	0.5991	0.5415	0.4878
3.05	.9690	.9212	.8645	.8036	.7416	.6806	.6216	.5656	.5129
3.10	.9716	.9275	.8746	.8174	.7587	.7003	.6436	.5892	.5378
3.15	.9741	.9334	.8842	.8305	.7750	.7194	.6649	.6124	.5623
3.20	.9763	.9388	.8931	.8429	.7905	.7377	.6856	.6350	.5864
3.25	0.9784	0.9439	0.9016	0.8546	0.8053	0.7553	0.7055	0.6569	0.6099
3.30	.9804	.9487	.9095	.8657	.8194	.7721	.7248	.6782	.6329
3.35	.9822	.9531	.9168	.8761	.8327	.7881	.7432	.6988	.6553
3.40	.9838	.9572	.9237	.8859	.8454	.8034	.7609	.7186	.6769
3.45	.9853	.9610	.9302	.8951	.8573	.8179	.7778	.7376	.6978
3.50	0.9867	0.9644	0.9361	0.9037	0.8685	0.8316	0.7938	0.7558	0.7180
3.55	.9879	.9677	.9417	.9117	.8790	.8446	.8091	.7732	.7373
3.60	.9891	.9706	.9468	.9192	.8889	.8568	.8236	.7898	.7558
3.65	.9901	.9734	.9516	.9261	.8981	.8683	.8372	.8055	.7735
3.70	.9911	.9759	.9560	.9326	.9067	.8790	.8501	.8204	.7903
3.75	0.9920	0.9782	0.9600	0.9386	0.9147	0.8891	0.8622	0.8345	0.8062
3.80	.9928	.9803	.9637	.9441	.9222	.8985	.8736	.8477	.8212
3.85	.9935	.9822	.9672	.9493	.9291	.9073	.8842	.8602	.8355
3.90	.9942	.9840	.9703	.9540	.9355	.9155	.8941	.8718	.8488
3.95	.9948	.9856	.9732	.9583	.9415	.9230	.9034	.8827	.8614
4.00	0.9953	0.9870	0.9758	0.9623	0.9469	0.9300	0.9120	0.8929	0.8731
4.05	.9958	.9883	.9782	.9660	.9520	.9365	.9199	.9024	.8841
4.10	.9963	.9895	.9804	.9693	.9566	.9425	.9273	.9112	.8943
4.15	.9967	.9906	.9824	.9724	.9608	.9480	.9341	.9193	.9038
4.20	.9970	.9916	.9842	.9752	.9647	.9530	.9404	.9268	.9126
4.25	0.9973	0.9925	0.9859	0.9777	0.9682	0.9576	0.9461	0.9338	0.9208
4.30	.9976	.9933	.9874	.9800	.9715	.9520	.9514	.9402	.9283
4.35	.9979	.9941	.9887	.9821	.9744	.9657	.9562	.9460	.9352
4.40	.9981	.9947	.9899	.9840	.9771	.9692	.9607	.9514	.9416
4.45	.9983	.9953	.9910	.9857	.9795	.9724	.9647	.9563	.9474
4.50	0.9985	0.9958	0.9920	0.9873	0.9817	0.9754	0.9684	0.9608	0.9527

PROBABILITY INTEGRAL OF THE RANGE

W \ n	11	12	13	14	15	16	17	18	19	20
2.25	0.1134	0.0872	0.0669	0.0511	0.0390	0.0297	0.0226	0.0172	0.0130	0.0099
2.30	.1286	.1003	.0779	.0604	.0468	.0361	.0279	.0214	.0165	.0127
2.35	.1450	.1145	.0902	.0709	.0556	.0435	.0340	.0265	.0207	.0161
2.40	.1624	.1299	.1036	.0825	.0655	.0519	.0411	.0325	.0256	.0202
2.45	.1810	.1466	.1183	.0953	.0766	.0615	.0493	.0394	.0315	.0251
2.50	0.2007	0.1643	0.1342	0.1094	0.0890	0.0722	0.0585	0.0474	0.0383	0.0309
2.55	.2213	.1833	.1513	.1247	.1025	.0842	.0690	.0565	.0462	.0377
2.60	.2429	.2032	.1696	.1413	.1174	.0974	.0807	.0668	.0552	.0455
2.65	.2653	.2243	.1891	.1590	.1335	.1119	.0937	.0783	.0654	.0545
2.70	.2885	.2462	.2096	.1780	.1509	.1278	.1080	.0911	.0768	.0647
2.75	0.3124	0.2690	0.2311	0.1981	0.1696	0.1449	0.1236	0.1053	0.0896	0.0761
2.80	.3368	.2926	.2536	.2194	.1894	.1632	.1405	.1208	.1037	.0889
2.85	.3618	.3169	.2770	.2416	.2103	.1828	.1587	.1376	.1191	.1031
2.90	.3870	.3417	.3011	.2647	.2323	.2036	.1782	.1557	.1360	.1186
2.95	.4125	.3670	.3258	.2887	.2553	.2255	.1989	.1752	.1541	.1355
3.00	0.4382	0.3927	0.3511	0.3134	0.2792	0.2484	0.2207	0.1959	0.1736	0.1537
3.05	.4639	.4186	.3769	.3387	.3039	.2723	.2436	.2177	.1944	.1733
3.10	.4895	.4446	.4029	.3645	.3292	.2969	.2675	.2407	.2163	.1942
3.15	.5150	.4706	.4291	.3907	.3551	.3223	.2922	.2646	.2394	.2163
3.20	.5401	.4965	.4554	.4171	.3814	.3483	.3177	.2894	.2634	.2395
3.25	0.5649	0.5222	0.4817	0.4437	0.4080	0.3748	0.3438	0.3151	0.2884	0.2638
3.30	.5893	.5475	.5078	.4703	.4348	.4016	.3704	.3413	.3142	.2890
3.35	.6131	.5725	.5337	.4967	.4617	.4286	.3974	.3681	.3407	.3150
3.40	.6363	.5970	.5592	.5230	.4885	.4557	.4246	.3953	.3676	.3416
3.45	.6589	.6209	.5842	.5489	.5150	.4827	.4519	.4227	.3950	.3688
3.50	0.6807	0.6442	0.6087	0.5744	0.5413	0.5096	0.4792	0.4502	0.4226	0.3964
3.55	.7017	.6668	.6326	.5994	.5672	.5362	.5063	.4777	.4504	.4242
3.60	.7220	.6886	.6558	.6237	.5926	.5624	.5332	.5051	.4781	.4522
3.65	.7414	.7096	.6782	.6474	.6173	.5881	.5597	.5322	.5056	.4801
3.70	.7600	.7298	.6999	.6704	.6414	.6132	.5856	.5588	.5329	.5078
3.75	0.7776	0.7491	0.7206	0.6925	0.6648	0.6376	0.6110	0.5850	0.5598	0.5352
3.80	.7944	.7675	.7406	.7138	.6874	.6613	.6357	.6106	.5861	.5622
3.85	.8103	.7850	.7596	.7342	.7090	.6842	.6596	.6355	.6118	.5887
3.90	.8254	.8016	.7777	.7537	.7298	.7062	.6827	.6596	.6369	.6145
3.95	.8395	.8173	.7948	.7723	.7497	.7273	.7050	.6829	.6611	.6397
4.00	0.8528	0.8321	0.8111	0.7899	0.7686	0.7474	0.7263	0.7053	0.6845	0.6640
4.05	.8653	.8460	.8264	.8066	.7866	.7666	.7466	.7268	.7070	.6874
4.10	.8769	.8590	.8408	.8223	.8036	.7848	.7660	.7472	.7285	.7099
4.15	.8878	.8712	.8543	.8371	.8196	.8021	.7844	.7667	.7491	.7315
4.20	.8978	.8826	.8669	.8509	.8347	.8183	.8018	.7852	.7686	.7520
4.25	0.9072	0.8931	0.8787	0.8639	0.8488	0.8336	0.8182	0.8027	0.7871	0.7715
4.30	.9158	.9029	.8896	.8760	.8620	.8479	.8336	.8191	.8046	.7899
4.35	.9238	.9120	.8998	.8872	.8744	.8613	.8480	.8346	.8210	.8074
4.40	.9312	.9204	.9092	.8976	.8858	.8737	.8615	.8490	.8364	.8237
4.45	.9379	.9281	.9178	.9073	.8964	.8853	.8740	.8625	.8508	.8391
4.50	0.9441	0.9352	0.9258	0.9162	0.9062	0.8960	0.8856	0.8750	0.8643	0.8534

PROBABILITY INTEGRAL OF THE RANGE

W \ n	2	3	4	5	6	7	8	9	10
4.50	0.9985	0.9958	0.9920	0.9873	0.9817	0.9754	0.9684	0.9608	0.9527
4.55	.9987	.9963	.9929	.9887	.9837	.9780	.9717	.9649	.9576
4.60	.9989	.9967	.9937	.9899	.9855	.9804	.9747	.9686	.9620
4.65	.9990	.9971	.9944	.9911	.9871	.9825	.9775	.9719	.9660
4.70	.9991	.9974	.9951	.9921	.9885	.9845	.9799	.9750	.9696
4.75	0.9992	0.9977	0.9956	0.9930	0.9898	0.9862	0.9822	0.9777	0.9729
4.80	.9993	.9980	.9962	.9938	.9910	.9878	.9842	.9802	.9759
4.85	.9994	.9982	.9966	.9945	.9920	.9892	.9860	.9824	.9786
4.90	.9995	.9985	.9970	.9952	.9930	.9904	.9876	.9844	.9810
4.95	.9995	.9986	.9974	.9958	.9938	.9916	.9890	.9862	.9832
5.00	0.9996	0.9988	0.9977	0.9963	0.9945	0.9926	0.9903	0.9878	0.9851
5.05	.9996	.9990	.9980	.9967	.9952	.9935	.9915	.9893	.9869
5.10	.9997	.9991	.9982	.9971	.9958	.9942	.9925	.9906	.9884
5.15	.9997	.9992	.9985	.9975	.9963	.9950	.9934	.9917	.9898
5.20	.9998	.9993	.9987	.9978	.9968	.9956	.9942	.9927	.9911
5.25	0.9998	0.9994	0.9988	0.9981	0.9972	0.9961	0.9949	0.9936	0.9922
5.30	.9998	.9995	.9990	.9983	.9975	.9966	.9956	.9944	.9931
5.35	.9998	.9995	.9991	.9985	.9979	.9971	.9961	.9951	.9940
5.40	.9999	.9996	.9992	.9987	.9981	.9974	.9966	.9957	.9948
5.45	.9999	.9997	.9993	.9989	.9984	.9978	.9971	.9963	.9954
5.50	0.9999	0.9997	0.9994	0.9990	0.9986	0.9981	0.9974	0.9968	0.9960
5.55	.9999	.9997	.9995	.9992	.9988	.9983	.9978	.9972	.9965
5.60	.9999	.9998	.9996	.9993	.9989	.9985	.9981	.9976	.9970
5.65	.9999	.9998	.9996	.9994	.9991	.9987	.9983	.9979	.9974
5.70	0.9999	.9998	.9997	.9995	.9992	.9989	.9986	.9982	.9977
5.75	1.0000	0.9999	0.9997	0.9995	0.9993	0.9991	0.9988	0.9984	0.9980
5.80		.9999	.9998	.9996	.9994	.9992	.9989	.9986	.9983
5.85		.9999	.9998	.9997	.9995	.9993	.9991	.9988	.9985
5.90		.9999	.9998	.9997	.9996	.9994	.9992	.9990	.9988
5.95		.9999	.9998	.9997	.9996	.9995	.9993	.9991	.9989
6.00		0.9999	0.9999	0.9998	0.9997	0.9996	0.9994	0.9993	0.9991

PROBABILITY INTEGRAL OF THE RANGE

W \ n	11	12	13	14	15	16	17	18	19	20
4.50	0.9441	0.9352	0.9258	0.9162	0.9062	0.8960	0.8856	0.8750	0.8643	0.8534
4.55	.9498	.9417	.9332	.9244	.9153	.9060	.8964	.8867	.8768	.8667
4.60	.9550	.9476	.9399	.9319	.9236	.9151	.9064	.8975	.8884	.8791
4.65	.9597	.9530	.9460	.9388	.9313	.9235	.9155	.9074	.8991	.8906
4.70	.9639	.9579	.9516	.9451	.9382	.9312	.9240	.9165	.9089	.9012
4.75	0.9678	0.9624	0.9567	0.9508	0.9446	0.9383	0.9317	0.9249	0.9180	0.9110
4.80	.9713	.9665	.9614	.9560	.9505	.9447	.9387	.9326	.9263	.9199
4.85	.9745	.9702	.9656	.9608	.9557	.9505	.9452	.9396	.9339	.9281
4.90	.9774	.9735	.9694	.9650	.9605	.9559	.9510	.9460	.9409	.9356
4.95	.9799	.9765	.9728	.9689	.9649	.9607	.9563	.9518	.9472	.9424
5.00	0.9822	0.9791	0.9759	0.9724	0.9688	0.9650	0.9611	0.9571	0.9529	0.9486
5.05	.9843	.9816	.9786	.9756	.9723	.9690	.9655	.9618	.9581	.9543
5.10	.9862	.9837	.9811	.9784	.9755	.9725	.9694	.9661	.9628	.9593
5.15	.9878	.9856	.9833	.9809	.9783	.9757	.9729	.9700	.9670	.9639
5.20	.9893	.9874	.9853	.9832	.9809	.9785	.9760	.9735	.9708	.9681
5.25	0.9906	0.9889	0.9871	0.9852	0.9832	0.9811	0.9789	0.9766	0.9742	0.9718
5.30	.9917	.9903	.9887	.9870	.9852	.9833	.9814	.9794	.9773	.9751
5.35	.9928	.9915	.9901	.9886	.9870	.9854	.9836	.9819	.9800	.9781
5.40	.9937	.9925	.9913	.9900	.9886	.9872	.9856	.9841	.9824	.9807
5.45	.9945	.9935	.9924	.9913	.9900	.9888	.9874	.9860	.9846	.9831
5.50	0.9952	0.9943	0.9934	0.9924	0.9913	0.9902	0.9890	0.9878	0.9865	0.9852
5.55	.9958	.9951	.9942	.9933	.9924	.9914	.9904	.9893	.9882	.9870
5.60	.9964	.9957	.9950	.9942	.9934	.9925	.9916	.9907	.9897	.9887
5.65	.9969	.9963	.9956	.9950	.9943	.9935	.9927	.9919	.9910	.9901
5.70	.9973	.9968	.9962	.9956	.9950	.9944	.9937	.9930	.9922	.9914
5.75	0.9970	0.9972	0.9907	0.9902	0.9957	0.9951	0.9945	0.9939	0.9932	0.9925
5.80	.9980	.9976	.9972	.9967	.9963	.9958	.9952	.9947	.9941	.9935
5.85	.9982	.9979	.9976	.9972	.9968	.9963	.9959	.9954	.9949	.9944
5.90	.9985	.9982	.9979	.9976	.9972	.9968	.9964	.9960	.9956	.9952
5.95	.9987	.9985	.9982	.9979	.9976	.9973	.9969	.9966	.9962	.9958
6.00	0.9989	0.9987	0.9984	0.9982	0.9979	0.9977	0.9974	0.9971	0.9967	0.9964

PROBABILITY INTEGRAL OF THE RANGE

W \ n	2	3	4	5	6	7	8	9	10
6.00		0.9999	0.9999	0.9998	0.9997	0.9996	0.9994	0.9993	0.9991
6.05		0.9999	.9999	.9998	.9997	.9996	.9995	.9994	.9992
6.10		1.0000	.9999	.9998	.9998	.9997	.9996	.9995	.9993
6.15			.9999	.9999	.9998	.9997	.9996	.9995	.9994
6.20			.9999	.9999	.9998	.9998	.9997	.9996	.9995
6.25			0.9999	0.9999	0.9999	0.9998	0.9997	0.9997	0.9996
6.30			1.0000	.9999	.9999	.9998	.9998	.9997	.9996
6.35				.9999	.9999	.9999	.9998	.9998	.9997
6.40				0.9999	.9999	.9999	.9998	.9998	.9997
6.45				0.9999	.9999	.9999	.9999	.9998	.9998
6.50				1.0000	0.9999	0.9999	0.9999	0.9999	0.9998
6.55					0.9999	.9999	.9999	.9999	.9998
6.60					1.0000	.9999	.9999	.9999	.9999
6.65						0.9999	.9999	.9999	.9999
6.70						1.0000	0.9999	.9999	.9999
6.75							1.0000	0.9999	0.9999
6.80								0.9999	.9999
6.85								1.0000	0.9999
6.90									1.0000
6.95									
7.00									
7.05									
7.10									
7.15									
7.20									
7.25									

PROBABILITY INTEGRAL OF THE RANGE

W \ n	11	12	13	14	15	16	17	18	19	20
6.00	0.9989	0.9987	0.9984	0.9982	0.9979	0.9977	0.9974	0.9971	0.9967	0.9964
6.05	.9990	.9989	.9987	.9985	.9982	.9980	.9977	.9975	.9972	.9969
6.10	.9992	.9990	.9989	.9987	.9985	.9983	.9981	.9978	.9976	.9973
6.15	.9993	.9992	.9990	.9989	.9987	.9985	.9983	.9981	.9979	.9977
6.20	.9994	.9993	.9992	.9990	.9989	.9987	.9986	.9984	.9982	.9980
6.25	0.9995	0.9994	0.9993	0.9992	0.9990	0.9989	0.9988	0.9986	0.9985	0.9983
6.30	.9996	.9995	.9994	.9993	.9992	.9991	.9990	.9988	.9987	.9986
6.35	.9996	.9996	.9995	.9994	.9993	.9992	.9991	.9990	.9989	.9988
6.40	.9997	.9996	.9996	.9995	.9994	.9993	.9992	.9992	.9991	.9990
6.45	.9997	.9997	.9996	.9996	.9995	.9994	.9994	.9993	.9992	.9991
6.50	0.9998	0.9997	0.9997	0.9996	0.9996	0.9995	0.9995	0.9994	0.9993	0.9993
6.55	.9998	.9998	.9997	.9997	.9996	.9996	.9995	.9995	.9994	.9994
6.60	.9998	.9998	.9998	.9997	.9997	.9997	.9996	.9996	.9995	.9995
6.65	.9999	.9998	.9998	.9998	.9997	.9997	.9997	.9996	.9996	.9995
6.70	.9999	.9999	.9998	.9998	.9998	.9998	.9997	.9997	.9997	.9996
6.75	0.9999	0.9999	0.9999	0.9998	0.9998	0.9998	0.9998	0.9997	0.9997	0.9997
6.80	.9999	.9999	.9999	.9999	.9998	.9998	.9998	.9998	.9998	.9997
6.85	.9999	.9999	.9999	.9999	.9999	.9999	.9998	.9998	.9998	.9998
6.90	0.9999	.9999	.9999	.9999	.9999	.9999	.9999	.9998	.9998	.9998
6.95	1.0000	0.9999	.9999	.9999	.9999	.9999	.9999	.9999	.9999	.9998
7.00		1.0000	0.9999	0.9999	0.9999	0.9999	0.9999	0.9999	0.9999	0.9999
7.05			1.0000	0.9999	.9999	.9999	.9999	.9999	.9999	.9999
7.10				1.0000	0.9999	0.9999	.9999	.9999	.9999	.9999
7.15					1.0000	1.0000	0.9999	0.9999	.9999	.9999
7.20							0.9999	0.9999	0.9999	0.9999
7.25							1.0000	1.0000	1.0000	0.9999
7.26										1.0000

VIII.2 PERCENTAGE POINTS, DISTRIBUTION OF THE RANGE

Percentage points of the range are found by the use of inverse interpolation in the table for the probability integral of the range.

Size of sample n	Factor $1/d_n$	Lower percentage points						Upper percentage points					
		0.1	**0.5**	**1.0**	**2.5**	**5.0**	**10.0**	**10.0**	**5.0**	**2.5**	**1.0**	**0.5**	**0.1**
2	0.8862	0.00	0.01	0.02	0.04	0.09	0.18	2.33	2.77	3.17	3.64	3.97	4.65
3	.5908	0.06	0.13	0.19	0.30	0.43	0.62	2.90	3.31	3.68	4.12	4.42	5.06
4	.4857	0.20	0.34	0.43	0.59	0.76	0.98	3.24	3.63	3.98	4.40	4.69	5.31
5	.4299	0.37	0.55	0.67	0.85	1.03	1.26	3.48	3.86	4.20	4.60	4.89	5.48
6	0.3946	0.53	0.75	0.87	1.07	1.25	1.49	3.66	4.03	4.36	4.76	5.03	5.62
7	.3698	0.69	0.92	1.05	1.25	1.44	1.68	3.81	4.17	4.49	4.88	5.15	5.73
8	.3512	0.83	1.08	1.20	1.41	1.60	1.84	3.93	4.29	4.60	4.99	5.25	5.82
9	.3367	0.97	1.21	1.34	1.55	1.74	1.97	4.04	4.39	4.70	5.08	5.34	5.90
10	0.3249	1.08	1.33	1.47	1.67	1.86	2.09	4.13	4.47	4.78	5.16	5.42	5.97
11	.3152	1.19	1.45	1.58	1.78	1.97	2.20	4.21	4.55	4.86	5.23	5.49	6.04
12	.3069	1.29	1.55	1.68	1.88	2.07	2.30	4.28	4.62	4.92	5.29	5.55	6.09
13	.2998	1.39	1.64	1.77	1.98	2.16	2.39	4.35	4.68	4.99	5.35	5.60	6.14
14	.2935	1.47	1.72	1.86	2.06	2.24	2.47	4.41	4.74	5.04	5.40	5.65	6.19
15	0.2880	1.55	1.80	1.93	2.14	2.32	2.54	4.47	4.80	5.09	5.45	5.70	6.23
16	.2831	1.63	1.88	2.01	2.21	2.39	2.61	4.52	4.85	5.14	5.49	5.74	6.27
17	.2787	1.69	1.94	2.07	2.27	2.45	2.67	4.57	4.89	5.18	5.54	5.78	6.31
18	.2747	1.76	2.01	2.14	2.34	2.52	2.73	4.61	4.93	5.22	5.57	5.82	6.35
19	.2711	1.82	2.07	2.20	2.39	2.57	2.79	4.65	4.97	5.26	5.61	5.86	6.38
20	0.2677	1.88	2.12	2.25	2.45	2.63	2.84	4.69	5.01	5.30	5.65	5.89	6.41

The unit is the population standard deviation.
Estimate of σ = range (or mean range) in a sample of n observations $\times 1/d_n$.

VIII.3 PERCENTAGE POINTS, STUDENTIZED RANGE

If in the standardized range $W = \frac{w}{\sigma}$, the unknown population standard deviation σ is replaced by s, the sample standard deviation computed from another sample from the same population, then the studentized range q is given by

$$q = \frac{w}{s},$$

where w is the range from a sample of size n and s is independent of w and is based on ν degrees of freedom. The probability integral of the studentized range is given by

$$\Pr\left\{\frac{w}{s} \leq q\right\} = \int_0^\infty \left[\Gamma\left(\frac{\nu}{2}\right)\right]^{-1} 2^{-\frac{1}{2}\nu+1}\nu^{\nu/2}s^{\nu-1}e^{-\frac{1}{2}\nu s^2}f(qs)\, ds$$

where $f(qs)$ is the probability integral of the range for samples of size n.

UPPER 1 PER CENT POINTS OF THE STUDENTIZED RANGE

The entries are $q_{.01}$, where $P(q < q_{.01}) = .99$

ν \ n	2	3	4	5	6	7	8	9	10
1	90.03	135.0	164.3	185.6	202.2	215.8	227.2	237.0	245.6
2	14.04	19.02	22.29	24.72	26.63	28.20	29.53	30.68	31.69
3	8.26	10.62	12.17	13.33	14.24	15.00	15.64	16.20	16.69
4	6.51	8.12	9.17	9.96	10.58	11.10	11.55	11.93	12.27
5	5.70	6.98	7.80	8.42	8.91	9.32	9.67	9.97	10.24
6	5.24	6.33	7.03	7.56	7.97	8.32	8.61	8.87	9.10
7	4.95	5.92	6.54	7.01	7.37	7.68	7.94	8.17	8.37
8	4.75	5.64	6.20	6.62	6.96	7.24	7.47	7.68	7.86
9	4.60	5.43	5.96	6.35	6.66	6.91	7.13	7.33	7.49
10	4.48	5.27	5.77	6.14	6.43	6.67	6.87	7.05	7.21
11	4.39	5.15	5.62	5.97	6.25	6.48	6.67	6.84	6.99
12	4.32	5.05	5.50	5.84	6.10	6.32	6.51	6.67	6.81
13	4.26	4.96	5.40	5.73	5.98	6.19	6.37	6.53	6.67
14	4.21	4.89	5.32	5.63	5.88	6.08	6.26	6.41	6.54
15	4.17	4.84	5.25	5.56	5.80	5.99	6.16	6.31	6.44
16	4.13	4.79	5.19	5.49	5.72	5.92	6.08	6.22	6.35
17	4.10	4.74	5.14	5.43	5.66	5.85	6.01	6.15	6.27
18	4.07	4.70	5.09	5.38	5.60	5.79	5.94	6.08	6.20
19	4.05	4.67	5.05	5.33	5.55	5.73	5.89	6.02	6.14
20	4.02	4.64	5.02	5.29	5.51	5.69	5.84	5.97	6.09
24	3.96	4.55	4.91	5.17	5.37	5.54	5.69	5.81	5.92
30	3.89	4.45	4.80	5.05	5.24	5.40	5.54	5.65	5.76
40	3.82	4.37	4.70	4.93	5.11	5.26	5.39	5.50	5.60
60	3.76	4.28	4.59	4.82	4.99	5.13	5.25	5.36	5.45
120	3.70	4.20	4.50	4.71	4.87	5.01	5.12	5.21	5.30
∞	3.64	4.12	4.40	4.60	4.76	4.88	4.99	5.08	5.16

UPPER 1 PER CENT POINTS OF THE STUDENTIZED RANGE

ν \ n	11	12	13	14	15	16	17	18	19	20
1	253.2	260.0	266.2	271.8	277.0	281.8	286.3	290.4	294.3	298.0
2	32.59	33.40	34.13	34.81	35.43	36.00	36.53	37.03	37.50	37.95
3	17.13	17.53	17.89	18.22	18.52	18.81	19.07	19.32	19.55	19.77
4	12.57	12.84	13.09	13.32	13.53	13.73	13.91	14.08	14.24	14.40
5	10.48	10.70	10.89	11.08	11.24	11.40	11.55	11.68	11.81	11.93
6	9.30	9.48	9.65	9.81	9.95	10.08	10.21	10.32	10.43	10.54
7	8.55	8.71	8.86	9.00	9.12	9.24	9.35	9.46	9.55	9.65
8	8.03	8.18	8.31	8.44	8.55	8.66	8.76	8.85	8.94	9.03
9	7.65	7.78	7.91	8.03	8.13	8.23	8.33	8.41	8.49	8.57
10	7.36	7.49	7.60	7.71	7.81	7.91	7.99	8.08	8.15	8.23
11	7.13	7.25	7.36	7.46	7.56	7.65	7.73	7.81	7.88	7.95
12	6.94	7.06	7.17	7.26	7.36	7.44	7.52	7.59	7.66	7.73
13	6.79	6.90	7.01	7.10	7.19	7.27	7.35	7.42	7.48	7.55
14	6.66	6.77	6.87	6.96	7.05	7.13	7.20	7.27	7.33	7.39
15	6.55	6.66	6.76	6.84	6.93	7.00	7.07	7.14	7.20	7.26
16	6.46	6.56	6.66	6.74	6.82	6.90	6.97	7.03	7.09	7.15
17	6.38	6.48	6.57	6.66	6.73	6.81	6.87	6.94	7.00	7.05
18	6.31	6.41	6.50	6.58	6.65	6.73	6.79	6.85	6.91	6.97
19	6.25	6.34	6.43	6.51	6.58	6.65	6.72	6.78	6.84	6.89
20	6.19	6.28	6.37	6.45	6.52	6.59	6.65	6.71	6.77	6.82
24	6.02	6.11	6.19	6.26	6.33	6.39	6.45	6.51	6.56	6.61
30	5.85	5.93	6.01	6.08	6.14	6.20	6.26	6.31	6.36	6.41
40	5.69	5.76	5.83	5.90	5.96	6.02	6.07	6.12	6.16	6.21
60	5.53	5.60	5.67	5.73	5.78	5.84	5.89	5.93	5.97	6.01
120	5.37	5.44	5.50	5.56	5.61	5.66	5.71	5.75	5.79	5.83
∞	5.23	5.29	5.35	5.40	5.45	5.49	5.54	5.57	5.61	5.65

UPPER 5 PER CENT POINTS OF THE STUDENTIZED RANGE

The entries are $q_{.05}$, where $P(q < q_{.05}) = .95$

ν \ n	2	3	4	5	6	7	8	9	10
1	17.97	26.98	32.82	37.08	40.41	43.12	45.40	47.36	49.07
2	6.08	8.33	9.80	10.88	11.74	12.44	13.03	13.54	13.99
3	4.50	5.91	6.82	7.50	8.04	8.48	8.85	9.18	9.46
4	3.93	5.04	5.76	6.29	6.71	7.05	7.35	7.60	7.83
5	3.64	4.60	5.22	5.67	6.03	6.33	6.58	6.80	6.99
6	3.46	4.34	4.90	5.30	5.63	5.90	6.12	6.32	6.49
7	3.34	4.16	4.68	5.06	5.36	5.61	5.82	6.00	6.16
8	3.26	4.04	4.53	4.89	5.17	5.40	5.60	5.77	5.92
9	3.20	3.95	4.41	4.76	5.02	5.24	5.43	5.59	5.74
10	3.15	3.88	4.33	4.65	4.91	5.12	5.30	5.46	5.60
11	3.11	3.82	4.26	4.57	4.82	5.03	5.20	5.35	5.49
12	3.08	3.77	4.20	4.51	4.75	4.95	5.12	5.27	5.39
13	3.06	3.73	4.15	4.45	4.69	4.88	5.05	5.19	5.32
14	3.03	3.70	4.11	4.41	4.64	4.83	4.99	5.13	5.25
15	3.01	3.67	4.08	4.37	4.59	4.78	4.94	5.08	5.20
16	3.00	3.65	4.05	4.33	4.56	4.74	4.90	5.03	5.15
17	2.98	3.63	4.02	4.30	4.52	4.70	4.86	4.99	5.11
18	2.97	3.61	4.00	4.28	4.49	4.67	4.82	4.96	5.07
19	2.96	3.59	3.98	4.25	4.47	4.65	4.79	4.92	5.04
20	2.95	3.58	3.96	4.23	4.45	4.62	4.77	4.90	5.01
24	2.92	3.53	3.90	4.17	4.37	4.54	4.68	4.81	4.92
30	2.89	3.49	3.85	4.10	4.30	4.46	4.60	4.72	4.82
40	2.86	3.44	3.79	4.04	4.23	4.39	4.52	4.63	4.73
60	2.83	3.40	3.74	3.98	4.16	4.31	4.44	4.55	4.65
120	2.80	3.36	3.68	3.92	4.10	4.24	4.36	4.47	4.56
∞	2.77	3.31	3.63	3.86	4.03	4.17	4.29	4.39	4.47

UPPER 5 PER CENT POINTS OF THE STUDENTIZED RANGE

ν \ n	11	12	13	14	15	16	17	18	19	20
1	50.59	51.96	53.20	54.33	55.36	56.32	57.22	58.04	58.83	59.56
2	14.39	14.75	15.08	15.38	15.65	15.91	16.14	16.37	16.57	16.77
3	9.72	9.95	10.15	10.35	10.53	10.69	10.84	10.98	11.11	11.24
4	8.03	8.21	8.37	8.52	8.66	8.79	8.91	9.03	9.13	9.23
5	7.17	7.32	7.47	7.60	7.72	7.83	7.93	8.03	8.12	8.21
6	6.65	6.79	6.92	7.03	7.14	7.24	7.34	7.43	7.51	7.59
7	6.30	6.43	6.55	6.66	6.76	6.85	6.94	7.02	7.10	7.17
8	6.05	6.18	6.29	6.39	6.48	6.57	6.65	6.73	6.80	6.87
9	5.87	5.98	6.09	6.19	6.28	6.36	6.44	6.51	6.58	6.64
10	5.72	5.83	5.93	6.03	6.11	6.19	6.27	6.34	6.40	6.47
11	5.61	5.71	5.81	5.90	5.98	6.06	6.13	6.20	6.27	6.33
12	5.51	5.61	5.71	5.80	5.88	5.95	6.02	6.09	6.15	6.21
13	5.43	5.53	5.63	5.71	5.79	5.86	5.93	5.99	6.05	6.11
14	5.36	5.46	5.55	5.64	5.71	5.79	5.85	5.91	5.97	6.03
15	5.31	5.40	5.49	5.57	5.65	5.72	5.78	5.85	5.90	5.96
16	5.26	5.35	5.44	5.52	5.59	5.66	5.73	5.79	5.84	5.90
17	5.21	5.31	5.39	5.47	5.54	5.61	5.67	5.73	5.79	5.84
18	5.17	5.27	5.35	5.43	5.50	5.57	5.63	5.69	5.74	5.79
19	5.14	5.23	5.31	5.39	5.46	5.53	5.59	5.65	5.70	5.75
20	5.11	5.20	5.28	5.36	5.43	5.49	5.55	5.61	5.66	5.71
24	5.01	5.10	5.18	5.25	5.32	5.38	5.44	5.49	5.55	5.59
30	4.92	5.00	5.08	5.15	5.21	5.27	5.33	5.38	5.43	5.47
40	4.82	4.90	4.98	5.04	5.11	5.16	5.22	5.27	5.31	5.36
60	4.73	4.81	4.88	4.94	5.00	5.06	5.11	5.15	5.20	5.24
120	4.64	4.71	4.78	4.84	4.90	4.95	5.00	5.04	5.09	5.13
∞	4.55	4.62	4.68	4.74	4.80	4.85	4.89	4.93	4.97	5.01

UPPER 10 PER CENT POINTS OF THE STUDENTIZED RANGE

The entries are $q_{.10}$, where $P(q < q_{.10}) = .90$

ν \ n	2	3	4	5	6	7	8	9	10
1	8.93	13.44	16.36	18.49	20.15	21.51	22.64	23.62	24.48
2	4.13	5.73	6.77	7.54	8.14	8.63	9.05	9.41	9.72
3	3.33	4.47	5.20	5.74	6.16	6.51	6.81	7.06	7.29
4	3.01	3.98	4.59	5.03	5.39	5.68	5.93	6.14	6.33
5	2.85	3.72	4.26	4.66	4.98	5.24	5.46	5.65	5.82
6	2.75	3.56	4.07	4.44	4.73	4.97	5.17	5.34	5.50
7	2.68	3.45	3.93	4.28	4.55	4.78	4.97	5.14	5.28
8	2.63	3.37	3.83	4.17	4.43	4.65	4.83	4.99	5.13
9	2.59	3.32	3.76	4.08	4.34	4.54	4.72	4.87	5.01
10	2.56	3.27	3.70	4.02	4.26	4.47	4.64	4.78	4.91
11	2.54	3.23	3.66	3.96	4.20	4.40	4.57	4.71	4.84
12	2.52	3.20	3.62	3.92	4.16	4.35	4.51	4.65	4.78
13	2.50	3.18	3.59	3.88	4.12	4.30	4.46	4.60	4.72
14	2.49	3.16	3.56	3.85	4.08	4.27	4.42	4.56	4.68
15	2.48	3.14	3.54	3.83	4.05	4.23	4.39	4.52	4.64
16	2.47	3.12	3.52	3.80	4.03	4.21	4.36	4.49	4.61
17	2.46	3.11	3.50	3.78	4.00	4.18	4.33	4.46	4.58
18	2.45	3.10	3.49	3.77	3.98	4.16	4.31	4.44	4.55
19	2.45	3.09	3.47	3.75	3.97	4.14	4.29	4.42	4.53
20	2.44	3.08	3.46	3.74	3.95	4.12	4.27	4.40	4.51
24	2.42	3.05	3.42	3.69	3.90	4.07	4.21	4.34	4.44
30	2.40	3.02	3.39	3.65	3.85	4.02	4.16	4.28	4.38
40	2.38	2.99	3.35	3.60	3.80	3.96	4.10	4.21	4.32
60	2.36	2.96	3.31	3.56	3.75	3.91	4.04	4.16	4.25
120	2.34	2.93	3.28	3.52	3.71	3.86	3.99	4.10	4.19
∞	2.33	2.90	3.24	3.48	3.66	3.81	3.93	4.04	4.13

UPPER 10 PER CENT POINTS OF THE STUDENTIZED RANGE

ν \ n	11	12	13	14	15	16	17	18	19	20
1	25.24	25.92	26.54	27.10	27.62	28.10	28.54	28.96	29.35	29.71
2	10.01	10.26	10.49	10.70	10.89	11.07	11.24	11.39	11.54	11.68
3	7.49	7.67	7.83	7.98	8.12	8.25	8.37	8.48	8.58	8.68
4	6.49	6.65	6.78	6.91	7.02	7.13	7.23	7.33	7.41	7.50
5	5.97	6.10	6.22	6.34	6.44	6.54	6.63	6.71	6.79	6.86
6	5.64	5.76	5.87	5.98	6.07	6.16	6.25	6.32	6.40	6.47
7	5.41	5.53	5.64	5.74	5.83	5.91	5.99	6.06	6.13	6.19
8	5.25	5.36	5.46	5.56	5.64	5.72	5.80	5.87	5.93	6.00
9	5.13	5.23	5.33	5.42	5.51	5.58	5.66	5.72	5.79	5.85
10	5.03	5.13	5.23	5.32	5.40	5.47	5.54	5.61	5.67	5.73
11	4.95	5.05	5.15	5.23	5.31	5.38	5.45	5.51	5.57	5.63
12	4.89	4.99	5.08	5.16	5.24	5.31	5.37	5.44	5.49	5.55
13	4.83	4.93	5.02	5.10	5.18	5.25	5.31	5.37	5.43	5.48
14	4.79	4.88	4.97	5.05	5.12	5.19	5.26	5.32	5.37	5.43
15	4.75	4.84	4.93	5.01	5.08	5.15	5.21	5.27	5.32	5.38
16	4.71	4.81	4.89	4.97	5.04	5.11	5.17	5.23	5.28	5.33
17	4.68	4.77	4.86	4.93	5.01	5.07	5.13	5.19	5.24	5.30
18	4.65	4.75	4.83	4.90	4.98	5.04	5.10	5.16	5.21	5.26
19	4.63	4.72	4.80	4.88	4.95	5.01	5.07	5.13	5.18	5.23
20	4.61	4.70	4.78	4.85	4.92	4.99	5.05	5.10	5.16	5.20
24	4.54	4.63	4.71	4.78	4.85	4.91	4.97	5.02	5.07	5.12
30	4.47	4.56	4.64	4.71	4.77	4.83	4.89	4.94	4.99	5.03
40	4.41	4.49	4.56	4.63	4.69	4.75	4.81	4.86	4.90	4.95
60	4.34	4.42	4.49	4.56	4.62	4.67	4.73	4.78	4.82	4.86
120	4.28	4.35	4.42	4.48	4.54	4.60	4.65	4.69	4.74	4.78
∞	4.21	4.28	4.35	4.41	4.47	4.52	4.57	4.61	4.65	4.69

VIII.4 CRITICAL VALUES FOR DUNCAN'S NEW MULTIPLE RANGE TEST

Let $q = \frac{w}{s}$, where w is the range of n independent normal variables having the same mean and unit standard deviation, and νs^2 is distributed as chi-square with ν degrees of freedom. This table lists the critical values for Duncan's New Multiple Range Test corresponding to protection level $P = \gamma_{p,\alpha} = (1 - \alpha)^{p-1}$ (Significance level α) for testing p successive values out of an ordered arrangement of m means of samples from a normal population, with ν degrees of freedom for the independent estimate s^2 of the population variance. The critical values for Duncan's test are percentage points of the studentized range of $n = p$ observations corresponding to cumulative probability $P = (1 - \alpha)^{p-1}$.

CRITICAL VALUES FOR DUNCAN'S NEW MULTIPLE RANGE TEST

PROTECTION LEVEL $P = (.90)^{p-1}$ SIGNIFICANCE LEVEL $\alpha = .10$

ν \ p	2	3	4	5	6	7	8	9	10
1	8.929	8.929	8.929	8.929	8.929	8.929	8.929	8.929	8.929
2	4.130	4.130	4.130	4.130	4.130	4.130	4.130	4.130	4.130
3	3.328	3.330	3.330	3.330	3.330	3.330	3.330	3.330	3.330
4	3.015	3.074	3.081	3.081	3.081	3.081	3.081	3.081	3.081
5	2.850	2.934	2.964	2.970	2.970	2.970	2.970	2.970	2.970
6	2.748	2.846	2.890	2.908	2.911	2.911	2.911	2.911	2.911
7	2.680	2.785	2.838	2.864	2.876	2.878	2.878	2.878	2.878
8	2.630	2.742	2.800	2.832	2.849	2.857	2.858	2.858	2.858
9	2.592	2.708	2.771	2.808	2.829	2.840	2.845	2.847	2.847
10	2.563	2.682	2.748	2.788	2.813	2.827	2.835	2.839	2.839
11	2.540	2.660	2.730	2.772	2.799	2.817	2.827	2.833	2.835
12	2.521	2.643	2.714	2.759	2.789	2.808	2.821	2.828	2.832
13	2.505	2.628	2.701	2.748	2.779	2.800	2.815	2.824	2.829
14	2.491	2.616	2.690	2.739	2.771	2.794	2.810	2.820	2.827
15	2.479	2.605	2.681	2.731	2.765	2.789	2.805	2.817	2.825
16	2.469	2.596	2.673	2.723	2.759	2.784	2.802	2.815	2.824
17	2.460	2.588	2.665	2.717	2.753	2.780	2.798	2.812	2.822
18	2.452	2.580	2.659	2.712	2.749	2.776	2.796	2.810	2.821
19	2.445	2.574	2.653	2.707	2.745	2.773	2.793	2.808	2.820
20	2.439	2.568	2.648	2.702	2.741	2.770	2.791	2.807	2.819
24	2.420	2.550	2.632	2.688	2.729	2.760	2.783	2.801	2.816
30	2.400	2.532	2.615	2.674	2.717	2.750	2.776	2.796	2.813
40	2.381	2.514	2.600	2.660	2.705	2.741	2.769	2.791	2.810
60	2.363	2.497	2.584	2.646	2.694	2.731	2.761	2.786	2.807
120	2.344	2.479	2.568	2.632	2.682	2.722	2.754	2.781	2.804
∞	2.326	2.462	2.552	2.619	2.670	2.712	2.746	2.776	2.801

ν \ p	11	12	13	14	15	16	17	18	19
1	8.929	8.929	8.929	8.929	8.929	8.929	8.929	8.929	8.929
2	4.130	4.130	4.130	4.130	4.130	4.130	4.130	4.130	4.130
3	3.330	3.330	3.330	3.330	3.330	3.330	3.330	3.330	3.330
4	3.081	3.081	3.081	3.081	3.081	3.081	3.081	3.081	3.081
5	2.970	2.970	2.970	2.970	2.970	2.970	2.970	2.970	2.970
6	2.911	2.911	2.911	2.911	2.911	2.911	2.911	2.911	2.911
7	2.878	2.878	2.878	2.878	2.878	2.878	2.878	2.878	2.878
8	2.858	2.858	2.858	2.858	2.858	2.858	2.858	2.858	2.858
9	2.847	2.847	2.847	2.847	2.847	2.847	2.847	2.847	2.847
10	2.839	2.839	2.839	2.839	2.839	2.839	2.839	2.839	2.839
11	2.835	2.835	2.835	2.835	2.835	2.835	2.835	2.835	2.835
12	2.833	2.833	2.833	2.833	2.833	2.833	2.833	2.833	2.833
13	2.832	2.832	2.832	2.832	2.832	2.832	2.832	2.832	2.832
14	2.831	2.832	2.833	2.833	2.833	2.833	2.833	2.833	2.833
15	2.830	2.833	2.834	2.834	2.834	2.834	2.834	2.834	2.834
16	2.829	2.833	2.835	2.836	2.836	2.836	2.836	2.836	2.836
17	2.829	2.834	2.836	2.838	2.838	2.838	2.838	2.838	2.838
18	2.828	2.834	2.838	2.840	2.840	2.840	2.840	2.840	2.840
19	2.828	2.834	2.839	2.841	2.842	2.843	2.843	2.843	2.843
20	2.828	2.834	2.839	2.843	2.845	2.845	2.845	2.845	2.845
24	2.827	2.835	2.842	2.848	2.851	2.854	2.856	2.857	2.857
30	2.826	2.837	2.846	2.853	2.859	2.863	2.867	2.869	2.871
40	2.825	2.838	2.849	2.858	2.866	2.873	2.878	2.883	2.887
60	2.825	2.839	2.853	2.864	2.874	2.883	2.890	2.897	2.903
120	2.824	2.842	2.857	2,871	2.883	2.893	2.903	2.912	2.920
∞	2.824	2.844	2.861	2.877	2.892	2.905	2.918	2.929	2.939

CRITICAL VALUES FOR DUNCAN'S NEW MULTIPLE RANGE TEST

PROTECTION LEVEL $P = (.90)^{p-1}$ SIGNIFICANCE LEVEL $\alpha = .10$

ν \ p	20	22	24	26	28	30	32	34	36
1	8.929	8.929	8.929	8.929	8.929	8.929	8.929	8.929	8.929
2	4.130	4.130	4.130	4.130	4.130	4.130	4.130	4.130	4.130
3	3.330	3.330	3.330	3.330	3.330	3.330	3.330	3.330	3.330
4	3.081	3.081	3.081	3.081	3.081	3.081	3.081	3.081	3.081
5	2.970	2.970	2.970	2.970	2.970	2.970	2.970	2.970	2.970
6	2.911	2.911	2.911	2.911	2.911	2.911	2.911	2.911	2.911
7	2.878	2.878	2.878	2.878	2.878	2.878	2.878	2.878	2.878
8	2.858	2.858	2.858	2.858	2.858	2.858	2.858	2.858	2.858
9	2.847	2.847	2.847	2.847	2.847	2.847	2.847	2.847	2.847
10	2.839	2.839	2.839	2.839	2.839	2.839	2.839	2.839	2.839
11	2.835	2.835	2.835	2.835	2.835	2.835	2.835	2.835	2.835
12	2.833	2.833	2.833	2.833	2.833	2.833	2.833	2.833	2.833
13	2.832	2.832	2.832	2.832	2.832	2.832	2.832	2.832	2.832
14	2.833	2.833	2.833	2.833	2.833	2.833	2.833	2.833	2.833
15	2.834	2.834	2.834	2.834	2.834	2.834	2.834	2.834	2.834
16	2.836	2.836	2.836	2.836	2.836	2.836	2.836	2.836	2.836
17	2.838	2.838	2.838	2.838	2.838	2.838	2.838	2.838	2.838
18	2.840	2.840	2.840	2.840	2.840	2.840	2.840	2.840	2.840
19	2.843	2.843	2.843	2.843	2.843	2.843	2.843	2.843	2.843
20	2.845	2.845	2.845	2.845	2.845	2.845	2.845	2.845	2.845
24	2.857	2.857	2.857	2.857	2.857	2.857	2.857	2.857	2.857
30	2.873	2.873	2.873	2.873	2.873	2.873	2.873	2.873	2.873
40	2.890	2.894	2.897	2.898	2.898	2.898	2.898	2.898	2.898
60	2.908	2.916	2.923	2.927	2.931	2.933	3.935	2.935	2.936
120	2.928	2.940	2.951	2.960	2.967	2.974	2.979	2.984	2.988
∞	2.949	2.966	2.982	2.995	3.008	3.019	3.029	3.038	3.047

ν \ p	38	40	50	60	70	80	90	100
1	8.929	8.929	8.929	8.929	8.929	8.929	8.929	8.929
2	4.130	4.130	4.130	4.130	4.130	4.130	4.130	4.130
3	3.330	3.330	3.330	3.330	3.330	3.330	3.330	3.330
4	3.081	3.081	3.081	3.081	3.081	3.081	3.081	3.081
5	2.970	2.970	2.970	2.970	2.970	2.970	2.970	2.970
6	2.911	2.911	2.911	2.911	2.911	2.911	2.911	2.911
7	2.878	2.878	2.878	2.878	2.878	2.878	2.878	2.878
7	2.858	2.858	2.858	2.858	2.858	2.858	2.858	2.858
9	2.847	2.847	2.847	2.847	2.847	2.847	2.847	2.847
10	2.839	2.839	2.839	2.839	2.839	2.839	2.839	2.839
11	2.835	2.835	2.835	2.835	2.835	2.835	2.835	2.835
12	2.833	2.833	2.833	2.833	2.833	2.833	2.833	2.833
13	2.832	2.832	2.832	2.832	2.832	2.832	2.832	2.832
14	2.833	2.833	2.833	2.833	2.833	2.833	2.833	2.833
15	2.834	2.834	2.834	2.834	2.834	2.834	2.834	2.834
16	2.836	2.836	2.836	2.836	2.836	2.836	2.836	2.836
17	2.838	2.838	2.838	2.838	2.838	2.838	2.838	2.838
18	2.840	2.840	2.840	2.840	2.840	2.840	2.840	2.840
19	2.843	2.843	2.843	2.843	2.843	2.843	2.843	2.843
20	2.845	2.845	2.845	2.845	2.845	2.845	2.845	2.845
24	2.857	2.857	2.857	2.857	2.857	2.857	2.857	2.857
30	2.873	2.873	2.873	2.873	2.873	2.873	2.873	2.873
40	2.898	2.898	2.898	2.898	2.898	2.898	2.898	2.898
60	2.936	2.936	2.936	2.936	2.936	2.936	2.936	2.936
120	2.991	2.994	3.001	3.001	3.001	3.001	3.001	3.001
∞	3.054	3.062	3.091	3.113	3.129	3.143	3.154	3.163

CRITICAL VALUES FOR DUNCAN'S NEW MULTIPLE RANGE TEST

PROTECTION LEVEL $P = (.95)^{p-1}$ SIGNIFICANCE LEVEL $\alpha = .05$

ν \ p	2	3	4	5	6	7	8	9	10
1	17.97	17.97	17.97	17.97	17.97	17.97	17.97	17.97	17.97
2	6.085	6.085	6.085	6.085	6.085	6.085	6.085	6.085	6.085
3	4.501	4.516	4.516	4.516	4.516	4.516	4.516	4.516	4.516
4	3.927	4.013	4.033	4.033	4.033	4.033	4.033	4.033	4.033
5	3.635	3.749	3.797	3.814	3.814	3.814	3.814	3.814	3.814
6	3.461	3.587	3.649	3.680	3.694	3.697	3.697	3.697	3.697
7	3.344	3.477	3.548	3.588	3.611	3.622	3.626	3.626	3.626
8	3.261	3.399	3.475	3.521	3.549	3.566	3.575	3.579	3.579
9	3.199	3.339	3.420	3.470	3.502	3.523	3.536	3.544	3.547
10	3.151	3.293	3.376	3.430	3.465	3.489	3.505	3.516	3.522
11	3.113	3.256	3.342	3.397	3.435	3.462	3.480	3.493	3.501
12	3.082	3.225	3.313	3.370	3.410	3.439	3.459	3.474	3.484
13	3.055	3.200	3.289	3.348	3.389	3.419	3.442	3.458	3.470
14	3.033	3.178	3.268	3.329	3.372	3.403	3.426	3.444	3.457
15	3.014	3.160	3.250	3.312	3.356	3.389	3.413	3.432	3.446
16	2.998	3.144	3.235	3.298	3.343	3.376	3.402	3.422	3.437
17	2.984	3.130	3.222	3.285	3.331	3.366	3.392	3.412	3.429
18	2.971	3.118	3.210	3.274	3.321	3.356	3.383	3.405	3.421
19	2.960	3.107	3.199	3.264	3.311	3.347	3.375	3.397	3.415
20	2.950	3.097	3.190	3.255	3.303	3.339	3.368	3.391	3.409
24	2.919	3.066	3.160	3.226	3.276	3.315	3.345	3.370	3.390
30	2.888	3.035	3.131	3.199	3.250	3.290	3.322	3.349	3.371
40	2.858	3.006	3.102	3.171	3.224	3.266	3.300	3.328	3.352
60	2.829	2.976	3.073	3.143	3.198	3.241	3.277	3.307	3.333
120	2.800	2.947	3.045	3.116	3.172	3.217	3.254	3.287	3.314
∞	2.772	2.918	3.017	3.089	3.146	3.193	3.232	3.265	3.294

ν \ p	11	12	13	14	15	16	17	18	19
1	17.97	17.97	17.97	17.97	17.97	17.97	17.97	17.97	17.97
2	6.085	6.085	6.085	6.085	6.085	6.085	6.085	6.085	6.085
3	4.516	4.516	4.516	4.516	4.516	4.516	4.516	4.516	4.516
4	4.033	4.033	4.033	4.033	4.033	4.033	4.033	4.033	4.033
5	3.814	3.814	3.814	3.814	3.814	3.814	3.814	3.814	3.814
6	3.697	3.697	3.697	3.697	3.697	3.697	3.697	3.697	3.697
7	3.626	3.626	3.626	3.626	3.626	3.626	3.626	3.626	3.626
8	3.579	3.579	3.579	3.579	3.579	3.579	3.579	3.579	3.579
9	3.547	3.547	3.547	3.547	3.547	3.547	3.547	3.547	3.547
10	3.525	3.526	3.526	3.526	3.526	3.526	3.526	3.526	3.526
11	3.506	3.509	3.510	3.510	3.510	3.510	3.510	3.510	3.510
12	3.491	3.496	3.498	3.499	3.499	3.499	3.499	3.499	3.499
13	3.478	3.484	3.488	3.490	3.490	3.490	3.490	3.490	3.490
14	3.467	3.474	3.479	3.482	3.484	3.484	3.485	3.485	3.485
15	3.457	3.465	3.471	3.476	3.478	3.480	3.481	3.481	3.481
16	3.449	3.458	3.465	3.470	3.473	3.477	3.478	3.478	3.478
17	3.441	3.451	3.459	3.465	3.469	3.473	3.475	3.476	3.476
18	3.435	3.445	3.454	3.460	3.465	3.470	3.472	3.474	3.474
19	3.429	3.440	3.449	3.456	3.462	3.467	3.470	3.472	3.473
20	3.424	3.436	3.445	3.453	3.459	3.464	3.467	3.470	3.472
24	3.406	3.420	3.432	3.441	3.449	3.456	3.461	3.465	3.469
30	3.389	3.405	3.418	3.430	3.439	3.447	3.454	3.460	3.466
40	3.373	3.390	3.405	3.418	3.429	3.439	3.448	3.456	3.463
60	3.355	3.374	3.391	3.406	3.419	3.431	3.442	3.451	3.460
120	3.337	3.359	3.377	3.394	3.409	3.423	3.435	3.446	3.457
∞	3.320	3.343	3.363	3.382	3.399	3.414	3.428	3.442	3.454

CRITICAL VALUES FOR DUNCAN'S NEW MULTIPLE RANGE TEST

PROTECTION LEVEL $P = (.95)^{p-1}$ SIGNIFICANCE LEVEL $\alpha = .05$

ν \ p	20	22	24	26	28	30	32	34	36
1	17.97	17.97	17.97	17.97	17.97	17.97	17.97	17.97	17.97
2	6.085	6.085	6.085	6.085	6.085	6.085	6.085	6.085	6.085
3	4.516	4.516	4.516	4.516	4.516	4.516	4.516	4.516	4.516
4	4.033	4.033	4.033	4.033	4.033	4.033	3.033	4.033	4.033
5	3.814	3.814	3.814	3.814	3.814	3.814	3.814	3.814	3.814
6	3.697	3.697	3.697	3.697	3.697	3.697	3.697	3.697	3.697
7	3.626	3.626	3.626	3.626	3.626	3.626	3.626	3.626	3.626
8	3.579	3.579	3.579	3.579	3.579	3.579	3.579	3.579	3.579
9	3.547	3.547	3.547	3.547	3.547	3.547	3.547	3.547	3.547
10	3.526	3.526	3.526	3.526	3.526	3.526	3.526	3.526	3.526
11	3.510	3.510	3.510	3.510	3.510	3.510	3.510	3.510	3.510
12	3.499	3.499	3.499	3.499	3.499	3.499	3.499	3.499	3.499
13	3.490	3.490	3.490	3.490	3.490	3.490	3.490	3.490	3.490
14	3.485	3.485	3.485	3.485	3.485	3.485	3.485	3.485	3.485
15	3.481	3.481	3.481	3.481	3.481	3.481	3.481	3.481	3.481
16	3.478	3.478	3.478	3.478	3.478	3.478	3.478	3.478	3.478
17	3.476	3.476	3.476	3.476	3.476	3.476	3.476	3.476	3.476
18	3.474	3.474	3.474	3.474	3.474	3.474	3.474	3.474	3.474
19	3.474	3.474	3.474	3.474	3.474	3.474	3.474	3.474	3.474
20	3.473	3.474	3.474	3.474	3.474	3.474	3.474	3.474	3.474
24	3.471	3.475	3.477	3.477	3.477	3.477	3.477	3.477	3.477
30	3.470	3.477	3.481	3.484	3.486	3.486	3.486	3.486	3.486
40	3.469	3.479	3.486	3.492	3.497	3.500	3.503	3.504	3.504
60	3.467	3.481	3.492	3.501	3.509	3.515	3.521	3.525	3.529
120	3.466	3.483	3.498	3.511	3.522	3.532	3.541	3.548	3.555
∞	3.466	3.486	3.505	3.522	3.536	3.550	3.562	3.574	3.584

ν \ p	38	40	50	60	70	80	90	100
1	17.97	17.97	17.97	17.97	17.97	17.97	17.97	17.97
2	6.085	6.085	6.085	6.085	6.085	6.085	6.085	6.085
3	4.516	4.516	4.516	4.516	4.516	4.516	4.516	4.516
4	4.033	4.033	4.033	4.033	4.033	4.033	4.033	4.033
5	3.814	3.814	3.814	3.814	3.814	3.814	3.814	3.814
6	3.697	3.697	3.697	3.697	3.697	3.697	3.697	3.697
7	3.626	3.626	3.626	3.626	3.626	3.626	3.626	3.626
8	3.579	3.579	3.579	3.579	3.579	3.579	3.579	3.579
9	3.547	3.547	3.547	3.547	3.547	3.547	3.547	3.547
10	3.526	3.526	3.526	3.526	3.526	3.526	3.526	3.526
11	3.510	3.510	3.510	3.510	3.510	3.510	3.510	3.510
12	3.499	3.499	3.499	3.499	3.499	3.499	3.499	3.499
13	3.490	3.490	3.490	3.490	3.490	3.490	3.490	3.490
14	3.485	3.485	3.485	3.485	3.485	3.485	3.485	3.485
15	3.481	3.481	3.481	3.481	3.481	3.481	3.481	3.481
16	3.478	3.478	3.478	3.478	3.478	3.478	3.478	3.478
17	3.476	3.476	3.476	3.476	3.476	3.476	3.476	3.476
18	3.474	3.474	3.474	3.474	3.474	3.474	3.474	3.474
19	3.474	3.474	3.474	3.474	3.474	3.474	3.474	3.474
20	3.474	3.474	3.474	3.474	3.474	3.474	3.474	3.474
24	3.477	3.477	3.477	3.477	3.477	3.477	3.477	3.477
30	3.486	3.486	3.486	3.486	3.486	3.486	3.486	3.486
40	3.504	3.504	3.504	3.504	3.504	3.504	3.504	3.504
60	3.531	3.534	3.537	3.537	3.537	3.537	3.537	3.537
120	3.561	3.566	3.585	3.596	3.600	3.601	3.601	3.601
∞	3.594	3.603	3.640	3.668	3.690	3.708	3.722	3.735

CRITICAL VALUES FOR DUNCAN'S NEW MULTIPLE RANGE TEST

PROTECTION LEVEL $P = (.99)^{p-1}$ SIGNIFICANCE LEVEL $\alpha = .01$

ν \ p	2	3	4	5	6	7	8	9	10
1	90.03	90.03	90.03	90.03	90.03	90.03	90.03	90.03	90.03
2	14.04	14.04	14.04	14.04	14.04	14.04	14.04	14.04	14.04
3	8.261	8.321	8.321	8.321	8.321	8.321	8.321	8.321	8.321
4	6.512	6.677	6.740	6.756	6.756	6.756	6.756	6.756	6.756
5	5.702	5.893	5.989	6.040	6.065	6.074	6.074	6.074	6.074
6	5.243	5.439	5.549	5.614	5.655	5.680	5.694	5.701	5.703
7	4.949	5.145	5.260	5.334	5.383	5.416	5.439	5.454	5.464
8	4.746	4.939	5.057	5.135	5.189	5.227	5.256	5.276	5.291
9	4.596	4.787	4.906	4.986	5.043	5.086	5.118	5.142	5.160
10	4.482	4.671	4.790	4.871	4.931	4.975	5.010	5.037	5.058
11	4.392	4.579	4.697	4.780	4.841	4.887	4.924	4.952	4.975
12	4.320	4.504	4.622	4.706	4.767	4.815	4.852	4.883	4.907
13	4.260	4.442	4.560	4.644	4.706	4.755	4.793	4.824	4.850
14	4.210	4.391	4.508	4.591	4.654	4.704	4.743	4.775	4.802
15	4.168	4.347	4.463	4.547	4.610	4.660	4.700	4.733	4.760
16	4.131	4.309	4.425	4.509	4.572	4.622	4.663	4.696	4.724
17	4.099	4.275	4.391	4.475	4.539	4.589	4.630	4.664	4.693
18	4.071	4.246	4.362	4.445	4.509	4.560	4.601	4.635	4.664
19	4.046	4.220	4.335	4.419	4.483	4.534	4.575	4.610	4.639
20	4.024	4.197	4.312	4.395	4.459	4.510	4.552	4.587	4.617
24	3.956	4.126	4.239	4.322	4.386	4.437	4.480	4.516	4.546
30	3.889	4.056	4.168	4.250	4.314	4.366	4.409	4.445	4.477
40	3.825	3.988	4.098	4.180	4.244	4.296	4.339	4.376	4.408
60	3.762	3.922	4.031	4.111	4.174	4.226	4.270	4.307	4.340
120	3.702	3.858	3.965	4.044	4.107	4.158	4.202	4.239	4.272
∞	3.643	3.796	3.900	3.978	4.040	4.091	4.135	4.172	4.205

ν \ p	11	12	13	14	15	16	17	18	19
1	90.03	90.03	90.03	90.03	90.03	90.03	90.03	90.03	90.03
2	14.04	14.04	14.04	14.04	14.04	14.04	14.04	14.04	14.04
3	8.321	8.321	8.321	8.321	8.321	8.321	8.321	8.321	8.321
4	6.756	6.756	6.756	6.756	6.756	6.756	6.756	6.756	6.756
5	6.074	6.074	6.074	6.074	6.074	6.074	6.074	6.074	6.074
6	5.703	5.703	5.703	5.703	5.703	5.703	5.703	5.703	5.703
7	5.470	5.472	5.472	5.472	5.472	5.472	5.472	5.742	5.472
8	5.302	5.309	5.314	5.316	5.317	5.317	5.317	5.317	5.317
9	5.174	5.185	5.193	5.199	5.203	5.205	5.206	5.206	5.206
10	5.074	5.088	5.098	5.106	5.112	5.117	5.120	5.122	5.124
11	4.994	5.009	5.021	5.031	5.039	5.045	5.050	5.054	5.057
12	4.927	4.944	4.958	4.969	4.978	4.986	4.993	4.998	5.002
13	4.872	4.889	4.904	4.917	4.928	4.937	4.944	4.950	4.956
14	4.824	4.843	4.859	4.872	4.884	4.894	4.902	4.910	4.916
15	4.783	4.803	4.820	4.834	4.846	4.857	4.866	4.874	4.881
16	4.748	4.768	4.786	4.800	4.813	4.825	4.835	4.844	4.851
17	4.717	4.738	4.756	4.771	4.785	4.797	4.807	4.816	4.824
18	4.689	4.711	4.729	4.745	4.759	4.772	4.783	4.792	4.801
19	4.665	4.686	4.705	4.722	4.736	4.749	4.761	4.771	4.780
20	4.642	4.664	4.684	4.701	4.716	4.729	4.741	4.751	4.761
24	4.573	4.596	4.616	4.634	4.651	4.665	4.678	4.690	4.700
30	4.504	4.528	4.550	4.569	4.586	4.601	4.615	4.628	4.640
40	4.436	4.461	4.483	4.503	4.521	4.537	4.553	4.566	4.579
60	4.368	4.394	4.417	4.438	4.456	4.474	4.490	4.504	4.518
120	4.301	4.327	4.351	4.372	4.392	4.410	4.426	4.442	4.456
∞	4.235	4.261	4.285	4.307	4.327	4.345	4.363	4.379	4.394

CRITICAL VALUES FOR DUNCAN'S NEW MULTIPLE RANGE TEST

PROTECTION LEVEL $P = (.99)^{p-1}$ SIGNIFICANCE LEVEL $\alpha = .01$

ν \ p	20	22	24	26	28	30	32	34	36
1	90.03	90.03	90.03	90.03	90.03	90.03	90.03	90.03	90.03
2	14.04	14.04	14.04	14.04	14.04	14.04	14.04	14.04	14.04
3	8.321	8.321	8.321	8.321	8.321	8.321	8.321	8.321	8.321
4	6.756	6.756	6.756	6.756	6.756	6.756	6.756	6.756	6.756
5	6.074	6.074	6.074	6.074	6.074	6.074	6.074	6.074	6.074
6	5.703	5.703	5.703	5.703	5.703	5.703	5.703	5.703	5.703
7	5.472	5.472	5.472	5.472	5.472	5.472	5.472	5.472	5.472
8	5.317	5.317	5.317	5.317	5.317	5.317	5.317	5.317	5.317
9	5.206	5.206	5.206	5.206	5.206	5.206	5.206	5.206	5.206
10	5.124	5.124	5.124	5.124	5.124	5.124	5.124	5.124	5.124
11	5.059	5.061	5.061	5.061	5.061	5.061	5.061	5.061	5.061
12	5.006	5.010	5.011	5.011	5.011	5.011	5.011	5.011	5.011
13	4.960	4.966	4.970	4.972	4.972	4.972	4.972	4.972	4.972
14	4.921	4.929	4.935	4.938	4.940	4.940	4.940	4.940	4.940
15	4.887	4.897	4.904	4.909	4.912	4.914	4.914	4.914	4.914
16	4.858	4.869	4.877	4.883	4.887	4.890	4.892	4.892	4.892
17	4.832	4.844	4.853	4.860	4.865	4.869	4.872	4.873	4.874
18	4.808	4.821	4.832	4.839	4.846	4.850	4.854	4.856	4.857
19	4.788	4.802	4.812	4.821	4.828	4.833	4.838	4.841	4.843
20	4.769	4.784	4.795	4.805	4.813	4.818	4.823	4.827	4.830
24	4.710	4.727	4.741	4.752	4.762	4.770	4.777	4.783	4.788
30	4.650	4.669	4.685	4.699	4.711	4.721	4.730	4.738	4.744
40	4.591	4.611	4.630	4.645	4.659	4.671	4.682	4.692	4.700
60	4.530	4.553	4.573	4.591	4.607	4.620	4.633	4.645	4.655
120	4.469	4.494	4.516	4.535	4.552	4.568	4.583	4.596	4.609
∞	4.408	4.434	4.457	4.478	4.497	4.514	4.530	4.545	4.559

ν \ p	38	40	50	60	70	80	90	100
1	90.03	90.03	90.03	90.03	90.03	90.03	90.03	90.03
2	14.04	14.04	14.04	14.04	14.04	14.04	14.04	14.04
3	8.321	8.321	8.321	8.321	8.321	8.321	8.321	8.321
4	6.756	6.756	6.756	6.756	6.756	6.756	6.756	6.756
5	6.074	6.074	6.074	6.074	6.074	6.074	6.074	6.074
6	5.703	5.703	5.703	5.703	5.703	5.703	5.703	5.703
7	5.472	5.472	5.472	5.472	5.472	5.472	5.472	5.472
8	5.317	5.317	5.317	5.317	5.317	5.317	5.317	5.317
9	5.206	5.206	5.206	5.206	5.206	5.206	5.206	5.206
10	5.124	5.124	5.124	5.124	5.124	5.124	5.124	5.124
11	5.061	5.061	5.061	5.061	5.061	5.061	5.061	5.061
12	5.011	5.011	5.011	5.011	5.011	5.011	5.011	5.011
13	4.972	4.972	4.972	4.972	4.972	4.972	4.972	4.972
14	4.940	4.940	4.940	4.940	4.940	4.940	4.940	4.940
15	4.914	4.914	4.914	4.914	4.914	4.914	4.914	4.914
16	4.892	4.892	4.892	4.892	4.892	4.892	4.892	4.892
17	4.874	4.874	4.874	4.874	4.874	4.874	4.874	4.874
18	4.858	4.858	4.858	4.858	4.858	4.858	4.858	4.858
19	4.844	4.845	4.845	4.845	4.845	4.845	4.845	4.845
20	4.832	4.833	4.833	4.833	4.833	4.833	4.833	4.833
24	4.791	4.794	4.802	4.802	4.802	4.802	4.802	4.802
30	4.750	4.755	4.772	4.777	4.777	4.777	4.777	4.777
40	4.708	4.715	4.740	4.754	4.761	4.764	4.764	4.764
60	4.665	4.673	4.707	4.730	4.745	4.755	4.761	4.765
120	4.619	4.630	4.673	4.703	4.727	4.745	4.759	4.770
∞	4.572	4.584	4.635	4.675	4.707	4.734	4.756	4.776

CRITICAL VALUES FOR DUNCAN'S NEW MULTIPLE RANGE TEST

PROTECTION LEVEL $P = (.995)^{p-1}$ SIGNIFICANCE LEVEL $\alpha = .005$

ν \ p	2	3	4	5	6	7	8	9	10
1	180.1	180.1	180.1	180.1	180.1	180.1	180.1	180.1	180.1
2	19.93	19.93	19.93	19.93	19.93	19.93	19.93	19.93	19.93
3	10.55	10.63	10.63	10.63	10.63	10.63	10.63	10.63	10.63
4	7.916	8.126	8.210	8.238	8.238	8.238	8.238	8.238	8.238
5	6.751	6.980	7.100	7.167	7.204	7.222	7.228	7.228	7.228
6	6.105	6.334	6.466	6.547	6.600	6.635	6.658	6.672	6.679
7	5.699	5.922	6.057	6.145	6.207	6.250	6.281	6.304	6.320
8	5.420	5.638	5.773	5.864	5.930	5.978	6.014	6.042	6.064
9	5.218	5.430	5.565	5.657	5.725	5.776	5.815	5.846	5.871
10	5.065	5.273	5.405	5.498	5.567	5.620	5.662	5.695	5.722
11	4.945	5.149	5.280	5.372	5.442	5.496	5.539	5.574	5.603
12	4.849	5.048	5.178	5.270	5.341	5.396	5.439	5.475	5.505
13	4.770	4.966	5.094	5.186	5.256	5.312	5.356	5.393	5.424
14	4.704	4.897	5.023	5.116	5.185	5.241	5.286	5.324	5.355
15	4.647	4.838	4.964	5.055	5.125	5.181	5.226	5.264	5.297
16	4.599	4.787	4.912	5.003	5.073	5.129	5.175	5.213	5.245
17	4.557	4.744	4.867	4.958	5.027	5.084	5.130	5.168	5.201
18	4.521	4.705	4.828	4.918	4.987	5.043	5.090	5.129	5.162
19	4.488	4.671	4.793	4.883	4.952	5.008	5.054	5.093	5.127
20	4.460	4.641	4.762	4.851	4.920	4.976	5.022	5.061	5.095
24	4.371	4.547	4.666	4.753	4.822	4.877	4.924	4.963	4.997
30	4.285	4.456	4.572	4.658	4.726	4.781	4.827	4.867	4.901
40	4.202	4.369	4.482	4.566	4.632	4.687	4.733	4.772	4.806
60	4.122	4.284	4.394	4.476	4.541	4.595	4.640	4.679	4.713
120	4.045	4.201	4.308	4.388	4.452	4.505	4.550	4.588	4.622
∞	3.970	4.121	4.225	4.303	4.365	4.417	4.461	4.499	4.532

ν \ p	11	12	13	14	15	16	17	18	19
1	180.1	180.1	180.1	180.1	180.1	180.1	180.1	180.1	180.1
2	19.93	19.93	19.93	19.93	19.93	19.93	19.93	19.93	19.93
3	10.63	10.63	10.63	10.63	10.63	10.63	10.63	10.63	10.63
4	8.238	8.238	8.238	8.238	8.238	8.238	8.238	8.238	8.238
5	7.228	7.228	7.228	7.228	7.228	7.228	7.228	7.228	7.228
6	6.682	6.682	6.682	6.682	6.682	6.682	6.682	6.682	6.682
7	6.331	6.339	6.343	6.345	6.345	6.345	6.345	6.345	6.345
8	6.080	6.092	6.101	6.108	6.113	6.116	6.118	6.119	6.119
9	5.891	5.907	5.920	5.930	5.938	5.944	5.949	5.952	5.955
10	5.744	5.762	5.777	5.790	5.800	5.809	5.816	5.821	5.826
11	5.626	5.646	5.663	5.678	5.690	5.700	5.709	5.716	5.722
12	5.531	5.552	5.570	5.585	5.599	5.610	5.620	5.629	5.636
13	5.450	5.472	5.492	5.508	5.523	5.535	5.546	5.556	5.564
14	5.382	5.405	5.425	5.442	5.458	5.471	5.483	5.494	5.503
15	5.324	5.348	5.368	5.386	5.402	5.416	5.429	5.440	5.450
16	5.273	5.298	5.319	5.338	5.354	5.368	5.381	5.393	5.404
17	5.229	5.254	5.275	5.295	5.311	5.327	5.340	5.352	5.363
18	5.190	5.215	5.237	5.256	5.274	5.289	5.303	5.316	5.327
19	5.156	5.181	5.203	5.222	5.240	5.256	5.270	5.283	5.295
20	5.124	5.150	5.172	5.193	5.210	5.226	5.241	5.254	5.266
24	5.027	5.053	5.076	5.097	5.116	5.133	5.148	5.162	5.175
30	4.931	4.958	4.981	5.003	5.022	5.040	5.056	5.071	5.085
40	4.837	4.864	4.888	4.910	4.930	4.948	4.965	4.980	4.995
60	4.744	4.771	4.796	4.818	4.838	4.857	4.874	4.890	4.905
120	4.652	4.679	4.704	4.726	4.747	4.766	4.784	4.800	4.815
∞	4.562	4.589	4.614	4.636	4.657	4.676	4.694	4.710	4.726

CRITICAL VALUES FOR DUNCAN'S NEW MULTIPLE RANGE TEST

PROTECTION LEVEL $P = (.995)^{p-1}$ SIGNIFICANCE LEVEL $\alpha = .005$

ν \ p	20	22	24	26	28	30	32	34	36
1	180.1	180.1	180.1	180.1	180.1	180.1	180.1	180.1	180.1
2	19.93	19.93	19.93	19.93	19.93	19.93	19.93	19.93	19.93
3	10.63	10.63	10.63	10.63	10.63	10.63	10.63	10.63	10.63
4	8.238	8.238	8.238	8.238	8.238	8.238	8.238	8.238	8.238
5	7.228	7.228	7.228	7.228	7.228	7.228	7.228	7.228	7.228
6	6.682	6.682	6.682	6.682	6.682	6.682	6.682	6.682	6.682
7	6.345	6.345	6.345	6.345	6.345	6.345	6.345	6.345	6.345
8	6.119	6.119	6.119	6.119	6.119	6.119	6.119	6.119	6.119
9	5.956	5.957	5.957	5.957	5.957	5.957	5.957	5.957	5.957
10	5.829	5.834	5.836	5.836	5.836	5.836	5.836	5.836	5.836
11	5.727	5.735	5.740	5.743	5.744	5.744	5.744	5.744	5.744
12	5.642	5.653	5.660	5.665	5.668	5.670	5.670	5.670	5.670
13	5.571	5.583	5.593	5.600	5.605	5.608	5.610	5.611	5.611
14	5.511	5.525	5.535	5.544	5.550	5.555	5.559	5.561	5.563
15	5.459	5.474	5.486	5.495	5.503	5.509	5.514	5.518	5.520
16	5.413	5.429	5.442	5.453	5.462	5.469	5.475	5.479	5.483
17	5.373	5.390	5.404	5.416	5.425	5.433	5.440	5.445	5.450
18	5.338	5.355	5.370	5.383	5.393	5.402	5.409	5.415	5.420
19	5.306	5.325	5.340	5.353	5.364	5.374	5.382	5.388	5.395
20	5.277	5.296	5.313	5.326	5.338	5.348	5.357	5.364	5.370
24	5.187	5.209	5.226	5.242	5.255	5.267	5.278	5.287	5.295
30	5.098	5.120	5.140	5.157	5.172	5.186	5.198	5.209	5.218
40	5.008	5.032	5.054	5.072	5.089	5.104	5.118	5.130	5.141
60	4.919	4.944	4.967	4.987	5.005	5.021	5.036	5.050	5.062
120	4.830	4.856	4.880	4.901	4.920	4.937	4.953	4.968	4.982
∞	4.740	4.767	4.792	4.813	4.833	4.852	4.869	4.885	4.899

ν \ p	38	40	50	60	70	80	90	100
1	180.1	180.1	180.1	180.1	180.1	180.1	180.0	180.1
2	19.93	19.93	19.93	19.93	19.93	19.93	19.93	19.93
3	10.63	10.63	10.63	10.63	10.63	10.63	10.63	10.63
4	8.238	8.238	8.238	8.238	8.238	8.238	8.238	8.238
5	7.228	7.228	7.228	7.228	7.228	7.228	7.228	7.228
6	6.682	6.682	6.682	6.682	6.682	6.682	6.682	6.682
7	6.345	6.345	6.345	6.345	6.345	6.345	6.345	6.345
8	6.119	6.119	6.119	6.119	6.119	6.119	6.119	6.119
9	5.957	5.957	5.957	5.957	5.957	5.957	5.957	5.957
10	5.836	5.836	5.836	5.836	5.836	5.836	5.836	5.836
11	5.744	5.744	5.744	5.744	5.744	5.744	5.744	5.744
12	5.670	5.670	5.670	5.670	5.670	5.670	5.670	5.670
13	5.611	5.611	5.611	5.611	5.611	5.611	5.611	5.611
14	5.563	5.563	5.563	5.563	5.563	5.563	5.563	5.563
15	5.522	5.523	5.523	5.523	5.523	5.523	5.523	5.523
16	5.485	5.488	5.489	5.489	5.489	5.489	5.489	5.489
17	5.453	5.456	5.461	5.461	5.461	5.461	5.461	5.461
18	5.425	5.428	5.436	5.436	5.436	5.436	5.436	5.436
19	5.399	5.403	5.414	5.415	5.415	5.415	5.415	5.415
20	5.376	5.380	5.394	5.397	5.397	5.397	5.397	5.397
24	5.302	5.308	5.329	5.340	5.343	5.343	5.343	5.343
30	5.227	5.235	5.264	5.281	5.292	5.297	5.298	5.298
40	5.151	5.160	5.197	5.221	5.238	5.249	5.257	5.261
60	5.074	5.084	5.128	5.159	5.182	5.199	5.213	5.223
120	4.995	5.007	5.056	5.094	5.123	5.146	5.166	5.182
∞	4.913	4.926	4.981	5.024	5.059	5.088	5.114	5.136

CRITICAL VALUES FOR DUNCAN'S NEW MULTIPLE RANGE TEST

PROTECTION LEVEL $P = (.999)^{p-1}$ SIGNIFICANCE LEVEL $\alpha = .001$

ν \ p	2	3	4	5	6	7	8	9	10
1	900.3	900.3	900.3	900.3	900.3	900.3	900.3	900.3	900.3
2	44.69	44.69	44.69	44.69	44.69	44.69	44.69	44.69	44.69
3	18.28	18.45	18.45	18.45	18.45	18.45	18.45	18.45	18.45
4	12.18	12.52	12.67	12.73	12.75	12.75	12.75	12.75	12.75
5	9.714	10.05	10.24	10.35	10.42	10.46	10.48	10.49	10.49
6	8.427	8.743	8.932	9.055	9.139	9.198	9.241	9.272	9.294
7	7.648	7.943	8.127	8.252	8.342	8.409	8.460	8.500	8.530
8	7.130	7.407	7.584	7.708	7.799	7.869	7.924	7.968	8.004
9	6.762	7.024	7.195	7.316	7.407	7.478	7.535	7.582	7.619
10	6.487	6.738	6.902	7.021	7.111	7.182	7.240	7.287	7.327
11	6.275	6.516	6.676	6.791	6.880	6.950	7.008	7.056	7.097
12	6.106	6.340	6.494	6.607	6.695	6.765	6.822	6.870	6.911
13	5.970	6.195	6.346	6.457	6.543	6.612	6.670	6.718	6.759
14	5.856	6.075	6.223	6.332	6.416	6.485	6.542	6.590	6.631
15	5.760	5.974	6.119	6.225	6.309	6.377	6.433	6.481	6.522
16	5.678	5.888	6.030	6.135	6.217	6.284	6.340	6.388	6.429
17	5.608	5.813	5.953	6.056	6.138	6.204	6.260	6.307	6.348
18	5.546	5.748	5.886	5.988	6.068	6.134	6.189	6.236	6.277
19	5.492	5.691	5.826	5.927	6.007	6.072	6.127	6.174	6.214
20	5.444	5.640	5.774	5.873	5.952	6.017	6.071	6.117	6.158
24	5.297	5.484	5.612	5.708	5.784	5.846	5.899	5.945	5.984
30	5.156	5.335	5.457	5.549	5.622	5.682	5.734	5.778	5.817
40	5.022	5.191	5.308	5.396	5.466	5.524	5.574	5.617	5.654
60	4.894	5.055	5.166	5.249	5.317	5.372	5.420	5.461	5.498
120	4.771	4.924	5.029	5.109	5.173	5.226	5.271	5.311	5.346
∞	4.654	4.798	4.898	4.974	5.034	5.085	5.128	5.166	5.199

ν \ p	11	12	13	14	15	16	17	18	19
1	900.3	900.3	900.3	900.3	900.3	900.3	900.3	900.3	900.3
2	44.69	44.69	44.69	44.69	44.69	44.69	44.69	44.69	44.69
3	18.45	18.45	18.45	18.45	18.45	18.45	18.45	18.45	18.45
4	12.75	12.75	12.75	12.75	12.75	12.75	12.75	12.75	12.75
5	10.49	10.49	10.49	10.49	10.49	10.49	10.49	10.49	10.49
6	9.309	9.319	9.325	9.328	9.329	9.329	9.329	9.329	9.329
7	8.555	8.574	8.589	8.600	8.609	8.616	8.621	8.624	8.626
8	8.033	8.057	8.078	8.094	8.108	8.119	8.129	8.137	8.143
9	7.652	7.679	7.702	7.722	7.739	7.753	7.766	7.777	7.786
10	7.361	7.390	7.415	7.437	7.456	7.472	7.487	7.500	7.511
11	7.132	7.162	7.188	7.211	7.231	7.250	7.266	7.280	7.293
12	6.947	6.978	7.005	7.029	7.050	7.069	7.086	7.102	7.116
13	6.795	6.826	6.854	6.878	6.900	6.920	6.937	6.954	6.968
14	6.667	6.699	6.727	6.752	6.774	6.794	6.812	6.829	6.844
15	6.558	6.590	6.619	6.644	6.666	6.687	6.706	6.723	6.739
16	6.465	6.497	6.525	6.551	6.574	6.595	6.614	6.631	6.647
17	6.384	6.416	6.444	6.470	6.493	6.514	6.533	6.551	6.567
18	6.313	6.345	6.373	6.399	6.422	6.443	6.462	6.480	6.497
19	6.250	6.281	6.310	6.336	6.359	6.380	6.400	6.418	6.434
20	6.193	6.225	6.254	6.279	6.303	6.324	6.344	6.362	6.379
24	6.020	6.051	6.079	6.105	6.129	6.150	6.170	6.188	6.205
30	5.851	5.882	5.910	5.935	5.958	5.980	6.000	6.018	6.036
40	5.688	5.718	5.745	5.770	5.793	5.814	5.834	5.852	5.869
60	5.530	5.559	5.586	5.610	5.632	5.653	5.672	5.690	5.707
120	5.377	5.405	5.341	5.454	5.476	5.496	5.515	5.532	5.549
∞	5.229	5.256	5.280	5.303	5.324	5.343	5.361	5.378	5.394

CRITICAL VALUES FOR DUNCAN'S NEW MULTIPLE RANGE TEST

PROTECTION LEVEL $P = (.999)^{p-1}$ SIGNIFICANCE LEVEL $\alpha = .001$

ν \ p	20	22	24	26	28	30	32	34	36
1	900.3	900.3	900.3	900.3	900.3	900.3	900.3	900.3	900.3
2	44.69	44.69	44.69	44.69	44.69	44.69	44.69	44.69	44.69
3	18.45	18.45	18.45	18.45	18.45	18.45	18.45	18.45	18.45
4	12.75	12.75	12.75	12.75	12.75	12.75	12.75	12.75	12.75
5	10.49	10.49	10.49	10.49	10.49	10.49	10.49	10.49	10.49
6	9.329	9.329	9.329	9.329	9.329	9.329	9.329	9.329	9.329
7	8.627	8.627	8.627	8.627	8.627	8.627	8.627	8.627	8.627
8	8.149	8.156	8.160	8.161	8.161	8.161	8.161	8.161	8.161
9	7.794	7.808	7.817	7.824	7.828	7.831	7.832	7.832	7.832
10	7.522	7.538	7.552	7.562	7.570	7.577	7.582	7.585	7.587
11	7.304	7.324	7.340	7.354	7.364	7.373	7.380	7.386	7.391
12	7.128	7.150	7.168	7.184	7.196	7.207	7.216	7.223	7.230
13	6.982	7.005	7.025	7.042	7.056	7.068	7.079	7.088	7.096
14	6.858	6.883	6.904	6.922	6.937	6.951	6.962	6.973	6.982
15	6.753	6.778	6.800	6.819	6.836	6.850	6.863	6.874	6.883
16	6.661	6.688	6.711	6.730	6.748	6.763	6.776	6.788	6.799
17	6.582	6.609	6.632	6.653	6.670	6.686	6.701	6.713	6.724
18	6.512	6.539	6.563	6.584	6.602	6.619	6.633	6.647	6.658
19	6.450	6.477	6.501	6.523	6.542	6.559	6.574	6.587	6.600
20	6.394	6.422	6.447	6.468	6.487	6.505	6.520	6.534	6.547
24	6.221	6.250	6.275	6.298	6.318	6.336	6.353	6.368	6.381
30	6.051	6.081	6.106	6.130	6.151	6.169	6.187	6.203	6.217
40	5.885	5.915	5.941	5.964	5.986	6.005	6.023	6.040	6.055
60	5.723	5.752	5.778	5.802	5.823	5.843	5.862	5.878	5.894
120	5.565	5.593	5.619	5.642	5.664	5.683	5.702	5.718	5.734
∞	5.409	5.437	5.462	5.485	5.506	5.525	5.543	5.560	5.576

ν \ p	38	40	50	60	70	80	90	100
1	900.3	900.3	900.3	900.3	900.3	900.3	900.3	900.3
2	44.69	44.69	44.69	44.69	44.69	44.69	44.69	44.69
3	18.45	18.45	18.45	18.45	18.45	18.45	18.45	18.45
4	12.75	12.75	12.75	12.75	12.75	12.75	12.75	12.75
5	10.49	10.49	10.49	10.49	10.49	10.49	10.49	10.49
6	9.329	9.329	9.329	9.329	9.329	9.329	9.329	9.329
7	8.627	8.627	8.627	8.627	8.627	8.627	8.627	8.627
8	8.161	8.161	8.161	8.161	8.161	8.161	8.161	8.161
9	7.832	7.832	7.832	7.832	7.832	7.832	7.832	7.832
10	7.588	7.588	7.588	7.588	7.588	7.588	7.588	7.588
11	7.394	7.397	7.400	7.400	7.400	7.400	7.400	7.400
12	7.235	7.239	7.251	7.251	7.251	7.251	7.251	7.251
13	7.102	7.108	7.126	7.132	7.132	7.132	7.132	7.132
14	6.989	6.996	7.019	7.030	7.034	7.034	7.034	7.034
15	6.892	6.900	6.927	6.942	6.949	6.951	6.951	6.951
16	6.808	6.816	6.848	6.865	6.875	6.880	6.881	6.881
17	6.734	6.743	6.777	6.798	6.811	6.818	6.821	6.821
18	6.669	6.679	6.715	6.738	6.753	6.762	6.767	6.770
19	6.611	6.621	6.660	6.685	6.702	6.713	6.719	6.723
20	6.558	6.569	6.610	6.637	6.655	6.668	6.676	6.681
24	6.394	6.405	6.451	6.484	6.507	6.525	6.538	6.547
30	6.231	6.243	6.294	6.331	6.360	6.381	6.399	6.412
40	6.069	6.082	6.137	6.178	6.210	6.236	6.257	6.274
60	5.909	5.922	5.980	6.024	6.059	6.088	6.113	6.134
120	5.749	5.763	5.822	5.868	5.906	5.938	5.965	5.988
∞	5.590	5.604	5.663	5.711	5.750	5.783	5.811	5.837

VIII.5 SUBSTITUTE *t*-RATIOS

A. The statistic $\tau_1 = \dfrac{\bar{x} - \mu}{w}$, where w is the range of the observations can be used to test hypotheses about μ. This table gives percentage points of the distribution of τ_1 for sample sizes up to 20. The percentage points at the top of the table are upper percentage points. Lower percentage points are obtained by entering the bottom of the table and prefixing the tabulated value with a minus sign.

B. The statistic $\tau_d = \dfrac{\bar{x}_1 - \bar{x}_2}{\frac{1}{2}(w_1 + w_2)}$ may be used to test hypotheses about the differences between means. Percentage points of the distribution of τ_d are given for samples of equal size up to 20.

C. The statistic $\tau_2 = \dfrac{\frac{1}{2}[x_{(1)} + x_{(n)}] - \mu}{w}$ can be used to test hypotheses about μ. This table gives percentage points of the distribution of τ_2 for samples of size 10 or less.

SUBSTITUTE *t*-RATIOS

A. Percentiles* for $\tau_1 = \dfrac{\bar{x} - \mu}{w}$

Sample size	P_{95}	$P_{97.5}$	P_{99}	$P_{99.5}$	$P_{99.9}$	$P_{99.95}$
2	3.175	6.353	15.910	31.828	159.16	318.31
3	.885	1.304	2.111	3.008	6.77	9.58
4	.529	.717	1.023	1.316	2.29	2.85
5	.388	.507	.685	.843	1.32	1.58
6	.312	.399	.523	.628	.92	1.07
7	.263	.333	.429	.507	.71	.82
8	.230	.288	.366	.429	.59	.67
9	.205	.255	.322	.374	.50	.57
10	.186	.230	.288	.333	.44	.50
11	.170	.210	.262	.302	.40	.44
12	.158	.194	.241	.277	.36	.40
13	.147	.181	.224	.256	.33	.37
14	.138	.170	.209	.239	.31	.34
15	.131	.160	.197	.224	.29	.32
16	.124	.151	.186	.212	.27	.30
17	.118	.144	.177	.201	.26	.28
18	.113	.137	.168	.191	.24	.26
19	.108	.131	.161	.182	.23	.25
20	.104	.126	.154	.175	.22	.24
	$-P_{05}$	$-P_{02.5}$	$-P_{01}$	$-P_{0.5}$	$-P_{0.1}$	$-P_{0.05}$

* When the table is read from the foot, the tabled values are to be prefixed with a negative sign.

SUBSTITUTE *t*-RATIOS

B. Percentiles* for $\tau_d = \dfrac{\bar{x}_1 - \bar{x}_2}{\frac{1}{2}(w_1 + w_2)}$

Sample sizes $N_1 = N_2$	P_{95}	$P_{97.5}$	P_{99}	$P_{99.5}$	$P_{99.9}$	$P_{99.95}$
2	2.322	3.427	5.553	7.916	17.81	25.23
3	.974	1.272	1.715	2.093	3.27	4.18
4	.644	.813	1.047	1.237	1.74	1.99
5	.493	.613	.772	.896	1.21	1.35
6	.405	.499	.621	.714	.94	1.03
7	.347	.426	.525	.600	.77	.85
8	.306	.373	.459	.521	.67	.73
9	.275	.334	.409	.464	.59	.64
10	.250	.304	.371	.419	.53	.58
11	.233	.280	.340	.384	.48	.52
12	.214	.260	.315	.355	.44	.48
13	.201	.243	.294	.331	.41	.45
14	.189	.228	.276	.311	.39	.42
15	.179	.216	.261	.293	.36	.39
16	.170	.205	.247	.278	.34	.37
17	.162	.195	.236	.264	.33	.35
18	.155	.187	.225	.252	.31	.34
19	.149	.179	.216	.242	.30	.32
20	.143	.172	.207	.232	.29	.31
	$-P_{05}$	$-P_{02.5}$	$-P_{01}$	$-P_{0.5}$	$-P_{0.1}$	$-P_{0.05}$

* When the table is read from the foot, the tabled values are to be prefixed with a negative sign.

C. Percentiles for $\tau_2 = \dfrac{\frac{1}{2}[x_{(1)} + x_{(n)}] - \mu}{w}$

Sample size	P_{95}	$P_{97.5}$	P_{99}	$P_{99.5}$
2	3.16	6.35	15.91	31.83
3	.90	1.30	2.11	3.02
4	.55	.74	1.04	1.37
5	.42	.52	.71	.85
6	.35	.43	.56	.66
7	.30	.37	.47	.55
8	.26	.33	.42	.47
9	.24	.30	.38	.42
10	.22	.27	.35	.39
	$-P_{05}$	$-P_{02.5}$	$-P_{01}$	$-P_{0.5}$

VIII.6 SUBSTITUTE F-RATIO

The ratio $F' = w_1/w_2$ of two ranges can be used as a substitute for the ratio of two variances. This table gives percentage points of the ratio of two ranges for respective sample sizes n_1 and n_2 less than or equal to 10. The hypothesis $\sigma_1 = \sigma_2$ is rejected if F' is significantly large or small. To test the hypothesis $\sigma_1 = \sigma_2$ at the α-level of significance, use the critical region $F' < F'_{\frac{1}{2}\alpha}$ and $F' > F'_{1-\frac{1}{2}\alpha}$. For a one-sided test $\sigma_1 \leq \sigma_2$ the α-critical region is $F' > F'_{1-\alpha}$.

SUBSTITUTE *F*-RATIO

Sample size for denominator	Cum. prop.	Sample size for numerator								
		2	3	4	5	6	7	8	9	10
2	.005	.0078	.096	.21	.30	.38	.44	.49	.54	.57
	.01	.0157	.136	.26	.38	.46	.53	.59	.64	.68
	.025	.039	.217	.37	.50	.60	.68	.74	.79	.83
	.05	.079	.31	.50	.62	.74	.80	.86	.91	.95
	.95	12.7	19.1	23	26	29	30	32	34	35
	.975	25.5	38.2	52	57	60	62	64	67	68
	.99	63.7	95	116	132	142	153	160	168	174
	.995	127	191	230	250	260	270	280	290	290
3	.005	.0052	.071	.16	.24	.32	.38	.43	.47	.50
	.01	.0105	.100	.20	.30	.37	.43	.49	.53	.57
	.025	.026	.160	.28	.39	.47	.54	.59	.64	.68
	.05	.052	.23	.37	.49	.57	.64	.70	.75	.80
	.95	3.19	4.4	5.0	5.7	6.2	6.6	6.9	7.2	7.4
	.975	4.61	6.3	7.3	8.0	8.7	9.3	9.8	10.2	10.5
	.99	7.37	10	12	13	14	15	15	16	17
	.995	10.4	14	17	18	20	21	22	23	25
4	.005	.0043	.059	.14	.22	.28	.34	.39	.43	.46
	.01	.0086	.084	.18	.26	.33	.39	.44	.48	.52
	.025	.019	.137	.25	.34	.42	.48	.53	.57	.61
	.05	.043	.20	.32	.42	.50	.57	.62	.67	.70
	.95	2.02	2.7	3.1	3.4	3.6	3.8	4.0	4.2	4.4
	.975	2.72	3.5	4.0	4.4	4.7	5.0	5.2	5.4	5.6
	.99	3.83	5.0	5.5	6.0	6.4	6.7	7.0	7.2	7.5
	.995	4.85	6.1	7.0	7.6	8.1	8.5	8.8	9.3	9.6
5	.005	.0039	.054	.13	.20	.26	.32	.36	.40	.44
	.01	.0076	.079	.17	.24	.31	.36	.41	.45	.49
	.025	.018	.124	.23	.32	.38	.44	.49	.53	.57
	.05	.038	.18	.29	.40	.46	.52	.57	.61	.65
	.95	1.61	2.1	2.4	2.6	2.8	2.9	3.0	3.1	3.2
	.975	2.01	2.6	2.9	3.2	3.4	3.6	3.7	3.8	3.9
	.99	2.64	3.4	3.8	4.1	4.3	4.6	4.7	4.9	5.0
	.995	3.36	4.1	4.6	4.9	5.2	5.5	5.7	5.9	6.1
6	.005	.0038	.051	.12	.19	.25	.30	.35	.38	.42
	.01	.0070	.073	.16	.23	.29	.34	.39	.43	.46
	.025	.017	.115	.21	.30	.36	.42	.46	.50	.54
	.05	.035	.16	.27	.36	.43	.49	.54	.58	.61
	.95	1.36	1.8	2.0	2.2	2.3	2.4	2.5	2.6	2.7
	.975	1.67	2.1	2.4	2.6	2.8	2.9	3.0	3.1	3.2
	.99	2.16	2.7	3.0	3.2	3.4	3.6	3.7	3.8	3.9
	.995	2.67	3.1	3.5	3.8	4.0	4.1	4.3	4.5	4.6

SUBSTITUTE *F*-RATIO

Sample size for denominator	Cum. prop.	Sample size for numerator								
		2	3	4	5	6	7	8	9	10
7	.005	.0037	.048	.12	.18	.24	.29	.33	.37	.40
	.01	.0066	.069	.15	.22	.28	.33	.37	.41	.45
	.025	.016	.107	.20	.28	.34	.40	.44	.48	.52
	.05	.032	.15	.26	.35	.41	.47	.51	.55	.59
	.95	1.26	1.6	1.8	1.9	2.0	2.1	2.2	2.3	2.4
	.975	1.48	1.9	2.1	2.3	2.4	2.5	2.6	2.7	2.8
	.99	1.87	2.3	2.6	2.8	2.9	3.0	3.1	3.2	3.3
	.995	2.28	2.7	2.9	2.9	3.3	3.5	3.6	3.7	3.8
8	.005	.0036	.045	.11	.18	.23	.28	.32	.36	.39
	.01	.0063	.065	.14	.21	.27	.32	.36	.40	.43
	.025	.016	.102	.19	.27	.33	.38	.43	.47	.50
	.05	.031	.14	.25	.33	.40	.45	.50	.53	.57
	.95	1.17	1.4	1.6	1.8	1.9	1.9	2.0	2.1	2.1
	.975	1.36	1.7	1.9	2.0	2.2	2.3	2.3	2.4	2.5
	.99	1.69	2.1	2.3	2.4	2.6	2.7	2.8	2.8	2.9
	.995	2.03	2.3	2.6	2.7	2.9	3.0	3.1	3.2	3.3
9	.005	.0035	.042	.11	.17	.22	.27	.31	.35	.38
	.01	.0060	.062	.14	.21	.26	.31	.35	.39	.42
	.025	.015	.098	.18	.26	.32	.37	.42	.46	.49
	.05	.030	.14	.24	.32	.38	.44	.48	.52	.55
	.95	1.10	1.3	1.5	1.6	1.7	1.8	1.9	1.9	2.0
	.975	1.27	1.6	1.8	1.9	2.0	2.1	2.1	2.2	2.3
	.99	1.56	1.9	2.1	2.2	2.3	2.4	2.5	2.6	2.6
	.995	1.87	2.1	2.3	2.5	2.6	2.7	2.8	2.9	3.0
10	.005	.0034	.041	.10	.16	.22	.26	.30	.34	.37
	.01	.0058	.060	.13	.20	.26	.30	.34	.38	.41
	.025	.015	.095	.18	.25	.31	.36	.41	.44	.48
	.05	.029	.13	.23	.31	.37	.43	.47	.51	.54
	.95	1.05	1.3	1.4	1.5	1.6	1.7	1.8	1.8	1.9
	.975	1.21	1.5	1.6	1.8	1.9	1.9	2.0	2.0	2.1
	.99	1.47	1.8	1.9	2.1	2.2	2.2	2.3	2.4	2.4
	.995	1.75	2.0	2.2	2.3	2.4	2.5	2.6	2.6	2.7

VIII.7 ANALYSIS OF VARIANCE BASED ON RANGE

Standard tests of significance in the analysis of variance are often F-tests based on the ratio of a "treatment" mean square to an error mean square s^2. If the treatment means $\bar{x}_t$, $(t = 1, 2, \ldots, k)$, are all calculated from the same number of observations n, a possible alternative criterion is

$$\sqrt{n} \text{ range } \bar{x}_t / s \ . \tag{1}$$

The independence of numerator and denominator may be proved, so that (1) is a studentized range q. In an overall analysis of variance its use would save very little work; however in procedures for ranking treatment means it plays a fundamental role.

For the case of a one-way classification a computationally simple criterion is obtained if s in (1) is replaced by $\frac{\bar{w}}{c}$. The ratio

$$c\sqrt{n} \text{ range } \bar{x}_t / \bar{w} \tag{2}$$

is then distributed approximately as q with degrees of freedom and scale factor c obtained from table (ii). Simpler still, an immediate test can be made with the help of table (i) which gives upper 5% and 1% points of

$$Q = \text{range } X_t / W,$$

where

$$X_t = \sum_{i=1}^{n} x_{ti} \quad \text{and} \quad W = \sum_{t=1}^{k} w_t \ .$$

ANALYSIS OF VARIANCE BASED ON RANGE

(i) UPPER PERCENTAGE POINTS OF Q = RANGE OF GROUP TOTALS/SUM OF GROUP RANGES IN A ONE-WAY CLASSIFICATION INTO k GROUPS OF n OBSERVATIONS

k \ n	2		3		4		5		6		7		8		9		10	
	5%	1%	5%	1%	5%	1%	5%	1%	5%	1%	5%	1%	5%	1%	5%	1%	5%	1%
2	3.5	8.3	1.91	3.2	1.63	2.5	1.54	2.3	1.50	2.2	1.49	2.1	1.49	2.1	1.51	2.1	1.52	2.1
3	2.4	4.4	1.44	2.1	1.26	1.74	1.19	1.61	1.17	1.55	1.17	1.53	1.17	1.53	1.19	1.54	1.20	1.55
4	1.75	2.9	1.14	1.57	1.01	1.33	0.97	1.24	0.95	1.21	0.95	1.20	0.96	1.20	0.97	1.21	0.98	1.22
5	1.40	2.1	0.94	1.25	0.84	1.07	.81	1.01	.80	1.00	.80	0.99	.81	0.99	.82	1.00	.83	1.01
6	1.16	1.68	.80	1.04	.72	0.90	.70	0.86	.69	0.84	.69	.84	.70	.84	.71	0.85	.72	0.86
7	1.00	1.39	.70	0.89	.64	.78	.61	.75	.61	.74	.61	.74	.62	.74	.62	.74	.63	.75
8	0.87	1.18	.62	.78	.57	.69	.55	.66	.55	.65	.55	.66	.56	.66	.56	.67	.57	.67
9	.78	1.03	.56	.69	.51	.62	.50	.59	.50	.59	.50	.59	.50	.59	.51	.60	.52	.61
10	.70	0.91	.51	.62	.47	.56	.46	.54	.45	.53	.45	.53	.46	.54	.47	.55	.47	.55

(ii) SCALE FACTOR, c, AND EQUIVALENT DEGREES OF FREEDOM, ν, APPROPRIATE TO A ONE-WAY CLASSIFICATION INTO k GROUPS OF n OBSERVATIONS

k \ n	2		3		4		5		6		7		8		9		10	
	ν	c	ν	c	ν	c	ν	c	ν	c	ν	c	ν	c	ν	c	ν	c
1	1.00	1.41	1.98	1.91	2.93	2.24	3.83	2.48	4.68	2.67	5.48	2.83	6.25	2.96	6.98	3.08	7.68	3.18
2	1.92	1.28	3.83	1.81	5.69	2.15	7.47	2.40	9.16	2.60	10.8	2.77	12.3	2.91	13.8	3.02	15.1	3.13
3	2.82	1.23	5.66	1.77	8.44	2.12	11.1	2.38	13.6	2.58	16.0	2.75	18.3	2.89	20.5	3.01	22.6	3.11
4	3.71	1.21	7.49	1.75	11.2	2.11	14.7	2.37	18.1	2.57	21.3	2.74	24.4	2.88	27.3	3.00	30.1	3.10
5	4.59	1.19	9.30	1.74	13.9	2.10	18.4	2.36	22.6	2.56	26.6	2.73	30.4	2.87	34.0	2.99	37.5	3.10
6	5.47	1.18	11.1	1.73	16.7	2.09	22.0	2.35	27.0	2.56	31.8	2.73	36.4	2.87	40.8	2.99	45.0	3.09
7	6.35	1.17	12.9	1.73	19.4	2.09	25.6	2.35	31.5	2.55	37.1	2.72	42.5	2.86	47.6	2.99	52.4	3.09
8	7.23	1.17	14.8	1.72	22.1	2.08	29.2	2.35	36.0	2.55	42.4	2.72	48.5	2.86	54.3	2.98	59.9	3.09
9	8.11	1.16	16.6	1.72	24.9	2.08	32.9	2.34	40.4	2.55	47.6	2.72	54.5	2.86	61.1	2.98	67.3	3.09
10	8.99	1.16	18.4	1.72	27.6	2.08	36.5	2.34	44.9	2.55	52.9	2.72	60.6	2.86	67.8	2.98	74.8	3.09
d_n		1.13		1.69		2.06		2.33		2.53		2.70		2.85		2.97		3.08
C.D.	0.88		1.82		2.74		3.62		4.47		5.27		6.03		6.76		7.45	

N.B.: C.D. = constant difference

VIII.8 CONFIDENCE INTERVALS FOR σ BASED ON MEAN RANGE

This table can be used to provide values of L, U by which the mean range $\bar{w}_{n,k} = \bar{w}$ has to be multiplied to give 95% and 99% confidence intervals ($L\bar{w}$, $U\bar{w}$) for σ. Small values of n have been included, as the table applies equally when σ is estimated from a one-way classification of k groups of n' observations.

CONFIDENCE INTERVALS FOR σ BASED ON MEAN RANGE

FACTORS TO BE APPLIED TO THE MEAN RANGE $\bar{w}_{n,k}$ TO GIVE 95 AND 99% CONFIDENCE INTERVALS $(L\bar{w}, U\bar{w})$ FOR σ

n	2		3		4		5		6		7		8		9		10	
k	L	U	L	U	L	U	L	U	L	U	L	U	L	U	L	U	L	U
1	0.32	23	0.27	3.3	0.25	1.69	0.24	1.18	0.23	0.94	0.22	0.80	0.22	0.71	0.21	0.65	0.21	0.60
	0.25	113	0.23	7.7	0.21	2.9	0.20	1.81	0.20	1.33	0.194	1.09	0.190	0.93	0.187	0.83	0.185	0.75
2	0.40	5.3	0.33	1.61	0.30	1.05	0.28	0.82	0.27	0.70	0.25	0.62	0.25	0.56	0.24	0.53	0.24	0.49
	0.34	9.8	0.28	4.7	0.26	1.44	0.25	1.06	0.24	0.87	0.23	0.75	0.22	0.67	0.22	0.62	0.22	0.58
3	0.45	3.8	0.36	1.28	0.32	0.89	0.30	0.71	0.28	0.62	0.27	0.55	0.26	0.51	0.25	0.48	0.25	0.45
	0.39	7.0	0.32	1.76	0.29	1.12	0.27	0.86	0.26	0.73	0.25	0.64	0.24	0.59	0.24	0.54	0.23	0.51
4	0.49	2.5	0.38	1.13	0.34	0.80	0.31	0.66	0.29	0.58	0.28	0.52	0.27	0.48	0.26	0.45	0.26	0.43
	0.42	4.9	0.34	1.45	0.30	0.97	0.28	0.77	0.27	0.66	0.26	0.59	0.25	0.54	0.25	0.50	0.24	0.48
5	0.52	2.2	0.40	1.04	0.35	0.75	0.32	0.62	0.30	0.55	0.29	0.50	0.28	0.47	0.27	0.44	0.26	0.42
	0.45	3.2	0.36	1.29	0.32	0.88	0.30	0.72	0.28	0.62	0.27	0.56	0.26	0.51	0.25	0.48	0.25	0.45
6	0.54	2.0	0.41	0.98	0.36	0.72	0.33	0.60	0.31	0.53	0.29	0.49	0.28	0.45	0.28	0.43	0.27	0.41
	0.47	2.7	0.37	1.18	0.33	0.83	0.30	0.68	0.29	0.59	0.28	0.54	0.27	0.49	0.26	0.46	0.25	0.44
7	0.55	1.82	0.42	0.93	0.36	0.70	0.33	0.59	0.31	0.52	0.30	0.47	0.29	0.44	0.28	0.42	0.27	0.40
	0.49	2.4	0.38	1.11	0.34	0.79	0.31	0.65	0.29	0.57	0.28	0.52	0.27	0.48	0.26	0.45	0.26	0.43
8	0.57	1.72	0.43	0.90	0.37	0.68	0.34	0.57	0.32	0.51	0.30	0.47	0.29	0.44	0.28	0.41	0.27	0.39
	0.50	2.2	0.39	1.06	0.34	0.77	0.32	0.63	0.30	0.56	0.29	0.51	0.28	0.47	0.27	0.44	0.26	0.42
9	0.58	1.64	0.43	0.88	0.38	0.66	0.34	0.56	0.32	0.50	0.31	0.46	0.29	0.43	0.29	0.41	0.28	0.39
	0.52	2.1	0.40	1.01	0.35	0.74	0.32	0.62	0.30	0.54	0.29	0.50	0.28	0.46	0.27	0.44	0.26	0.41
10	0.59	1.58	0.44	0.86	0.38	0.65	0.35	0.55	0.33	0.49	0.31	0.45	0.30	0.43	0.29	0.40	0.28	0.39
	0.53	1.97	0.41	0.98	0.36	0.72	0.33	0.61	0.31	0.53	0.29	0.49	0.28	0.45	0.27	0.43	0.27	0.41

IX. Correlation Coefficient

IX.1 PERCENTAGE POINTS, DISTRIBUTION OF THE CORRELATION COEFFICIENT, WHEN $\rho = 0$

The bivariate normal probability function is given by

$$f(x,y) = \frac{1}{2\pi\sigma_x\sigma_y\sqrt{1-\rho^2}} \exp\left\{-\frac{1}{2(1-\rho^2)}\left[\left(\frac{x-\mu_x}{\sigma_x}\right)^2 - 2\rho\left(\frac{x-\mu_x}{\sigma_x}\right)\left(\frac{y-\mu_y}{\sigma_y}\right) + \left(\frac{y-\mu_y}{\sigma_y}\right)^2\right]\right\},$$

where μ_x = mean of x
μ_y = mean of y
σ_x = standard deviation of x
σ_y = standard deviation of y
ρ = correlation coefficient between x and y.

If (x_i,y_i) $(i = 1, 2, \ldots, n)$ denote a random sample of n ordered observations drawn from a bivariate normal distribution, then an estimate of ρ is given by the sample product-moment correlation coefficient r, given by

$$r = \frac{\sum_i (x_i - \bar{x})(y_i - \bar{y})}{\sqrt{\sum_i (x_i - \bar{x})^2 \cdot \sum_i (y_i - \bar{y})^2}}.$$

The frequency function of r is given by

$$f(r) = \frac{(1-\rho^2)^{\frac{n-1}{2}}}{\pi(n-3)!}(1-r^2)^{\frac{n-4}{2}} \frac{d^{n-2}}{d(r\rho)^{n-2}}\left[\frac{\text{Arccos}\,(-r\rho)}{\sqrt{1-r^2\rho^2}}\right]$$

which can also be written as

$$f(r) = \frac{(1-\rho^2)^{\frac{n-1}{2}}(1-r^2)^{\frac{n-4}{2}}}{\sqrt{\pi}\,\Gamma\left(\frac{n-1}{2}\right)\Gamma\left(\frac{n-2}{2}\right)} \sum_{i=0}^{\infty} \frac{(2r\rho)^i}{i!}\Gamma^2\left(\frac{n-1+i}{2}\right).$$

In the special case where $\rho = 0$, the frequency function of r becomes

$$f(r) = \frac{\Gamma\left(\frac{n-1}{2}\right)}{\sqrt{\pi}\,\Gamma\left(\frac{n}{2}-1\right)}(1-r^2)^{\frac{n-4}{2}}.$$

Under the transformation

$$r^2 = \frac{t^2}{t^2+\nu},$$

$f(r)$ is transformed into the t-distribution with $\nu = n - 2$ degrees of freedom. This table gives percentage points of the distribution of the correlation coefficient when $\rho = 0$.

PERCENTAGE POINTS, DISTRIBUTION OF THE CORRELATION COEFFICIENT, WHEN $\rho = 0$

$\Pr\{r \leq \text{tabular value} | \rho = 0\} = 1 - \alpha$

ν	$\alpha =$ 0.05	0.025	0.01	0.005	0.0025	0.0005	ν	$\alpha =$ 0.05	0.025	0.01	0.005	0.0025	0.0005
	$2\alpha =$ 0.1	0.05	0.02	0.01	0.005	0.001		$2\alpha =$ 0.1	0.05	0.02	0.01	0.005	0.001
1	0.9877	$0.9^{2}692$	$0.9^{3}507$	$0.9^{3}877$	$0.9^{4}692$	$0.9^{5}877$	16	0.400	0.468	0.543	0.590	0.631	0.708
2	.9000	.9500	.9800	$.9^{2}000$	$.9^{2}500$	$.9^{3}000$	17	.389	.456	.529	.575	.616	.693
3	.805	.878	.9343	.9587	.9740	$.9^{2}114$	18	.378	.444	.516	.561	.602	.679
4	.729	.811	.882	.9172	.9417	.9741	19	.369	.433	.503	.549	.589	.665
5	.669	.754	.833	.875	.9056	.9509	20	.360	.423	.492	.537	.576	.652
6	0.621	0.707	0.789	0.834	0.870	0.9249	25	0.323	0.381	0.445	0.487	0.524	0.597
7	.582	.666	.750	.798	.836	.898	30	.296	.349	.409	.449	.484	.554
8	.549	.632	.715	.765	.805	.872	35	.275	.325	.381	.418	.452	.519
9	.521	.602	.685	.735	.776	.847	40	.257	.304	.358	.393	.425	.490
10	.497	.576	.658	.708	.750	.823	45	.243	.288	.338	.372	.403	.465
11	0.476	0.553	0.634	0.684	0.726	0.801	50	0.231	0.273	0.322	0.354	0.384	0.443
12	.457	.532	.612	.661	.703	.780	60	.211	.250	.295	.325	.352	.408
13	.441	.514	.592	.641	.683	.760	70	.195	.232	.274	.302	.327	.380
14	.426	.497	.574	.623	.664	.742	80	.183	.217	.257	.283	.307	.357
15	.412	.482	.558	.606	.647	.725	90	.173	.205	.242	.267	.290	.338
							100	.164	.195	.230	.254	.276	.321

$\alpha = 1 - F(r|\nu, \rho = 0)$ is the upper-tail area of the distribution of r appropriate for use in a single-tail test. For a two-tail test, 2α must be used. If r is calculated from n paired observations, enter the table with $\nu = n - 2$. For partial correlations enter with $\nu = n - k - 2$, where k is the number of variables held constant.

IX.2 CONFIDENCE LIMITS FOR THE POPULATION CORRELATION COEFFICIENT

The cumulative distribution of the correlation coefficient is given by

$$F(r;n,\rho) = \int_{-1}^{r} \frac{(1-\rho^2)^{\frac{n-1}{2}}}{\pi(n-3)!} (1-u^2)^{\frac{n-4}{2}} \frac{d^{n-2}}{d(u\rho)^{n-2}} \left[\frac{\text{Arccos}\,(-u\rho)}{\sqrt{1-u^2\rho^2}} \right] du \; .$$

This table shows graphically the roots ρ_1 and $\rho_2 (\rho_2 > \rho_1)$ of

$$\alpha = F(r;n,\rho_2) \qquad \text{and} \qquad 1-\alpha = F(r;n,\rho_1)$$

plotted against r for selected sample sizes n for the values $\alpha = 0.025$ and 0.005.

GRAPHS SHOWING CONFIDENCE LIMITS FOR THE POPULATION CORRELATION COEFFICIENT, ρ, GIVEN THE SAMPLE COEFFICIENT, r. CONFIDENCE COEFFICIENT, $1 - 2\alpha = 0.95$

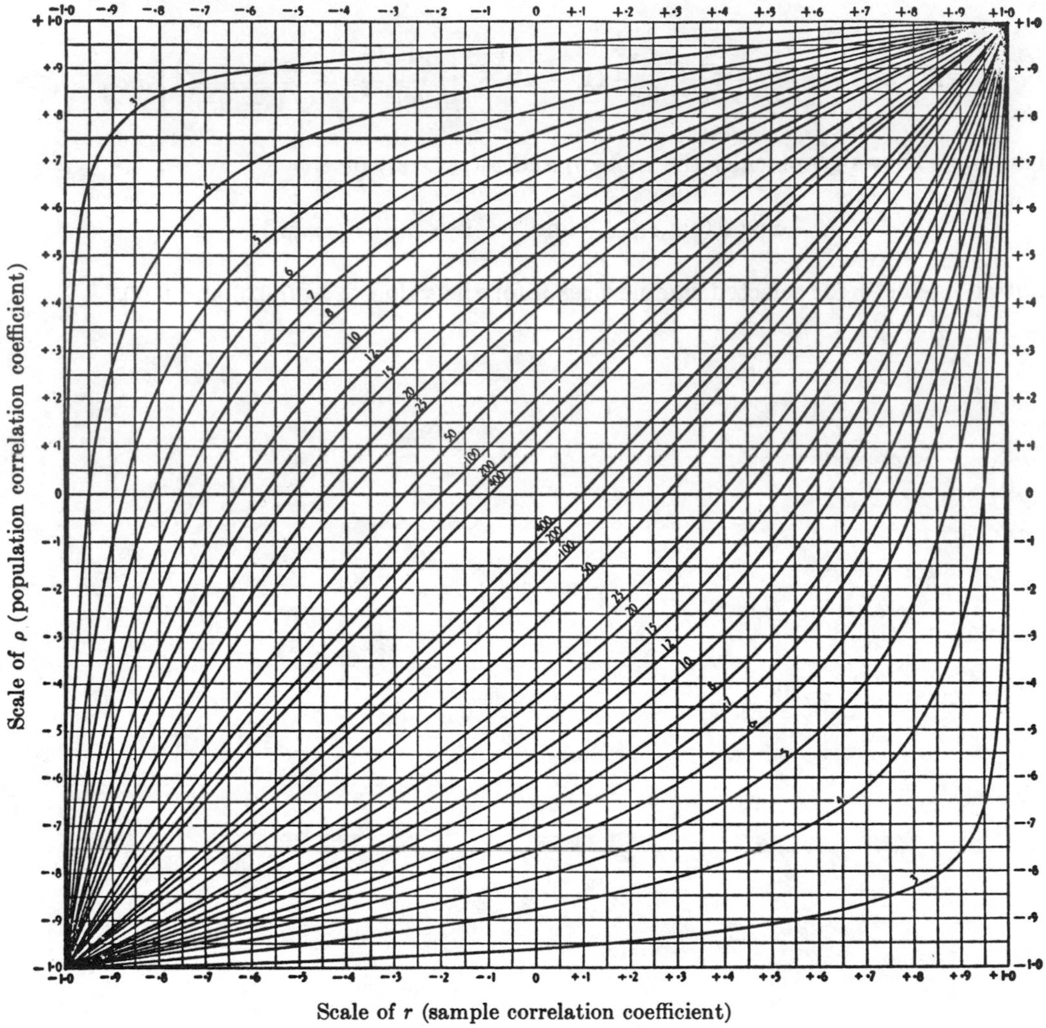

The numbers on the curves indicate sample size. The chart can also be used to determine upper and lower 2.5% significance points for r, given ρ.

GRAPHS SHOWING CONFIDENCE LIMITS FOR THE POPULATION CORRELATION COEFFICIENT, ρ, GIVEN THE SAMPLE COEFFICIENT, r. CONFIDENCE COEFFICIENT, $1 - 2\alpha = 0.99$

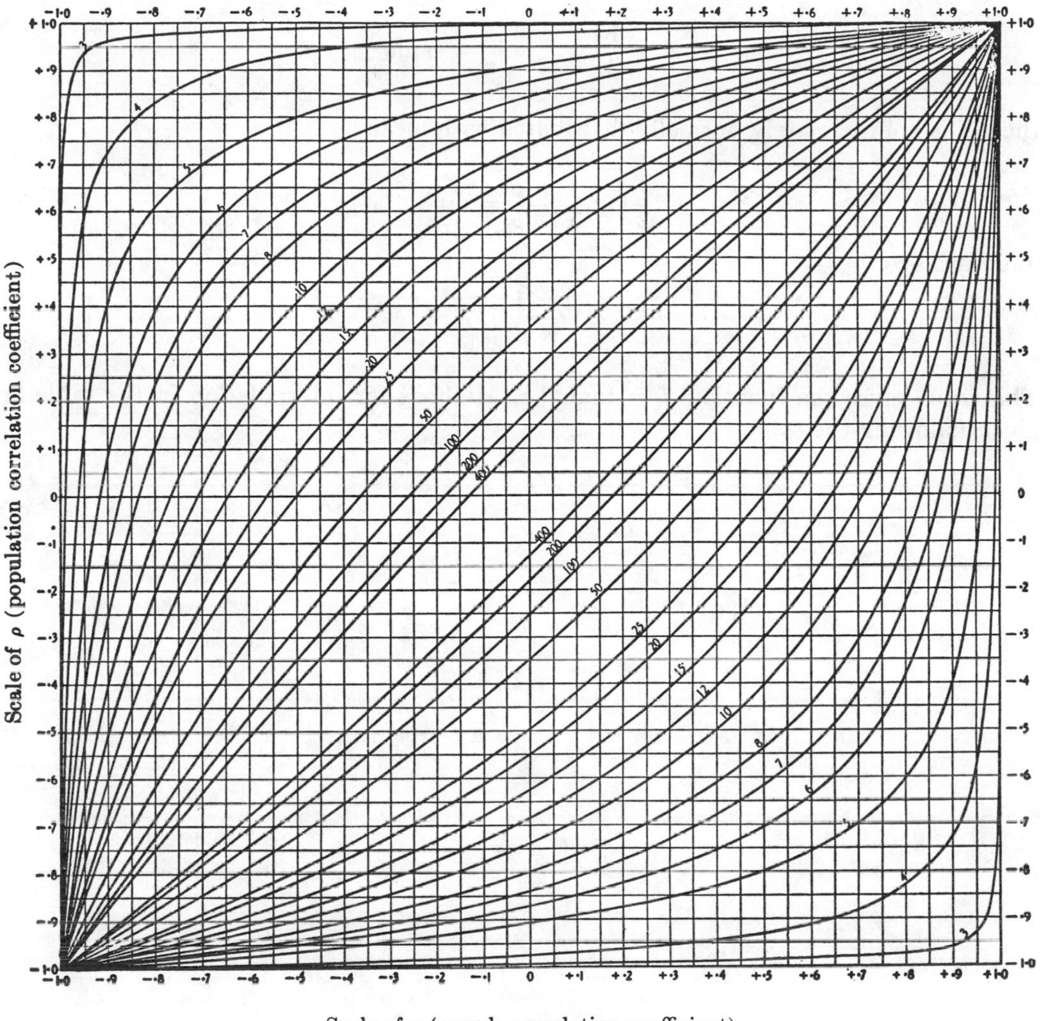

The numbers on the curves indicate sample size. The chart can also be used to determine upper and lower 0.5% significance points for r, given ρ.

IX.3 THE TRANSFORMATION $Z = \text{TANH}^{-1}\,r$ FOR THE CORRELATION COEFFICIENT

If one introduces the transformation

$$Z = \frac{1}{2}\log_e \frac{1+r}{1-r} = \tanh^{-1} r,$$

then Z is approximately normally distributed with mean

$$\frac{1}{2}\log_e \frac{1+\rho}{1-\rho} = \tanh^{-1} \rho$$

and variance

$$\frac{1}{n-3}\,.$$

This table gives the function $Z = \tanh^{-1} r$. Methods for interpolation in the table are given following the table.

THE TRANSFORMATION $Z = \text{TANH}^{-1}\, r$ FOR THE CORRELATION COEFFICIENT

	r (3rd decimal)					Proportional parts, for right side→										r (3rd decimal)					
r	**.000**	**.002**	**.004**	**.006**	**.008**	**1**	**2**	**3**	**4**	**5**	**6**	**7**	**8**	**9**	**10**	**.000**	**.002**	**.004**	**.006**	**.008**	r
.00	.0000	.0020	.0040	.0060	.0080	1	3	4	5	7	8	9	11	12	13	.5493	.5520	.5547	.5573	.5600	**.50**
1	.0100	.0120	.0140	.0160	.0180	1	3	4	5	7	8	10	11	12	14	.5627	.5654	.5682	.5709	.5736	**1**
2	.0200	.0220	.0240	.0260	.0280	1	3	4	6	7	8	10	11	13	14	.5763	.5791	.5818	.5846	.5874	**2**
3	.0300	.0320	.0340	.0360	.0380	1	3	4	6	7	8	10	11	13	14	.5901	.5929	.5957	.5985	.6013	**3**
4	.0400	.0420	.0440	.0460	.0480	1	3	4	6	7	9	10	11	13	14	.6042	.6070	.6098	.6127	.6155	**4**
.05	.0500	.0520	.0541	.0561	.0581	1	3	4	6	7	9	10	12	13	14	.6184	.6213	.6241	.6270	.6299	**.55**
6	.0601	.0621	.0641	.0661	.0681	1	3	4	6	7	9	10	12	13	15	.6328	.6358	.6387	.6416	.6446	**6**
7	.0701	.0721	.0741	.0761	.0782	1	3	4	6	7	9	10	12	14	15	.6475	.6505	.6535	.6565	.6595	**7**
8	.0802	.0822	.0842	.0862	.0882	2	3	5	6	8	9	11	12	14	15	.6625	.6655	.6685	.6716	.6746	**8**
9	.0902	.0923	.0943	.0963	.0983	2	3	5	6	8	9	11	12	14	15	.6777	.6807	.6838	.6869	.6900	**9**
.10	.1003	.1024	.1044	.1064	.1084	2	3	5	6	8	9	11	13	14	16	.6931	.6963	.6994	.7026	.7057	**.60**
1	.1104	.1125	.1145	.1165	.1186	2	3	5	6	8	10	11	13	14	16	.7089	.7121	.7153	.7185	.7218	**1**
2	.1206	.1226	.1246	.1267	.1287	2	3	5	7	8	10	11	13	15	16	.7250	.7283	.7315	.7348	.7381	**2**
3	.1307	.1328	.1348	.1368	.1389	2	3	5	7	8	10	12	13	15	17	.7414	.7447	.7481	.7514	.7548	**3**
4	.1409	.1430	.1450	.1471	.1491	2	3	5	7	9	10	12	14	15	17	.7582	.7616	.7650	.7684	.7718	**4**
.15	.1511	.1532	.1552	.1573	.1593	2	4	5	7	9	11	12	14	16	18	.7753	.7788	.7823	.7858	.7893	**.65**
6	.1614	.1634	.1655	.1676	.1696	2	4	5	7	9	11	13	14	16	18	.7928	.7964	.7999	.8035	.8071	**6**
7	.1717	.1737	.1758	.1779	.1799	2	4	6	7	9	11	13	15	17	18	.8107	.8144	.8180	.8217	.8254	**7**
8	.1820	.1841	.1861	.1882	.1903	2	4	6	8	9	11	13	15	17	19	.8291	.8328	.8366	.8404	.8441	**8**
9	.1923	.1944	.1965	.1986	.2007	2	4	6	8	10	12	14	15	17	19	.8480	.8518	.8556	.8595	.8634	**9**
.20	.2027	.2048	.2069	.2090	.2111	2	4	6	8	10	12	14	16	18	20	.8673	.8712	.8752	.8792	.8832	**.70**
1	.2132	.2153	.2174	.2195	.2216	2	4	6	8	10	12	15	16	18	20	.8872	.8912	.8953	.8994	.9035	**1**
2	.2237	.2258	.2279	.2300	.2321	2	4	6	8	11	13	15	17	19	21	.9076	.9118	.9160	.9202	.9245	**2**
3	.2342	.2363	.2384	.2405	.2427	2	4	7	9	11	13	15	17	20	22	.9287	.9330	.9373	.9417	.9461	**3**
4	.2448	.2469	.2490	.2512	.2533	2	4	7	9	11	13	16	18	20	22	.9505	.9549	.9594	.9639	.9684	**4**
r	**.000**	**.002**	**.004**	**.006**	**.008**	**1**	**2**	**3**	**4**	**5**	**6**	**7**	**8**	**9**	**10**	**.000**	**.002**	**.004**	**.006**	**.008**	r
	r (3rd decimal)					←Proportional parts, for left side										r (3rd decimal)					

Interpolation

(1) $0 \leq r \leq 0.25$: find argument r_0 nearest to r and form $z = z(r_0) + \Delta r$ (where $\Delta r = r - r_0$), e.g. for $r = 0.2042$, $z = 0.2069 + 0.0002 = 0.2071$.

(2) $0.25 \leq r \leq 0.75$: find argument r_0 nearest to r and form $z = z(r_0) \pm P$, where P is the proportional part for $\Delta r = r - r_0$, e.g. for $r = 0.5146$, $z = 0.5682 + 0.0008 = 0.5690$; for $r = 0.5372$, $z = 0.6013 - 0.0011 = 0.6002$.

(3) $0.75 \leq r \leq 0.98$: use linear interpolation to get 3-decimal place accuracy.

(4) $0.98 \leq r < 1$: form $z = -\frac{1}{2}\log_e\,(1 - r) + 0.097 + \frac{1}{4}r$, with the help of table of natural logarithms.

THE TRANSFORMATION $Z = \tanh^{-1} r$ FOR THE CORRELATION COEFFICIENT

	r (3rd decimal)					Proportional parts, for right side→										*r* (3rd decimal)					
r	.000	.002	.004	.006	.008	1	2	3	4	5	6	7	8	9	10	.000	.002	.004	.006	.008	*r*
.25	.2554	.2575	.2597	.2618	.2640	1	2	3	4	5	6	7	9	10	11	0.973	0.978	0.982	0.987	0.991	.75
6	.2661	.2683	.2704	.2726	.2747	1	2	3	4	5	6	8	9	10	11	0.996	1.001	1.006	1.011	1.015	6
7	.2769	.2790	.2812	.2833	.2855	1	2	3	4	5	6	8	9	10	11	1.020	1.025	1.030	1.035	1.040	7
8	.2877	.2899	.2920	.2942	.2964	1	2	3	4	5	7	8	9	10	11	1.045	1.050	1.056	1.061	1.066	8
9	.2986	.3008	.3029	.3051	.3073	1	2	3	4	5	7	8	9	10	11	1.071	1.077	1.082	1.088	1.093	9
.30	.3095	.3117	.3139	.3161	.3183	1	2	3	4	6	7	8	9	10	11	1.099	1.104	1.110	1.116	1.121	.80
1	.3205	.3228	.3250	.3272	.3294	1	2	3	4	6	7	8	9	10	11	1.127	1.133	1.139	1.145	1.151	1
2	.3316	.3339	.3361	.3383	.3406	1	2	3	4	6	7	8	9	10	11	1.157	1.163	1.169	1.175	1.182	2
3	.3428	.3451	.3473	.3496	.3518	1	2	3	5	6	7	8	9	10	11	1.188	1.195	1.201	1.208	1.214	3
4	.3541	.3564	.3586	.3609	.3632	1	2	3	5	6	7	8	9	10	11	1.221	1.228	1.235	1.242	1.249	4
.35	.3654	.3677	.3700	.3723	.3746	1	2	3	5	6	7	8	9	10	11	1.256	1.263	1.271	1.278	1.286	.85
6	.3769	.3792	.3815	.3838	.3861	1	2	3	5	6	7	8	9	10	12	1.293	1.301	1.309	1.317	1.325	6
7	.3884	.3907	.3931	.3954	.3977	1	2	3	5	6	7	8	9	10	12	1.333	1.341	1.350	1.358	1.367	7
8	.4001	.4024	.4047	.4071	.4094	1	2	4	5	6	7	8	9	11	12	1.376	1.385	1.394	1.403	1.412	8
9	.4118	.4142	.4165	.4189	.4213	1	2	4	5	6	7	8	9	11	12	1.422	1.432	1.442	1.452	1.462	9
.40	.4236	.4260	.4284	.4308	.4332	1	2	4	5	6	7	8	10	11	12	1.472	1.483	1.494	1.505	1.516	.90
1	.4356	.4380	.4404	.4428	.4453	1	2	4	5	6	7	8	10	11	12	1.528	1.539	1.551	1.564	1.576	1
2	.4477	.4501	.4526	.4550	.4574	1	2	4	5	6	7	9	10	11	12	1.589	1.602	1.616	1.630	1.644	2
3	.4599	.4624	.4648	.4673	.4698	1	2	4	5	6	7	9	10	11	12	1.658	1.673	1.689	1.705	1.721	3
4	.4722	.4747	.4772	.4797	.4822	1	2	4	5	6	7	9	10	11	12	1.738	1.756	1.774	1.792	1.812	4
.45	.4847	.4872	.4897	.4922	.4948	1	3	4	5	6	8	9	10	11	13	1.832	1.853	1.874	1.897	1.921	.95
6	.4973	.4999	.5024	.5049	.5075	1	3	4	5	6	8	9	10	11	13	1.946	1.972	2.000	2.029	2.060	6
7	.5101	.5126	.5152	.5178	.5204	1	3	4	5	6	8	9	10	12	13	2.092	2.127	2.165	2.205	2.249	7
8	.5230	.5256	.5282	.5308	.5334	1	3	4	5	7	8	9	10	12	13	2.298	2.351	2.410	2.477	2.555	8
9	.5361	.5387	.5413	.5440	.5466	1	3	4	5	7	8	9	11	12	13	2.647	2.759	2.903	3.106	3.453	9
r	.000	.002	.004	.006	.008	1	2	3	4	5	6	7	8	9	10	.000	.002	.004	.006	.008	*r*
	r (3rd decimal)					←Proportional parts, for left side										*r* (3rd decimal)					

Interpolation

(1) $0 \leq r \leq 0.25$: find argument r_0 nearest to r and form $z = z(r_0) + \Delta r$ (where $\Delta r = r - r_0$), e.g. for $r = 0.2042$, $z = 0.2069 + 0.0002 = 0.2071$.

(2) $0.25 \leq r \leq 0.75$: find argument r_0 nearest to r and form $z = z(r_0) \pm P$, where P is the proportional part for $\Delta r = r - r_0$, e.g. for $r = 0.5146$, $z = 0.5682 + 0.0008 = 0.5690$; for $r = 0.5372$, $z = 0.6013 - 0.0011 = 0.6002$.

(3) $0.75 \leq r \leq 0.98$: use linear interpolation to get 3-decimal place accuracy.

(4) $0.98 \leq r < 1$: form $z = -\frac{1}{2} \log_e (1 - r) + 0.097 + \frac{1}{4}r$, with the help of table of natural logarithms.

X. Non-Parametric Statistics

X.1 CRITICAL VALUES FOR THE SIGN TEST

The observations in a random sample of size n from X and those of the same size from Y are paired according to the order of observation: (X_i, Y_i), $i = 1, 2, \ldots, n$. The differences $d_i = X_i - Y_i$ are calculated for each of the n pairs. The null hypothesis is that the difference d_i has a distribution with median zero, i.e., the true proportion of positive (negative) signs is equal to $p = \frac{1}{2}$. Thus the test is whether X and Y have the same median. The probability of x positive (negative) signs is given by the binomial probability function

$$f(x) = f(x;n, p = \tfrac{1}{2}) = \binom{n}{x}\left(\frac{1}{2}\right)^n .$$

This table gives the critical value k such that

$$P(x \le k) = \sum_{x=0}^{k} \binom{n}{x}\left(\frac{1}{2}\right)^n < \frac{\alpha}{2} .$$

For a one-tailed test with significance level α enter the table in the column headed by 2α.

CRITICAL VALUES FOR THE SIGN TEST

(Two-tail percentage points for the binomial for $p = .5$)

n	1%	5%	10%	25%	n	1%	5%	10%	25%
1					46	13	15	16	18
2					47	14	16	17	19
3				0	48	14	16	17	19
4				0	49	15	17	18	19
5			0	0	50	15	17	18	20
6		0	0	1	51	15	18	19	20
7		0	0	1	52	16	18	19	21
8	0	0	1	1	53	16	18	20	21
9	0	1	1	2	54	17	19	20	22
10	0	1	1	2	55	17	19	20	22
11	0	1	2	3	56	17	20	21	23
12	1	2	2	3	57	18	20	21	23
13	1	2	3	3	58	18	21	22	24
14	1	2	3	4	59	19	21	22	24
15	2	3	3	4	60	19	21	23	25
16	2	3	4	5	61	20	22	23	25
17	2	4	4	5	62	20	22	24	25
18	3	4	5	6	63	20	23	24	26
19	3	4	5	6	64	21	23	24	26
20	3	5	5	6	65	21	24	25	27
21	4	5	6	7	66	22	24	25	27
22	4	5	6	7	67	22	25	26	28
23	4	6	7	8	68	22	25	26	28
24	5	6	7	8	69	23	25	27	29
25	5	7	7	9	70	23	26	27	29
26	6	7	8	9	71	24	26	28	30
27	6	7	8	10	72	24	27	28	30
28	6	8	9	10	73	25	27	28	31
29	7	8	9	10	74	25	28	29	31
30	7	9	10	11	75	25	28	29	32
31	7	9	10	11	76	26	28	30	32
32	8	9	10	12	77	26	29	30	32
33	8	10	11	12	78	27	29	31	33
34	9	10	11	13	79	27	30	31	33
35	9	11	12	13	80	28	30	32	34
36	9	11	12	14	81	28	31	32	34
37	10	12	13	14	82	28	31	33	35
38	10	12	13	14	83	29	32	33	35
39	11	12	13	15	84	29	32	33	36
40	11	13	14	15	85	30	32	34	36
41	11	13	14	16	86	30	33	34	37
42	12	14	15	16	87	31	33	35	37
43	12	14	15	17	88	31	34	35	38
44	13	15	16	17	89	31	34	36	38
45	13	15	16	18	90	32	35	36	39

For values of n larger than 90, approximate values of r may be found by taking the nearest integer less than $(n - 1)/2 - k\sqrt{n + 1}$, where k is 1.2879, 0.9800, 0.8224, 0.5752 for the 1, 5, 10, 25% values, respectively.

X.2 CRITICAL VALUES OF T IN THE WILCOXON MATCHED-PAIRS SIGNED-RANKS TEST

Let d_i denote the difference score for any matched pair of a set of n pairs of observations: $d_i = x_i - y_i$. Rank all the d_i's without regard to sign: give the rank of 1 to the smallest d_i, the rank of 2 to the next smallest, etc. After the ranking is completed, affix the sign of the difference to each rank. Let T equal the smaller sum of the like-signed ranks. This table gives approximate 1%, 2%, and 5% points of T for various values of n. The hypothesis tested is that there is no difference between the distributions of x and y. The table is adapted for use with both one-tailed and two-tailed tests.

CRITICAL VALUES OF *T* IN THE WILCOXON MATCHED-PAIRS SIGNED-RANKS TEST

$n = 5(1)50$

One-sided	Two-sided	$n = 5$	$n = 6$	$n = 7$	$n = 8$	$n = 9$	$n = 10$
$P = .05$	$P = .10$	1	2	4	6	8	11
$P = .025$	$P = .05$		1	2	4	6	8
$P = .01$	$P = .02$			0	2	3	5
$P = .005$	$P = .01$				0	2	3
One-sided	**Two-sided**	$n = 11$	$n = 12$	$n = 13$	$n = 14$	$n = 15$	$n = 16$
$P = .05$	$P = .10$	14	17	21	26	30	36
$P = .025$	$P = .05$	11	14	17	21	25	30
$P = .01$	$P = .02$	7	10	13	16	20	24
$P = .005$	$P = .01$	5	7	10	13	16	19
One-sided	**Two-sided**	$n = 17$	$n = 18$	$n = 19$	$n = 20$	$n = 21$	$n = 22$
$P = .05$	$P = .10$	41	47	54	60	68	75
$P = .025$	$P = .05$	35	40	46	52	59	66
$P = .01$	$P = .02$	28	33	38	43	49	56
$P = .005$	$P = .01$	23	28	32	37	43	49
One-sided	**Two-sided**	$n = 23$	$n = 24$	$n = 25$	$n = 26$	$n = 27$	$n = 28$
$P = .05$	$P = .10$	83	92	101	110	120	130
$P = .025$	$P = .05$	73	81	90	98	107	117
$P = .01$	$P = .02$	62	69	77	85	93	102
$P = .005$	$P = .01$	55	61	68	76	84	92
One-sided	**Two-sided**	$n = 29$	$n = 30$	$n = 31$	$n = 32$	$n = 33$	$n = 34$
$P = .05$	$P = .10$	141	152	163	175	188	201
$P = .025$	$P = .05$	127	137	148	159	171	183
$P = .01$	$P = .02$	111	120	130	141	151	162
$P = .005$	$P = .01$	100	109	118	128	138	149
One-sided	**Two-sided**	$n = 35$	$n = 36$	$n = 37$	$n = 38$	$n = 39$	
$P = .05$	$P = .10$	214	228	242	256	271	
$P = .025$	$P = .05$	195	208	222	235	250	
$P = .01$	$P = .02$	174	186	198	211	224	
$P = .005$	$P = .01$	160	171	183	195	208	
One-sided	**Two-sided**	$n = 40$	$n = 41$	$n = 42$	$n = 43$	$n = 44$	$n = 45$
$P = .05$	$P = .10$	287	303	319	336	353	371
$P = .025$	$P = .05$	264	279	295	311	327	344
$P = .01$	$P = .02$	238	252	267	281	297	313
$P = .005$	$P = .01$	221	234	248	262	277	292
One-sided	**Two-sided**	$n = 46$	$n = 47$	$n = 48$	$n = 49$	$n = 50$	
$P = .05$	$P = .10$	389	408	427	446	466	
$P = .025$	$P = .05$	361	379	397	415	434	
$P = .01$	$P = .02$	329	345	362	380	398	
$P = .005$	$P = .01$	307	323	339	356	373	

X.3 PROBABILITIES FOR THE WILCOXON (MANN-WHITNEY) TWO-SAMPLE STATISTIC

Given two samples of size m and n, $m \leq n$, the Mann-Whitney U-Statistic is used to test the hypothesis that the two samples are from populations with the same median. Rank all the observations in ascending order of magnitude. Let T be the sum of the ranks assigned to the sample of size m. Then U is defined as

$$U = mn + \frac{m(m+1)}{2} - T\,.$$

This table is used to determine the exact probability associated with the occurrence under the null hypothesis of any U as extreme as an observed value of U.

The probabilities given in this table are one-tailed. For a two-tailed test, the value of p given in the table should be doubled. The table is made up of six separate subtables, one for each value of n.

PROBABILITIES ASSOCIATED WITH VALUES AS SMALL AS OBSERVED VALUES OF U IN THE MANN-WHITNEY TEST

$n = 3$

U \ m	1	2	3
0	.250	.100	.050
1	.500	.200	.100
2	.750	.400	.200
3		.600	.350
4			.500
5			.650

$n = 4$

U \ m	1	2	3	4
0	.200	.067	.028	.014
1	.400	.133	.057	.029
2	.600	.267	.114	.057
3		.400	.200	.100
4		.600	.314	.171
5			.429	.243
6			.571	.343
7				.443
8				.557

$n = 5$

U \ m	1	2	3	4	5
0	.167	.047	.018	.008	.004
1	.333	.095	.036	.016	.008
2	.500	.190	.071	.032	.016
3	.667	.286	.125	.056	.028
4		.429	.196	.095	.048
5		.571	.286	.143	.075
6			.393	.206	.111
7			.500	.278	.155
8			.607	.365	.210
9				.452	.274
10				.548	.345
11					.421
12					.500
13					.579

$n = 6$

U \ m	1	2	3	4	5	6
0	.143	.036	.012	.005	.002	.001
1	.286	.071	.024	.010	.004	.002
2	.428	.143	.048	.019	.009	.004
3	.571	.214	.083	.033	.015	.008
4		.321	.131	.057	.026	.013
5		.429	.190	.086	.041	.021
6		.571	.274	.129	.063	.032
7			.357	.176	.089	.047
8			.452	.238	.123	.066
9			.548	.305	.165	.090
10				.381	.214	.120
11				.457	.268	.155
12				.545	.331	.197
13					.396	.242
14					.465	.294
15					.535	.350
16						.409
17						.469
18						.531

PROBABILITIES ASSOCIATED WITH VALUES AS SMALL AS OBSERVED VALUES OF U IN THE MANN-WHITNEY TEST

$n = 7$

U \ m	1	2	3	4	5	6	7
0	.125	.028	.008	.003	.001	.001	.000
1	.250	.056	.017	.006	.003	.001	.001
2	.375	.111	.033	.012	.005	.002	.001
3	.500	.167	.058	.021	.009	.004	.002
4	.625	.250	.092	.036	.015	.007	.003
5		.333	.133	.055	.024	.011	.006
6		.444	.192	.082	.037	.017	.009
7		.556	.258	.115	.053	.026	.013
8			.333	.158	.074	.037	.019
9			.417	.206	.101	.051	.027
10			.500	.264	.134	.069	.036
11			.583	.324	.172	.090	.049
12				.394	.216	.117	.064
13				.464	.265	.147	.082
14				.538	.319	.183	.104
15					.378	.223	.130
16					.438	.267	.159
17					.500	.314	.191
18					.562	.365	.228
19						.418	.267
20						.473	.310
21						.527	.355
22							.402
23							.451
24							.500
25							.549

PROBABILITIES ASSOCIATED WITH VALUES AS SMALL AS OBSERVED VALUES OF U IN THE MANN-WHITNEY TEST

$n = 8$

U \ m	1	2	3	4	5	6	7	8	t	Normal
0	.111	.022	.006	.002	.001	.000	.000	.000	3.308	.001
1	.222	.044	.012	.004	.002	.001	.000	.000	3.203	.001
2	.333	.089	.024	.008	.003	.001	.001	.000	3.098	.001
3	.444	.133	.042	.014	.005	.002	.001	.001	2.993	.001
4	.556	.200	.067	.024	.009	.004	.002	.001	2.888	.002
5		.267	.097	.036	.015	.006	.003	.001	2.783	.003
6		.356	.139	.055	.023	.010	.005	.002	2.678	.004
7		.444	.188	.077	.033	.015	.007	.003	2.573	.005
8		.556	.248	.107	.047	.021	.010	.005	2.468	.007
9			.315	.141	.064	.030	.014	.007	2.363	.009
10			.387	.184	.085	.041	.020	.010	2.258	.012
11			.461	.230	.111	.054	.027	.014	2.153	.016
12			.539	.285	.142	.071	.036	.019	2.048	.020
13				.341	.177	.091	.047	.025	1.943	.026
14				.404	.217	.114	.060	.032	1.838	.033
15				.467	.262	.141	.076	.041	1.733	.041
16				.533	.311	.172	.095	.052	1.628	.052
17					.362	.207	.116	.065	1.523	.064
18					.416	.245	.140	.080	1.418	.078
19					.472	.286	.168	.097	1.313	.094
20					.528	.331	.198	.117	1.208	.113
21						.377	.232	.139	1.102	.135
22						.426	.268	.164	.998	.159
23						.475	.306	.191	.893	.185
24						.525	.347	.221	.788	.215
25							.389	.253	.683	.247
26							.433	.287	.578	.282
27							.478	.323	.473	.318
28							.522	.360	.368	.356
29								.399	.263	.396
30								.439	.158	.437
31								.480	.052	.481
32								.520		

X.4 CRITICAL VALUES OF *U* IN THE WILCOXON (MANN-WHITNEY) TWO-SAMPLE STATISTIC

This table gives critical values of U for significance levels 0.001, 0.005, 0.01, 0.025, 0.05 and 0.10 for a one-tailed test. For a two-tailed test, the significance levels are 0.002, 0.01, 0.02, 0.05, 0.10 and 0.20. If an observed U is equal to or less than the tabular value, the null hypothesis may be rejected at the level of significance indicated at the head of that table.

CRITICAL VALUES OF U IN THE MANN-WHITNEY TEST

Critical Values of U for the .10 Level of Significance

m \ n	1	2	3	4	5	6	7	8	9	10	11	12	13	14	15	16	17	18	19	20
1									0	0	0	0	0	0	0	0	0	0	1	1
2			0	0	1	1	1	2	2	3	3	4	4	4	5	5	6	6	7	7
3		0	1	1	2	3	4	5	5	6	7	8	9	10	10	11	12	13	14	15
4		0	1	3	4	5	6	7	9	10	11	12	13	15	16	17	18	20	21	22
5		1	2	4	5	7	8	10	12	13	15	17	18	20	22	23	25	27	28	30
6		1	3	5	7	9	11	13	15	17	19	21	23	25	27	29	31	34	36	38
7		1	4	6	8	11	13	16	18	21	23	26	28	31	33	36	38	41	43	46
8		2	5	7	10	13	16	19	22	24	27	30	33	36	39	42	45	48	51	54
9	0	2	5	9	12	15	18	22	25	28	31	35	38	41	45	48	52	55	58	62
10	0	3	6	10	13	17	21	24	28	32	36	39	43	47	51	54	58	62	66	70
11	0	3	7	11	15	19	23	27	31	36	40	44	48	52	57	61	65	69	73	78
12	0	4	8	12	17	21	26	30	35	39	44	49	53	58	63	67	72	77	81	86
13	0	4	9	13	18	23	28	33	38	43	48	53	58	63	68	74	79	84	89	94
14	0	4	10	15	20	25	31	36	41	47	52	58	63	69	74	80	85	91	97	102
15	0	5	10	16	22	27	33	39	45	51	57	63	68	74	80	86	92	98	104	110
16	0	5	11	17	23	29	36	42	48	54	61	67	74	80	86	93	99	106	112	119
17	0	6	12	18	25	31	38	45	52	58	65	72	79	85	92	99	106	113	120	127
18	0	6	13	20	27	34	41	48	55	62	69	77	84	91	98	106	113	120	128	135
19	1	7	14	21	28	36	43	51	58	66	73	81	89	97	104	112	120	128	135	143
20	1	7	15	22	30	38	46	54	62	70	78	86	94	102	110	119	127	135	143	151

Critical Values of U for the .05 Level of Significance

m \ n	1	2	3	4	5	6	7	8	9	10	11	12	13	14	15	16	17	18	19	20
1																			0	0
2					0	0	0	1	1	1	1	2	2	2	3	3	3	4	4	4
3			0	0	1	2	2	3	3	4	5	5	6	7	7	8	9	9	10	11
4			0	1	2	3	4	5	6	7	8	9	10	11	12	14	15	16	17	18
5		0	1	2	4	5	6	8	9	11	12	13	15	16	18	19	20	22	23	25
6		0	2	3	5	7	8	10	12	14	16	17	19	21	23	25	26	28	30	32
7		0	2	4	6	8	11	13	15	17	19	21	24	26	28	30	33	35	37	39
8		1	3	5	8	10	13	15	18	20	23	26	28	31	33	36	39	41	44	47
9		1	3	6	9	12	15	18	21	24	27	30	33	36	39	42	45	48	51	54
10		1	4	7	11	14	17	20	24	27	31	34	37	41	44	48	51	55	58	62
11		1	5	8	12	16	19	23	27	31	34	38	42	46	50	54	57	61	65	69
12		2	5	9	13	17	21	26	30	34	38	42	47	51	55	60	64	68	72	77
13		2	6	10	15	19	24	28	33	37	42	47	51	56	61	65	70	75	80	84
14		2	7	11	16	21	26	31	36	41	46	51	56	61	66	71	77	82	87	92
15		3	7	12	18	23	28	33	39	44	50	55	61	66	72	77	83	88	94	100
16		3	8	14	19	25	30	36	42	48	54	60	65	71	77	83	89	95	101	107
17		3	9	15	20	26	33	39	45	51	57	64	70	77	83	89	96	102	109	115
18		4	9	16	22	28	35	41	48	55	61	68	75	82	88	95	102	109	116	123
19	0	4	10	17	23	30	37	44	51	58	65	72	80	87	94	101	109	116	123	130
20	0	4	11	18	25	32	39	47	54	62	69	77	84	92	100	107	115	123	130	138

CRITICAL VALUES OF U IN THE MANN-WHITNEY TEST

Critical Values of U for the .025 Level of Significance

$m \backslash n$	1	2	3	4	5	6	7	8	9	10	11	12	13	14	15	16	17	18	19	20
1																				
2								0	0	0	0	1	1	1	1	1	2	2	2	2
3					0	1	1	2	2	3	3	4	4	5	5	6	6	7	7	8
4				0	1	2	3	4	4	5	6	7	8	9	10	11	11	12	13	13
5			0	1	2	3	5	6	7	8	9	11	12	13	14	15	17	18	19	20
6			1	2	3	5	6	8	10	11	13	14	16	17	19	21	22	24	25	27
7			1	3	5	6	8	10	12	14	16	18	20	22	24	26	28	30	32	34
8		0	2	4	6	8	10	13	15	17	19	22	24	26	29	31	34	36	38	41
9		0	2	4	7	10	12	15	17	20	23	26	28	31	34	37	39	42	45	48
10		0	3	5	8	11	14	17	20	23	26	29	33	36	39	42	45	48	52	55
11		0	3	6	9	13	16	19	23	26	30	33	37	40	44	47	51	55	58	62
12		1	4	7	11	14	18	22	26	29	33	37	41	45	49	53	57	61	65	69
13		1	4	8	12	16	20	24	28	33	37	41	45	50	54	59	63	67	72	76
14		1	5	9	13	17	22	26	31	36	40	45	50	55	59	64	67	74	78	83
15		1	5	10	14	19	24	29	34	39	44	49	54	59	64	70	75	80	85	90
16		1	6	11	15	21	26	31	37	42	47	53	59	64	70	75	81	86	92	98
17		2	6	11	17	22	28	34	39	45	51	57	63	67	75	81	87	93	99	105
18		2	7	12	18	24	30	36	42	48	55	61	67	74	80	86	93	99	106	112
19		2	7	13	19	25	32	38	45	52	58	65	72	78	85	92	99	106	113	119
20		2	8	13	20	27	34	41	48	55	62	69	76	83	90	98	105	112	119	127

Critical Values of U for the .01 Level of Significance

$m \backslash n$	1	2	3	4	5	6	7	8	9	10	11	12	13	14	15	16	17	18	19	20
1																				
2													0	0	0	0	0	0	1	1
3							0	0	1	1	1	2	2	2	3	3	4	4	4	5
4					0	1	1	2	3	3	4	5	5	6	7	7	8	9	9	10
5				0	1	2	3	4	5	6	7	8	9	10	11	12	13	14	15	16
6				1	2	3	4	6	7	8	9	11	12	13	15	16	18	19	20	22
7			0	1	3	4	6	7	9	11	12	14	16	17	19	21	23	24	26	28
8			0	2	4	6	7	9	11	13	15	17	20	22	24	26	28	30	32	34
9			1	3	5	7	9	11	14	16	18	21	23	26	28	31	33	36	38	40
10			1	3	6	8	11	13	16	19	22	24	27	30	33	36	38	41	44	47
11			1	4	7	9	12	15	18	22	25	28	31	34	37	41	44	47	50	53
12			2	5	8	11	14	17	21	24	28	31	35	38	42	46	49	53	56	60
13		0	2	5	9	12	16	20	23	27	31	35	39	43	47	51	55	59	63	67
14		0	2	6	10	13	17	22	26	30	34	38	43	47	51	56	60	65	69	73
15		0	3	7	11	15	19	24	28	33	37	42	47	51	56	61	66	70	75	80
16		0	3	7	12	16	21	26	31	36	41	46	51	56	61	66	71	76	82	87
17		0	4	8	13	18	23	28	33	38	44	49	55	60	66	71	77	82	88	93
18		0	4	9	14	19	24	30	36	41	47	53	59	65	70	76	82	88	94	100
19		1	4	9	15	20	26	32	38	44	50	56	63	69	75	82	88	94	101	107
20		1	5	10	16	22	28	34	40	47	53	60	67	73	80	87	93	100	107	114

CRITICAL VALUES OF U IN THE MANN-WHITNEY TEST

Critical Values of U for the .005 Level of Significance

m \ n	1	2	3	4	5	6	7	8	9	10	11	12	13	14	15	16	17	18	19	20
1																				
2																			0	0
3									0	0	0	1	1	1	2	2	2	2	3	3
4						0	0	1	1	2	2	3	3	4	5	5	6	6	7	8
5					0	1	1	2	3	4	5	6	7	7	8	9	10	11	12	13
6				0	1	2	3	4	5	6	7	9	10	11	12	13	15	16	17	18
7				0	1	3	4	6	7	9	10	12	13	15	16	18	19	21	22	24
8				1	2	4	6	7	9	11	13	15	17	18	20	22	24	26	28	30
9			0	1	3	5	7	9	11	13	16	18	20	22	24	27	29	31	33	36
10			0	2	4	6	9	11	13	16	18	21	24	26	29	31	34	37	39	42
11			0	2	5	7	10	13	16	18	21	24	27	30	33	36	39	42	45	48
12			1	3	6	9	12	15	18	21	24	27	31	34	37	41	44	47	51	54
13			1	3	7	10	13	17	20	24	27	31	34	38	42	45	49	53	56	60
14			1	4	7	11	15	18	22	26	30	34	38	42	46	50	54	58	63	67
15			2	5	8	12	16	20	24	29	33	37	42	46	51	55	60	64	69	73
16			2	5	9	13	18	22	27	31	36	41	45	50	55	60	65	70	74	79
17			2	6	10	15	19	24	29	34	39	44	49	54	60	65	70	75	81	86
18			2	6	11	16	21	26	31	37	42	47	53	58	64	70	75	81	87	92
19		0	3	7	12	17	22	28	33	39	45	51	56	63	69	74	81	87	93	99
20		0	3	8	13	18	24	30	36	42	48	54	60	67	73	79	86	92	99	105

Critical Values of U for the .001 Level of Significance

m \ n	1	2	3	4	5	6	7	8	9	10	11	12	13	14	15	16	17	18	19	20
1																				
2																				
3																	0	0	0	0
4										0	0	0	1	1	1	2	2	3	3	3
5								0	1	1	2	2	3	3	4	5	5	6	7	7
6							0	1	2	3	4	4	5	6	7	8	9	10	11	12
7						0	1	2	3	5	6	7	8	9	10	11	13	14	15	16
8					0	1	2	4	5	6	8	9	11	12	14	15	17	18	20	21
9					1	2	3	5	7	8	10	12	14	15	17	19	21	23	25	26
10				0	1	3	5	6	8	10	12	14	17	19	21	23	25	27	29	32
11				0	2	4	6	8	10	12	15	17	20	22	24	27	29	32	34	37
12				0	2	4	7	9	12	14	17	20	23	25	28	31	34	37	40	42
13				1	3	5	8	11	14	17	20	23	26	29	32	35	38	42	45	48
14				1	3	6	9	12	15	19	22	25	29	32	36	39	43	46	50	54
15				1	4	7	10	14	17	21	24	28	32	36	40	43	47	51	55	59
16				2	5	8	11	15	19	23	27	31	35	39	43	48	52	56	60	65
17			0	2	5	9	13	17	21	25	29	34	38	43	47	52	57	61	66	70
18			0	3	6	10	14	18	23	27	32	37	42	46	51	56	61	66	71	76
19			0	3	7	11	15	20	25	29	34	40	45	50	55	60	66	71	77	82
20			0	3	7	12	16	21	26	32	37	42	48	54	59	65	70	76	82	88

X.5 CRITICAL VALUES FOR THE WILCOXON RANK SUM TEST

Given two samples of size m and n, $m \leq n$, the Wilcoxon rank sum test is used to test the hypothesis that the two samples are from populations with the same mean. Rank all the observations in ascending order of magnitude. Assigned tied values the average rank. Let T be the sum of the ranks assigned to the sample of size m. This table gives, for specified m and n, the critical upper and lower rank sums, T_u and T_l, respectively, associated with specific probabilities. If $T \geq T_u$, then the mean of the smaller sample is said to be significantly larger than the mean of the other sample at the specified probability level. If $T \leq T_l$, then the mean of the smaller sample is said to be significantly smaller than the mean of the other sample at the specified probability level. If $T_l \leq T \leq T_u$, then there is not sufficient evidence at the specified probability level to say that the means of the two samples differ.

The relationship between T and the Mann-Whitney U-Statistic is given by

$$U = mn + \frac{m(m+1)}{2} - T\,.$$

CRITICAL VALUES FOR THE WILCOXON RANK SUM TEST

$m = 3(1)25$ and $n = m(1)m + 25$
$P = .05$ one-sided; $P = .10$ two-sided

n	$m = 3$	$m = 4$	$m = 5$	$m = 6$	$m = 7$	$m = 8$	$m = 9$	$m = 10$	$m = 11$	$m = 12$	$m = 13$	$m = 14$
$n = m$	6,15	12,24	19,36	28,50	39,66	52,84	66,105	83,127	101,152	121,179	143,208	167,239
$n = m + 1$	7,17	13,27	20,40	30,54	41,71	54,90	69,111	86,134	105,159	125,187	148,216	172,248
$n = m + 2$	7,20	14,30	22,43	32,58	43,76	57,95	72,117	89,141	109,166	129,195	152,225	177,257
$n = m + 3$	8,22	15,33	24,46	33,63	46,80	60,100	75,123	93,147	112,174	134,202	157,233	182,266
$n = m + 4$	9,24	16,36	25,50	35,67	48,85	62,106	78,129	96,154	116,181	138,210	162,241	187,275
$n = m + 5$	9,27	17,39	26,54	37,71	50,90	65,111	81,135	100,160	120,188	142,218	166,250	192,284
$n = m + 6$	10,29	18,42	27,58	39,75	52,95	67,117	84,141	103,167	124,195	147,225	171,258	197,293
$n = m + 7$	11,31	19,45	29,61	41,79	54,100	70,122	87,147	107,173	128,202	151,233	176,266	203,301
$n = m + 8$	11,34	20,48	30,65	42,84	57,104	73,127	90,153	110,180	132,209	155,241	181,274	208,310
$n = m + 9$	12,36	21,51	32,68	44,88	59,109	75,133	93,159	114,186	136,216	159,249	185,283	213,319
$n = m + 10$	13,38	22,54	33,72	46,92	61,114	78,138	96,165	117,193	139,224	164,256	190,291	218,328
$n = m + 11$	13,41	23,57	34,76	48,96	63,119	80,144	100,170	120,200	143,231	168,264	195,299	223,337
$n = m + 12$	14,43	24,60	36,79	50,100	65,124	83,149	103,176	124,206	147,238	172,272	199,308	228,346
$n = m + 13$	15,45	25,63	37,83	52,104	68,128	86,154	106,182	127,213	151,245	177,279	204,316	234,354
$n = m + 14$	15,48	26,66	39,86	53,109	70,133	88,160	109,188	131,219	155,252	181,287	209,324	239,363
$n = m + 15$	16,50	27,69	40,90	55,113	72,138	91,165	112,194	134,226	159,259	185,295	214,332	244,372
$n = m + 16$	17,52	28,72	42,93	57,117	74,143	94,170	115,200	138,232	163,266	190,302	218,341	249,381
$n = m + 17$	17,55	29,75	43,97	59,121	77,147	96,176	118,206	141,239	167,273	194,310	223,349	254,390
$n = m + 18$	18,57	30,78	44,101	61,125	79,152	99,181	121,212	145,245	171,280	198,318	228,357	260,398
$n = m + 19$	19,59	31,81	46,104	62,130	81,157	102,186	124,218	148,252	175,287	203,325	233,365	265,407
$n = m + 20$	19,62	32,84	47,108	64,134	83,162	104,192	127,224	152,258	178,295	207,333	237,374	270,416
$n = m + 21$	20,64	33,87	49,111	66,138	86,166	107,197	130,230	155,265	182,302	211,341	242,382	275,425
$n = m + 22$	21,66	34,90	50,115	68,142	88,171	109,203	133,236	159,271	186,309	216,348	247,390	280,434
$n = m + 23$	21,69	35,93	52,118	70,146	90,176	112,208	136,242	162,278	190,316	220,356	252,398	285,443
$n = m + 24$	22,71	37,95	53,122	72,150	92,181	115,213	139,248	166,284	194,323	224,364	257,406	291,451
$n = m + 25$	23,73	38,98	54,126	73,155	94,186	117,219	142,254	169,291	198,330	229,371	261,415	296,460

$m = 3(1)25$ and $n = m(1)m + 25$
$P = .05$ one-sided; $P = .10$ two-sided

n	$m = 15$	$m = 16$	$m = 17$	$m = 18$	$m = 19$	$m = 20$	$m = 21$	$m = 22$	$m = 23$	$m = 24$	$m = 25$
$n = m$	192,273	220,308	249,346	280,386	314,427	349,471	386,517	424,566	465,616	508,668	552,723
$n = m + 1$	198,282	226,318	256,356	287,397	321,439	356,484	394,530	433,579	474,630	517,683	562,738
$n = m + 2$	203,292	232,328	262,367	294,408	328,451	364,496	402,543	442,592	483,644	527,697	572.753
$n = m + 3$	209,301	238,338	268,378	301,419	336,462	372,508	410,556	450,606	492,658	536,712	582,768
$n = m + 4$	215,310	244,348	275,388	308,430	343,474	380,520	418,569	459,619	501,672	546,726	592,783
$n = m + 5$	220,320	250,358	281,399	315,441	350,486	387,533	427,581	468,632	511,685	555,741	602,798
$n = m + 6$	226,329	256,368	288,409	322,452	358,497	395,545	435,594	476,646	520,699	565,755	612,813
$n = m + 7$	231,339	262,378	294,420	329,463	365,509	403,557	443,607	485,659	529,713	574,770	622,828
$n = m + 8$	237,348	268,388	301,430	336,474	372,521	411,569	451,620	494,672	538,727	584,784	632,843
$n = m + 9$	242,358	274,398	307,441	342,486	380,532	419,581	459,633	502,686	547,741	594,798	642,858
$n = m + 10$	248,367	280,408	314,451	349,497	387,544	426,594	468,645	511,699	556,755	603,813	652,873
$n = m + 11$	254,376	286,418	320,462	356,508	394,556	434,606	476,658	520,712	565,769	613,827	662,888
$n = m + 12$	259,386	292,428	327,472	363,519	402,567	442,618	484,671	528,726	574,783	622,842	672,903
$n = m + 13$	265,395	298,438	333,483	370,530	409,579	450,630	492,684	537,739	584,796	632,856	682,918
$n = m + 14$	270,405	304,448	340,493	377,541	416,591	458,642	501,696	546,752	593,810	642,870	692,933
$n = m + 15$	276,414	310,458	346,504	384,552	424,602	465,655	509,709	554,766	602,824	651,885	702,948
$n = m + 16$	282,423	316,468	353,514	391,563	431,614	473,667	517,722	563,779	611,838	661,899	712,963
$n = m + 17$	287,433	322,478	359,525	398,574	438,626	481,679	526,734	572,792	620,852	670,914	723,977
$n = m + 18$	293,442	328,488	366,535	405,585	446,637	489,691	534,747	581,805	629,866	680,928	733,992
$n = m + 19$	299,451	334,498	372,546	412,596	453,649	497,703	542,760	589,819	639,879	690,942	743,1007
$n = m + 20$	304,461	340,508	379,556	419,607	461,660	505,715	550,773	598,832	648,893	699,957	753,1022
$n = m + 21$	310,470	347,517	385,568	426,618	468,672	512,728	559,785	607,845	657,907	709,971	763,1037
$n = m + 22$	315,480	353,527	392,577	433,629	475,684	520,740	567,798	615,859	666,921	718,986	773,1052
$n = m + 23$	321,489	359,537	398,588	439,641	483,695	528,752	575,811	624,872	675,935	728,1000	783,1067
$n = m + 24$	327,498	365,547	405,598	446,652	490,707	536,764	583,824	633,885	684,949	738,1014	793,1082
$n = m + 25$	332,508	371,557	411,609	453,663	498,718	544,776	592,836	642,898	694,962	747,1029	803,1097

CRITICAL VALUES FOR THE WILCOXON RANK SUM TEST

$m = 3(1)25$ and $n = m(1)m + 25$

$P = .025$ one-sided; $P = .05$ two-sided

n	$m = 3$	$m = 4$	$m = 5$	$m = 6$	$m = 7$	$m = 8$	$m = 9$	$m = 10$	$m = 11$	$m = 12$	$m = 13$	$m = 14$
$n = m$	5,16	11,25	18,37	26,52	37,68	49,87	63,108	79,131	96,157	116,184	137,214	160,246
$n = m + 1$	6,18	12,28	19,41	28,56	39,73	51,93	66,114	82,138	100,164	120,192	141,223	165,255
$n = m + 2$	6,21	12,32	20,45	29,61	41,78	54,98	68,121	85,145	103,172	124,200	146,231	170,264
$n = m + 3$	7,23	13,35	21,49	31,65	43,83	56,104	71,127	88,152	107,179	128,208	150,240	174,274
$n = m + 4$	7,26	14,38	22,53	32,70	45,88	58,110	74,133	91,159	110,187	131,217	154,249	179,283
$n = m + 5$	8,28	15,41	24,56	34,74	46,94	61,115	77,139	94,166	114,194	135,225	159,257	184,292
$n = m + 6$	8,31	16,44	25,60	36,78	48,99	63,121	79,146	97,173	118,201	139,233	163,266	189,301
$n = m + 7$	9,33	17,47	26,64	37,83	50,104	65,127	82,152	101,179	121,209	143,241	168,274	194,310
$n = m + 8$	10,35	17,51	27,68	39,87	52,109	68,132	85,158	104,186	125,216	147,249	172,283	198,320
$n = m + 9$	10,38	18,54	29,71	41,91	54,114	70,138	88,164	107,193	128,224	151,257	176,292	203,329
$n = m + 10$	11,40	19,57	30,75	42,96	56,119	72,144	90,171	110,200	132,231	155,265	181,300	208,338
$n = m + 11$	11,43	20,60	31,79	44,100	58,124	75,149	93,177	113,207	135,239	159,273	185,309	213,347
$n = m + 12$	12,45	21,63	32,83	45,105	60,129	77,155	96,183	117,213	139,246	163,281	190,317	218,356
$n = m + 13$	12,48	22,66	33,87	47,109	62,134	80,160	99,189	120,220	143,253	167,289	194,326	222,366
$n = m + 14$	13,50	23,69	35,90	49,113	64,139	82,166	101,196	123,227	146,261	171,297	198,335	227,375
$n = m + 15$	13,53	24,72	36,94	50,118	66,144	84,172	104,202	126,234	150,268	175,305	203,343	232,384
$n = m + 16$	14,55	24,76	37,98	52,122	68,149	87,177	107,208	129,241	153,276	179,313	207,352	237,393
$n = m + 17$	14,58	25,79	38,102	53,127	70,154	89,183	110,214	132,248	157,283	183,321	212,360	242,402
$n = m + 18$	15,60	26,82	40,105	55,131	72,159	92,188	113,220	136,254	161,290	187,329	216,369	247,411
$n = m + 19$	15,63	27,85	41,109	57,135	74,164	94,194	115,227	139,261	164,298	191,337	221,377	252,420
$n = m + 20$	16,65	28,88	42,113	58,140	76,169	96,200	118,233	142,268	168,305	195,345	225,386	256,430
$n = m + 21$	16,68	29,91	43,117	60,144	78,174	99,205	121,239	145,275	171,313	199,353	229,395	261,439
$n = m + 22$	17,70	30,94	45,120	61,149	80,179	101,211	124,245	148,282	175,320	203,361	234,403	266,448
$n = m + 23$	17,73	31,97	46,124	63,153	82,184	103,217	127,251	152,288	179,327	207,369	238,412	271,457
$n = m + 24$	18,75	31,101	47,128	65,157	84,189	106,222	129,258	155,295	182,335	211,377	243,420	276,466
$n = m + 25$	18,78	32,104	48,132	66,162	86,194	108,228	132,264	158,302	186,342	216,384	247,429	281,475

$m = 3(1)25$ and $n = m(1)m + 25$

$P = .025$ one-sided; $P = .05$ two-sided

n	$m = 15$	$m = 16$	$m = 17$	$m = 18$	$m = 19$	$m = 20$	$m = 21$	$m = 22$	$m = 23$	$m = 24$	$m = 25$
$n = m$	185,280	212,316	240,355	271,395	303,438	337,483	373,530	411,579	451,630	493,683	536,739
$n = m + 1$	190,290	217,327	246,366	277,407	310,450	345,495	381,543	419,593	460,644	502,698	546,754
$n = m + 2$	195,300	223,337	252,377	284,418	317,462	352,508	389,556	428,606	468,659	511,713	555,770
$n = m + 3$	201,309	229,347	258,388	290,430	324,474	359,521	397,569	436,620	477,673	520,728	565,785
$n = m + 4$	206,319	234,358	264,399	297,441	331,486	367,533	404,583	444,634	486,687	529,743	574,801
$n = m + 5$	211,329	240,368	271,409	303,453	338,498	374,546	412,596	452,648	494,702	538,758	584,816
$n = m + 6$	216,339	245,379	277,420	310,464	345,510	381,559	420,609	460,662	503,716	547,773	593,832
$n = m + 7$	221,349	251,389	283,431	316,476	351,523	389,571	428,622	469,675	512,730	556,788	603,847
$n = m + 8$	227,358	257,399	289,442	323,487	358,535	396,584	436,635	477,689	520,745	565,803	612,863
$n = m + 9$	232,368	262,410	295,453	329,499	365,547	403,597	443,649	485,703	529,759	575,817	622,878
$n = m + 10$	237,378	268,420	301,464	336,510	372,559	411,609	451,662	493,717	538,773	584,832	632,893
$n = m + 11$	242,388	274,430	307,475	342,522	379,571	418,622	459,675	502,730	546,788	593,847	641,909
$n = m + 12$	248,397	279,441	313,486	349,533	386,583	426,634	467,688	510,744	555,802	602,862	651,924
$n = m + 13$	253,407	285,451	319,497	355,545	393,595	433,647	475,701	518,758	564,816	611,877	660,940
$n = m + 14$	258,417	291,461	325,508	362,556	400,607	440,660	482,715	526,772	572,831	620,892	670,955
$n = m + 15$	263,427	296,472	331,519	368,568	407,619	448,672	490,728	535,785	581,845	629,907	679,971
$n = m + 16$	269,436	302,482	338,529	375,579	414,631	455,685	498,741	543,799	590,859	638,922	689,986
$n = m + 17$	274,446	308,492	344,540	381,591	421,643	463,697	506,754	551,813	599,873	648,936	699,1001
$n = m + 18$	279,456	314,502	350,551	388,602	428,655	470,710	514,767	560,826	607,888	657,951	708,1017
$n = m + 19$	284,466	319,513	356,562	395,613	435,667	477,723	522,780	568,840	616,902	666,966	718,1032
$n = m + 20$	290,475	325,523	362,573	401,625	442,679	485,735	530,793	576,854	625,916	675,981	727,1048
$n = m + 21$	295,485	331,533	368,584	408,636	449,691	492,748	537,807	584,868	633,931	684,996	737,1063
$n = m + 22$	300,495	336,544	374,595	414,648	456,703	500,760	545,820	593,881	642,945	693,1011	747,1078
$n = m + 23$	306,504	342,554	380,606	421,659	463,715	507,773	553,833	601,895	651,959	703,1025	756,1094
$n = m + 24$	311,514	348,564	387,616	427,671	470,727	515,785	561,846	609,909	660,973	712,1040	766,1109
$n = m + 25$	316,524	353,575	393,627	434,682	477,739	522,798	569,859	618,922	668,988	721,1055	775,1125

CRITICAL VALUES FOR THE WILCOXON RANK SUM TEST

$m = 3(1)25$ and $n = m(1)m + 25$

$P = .01$ one-sided; $P = .02$ two-sided

n	$m = 3$	$m = 4$	$m = 5$	$m = 6$	$m = 7$	$m = 8$	$m = 9$	$m = 10$	$m = 11$	$m = 12$	$m = 13$	$m = 14$
$n = m$	5,16	10,26	16,39	24,54	34,71	46,90	59,112	74,136	91,162	110,190	130,221	153,253
$n = m + 1$	5,19	10,30	17,43	26,58	36,76	48,96	62,118	77,143	94,170	113,199	134,230	157,263
$n = m + 2$	6,21	11,33	18,47	27,63	38,81	50,102	64,125	80,150	97,178	117,207	138,239	161,273
$n = m + 3$	6,24	12,36	19,51	28,68	39,87	52,108	66,132	83,157	101,185	120,216	142,248	166,282
$n = m + 4$	6,27	12,40	20,55	30,72	41,92	54,114	69,138	85,165	104,193	124,224	146,257	170,292
$n = m + 5$	7,29	13,43	21,59	31,77	43,97	56,120	71,145	88,172	107,201	128,232	150,266	174,302
$n = m + 6$	7,32	14,46	22,63	32,82	44,103	58,126	74,151	91,179	110,209	131,241	154,275	179,311
$n = m + 7$	7,35	14,50	23,67	34,86	46,108	60,132	76,158	94,186	113,217	135,249	158,284	183,321
$n = m + 8$	8,37	15,53	24,71	35,91	48,113	62,138	79,164	97,193	117,224	138,258	162,293	188,330
$n = m + 9$	8,40	16,56	25,75	36,96	49,119	64,144	81,171	100,200	120,232	142,266	166,302	192,340
$n = m + 10$	9,42	16,60	26,79	38,100	51,124	66,150	83,178	102,208	123,240	146,274	170,311	196,350
$n = m + 11$	9,45	17,63	27,83	39,105	53,129	68,156	86,184	105,215	126,248	149,283	174,320	201,359
$n = m + 12$	9,48	18,66	28,87	40,110	55,134	71,161	88,191	108,222	130,255	153,291	178,329	205,369
$n = m + 13$	10,50	18,70	29,91	42,114	56,140	73,167	91,197	111,229	133,263	157,299	182,338	210,378
$n = m + 14$	10,53	19,73	30,95	43,119	58,145	75,173	93,204	114,236	136,271	160,308	186,347	214,388
$n = m + 15$	10,56	20,76	31,99	45,123	60,150	77,179	96,210	117,243	139,279	164,316	190,356	219,397
$n = m + 16$	11,58	20,80	32,103	46,128	61,156	79,185	98,217	120,250	143,286	168,324	194,365	223,407
$n = m + 17$	11,61	21,83	33,107	47,133	63,161	81,191	101,223	122,258	146,294	171,333	198,374	228,416
$n = m + 18$	12,63	22,86	34,111	49,137	65,166	83,197	103,230	125,265	149,302	175,341	203,382	232,426
$n = m + 19$	12,66	23,89	35,115	50,142	67,171	85,203	106,236	128,272	152,310	179,349	207,391	236,436
$n = m + 20$	12,69	23,93	36,119	51,147	68,177	87,209	108,243	131,279	156,317	182,358	211,400	241,445
$n = m + 21$	13,71	24,96	37,123	53,151	70,182	90,214	111,249	134,286	159,325	186,366	215,409	245,455
$n = m + 22$	13,74	25,99	38,127	54,156	72,187	92,220	113,256	137,293	162,333	190,374	219,418	250,464
$n = m + 23$	14,76	25,103	39,131	56,160	74,192	94,226	116,262	140,300	165,341	193,383	223,427	254,474
$n = m + 24$	14,79	26,106	40,135	57,165	75,198	96,232	118,269	143,307	169,348	197,391	227,436	259,483
$n = m + 25$	14,82	27,109	41,139	58,170	77,203	98,238	121,275	145,315	172,356	201,399	231,445	263,493

$m = 3(1)25$ and $n = m(1)m + 25$

$P = .01$ one-sided; $P = .02$ two-sided

n	$m = 15$	$m = 16$	$m = 17$	$m = 18$	$m = 19$	$m = 20$	$m = 21$	$m = 22$	$m = 23$	$m = 24$	$m = 25$
$n = m$	177,288	202,326	230,365	260,406	291,450	324,496	359,544	396,594	435,646	476,700	518,757
$n = m + 1$	181,299	208,336	236,376	266,418	297,463	331,509	367,557	404,608	443,661	484,716	527,773
$n = m + 2$	186,309	213,347	241,388	272,430	304,475	338,522	374,571	412,622	451,676	493,731	536,789
$n = m + 3$	191,319	218,358	247,399	278,442	310,488	345,535	381,585	419,637	459,691	501,747	545,805
$n = m + 4$	196,329	223,369	253,410	284,454	317,500	352,548	388,599	427,651	467,706	510,762	554,821
$n = m + 5$	200,340	228,380	258,422	290,466	323,513	359,561	396,612	435,665	476,720	518,778	563,837
$n = m + 6$	205,350	234,390	264,433	296,478	330,525	365,575	403,626	442,680	484,735	527,793	572,853
$n = m + 7$	210,360	239,401	269,445	302,490	336,538	372,588	410,640	450,694	492,750	535,809	581,869
$n = m + 8$	215,370	244,412	275,456	308,502	343,550	379,601	418,653	458,708	500,765	544,824	590,885
$n = m + 9$	220,380	249,423	281,467	314,514	349,563	386,614	425,667	466,722	508,780	553,839	599,901
$n = m + 10$	225,390	255,433	286,479	320,526	356,575	393,627	432,681	473,737	516,795	561,855	608,917
$n = m + 11$	229,401	260,444	292,490	326,538	362,588	400,640	440,694	481,751	524,810	570,870	617,933
$n = m + 12$	234,411	265,455	298,501	332,550	369,600	407,653	447,708	489,765	533,824	578,886	626,949
$n = m + 13$	239,421	270,466	303,513	338,562	375,613	414,666	454,722	497,779	541,839	587,901	635,965
$n = m + 14$	244,431	276,476	309,524	344,574	382,625	421,679	462,735	504,794	549,854	596,916	644,981
$n = m + 15$	249,441	281,487	315,535	350,586	388,638	428,692	469,749	512,808	557,869	604,932	653,997
$n = m + 16$	254,451	286,498	320,547	357,597	395,650	434,706	476,763	520,822	565,884	613,947	662,1013
$n = m + 17$	259,461	291,509	326,558	363,609	401,663	441,719	484,776	528,836	574,898	621,963	671,1029
$n = m + 18$	263,472	297,519	332,569	369,621	408,675	448,732	491,790	535,851	582,913	630,978	680,1045
$n = m + 19$	268,482	302,530	337,581	375,633	414,688	455,745	498,804	543,865	590,928	639,993	689,1061
$n = m + 20$	273,492	307,541	343,592	381,645	421,700	462,758	506,817	551,879	598,943	647,1009	698,1077
$n = m + 21$	278,502	312,552	349,603	387,657	427,713	469,771	513,831	559,893	606,958	656,1024	707,1093
$n = m + 22$	283,512	318,562	355,614	393,669	434,725	476,784	520,845	567,907	615,972	665,1039	716,1109
$n = m + 23$	288,522	323,573	360,626	399,681	440,738	483,797	528,858	574,922	623,987	673,1055	726,1124
$n = m + 24$	293,532	328,584	366,637	405,693	447,750	490,810	535,872	582,936	631,1002	682,1070	735,1140
$n = m + 25$	298,542	334,594	372,648	412,704	453,763	497,823	543,885	590,950	639,1017	691,1085	744,1156

CRITICAL VALUES FOR THE WILCOXON RANK SUM TEST

$m = 3(1)25$ and $n = m(1)m + 25$
$P = .005$ one-sided; $P = .01$ two-sided

n	$m = 3$	$m = 4$	$m = 5$	$m = 6$	$m = 7$	$m = 8$	$m = 9$	$m = 10$	$m = 11$	$m = 12$	$m = 13$	$m = 14$
$n = m$	5,16	9,27	15,40	23,55	33,72	44,92	57,114	71,139	88,165	106,194	126,225	148,258
$n = m + 1$	5,19	10,30	16,44	24,60	34,78	46,98	59,121	74,146	91,173	109,203	130,234	152,268
$n = m + 2$	5,22	10,34	17,48	25,65	36,83	47,105	61,128	76,154	94,181	113,211	133,244	156,278
$n = m + 3$	5,25	11,37	18,52	27,69	37,89	49,111	63,135	79,161	97,189	116,220	137,253	160,288
$n = m + 4$	6,27	11,41	19,56	28,74	39,94	51,117	65,142	82,168	100,197	119,229	141,262	164,298
$n = m + 5$	6,30	12,44	19,61	29,79	40,100	53,123	68,148	84,176	102,206	123,237	144,272	168,308
$n = m + 6$	6,33	12,48	20,65	30,84	42,105	55,129	70,155	87,183	105,214	126,246	148,281	172,318
$n = m + 7$	6,36	13,51	21,69	31,89	43,111	57,135	72,162	89,191	108,222	129,255	152,290	176,328
$n = m + 8$	7,38	13,55	22,73	32,94	45,116	59,141	74,169	92,198	111,230	133,263	156,299	180,338
$n = m + 9$	7,41	14,58	23,77	34,98	46,122	61,147	77,175	95,205	114,238	136,272	159,309	185,347
$n = m + 10$	7,44	15,61	24,81	35,103	48,127	62,154	79,182	97,213	117,246	139,281	163,318	189,357
$n = m + 11$	8,46	15,65	25,85	36,108	49,133	64,160	81,189	100,220	120,254	143,289	167,327	193,367
$n = m + 12$	8,49	16,68	26,89	37,113	51,138	66,166	83,196	103,227	123,262	146,298	171,336	197,377
$n = m + 13$	8,52	16,72	26,94	38,118	52,144	68,172	86,202	105,235	126,270	150,306	175,345	201,387
$n = m + 14$	9,54	17,75	27,98	40,122	54,149	70,178	88,209	108,242	129,278	153,315	178,355	205,397
$n = m + 15$	9,57	17,79	28,102	41,127	55,155	72,184	90,216	110,250	132,286	156,324	182,364	210,406
$n = m + 16$	9,60	18,82	29,106	42,132	57,160	74,190	93,222	113,257	136,293	160,332	186,373	214,416
$n = m + 17$	9,63	19,85	30,110	43,137	59,165	76,196	95,229	116,264	139,301	163,341	190,382	218,426
$n = m + 18$	10,65	19,89	31,114	45,141	60,171	78,202	97,236	118,272	142,309	167,349	194,391	222,436
$n = m + 19$	10,68	20,92	32,118	46,146	62,176	80,208	99,243	121,279	145,317	170,358	197,401	226,446
$n = m + 20$	10,71	20,96	33,122	47,151	63,182	82,214	102,249	124,286	148,325	173,367	201,410	231,455
$n = m + 21$	11,73	21,99	33,127	48,156	65,187	83,221	104,256	126,294	151,333	177,375	205,419	235,465
$n = m + 22$	11,76	21,103	34,131	49,161	66,193	85,227	106,263	129,301	154,341	180,384	209,428	239,475
$n = m + 23$	11,79	22,106	35,135	51,165	68,198	87,233	109,269	132,308	157,349	184,392	213,437	243,485
$n = m + 24$	12,81	23,109	36,139	52,170	70,203	89,239	111,276	134,316	160,357	187,401	216,447	247,495
$n = m + 25$	12,84	23,113	37,143	53,175	71,209	91,245	113,283	137,323	163,365	191,409	220,456	252,504

$m = 3(1)25$ and $n = m(1)m + 25$
$P = .005$ one-sided; $P = .01$ two-sided

n	$m = 15$	$m = 16$	$m = 17$	$m = 18$	$m = 19$	$m = 20$	$m = 21$	$m = 22$	$m = 23$	$m = 24$	$m = 25$
$n = m$	171,294	196,332	223,372	252,414	283,458	316,504	350,553	386,604	424,657	464,712	506,769
$n = m + 1$	176,304	201,343	229,383	258,426	289,471	322,518	357,567	393,619	432,672	472,728	514,786
$n = m + 2$	180,315	206,354	234,395	264,438	295,484	329,531	364,581	401,633	440,687	480,744	523,802
$n = m + 3$	184,326	211,365	239,407	269,451	301,497	335,545	371,595	408,648	447,703	489,759	531,819
$n = m + 4$	189,336	216,376	245,418	275,463	307,510	342,558	378,609	415,663	455,718	497,775	540,835
$n = m + 5$	194,346	221,387	250,430	281,475	314,522	348,572	385,623	423,677	463,733	505,791	549,851
$n = m + 6$	198,357	226,398	255,442	287,487	320,535	355,585	392,637	430,692	471,748	513,807	557,868
$n = m + 7$	203,367	231,409	261,453	292,500	326,548	361,599	399,651	438,706	479,763	521,823	566,884
$n = m + 8$	207,378	236,420	266,465	298,512	332,561	368,612	405,666	445,721	486,779	530,838	575,900
$n = m + 9$	212,388	241,431	271,477	304,524	338,574	374,626	412,680	452,736	494,794	538,854	583,917
$n = m + 10$	216,399	245,443	277,488	310,536	344,587	381,639	419,694	460,750	502,809	546,870	592,933
$n = m + 11$	221,409	250,454	282,500	315,549	351,599	388,652	426,708	467,765	510,824	554,886	601,949
$n = m + 12$	225,420	255,465	287,512	321,561	357,612	394,666	433,722	475,779	518,839	563,901	609,966
$n = m + 13$	230,430	260,476	293,523	327,573	363,625	401,679	440,736	482,794	526,854	571,917	618,982
$n = m + 14$	235,440	265,487	298,535	333,585	369,638	407,693	447,750	490,808	533,870	579,933	627,998
$n = m + 15$	239,451	270,498	303,547	338,598	375,651	414,706	454,764	497,823	541,885	587,949	635,1015
$n = m + 16$	244,461	275,509	309,558	344,610	381,664	421,719	462,777	504,838	549,900	596,964	644,1031
$n = m + 17$	248,472	280,520	314,570	350,622	388,676	427,733	469,791	512,852	557,915	604,980	653,1047
$n = m + 18$	253,482	285,531	320,581	356,634	394,689	434,746	476,805	519,867	565,930	612,996	661,1064
$n = m + 19$	257,493	290,542	325,593	362,646	400,702	440,760	483,819	527,881	573,945	620,1012	670,1080
$n = m + 20$	262,503	295,553	330,605	367,659	406,715	447,773	490,833	534,896	580,961	629,1027	679,1096
$n = m + 21$	267,513	300,564	336,616	373,671	413,727	454,786	497,847	542,910	588,976	637,1043	687,1113
$n = m + 22$	271,524	305,575	341,628	379,683	419,740	460,800	504,861	549,925	596,991	645,1059	696,1129
$n = m + 23$	276,534	310,586	347,639	385,695	425,753	467,813	511,875	556,940	604,1006	654,1074	705,1145
$n = m + 24$	280,545	315,597	352,651	391,707	431,766	474,826	518,889	564,954	612,1021	662,1090	714,1161
$n = m + 25$	285,555	320,608	357,663	397,719	438,778	480,840	525,903	571,969	620,1036	670,1106	722,1178

X.6 DISTRIBUTION OF THE TOTAL NUMBER OF RUNS FOR UNEQUAL-SIZE SAMPLES

The theory of runs can be used to test data for randomness or to test the hypothesis that two samples come from the same population. A run is defined as a succession of identical elements which are followed and preceded by different elements or by no elements at all. Let N_1 be the number of elements of one kind and N_2 be the number of elements of the other kind. Let u equal the total number of runs among the $N_1 + N_2$ elements. Table (a) gives the sampling distribution for u for values of N_1 and N_2 less than or equal to 20 and Table (b) gives a number of percentage points of the distribution for larger sample sizes. The values listed in Table (a) give the probability that u or fewer runs will occur. In Table (b), the columns headed 0.5, 1, 2.5, 5 gives values of u such that u or fewer runs occur with probability less than that indicated; the columns headed 95, 97.5, 99, 99.5 gives values of u for which the probability of u or more runs is less than 0.05, 0.025, 0.01, 0.005. For large values of N_1 and N_2, particularly for $N_1 = N_2$ greater than 10, a normal approximation may be used, with

$$\text{mean} = \frac{2N_1N_2}{N_1 + N_2} + 1$$

and

$$\text{variance} = \frac{2N_1N_2(2N_1N_2 - N_1 - N_2)}{(N_1 + N_2)^2(N_1 + N_2 - 1)}$$

a) DISTRIBUTION OF THE TOTAL NUMBER OF RUNS u IN SAMPLES OF SIZE (N_1, N_2)

N_1, N_2 \ u	2	3	4	5	6	7	8	9	10
2,2	0.3333	0.6667	1.0000						
2,3	.2000	.5000	0.9000	1.0000					
2,4	.1333	.4000	.8000	1.0000					
2,5	.0952	.3333	.7143	1.0000					
2,6	.0714	.2857	.6429	1.0000					
2,7	.0556	.2500	.5833	1.0000					
2,8	.0444	.2222	.5333	1.0000					
2,9	.0364	.2000	.4909	1.0000					
2,10	.0303	.1818	.4545	1.0000					
2,11	.0256	.1667	.4231	1.0000					
2,12	.0220	.1538	.3956	1.0000					
2,13	.0190	.1429	.3714	1.0000					
2,14	.0167	.1333	.3500	1.0000					
2,15	.0147	.1250	.3309	1.0000					
2,16	.0131	.1176	.3137	1.0000					
2,17	.0117	.1111	.2982	1.0000					
2,18	.0105	.1053	.2842	1.0000					
2,19	.0095	.1000	.2714	1.0000					
2,20	.0087	.0952	.2597	1.0000					
3,3	0.1000	0.3000	0.7000	0.9000	1.0000				
3,4	.0571	.2000	.5429	.8000	0.9714	1.0000			
3,5	.0357	.1429	.4286	.7143	.9286	1.0000			
3,6	.0238	.1071	.3452	.6429	.8810	1.0000			
3,7	.0167	.0833	.2833	.5833	.8333	1.0000			
3,8	.0121	.0667	.2364	.5333	.7879	1.0000			
3,9	.0091	.0545	.2000	.4909	.7454	1.0000			
3,10	.0070	.0454	.1713	.4545	.7063	1.0000			
3,11	.0055	.0385	.1484	.4231	.6703	1.0000			
3,12	.0044	.0330	.1297	.3956	.6374	1.0000			
3,13	.0036	.0286	.1143	.3714	.6071	1.0000			
3,14	.0029	.0250	.1015	.3500	.5794	1.0000			
3,15	.0024	.0221	.0907	.3309	.5539	1.0000			
3,16	.0021	.0196	.0815	.3137	.5304	1.0000			
3,17	.0018	.0175	.0737	.2982	.5088	1.0000			
3,18	.0015	.0158	.0669	.2842	.4887	1.0000			
3,19	.0013	.0143	.0610	.2714	.4701	1.0000			
3,20	.0011	.0130	.0559	.2597	.4528	1.0000			

a) DISTRIBUTION OF THE TOTAL NUMBER OF RUNS u IN SAMPLES OF SIZE (N_1,N_2)

N_1,N_2 \ u	2	3	4	5	6	7	8	9	10
4,4	0.0286	0.1143	0.3714	0.6286	0.8857	0.9714	1.0000		
4,5	.0159	.0714	.2619	.5000	.7857	.9286	0.9921	1.0000	
4,6	.0095	.0476	.1905	.4048	.6905	.8810	.9762	1.0000	
4,7	.0061	.0333	.1424	.3333	.6061	.8333	.9545	1.0000	
4,8	.0040	.0242	.1091	.2788	.5333	.7879	.9293	1.0000	
4,9	.0028	.0182	.0853	.2364	.4713	.7454	.9021	1.0000	
4,10	.0020	.0140	.0679	.2028	.4186	.7063	.8741	1.0000	
4,11	.0015	.0110	.0549	.1758	.3736	.6703	.8462	1.0000	
4,12	.0011	.0088	.0451	.1538	.3352	.6374	.8187	1.0000	
4,13	$.0^{3}840$	.0071	.0374	.1357	.3021	.6071	.7920	1.0000	
4,14	$.0^{3}654$	.0059	.0314	.1206	.2735	.5794	.7663	1.0000	
4,15	$.0^{3}516$	.0049	.0266	.1078	.2487	.5539	.7417	1.0000	
4,16	$.0^{3}413$	.0041	.0227	.0970	.2270	.5304	.7183	1.0000	
4,17	$.0^{3}334$	.0035	.0195	.0877	.2080	.5088	.6959	1.0000	
4,18	$.0^{3}273$	.0030	.0170	.0797	.1912	.4887	.6746	1.0000	
4,19	$.0^{3}226$	.0026	.0148	.0727	.1764	.4701	.6544	1.0000	
4,20	$.0^{3}188$	.0023	.0130	.0666	.1632	.4528	.6352	1.0000	
5,5	$0.0^{2}794$	0.0397	0.1667	0.3571	0.6429	0.8333	0.9603	0.9921	1.0000
5,6	$.0^{2}433$	.0238	.1104	.2619	.5216	.7381	.9112	.9762	0.9978
5,7	$.0^{2}252$	.0152	.0758	.1970	.4242	.6515	.8535	.9545	.9924
5,8	$.0^{2}155$	.0101	.0536	.1515	.3473	.5758	.7933	.9293	.9837
5,9	$.0^{3}999$	$.0^{2}699$	.0390	.1189	.2867	.5105	.7343	.9021	.9720
5,10	$.0^{3}666$	$.0^{2}500$	.0290	.0949	.2388	.4545	.6783	.8741	.9580
5,11	$.0^{3}458$	$.0^{2}366$	.0220	.0769	.2005	.4066	.6264	.8462	.9423
5,12	$.0^{3}323$	$.0^{2}275$	.0170	.0632	.1698	.3654	.5787	.8187	.9253
5,13	$.0^{3}233$	$.0^{2}210$	.0133	.0525	.1450	.3298	.5352	.7920	.9076
5,14	$.0^{3}172$	$.0^{2}163$	.0106	.0441	.1246	.2990	.4958	.7663	.8893
5,15	$.0^{3}129$	$.0^{2}129$	$.0^{2}851$	.0374	.1078	.2722	.4600	.7417	.8709
5,16	$.0^{4}983$	$.0^{2}103$	$.0^{2}693$	.0320	.0939	.2487	.4276	.7183	.8524
5,17	$.0^{4}759$	$.0^{3}835$	$.0^{2}570$	.0276	.0822	.2281	.3982	.6959	.8341
5,18	$.0^{4}594$	$.0^{3}684$	$.0^{2}472$	.0239	.0724	.2098	.3715	.6746	.8161
5,19	$.0^{4}471$	$.0^{3}565$	$.0^{2}395$	.0209	.0641	.1937	.3473	.6544	.7984
5,20	$.0^{4}376$	$.0^{3}470$	$.0^{2}333$	.0184	.0570	.1793	.3252	.6352	.7811
6,6	$0.0^{2}216$	0.0130	0.0671	0.1753	0.3918	0.6082	0.8247	0.9329	0.9870
6,7	$.0^{2}117$	$.0^{2}758$	.0425	.1212	.2960	.5000	.7331	.8788	.9662
6,8	$.0^{3}666$	$.0^{2}466$	.0280	.0862	.2261	.4126	.6457	.8205	.9371
6,9	$.0^{3}400$	$.0^{2}300$	.0190	.0629	.1748	.3427	.5664	.7622	.9021
6,10	$.0^{3}250$	$.0^{2}200$	.0132	.0470	.1369	.2867	.4965	.7063	.8636
6,11	$.0^{3}162$	$.0^{2}137$	$.0^{2}945$	.0357	.1084	.2418	.4357	.6538	.8235
6,12	$.0^{3}108$	$.0^{3}970$	$.0^{2}690$	.0276	.0869	.2054	.3832	.6054	.7831
6,13	$.0^{4}737$	$.0^{3}700$	$.0^{2}512$	.0217	.0704	.1758	.3379	.5609	.7434
6,14	$.0^{4}516$	$.0^{3}516$	$.0^{2}387$	.0173	.0575	.1514	.2990	.5204	.7048
6,15	$.0^{4}369$	$.0^{3}387$	$.0^{2}297$	.0139	.0475	.1313	.2655	.4835	.6680
6,16	$.0^{4}268$	$.0^{3}295$	$.0^{2}230$	.0114	.0395	.1146	.2365	.4500	.6329
6,17	$.0^{4}198$	$.0^{3}228$	$.0^{2}181$	$.0^{2}934$	.0331	.1005	.2114	.4195	.5998
6,18	$.0^{4}149$	$.0^{3}178$	$.0^{2}144$	$.0^{2}776$	.0280	.0886	.1896	.3917	.5685
6,19	$.0^{4}113$	$.0^{3}141$	$.0^{2}116$	$.0^{2}649$	.0238	.0785	.1706	.3665	.5392
6,20	$.0^{5}087$	$.0^{3}113$	$.0^{3}938$	$.0^{2}548$	.0203	.0698	.1540	.3434	.5118

a) DISTRIBUTION OF THE TOTAL NUMBER OF RUNS u IN SAMPLES OF SIZE (N_1, N_2)

11	12	13	14	15	16	17	18	19	20	21
1.0000										
1.0000										
1.0000										
1.0000										
1.0000										
1.0000										
1.0000										
1.0000										
1.0000										
1.0000										
1.0000										
1.0000										
1.0000										
1.0000										
1.0000										
0.9978	1.0000									
.9924	0.9994	1.0000								
.9837	.9977	1.0000								
.9720	.9944	1.0000								
.9580	.9895	1.0000								
.9423	.9830	1.0000								
.9253	.9751	1.0000								
.9076	.9659	1.0000								
.8893	.9557	1.0000								
.8709	.9447	1.0000								
.8524	.9329	1.0000								
.8341	.9207	1.0000								
.8161	.9080	1.0000								
.7984	.8952	1.0000								
.7811	.8822	1.0000								

a) DISTRIBUTION OF THE TOTAL NUMBER OF RUNS u IN SAMPLES OF SIZE (N_1, N_2)

N_1, N_2 \ u	2	3	4	5	6	7	8	9	10
7,7	0.0^{3}583	0.0^{2}408	0.0251	0.0775	0.2086	0.3834	0.6166	0.7914	0.9225
7,8	.0^{3}311	.0^{2}233	.0154	.0513	.1492	.2960	.5136	.7040	.8671
7,9	.0^{3}175	.0^{2}140	.0^{2}979	.0350	.1084	.2308	.4266	.6224	.8059
7,10	.0^{3}103	.0^{3}874	.0^{2}643	.0245	.0800	.1818	.3546	.5490	.7433
7,11	.0^{4}628	.0^{3}566	.0^{2}434	.0175	.0600	.1448	.2956	.4842	.6821
7,12	.0^{4}397	.0^{3}377	.0^{2}300	.0128	.0456	.1165	.2475	.4276	.6241
7,13	.0^{4}258	.0^{3}258	.0^{2}212	.0^{2}955	.0351	.0947	.2082	.3785	.5700
7,14	.0^{4}172	.0^{3}181	.0^{2}152	.0^{2}722	.0273	.0777	.1760	.3359	.5204
7,15	.0^{4}117	.0^{3}129	.0^{2}111	.0^{2}555	.0216	.0642	.1496	.2990	.4751
7,16	.0^{4}082	.0^{4}938	.0^{3}828	.0^{2}432	.0172	.0536	.1278	.2670	.4340
7,17	.0^{4}058	.0^{4}693	.0^{3}624	.0^{2}340	.0138	.0450	.1097	.2392	.3969
7,18	.0^{4}042	.0^{4}520	.0^{3}476	.0^{2}270	.0112	.0381	.0946	.2149	.3634
7,19	.0^{4}030	.0^{4}395	.0^{3}368	.0^{2}217	.0^{2}915	.0324	.0820	.1937	.3332
7,20	.0^{4}023	.0^{4}304	.0^{3}287	.0^{2}176	.0^{2}754	.0278	.0714	.1751	.3060
8,8	0.0^{3}155	0.0^{2}124	0.0^{2}886	0.03170	0.1002	0.2144	0.4048	0.5952	0.7855
8,9	.0^{4}823	.0^{3}6993	.0^{2}5306	.02028	.06865	.1573	.3186	.5000	.7016
8,10	.0^{4}457	.0^{3}4114	.0^{2}3291	.01337	.04792	.1170	.2514	.4194	.6209
8,11	.0^{4}265	.0^{3}2514	.0^{2}2104	.0^{2}9050	.03406	.08824	.1994	.3522	.5467
8,12	.0^{4}159	.0^{3}1588	.0^{2}1381	.0^{2}6271	.02461	.06740	.1591	.2966	.4800
8,13	.0^{4}098	.0^{3}1032	.0^{3}9288	.0^{2}4438	.01806	.05212	.1278	.2508	.4210
8,14	.0^{4}063	.0^{4}688	.0^{3}6380	.0^{2}3199	.01344	.04076	.1034	.2129	.3694
8,15	.0^{4}041	.0^{4}469	.0^{3}4467	.0^{2}2345	.01014	.03223	.08419	.1816	.3245
8,16	.0^{4}027	.0^{4}326	.0^{3}3182	.0^{2}1746	.0^{2}7742	.02573	.06904	.1556	.2856
8,17	.0^{4}018	.0^{4}231	.0^{3}2302	.0^{2}1318	.0^{2}5977	.02073	.05698	.1340	.2518
8,18	.0^{4}013	.0^{4}166	.0^{3}1690	.0^{2}1007	.0^{2}4663	.01685	.04732	.1159	.2225
8,19	.0^{4}009	.0^{4}122	.0^{3}1257	.0^{3}7784	.0^{2}3673	.01380	.03953	.1006	.1971
8,20	.0^{4}006	.0^{4}090	.0^{4}946	.0^{3}6081	.0^{2}2919	.01139	.03322	.08777	.1751
9,9	0.0^{4}411	0.0^{3}3702	0.0^{2}3003	0.01222	0.04447	0.1090	0.2380	0.3992	0.6008
9,10	.0^{4}217	.0^{3}2057	.0^{2}1764	.0^{2}7610	.02943	.07672	.1786	.3186	.5095
9,11	.0^{4}119	.0^{3}1191	.0^{2}1072	.0^{2}4882	.01989	.05489	.1349	.2549	.4300
9,12	.0^{4}068	.0^{4}714	.0^{3}6702	.0^{2}3215	.01369	.03989	.1028	.2049	.3621
9,13	.0^{4}040	.0^{4}442	.0^{3}4302	.0^{2}2167	.0^{2}9598	.02941	.07895	.1656	.3050
9,14	.0^{4}024	.0^{4}281	.0^{3}2827	.0^{2}1492	.0^{2}6837	.02198	.06118	.1347	.2572
9,15	.0^{4}015	.0^{4}184	.0^{3}1897	.0^{2}1046	.0^{2}4944	.01664	.04782	.1102	.2174
9,16	.0^{4}010	.0^{4}122	.0^{3}1297	.0^{3}7465	.0^{2}3625	.01274	.03768	.09069	.1842
9,17	.0^{4}006	.0^{4}083	.0^{4}903	.0^{3}5409	.0^{2}2692	.0^{2}9861	.02993	.07510	.1566
9,18	.0^{4}004	.0^{4}058	.0^{4}638	.0^{3}3975	.0^{2}2022	.0^{2}7710	.02396	.06255	.1336
9,19	.0^{4}003	.0^{4}041	.0^{4}458	.0^{3}2959	.0^{2}1536	.0^{2}6085	.01932	.05240	.1144
9,20	.0^{4}002	.0^{4}029	.0^{4}333	.0^{3}2230	.0^{2}1179	.0^{2}4844	.01568	.04413	.09831
10,10	0.0^{4}108	0.0^{3}1083	0.0^{3}9851	0.0^{2}4492	0.01852	0.05126	0.1276	0.2422	0.4141
10,11	.0^{4}057	.0^{4}595	.0^{3}5699	.0^{2}2739	.01192	.03489	.09205	.1849	.3350
10,12	.0^{4}031	.0^{4}340	.0^{3}3402	.0^{2}1718	.0^{2}7842	.02417	.06704	.1421	.2707
10,13	.0^{4}017	.0^{4}201	.0^{3}2089	.0^{2}1106	.0^{2}5259	.01703	.04933	.1099	.2189
10,14	.0^{4}010	.0^{4}122	.0^{3}1315	.0^{3}7281	.0^{2}3592	.01218	.03668	.08568	.1775
10,15	.0^{4}006	.0^{4}076	.0^{4}847	.0^{3}4895	.0^{2}2494	.0^{2}8841	.02755	.06731	.1445
10,16	.0^{4}004	.0^{4}049	.0^{4}557	.0^{3}3353	.0^{2}1759	.0^{2}6503	.02089	.05327	.1180
10,17	.0^{4}002	.0^{4}032	.0^{4}373	.0^{3}2336	.0^{2}1258	.0^{2}4842	.01599	.04248	.09684
10,18	.0^{4}002	.0^{4}021	.0^{4}255	.0^{3}1654	.0^{3}9115	.0^{2}3648	.01235	.03412	.07982
10,19	.0^{4}001	.0^{4}014	.0^{4}176	.0^{3}1187	.0^{3}6687	.0^{2}2777	.0^{2}9621	.02759	.06608
10,20	.0^{5}001	.0^{4}010	.0^{4}124	.0^{4}864	.0^{3}4962	.0^{2}2135	.0^{2}7554	.02245	.05496

a) DISTRIBUTION OF THE TOTAL NUMBER OF RUNS u IN SAMPLES OF SIZE (N_1, N_2)

11	12	13	14	15	16	17	18	19	20	21
0.9749	0.9959	0.9994	1.0000							
.9487	.9879	.9977	0.9998	1.0000						
.9161	.9748	.9944	.9993	1.0000						
.8794	.9571	.9895	.9981	1.0000						
.8405	.9355	.9830	.9962	1.0000						
.8009	.9109	.9751	.9934	1.0000						
.7616	.8842	.9659	.9898	1.0000						
.7233	.8561	.9557	.9852	1.0000						
.6864	.8273	.9447	.9799	1.0000						
.6512	.7982	.9329	.9738	1.0000						
.6178	.7692	.9207	.9669	1.0000						
.5862	.7407	.9081	.9595	1.0000						
.5565	.7128	.8952	.9516	1.0000						
.5286	.6857	.8822	.9433	1.0000						
0.8998	0.9683	0.9911	0.9988	0.9998	1.0000					
.8427	.9394	.9797	.9958	.9993	0.99996	1.0000				
.7822	.9031	.9636	.9905	.9981	.99979	1.0000				
.7217	.8618	.9434	.9823	.9962	.99940	1.0000				
.6634	.8174	.9201	.9714	.9934	.99869	1.0000				
.6084	.7718	.8944	.9580	.9898	.99757	1.0000				
.5573	.7263	.8672	.9423	.9852	.99598	1.0000				
.5103	.6818	.8390	.9248	.9799	.99388	1.0000				
.4674	.6389	.8104	.9057	.9738	.99125	1.0000				
.4285	.5981	.7818	.8855	.9670	.9881	1.0000				
.3931	.5595	.7536	.8645	.9595	.9844	1.0000				
.3611	.5232	.7258	.8429	.9516	.9803	1.0000				
.3322	.4893	.6988	.8210	.9433	.9757	1.0000				
0.7620	0.8910	0.9555	0.9878	0.9970	0.9997	0.99996	1.0000			
.6814	.8342	.9233	.9742	.9924	.9986	.9998	0.99999	1.0000		
.6050	.7731	.8851	.9551	.9851	.9966	.9994	.99994	1.0000		
.5350	.7110	.8431	.9311	.9751	.9931	.9987	.99981	1.0000		
.4721	.6505	.7991	.9031	.9625	.9880	.9976	.99956	1.0000		
.4164	.5928	.7545	.8721	.9477	.9813	.9960	.99912	1.0000		
.3674	.5389	.7104	.8390	.9309	.9729	.9939	.99847	1.0000		
.3245	.4892	.6675	.8047	.9125	.9629	.9912	.99755	1.0000		
.2871	.4437	.6264	.7699	.8929	.9515	.9881	.99634	1.0000		
.2545	.4024	.5872	.7351	.8724	.9388	.9844	.99481	1.0000		
.2261	.3650	.5502	.7008	.8513	.9250	.9803	.99296	1.0000		
.2013	.3313	.5155	.6672	.8298	.9103	.9757	.99078	1.0000		
0.5859	0.7578	0.8724	0.9487	0.9815	0.9955	0.9990	0.9999	0.99999	1.0000	
.5000	.6800	.8151	.9151	.9651	.9896	.9973	.9996	.99994	0.999997	1.0000
.4250	.6050	.7551	.8751	.9437	.9804	.9942	.9988	.9998	.99998	1.0000
.3607	.5351	.6950	.8370	.9180	.9678	.9896	.9974	.9996	.99994	1.0000
.3062	.4715	.6369	.7839	.8889	.9519	.9834	.9952	.9991	.99985	1.0000
.2602	.4146	.5818	.7361	.8574	.9330	.9755	.9920	.9985	.99969	1.0000
.2216	.3641	.5303	.6886	.8243	.9115	.9660	.9879	.9976	.99943	1.0000
.1893	.3197	.4828	.6423	.7904	.8880	.9552	.9826	.9963	.99905	1.0000
.1621	.2809	.4393	.5978	.7562	.8629	.9429	.9763	.9948	.99852	1.0000
.1392	.2470	.3997	.5554	.7223	.8367	.9296	.9689	.9930	.99782	1.0000
.1200	.2175	.3638	.5155	.6889	.8096	.9153	.9606	.9908	.99692	1.0000

a) DISTRIBUTION OF THE TOTAL NUMBER OF RUNS u IN SAMPLES OF SIZE (N_1,N_2)

N_1,N_2 \ u	2	3	4	5	6	7	8	9	10
11,11	0.0^{4}028	0.0^{4}312	0.0^{3}3147	0.0^{2}1590	0.0^{2}7332	0.02264	0.06347	0.1349	0.2599
11,12	.0^{4}015	.0^{4}170	.0^{3}1797	.0^{3}9526	.0^{2}4614	.01499	.04427	.09919	.2017
11,13	.0^{4}008	.0^{4}096	.0^{3}1058	.0^{3}5865	.0^{2}2966	.01010	.03126	.07356	.1568
11,14	.0^{4}004	.0^{4}056	.0^{4}639	.0^{3}3702	.0^{2}1945	.0^{2}6932	.02233	.05505	.1224
11,15	.0^{4}003	.0^{4}034	.0^{4}346	.0^{3}2389	.0^{2}1299	.0^{2}4832	.01614	.04158	.09600
11,16	.0^{4}002	.0^{4}021	.0^{4}251	.0^{3}1574	.0^{3}8822	.0^{2}3419	.01180	.03169	.07566
11,17	.0^{4}001	.0^{4}013	.0^{4}162	.0^{3}1056	.0^{3}6085	.0^{2}2453	.0^{2}8711	.02436	.05995
11,18	.0^{4}001	.0^{4}008	.0^{4}107	.0^{4}721	.0^{3}4259	.0^{2}1782	.0^{2}6499	.01888	.04777
11,19		.0^{4}005	.0^{4}071	.0^{4}500	.0^{3}3020	.0^{2}1310	.0^{2}4895	.01475	.03828
11,20		.0^{4}004	.0^{4}049	.0^{4}351	.0^{3}2169	.0^{3}9742	.0^{2}3721	.01162	.03084
12,12	0.0^{4}007	0.0^{4}089	0.0^{4}984	0.0^{3}5458	0.0^{2}2783	0.0^{2}9495	0.02963	0.06990	0.1504
12,13	.0^{4}004	.0^{4}048	.0^{4}556	.0^{3}3221	.0^{2}1718	.0^{2}6139	.02010	.04977	.1126
12,14	.0^{4}002	.0^{4}027	.0^{4}323	.0^{3}1952	.0^{2}1084	.0^{2}4045	.01382	.03581	.08467
12,15	.0^{4}001	.0^{4}016	.0^{4}193	.0^{3}1211	.0^{3}6970	.0^{2}2712	.0^{2}9622	.02603	.06404
12,16	.0^{4}001	.0^{4}009	.0^{4}118	.0^{4}769	.0^{3}4565	.0^{2}1849	.0^{2}6784	.01912	.04874
12,17		.0^{4}006	.0^{4}073	.0^{4}497	.0^{3}3041	.0^{2}1279	.0^{2}4840	.01419	.03733
12,18		.0^{4}003	.0^{4}047	.0^{4}328	.0^{3}2057	.0^{3}8976	.0^{2}3492	.01063	.02879
12,19		.0^{4}002	.0^{4}030	.0^{4}220	.0^{3}1412	.0^{3}6381	.0^{2}2546	.0^{2}8032	.02234
12,20		.0^{4}001	.0^{4}020	.0^{4}150	.0^{4}983	.0^{3}4593	.0^{2}1876	.0^{2}6124	.01745
13,13	0.0^{4}002	0.0^{4}025	0.0^{4}302	0.0^{3}1825	0.0^{2}1020	0.0^{2}3812	0.01312	0.03406	0.08118
13,14	.0^{4}001	.0^{4}013	.0^{4}169	.0^{3}1063	.0^{3}6196	.0^{2}2416	.0^{2}8690	.02359	.05888
13,15	.0^{4}001	.0^{4}007	.0^{4}097	.0^{4}636	.0^{3}3844	.0^{2}1561	.0^{2}5838	.01653	.04300
13,16		.0^{4}004	.0^{4}057	.0^{4}389	.0^{3}2431	.0^{2}1026	.0^{2}3976	.01172	.03168
13,17		.0^{4}003	.0^{4}035	.0^{4}243	.0^{3}1566	.0^{3}6856	.0^{2}2743	.0^{2}8401	.02345
13,18		.0^{4}002	.0^{4}021	.0^{4}155	.0^{3}1025	.0^{3}4652	.0^{2}1916	.0^{2}6086	.01751
13,19		.0^{4}001	.0^{4}013	.0^{4}100	.0^{4}682	.0^{3}3201	.0^{2}1354	.0^{2}4454	.01318
13,20		.0^{4}001	.0^{4}009	.0^{4}066	.0^{4}460	.0^{3}2232	.0^{3}9671	.0^{2}3292	.0^{2}9986
14,14		0.0^{4}007	0.0^{4}095	0.0^{4}597	0.0^{3}3630	0.0^{2}1475	0.0^{2}5553	0.01575	0.04123
14,15		.0^{4}004	.0^{4}051	.0^{4}344	.0^{3}2174	.0^{3}9191	.0^{2}3604	.01065	.02911
14,16		.0^{4}002	.0^{4}029	.0^{4}203	.0^{3}1330	.0^{3}5835	.0^{2}2373	.0^{2}7295	.02072
14,17		.0^{4}001	.0^{4}017	.0^{4}123	.0^{4}829	.0^{3}3770	.0^{2}1585	.0^{2}5058	.01487
14,18		.0^{4}001	.0^{4}010	.0^{4}076	.0^{4}526	.0^{3}2476	.0^{2}1073	.0^{2}3548	.01077
14,19			.0^{4}006	.0^{4}048	.0^{4}339	.0^{3}1651	.0^{3}7351	.0^{2}2516	.0^{2}7861
14,20			.0^{4}004	.0^{4}030	.0^{4}222	.0^{3}1116	.0^{3}5098	.0^{2}1804	.0^{2}5786
15,15		0.0^{4}002	0.0^{4}027	0.0^{4}191	0.0^{3}1259	0.0^{3}5530	0.0^{2}2261	0.0^{2}6959	0.01988
15,16		.0^{4}001	.0^{4}015	.0^{4}109	.0^{4}745	.0^{3}3395	.0^{2}1442	.0^{2}4610	.01370
15,17		.0^{4}001	.0^{4}008	.0^{4}064	.0^{4}450	.0^{3}2123	.0^{3}9329	.0^{2}3095	.0^{2}9536
15,18			.0^{4}005	.0^{4}038	.0^{4}277	.0^{3}1351	.0^{3}6124	.0^{2}2104	.0^{2}6698
15,19			.0^{4}003	.0^{4}023	.0^{4}173	.0^{4}873	.0^{3}4074	.0^{2}1448	.0^{2}4748
15,20			.0^{4}002	.0^{4}014	.0^{4}110	.0^{4}573	.0^{3}2745	.0^{2}1008	.0^{2}3397
16,16		0.0^{4}001	0.0^{4}008	0.0^{4}060	0.0^{4}427	0.0^{3}2017	0.0^{3}8905	0.0^{2}2957	0.0^{2}9157
16,17			.0^{4}004	.0^{4}034	.0^{4}250	.0^{3}1222	.0^{3}5590	0.0^{2}1924	.0^{2}6182
16,18			.0^{4}002	.0^{4}020	.0^{4}149	.0^{4}754	.0^{3}3562	.0^{2}1269	.0^{2}4217
16,19			.0^{4}001	.0^{4}012	.0^{4}091	.0^{4}473	.0^{3}2302	.0^{3}8475	.0^{2}2905
16,20			.0^{4}001	.0^{4}007	.0^{4}056	.0^{4}302	.0^{3}1509	.0^{3}5732	.0^{2}2021
17,17			0.0^{4}002	0.0^{4}019	0.0^{4}142	0.0^{4}718	0.0^{3}3406	0.0^{2}1214	0.0^{2}4053
17,18			.0^{4}001	.0^{4}011	.0^{4}083	.0^{4}430	.0^{3}2109	.0^{3}7773	.0^{2}2686
17,19			.0^{4}001	.0^{4}006	.0^{4}049	.0^{4}262	.0^{3}1325	.0^{3}5046	.0^{2}1800
17,20				.0^{4}004	.0^{4}029	.0^{4}163	.0^{4}845	.0^{3}3318	.0^{2}1219
18,18			0.0^{4}001	0.0^{4}006	0.0^{4}047	0.0^{4}250	0.0^{3}1269	0.0^{3}4836	0.0^{2}1732
18,19				.0^{4}003	.0^{4}027	.0^{4}148	.0^{4}776	.0^{3}3053	.0^{2}1130
18,20				.0^{4}002	.0^{4}016	.0^{4}090	.0^{4}482	.0^{3}1954	.0^{3}7448
19,19				0.0^{4}002	0.0^{4}015	0.0^{4}086	0.0^{4}462	0.0^{3}1875	0.0^{3}7174
19,20				.0^{4}001	.0^{4}009	.0^{4}050	.0^{4}280	.0^{3}1169	.0^{3}4611
20,20				0.0^{4}001	0.0^{4}005	0.0^{4}029	0.0^{4}165	0.0^{4}710	0.0^{3}2890

a) DISTRIBUTION OF THE TOTAL NUMBER OF RUNS u IN SAMPLES OF SIZE (N_1, N_2)

11	12	13	14	15	16	17	18	19	20	21
0.4100	0.5900	0.7401	0.8651	0.9365	0.9774	0.9927	0.9984	0.9997	0.99997	0.999997
.3350	.5072	.6650	.8086	.9008	.9594	.9850	.9960	.9990	.9999	.99998
.2735	.4335	.5933	.7488	.8598	.9360	.9740	.9919	.9978	.9996	.9999
.2235	.3690	.5266	.6883	.8154	.9078	.9598	.9857	.9958	.9990	.9998
.1831	.3137	.4660	.6293	.7692	.8758	.9424	.9774	.9930	.9981	.9997
.1504	.2665	.4116	.5728	.7225	.8410	.9224	.9669	.9891	.9967	.9994
.1240	.2265	.3632	.5199	.6765	.8043	.9002	.9542	.9841	.9948	.9990
.1027	.1928	.3205	.4708	.6317	.7666	.8763	.9395	.9781	.9922	.9985
.08533	.1644	.2830	.4257	.5888	.7286	.8510	.9230	.9711	.9890	.9978
.07122	.1404	.2500	.3846	.5480	.6908	.8247	.9051	.9631	.9849	.9969
0.2632	0.4211	0.5789	0.7368	0.8496	0.9301	0.9704	0.9905	0.9972	0.9994	0.9999
.2068	.3475	.5000	.6642	.7932	.8937	.9502	.9816	.9939	.9985	.9997
.1628	.2860	.4296	.5938	.7345	.8518	.9251	.9691	.9886	.9968	.9992
.1286	.2351	.3681	.5277	.6759	.8062	.8958	.9528	.9813	.9940	.9984
.1020	.1932	.3149	.4669	.6189	.7585	.8632	.9330	.9718	.9899	.9971
.08131	.1591	.2693	.4118	.5646	.7101	.8283	.9101	.9602	.9844	.9953
.06511	.1312	.2304	.3626	.5137	.6621	.7919	.8847	.9465	.9774	.9929
.05240	.1085	.1973	.3189	.4665	.6153	.7548	.8572	.9311	.9690	.9898
.04238	.08996	.1693	.2803	.4231	.5703	.7176	.8281	.9140	.9590	.9860
0.1566	0.2772	0.4179	0.5821	0.7228	0.8434	0.9188	0.9659	0.9869	0.9962	0.9990
.1189	.2205	.3475	.5056	.6524	.7880	.8811	.9446	.9764	.9921	.9976
.09064	.1753	.2883	.4365	.5847	.7299	.8388	.9182	.9623	.9858	.9952
.06947	.1396	.2389	.3751	.5212	.6714	.7934	.8873	.9446	.9771	.9917
.05354	.1113	.1980	.3215	.4628	.6141	.7465	.8529	.9238	.9658	.9868
.04150	.08902	.1643	.2752	.4098	.5592	.6692	.8159	.9001	.9520	.9805
.03236	.07143	.1366	.2353	.3623	.5074	.6525	.7772	.8742	.9358	.9728
.02538	.05752	.1138	.2012	.3200	.4592	.6072	.7377	.8465	.9174	.9635
0.08711	0.1697	0.2798	0.4266	0.5734	0.7202	0.8303	0.9129	0.9588	0.9842	0.9944
.06417	.1306	.2247	.3576	.5000	.6519	.7753	.8749	.9358	.9727	.9893
.04756	.1007	.1804	.2986	.4336	.5854	.7183	.8322	.9081	.9574	.9820
.03548	.07788	.1450	.2486	.3745	.5226	.6614	.7863	.8765	.9382	.9721
.02665	.06044	.1168	.2068	.3227	.4643	.6058	.7386	.8418	.9155	.9598
.02015	.04709	.09422	.1720	.2776	.4110	.5527	.6903	.8049	.8898	.9450
.01534	.03684	.07626	.1432	.2387	.3640	.5027	.6425	.7667	.8616	.9281
0.04572	0.09739	0.1749	0.2912	0.4241	0.5759	0.7088	0.8251	0.9026	0.9543	0.9801
.03280	.07281	.1362	.2362	.3576	.5046	.6424	.7710	.8638	.9305	.9672
.02370	.05462	.1062	.1912	.3005	.4393	.5781	.7147	.8210	.9020	.9505
.01726	.04115	.08296	.1546	.2519	.3806	.5174	.6581	.7754	.8693	.9303
.01267	.03115	.06504	.1251	.2109	.3286	.4610	.6026	.7285	.8334	.9068
.$0^{2}9370$	.02370	.05118	.1014	.1766	.2831	.4095	.5493	.6813	.7952	.8806
0.02280	0.05280	0.1028	0.1862	0.2933	0.4311	0.5689	0.7067	0.8138	0.8972	0.9472
.01598	.03846	.07781	.1465	.2397	.3659	.5000	.6420	.7603	.8584	.9222
.01129	.02816	.05907	.1153	.1956	.3091	.4369	.5789	.7050	.8155	.8928
.$0^{2}8049$	.02072	.04502	.09079	.1594	.2603	.3801	.5188	.6498	.7697	.8596
.$0^{2}5786$	.01534	.03446	.07162	.1300	.2188	.3297	.4628	.5959	.7224	.8237
0.01087	0.02722	0.05720	0.1122	0.1907	0.3028	0.4290	0.5710	0.6972	0.8093	0.8878
.$0^{2}7460$	.01937	.04221	.08589	.1514	.2495	.3659	.5038	.6341	.7566	.8486
.$0^{2}5168$	.01388	.03129	.06587	.1202	.2049	.3108	.4418	.5728	.7022	.8057
.$0^{2}3614$	.01000	.02331	.05063	.09551	.1680	.2631	.3854	.5146	.6474	.7604
0.$0^{2}4978$	0.01342	0.03029	0.06405	0.1171	0.2004	0.3046	0.4349	0.5651	0.6954	0.7996
.$0^{2}3355$	.$0^{2}9355$	.02186	.04786	.09057	.1606	.2525	.3729	.5000	.6338	.7475
.$0^{2}2283$	.$0^{2}6569$	.01586	.03586	.07014	.1285	.2088	.3182	.4398	.5736	.6940
0.$0^{2}2201$	0.$0^{2}6355$	0.01536	0.03486	0.06828	0.1256	0.2044	0.3127	0.4331	0.5669	0.6873
.$0^{2}1459$	.$0^{2}4350$	.01086	.02547	.05157	.09810	.1650	.2610	.3729	.5033	.6271
0.$0^{3}9429$	0.$0^{2}2905$	0.$0^{2}7482$	0.01816	0.03800	0.07484	0.1301	0.2130	0.3143	0.4381	0.5619

a) DISTRIBUTION OF THE TOTAL NUMBER OF RUNS u IN SAMPLES OF SIZE (N_1, N_2)

N_1, N_2 \ u	22	23	24	25	26	27	28	29
11,11	1.0000							
11,12	0.999999	1.0000						
11,13	.99999	1.0000						
11,14	.99998	1.0000						
11,15	.99995	1.0000						
11,16	.99989	1.0000						
11,17	.9998	1.0000						
11,18	.9996	1.0000						
11,19	.9994	1.0000						
11,20	.9991	1.0000						
12,12	0.99999	0.999999	1.0000					
12,13	.99996	.99999	0.999999	1.0000				
12,14	.99986	.99998	.999999	1.0000				
12,15	.99966	.99995	.999995	1.0000				
12,16	.99930	.9999	.999985	1.0000				
12,17	.99872	.9998	.99996	1.0000				
12,18	.9978	.9996	.99993	1.0000				
12,19	.9966	.9994	.99987	1.0000				
12,20	.9950	.9991	.99978	1.0000				
13,13	0.9998	0.99997	0.999998	0.9999998	1.0000			
13,14	.9995	.9999	.99999	.999999	0.9999999	1.0000		
13,15	.9988	.9997	.99996	.999995	.9999996	1.0000		
13,16	.9975	.9994	.99988	.99999	.999998	1.0000		
13,17	.9957	.9989	.99975	.99996	.999995	1.0000		
13,18	.9930	.9981	.99951	.99993	.99999	1.0000		
13,19	.9894	.9969	.99914	.99987	.99998	1.0000		
13,20	.9848	.9954	.9986	.99978	.99995	1.0000		
14,14	0.9985	0.9996	0.9999	0.99999	0.999999	0.9999999	1.0000	
14,15	.9967	.9991	.9998	.99997	.999996	.9999996	0.99999999	1.0000
14,16	.9938	.9981	.9995	.99990	.999986	.9999985	.9999999	1.0000
14,17	.9894	.9965	.9990	.99978	.999961	.9999953	.9999995	1.0000
14,18	.9834	.9941	.9982	.99957	.999910	.9999885	.9999986	1.0000
14,19	.9756	.9909	.9970	.99923	.999817	.9999753	.9999963	1.0000
14,20	.9660	.9867	.9952	.99872	.999663	.9999527	.9999916	1.0000
15,15	0.9930	0.9977	0.9994	0.9999	0.99998	0.999997	0.9999998	0.9999999
15,16	.9872	.9954	.9987	.9997	.99994	.999989	.9999988	.9999999
15,17	.9789	.9918	.9974	.9992	.99983	.999968	.9999956	.9999995
15,18	.9678	.9866	.9953	.9985	.99963	.999923	.9999871	.9999986
15,19	.9540	.9798	.9923	.9975	.99928	.999839	.9999686	.9999963
15,20	.9375	.9712	.9881	.9959	.99872	.999699	.9999332	.9999916
16,16	0.9772	0.9908	0.9970	0.9991	0.9998	0.99996	0.99999	0.999999
16,17	.9634	.9840	.9942	.9981	.9995	.99988	.99998	.999997
16,18	.9457	.9747	.9900	.9964	.9989	.99971	.99994	.999989
16,19	.9244	.9626	.9840	.9938	.9980	.99942	.99986	.999973
16,20	.8996	.9479	.9761	.9902	.9965	.99894	.99972	.999942
17,17	0.9428	0.9728	0.9891	0.9959	0.9988	0.9997	0.9999	0.99999
17,18	.9172	.9578	.9816	.9925	.9975	.9992	.9998	.99996
17,19	.8872	.9391	.9714	.9876	.9954	.9985	.9996	.99989
17,20	.8534	.9168	.9584	.9808	.9924	.9972	.9992	.99977
18,18	0.8829	0.9360	0.9697	0.9866	0.9950	0.9983	0.9995	0.9999
18,19	.8438	.9094	.9540	.9782	.9911	.9966	.9990	.9997
18,20	.8010	.8788	.9345	.9670	.9856	.9941	.9980	.9994
19,19	0.7956	0.8744	0.9317	0.9651	0.9846	0.9936	0.9978	0.9993
19,20	.7444	.8350	.9048	.9484	.9756	.9891	.9959	.9985
20,20	0.6857	0.7870	0.8699	0.9252	0.9620	0.9818	0.9925	0.9971

a) DISTRIBUTION OF THE TOTAL NUMBER OF RUNS u IN SAMPLES OF SIZE (N_1,N_2)

30	31	32	33	34	35	36	37
1.0000							
1.0000							
1.0000							
0.9999999	1.0000						
.9999996	1.0000						
.9999988	1.0000						
0.9999999	1.0000						
.9999997	1.0000						
.9999986	0.9999999	1.0000					
.9999958	.9999996	1.0000					
.9999893	.9999988	0.9999999	1.0000				
0.9999981	0.9999998	1.0000					
.9999929	.9999989	0.9999999	1.0000				
.9999795	.9999965	.9999996	1.0000				
.9999499	.9999909	.9999986	0.9999999	1.0000			
0.99998	0.999995	0.999999	0.9999999	1.0000			
.99993	.999985	.999998	.9999997	1.0000			
.99984	.999962	.999993	.9999989	0.9999999	0.99999999	1.0000	
0.9998	0.99995	0.99999	0.999999	.9999998	0.9999999	1.0000	
.9996	.99988	.99997	.999995	.9999993	.9999999	1.0000	
0.9990	0.9997	0.99993	0.99998	0.999997	0.9999995	0.9999999	1.0000

b) DISTRIBUTION OF THE TOTAL NUMBER OF RUNS u IN SAMPLES OF SIZE (N_1,N_2)

The values listed on the previous pages give the chance that u or fewer runs will occur. For example, for two samples of size 4, the chance of three or fewer runs is .114. For sample sizes $N_1 = N_2$ larger than 10 the following table can be used. The columns headed 0.5, 1, 2.5, 5 give values of u such that u or fewer-runs occur with chance less than the indicated percentage. For example, for $N_1 = N_2 = 12$ the chance of 8 or fewer runs is about .05. The columns headed 95, 97.5, 99, 99.5 give values of u for which the chance of u or more runs is less than 5, 2.5, 1, 0.5 per cent.

$N_1 = N_2$	0.5	1	2.5	5	95	97.5	99	99.5	Mean	Var.	s.d.
11	5	6	7	7	16	16	17	18	12	5.24	2.29
12	6	7	7	8	17	18	18	19	13	5.74	2.40
13	7	7	8	9	18	19	20	20	14	6.24	2.50
14	7	8	9	10	19	20	21	22	15	6.74	2.60
15	8	9	10	11	20	21	22	23	16	7.24	2.69
16	9	10	11	11	22	22	23	24	17	7.74	2.78
17	10	10	11	12	23	24	25	25	18	8.24	2.87
18	10	11	12	13	24	25	26	27	19	8.74	2.96
19	11	12	13	14	25	26	27	28	20	9.24	3.04
20	12	13	14	15	26	27	28	29	21	9.74	3.12
25	16	17	18	19	32	33	34	35	26	12.24	3.50
30	20	21	22	24	37	39	40	41	31	14.75	3.84
35	24	25	27	28	43	44	46	47	36	17.25	4.15
40	29	30	31	33	48	50	51	52	41	19.75	4.44
45	33	34	36	37	54	55	57	58	46	22.25	4.72
50	37	38	40	42	59	61	63	64	51	24.75	4.97
55	42	43	45	46	65	66	68	69	56	27.25	5.22
60	46	47	49	51	70	72	74	75	61	29.75	5.45
65	50	52	54	56	75	77	79	81	66	32.25	5.68
70	55	56	58	60	81	83	85	86	71	34.75	5.89
75	59	61	63	65	86	88	90	92	76	37.25	6.10
80	64	65	68	70	91	93	96	97	81	39.75	6.30
85	68	70	72	74	97	99	101	103	86	42.25	6.50
90	73	74	77	79	102	104	107	108	91	44.75	6.69
95	77	79	82	84	107	109	112	114	96	47.25	6.87
100	82	84	86	88	113	115	117	119	101	49.75	7.05

X.7 CRITICAL VALUES FOR THE KOLMOGOROV-SMIRNOV ONE-SAMPLE STATISTIC

A sample of size n is drawn from a population with cumulative distribution function $F(x)$. Define the empirical distribution function $F_n(x)$ to be the step function

$$F_n(x) = \frac{k}{n} \qquad \text{for} \qquad x_{(i)} \leq x \leq x_{(i+1)} \ ,$$

where k is the number of observations not greater than x. $x_{(1)} \ . \ . \ . \ , x_{(n)}$ denote the sample values arranged in ascending order. Under the null hypothesis that the sample has been drawn from the specified distribution, $F_n(x)$ should be fairly close to $F(x)$. Define

$$D = \max |F_n(x) - F(x)| \ .$$

For a two-tailed test this table gives critical values of the sampling distribution of D under the null hypothesis. Reject the hypothetical distribution if D exceeds the tabulated value. If n is over 35, determine the critical values of D by the divisions indicated in the table.

A one-tailed test is provided by the statistic

$$D^+ = \max [F_n(x) - F(x)] \ .$$

CRITICAL VALUES FOR THE KOLMOGOROV-SMIRNOV TEST OF GOODNESS OF FIT

Sample Size (n)	Significance Level .20	.15	.10	.05	.01
1	.900	.925	.950	.975	.995
2	.684	.726	.776	.842	.929
3	.565	.597	.642	.708	.829
4	.494	.525	.564	.624	.734
5	.446	.474	.510	.563	.669
6	.410	.436	.470	.521	.618
7	.381	.405	.438	.486	.577
8	.358	.381	.411	.457	.543
9	.339	.360	.388	.432	.514
10	.322	.342	.368	.409	.486
11	.307	.326	.352	.391	.468
12	.295	.313	.338	.375	.450
13	.284	.302	.325	.361	.433
14	.274	.292	.314	.349	.418
15	.266	.283	.304	.338	.404
16	.258	.274	.295	.328	.391
17	.250	.266	.286	.318	.380
18	.244	.259	.278	.309	.370
19	.237	.252	.272	.301	.361
20	.231	.246	.264	.294	.352
25	.21	.22	.24	.264	.32
30	.19	.20	.22	.242	.29
35	.18	.19	.21	.23	.27
40				.21	.25
50				.19	.23
60				.17	.21
70				.16	.19
80				.15	.18
90				.14	
100				.14	
Asymptotic Formula:	$\frac{1.07}{\sqrt{n}}$	$\frac{1.14}{\sqrt{n}}$	$\frac{1.22}{\sqrt{n}}$	$\frac{1.36}{\sqrt{n}}$	$\frac{1.63}{\sqrt{n}}$

Reject the hypothetical distribution $F(x)$ if $D_n = \max |F_n(x) - F(x)|$ exceeds the tabulated value. (For $\alpha = .01$ and .05, asymptotic formulas give values which are too high—by 1.5 per cent for $n = 80$.)

X.8 CRITICAL VALUES FOR THE KOLMOGOROV-SMIRNOV TWO-SAMPLE STATISTIC

A sample of size n_1 is drawn from a population with cumulative distribution function $F(x)$. Define the empirical distribution function $F_{n_1}(x)$ to be the step function

$$F_{n_1}(x) = \frac{k}{n_1},$$

where k is the number of observations not greater than x. A second sample of size n_2 is drawn with empirical distribution function $F_{n_2}(x)$. Define

$$D_{n_1,n_2} = \max |F_{n_1}(x) - F_{n_2}(x)|$$

for a two-tailed test. This table gives critical values of the sampling distribution of D under the null hypothesis that two independent samples have been drawn from the same population or from populations with the same distribution. Reject the null hypothesis if D exceeds the tabulated value.

A one-tailed test is provided by the statistic

$$D^+ = \max [F_{n_1}(x) - F_{n_2}(x)] .$$

For large values of n_1 and n_2, approximate formulas to be used are given at the bottom of the table.

CRITICAL VALUES FOR THE KOLMOGOROV-SMIRNOV TEST OF H_0: $F_1(x) = F_2(x)$

Sample size n_2	Sample size n_1: 1	2	3	4	5	6	7	8	9	10	12	15
1	* *	* *	* *	* *	* *	* *	* *	* *	* *	* *		
2		* *	* *	* *	* *	* *	* *	7/8 *	16/18 *	9/10 *		
3			* *	* *	12/15 *	5/6 *	18/21 *	18/24 *	7/9 8/9		9/12 11/12	
4				3/4 *	16/20 *	9/12 10/12	21/28 24/28	6/8 7/8	27/36 32/36	14/20 16/20	8/12 10/12	
5					4/5 4/5	20/30 25/30	25/35 30/35	27/40 32/40	31/45 36/45	7/10 8/10		10/15 11/15
6						4/6 5/6	29/42 35/42	16/24 18/24	12/18 14/18	19/30 22/30	7/12 9/12	
7							5/7 5/7	35/56 42/56	40/63 47/63	43/70 53/70		
8								5/8 6/8	45/72 54/72	23/40 28/40	14/24 16/24	
9									5/9 6/9	52/90 62/90	20/36 24/36	
10										6/10 7/10		15/30 19/30
12											6/12 7/12	30/60 35/60
15												7/15 8/15

Reject H_0 if

$$D = \max |F_{n_1}(x) - F_{n_2}(x)|$$

exceeds the tabulated value. The upper value gives a level at most .05 and the lower value gives a level at most .01.

Note 1: Where * appears, do not reject H_0 at the given level.
Note 2: For large values of n_1 and n_2, the following approximate formulas may be used:

$$\alpha = .05: \quad 1.36\sqrt{\frac{n_1 + n_2}{n_1 n_2}}$$

$$\alpha = .01: \quad 1.63\sqrt{\frac{n_1 + n_2}{n_1 n_2}}$$

CRITICAL VALUES OF D IN THE KOLMOGOROV-SMIRNOV TWO-SAMPLE TEST

(Large samples: two-tailed test)

Level of significance	Value of D so large as to call for rejection of H_0 at the indicated level of significance, where $D = \text{maximum } \lvert F_{n_1}(X) - F_{n_2}(X)\rvert$
.10	$1.22\sqrt{\frac{n_1+n_2}{n_1n_2}}$
.05	$1.36\sqrt{\frac{n_1+n_2}{n_1n_2}}$
.025	$1.48\sqrt{\frac{n_1+n_2}{n_1n_2}}$
.01	$1.63\sqrt{\frac{n_1+n_2}{n_1n_2}}$
.005	$1.73\sqrt{\frac{n_1+n_2}{n_1n_2}}$
.001	$1.95\sqrt{\frac{n_1+n_2}{n_1n_2}}$

X.9 KRUSKAL-WALLIS ONE-WAY ANALYSIS OF VARIANCE BY RANKS. PROBABILITIES ASSOCIATED WITH VALUES AS LARGE AS OBSERVED VALUES OF H

Three samples of sizes n_1, n_2, and n_3 are combined and ranked in ascending order of magnitude: numbers from 1 up to $N = n_1 + n_2 + n_3$ are attached to the ranks. To test whether the three samples come from the same population, the test statistic is

$$H = \frac{12}{N(N+1)} \sum_{j=1}^{3} \frac{R_j^2}{n_j} - 3(N+1),$$

where n_j = number of observations in j^{th} sample, $j = 1, 2, 3$,

$N = \sum_{j=1}^{3} n_j$ = number of observations in all samples combined ,

R_j = sum of ranks in j^{th} sample.

Large values of H lead to rejection of the null hypothesis. If the three samples are from identical populations and the sample sizes are not too small, then H is approximately distributed as chi-square with two degrees of freedom. The first column in the table gives the sizes of the three samples. The second gives various values of H. The third gives the probability associated with the occurrence under the null hypothesis of values as large as an observed H.

PROBABILITIES ASSOCIATED WITH VALUES AS LARGE AS OBSERVED VALUES OF *H* IN THE KRUSKAL-WALLIS ONE-WAY ANALYSIS OF VARIANCE BY RANKS

Sample sizes			H	p
n_1	n_2	n_3		
2	1	1	2.7000	.500
2	2	1	3.6000	.200
2	2	2	4.5714	.067
			3.7143	.200
3	1	1	3.2000	.300
3	2	1	4.2857	.100
			3.8571	.133
3	2	2	5.3572	.029
			4.7143	.048
			4.5000	.067
			4.4643	.105
3	3	1	5.1429	.043
			4.5714	.100
			4.0000	.129
3	3	2	6.2500	.011
			5.3611	.032
			5.1389	.061
			4.5556	.100
			4.2500	.121
3	3	3	7.2000	.004
			6.4889	.011
			5.6889	.029
			5.6000	.050
			5.0667	.086
			4.6222	.100
4	1	1	3.5714	.200
4	2	1	4.8214	.057
			4.5000	.076
			4.0179	.114
4	2	2	6.0000	.014
			5.3333	.033
			5.1250	.052
			4.4583	.100
			4.1667	.105
4	3	1	5.8333	.021
			5.2083	.050
			5.0000	.057
			4.0556	.093
			3.8889	.129
4	3	2	6.4444	.008
			6.3000	.011
			5.4444	.046
			5.4000	.051
			4.5111	.098
			4.4444	.102
4	3	3	6.7455	.010
			6.7091	.013
			5.7909	.046
			5.7273	.050
			4.7091	.092
			4.7000	.101
4	4	1	6.6667	.010
			6.1667	.022
			4.9667	.048
			4.8667	.054
			4.1667	.082
			4.0667	.102
4	4	2	7.0364	.006
			6.8727	.011
			5.4545	.046
			5.2364	.052
			4.5545	.098
			4.4455	.103
4	4	3	7.1439	.010
			7.1364	.011
			5.5985	.049
			5.5758	.051
			4.5455	.099
			4.4773	.102
4	4	4	7.6538	.008
			7.5385	.011
			5.6923	.049
			5.6538	.054
			4.6539	.097
			4.5001	.104
5	1	1	3.8571	.143
5	2	1	5.2500	.036
			5.0000	.048
			4.4500	.071
			4.2000	.095
			4.0500	.119

PROBABILITIES ASSOCIATED WITH VALUES AS LARGE AS OBSERVED VALUES OF H IN THE KRUSKAL-WALLIS ONE-WAY ANALYSIS OF VARIANCE BY RANKS

Sample sizes			H	p
n_1	n_2	n_3		
5	2	2	6.5333	.008
			6.1333	.013
			5.1600	.034
			5.0400	.056
			4.3733	.090
			4.2933	.122
5	3	1	6.4000	.012
			4.9600	.048
			4.8711	.052
			4.0178	.095
			3.8400	.123
5	3	2	6.9091	.009
			6.8218	.010
			5.2509	.049
			5.1055	.052
			4.6509	.091
			4.4945	.101
5	3	3	7.0788	.009
			6.9818	.011
			5.6485	.049
			5.5152	.051
			4.5333	.097
			4.4121	.109
5	4	1	6.9545	.008
			6.8400	.011
			4.9855	.044
			4.8600	.056
			3.9873	.098
			3.9600	.102
5	4	2	7.2045	.009
			7.1182	.010
			5.2727	.049
			5.2682	.050
			4.5409	.098
			4.5182	.101
5	4	3	7.4449	.010
			7.3949	.011
			5.6564	.049
			5.6308	.050
			4.5487	.099
			4.5231	.103
5	4	4	7.7604	.009
			7.7440	.011
			5.6571	.049
			5.6176	.050
			4.6187	.100
			4.5527	.102
5	5	1	7.3091	.009
			6.8364	.011
			5.1273	.046
			4.9091	.053
			4.1091	.086
			4.0364	.105
5	5	2	7.3385	.010
			7.2692	.010
			5.3385	.047
			5.2462	.051
			4.6231	.097
			4.5077	.100
5	5	3	7.5780	.010
			7.5429	.010
			5.7055	.046
			5.6264	.051
			4.5451	.100
			4.5363	.102
5	5	4	7.8229	.010
			7.7914	.010
			5.6657	.049
			5.6429	.050
			4.5229	.099
			4.5200	.101
5	5	5	8.0000	.009
			7.9800	.010
			5.7800	.049
			5.6600	.051
			4.5600	.100
			4.5000	.102

X.10 CRITICAL VALUES FOR A SUM OF RANKS PROCEDURE FOR RELATIVE SPREAD IN UNPAIRED SAMPLES

Let x and y be independent random variables with continuous cumulative distribution functions. Let $m \leq n$ be the sizes of the two samples. Rank all the observations in ascending order of magnitude. Let R_1 be the sum of the ranks for the sample of size m. This table gives critical values of R_1 for $m \leq n \leq 20$ associated for specific probabilities. The null-hypothesis probability of obtaining a smaller sample rank sum less than or equal to any entry in the left half of the table is not greater than the smaller percentage at the head of the column containing the entry. The null-hypothesis probability of obtaining a smaller-sample rank sum greater than or equal to any entry in the right half of the table is not greater than the smaller percentage at the head of the column containing the entry. Where the least extreme rank sum which is significant at a given tabular level is also significant at a more extreme level, this fact is indicated by the entry of an arrow.

This table is related to the Mann-Whitney U-statistic in the same way that the Wilcoxon T-statistic is related to U. Thus this table is equally applicable to the ordinary rank sum procedure for relative location of two unpaired samples.

TABLES OF EXACT CRITICAL VALUES FOR R_1

R_1 = sum of ranks for smaller sample, m = size of smaller sample, n = size of larger sample. One-tail % given above blocks; two-tail % given below blocks. (Also applicable to the Wilcoxon test in its original form.)

$m = 1$

n	100	99.9	99.5	99	97.5	95	90	%→	10	5	2.5	1	0.5	0.1	0
	0	0.1	0.5	1	2.5	5	10	←%	90	95	97.5	99	99.5	99.9	100
≤8	(R_1 never reaches a one-sided 10% level of significance for $n \leq 8$)														
9	0						1		10						11
10	0						1		11						12
11	0						1		12						13
12	0						1		13						14
13	0						1		14						15
14	0						1		15						16
15	0						1		16						17
16	0						1		17						18
17	0					—	1		18	—					19
18	0					—	1		19	—					20
19	0	—	—	—	—	1	2		19	20	—	—	—	—	21
20	0	—	—	—	—	1	2		20	20	—	—	—	—	22
%	0	0.2	1	2	5	10	20	↔	20	10	5	2	1	0.2	0

$m = 2$

n	100	99.9	99.5	99	97.5	95	90	%→	10	5	2.5	1	0.5	0.1	0
	0	0.1	0.5	1	2.5	5	10	←%	90	95	97.5	99	99.5	99.9	100
2	2						—		—						8
3	2					—	3		9	—					10
4	2					—	3		11	—					12
5	2					3	4		12	13					14
6	2				—	3	4		14	15	—				16
7	2				—	3	4		16	17	—				18
8	2				3	4	5		17	18	19				20
9	2				3	4	5		19	20	21				22
10	2				3	4	6		20	22	23				24
11	2			—	3	4	6		22	24	25	—			26
12	2			—	4	5	7		23	25	26	—			28
13	2			3	4	5	7		25	27	28	29			30
14	2			3	4	5	7		27	29	30	31			32
15	2			3	4	6	8		28	30	32	33			34
16	2			3	4	6	8		30	32	34	35			36
17	2		—	3	5	6	9		31	34	35	37	—		38
18	2		—	3	5	7	9		33	35	37	39	—		40
19	2	—	3	4	5	7	10		34	37	39	40	41	—	42
20	2	—	3	4	5	7	10		36	39	41	42	43	—	44
%	0	0.2	1	2	5	10	20	↔	20	10	5	2	1	0.2	0

TABLES OF EXACT CRITICAL VALUES FOR R_1

$m = 3$

n	100 1	99.9 0.1	99.5 0.5	99 1	97.5 2.5	95 5	90 10	%→ ←%	10 90	5 95	2.5 97.5	1 99	0.5 99.5	0.1 99.9	0 100
3	5				—	6	7		14	15	—				16
4	5				—	6	7		17	18	—				19
5	5			—	6	7	8		19	20	21	—			22
6	5			—	7	8	9		21	22	23	—			25
7	5		—	6	7	8	10		23	25	26	27	—		28
8	5		—	6	8	9	11		25	27	28	30	—		31
9	5		6	7	8	9	11		28	30	31	32	33		34
10	5		6	7	9	10	12		30	32	33	35	36		37
11	5		6	7	9	11	13		32	34	36	38	39		40
12	5		7	8	10	11	14		34	37	38	40	41		43
13	5		7	8	10	12	15		36	39	41	43	44		46
14	5		7	8	11	13	16		38	41	43	46	47		49
15	5	—	8	9	11	13	16		41	44	46	48	49	—	52
16	5	—	8	9	12	14	17		43	46	48	51	52	—	55
17	5	6	8	10	12	15	18		45	48	51	53	55	57	58
18	5	6	8	10	13	15	19		47	51	53	56	58	60	61
19	5	6	9	10	13	16	20		49	53	56	59	60	63	64
20	5	6	9	11	14	17	21		51	55	58	61	63	66	67
%	0	0.2	1	2	5	10	20	↔	20	10	5	2	1	0.2	0

$m = 4$

n	100 1	99.9 0.1	99.5 0.5	99 1	97.5 2.5	95 5	90 10	%→ ←%	10 90	5 95	2.5 97.5	1 99	0.5 99.5	0.1 99.9	0 100
4	9		—	—	10	11	13		23	25	26	—	—		27
5	9		—	10	11	12	14		26	28	29	30	—		31
6	9		10	11	12	13	15		29	31	32	33	34		35
7	9		10	11	13	14	16		32	34	35	37	38		39
8	9	—	11	12	14	15	17		35	37	38	40	41	—	43
9	9	—	11	13	14	16	19		37	40	42	43	45	—	47
10	9	10	12	13	15	17	20		40	43	45	47	48	50	51
11	9	10	12	14	16	18	21		43	46	48	50	52	54	55
12	9	10	13	15	17	19	22		46	49	51	53	55	58	59
13	9	11	13	15	18	20	23		49	52	54	57	59	61	63
14	9	11	14	16	19	21	25		51	55	57	60	62	65	67
15	9	11	15	17	20	22	26		54	58	60	63	65	69	71
16	9	12	15	17	21	24	27		57	60	63	67	69	72	75
17	9	12	16	18	21	25	28		60	63	67	70	72	76	79
18	9	13	16	19	22	26	30		62	66	70	73	76	79	83
19	9	13	17	19	23	27	31		65	69	73	77	79	83	87
20	9	13	18	20	23	28	32		68	72	77	80	82	87	91
%	0	0.2	1	2	5	10	20	↔	20	10	5	2	1	0.2	0

TABLES OF EXACT CRITICAL VALUES FOR R_1

$m = 5$

n	100 0	99.9 0.1	99.5 0.5	99 1	97.5 2.5	95 5	90 10	%→ ←%	10 90	5 95	2.5 97.5	1 99	0.5 99.5	0.1 99.9	0 100
5	14		15	16	17	19	20		35	36	38	39	40		41
6	14	—	16	17	18	20	22		38	40	42	43	44	—	46
7	14	—	16	18	20	21	23		42	44	45	47	49	—	51
8	14	15	17	19	21	23	25		45	47	49	51	53	55	56
9	14	16	18	20	22	24	27		48	51	53	55	57	59	61
10	14	16	19	21	23	26	28		52	54	57	59	61	64	66
11	14	17	20	22	24	27	30		55	58	61	63	65	68	71
12	14	17	21	23	26	28	32		58	62	64	67	69	73	76
13	14	18	22	24	27	30	33		62	65	68	71	73	77	81
14	14	18	22	25	28	31	35		65	69	72	75	78	82	86
15	14	19	23	26	29	33	37		68	72	76	79	82	86	91
16	14	20	24	27	30	34	38		72	76	80	83	86	90	96
17	14	20	25	28	32	35	40		75	80	83	87	90	95	101
18	14	21	26	29	33	37	42		78	83	87	91	94	99	106
19	14	22	27	30	34	38	43		82	87	91	95	98	103	111
20	14	22	28	31	35	40	45		85	90	95	99	102	108	116
%	0	0.2	1	2	5	10	20	↔	20	10	5	2	1	0.2	0

$m = 6$

n	100 1	99.9 0.1	99.5 0.5	99 1	97.5 2.5	95 5	90 10	%→ ←%	10 90	5 95	2.5 97.5	1 99	0.5 99.5	0.1 99.9	0 100
6	20	—	23	24	26	28	30		48	50	52	54	55	—	58
7	20	21	24	25	27	29	32		52	55	57	59	60	63	64
8	20	22	25	27	29	31	34		56	59	61	63	65	68	70
9	20	23	26	28	31	33	36		60	63	65	68	70	73	76
10	20	24	27	29	32	35	38		64	67	70	73	75	78	82
11	20	25	28	30	34	37	40		68	71	74	78	80	83	88
12	20	25	30	32	35	38	42		72	76	79	82	84	89	94
13	20	26	31	33	37	40	44		76	80	83	87	89	95	100
14	20	27	32	34	38	42	46		80	84	88	92	94	99	106
15	20	28	33	36	40	44	48		84	88	92	96	99	104	112
16	20	29	34	37	42	46	50		88	92	96	101	104	109	118
17	20	30	36	39	43	47	52		92	97	101	105	108	114	124
18	20	31	37	40	45	49	55		95	101	105	110	113	119	130
19	20	32	38	41	46	51	57		99	105	110	115	118	124	136
20	20	33	39	43	48	53	59		103	109	114	119	123	129	142
%	0	0.2	1	2	5	10	20	↔	20	10	5	2	1	0.2	0

TABLES OF EXACT CRITICAL VALUES FOR R_1

$m = 7$

n	100 0	99.9 0.1	99.5 0.5	99 1	97.5 2.5	95 5	90 10	%→ ←%	10 90	5 95	2.5 97.5	1 99	0.5 99.5	0.1 99.9	0 100
7	27	29	32	34	36	39	41		64	66	69	71	73	76	78
8	27	30	34	35	38	41	44		68	71	74	77	78	82	85
9	27	31	35	37	40	43	46		73	76	79	82	84	88	92
10	27	33	37	39	42	45	49		77	81	84	87	89	93	99
11	27	34	38	40	44	47	51		82	86	89	93	95	99	106
12	27	35	40	42	46	49	54		86	91	94	98	100	105	113
13	27	36	41	44	48	52	56		91	95	99	103	106	111	120
14	27	37	43	45	50	54	59		95	100	104	109	111	117	127
15	27	38	44	47	52	56	61		100	105	109	114	117	123	134
16	27	39	46	49	54	58	64		104	110	114	119	122	129	141
17	27	41	47	51	56	61	66		109	114	119	124	128	134	148
18	27	42	49	52	58	63	69		113	119	124	130	133	140	155
19	27	43	50	54	60	65	71		118	124	129	135	139	146	162
20	27	44	52	56	62	67	74		122	129	134	140	144	152	169
%	0	0.2	1	2	5	10	20	↔	20	10	5	2	1	0.2	0

$m = 8$

n	100 0	99.9 0.1	99.5 0.5	99 1	97.5 2.5	95 5	90 10	%→ ←%	10 90	5 95	2.5 97.5	1 99	0.5 99.5	0.1 99.9	0 100
8	35	40	43	45	49	51	55		81	85	87	91	93	96	101
9	35	41	45	47	51	54	58		86	90	93	97	99	103	109
10	35	42	47	49	53	56	60		92	96	99	103	105	110	117
11	35	44	49	51	55	59	63		97	101	105	109	111	116	125
12	35	45	51	53	58	62	66		102	106	110	115	117	123	133
13	35	47	53	56	60	64	69		107	112	116	120	123	129	141
14	35	48	54	58	62	67	72		112	117	122	126	130	136	149
15	35	50	56	60	65	69	75		117	123	127	132	136	142	157
16	35	51	58	62	67	72	78		122	128	133	138	142	149	165
17	35	53	60	64	70	75	81		127	133	138	144	148	155	173
18	35	54	62	66	72	77	84		132	139	144	150	154	162	181
19	35	56	64	68	74	80	87		137	144	150	156	160	168	189
20	35	57	66	70	77	83	90		142	149	155	162	166	175	197
%	0	0.2	1	2	5	10	20	↔	20	10	5	2	1	0.2	0

TABLES OF EXACT CRITICAL VALUES FOR R_1

$m = 9$

n	100 0	99.9 0.1	99.5 0.5	99 1	97.5 2.5	95 5	90 10	%→ ←%	10 90	5 95	2.5 97.5	1 99	0.5 99.5	0.1 99.9	0 100
9	44	52	56	59	62	66	70		101	105	109	112	115	119	127
10	44	53	58	61	65	69	73		107	111	115	119	122	127	136
11	44	55	61	63	68	72	76		113	117	121	126	128	134	145
12	44	57	63	66	71	75	80		118	123	127	132	135	141	154
13	44	59	65	68	73	78	83		124	129	134	139	142	148	163
14	44	60	67	71	76	81	86		130	135	140	145	149	156	172
15	44	62	69	73	79	84	90		135	141	146	152	156	163	181
16	44	64	72	76	82	87	93		141	147	152	158	162	170	190
17	44	66	74	78	84	90	97		146	153	159	165	169	177	199
18	44	68	76	81	87	93	100		152	159	165	171	176	184	208
19	44	70	78	83	90	96	103		158	165	171	178	183	191	217
20	44	71	81	85	93	99	107		163	171	177	185	189	199	226
%	0	0.2	1	2	5	10	20	↔	20	10	5	2	1	0.2	0

$m = 10$

n	100 0	99.9 0.1	99.5 0.5	99 1	97.5 2.5	95 5	90 10	%→ ←%	10 90	5 95	2.5 97.5	1 99	0.5 99.5	0.1 99.9	0 100
10	54	65	71	74	78	82	87		123	128	132	136	139	145	156
11	54	67	73	77	81	86	91		129	134	139	143	147	153	166
12	54	69	76	79	84	89	94		136	141	146	151	154	161	176
13	54	72	79	82	88	92	98		142	148	152	158	161	168	186
14	54	74	81	85	91	96	102		148	154	159	165	169	176	196
15	54	76	84	88	94	99	106		154	161	166	172	176	184	206
16	54	78	86	91	97	103	109		161	167	173	179	184	192	216
17	54	80	89	93	100	106	113		167	174	180	187	191	200	226
18	54	82	92	96	103	110	117		173	178	187	194	198	208	236
19	54	84	94	99	107	113	121		179	187	193	201	206	216	246
20	54	87	97	102	110	117	125		185	193	200	208	213	223	256
%	0	0.2	1	2	5	10	20	↔	20	10	5	2	1	0.2	0

$m = 11$

n	100 0	99.9 0.1	99.5 0.5	99 1	97.5 2.5	95 5	90 10	%→ ←%	10 90	5 95	2.5 97.5	1 99	0.5 99.5	0.1 99.9	0 100
11	65	81	87	91	96	100	106		147	153	157	162	166	172	188
12	65	83	90	94	99	104	110		154	160	165	170	174	181	199
13	65	86	93	97	103	108	114		161	167	172	178	182	189	210
14	65	88	96	100	106	112	118		168	174	180	186	190	198	221
15	65	90	99	103	110	116	123		174	181	187	194	198	207	232
16	65	93	102	107	113	120	127		181	188	195	201	206	215	243
17	65	95	105	110	117	123	131		188	196	202	209	214	224	254
18	65	98	108	113	121	127	135		195	203	209	217	222	232	265
19	65	100	111	116	124	131	139		202	210	217	225	230	241	276
20	65	103	114	119	128	135	144		208	217	224	233	238	249	287
%	0	0.2	1	2	5	10	20	↔	20	10	5	2	1	0.2	0

TABLES OF EXACT CRITICAL VALUES FOR R_1

$m = 12$

n	100	99.9	99.5	99	97.5	95	90	%→	10	5	2.5	1	0.5	0.1	0
	0	0.1	0.5	1	2.5	5	10	←%	90	95	97.5	99	99.5	99.9	100
12	77	98	105	109	115	120	127		173	180	185	191	195	202	223
13	77	101	109	113	119	125	131		181	187	193	199	203	211	235
14	77	103	112	116	123	129	136		188	195	201	208	212	221	247
15	77	106	115	120	127	133	141		195	203	209	216	221	230	259
16	77	109	119	124	131	138	145		203	210	217	224	229	239	271
17	77	112	122	127	135	142	150		210	218	225	233	238	248	283
18	77	115	125	131	139	146	155		217	226	233	241	247	257	295
19	77	118	129	134	143	150	159		225	234	241	250	255	266	307
20	77	120	132	138	147	155	164		232	241	249	258	264	276	319
%	0	0.2	1	2	5	10	20	↔	20	10	5	2	1	0.2	0

$m = 13$

n	100	99.9	99.5	99	97.5	95	90	%→	10	5	2.5	1	0.5	0.1	0
	0	0.1	0.5	1	2.5	5	10	←%	90	95	97.5	99	99.5	99.9	100
13	90	117	125	130	136	142	149		202	209	215	221	226	234	261
14	90	120	129	134	141	147	154		210	217	223	230	235	244	274
15	90	123	133	138	145	152	159		218	225	232	239	244	254	287
16	90	126	136	142	150	156	165		225	234	240	248	254	264	300
17	90	129	140	146	154	161	170		233	242	249	257	263	274	313
18	90	130	144	150	158	166	175		241	250	258	266	272	283	326
19	90	136	147	154	163	171	180		249	258	266	275	282	293	339
20	90	139	151	158	167	175	185		257	267	275	284	291	303	352
%	0	0.2	1	2	5	10	20	↔	20	10	5	2	1	0.2	0

$m = 14$

n	100	99.9	99.5	99	97.5	95	90	%→	10	5	2.5	1	0.5	0.1	0
	0	0.1	0.5	1	2.5	5	10	←%	90	95	97.5	99	99.5	99.9	100
14	104	137	147	152	160	166	174		232	240	246	254	259	269	302
15	104	141	151	156	164	171	179		241	249	256	264	269	279	316
16	104	144	155	161	169	176	185		249	258	265	273	279	290	330
17	104	148	159	165	172	182	190		258	266	276	283	289	300	344
18	104	151	163	170	179	187	196		266	275	283	292	299	311	358
19	104	155	168	174	183	192	202		274	284	293	302	308	321	372
20	104	159	172	178	188	197	207		283	293	302	312	318	331	386
%	0	0.2	1	2	5	10	20	↔	20	10	5	2	1	0.2	0

TABLES OF EXACT CRITICAL VALUES FOR R_1

$m = 15$

n	100 0	99.9 0.1	99.5 0.5	99 1	97.5 2.5	95 5	90 10	%→ ←%	10 90	5 95	2.5 97.5	1 99	0.5 99.5	0.1 99.9	0 100
15	119	160	171	176	184	192	200		265	273	281	289	294	305	346
16	119	163	175	181	190	197	206		274	283	290	299	305	317	361
17	119	167	180	186	195	203	212		283	292	300	309	315	328	376
18	119	171	184	190	200	206	218		292	302	310	320	326	339	391
19	119	175	189	195	205	214	224		301	311	320	330	336	350	406
20	119	179	193	200	210	220	230		310	320	330	340	347	361	421
%	0	0.2	1	2	5	10	20	↔	20	10	5	2	1	0.2	0

$m = 16$

n	100 0	99.9 0.1	99.5 0.5	99 1	97.5 2.5	95 5	90 10	%→ ←%	10 90	5 95	2.5 97.5	1 99	0.5 99.5	0.1 99.9	0 100
16	135	184	196	202	211	219	229		299	309	317	326	332	344	393
17	135	188	201	207	217	225	235		309	319	327	337	343	356	409
18	135	192	206	212	222	231	242		318	329	338	348	354	368	425
19	135	196	210	218	228	237	248		328	339	348	358	366	380	441
20	135	201	215	223	234	243	255		337	349	358	369	377	391	457
%	0	0.2	1	2	5	10	20	↔	20	10	5	2	1	0.2	0

$m = 17$

n	100 0	99.9 0.1	99.5 0.5	99 1	97.5 2.5	95 5	90 10	%→ ←%	10 90	5 95	2.5 97.5	1 99	0.5 99.5	0.1 99.9	0 100
17	152	210	223	230	240	249	259		336	346	355	365	372	385	443
18	152	214	228	235	246	255	266		346	357	366	377	384	398	460
19	152	219	234	241	252	262	273		356	367	377	388	395	410	477
20	152	223	239	246	258	268	280		366	378	388	400	407	423	494
%	0	0.2	1	2	5	10	20	↔	20	10	5	2	1	0.2	0

$m = 18$

n	100 0	99.9 0.1	99.5 0.5	99 1	97.5 2.5	95 5	90 10	%→ ←%	10 90	5 95	2.5 97.5	1 99	0.5 99.5	0.1 99.9	0 100
18	170	237	252	259	270	280	291		375	386	396	407	414	429	496
19	170	242	258	265	277	287	299		385	397	407	419	426	442	514
20	170	247	263	271	283	294	306		396	408	419	431	439	455	532
%	0	0.2	1	2	5	10	20	↔	20	10	5	2	1	0.2	0

TABLES OF EXACT CRITICAL VALUES FOR R_1

$m = 19$

n	100 0	99.9 0.1	99.5 0.5	99 1	97.5 2.5	95 5	90 10	%→ ←%	10 90	5 95	2.5 97.5	1 99	0.5 99.5	0.1 99.9	0 100
19	189	267	283	291	303	313	325		416	428	438	450	458	474	552
20	189	272	289	297	309	320	333		427	440	451	463	471	488	571
%	0	0.2	1	2	5	10	20	↔	20	10	5	2	1	0.2	0

$m = 20$

n	100 0	99.9 0.1	99.5 0.5	99 1	97.5 2.5	95 5	90 10	%→ ←%	10 90	5 95	2.5 97.5	1 99	0.5 99.5	0.1 99.9	0 100
20	209	298	315	324	337	348	361		459	472	483	496	505	522	610
%	0	0.2	1	2	5	10	20	↔	20	10	5	2	1	0.2	0

X.11 SIGNIFICANT VALUES FOR A RANK-SUM TEST FOR DISPERSION

Two samples, x- and y-samples of m and n independent observations from populations with continuous cumulative distribution functions $F(u)$ and $G(u)$, respectively, are considered. It is required for the basic test that the difference in locations (medians), $\mu_x - \mu_y$, of the two populations be known, and the difference may be taken to be zero as the initial samples may be adjusted by subtracting $\mu_x - \mu_y$ from each x-observation. The parameters μ_x and μ_y need not be known. The hypothesis to be tested is $G(u) = F(u)$ against alternatives of the form $G(u) = F(\theta u)$, $\theta \neq 1$. The two samples are ordered in a single joint array and ranks are assigned from each end of the joint array towards the middle. The statistic used is W, the sum of the ranks for the x-sample. Small values of W indicate larger dispersion for the x-sample and large values of W indicate larger dispersion for the y-sample. This table gives critical values of W for $m + n \leq 20$ for both upper- and lower-tail significance levels.

If $W_0(\alpha)$ is a critical value of W with significance level α,

$$P[W \geq W_0(\alpha)|H_0] \leq \alpha$$

for $\alpha \leq .05$ and

$$P[W \leq W_0(\alpha)|H_0] \leq 1 - \alpha \text{ for } \alpha \geq .95.$$

LOWER AND UPPER SIGNIFICANCE LEVELS OF ***W***

Sample Sizes		Significance Levels							
m	n	.995	.99	.975	.95	.05	.025	.01	.005
2	5	—	—	—	2	—	—	—	—
2	6	—	—	—	2	8	—	—	—
2	7	—	—	—	2	9	—	—	—
2	8	—	—	2	2	10	10	—	—
2	9	—	—	2	2	11	11	—	—
2	10	—	—	2	2	12	12	—	—
2	11	—	—	2	2	13	13	—	—
2	12	—	—	2	2	14	14	—	—
2	13	—	2	2	3	14	15	—	—
2	14	—	2	2	3	15	16	16	—
2	15	—	2	2	3	16	17	—	—
2	16	—	2	2	3	17	17	18	—
2	17	—	2	2	3	18	19	—	—
2	18	—	2	2	3	19	19	20	—
3	5	—	—	—	4	11	—	—	—
3	6	—	—	4	4	13	13	—	—
3	7	—	—	4	5	13	14	—	—
3	8	—	—	4	5	15	16	16	—
3	9	—	4	4	5	16	17	17	—
3	10	—	4	5	5	17	18	18	19
3	11	—	4	5	6	18	19	20	—
3	12	4	4	5	6	20	21	22	22
3	13	4	4	5	6	21	22	23	23
3	14	4	5	6	7	22	23	24	25
3	15	4	5	6	7	23	24	25	26
3	16	4	5	6	7	24	25	27	28
3	17	4	5	6	8	25	26	28	29
4	4			6	6	14	14	—	—
4	5	—	6	6	7	14	16	—	—
4	6	6	6	7	7	17	17	18	18
4	7	6	6	7	8	19	19	20	—
4	8	6	6	7	8	20	21	22	22
4	9	6	7	8	9	21	22	23	24
4	10	7	7	8	9	23	24	25	25
4	11	7	7	9	10	24	26	27	27
4	12	7	8	9	10	26	27	28	29
4	13	7	8	9	11	27	29	30	31
4	14	8	9	10	11	29	30	31	32
4	15	8	9	10	12	30	32	33	34
4	16	8	9	11	12	32	33	35	36

LOWER AND UPPER SIGNIFICANCE LEVELS OF *W*

Sample Sizes		Significance Levels							
m	*n*	.995	.99	.975	.95	.05	.025	.01	.005
5	5	—	9	10	10	20	20	21	—
5	6	9	9	10	11	22	23	24	24
5	7	9	10	11	11	24	24	25	26
5	8	10	10	11	12	26	26	28	29
5	9	10	11	12	13	27	28	29	30
5	10	10	11	12	14	29	30	32	32
5	11	11	12	13	14	31	32	33	34
5	12	11	12	14	15	33	34	36	37
5	13	12	13	14	16	34	36	37	38
5	14	12	13	15	16	36	38	40	41
5	15	12	14	15	17	38	40	41	43
6	6	12	13	14	15	27	28	29	30
6	7	13	14	15	16	29	30	32	32
6	8	14	14	16	17	31	32	34	34
6	9	14	15	16	18	34	35	36	37
6	10	15	16	17	18	36	37	38	39
6	11	15	16	18	19	38	40	41	42
6	12	16	17	19	20	40	41	43	44
6	13	16	18	19	21	42	44	46	47
6	14	17	18	20	22	44	46	48	49
7	7	17	18	19	21	35	37	38	39
7	8	18	19	20	22	38	39	41	42
7	9	19	20	21	23	40	42	43	44
7	10	20	21	22	24	43	44	46	47
7	11	20	22	23	25	45	47	48	50
8	8	23	24	26	27	45	46	48	49
8	9	24	25	27	29	48	49	51	52
8	10	25	26	28	30	50	52	54	55
8	11	26	27	29	31	53	55	57	58
8	12	27	28	30	32	56	58	60	61
9	9	30	31	33	35	55	57	59	60
9	10	31	32	34	36	58	60	62	64
9	11	32	34	36	38	61	63	65	67
10	10	38	39	41	43	67	69	71	72

X.12 CRITICAL VALUES OF SPEARMAN'S RANK CORRELATION COEFFICIENT

Spearman's coefficient of rank correlation, denoted by the letter ρ_s measures the correspondence between two rankings. If d_i is the difference between the ranks of the ith pair of a set of n pairs of elements, then Spearman's Rho is defined as

$$\rho_s = 1 - \frac{6 \sum_{i=1}^{n} d_i^2}{n^3 - n}$$

$$= 1 - \frac{6S_r}{n^3 - n}, \qquad \text{where } S_r = \sum_{i=1}^{n} d_i^2.$$

The exact distribution of S_r has been studied, and critical values when there is complete independence are given in Table X.12a).

Table X.12b) gives the distribution of Σd_i^2. These values are such that Σd_i^2 computed for a sample will equal or exceed the tabulated value with probability as given in the table.

a) **CRITICAL VALUES OF SPEARMAN'S RANK CORRELATION COEFFICIENT**

n	$\gamma = 0.10$	$\gamma = 0.05$	$\gamma = 0.02$	$\gamma = 0.01$
5	0.900	—	—	—
6	0.829	0.886	0.943	—
7	0.714	0.786	0.893	0.929
8	0.643	0.738	0.833	0.881
9	0.600	0.700	0.783	0.833
10	0.564	0.648	0.745	0.794
11	0.536	0.618	0.709	0.818
12	0.497	0.591	0.703	0.780
13	0.475	0.566	0.673	0.745
14	0.457	0.545	0.646	0.716
15	0.441	0.525	0.623	0.689
16	0.425	0.507	0.601	0.666
17	0.412	0.490	0.582	0.645
18	0.399	0.476	0.564	0.625
19	0.388	0.462	0.549	0.608
20	0.377	0.450	0.534	0.591
21	0.368	0.438	0.521	0.576
22	0.359	0.428	0.508	0.562
23	0.351	0.418	0.496	0.549
24	0.343	0.409	0.485	0.537
25	0.336	0.400	0.475	0.526
26	0.329	0.392	0.465	0.515
27	0.323	0.385	0.456	0.505
28	0.317	0.377	0.448	0.496
29	0.311	0.370	0.440	0.487
30	0.305	0.364	0.432	0.478

b) EXACT VALUES OF Σd_i^2 FOR SPEARMAN'S RANK CORRELATION

The probability that $\Sigma d^2 \geq S$ for $S \geq \Sigma m$, or that $\Sigma d^2 \leq S$ for $S \leq \Sigma m$
(where Σm represents mean value of sum of squares)

	$n = 2$	3	4	5	6	7	8	9	10
S \ Σm	1	4	10	20	35	56	84	120	165
0	0.5000	0.1667	0.0417	0.0083	0.0014	0.0002	0.0003	0.0001	0.0000
2	.5000	.5000	.1667	.0417	.0083	.0014	.0006	.0002	.0001
4		.5000	.2083	.0667	.0167	.0034	.0011	.0003	.0001
6		.5000	.3750	.1167	.0292	.0062	.0018	.0005	.0001
8		.1667	.4583	.1750	.0514	.0119	.0028	.0007	.0002
10			0.5417	0.2250	0.0681	0.0171	0.0042	0.0010	0.0003
12			.4583	.2583	.0875	.0240	.0059	.0015	.0004
14			.3750	.3417	.1208	.0331	.0081	.0020	.0005
16			.2083	.3917	.1486	.0440	.0108	.0027	.0007
18			.1667	.4750	.1778	.0548	.0141	.0035	.0009
20			0.0417	0.5250	0.2097	0.0694	0.0179	0.0045	0.0011
22				.4750	.2486	.0833	.0224	.0057	.0014
24				.3917	.2819	.1000	.0275	.0071	.0018
26				.3417	.3292	.1179	.0331	.0087	.0022
28				.2583	.3569	.1333	.0396	.0106	.0027
30				0.2250	0.4014	0.1512	0.0469	0.0127	0.0032
32				.1750	.4597	.1768	.0550	.0152	.0039
34				.1167	.5000	.1978	.0639	.0179	.0046
36				.0667	.5000	.2222	.0736	.0210	.0054
38				.0417	.4597	.2488	.0841	.0244	.0064
40				0.0083	0.4014	0.2780	0.0956	0.0281	0.0075
42					.3569	.2974	.1078	.0323	.0086
44					.3292	.3308	.1207	.0368	.0100
46					.2819	.3565	.1345	.0417	.0114
48					.2486	.3913	.1491	.0470	.0130
50					0.2097	0.4198	0.1645	0.0528	0.0148
52					.1778	.4532	.1806	.0589	.0168
54					.1486	.4817	.1974	.0656	.0189
56					.1208	.5183	.2150	.0726	.0212
58					.0875	.4817	.2332	.0802	.0237
60					0.0681	0.4532	0.2520	0.0882	0.0264
62					.0514	.4198	.2715	.0966	.0293
64					.0292	.3913	.2915	.1056	.0324
66					.0167	.3565	.3120	.1149	.0358
68					.0083	.3308	.3330	.1248	.0394
70					0.0014	0.2974	0.3544	0.1351	0.0432
72						.2780	.3761	.1459	.0472
74						.2488	.3982	.1571	.0515
76						.2222	.4205	.1688	.0561
78						.1978	.4431	.1809	.0609

b) EXACT VALUES OF Σd_i^2 FOR SPEARMAN'S RANK CORRELATION

The probability that $\Sigma d^2 \geq S$ for $S \geq \Sigma m$, or that $\Sigma d^2 \leq S$ for $S \leq \Sigma m$ (where Σm represents mean value of sum of squares)

	$n = 2$	3	4	5	6	7	8	9	10
S \ Σm	1	4	10	20	35	56	84	120	165
80						0.1768	0.4657	0.1935	0.0659
82						.1512	.4885	.2065	.0713
84						.1333	.5113	.2198	.0769
86						.1179	.4885	.2336	.0828
88						.1000	.4657	.2477	.0889
90						0.0833	0.4431	0.2622	0.0954
92						.0694	.4205	.2770	.1021
94						.0548	.3982	.2922	.1091
96						.0440	.3761	.3077	.1164
98						.0331	.3544	.3234	.1239
100						0.0240	0.3330	0.3394	0.1318
102						.0171	.3120	.3557	.1399
104						.0119	.2915	.3721	.1483
106						.0062	.2715	.3888	.1570
108						.0034	.2520	.4056	.1659
110						0.0014	0.2332	0.4226	0.1751
112						.0002	.2150	.4397	.1846
114							.1974	.4568	.1944
116							.1806	.4741	.2044
118							.1645	.4914	.2146
120							0.1491	0.5086	0.2251
122							.1345	.4914	.2358
124							.1207	.4741	.2468
126							.1078	.4568	.2580
128							.0956	.4397	.2694
130							0.0841	0.4226	0.2810
132							.0736	.4056	.2928
134							.0639	.3888	.3048
136							.0550	.3721	.3169
138							.0469	.3557	.3293
140							0.0396	0.3394	0.3418
142							.0331	.3234	.3545
144							.0275	.3077	.3673
146							.0224	.2922	.3802
148							.0179	.2770	.3932
150							0.0141	0.2622	0.4063
152							.0108	.2477	.4196
154							.0081	.2336	.4328
156							.0059	.2198	.4462
158							.0042	.2065	.4596
160							0.0028	0.1935	0.4731
162							.0018	.1809	.4865
164							.0011	.1688	.5000
166							.0006	.1571	.5000
168							.0003	.1459	.4865

(Tables for cases of $n = 9$ and $n = 10$ can be completed by symmetry)

X.13 DISTRIBUTION OF KENDALL'S RANK CORRELATION COEFFICIENT

Consider any one of the $\frac{n}{2}(n-1)$ possible pairs for two sets of ranked elements. Associate with this pair (*a*) a score of $+1$ if the ranking for both sets is the same order or (*b*) a score of -1 if the ranking is in different order. Kendall's score S_t is then defined as the total of these $\frac{n}{2}(n-1)$ individual pairs. S_t will have a maximum value of $\frac{n}{2}(n-1)$ if the two rankings are identical and a minimum value of $-\frac{n}{2}(n-1)$ if the sets are ranked in exactly opposite order. Kendall's Tau is defined as

$$\tau = \frac{S_t}{\frac{n}{2}(n-1)},$$

and has the range $-1 \leq \tau \leq 1$. This table may be used to determine the exact probability associated with the occurrence (one-tailed) under the null hypothesis that the observed value of Kendall's Tau indicates the existence of an association between the two sets of any value as extreme as an observed S_t. The tabled value is the probability that S_t is equalled or exceeded.

DISTRIBUTION OF KENDALL'S RANK CORRELATION COEFFICIENT, t_k, IN RANDOM RANKINGS

S_t	Values of n				S_t	Values of n		
	4	5	8	9		6	7	10
0	0.625	0.592	0.548	0.540	1	0.500	0.500	0.500
2	.375	.408	.452	.460	3	.360	.386	.431
4	.167	.242	.360	.381	5	.235	.281	.364
6	.042	.117	.274	.306	7	.136	.191	.300
8		.042	.199	.238	9	.068	.119	.242
10		0.0083	0.138	0.179	11	0.028	0.068	0.190
12			.089	.130	13	.0083	.035	.146
14			.054	.090	15	.0014	.015	.108
16			.031	.060	17		.0054	.078
18			.016	.038	19		.0014	.054
20			0.0071	0.022	21		0.0002	0.036
22			.0028	.012	23			.023
24			.0009	.0063	25			.014
26			.0002	.0029	27			.0083
28				.0012	29			.0046
30				0.0004	31			0.0023
					33			.0011
					35			.0005

The distribution of S_t is symmetrical so that values of the probability for negative S_t can be obtained by appropriate subtraction from unity; e.g. for $n = 9$,

$$\Pr\{S_t \geq -14\} = 1 - \Pr\{S_t \geq 16\} = 1 - 0.060 = 0.940 .$$

XI. Quality Control

XI.1 FACTORS FOR COMPUTING CONTROL LIMITS

A. Control Charts for Measurement

If the process mean and standard deviation, μ and σ, are known, and it is assumed that the underlying distribution is normal, it is possible to assert with probability $1 - \alpha$ that the mean of a random sample of size n will fall between $\bar{x} - z_{\alpha/2}\frac{\sigma}{\sqrt{n}}$ and $\bar{x} + z_{\alpha/2}\frac{\sigma}{\sqrt{n}}$. These two limits on $\bar{x}$ provide upper and lower control limits. In actual practice, μ and σ are usually unknown and it is necessary to estimate their values from a large sample taken while the process is "in control". The central line of an $\bar{x}$-chart is given by μ and the lower and upper three-sigma control limits are given by $\mu - A\sigma$ and $\mu + A\sigma$, respectively, where $A = \frac{3}{\sqrt{n}}$ and n is the sample size. Where the population parameters are unknown, it is necessary to estimate these parameters on the basis of preliminary samples. If k samples are used, each of size n, denote the mean of the ith sample by $\bar{x}_i$ and the grand mean of the k sample means by $\bar{\bar{x}}$, i.e.

$$\bar{\bar{x}} = \frac{1}{k}\sum_{i=1}^{k} \bar{x}_i \, .$$

Denote the range of the ith sample by R_i and by $\bar{R}$ the mean of the k sample ranges, i.e.

$$\bar{R} = \frac{1}{k}\sum_{i=1}^{k} R_i \, .$$

Since $\bar{\bar{x}}$ is an unbiased estimate of the population mean μ, the central line for the $\bar{x}$-chart is given by $\bar{\bar{x}}$. The statistic R does not provide an unbiased estimate of σ, but $A_2\bar{R}$ is an unbiased estimate of $\frac{3\sigma}{\sqrt{n}}$. The constant multiplier A_2 depends on the assumption of normality. Thus, the central line and the lower and upper three sigma limits, LCL and UCL, for an $\bar{x}$-chart (with μ and σ estimated from past date) are given by

$$\begin{aligned} \text{central line} &= \bar{\bar{x}} \\ \text{LCL} &= \bar{\bar{x}} - A_2\bar{R} \\ \text{UCL} &= \bar{\bar{x}} + A_2\bar{R} \, . \end{aligned}$$

The central line and control limits of an R chart are based on the distribution of the range of samples of size n from a normal population. The mean and standard deviation of the sampling distribution of R are given by $d_2\sigma$ and $d_3\sigma$, respectively, when σ is known. Here d_2 and d_3 are constants which depend on the size of the sample. The set of control chart values for an R chart (with σ known) is given by

$$\begin{aligned} \text{central line} &= d_2\sigma \\ \text{LCL} &= D_1\sigma \\ \text{UCL} &= D_2\sigma, \end{aligned}$$

where $D_1 = d_2 - 3d_3$ and $D_2 = d_2 + 3d_3$.

If σ is unknown, the control chart values for an R chart are given by

$$\begin{aligned} \text{central line} &= \bar{R} \\ \text{LCL} &= D_3\bar{R} \\ \text{UCL} &= D_4\bar{R}, \end{aligned}$$

where $D_3 = \frac{D_1}{d_2}$ and $D_4 = \frac{D_2}{d_2}$.

The central line and control limits of an s-chart are based on estimates obtained from the samples. A pooled estimate of the population variance is obtained from the k samples, i.e.

$$s_p^2 = \frac{\sum_i (n_i - 1)s_i^2}{\sum_i (n_i - 1)}, \qquad i = 1, 2, \ldots, k .$$

If the sample sizes are all equal, the pooled estimate is

$$s_p^2 = \frac{1}{k}\sum_i s_i^2 .$$

The control chart values for an s-chart are given by

$$\begin{aligned} \text{central line} &= C_2' s_p \\ \text{LCL} &= B_2' s_p \\ \text{UCL} &= B_4' s_p . \end{aligned}$$

If one uses the biased estimator of the variance s_p', as is often done in quality control work, the control chart values are given by

$$\begin{aligned} \text{central line} &= c_2 s_p' \\ \text{LCL} &= B_2 s_p' \\ \text{UCL} &= B_4 s_p' . \end{aligned}$$

B. Control Charts for Attributes

Control limits for a fraction-defective chart are based on the sampling theory for proportions, using the normal curve approximation to the binomial. If k samples are taken, the estimator of p is given by

$$\bar{p} = \frac{\sum_i x_i}{\sum_i n_i}, \qquad i = 1, 2, \ldots, k$$

where x_i is the number of defectives in the ith sample of size n_i. The central line and control limits of a fraction defective chart based on analysis of past data are given by

$$\begin{aligned} \text{central line} &= \bar{p} \\ \text{LCL} &= \bar{p} - 3\sqrt{\frac{\bar{p}(1-\bar{p})}{n_i}} \\ \text{UCL} &= \bar{p} + 3\sqrt{\frac{\bar{p}(1-\bar{p})}{n_i}} . \end{aligned}$$

When the sample sizes are approximately equal, n_i is replaced by $\bar{n} = \frac{1}{k}\sum_i n_i$.

Equivalent to the p chart for the fraction defective is the control chart for the number of defective. Here, if p is estimated by $\bar{p}$, the control chart values for a number-of-defectives chart are given by

$$\begin{aligned} \text{central line} &= \bar{n}\bar{p} \\ \text{LCL} &= \bar{n}\bar{p} - 3\sqrt{\bar{n}\bar{p}(1-\bar{p})} \\ \text{UCL} &= \bar{n}\bar{p} + 3\sqrt{\bar{n}\bar{p}(1-\bar{p})}\ . \end{aligned}$$

In many cases it is necessary to control the number of defects per unit C, where C is taken to be a value of a random variable having a Poisson distribution. If k is the number of units available for estimating λ, the parameter of the Poisson distribution, and if C_i is the number of defects in the ith unit, then λ is estimated by

$$\bar{C} = \frac{1}{k}\sum_{i=1}^{k} C_i\ ,$$

and the control-chart values for the C-chart are

$$\begin{aligned} \text{central line} &= \bar{C} \\ \text{LCL} &= \bar{C} - 3\sqrt{\bar{C}} \\ \text{UCL} &= \bar{C} + 3\sqrt{\bar{C}} \end{aligned}$$

This table presents values of the factors for computing control limits for various sample sizes n.

FACTORS FOR COMPUTING CONTROL LIMITS

Number of observations in sample, n	$\bar{X}$ chart		R chart			s chart			$\hat{\sigma}$ chart (biased)		
	Factors for control limits		Factor for central line	Factors for control limits		Factor for central line	Factors for control limits		Factor for central line	Factors for control limits	
	A	A_2	d_2	D_3	D_4	c_2'	B_2'	B_4'	c_2	B_2	B_4
2	2.121	1.880	1.128	0	3.267	0.798	0	2.298	0.5642	0	3.267
3	1.732	1.023	1.693	0	2.575	0.886	0	2.111	0.7236	0	2.568
4	1.500	0.729	2.059	0	2.282	0.921	0	1.982	0.7979	0	2.266
5	1.342	0.577	2.326	0	2.115	0.940	0	1.889	0.8407	0	2.089
6	1.225	0.483	2.534	0	2.004	0.951	0.085	1.817	0.8686	0.030	1.970
7	1.134	0.419	2.704	0.076	1.924	0.960	0.158	1.762	0.8882	0.118	1.882
8	1.061	0.373	2.847	0.136	1.864	0.965	0.215	1.715	0.9027	0.185	1.815
9	1.000	0.337	2.970	0.184	1.816	0.969	0.262	1.676	0.9139	0.239	1.761
10	0.949	0.308	3.078	0.223	1.777	0.973	0.302	1.644	0.9227	0.284	1.716
11	0.905	0.285	3.173	0.256	1.744	0.976	0.336	1.616	0.9300	0.321	1.679
12	0.866	0.266	3.258	0.284	1.716	0.977	0.365	1.589	0.9359	0.354	1.646
13	0.832	0.249	3.336	0.308	1.692	0.980	0.392	1.568	0.9410	0.382	1.618
14	0.802	0.235	3.407	0.329	1.671	0.981	0.414	1.548	0.9453	0.406	1.594
15	0.775	0.223	3.472	0.348	1.652	0.982	0.434	1.530	0.9490	0.428	1.572
16	0.750	0.212	3.532	0.364	1.636	0.984	0.454	1.514	0.9523	0.448	1.552
17	0.728	0.203	3.588	0.379	1.621	0.984	0.469	1.499	0.9551	0.466	1.534
18	0.707	0.194	3.640	0.392	1.608	0.986	0.486	1.486	0.9576	0.482	1.518
19	0.688	0.187	3.689	0.404	1.596	0.986	0.500	1.472	0.9599	0.497	1.503
20	0.671	0.180	3.735	0.414	1.586	0.987	0.513	1.461	0.9619	0.510	1.490
21	0.655	0.173	3.778	0.425	1.575	0.988	0.525	1.451	0.9638	0.523	1.477
22	0.640	0.167	3.819	0.434	1.566	0.988	0.536	1.440	0.9655	0.534	1.466
23	0.626	0.162	3.858	0.443	1.557	0.989	0.546	1.432	0.9670	0.545	1.455
24	0.612	0.157	3.895	0.452	1.548	0.989	0.556	1.422	0.9684	0.555	1.445
25	0.600	0.153	3.931	0.459	1.541	0.990	0.566	1.414	0.9696	0.565	1.435

XI.2 PERCENTAGE POINTS OF THE DISTRIBUTION OF THE MEAN DEVIATION

If $x_1, x_2, \ldots, x_n$ is a random sample of n observations, the mean deviation is given by

$$\text{M.D.} = \frac{1}{n}\sum_{i=1}^{n} |x_i - \bar{x}|$$

where $\bar{x}$ is the sample mean. This table gives certain lower and upper percentage points of the standardized mean deviation $\frac{\text{M.D.}}{\sigma}$.

PERCENTAGE POINTS OF THE DISTRIBUTION OF THE MEAN DEVIATION

Lower percentage points

Size of sample n	0.1	0.5	1.0	2.5	5.0	10.0
2	0.001	0.004	0.009	0.022	0.044	0.089
3	0.022	0.052	0.073	0.116	0.166	0.238
4	0.066	0.114	0.145	0.199	0.254	0.328
5	0.112	0.170	0.203	0.260	0.315	0.386
6	0.153	0.215	0.250	0.306	0.360	0.428
7	0.190	0.252	0.287	0.342	0.394	0.459
8	0.220	0.283	0.318	0.372	0.422	0.484
9	0.247	0.310	0.344	0.396	0.445	0.504
10	0.271	0.333	0.366	0.417	0.464	0.521
Normal approximation						
10	0.171	0.269	0.316	0.386	0.445	0.514

Upper percentage points

Size of sample n	10.0	5.0	2.5	1.0	0.5	0.1
2	1.163	1.386	1.585	1.821	1.985	2.327
3	1.117	1.276	1.417	1.586	1.703	1.949
4	1.089	1.224	1.344	1.489	1.590	1.806
5	1.069	1.187	1.292	1.419	1.507	1.693
6	1.052	1.158	1.253	1.366	1.445	1.613
7	1.038	1.135	1.222	1.325	1.397	1.550
8	1.026	1.116	1.196	1.292	1.358	1.499
9	1.016	1.100	1.175	1.264	1.326	1.457
10	1.007	1.086	1.156	1.240	1.299	1.422
Normal approximation						
10	1.000	1.069	1.128	1.198	1.245	1.342

The unit is the population standard deviation.

XI.3 CUMULATIVE SUM CONTROL CHARTS (CSCC)

Another form of control chart which has gained wide applicability in the last few years is the cumulative sum control chart (CSCC). CSCC for means, ranges, variances, *np*, and *c* are presented here.

A. CSCC for the Mean

The mean of the *i*th sample of size *n* is denoted by $\bar{x}_i$. We plot on the control chart points with the coordinates (m, Y_m) where m is the sample number and

$$Y_m = \sigma_{\bar{x}}^{-1} \sum_i (\bar{x}_i - \mu_0)$$

with μ_0 equal to the proposed "target mean". The chart is interpreted by placing a mask, which is the shaded area of Figure a, over the chart with the point O over the last point

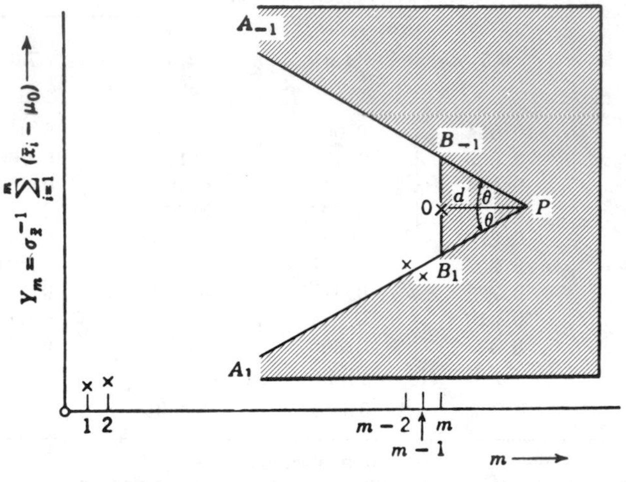

Figure a: Mask for cumulative sum control chart for the mean.

plotted on the chart, with the line OP horizontal. The process is said to be out of control if any points of the CSCC are covered by the mask. If any points lie below the straight line A_1B_1 it is regarded as an indication of increase in the process average; if any points lie above $A_{-1}B_{-1}$ a decrease is indicated. (For each chart an appropriate scaling factor is utilized. This will be considered later in the section.)

In order to determine the dimensions of the mask we must calculate the size 2θ of the angle $B_{-1}PB_1$, and the length, d, from O to the vertex, P, of this angle in Figure a. To do so we first decide on the size of errors of the first and second kind. (As long as β is very small, less than 0.01, say, this can be deleted from the exact formula.) The approximate formulas for θ and d are

$$(1) \qquad \begin{cases} \theta = \arctan(\delta/2) \\ d = -2\delta^{-2} \ln \alpha \end{cases}$$

where $\delta = D/\sigma_{\bar{x}}$ and "D" is the least size shift (in either direction) which it is desired to detect with fair certainty ($1 - \beta$, or power). The probability of error of the first kind for a *two-sided test* is taken here as 2α and for a *one-sided test* as α.

The procedure for a CSCC on means is as follows:

1. Decide on α (or 2α) and D.
2. Determine θ and d from equation (1).
3. Plot the sequential points Y_m moving the mask with each successive point.

4. At each step make a decision to
   a. continue the test
   b. accept a shift of $\mu_0 + D$, or
   c. accept a shift of $\mu_0 - D$.

If σ (and hence $\sigma_{\bar{x}}$) is not known or assumed before the test, this can be estimated by

$$s_p = \sqrt{\Sigma s_i^2/m}$$

where s_i^2 is the variance from sample i, and m is the number of samples. As long as the number of degrees of freedom $\nu = m(n - 1)$ is greater than 30 or 40, this estimate by s_p is quite reliable.

An alternative to calculating the values of θ and d is to make use of Table a. For selected values of δ and α, the values of θ and d can be taken directly from this table.

To attempt to calculate the dimensions of the mask is somewhat meaningless unless the appropriate *scaling factor* is brought into these dimensions. This is different from the Shewhart chart where only the vertical scale is important. Let k units for the ordinate be equal to one unit for the abscissa. Then the equations for θ^* and d^* become

$$\begin{cases} \theta^* = \text{arc tan } (D/2k) \\ d^* = -2\delta^{-2} \ln \alpha = d\,. \end{cases}$$

Note that if Table a be used for the determination of the dimensions of the mask for θ^* and d^*, it must be entered twice as follows:

1. To select θ^*, choose the row for D/k rather than δ.
2. To select d^* (for a designated α or 2α) choose the appropriate row for δ and appropriate column for α or 2α.

TABLE *a*

CUMULATIVE SUM CONTROL LIMITS FOR SAMPLE MEANS

		Values of d						
δ	θ	$2\alpha = 0.10$* $\alpha = 0.05$†	$2\alpha = 0.05$ $\alpha = 0.025$	$2\alpha = 0.02$ $\alpha = 0.01$	$2\alpha = 0.01$ $\alpha = 0.005$	$2\alpha = 0.0027$ $\alpha = 0.00135$‡	$2\alpha = 0.002$ $\alpha = 0.001$	$2\alpha = 0.001$ $\alpha = 0.0005$
0.2	5° 43′	149.8	184.4	230.6	264.9	330.4	345.4	380.0
0.4	11° 19′	37.4	46.1	57.6	66.2	82.6	86.3	95.0
0.6	16° 42′	16.6	20.5	25.6	29.4	36.7	38.4	42.2
0.8	21° 48′	9.36	11.5	14.4	16.6	20.6	21.6	23.8
1.0	26° 34′	5.99	7.38	9.21	10.6	13.2	13.8	15.2
1.2	30° 58′	4.16	5.12	6.40	7.36	9.18	9.59	10.6
1.4	35° 0′	3.06	3.76	4.70	5.41	6.74	7.05	7.76
1.6	38° 40′	2.34	2.88	3.60	4.14	5.16	5.40	5.94
1.8	41° 59′	1.85	2.28	2.84	3.27	4.08	4.26	4.69
2.0	45° 0′	1.50	1.84	2.30	2.65	3.30	3.45	3.80
2.2	47° 44′	1.24	1.52	1.90	2.19	2.73	2.85	3.14
2.4	50° 12′	1.04	1.28	1.60	1.84	2.29	2.40	2.64
2.6	52° 26′	0.89	1.09	1.36	1.57	1.95	2.04	2.25
2.8	54° 28′	0.76	0.94	1.17	1.35	1.69	1.76	1.94
3.0	56° 19′	0.67	0.82	1.02	1.18	1.47	1.54	1.69

* Two-sided test.

† One-sided test.

‡ These are comparable to the "3σ" limits used in the Shewhart chart, i.e. $2\alpha = 0.0027$ and $\alpha = 0.00135$.

B. CSCC for Sample Ranges

In constructing a CSCC on sample ranges, we utilize the distribution of the sample range, using two approximations for the distribution of the sample range from samples of size n from a normal population, with variance equal to 1. These are

(*a*) $c \times$ (χ with ν_1 degrees of freedom)
(*b*) $c' \times$ (χ^2 with ν_1' degrees of freedom)

The first of these is a better approximation if n is less than 10; otherwise (*b*) is better. Again we retain a constant sample size (n) with c, c', ν_1 and ν_1' dependent upon n.

For approximation (*a*) one plots the point

$$\left(m\nu_1, (\sigma c)^{-2} \sum_i R_i^2\right).$$

The corresponding values of θ and d are

$$\begin{cases} \theta = \text{arc tan}\left[\dfrac{2 \ln \sigma_1/\sigma_0}{1 - (\sigma_0/\sigma_1)^2}\right] \\ d = -\ln \alpha / \ln (\sigma_1/\sigma_0) . \end{cases}$$

In approximation (*b*) the coordinates of the point and the values of d and θ as shown in Figure b.1, are

$$\begin{cases} \left(m\nu_1', (\sigma_0 c')^{-1} \sum_i R_i\right) \\ \theta = \text{arc tan}\left[\dfrac{\ln (\sigma_1/\sigma_0)}{1 - (\sigma_0/\sigma_1)}\right] \\ d = -2 \ln \alpha / \ln (\sigma_1/\sigma_0) . \end{cases}$$

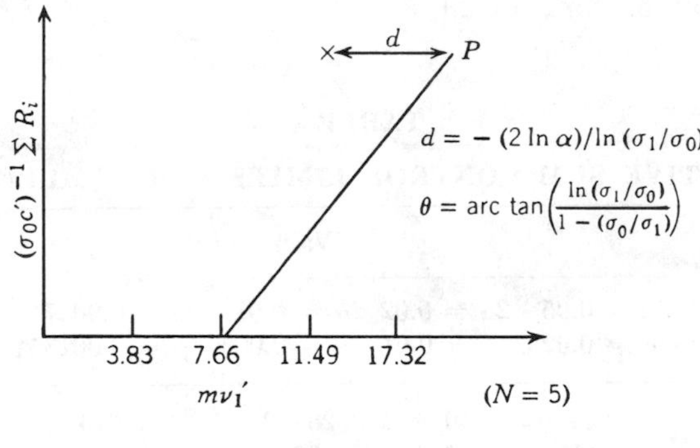

Figure *b*.1: CSCC for sample ranges of samples of size 5.

Here σ_0^2 is the proposed variance in the null hypothesis, for which the risk of rejection, if true, is α and σ_1^2 is the alternative variance which we wish to detect. Values of c, c', ν_1 and ν_1' are given in Table b for sample sizes from 3 to 10.

In order to construct a CSCC based on sample ranges it is again desirable to introduce a scaling factor. By so doing we can plot

$$m, \Sigma R_i$$

with a scale factor k (that is, k units on the ordinate is the same length as one unit on the abscissa). For approximation (*b*) the critical values for the mask as shown in Figure b.2 are

$$\begin{cases} \theta^* = \text{arc tan}\left[\dfrac{\sigma_0 c' \nu_1'}{k} \cdot \dfrac{\ln (\sigma_1/\sigma_0)}{1 - (\sigma_0/\sigma_1)}\right] \\ d^* = -2 \ln \alpha / [\nu_1' \ln (\sigma_1/\sigma_0)] = d/\nu_1' \end{cases}$$

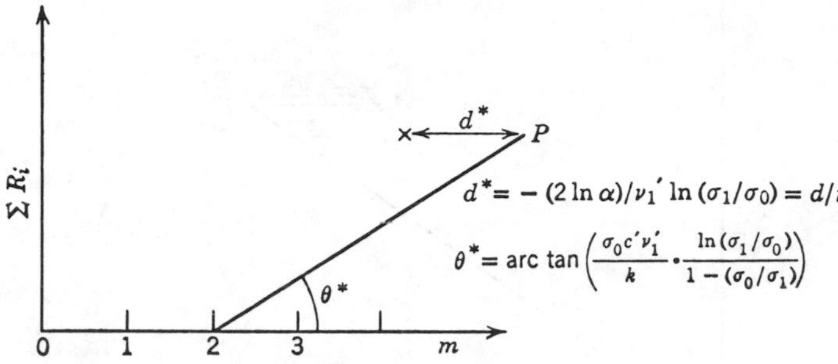

Figure b.2: Scaling in CSCC on sample ranges.

TABLE b

SCALE VALUES FOR CSCC ON SAMPLE RANGES*

Sample Size	Approximation (a)		Approximation (b)	
n	c	ν_1	c'	ν_1'
3	1.378	1.93	0.233	7.27
4	1.302	2.95	0.188	10.95
5	1.268	2.83	0.160	14.49
6	1.237	4.69	0.142	17.86
7	1.207	5.50	0.128	21.08
8	1.184	6.26	0.118	24.11
9	1.164	6.99	0.110	27.01
10	1.146	7.69	0.103	29.82

* c and ν are based on the work of P. B. Patnaik, "The Use of the Mean Range in Statistical Tests", *Biometrika,* **37** (1950). c' and ν' are based on the work of D. R. Cox, "The Use of Range in Sequential Analysis", *Journal of the Royal Statistical Society Series B,* **11** (1949).

C. CSCC for Sample Variances

Let us consider a two-sided control chart where H_0 is $\sigma^2 = \sigma_0^2$, H_1 is $\sigma^2 = \sigma_1^2$ ($> \sigma_0^2$), and H_{-1} is $\sigma^2 = \sigma_1'^2$ ($< \sigma_0^2$). Again let the probability of error of the first kind be α. If the scale of the control chart has length of k units on the ordinate equal to the length of 1 unit on the abscissa, then the values for θ^* and d^* are

$$\begin{cases} \theta^* = \text{arc tan}\left[\dfrac{2(\sigma_0^2/k)\ \ln\ (\sigma_1/\sigma_0)}{1 - (\sigma_0/\sigma_1)^2}\right] \\ d^* = -\ \ln\ \alpha/\ln\ (\sigma_1/\sigma_0) \end{cases}$$

These values can be read directly from Table c for both a two-sided and one-sided test. In plotting the points on a CSCC chart for sample variances, the coordinates of each point are

$$\sum_{i=1}^{m} \nu_i, \sum_{i=1}^{m} \nu_i s_i^2$$

where ν_i and s_i^2 are the degrees of freedom and variance, respectively, of sample i. An illustration of a one-sided CSCC for variances is given in Figure c.1. A two-sided test is shown in Figure c.2, in which $d^{*\prime}$ and $\theta^{*\prime}$ are the critical values for acceptance of the hypothesis, H_{-1}. Note that if $\sigma_1/\sigma_0 < 1$, d is measured in the negative direction, that is, from right to left. Table d.2 can also be used to evaluate d, if

$$\frac{\sigma_1}{\sigma_0} = \frac{1 - p_0}{1 - p_1}.$$

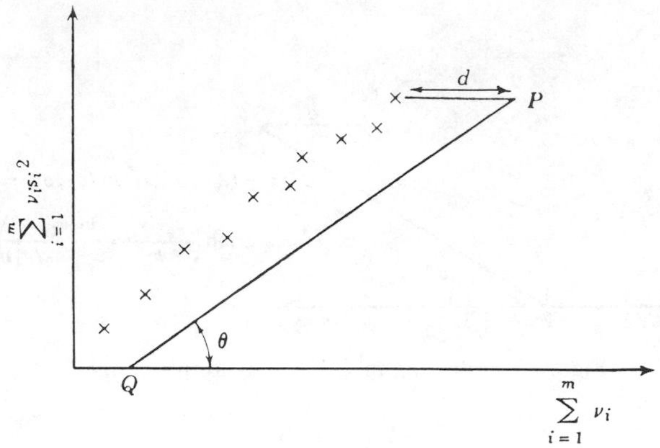

Figure c.1: CSCC for sample variances (one-sided limit to detect increase in variance).

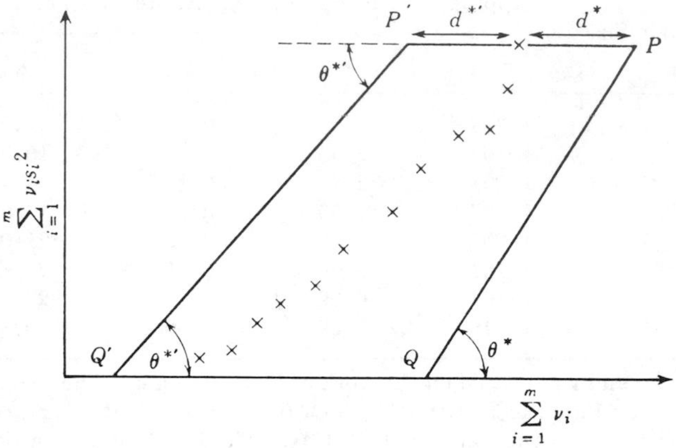

Figure c.2: CSCC for sample variances (two-sided limits).

TABLE *c*

CUMULATIVE SUM CONTROL LIMITS FOR SAMPLE VARIANCES

		Values of d						
σ_1/σ_0	θ	$2\alpha = 0.10$* $\alpha = 0.05$†	$2\alpha = 0.05$ $\alpha = 0.025$	$2\alpha = 0.02$ $\alpha = 0.01$	$2\alpha = 0.01$ $\alpha = 0.005$	$2\alpha = 0.0027$ $\alpha = 0.00135$‡	$2\alpha = 0.002$ $\alpha = 0.001$	$2\alpha = 0.001$ $\alpha = 0.0005$
0.25	10° 28′	2.16	2.66	3.32	3.82	4.77	4.98	5.48
0.5	24° 48′	4.32	5.32	6.64	7.64	9.53	9.93	11.0
0.75	36° 31′	10.4	12.8	16.0	18.4	23.0	24.0	26.4
1.2	50° 2′	16.4	20.2	25.3	29.1	36.2	37.9	41.7
1.4	52° 37′	8.90	11.0	13.7	15.7	19.6	20.5	22.6
1.6	57° 2′	6.37	7.85	9.80	11.3	14.1	14.7	16.2
1.8	59° 32′	5.10	6.28	7.83	9.01	11.2	11.8	12.9
2.0	61° 35′	4.32	5.32	6.64	7.64	9.53	9.97	11.0
2.5	65° 23′	3.27	4.03	5.03	5.78	7.21	7.54	8.30
3.0	67° 57′	2.73	3.36	4.19	4.82	6.01	6.29	6.92
3.5	69° 52′	2.39	2.94	3.68	4.23	5.27	5.51	6.07
4.0	71° 19′	2.16	2.66	3.32	3.82	4.77	4.98	5.48

Note that if $\sigma_1/\sigma_0 < 1$, d is measured in negative direction, that is, from right to left. Table d.2 can also be used to evaluate d, if $\frac{\sigma_1}{\sigma_0} = \frac{1 - p_0}{1 - p_1}$.

* Two-sided test.
† One-sided test.
‡ "3σ" limits.

D. CSCC for Number of Defectives, np, or Fraction Defective, p

The control limit diagram is similar in appearance to those for the range and variance. The line PQ in a figure similar to Figure d is inclined at an angle θ^* to the sample number axis, and P is at a distance d^* to the right of the last plotted point with

$$\begin{cases} \theta^* = \arc\tan\left[\dfrac{\ln[(1-p_0)/(1-p_1)]}{k\ln[p_1(1-p_0)/p_0(1-p_1)]}\right] \\ d^* = -\dfrac{\ln\alpha}{\ln[(1-p_0)/(1-p_1)]} \end{cases}$$

Again, k units on the ordinate are equal in length to one unit on the abscissa. The coordinates plotted on the CSCC chart are

$$\left(\sum_{i=1}^{m} n_i,\ X_m = \sum_{i=1}^{m} x_i\right)$$

where n_i and x_i are the sample size and number of defectives, respectively, of sample i. Figure d presents an illustration of a CSCC for fraction defective, p, where the coordinates of the point are

$$(m, \Sigma x_i)$$

and all of the sample sizes, n_i, are equal to n, say. Given this latter scale, the values of θ^{**} and d^{**} become

$$\begin{cases} \theta^{**} = \arc\tan(n\tan\theta^*) \\ d^{**} = d^*/n \end{cases}$$

In order to obtain θ^* and d^* we may make use of Tables d.1 (A and B) and d.2 and read off approximately the values of θ and d respectively. These are related to θ and d by the equations

$$\begin{cases} \theta^* = \arc\tan[(\tan\theta)/k] \\ d^* = d \end{cases}$$

or, in the case of θ^{**} and d^{**},

$$\begin{cases} \theta^{**} = \arc\tan[n(\tan\theta)/k] \\ d^{**} = d/n \end{cases}$$

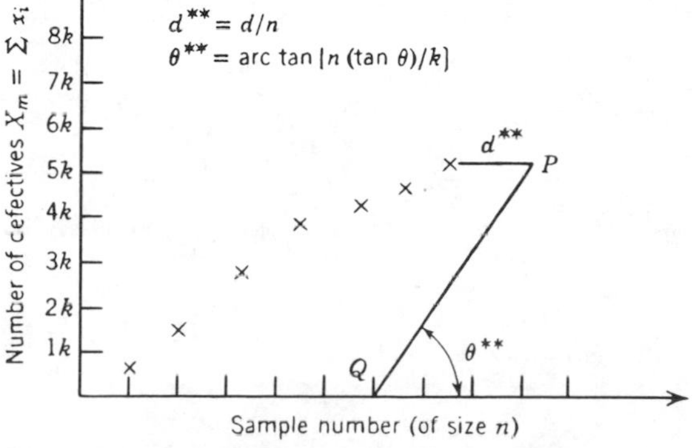

Figure d: CSCC for number of defectives.

TABLE *d*.1

CUMULATIVE SUM CONTROL LIMITS FOR BINOMIAL VARIABLES*

VALUES OF θ (FOR ANY α)

TABLE A

	p_1			
p_0	0.025	0.05	0.075	0.10
0.005	0° 43′	1° 8′	1° 30′	1° 51′
0.01	0° 56′	1° 26′	1° 52′	2° 17′
0.015	1° 7′	1° 40′	2° 9′	2° 36′
0.02	1° 17′	1° 53′	2° 24′	2° 53′
0.025	—	2° 4′	2° 37′	3° 8′
0.03	—	2° 15′	2° 49′	3° 21′
0.035	—	2° 25′	3° 1′	3° 34′
0.04	—	3° 34′	3° 12′	3° 46′
0.045	—	2° 43′	3° 22′	3° 58′
0.05	—	—	3° 32′	4° 8′
0.06	—	—	3° 51′	4° 29′
0.07	—	—	4° 9′	4° 49′
0.08	—	—	—	5° 8′
0.09	—	—	—	5° 25′

TABLE B

	p_1				
p_0	0.15	0.20	0.25	0.30	0.35
0.10	7° 3′	8° 16′	9° 25′	10° 33′	11° 39′
0.12	7° 40′	8° 56′	10° 8′	11° 18′	12° 26′
0.14	8° 15′	9° 34′	10° 49′	12° 0′	13° 10′
0.16	—	10° 10′	11° 27′	12° 40′	13° 52′
0.18	—	10° 45′	12° 3′	13° 18′	14° 31′
0.20	—	—	12° 39′	13° 55′	15° 9′
0.25	—	—	—	15° 21′	16° 38′

* p (or Np) charts.

TABLE d.2

CUMULATIVE SUM CONTROL LIMITS FOR BINOMIAL VARIABLES*

		Values of d						
		$2\alpha = 0.10$†	$2\alpha = 0.05$	$2\alpha = 0.02$	$2\alpha = 0.01$	$2\alpha = 0.0027$	$2\alpha = 0.002$	$2\alpha = 0.001$
p_0	p_1	$\alpha = 0.05$‡	$\alpha = 0.025$	$\alpha = 0.01$	$\alpha = 0.005$	$\alpha = 0.00135$§	$\alpha = 0.001$	$\alpha = 0.0005$
0.02	0.05	96.3	119	148	170	212	222	244
0.04	0.05	286	352	440	506	631	659	726
0.04	0.075	80.7	99.3	124	143	178	186	205
0.06	0.10	186	229	286	329	411	429	472
0.08	0.10	136	168	209	241	300	314	346
0.10	0.15	52.3	64.4	80.4	92.5	115	121	133
0.15	0.20	49.4	60.8	76.0	87.4	109	114	125
0.15	0.25	23.9	29.5	36.8	42.3	52.8	55.2	60.7
0.20	0.25	46.4	57.2	71.4	82.1	102	107	118
0.20	0.30	22.4	27.6	34.5	39.7	49.5	51.7	56.9
0.25	0.30	43.4	53.5	66.8	86.9	95.8	100	110
0.30	0.35	40.4	49.8	62.1	71.5	89.1	93.2	103

* Table c can also be used if $\dfrac{1 - p_0}{1 - p_1} = \dfrac{\sigma_1}{\sigma_0}$.

† Two sided test.
‡ One-sided test.
§ "3σ" limits.

E. CSCC for Number of Defects, c

The control limits for a CSCC for the number of defects are based on the constants

$$(1)\quad \begin{cases} \theta = \arctan\,[(\mu_1 - \mu_0)/\ln\,(\mu_1/\mu_0)] \\ d = -\ln\,\alpha/(\mu_1 - \mu_0) \end{cases}$$

The coordinates of the points on the control chart are

$$\left(m, \sum_{i=1}^{m} x_i\right)$$

where x_i is the number of defects in sample i. Figure e presents an example of a CSCC for number of defects for a 2-sided test. In order to calculate θ' and d', we substitute μ_1' ($<\mu_0$) for μ, in equations (1) above. Tables e.1 and e.2 can be used to obtain the values of θ and d, respectively.

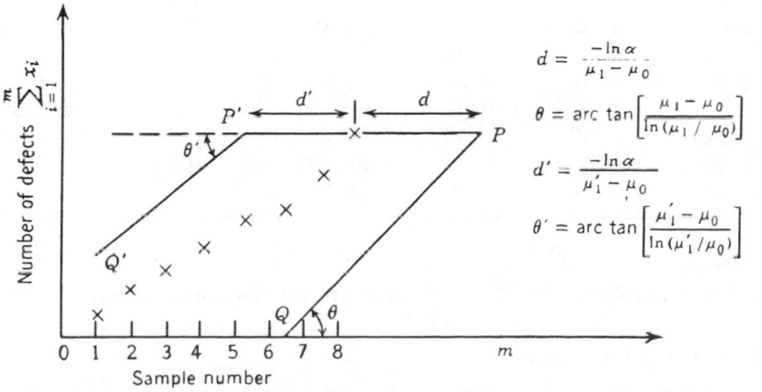

Figure e: CSCC for number of defects (c).

TABLE e.1

CUMULATIVE SUM CONTROL LIMITS FOR POISSON VARIABLE (c-CHARTS) VALUES OF θ (FOR ANY α)

μ_0	μ_1 = 1	2	3	4	5	6	8	10	12	15
0.5	35° 48′	47° 15′	54° 22′	59° 17′	62° 54′	65° 41′	69° 43′	72° 30′	74° 33′	76° 48′
1.0	—	55° 16′	61° 13′	65° 12′	68° 5′	70° 17′	73° 27′	75° 39′	77° 16′	79° 3′
1.5	—	60° 5′	65° 12′	68° 35′	71° 1′	72° 53′	75° 33′	77° 25′	78° 48′	80° 19′
2.0	—	—	67° 56′	70° 53′	73° 1′	74° 39′	76° 59′	78° 38′	79° 51′	81° 11′
2.5	—	—	69° 58′	72° 36′	74° 30′	75° 57′	78° 4′	79° 32′	80° 37′	81° 51′
3.0	—	—	—	73° 57′	75° 40′	76° 59′	78° 54′	80° 14′	81° 15′	82° 22′
3.5	—	—	—	75° 3′	76° 37′	77° 50′	79° 35′	80° 50′	81° 45′	82° 47′
4.0	—	—	—	—	77° 25′	78° 32′	80° 10′	81° 19′	82° 11′	83° 9′
4.5	—	—	—	—	78° 6′	79° 9′	80° 40′	81° 45′	82° 33′	83° 28′
5	—	—	—	—	—	79° 40′	81° 6′	82° 6′	82° 52′	83° 44′
6	—	—	—	—	—	—	81° 49′	82° 43′	83° 25′	84° 11′
7	—	—	—	—	—	—	82° 24′	83° 13′	83° 51′	84° 33′
8	—	—	—	—	—	—	—	83° 38′	84° 13′	84° 52′
9	—	—	—	—	—	—	—	83° 59′	84° 31′	85° 8′
10	—	—	—	—	—	—	—	—	84° 47′	85° 22′

TABLE e.2

CUMULATIVE SUM CONTROL LIMITS FOR POISSON VARIABLES (c-CHARTS) VALUES OF d

$\mu_1 - \mu_0$	$2\alpha_0 = 0.10$* $\alpha_0 = 0.05$†	$2\alpha = 0.05$ $\alpha_0 = 0.025$	$2\alpha_0 = 0.02$ $\alpha_0 = 0.01$	$2\alpha_0 = 0.01$ $\alpha_0 = 0.005$	$2\alpha_0 = 0.0027$ $\alpha_0 = 0.00135$‡	$2\alpha_0 = 0.002$ $\alpha_0 = 0.001$	$2\alpha_0 = 0.001$ $\alpha_0 = 0.0005$
0.5	6.00	7.38	9.21	10.6	13.2	13.8	15.2
1.0	3.00	3.69	4.61	5.30	6.61	6.91	7.60
1.5	2.00	2.46	3.07	3.53	4.40	4.61	5.07
2.0	1.50	1.84	2.30	2.65	3.30	3.45	3.80
2.5	1.20	1.48	1.84	2.12	2.64	2.76	3.04
3.0	1.00	1.23	1.54	1.77	2.20	2.30	2.53
3.5	0.86	1.05	1.32	1.51	1.89	1.97	2.03
4.0	0.75	0.92	1.15	1.32	1.65	1.73	1.90
4.5	0.68	0.82	1.02	1.18	1.47	1.53	1.69
5.0	0.60	0.74	0.92	1.06	1.32	1.38	1.52
6.0	0.50	0.61	0.77	0.88	1.10	1.15	1.27
7.0	0.43	0.53	0.66	0.76	0.94	0.99	1.09
8.0	0.37	0.46	0.58	0.66	0.83	0.86	0.95
9.0	0.33	0.41	0.51	0.59	0.73	0.77	0.84
10.0	0.30	0.37	0.46	0.53	0.66	0.69	0.76

* Two-sided test.
† One-sided test.
‡ These are comparable to the "3σ" limits used in the Shewhart chart.

F. Summary of CSCC Limits

The formulas for θ and α for the various CSCC are given in Table f for both the case of a scaling factor k and when no scaling factor is used.

TABLE *f*

FORMULAS FOR CSCC LIMITS (ONE-SIDED: α)

Sample Statistic	Coordinates	(No Scaling Factor) d	$\tan\theta$	Coordinates	(Including Scaling Factor, k) d^*	$\tan\theta^*$
Mean $\bar{x}$	$m,\ \sigma_{\bar{x}}^{-1}\Sigma(\bar{x}_i - \mu_0)$	$(-2\ln\alpha)/\delta^2$ $[\delta = (\mu_1 - \mu_0)/\sigma_{\bar{x}}]$	$\frac{1}{2}\delta$	$m,\ \Sigma(x_i - \mu_0)$	$(-2\ln\alpha)/\delta$	$D/2k$ $[D = \mu_1 - \mu_0]$
Variance s^2	$\Sigma\nu_i,\ \dfrac{\Sigma\nu_i s_i^2}{\sigma_0^2}$	$\dfrac{-\ln\alpha}{\ln(\sigma_1/\sigma_0)}$	$\dfrac{2\ln(\sigma_1/\sigma_0)}{1-(\sigma_0/\sigma_1)^2}$	$\Sigma\nu_i,\ \Sigma\nu_i s_i^2$	$\dfrac{-\ln\alpha}{\ln(\sigma_1/\sigma_0)}$	$\dfrac{2(\sigma_0^2/k)\ln(\sigma_1/\sigma_0)}{1-(\sigma_0/\sigma_1)^2}$
Range R*	$m\nu_1',\ (\sigma_0 c_1')^{-1}\Sigma R_i$	$\dfrac{-2\ln\alpha}{\ln(\sigma_1/\sigma_0)}$	$\dfrac{\ln(\sigma_1/\sigma_0)}{1-(\sigma_0/\sigma_1)}$	$m,\ \Sigma R_i$	$\dfrac{-2\ln\alpha}{\nu_1'\ln(\sigma_1/\sigma_0)}$	$\dfrac{\sigma_0 c'\nu_1'}{k}\cdot\dfrac{\ln(\sigma_1/\sigma_0)}{1-(\sigma_0/\sigma_1)}$
Number of Defects c	$m,\ \Sigma x_i$	$\dfrac{-\ln\alpha}{\mu_1-\mu_0}$	$\dfrac{(\mu_1-\mu_0)}{\ln(\mu_1/\mu_0)}$	$m,\ \Sigma x_i$ $(x_i = 0 \text{ or } 1)$	$\dfrac{-\ln\alpha}{\mu_1-\mu_0}$	$\dfrac{\mu_1-\mu_0}{k\ln(\mu_1/\mu_0)}$
Number of Defectives Np	$m,\ \Sigma x_i$ (sample of size 1)	$\dfrac{-\ln\alpha}{\ln\left(\dfrac{1-p_0}{1-p_1}\right)}$	$\dfrac{\ln\left(\dfrac{1-p_0}{1-p_1}\right)}{\ln\left(\dfrac{p_1(1-p_0)}{p_0(1-p_1)}\right)}$	$m,\ \Sigma x_i$ $(x_i = 0 \text{ or } 1)$ m = sample number n = fixed sample size	$\dfrac{-\ln\alpha}{n\ln\left(\dfrac{1-p_0}{1-p_1}\right)}$	$\dfrac{\ln\left(\dfrac{1-p_0}{1-p_1}\right)}{k\ln\left(\dfrac{p_1(1-p_0)}{p_0(1-p_1)}\right)}$
"Np" (unequal sample sizes)				$\Sigma n_i,\ \Sigma x_i$ $(x_i = 0 \text{ or } 1)$	$\dfrac{-\ln\alpha}{\ln\left(\dfrac{1-p_0}{1-p_1}\right)}$	$\dfrac{\ln\left(\dfrac{1-p_0}{1-p_1}\right)}{k\ln\left(\dfrac{p_1(1-p_0)}{p_0(1-p_1)}\right)}$

* Approximation b (see Section B).

XII. Miscellaneous Statistical Tables

XII.1 NUMBER OF PERMUTATIONS $P(n,m)$

This table contains the number of permutations of n distinct things taken m at a time, given by

$$P(n,m) = \frac{n!}{(n-m)!} = n(n-1) \cdots (n-m+1)$$

n \ m	0	1	2	3	4	5	6	7	8	9	10
0	1										
1	1	1									
2	1	2	2								
3	1	3	6	6							
4	1	4	12	24	24						
5	1	5	20	60	120	120					
6	1	6	30	120	360	720	720				
7	1	7	42	210	840	2520	5040	5040			
8	1	8	56	336	1680	6720	20160	40320	40320		
9	1	9	72	504	3024	15120	60480	1 81440	3 62880	3 62880	
10	1	10	90	720	5040	30240	1 51200	6 04800	18 14400	36 28800	36 28800
11	1	11	110	990	7920	55440	3 32640	16 63200	66 52800	199 58400	399 16800
12	1	12	132	1320	11880	95040	6 65280	39 91680	199 58400	798 33600	2395 00800
13	1	13	156	1716	17160	1 54440	12 35520	86 48640	518 91840	2594 59200	10378 36800
14	1	14	182	2184	24024	2 40240	21 62160	172 97280	1210 80960	7264 85760	36324 28800
15	1	15	210	2730	32760	3 60360	36 03600	324 32400	2594 59200	18162 14400	1 08972 86400

n \ m	11	12	13	14	15
8					
9					
10					
11	399 16800				
12	4790 01600	4790 01600			
13	31135 10400	62270 20800	62270 20800		
14	1 45297 15200	4 35891 45600	8 71782 91200	8 71782 91200	
15	5 44864 32000	21 79457 28000	65 38371 84000	130 76743 68000	130 76743 68000

XII.2 NUMBER OF COMBINATIONS $C(n,m)$

This table contains the number of combinations of n distinct things taken m at a time, given by

$$\binom{n}{m} = C(n,m) = \frac{n!}{m!(n-m)!} = \frac{P(n,r)}{m!}\ .$$

For values missing from the above table, use the relation $\binom{n}{m} = \binom{n}{n-m}$, e.g. $\binom{20}{12} = \binom{20}{8} = 125970$. $\binom{n}{m}$ is also referred to as a binomial coefficient. A recursion relation for the binomial coefficients is

$$\binom{n+1}{m+1} = \binom{n}{m} + \binom{n}{m+1}\ .$$

NUMBER OF COMBINATIONS

$$\binom{n}{m} = C(n,m)$$

n \ m	0	1	2	3	4	5	6	7	8
1	1	1							
2	1	2	1						
3	1	3	3	1					
4	1	4	6	4	1				
5	1	5	10	10	5	1			
6	1	6	15	20	15	6	1		
7	1	7	21	35	35	21	7	1	
8	1	8	28	56	70	56	28	8	1
9	1	9	36	84	126	126	84	36	9
10	1	10	45	120	210	252	210	120	45
11	1	11	55	165	330	462	462	330	165
12	1	12	66	220	495	792	924	792	495
13	1	13	78	286	715	1287	1716	1716	1287
14	1	14	91	364	1001	2002	3003	3432	3003
15	1	15	105	455	1365	3003	5005	6435	6435
16	1	16	120	560	1820	4368	8008	11440	12870
17	1	17	136	680	2380	6188	12376	19448	24310
18	1	18	153	816	3060	8568	18564	31824	43758
19	1	19	171	969	3876	11628	27132	50388	75582
20	1	20	190	1140	4845	15504	38760	77520	1 25970
21	1	21	210	1330	5985	20349	54264	1 16280	2 03490
22	1	22	231	1540	7315	26334	74613	1 70544	3 19770
23	1	23	253	1771	8855	33649	1 00947	2 45157	4 90314
24	1	24	276	2024	10626	42504	1 34596	3 46104	7 35471
25	1	25	300	2300	12650	53130	1 77100	4 80700	10 81575
26	1	26	325	2600	14950	65780	2 30230	6 57800	15 62275
27	1	27	351	2925	17550	80730	2 96010	8 88030	22 20075
28	1	28	378	3276	20475	98280	3 76740	11 84040	31 08105
29	1	29	406	3654	23751	1 18755	4 75020	15 60780	42 92145
30	1	30	435	4060	27405	1 42506	5 93775	20 35800	58 52925
31	1	31	465	4495	31465	1 69911	7 36281	26 29575	78 88725
32	1	32	496	4960	35960	2 01376	9 06192	33 65856	105 18300
33	1	33	528	5456	40920	2 37336	11 07568	42 72048	138 84156
34	1	34	561	5984	46376	2 78256	13 44904	53 79616	181 56204
35	1	35	595	6545	52360	3 24632	16 23160	67 24520	235 35820
36	1	36	630	7140	58905	3 76992	19 47792	83 47680	302 60340
37	1	37	666	7770	66045	4 35897	23 24784	102 95472	386 08020
38	1	38	703	8436	73815	5 01942	27 60681	126 20256	489 03492
39	1	39	741	9139	82251	5 75757	32 62623	153 80937	615 23748
40	1	40	780	9880	91390	6 58008	38 38380	186 43560	769 04685
41	1	41	820	10660	101270	7 49398	44 96388	224 81940	955 48245
42	1	42	861	11480	111930	8 50668	52 45786	269 78328	1180 30185
43	1	43	903	12341	123410	9 62598	60 96454	322 24114	1450 08513
44	1	44	946	13244	135751	10 86008	70 59052	383 20568	1772 32627
45	1	45	990	14190	148995	12 21759	81 45060	453 79620	2155 53195
46	1	46	1035	15180	163185	13 70754	93 66819	535 24680	2609 32815
47	1	47	1081	16215	178365	15 33939	107 37573	628 91499	3144 57495
48	1	48	1128	17296	194580	17 12304	122 71512	736 29072	3773 48994
49	1	49	1176	18424	211876	19 06884	139 83816	859 00584	4509 78066
50	1	50	1225	19600	230300	21 18760	158 90700	998 84400	5368 78650

NUMBER OF COMBINATIONS

$$\binom{n}{m} = C(n,m)$$

n \ m	9	10	11	12	13
9	1				
10	10	1			
11	55	11	1		
12	220	66	12	1	
13	715	286	78	13	1
14	2002	1001	364	91	14
15	5005	3003	1365	455	105
16	11440	8008	4368	1820	560
17	24310	19448	12376	6188	2380
18	48620	43758	31824	18564	8568
19	92378	92378	75582	50388	27132
20	1 67960	1 84756	1 67960	1 25970	77520
21	2 93930	3 52716	3 52716	2 93930	2 03490
22	4 97420	6 46646	7 05432	6 46646	4 97420
23	8 17190	11 44066	13 52078	13 52078	11 44066
24	13 07504	19 61256	24 96144	27 04156	24 96144
25	20 42975	32 68760	44 57400	52 00300	52 00300
26	31 24550	53 11735	77 26160	96 57700	104 00600
27	46 86825	84 36285	130 37895	173 83860	200 58300
28	69 06900	131 23110	214 74180	304 21755	374 42160
29	100 15005	200 30010	345 97290	518 95935	678 63915
30	143 07150	300 45015	546 27300	864 93225	1197 59850
31	201 60075	443 52165	846 72315	1411 20525	2062 53075
32	280 48800	645 12240	1290 24480	2257 92840	3474 73600
33	385 67100	925 61040	1935 36720	3548 17320	5731 66440
34	524 51256	1311 28140	2860 97760	5483 54040	9279 83760
35	706 07460	1835 79396	4172 25900	8344 51800	14763 37800
36	941 43280	2541 86856	6008 05296	12516 77700	23107 89600
37	1244 03620	3483 30136	8549 92152	18524 82996	35624 67300
38	1630 11640	4727 33756	12033 22288	27074 75148	54149 50296
39	2119 15132	6357 45396	16760 56044	39107 97436	81224 25444
40	2734 38880	8476 60528	23118 01440	55868 53480	1 20332 22880
41	3503 43565	11210 99408	31594 61968	78986 54920	1 76200 76360
42	4458 91810	14714 42973	42805 61376	1 10581 16888	2 55187 31280
43	5639 21995	19173 34783	57520 04349	1 53386 78264	3 65768 48168
44	7098 30508	24812 56778	76693 39132	2 10906 82613	5 19155 26432
45	8861 63135	31901 87286	1 01505 95910	2 87600 21745	7 30062 09045
46	11017 16330	40763 50421	1 33407 83196	3 89106 17655	10 17662 30790
47	13626 49145	51780 66751	1 74171 33617	5 22514 00851	14 06768 48445
48	16771 06640	65407 15896	2 25952 00368	6 96685 34468	19 29282 49296
49	20544 55634	82178 22536	2 91359 16264	9 22637 34836	26 25967 83764
50	25054 33700	1 02722 78170	3 73537 38800	12 13996 51100	35 48605 18600

NUMBER OF COMBINATIONS

$$\binom{n}{m} = C(n,m)$$

n \ m	14	15	16	17	18	19
14	1					
15	15	1				
16	120	16	1			
17	680	136	17	1		
18	3060	816	153	18	1	
19	11628	3876	969	171	19	1
20	38760	15504	4845	1140	190	20
21	1 16280	54264	20349	5985	1330	210
22	3 19770	1 70544	74613	26334	7315	1540
23	8 17190	4 90314	2 45157	1 00947	33649	8855
24	19 61256	13 07504	7 35471	3 46104	1 34596	42504
25	44 57400	32 68760	20 42975	10 81575	4 80700	1 77100
26	96 57700	77 26160	53 11735	31 24550	15 62275	6 57800
27	200 58300	173 83860	130 37895	84 36285	46 86825	22 20075
28	401 16600	374 42160	304 21755	214 74180	131 23110	69 06900
29	775 58760	775 58760	678 63915	518 95935	345 97290	200 30010
30	1454 22675	1551 17520	1454 22675	1197 59850	864 93225	546 27300
31	2651 82525	3005 40195	3005 40195	2651 82525	2062 53075	1411 20525
32	4714 35600	5657 22720	6010 80390	5657 22720	4714 35600	3473 73600
33	8188 09200	10371 58320	11668 03110	11668 03110	10371 58320	8188 09200
34	13919 75640	18559 67520	22039 61430	23336 06220	22039 61430	18559 67520
35	23199 59400	32479 43160	40599 28950	45375 67650	45375 67650	40599 28950
36	37962 97200	55679 02560	73078 72110	85974 96600	90751 35300	85974 96600
37	61070 86800	93641 99760	1 28757 74670	1 59053 68710	1 76726 31900	1 76726 31900
38	96695 54100	1 54712 86560	2 22399 74430	2 87811 43380	3 35780 00610	3 53452 63800
39	1 50845 04396	2 51408 40660	3 77112 60990	5 10211 17810	6 23591 43990	6 89232 64410
40	2 32069 29840	4 02253 45056	6 28521 01650	8 87323 78800	11 33802 61800	13 12824 08400
41	3 52401 52720	6 34322 74896	10 30774 46706	15 15844 80450	20 21126 40600	24 46626 70200
42	5 28602 29080	9 86724 27616	16 65097 21602	25 46619 27156	35 36971 21050	44 67753 10800
43	7 83789 60360	15 15326 56696	26 51821 49218	42 11716 48758	60 83590 48206	80 04724 31850
44	11 49558 08528	22 99116 17056	41 67148 05914	68 63537 97976	102 95306 96964	140 88314 80056
45	16 68713 34960	34 48674 25584	64 66264 22970	110 30686 03890	171 58844 94940	243 83621 77020
46	23 98775 44005	51 17387 60544	99 14938 48554	174 96950 26860	281 89530 98830	415 42466 71960
47	34 16437 74795	75 16163 04549	150 32326 09098	274 11888 75414	456 86481 25690	697 31997 70790
48	48 23206 23240	109 32600 79344	225 48489 13647	424 44214 84512	730 98370 01104	1154 18478 96480
49	67 52488 72536	157 55807 02584	334 81089 92991	649 92703 98159	1155 42584 85616	1885 16848 97584
50	93 78456 56300	225 08295 75120	492 36896 95575	984 73793 91150	1805 35288 83775	3040 59433 83200

NUMBER OF COMBINATIONS

$$\binom{n}{m} = C(n,m)$$

n \ m	20	21	22	23	24	25
20	1					
21	21	1				
22	231	22	1			
23	1771	253	23	1		
24	10626	2024	276	24	1	
25	53130	12650	2300	300	25	1
26	2 30230	65780	14950	2600	325	26
27	8 88030	2 96010	80730	17550	2925	351
28	31 08105	11 84040	3 76740	98280	20475	3276
29	100 15005	42 92145	15 60780	4 75020	1 18755	23751
30	300 45015	143 07150	58 52925	20 35800	5 93775	1 42506
31	846 72315	443 52165	201 60075	78 88725	26 29575	7 36281
32	2257 92840	1290 24480	645 12240	280 48800	105 18300	33 65856
33	5731 66440	3548 17320	1935 36720	925 61040	385 67100	138 84156
34	13919 75640	9279 83760	5483 54040	2860 97760	1311 28140	524 51256
35	32479 43160	23199 59400	14763 37800	8344 51800	4172 25900	1835 79396
36	73078 72110	55679 02560	37962 97200	23107 89600	12516 77700	6008 05296
37	1 59053 68710	1 28757 74670	93641 99760	61070 86800	35624 67300	18524 82996
38	3 35780 00610	2 87811 43380	2 22399 74430	1 54712 86560	96695 54100	54149 50296
39	6 89232 64410	6 23591 43990	5 10211 17810	3 77112 60990	2 51408 40660	1 50845 04396
40	13 78465 28820	13 12824 08400	11 33802 61800	8 87323 78800	6 28521 01650	4 02253 45056
41	26 91289 37220	26 91289 37220	24 46626 70200	20 21126 40600	15 15844 80450	10 30774 46706
42	51 37916 07420	53 82578 74440	51 37916 07420	44 67753 10800	35 36971 21050	25 46619 27156
43	96 05669 18220	105 20494 81860	105 20494 81860	96 05669 18220	80 04724 31850	60 83590 48206
44	176 10393 50070	201 26164 00080	210 40989 63720	201 26164 00080	176 10393 50070	140 88314 80056
45	316 98708 30126	377 36557 50150	411 67153 63800	411 67153 63800	377 36557 50150	316 98708 30126
46	560 82330 07146	694 35265 80276	789 03711 13950	823 34307 27600	789 03711 13950	694 35265 80276
47	976 24796 79106	1255 17595 87422	1483 38976 94226	1612 38018 41550	1612 38018 41550	1483 38976 94226
48	1673 56794 49896	2231 42392 66528	2738 56572 81648	3095 76995 35776	3224 76036 83100	3095 76995 35776
49	2827 75273 46376	3904 99187 16424	4969 98965 48176	5834 33568 17424	6320 53032 18876	6320 53032 18876
50	4712 92122 43960	6732 74460 62800	8874 98152 64600	10804 32533 65600	12154 86600 36300	12641 06064 37752

XII.3 LOGARITHMS OF THE BINOMIAL COEFFICIENTS

This table contains the logarithms of the binomial coefficients $\binom{n}{m}$; also referred to as the number of combinations of n distinct things taken m at a time. For values missing from the table, use the relation

$$\binom{n}{m} = \frac{n!}{m!(n-m)!} = \binom{n}{n-m}$$

LOGARITHMS OF THE BINOMIAL COEFFICIENTS

m	$n = 1$	$n = 2$	$n = 3$	$n = 4$	$n = 5$	$n = 6$	$n = 7$	$n = 8$	$n = 9$	$n = 10$
1	.0000	.3010	.4771	.6021	.6990	.7782	.8451	.9031	.9542	1.0000
2			.4771	.7782	1.0000	1.1761	1.3222	1.4472	1.5563	1.6532
3					1.0000	1.3010	1.5441	1.7482	1.9243	2.0792
4							1.5441	1.8451	2.1004	2.3222
5									2.1004	2.4014

m	$n = 11$	$n = 12$	$n = 13$	$n = 14$	$n = 15$	$n = 16$	$n = 17$	$n = 18$	$n = 19$	$n = 20$
1	1.0414	1.0792	1.1139	1.1461	1.1761	1.2041	1.2304	1.2553	1.2788	1.3010
2	1.7404	1.8195	1.8921	1.9590	2.0212	2.0792	2.1335	2.1847	2.2330	2.2788
3	2.2175	2.3424	2.4564	2.5611	2.6580	2.7482	2.8325	2.9117	2.9863	3.0569
4	2.5185	2.6946	2.8543	3.0004	3.1351	3.2601	3.3766	3.4857	3.5884	3.6853
5	2.6646	2.8987	3.1096	3.3015	3.4776	3.6403	3.7910	3.9329	4.0055	4.1904
6	2.6646	2.9657	3.2345	3.4776	3.6994	3.9035	4.0926	4.2687	4.4335	4.5884
7			3.2345	3.5355	3.8085	4.0584	4.2889	4.5028	4.7023	4.8894
8					3.8085	4.1096	4.3858	4.6411	4.8784	5.1003
9							4.3858	4.6868	4.9656	5.2252
10									4.9656	5.2666

m	$n = 21$	$n = 22$	$n = 23$	$n = 24$	$n = 25$	$n = 26$	$n = 27$	$n = 28$	$n = 29$	$n = 30$
1	1.3222	1.3424	1.3617	1.3802	1.3979	1.4150	1.4314	1.4472	1.4624	1.4771
2	2.3222	2.3636	2.4031	2.4409	2.4771	2.5119	2.5453	2.5775	2.6085	2.6385
3	3.1239	3.1875	3.2482	3.3062	3.3617	3.4150	3.4661	3.5153	3.5628	3.6085
4	3.7771	3.8642	3.9472	4.0264	4.1021	4.1746	4.2443	4.3112	4.3757	4.4378
5	4.3085	4.4205	4.5270	4.6284	4.7253	4.8181	4.9070	4.9925	5.0747	5.1538
6	4.7345	4.8728	5.0041	5.1290	5.2482	5.3622	5.4713	5.5760	5.6767	5.7736
7	5.0655	5.2318	5.3894	5.5392	5.6819	5.8181	5.9484	6.0734	6.1933	6.3087
8	5.3085	5.5048	5.6905	5.8666	6.0341	6.1938	6.3464	6.4925	6.6327	6.7674
9	5.4682	5.6967	5.9123	6.1164	6.3103	6.4948	6.6709	6.8393	7.0007	7.1556
10	5.5474	5.8107	6.0585	6.2925	6.5144	6.7252	6.9262	7.1180	7.3017	7.4778
11	5.5474	5.8485	6.1310	6.3973	6.6491	6.8880	7.1152	7.3319	7.5390	7.7374
12			6.1310	6.4320	6.7160	6.9849	7.2401	7.4832	7.7151	7.9370
13					6.7160	7.0171	7.3023	7.5734	7.8316	8.0783
14							7.3023	7.6033	7.8896	8.1626
15									7.8896	8.1907

LOGARITHMS OF THE BINOMIAL COEFFICIENTS

m	$n = 31$	$n = 32$	$n = 33$	$n = 34$	$n = 35$	$n = 36$	$n = 37$	$n = 38$	$n = 39$	$n = 40$
1	1.4914	1.5052	1.5185	1.5315	1.5441	1.5563	1.5682	1.5798	1.5911	1.6021
2	2.6675	2.6955	2.7226	2.7490	2.7745	2.7993	2.8235	2.8470	2.8698	2.8921
3	3.6527	3.6955	3.7369	3.7770	3.8159	3.8537	3.8904	3.9261	3.9609	3.9948
4	4.4978	4.5558	4.6119	4.6663	4.7190	4.7702	4.8198	4.8681	4.9151	4.9609
5	5.2302	5.3040	5.3754	5.4444	5.5114	5.5763	5.6394	5.7007	5.7602	5.8182
6	5.8670	5.9572	6.0444	6.1287	6.2104	6.2895	6.3664	6.4410	6.5136	6.5841
7	6.4199	6.5271	6.6306	6.7308	6.8277	6.9216	7.0126	7.1011	7.1870	7.2705
8	6.8970	7.0219	7.1425	7.2590	7.3717	7.4809	7.5867	7.6893	7.7890	7.8860
9	7.3045	7.4479	7.5862	7.7198	7.8489	7.9738	8.0948	8.2122	8.3262	8.4369
10	7.6469	7.8096	7.9664	8.1177	8.2638	8.4052	8.5420	8.6746	8.8033	8.9282
11	7.9277	8.1107	8.2868	8.4565	8.6204	8.7787	8.9320	9.0804	9.2243	9.3640
12	8.1496	8.3537	8.5500	8.7391	8.9214	9.0975	9.2678	9.4326	9.5923	9.7472
13	8.3144	8.5408	8.7583	8.9675	9.1692	9.3638	9.5518	9.7336	9.9097	10.0804
14	8.4235	8.6734	8.9132	9.1436	9.3655	9.5794	9.7858	9.9854	10.1785	10.3656
15	8.4779	8.7526	9.0158	9.2686	9.5116	9.7457	9.9715	10.1895	10.4004	10.6045
16	8.4779	8.7789	9.0670	9.3432	9.6085	9.8638	10.1098	10.3471	10.5765	10.7983
17			9.0670	9.3680	9.6568	9.9344	10.2015	10.4591	10.7078	10.9481
18					9.6568	9.9579	10.2473	10.5261	10.7949	11.0545
19							10.2473	10.5483	10.8384	11.1182
20									10.8384	11.1394

m	$n = 41$	$n = 42$	$n = 43$	$n = 44$	$n = 45$	$n = 46$	$n = 47$	$n = 48$	$n = 49$	$n = 50$
1	1.6128	1.6232	1.6335	1.6435	1.6532	1.6628	1.6721	1.6812	1.6902	1.6990
2	2.9138	2.9350	2.9557	2.9759	2.9956	3.0149	3.0338	3.0523	3.0704	3.0881
3	4.0278	4.0599	4.0914	4.1220	4.1520	4.1813	4.2099	4.2379	4.2654	4.2923
4	5.0055	5.0489	5.0914	5.1327	5.1732	5.2127	5.2513	5.2891	5.3261	5.3623
5	5.8747	5.9298	5.9834	6.0358	6.0870	6.1370	6.1858	6.2336	6.2803	6.3261
6	6.6529	6.7198	6.7851	6.8487	6.9109	6.9716	7.0309	7.0889	7.1456	7.2011
7	7.3518	7.4310	7.5082	7.5834	7.6569	7.7286	7.7986	7.8670	7.9340	7.9995
8	7.9802	8.0720	8.1614	8.2485	8.3336	8.4165	8.4976	8.5767	8.6542	8.7299
9	8.5445	8.6492	8.7512	8.8506	8.9475	9.0421	9.1344	9.2246	9.3127	9.3989
10	9.0496	9.1677	9.2827	9.3947	9.5038	9.6103	9.7142	9.8156	9.9148	10.0117
11	9.4996	9.6315	9.7598	9.8848	10.0065	10.1252	10.2410	10.3540	10.4644	10.5723
12	9.8976	10.0437	10.1858	10.3241	10.4588	10.5901	10.7181	10.8430	10.9650	11.0842
13	10.2460	10.4069	10.5632	10.7153	10.8634	11.0076	11.1482	11.2854	11.4193	11.5501
14	10.5470	10.7231	10.8942	11.0605	11.2224	11.3800	11.5336	11.6833	11.8295	11.9721
15	10.8023	10.9942	11.1805	11.3616	11.5377	11.7090	11.8760	12.0387	12.1974	12.3523
16	11.0132	11.2214	11.4235	11.6198	11.8107	11.9963	12.1770	12.3531	12.5248	12.6923
17	11.1807	11.4060	11.6245	11.8365	12.0426	12.2430	12.4379	12.6278	12.8129	12.9933
18	11.3056	11.5486	11.7842	12.0126	12.2345	12.4501	12.6598	12.8639	13.0627	13.2566
19	11.3886	11.6501	11.9033	12.1489	12.3871	12.6185	12.8434	13.0623	13.2754	13.4830
20	11.4300	11.7108	11.9825	12.2458	12.5010	12.7488	12.9896	13.2236	13.4514	13.6733
21	11.4300	11.7310	12.0220	12.3038	12.5768	12.8416	13.0987	13.3486	13.5916	13.8282
22			12.0220	12.3231	12.6146	12.8971	13.1713	13.4375	13.6964	13.9482
23					12.6146	12.9156	13.2075	13.4908	13.7660	14.0336
24							13.2075	13.5085	13.8008	14.0848
25									13.8008	14.1018

LOGARITHMS OF THE BINOMIAL COEFFICIENTS

m	$n = 51$	$n = 52$	$n = 53$	$n = 54$	$n = 55$	$n = 56$	$n = 57$	$n = 58$	$n = 59$	$n = 60$
1	1.7076	1.7160	1.7243	1.7324	1.7404	1.7482	1.7559	1.7634	1.7709	1.7782
2	3.1055	3.1225	3.1392	3.1556	3.1717	3.1875	3.2030	3.2183	3.2333	3.2480
3	4.3186	4.3444	4.3697	4.3945	4.4189	4.4428	4.4663	4.4893	4.5120	4.5343
4	5.3978	5.4325	5.4666	5.5000	5.5328	5.5650	5.5966	5.6276	5.6581	5.6881
5	6.3709	6.4148	6.4578	6.5000	6.5414	6.5820	6.6219	6.6611	6.6995	6.7373
6	7.2555	7.3087	7.3609	7.4121	7.4622	7.5115	7.5598	7.6072	7.6538	7.6995
7	8.0636	8.1264	8.1879	8.2482	8.3073	8.3653	8.4222	8.4781	8.5329	8.5868
8	8.8040	8.8765	8.9476	9.0172	9.0855	9.1524	9.2181	9.2826	9.3459	9.4080
9	9.4832	9.5657	9.6466	9.7257	9.8033	9.8794	9.9541	10.0273	10.0992	10.1698
10	10.1065	10.1992	10.2900	10.3790	10.4661	10.5515	10.6353	10.7175	10.7982	10.8773
11	10.6778	10.7811	10.8821	10.9810	11.0779	11.1729	11.2660	11.3573	11.4470	11.5349
12	11.2007	11.3147	11.4262	11.5353	11.6422	11.7469	11.8496	11.9503	12.0490	12.1459
13	11.6778	11.8028	11.9250	12.0446	12.1617	12.2764	12.3889	12.4991	12.6072	12.7132
14	12.1115	12.2477	12.3809	12.5113	12.6388	12.7638	12.8862	13.0062	13.1238	13.2392
15	12.5036	12.6514	12.7959	12.9372	13.0755	13.2109	13.3436	13.4735	13.6009	13.7259
16	12.8558	13.0155	13.1716	13.3242	13.4735	13.6196	13.7627	13.9029	14.0403	14.1750
17	13.1694	13.3413	13.5093	13.6735	13.8341	13.9912	14.1450	14.2957	14.4433	14.5880
18	13.4456	13.6301	13.8104	13.9864	14.1586	14.3270	14.4918	14.6532	14.8113	14.9662
19	13.6854	13.8829	14.0757	14.2640	14.4481	14.6280	14.8041	14.9765	15.1453	15.3107
20	13.8895	14.1004	14.3061	14.5070	14.7033	14.8952	15.0829	15.2665	15.4463	15.6224
21	14.0586	14.2833	14.5024	14.7163	14.9252	15.1293	15.3289	15.5241	15.7152	15.9022
22	14.1933	14.4322	14.6651	14.8924	15.1142	15.3309	15.5427	15.7499	15.9525	16.1509
23	14.2940	14.5476	14.7948	15.0358	15.2710	15.5007	15.7251	15.9444	16.1590	16.3689
24	14.3610	14.6298	14.8917	15.1470	15.3960	15.6390	15.8764	16.1083	16.3351	16.5569
25	14.3944	14.6790	14.9561	15.2261	15.4894	15.7462	15.9969	16.2418	16.4812	16.7153
26	14.3944	14.6954	14.9883	15.2736	15.5515	15.8226	16.0871	16.3454	16.5977	16.8444
27			14.9883	15.2894	15.5826	15.8683	16.1471	16.4192	16.6849	16.9445
28					15.5826	15.8836	16.1771	16.4634	16.7429	17.0159
29							16.1771	16.4781	16.7718	17.0586
30									16.7718	17.0729

m	$n = 61$	$n = 62$	$n = 63$	$n = 64$	$n = 65$	$n = 66$	$n = 67$	$n = 68$	$n = 69$	$n = 70$
1	1.7853	1.7924	1.7993	1.8062	1.8129	1.8195	1.8261	1.8325	1.8388	1.8451
2	3.2625	3.2767	3.2907	3.3045	3.3181	3.3314	3.3446	3.3576	3.3703	3.3829
3	4.5562	4.5777	4.5989	4.6198	4.6403	4.6605	4.6804	4.7000	4.7193	4.7383
4	5.7175	5.7465	5.7750	5.8030	5.8306	5.8578	5.8845	5.9108	5.9368	5.9623
5	6.7745	6.8110	6.8469	6.8822	6.9170	6.9512	6.9849	7.0180	7.0507	7.0829
6	7.7445	7.7887	7.8322	7.8749	7.9170	7.9584	7.9991	8.0392	8.0787	8.1177
7	8.6398	8.6918	8.7429	8.7932	8.8427	8.8914	8.9393	8.9865	9.0330	9.0787
8	9.4691	9.5291	9.5880	9.6460	9.7031	9.7592	9.8144	9.8688	9.9223	9.9750
9	10.2391	10.3072	10.3742	10.4400	10.5047	10.5684	10.6310	10.6927	10.7534	10.8131
10	10.9551	11.0315	11.1066	11.1803	11.2529	11.3242	11.3944	11.4635	11.5315	11.5985
11	11.6213	11.7061	11.7894	11.8713	11.9519	12.0310	12.1089	12.1856	12.2610	12.3352
12	12.2411	12.3345	12.4263	12.5164	12.6051	12.6922	12.7779	12.8623	12.9452	13.0269
13	12.8173	12.9195	13.0199	13.1185	13.2154	13.3107	13.4044	13.4965	13.5872	13.6764
14	13.3524	13.4636	13.5727	13.6799	13.7853	13.8888	13.9906	14.0907	14.1892	14.2861
15	13.8484	13.9687	14.0868	14.2028	14.3168	14.4287	14.5388	14.6470	14.7535	14.8582
16	14.3071	14.4367	14.5640	14.6889	14.8116	14.9322	15.0507	15.1672	15.2818	15.3945
17	14.7298	14.8690	15.0056	15.1397	15.2714	15.4007	15.5278	15.6527	15.7756	15.8964
18	15.1180	15.2670	15.4131	15.5565	15.6973	15.8356	15.9715	16.1050	16.2363	16.3654
19	15.4727	15.6317	15.7875	15.9405	16.0907	16.2381	16.3829	16.5253	16.6651	16.8027
20	15.7950	15.9641	16.1300	16.2927	16.4524	16.6092	16.7632	16.9144	17.0631	17.2092

LOGARITHMS OF THE BINOMIAL COEFFICIENTS

m	$n = 61$	$n = 62$	$n = 63$	$n = 64$	$n = 65$	$n = 66$	$n = 67$	$n = 68$	$n = 69$	$n = 70$
21	16.0855	16.2651	16.4412	16.6139	16.7834	16.9497	17.1130	17.2734	17.4311	17.5860
22	16.3452	16.5355	16.7220	16.9050	17.0844	17.2605	17.4334	17.6031	17.7699	17.9337
23	16.5745	16.7758	16.9731	17.1665	17.3562	17.5422	17.7249	17.9042	18.0802	18.2532
24	16.7741	16.9867	17.1949	17.3991	17.5992	17.7955	17.9881	18.1772	18.3628	18.5451
25	16.9443	17.1685	17.3881	17.6032	17.8140	18.0208	18.2236	18.4227	18.6181	18.8099
26	17.0857	17.3217	17.5529	17.7793	18.0011	18.2186	18.4319	18.6412	18.8465	19.0482
27	17.1984	17.4467	17.6897	17.9277	18.1608	18.3893	18.6133	18.8330	19.0486	19.2603
28	17.2827	17.5436	17.7989	18.0487	18.2935	18.5332	18.7682	18.9987	19.2247	19.4466
29	17.3388	17.6127	17.8805	18.1426	18.3993	18.6506	18.8969	19.1383	19.3751	19.6074
30	17.3668	17.6541	17.9349	18.2096	18.4784	18.7417	18.9996	19.2523	19.5001	19.7431
31	17.3668	17.6679	17.9620	18.2497	18.5311	18.8066	19.0764	19.3407	19.5998	19.8538
32			17.9620	18.2631	18.5575	18.8455	19.1275	19.4038	19.6744	19.9397
33					18.5575	18.8585	19.1531	19.4415	19.7241	20.0010
34							19.1531	19.4541	19.7489	20.0377
35									19.7489	20.0499

m	$n = 71$	$n = 72$	$n = 73$	$n = 74$	$n = 75$	$n = 76$	$n = 77$	$n = 78$	$n = 79$	$n = 80$
1	1.8513	1.8573	1.8633	1.8692	1.8751	1.8808	1.8865	1.8921	1.8976	1.9031
2	3.3953	3.4076	3.4196	3.4315	3.4433	3.4548	3.4663	3.4776	3.4887	3.4997
3	4.7571	4.7755	4.7938	4.8117	4.8295	4.8470	4.8642	4.8812	4.8981	4.9147
4	5.9875	6.0123	6.0368	6.0609	6.0847	6.1082	6.1314	6.1542	6.1768	6.1991
5	7.1146	7.1459	7.1767	7.2071	7.2370	7.2666	7.2957	7.3245	7.3529	7.3809
6	8.1560	8.1938	8.2310	8.2678	8.3040	8.3397	8.3749	8.4097	8.4440	8.4778
7	9.1238	9.1682	9.2120	9.2552	9.2977	9.3397	9.3811	9.4219	9.4622	9.5020
8	10.0269	10.0781	10.1285	10.1782	10.2271	10.2754	10.3231	10.3701	10.4165	10.4622
9	10.8720	10.9300	10.9871	11.0435	11.0990	11.1537	11.2077	11.2609	11.3135	11.3653
10	11.6644	11.7293	11.7933	11.8564	11.9185	11.9798	12.0402	12.0998	12.1586	12.2166
11	12.4083	12.4803	12.5513	12.6212	12.6900	12.7579	12.8249	12.8909	12.9560	13.0203
12	13.1073	13.1865	13.2645	13.3413	13.4170	13.4917	13.5652	13.6378	13.7094	13.7799
13	13.7642	13.8507	13.9359	14.0198	14.1024	14.1839	14.2642	14.3434	14.4215	14.4985
14	14.3815	14.4754	14.5679	14.6590	14.7487	14.8371	14.9243	15.0102	15.0949	15.1784
15	14.9613	15.0628	15.1626	15.2610	15.3579	15.4534	15.5475	15.6403	15.7317	15.8219
16	15.5054	15.6145	15.7220	15.8278	15.9320	16.0346	16.1358	16.2355	16.3338	16.4307
17	16.0153	16.1322	16.2474	16.3607	16.4724	16.5823	16.6907	16.7974	16.9027	17.0064
18	16.4924	16.6173	16.7403	16.8613	16.9805	17.0979	17.2136	17.3275	17.4398	17.5505
19	16.9379	17.0710	17.2019	17.3308	17.4576	17.5826	17.7057	17.8269	17.9464	18.0641
20	17.3529	17.4942	17.6333	17.7701	17.9048	18.0374	18.1680	18.2967	18.4235	18.5484
21	17.7382	17.8880	18.0353	18.1803	18.3230	18.4634	18.6017	18.7379	18.8721	19.0044
22	18.0948	18.2532	18.4089	18.5621	18.7129	18.8613	19.0075	19.1514	19.2931	19.4328
23	18.4233	18.5904	18.7547	18.9164	19.0755	19.2320	19.3861	19.5378	19.6873	19.8345
24	18.7243	18.9004	19.0735	19.2438	19.4113	19.5761	19.7383	19.8980	20.0553	20.2102
25	18.9984	19.1837	19.3568	19.5448	19.7209	19.8941	20.0646	20.2324	20.3977	20.5604
26	19.2462	19.4408	19.6320	19.8200	20.0049	20.1867	20.3657	20.5417	20.7151	20.8858
27	19.4681	19.6722	19.8728	20.0699	20.2637	20.4543	20.6419	20.8264	21.0080	21.1868
28	19.6644	19.8783	20.0884	20.2948	20.4978	20.6974	20.8937	21.0868	21.2769	21.4639
29	19.8354	20.0593	20.2792	20.4952	20.7075	20.9162	21.1215	21.3234	21.5220	21.7175
30	19.9816	20.2157	20.4455	20.6713	20.8931	21.1112	21.3256	21.5364	21.7439	21.9480
31	20.1030	20.3475	20.5876	20.8234	21.0550	21.2826	21.5063	21.7263	21.9427	22.1556
32	20.1999	20.4552	20.7057	20.9517	21.1933	21.4307	21.6639	21.8933	22.1188	22.3406
33	20.2725	20.5387	20.8000	21.0564	21.3082	21.5556	21.7986	22.0375	22.2724	22.5034
34	20.3208	20.5983	20.8706	21.1377	21.4000	21.6576	21.9106	22.1592	22.4037	22.6440
35	20.3449	20.6340	20.9176	21.1957	21.4687	21.7368	22.0000	22.2586	22.5128	22.7627

LOGARITHMS OF THE BINOMIAL COEFFICIENTS

m	$n = 71$	$n = 72$	$n = 73$	$n = 74$	$n = 75$	$n = 76$	$n = 77$	$n = 78$	$n = 79$	$n = 80$
36	20.3449	20.6459	20.9410	21.2305	21.5145	21.7932	22.0670	22.3358	22.6000	22.8596
37			20.9410	21.2421	21.5374	21.8271	22.1115	22.3908	22.6652	22.9348
38					21.5374	21.8384	22.1338	22.4238	22.7087	22.9885
39							22.1338	22.4348	22.7304	23.0207
40									22.7304	23.0314

m	$n = 81$	$n = 82$	$n = 83$	$n = 84$	$n = 85$	$n = 86$	$n = 87$	$n = 88$	$n = 89$	$n = 90$
1	1.9085	1.9138	1.9191	1.9243	1.9294	1.9345	1.9395	1.9445	1.9494	1.9542
2	3.5105	3.5213	3.5319	3.5423	3.5527	3.5629	3.5730	3.5830	3.5928	3.6026
3	4.9311	4.9472	4.9632	4.9790	4.9946	5.0100	5.0253	5.0403	5.0552	5.0700
4	6.2211	6.2428	6.2643	6.2854	6.3064	6.3271	6.3475	6.3677	6.3877	6.4074
5	7.4086	7.4359	7.4629	7.4896	7.5159	7.5419	7.5676	7.5930	7.6181	7.6430
6	8.5113	8.5443	8.5769	8.6090	8.6408	8.6722	8.7033	8.7339	8.7643	8.7942
7	9.5412	9.5800	9.6182	9.6560	9.6934	9.7302	9.7667	9.8027	9.8382	9.8734
8	10.5074	10.5520	10.5960	10.6394	10.6824	10.7248	10.7667	10.8081	10.8490	10.8894
9	11.4165	11.4669	11.5168	11.5660	11.6146	11.6626	11.7100	11.7569	11.8032	11.8490
10	12.2738	12.3303	12.3860	12.4411	12.4954	12.5491	12.6021	12.6545	12.7063	12.7574
11	13.0837	13.1462	13.2080	13.2689	13.3291	13.3885	13.4472	13.5052	13.5625	13.6191
12	13.8496	13.9183	13.9861	14.0531	14.1191	14.1844	14.2489	14.3125	14.3754	14.4376
13	14.5745	14.6494	14.7234	14.7964	14.8685	14.9397	15.0100	15.0794	15.1480	15.2157
14	15.2609	15.3422	15.4224	15.5016	15.5797	15.6569	15.7331	15.8083	15.8827	15.9561
15	15.9108	15.9986	16.0851	16.1706	16.2549	16.3381	16.4203	16.5015	16.5816	16.6608
16	16.5263	16.6205	16.7135	16.8053	16.8959	16.9853	17.0735	17.1607	17.2468	17.3318
17	17.1087	17.2096	17.3092	17.4074	17.5043	17.5999	17.6943	17.7876	17.8796	17.9705
18	17.6596	17.7673	17.8734	17.9782	18.0815	18.1835	18.2842	18.3836	18.4817	18.5786
19	18.1802	18.2947	18.4076	18.5190	18.6288	18.7373	18.8443	18.9499	19.0542	19.1572
20	18.6716	18.7930	18.9127	19.0308	19.1473	19.2623	19.3757	19.4877	19.5983	19.7074
21	19.1347	19.2632	19.3899	19.5148	19.6380	19.7596	19.8796	19.9980	20.1149	20.2303
22	19.5704	19.7061	19.8398	19.9717	20.1018	20.2301	20.3567	20.4817	20.6050	20.7267
23	19.9795	20.1225	20.2634	20.4024	20.5394	20.6746	20.8079	20.9395	21.0693	21.1975
24	20.3628	20.5131	20.6614	20.8075	20.9516	21.0937	21.2339	21.3722	21.5087	21.6434
25	20.7207	20.8786	21.0343	21.1877	21.3390	21.4882	21.6353	21.7804	21.9236	22.0650
26	21.0539	21.2195	21.3827	21.5436	21.7022	21.8585	22.0127	22.1648	22.3148	22.4629
27	21.3629	21.5364	21.7073	21.8757	22.0416	22.2053	22.3667	22.5258	22.6828	22.8377
28	21.6481	21.8296	22.0083	22.1844	22.3579	22.5290	22.6977	22.8640	23.0280	23.1899
29	21.9100	22.0996	22.2862	22.4702	22.6514	22.8300	23.0061	23.1797	23.3510	23.5199
30	22.1489	22.3467	22.5415	22.7334	22.9225	23.1088	23.2924	23.4735	23.6520	23.8281
31	22.3651	22.5714	22.7744	22.9744	23.1715	23.3656	23.5569	23.7455	23.9315	24.1149
32	22.5589	22.7738	22.9853	23.1936	23.3987	23.6008	23.8000	23.9963	24.1898	24.3806
33	22.7306	22.9542	23.1743	23.3911	23.6045	23.8147	24.0218	24.2259	24.4271	24.6255
34	22.8804	23.1130	23.3418	23.5671	23.7890	24.0075	24.2227	24.4348	24.6438	24.8499
35	23.0084	23.2501	23.4880	23.7220	23.9525	24.1794	24.4029	24.6231	24.8401	25.0540
36	23.1149	23.3659	23.6129	23.8559	24.0952	24.3307	24.5626	24.7911	25.0162	25.2381
37	23.1999	23.4605	23.7168	23.9690	24.2172	24.4615	24.7020	24.9389	25.1723	25.4023
38	23.2635	23.5339	23.7998	24.0613	24.3186	24.5719	24.8212	25.0667	25.3085	25.5468
39	23.3060	23.5863	23.8619	24.1330	24.3996	24.6620	24.9203	25.1746	25.4250	25.6717
40	23.3271	23.6177	23.9033	24.1841	24.4603	24.7321	24.9995	25.2627	25.5219	25.7772
41	23.3271	23.6828	23.9240	24.2148	24.5008	24.7821	25.0588	25.3312	25.5994	25.8634
42			23.9240	24.2250	24.5210	24.8120	25.0983	25.3801	25.6573	25.9303
43					24.5210	24.8220	25.1181	25.4093	25.6960	25.9781
44							25.1181	25.4191	25.7153	26.0068
45									25.7153	26.0163

LOGARITHMS OF THE BINOMIAL COEFFICIENTS

m	$n = 91$	$n = 92$	$n = 93$	$n = 94$	$n = 95$	$n = 96$	$n = 97$	$n = 98$	$n = 99$	$n = 100$
1	1.9590	1.9638	1.9685	1.9731	1.9777	1.9823	1.9868	1.9912	1.9956	2.0000
2	3.6123	3.6218	3.6312	3.6406	3.6498	4.6590	3.6680	3.6770	3.6858	3.6946
3	5.0845	5.0989	5.1132	5.1272	5.1412	5.1550	5.1686	5.1821	5.1955	5.2087
4	6.4269	6.4463	6.4653	6.4842	6.5029	6.5214	6.5397	6.5578	6.5757	6.5934
5	7.6675	7.6918	7.7158	7.7395	7.7630	7.7862	7.8092	7.8319	7.8544	7.8767
6	8.8238	8.8531	8.8821	8.9107	8.9391	8.9671	8.9948	9.0223	9.0494	9.0763
7	9.9082	9.9425	9.9765	10.0101	10.0434	10.0762	10.1088	10.1410	10.1728	10.2043
8	10.9294	10.9689	11.0079	11.0466	11.0848	11.1225	11.1599	11.1969	11.2335	11.2697
9	11.8942	11.9389	11.9831	12.0268	12.0700	12.1128	12.1551	12.1969	12.2383	12.2793
10	12.8080	12.8580	12.9074	12.9562	13.0045	13.0523	13.0996	13.1463	13.1925	13.2383
11	13.6751	13.7304	13.7851	13.8391	13.8926	13.9454	13.9977	14.0494	14.1005	14.1512
12	14.4990	14.5597	14.6197	14.6790	14.7377	14.7956	14.8530	14.9097	14.9658	15.0214
13	15.2827	15.3488	15.4142	15.4789	15.5428	15.6060	15.6685	15.7303	15.7914	15.8519
14	16.0287	16.1003	16.1712	16.2412	16.3105	16.3789	16.4466	16.5136	16.5798	16.6453
15	16.7391	16.8163	16.8927	16.9682	17.0429	17.1167	17.1896	17.2618	17.3331	17.4037
16	17.4157	17.4987	17.5807	17.6617	17.7418	17.8210	17.8993	17.9767	18.0533	18.1290
17	18.0604	18.1491	18.2368	18.3234	18.4090	18.4937	18.5773	18.6601	18.7419	18.8228
18	18.6743	18.7689	18.8623	18.9546	19.0458	19.1360	19.2252	19.3133	19.4005	19.4866
19	19.2589	19.3594	19.4586	19.5567	19.6536	19.7494	19.8440	19.9376	20.0302	20.1217
20	19.8152	19.9216	20.0268	20.1307	20.2334	20.3348	20.4351	20.5342	20.6322	20.7292
21	20.3442	20.4568	20.5679	20.6777	20.7862	20.8934	20.9994	21.1041	21.2076	21.3100
22	20.8469	20.9656	21.0828	21.1986	21.3130	21.4261	21.5378	21.6482	21.7573	21.8652
23	21.3240	21.4490	21.5723	21.6942	21.8146	21.9336	22.0511	22.1673	22.2821	22.3956
24	21.7763	21.9076	22.0372	22.1653	22.2917	22.4167	22.5401	22.6621	22.7827	22.9019
25	22.2045	22.3422	22.4781	22.6124	22.7450	22.8761	23.0055	23.1334	23.2598	23.3847
26	22.6090	22.7533	22.8957	23.0363	23.1752	23.3123	23.4479	23.5818	23.7141	23.8448
27	22.9906	23.1415	23.2904	23.4374	23.5827	23.7261	23.8678	24.0077	24.1460	24.2827
28	23.3496	23.5072	23.6628	23.8164	23.9680	24.1178	24.2657	24.4118	24.5562	24.6989
29	23.6865	23.8510	24.0133	24.1735	24.3317	24.4879	24.6421	24.7945	24.9451	25.0938
30	24.0018	24.1732	24.3423	24.5093	24.6741	24.8368	24.9975	25.1563	25.3130	25.4679
31	24.2958	24.4742	24.6503	24.8241	24.9957	25.1650	25.3322	25.4974	25.6605	25.8217
32	24.5688	24.7544	24.9376	25.1183	25.2967	25.4728	25.6466	25.8183	25.9879	26.1554
33	24.9211	25.0141	25.2044	25.3922	25.5775	25.7604	25.9410	26.1194	26.2954	26.4694
34	25.0531	25.2534	25.4511	25.6460	25.8384	26.0283	26.2157	26.4008	26.5835	26.7640
35	25.2649	25.4728	25.6778	25.8801	26.0797	26.2766	26.4710	26.6629	26.8524	27.0394
36	25.4568	25.6724	25.8850	26.0947	26.3015	26.5057	26.7071	26.9059	27.1022	27.2961
37	25.6289	25.8523	26.0726	26.2899	26.5042	26.7156	26.9242	27.1301	27.3334	27.5340
38	25.7815	26.0129	26.2410	26.4660	26.6878	26.9067	27.1226	27.3357	27.5460	27.7536
39	25.9147	26.1543	26.3903	26.6231	26.8526	27.0790	27.3024	27.5228	27.7402	27.9549
40	26.0287	26.2765	26.5207	26.7614	26.9988	27.2329	27.4638	27.6916	27.9163	28.1382
41	26.1235	26.3797	26.6322	26.8810	27.1264	27.3683	27.6068	27.8422	28.0744	28.3036
42	26.1992	26.4640	26.7249	26.9820	27.2355	27.4854	27.7318	27.9748	28.2146	28.4512
43	26.2559	26.5295	26.7990	27.0646	27.3263	27.5843	27.8387	28.0895	28.3370	28.5811
44	26.2937	26.5763	26.8545	27.1287	27.3989	27.6651	27.9276	28.1865	28.4417	28.6935
45	26.3126	26.6043	26.8915	27.1745	27.4532	27.7279	27.9987	28.2656	28.5289	28.7885
46	26.3126	26.6136	26.9100	27.2019	27.3894	27.7727	28.0519	28.3272	28.5985	28.8661
47			26.9100	27.2110	27.5075	27.7996	28.0874	28.3711	28.6507	28.9264
48					27.5075	27.8086	28.1051	28.3974	28.6855	28.9694
49							28.1051	28.4062	28.7028	28.9953
50									28.7028	29.0039

XII.4 RANDOM UNITS

Use of Table. If one wishes to select a random sample of N items from a universe of M items, the following procedure may be applied. ($M > N$.)

1. Decide upon some arbitrary scheme of selecting entries from the table. For example, one may decide to use the entries in the first line, second column; second line, third column; third line, fourth column; etc.

2. Assign numbers to each of the items in the universe from 1 to M. Thus, if $M = 500$, the items would be numbered from 001 to 500, and therefore, each designated item is associated with a three digit number.

3. Decide upon some arbitrary scheme of selecting positional digits from each entry chosen according to Step 1. Thus, if $M = 500$, one may decide to use the first, third, and fourth digit of each entry selected, and as a consequence a three digit number is created for each entry choice.

4. If the number formed is $\leqq M$, the correspondingly designated item in the universe is chosen for the random sample of N items. If a number formed is $> M$ or is a repeated number of one already chosen, it is passed over and the next desirable number is taken. This process is continued until the random sample of N items if selected.

A TABLE OF 14,000 RANDOM UNITS

Line/Col.	(1)	(2)	(3)	(4)	(5)	(6)	(7)	(8)	(9)	(10)	(11)	(12)	(13)	(14)
1	10480	15011	01536	02011	81647	91646	69179	14194	62590	36207	20969	99570	91291	90700
2	22368	46573	25595	85393	30995	89198	27982	53402	93965	34095	52666	19174	39615	99505
3	24130	48360	22527	97265	76393	64809	15179	24830	49340	32081	30680	19655	63348	58629
4	42167	93093	06243	61680	07856	16376	39440	53537	71341	57004	00849	74917	97758	16379
5	37570	39975	81837	16656	06121	91782	60468	81305	49684	60672	14110	06927	01263	54613
6	77921	06907	11008	42751	27756	53498	18602	70659	90655	15053	21916	81825	44394	42880
7	99562	72905	56420	69994	98872	31016	71194	18738	44013	48840	63213	21069	10634	12952
8	96301	91977	05463	07972	18876	20922	94595	56869	69014	60045	18425	84903	42508	32307
9	89579	14342	63661	10281	17453	18103	57740	84378	25331	12566	58678	44947	05585	56941
10	85475	36857	43342	53988	53060	59533	38867	62300	08158	17983	16439	11458	18593	64952
11	28918	69578	88231	33276	70997	79936	56865	05859	90106	31595	01547	85590	91610	78188
12	63553	40961	48235	03427	49626	69445	18663	72695	52180	20847	12234	90511	33703	90322
13	09429	93969	52636	92737	88974	33488	36320	17617	30015	08272	84115	27156	30613	74952
14	10365	61129	87529	85689	48237	52267	67689	93394	01511	26358	85104	20285	29975	89868
15	07119	97336	71048	08178	77233	13916	47564	81056	97735	85977	29372	74461	28551	90707
16	51085	12765	51821	51259	77452	16308	60756	92144	49442	53900	70960	63990	75601	40719
17	02368	21382	52404	60268	89368	19885	55322	44819	01188	65255	64835	44919	05944	55157
18	01011	54092	33362	94904	31273	04146	18594	29852	71585	85030	51132	01915	92747	64951
19	52162	53916	46369	58586	23216	14513	83149	98736	23495	64350	94738	17752	35156	35749
20	07056	97628	33787	09998	42698	06691	76988	13602	51851	46104	88916	19509	25625	58104
21	48663	91245	85828	14346	09172	30168	90229	04734	59193	22178	30421	61666	99904	32812
22	54164	58492	22421	74103	47070	25306	76468	26384	58151	06646	21524	15227	96909	44592
23	32639	32363	05597	24200	13363	38005	94342	28728	35806	06912	17012	64161	18296	22851
24	29334	27001	87637	87308	58731	00256	45834	15398	46557	41135	10367	07684	36188	18510
25	02488	33062	28834	07351	19731	92420	60952	61280	50001	67658	32586	86679	50720	94953
26	81525	72295	04839	96423	24878	82651	66566	14778	76797	14780	13300	87074	79666	95725
27	29676	20591	68086	26432	46901	20849	89768	81536	86645	12659	92259	57102	80428	25280
28	00742	57392	39064	66432	84673	40027	32832	61362	98947	96067	64760	64584	96096	98253
29	05366	04213	25669	26422	44407	44048	37937	63904	45766	66134	75470	66520	34693	90449
30	91921	26418	64117	94305	26766	25940	39972	22209	71500	64568	91402	42416	07844	69618
31	00582	04711	87917	77341	42206	35126	74087	99547	81817	42607	43808	76655	62028	76630
32	00725	69884	62797	56170	86324	88072	76222	36086	84637	93161	76038	65855	77919	88006
33	69011	65797	95876	55293	18988	27354	26575	08625	40801	59920	29841	80150	12777	48501
34	25976	57948	29888	88604	67917	48708	18912	82271	65424	69774	33611	54262	85963	03547
35	09763	83473	73577	12908	30883	18317	28290	35797	05998	41688	34952	37888	38917	88050
36	91567	42595	27958	30134	04024	86385	29880	99730	55536	84855	29080	09250	79656	73211
37	17955	56349	90999	49127	20044	59931	06115	20542	18059	02008	73708	83517	36103	42791
38	46503	18584	18845	49618	02304	51038	20655	58727	28168	15475	56942	53389	20562	87338
39	92157	89634	94824	78171	84610	82834	09922	25417	44137	48413	25555	21246	35509	20468
40	14577	62765	35605	81263	39667	47358	56873	56307	61607	49518	89656	20103	77490	18062
41	98427	07523	33362	64270	01638	92477	66969	98420	04880	45585	46565	04102	46880	45709
42	34914	63976	88720	82765	34476	17032	87589	40836	32427	70002	70663	88863	77775	69348
43	70060	28277	39475	46473	23219	53416	94970	25832	69975	94884	19661	72828	00102	66794
44	53976	54914	06990	67245	68350	82948	11398	42878	80287	88267	47363	46634	06541	97809
45	76072	29515	40980	07391	58745	25774	22987	80059	39911	96189	41151	14222	60697	59583
46	90725	52210	83974	29992	65831	38857	50490	83765	55657	14361	31720	57375	56228	41546
47	64364	67412	33339	31926	14883	24413	59744	92351	97473	89286	35931	04110	23726	51900
48	08962	00358	31662	25388	61642	34072	81249	35648	56891	69352	48373	45578	78547	81788
49	95012	68379	93526	70765	10593	04542	76463	54328	02349	17247	28865	14777	62730	92277
50	15664	10493	20492	38391	91132	21999	59516	81652	27195	48223	46751	22923	32261	85653

A TABLE OF 14,000 RANDOM UNITS

Line/Col.	(1)	(2)	(3)	(4)	(5)	(6)	(7)	(8)	(9)	(10)	(11)	(12)	(13)	(14)
51	16408	81899	04153	53381	79401	21438	83035	92350	36693	31238	59649	91754	72772	02338
52	18629	81953	05520	91962	04739	13092	97662	24822	94730	06496	35090	04822	86772	98289
53	73115	35101	47498	87637	99016	71060	88824	71013	18735	20286	23153	72924	35165	43040
54	57491	16703	23167	49323	45021	33132	12544	41035	80780	45393	44812	12515	98931	91202
55	30405	83946	23792	14422	15059	45799	22716	19792	09983	74353	68668	30429	70735	25499
56	16631	35006	85900	98275	32388	52390	16815	69298	82732	38480	73817	32523	41961	44437
57	96773	20206	42559	78985	05300	22164	24369	54224	35083	19687	11052	91491	60383	19746
58	38935	64202	14349	82674	66523	44133	00697	35552	35970	19124	63318	29686	03387	59846
59	31624	76384	17403	53363	44167	64486	64758	75366	76554	31601	12614	33072	60332	92325
60	78919	19474	23632	27889	47914	02584	37680	20801	72152	39339	34806	08930	85001	87820
61	03931	33309	57047	74211	63445	17361	62825	39908	05607	91284	68833	25570	38818	46920
62	74426	33278	43972	10119	89917	15665	52872	73823	73144	88662	88970	74492	51805	99378
63	09066	00903	20795	95452	92648	45454	09552	88815	16553	51125	79375	97596	16296	66092
64	42238	12426	87025	14267	20979	04508	64535	31355	86064	29472	47689	05974	52468	16834
65	16153	08002	26504	41744	81959	65642	74240	56302	00033	67107	77510	70625	28725	34191
66	21457	40742	29820	96783	29400	21840	15035	34537	33310	06116	95240	15957	16572	06004
67	21581	57802	02050	89728	17937	37621	47075	42080	97403	48626	68995	43805	33386	21597
68	55612	78095	83197	33732	05810	24813	86902	60397	16489	03264	88525	42786	05269	92532
69	44657	66999	99324	51281	84463	60563	79312	93454	68876	25471	93911	25650	12682	73572
70	91340	84979	46949	81973	37949	61023	43997	15263	80644	43942	89203	71795	99533	50501
71	91227	21199	31935	27022	84067	05462	35216	14486	29891	68607	41867	14951	91696	85065
72	50001	38140	66321	19924	72163	09538	12151	06878	91903	18749	34405	56087	82790	70925
73	65390	05224	72958	28609	81406	39147	25549	48542	42627	45233	57202	94617	23772	07896
74	27504	96131	83944	41575	10573	08619	64482	73923	36152	05184	94142	25299	84387	34925
75	37169	94851	39117	89632	00959	16487	65536	49071	39782	17095	02330	74301	00275	48280
76	11508	70225	51111	38351	19444	66499	71945	05422	13442	78675	84081	66938	93654	59894
77	37449	30362	06694	54690	04052	53115	62757	95348	78662	11163	81651	50245	34971	52924
78	46515	70331	85922	38329	57015	15765	97161	17860	45340	61796	66345	81073	49106	79860
79	30986	81223	42416	58353	21532	30502	32305	86482	05174	07901	54339	58861	74818	46942
80	63798	64995	46583	09765	44160	78128	83991	42865	92520	83531	80377	35909	81250	54238
81	82486	84846	99254	67632	43218	50076	21361	64816	51202	88124	41870	52689	51275	83556
82	21885	32906	92431	09060	64297	51674	64126	62570	26123	05155	59194	52799	28225	85762
83	60336	98782	07408	53458	13564	59089	26445	29789	85205	41001	12535	12133	14645	23541
84	43937	46891	24010	25560	86355	33941	25786	54990	71899	15475	95434	98227	21824	19585
85	97656	63175	89303	16275	07100	92063	21942	18611	47348	20203	18534	03862	78095	50136
86	03299	01221	05418	38982	55758	92237	26759	86367	21216	98442	08303	56613	91511	75928
87	79626	06486	03574	17668	07785	76020	79924	25651	83325	88428	85076	72811	22717	50585
88	85636	68335	47539	03129	65651	11977	02510	26113	99447	68645	34327	15152	55230	93448
89	18039	14367	61337	06177	12143	46609	32989	74014	64708	00533	35398	58408	13261	47908
90	08362	15656	60627	36478	65648	16764	53412	09013	07832	41574	17639	82163	60859	75567
91	79556	29068	04142	16268	15387	12856	66227	38358	22478	73373	88732	09443	82558	05250
92	92608	82674	27072	32534	17075	27698	98204	63863	11951	34648	88022	56148	34925	57031
93	23982	25835	40055	67006	12293	02753	14827	22235	35071	99704	37543	11601	35503	85171
94	09915	96306	05908	97901	28395	14186	00821	80703	70426	75647	76310	88717	37890	40129
95	50937	33300	26695	62247	69927	76123	50842	43834	86654	70959	79725	93872	28117	19233
96	42488	78077	69882	61657	34136	79180	97526	43092	04098	73571	80799	76536	71255	64239
97	46764	86273	63003	93017	31204	36692	40202	35275	57306	55543	53203	18098	47625	88684
98	03237	45430	55417	63282	90816	17349	88298	90183	36600	78406	06216	95787	42579	90730
99	86501	81482	52667	61583	14972	90053	89534	76036	49199	43716	97548	04379	46370	28672
100	38534	01715	94964	87288	65680	43772	39560	12918	86537	62738	19636	51132	25739	56947

A TABLE OF 14,000 RANDOM UNITS

Line/Col.	(1)	(2)	(3)	(4)	(5)	(6)	(7)	(8)	(9)	(10)	(11)	(12)	(13)	(14)
101	13284	16834	74151	92027	24670	36665	00770	22878	02179	51602	07270	76517	97275	45960
102	21224	00370	30420	03883	96648	89428	41583	17564	27395	63904	41548	49197	82277	24120
103	99052	47887	81085	64933	66279	80432	65793	83287	34142	13241	30590	97760	35848	91983
104	00199	50993	98603	38452	87890	94624	69721	57484	67501	77638	44331	11257	71131	11059
105	60578	06483	28733	37867	07936	98710	98539	27186	31237	80612	44488	97819	70401	95419
106	91240	18312	17441	01929	18163	69201	31211	54288	39296	37318	65724	90401	79017	62077
107	97458	14229	12063	59611	32249	90466	33216	19358	02591	54263	88449	01912	07436	50813
108	35249	38646	34475	72417	60514	69257	12489	51924	86871	92446	36607	11458	30440	52639
109	38980	46600	11759	11900	46743	27860	77940	39298	97838	95145	32378	68038	89351	37005
110	10750	52745	38749	87365	58959	53731	89295	59062	39404	13198	59960	70408	29812	83126
111	36247	27850	73958	20673	37800	63835	71051	84724	52492	22342	78071	17456	96104	18327
112	70994	66986	99744	72438	01174	42159	11392	20724	54322	36923	70009	23233	65438	59685
113	99638	94702	11463	18148	81386	80431	90628	52506	02016	85151	88598	47821	00265	82525
114	72055	15774	43857	99805	10419	76939	25993	03544	21560	83471	43989	90770	22965	44247
115	24038	65541	85788	55835	38835	59399	13790	35112	01324	39520	76210	22467	83275	32286
116	74976	14631	35908	28221	39470	91548	12854	30166	09073	75887	36782	00268	97121	57676
117	35553	71628	70189	26436	63407	91178	90348	55359	80392	41012	36270	77786	89578	21059
118	35676	12797	51434	82976	42010	26344	92920	92155	58807	54644	58581	95331	78629	73344
119	74815	67523	72985	23183	02446	63594	98924	20633	58842	85961	07648	70164	34994	67662
120	45246	88048	65173	50989	91060	89894	36063	32819	68559	99221	49475	50558	34698	71800
121	76509	47069	86378	41797	11910	49672	88575	97966	32466	10083	54728	81972	58975	30761
122	19689	90332	04315	21358	97248	11188	39062	63312	52496	07349	79178	33692	57352	72862
123	42751	35318	97513	61537	54955	08159	00337	80778	27507	95478	21252	12746	37554	97775
124	11946	22681	45045	13964	57517	59419	58045	44067	58716	58840	45557	96345	33271	53464
125	96518	48688	20996	11090	48396	57177	83867	86464	14342	21545	46717	72364	86954	55580
126	35726	58643	76869	84622	39098	36083	72505	92265	23107	60278	05822	46760	44294	07672
127	39737	42750	48968	70536	84864	64952	38404	94317	65402	13589	01055	79044	19308	83623
128	97025	66492	56177	04049	80312	48028	26408	43591	75528	65341	49044	95495	81256	53214
129	62814	08075	09788	56350	76787	51591	54509	49295	85830	59860	30883	89660	96142	18354
130	25578	22950	15227	83291	41737	79599	96191	71845	86899	70694	24290	01551	80092	82118
131	68763	69576	88991	49662	46704	63362	56625	00481	73323	91427	15264	06969	57048	54149
132	17900	00813	64361	60725	88974	61005	99709	30666	26451	11528	44323	34778	60342	60388
133	71944	60227	63551	71109	05624	43836	58254	26160	32116	63403	35404	57146	10909	07346
134	54684	93691	85132	64399	29182	44324	14491	55226	78793	34107	30374	48429	51376	09559
135	25946	27623	11258	65204	52832	50880	22273	05554	99521	73791	85744	29276	70326	60251
136	01353	39318	44961	44972	91766	90262	56073	06606	51826	18893	83448	31915	97764	75091
137	99083	88191	27662	99113	57174	35571	99884	13951	71057	53961	61448	74909	07322	80960
138	52021	45406	37945	75234	24327	86978	22644	87779	23753	99926	63898	54886	18051	96314
139	78755	47744	43776	83098	03225	14281	83637	55984	13300	52212	58781	14905	46502	04472
140	25282	69106	59180	16257	22810	43609	12224	25643	89884	31149	85423	32581	34374	70873
141	11959	94202	02743	86847	79725	51811	12998	76844	05320	54236	53891	70226	38632	84776
142	11644	13792	98190	01424	30078	28197	55583	05197	47714	68440	22016	79204	06862	94451
143	06307	97912	68110	59812	95448	43244	31262	88880	13040	16458	43813	89416	42482	33939
144	76285	75714	89585	99296	52640	46518	55486	90754	88932	19937	57119	23251	55619	23679
145	55322	07589	39600	60866	63007	20007	66819	84164	61131	81429	60676	42807	78286	29015
146	78017	90928	90220	92503	83375	26986	74399	30885	88567	29169	72816	53357	15428	86932
147	44768	43342	20696	26331	43140	69744	82928	24988	94237	46138	77426	39039	55596	12655
148	25100	19336	14605	86603	51680	97678	24261	02464	86563	74812	60069	71674	15478	47642
149	83612	46623	62876	85197	07824	91392	58317	37726	84628	42221	10268	20692	15699	29167
150	41347	81666	82961	60413	71020	83658	02415	33322	66036	98712	46795	16308	28413	05417

A TABLE OF 14,000 RANDOM UNITS

Line/Col.	(1)	(2)	(3)	(4)	(5)	(6)	(7)	(8)	(9)	(10)	(11)	(12)	(13)	(14)
151	38128	51178	75096	13609	16110	73533	42564	59870	29399	67834	91055	89917	51096	89011
152	60950	00455	73254	96067	50717	13878	03216	78274	65863	37011	91283	33914	91303	49326
153	90524	17320	29832	96118	75792	25326	22940	24904	80523	38928	91374	55597	97567	38914
154	49897	18278	67160	39408	97056	43517	84426	59650	20247	19293	02019	14790	02852	05819
155	18494	99209	81060	19488	65596	59787	47939	91225	98768	43688	00438	05548	09443	82897
156	65373	72984	30171	37741	70203	94094	87261	30056	58124	70133	18936	02138	59372	09075
157	40653	12843	04213	70925	95360	55774	76439	61768	52817	81151	52188	31940	54273	49032
158	51638	22238	56344	44587	83231	50317	74541	07719	25472	41602	77318	15145	57515	07633
159	69742	99303	62578	83575	30337	07488	51941	84316	42067	49692	28616	29101	03013	73449
160	58012	74072	67488	74580	47992	69482	58624	17106	47538	13452	22620	24260	40155	74716
161	18348	19855	42887	08279	43206	47077	42637	45606	00011	20662	14642	49984	94509	56380
162	59614	09193	58064	29086	44385	45740	70752	05663	49081	26960	57454	99264	24142	74648
163	75688	28630	39210	52897	62748	72658	98059	67202	72789	01869	13496	14663	87645	89713
164	13941	77802	69101	70061	35460	34576	15412	81304	58757	35498	94830	75521	00603	97701
165	96656	86420	96475	86458	54463	96419	55417	41375	76886	19008	66877	35934	59801	00497
166	03363	82042	15942	14549	38324	87094	19069	67590	11087	68570	22591	65232	85915	91499
167	70366	08390	69155	25496	13240	57407	91407	49160	07379	34444	94567	66035	38918	65708
168	47870	36605	12927	16043	53257	93796	52721	73120	48025	76074	95605	67422	41646	14557
169	79504	77606	22761	30518	28373	73898	30550	76684	77366	32276	04690	61667	64798	66276
170	46967	74841	50923	15339	37755	98995	40162	89561	69199	42257	11647	47603	48779	97907
171	14558	50769	35444	59030	87516	48193	02945	00922	48189	04724	21263	20892	92955	90251
172	12440	25057	01132	38611	28135	68089	10954	10097	54243	06460	50856	65435	79377	53890
173	32293	29938	68653	10497	98919	46587	77701	99119	93165	67788	17638	23097	21468	30992
174	10640	21875	72462	77981	56550	55999	87310	69643	45124	00349	25748	00844	96831	30651
175	47615	23169	39571	56972	20628	21788	51736	33133	72696	32605	41569	76148	91544	21121
176	16948	11128	71624	72754	49084	96303	27830	45817	67867	18062	87453	17226	72904	71474
177	21258	61092	66634	70335	92448	17354	83432	49608	66520	06442	59664	20420	39201	69549
178	15072	48853	15178	30730	47481	48490	41430	25015	49932	20474	53821	51015	70841	32105
179	99154	57412	09858	65671	70655	71479	63520	31357	56968	06729	34465	70685	04184	25250
180	08759	61089	23706	32994	35426	36666	63988	98844	37533	08269	27021	45886	22835	78451
181	67323	57839	61114	62192	47547	58023	64630	34886	98777	75442	95592	06141	45096	73117
182	09255	13986	84834	20764	72206	89393	34548	93438	88730	61805	78955	18952	46436	58740
183	36304	74712	00374	10107	85061	69228	81969	92216	03568	39630	81869	52824	50937	27954
184	15884	67429	86612	47367	10242	44880	12060	44309	46629	55105	66793	93173	00480	13311
185	18745	32031	35303	08134	33925	03044	59929	95418	04917	57590	24078	61703	02834	64154
186	72934	40086	88292	65728	38300	42323	64068	98373	48971	09049	59943	36538	05976	82118
187	17626	02944	20910	57662	80181	38579	24580	90529	52303	50436	29401	57824	86039	81062
188	27117	61399	50967	41399	81636	16663	15634	79717	94696	59240	25543	97989	63306	90946
189	93995	18678	90012	63645	85701	85269	62263	68331	00389	72571	15210	20769	44686	96176
190	67392	89421	09623	80725	62620	84162	87368	29560	00519	84545	08004	24526	41252	14521
191	04910	12261	37566	80016	21245	69377	50420	85658	55263	68667	78770	04533	14513	18099
192	81453	20283	79929	59839	23875	13245	46808	74124	74703	35769	95588	21014	37078	39170
193	19480	75790	48539	23703	15537	48885	02861	86587	74539	65227	90799	58789	96257	02708
194	21456	13162	74608	81011	55512	07481	93551	72189	76261	91206	89941	15132	37738	59284
195	89406	20912	46189	76376	25538	87212	20748	12831	57166	35026	16817	79121	18929	40628
196	09866	07414	55977	16419	01101	69343	13305	94302	80703	57910	36933	57771	42546	03003
197	86541	24681	23421	13521	28000	94917	07423	57523	97234	63951	42876	46829	09781	58160
198	10414	96941	06205	72222	57167	83902	07460	69507	10600	08858	07685	44472	64220	27040
199	49942	06683	41479	58982	56288	42853	92196	20632	62045	78812	35895	51851	83534	10689
200	23995	68882	42291	23374	24299	27024	67460	94783	40937	16961	26053	78749	46704	21983

XII.5 RANDOM NORMAL NUMBERS, $\mu = 0$, $\sigma = 1$

01	02	03	04	05	06	07	08	09	10
0.464	0.137	2.455	−0.323	−0.068	0.296	−0.288	1.298	0.241	−0.957
0.060	−2.526	−0.531	−0.194	0.543	−1.558	0.187	−1.190	0.022	0.525
1.486	−0.354	−0.634	0.697	0.926	1.375	0.785	−0.963	−0.853	−1.865
1.022	−0.472	1.279	3.521	0.571	−1.851	0.194	1.192	−0.501	−0.273
1.394	−0.555	0.046	0.321	2.945	1.974	−0.258	0.412	0.439	−0.035
0.906	−0.513	−0.525	0.595	0.881	−0.934	1.579	0.161	−1.885	0.371
1.179	−1.055	0.007	0.769	0.971	0.712	1.090	−0.631	−0.255	−0.702
−1.501	−0.488	−0.162	−0.136	1.033	0.203	0.448	0.748	−0.423	−0.432
−0.690	0.756	−1.618	−0.345	−0.511	−2.051	−0.457	−0.218	0.857	−0.465
1.372	0.225	0.378	0.761	0.181	−0.736	0.960	−1.530	−0.260	0.120
−0.482	1.678	−0.057	−1.229	−0.486	0.856	−0.491	−1.983	−2.830	−0.238
−1.376	−0.150	1.356	−0.561	−0.256	−0.212	0.219	0.779	0.953	−0.869
−1.010	0.598	−0.918	1.598	0.065	0.415	−0.169	0.313	−0.973	−1.016
−0.005	−0.899	0.012	−0.725	1.147	−0.121	1.096	0.481	−1.691	0.417
1.393	−1.163	−0.911	1.231	−0.199	−0.246	1.239	−2.574	−0.558	0.056
−1.787	−0.261	1.237	1.046	−0.508	−1.630	−0.146	−0.392	−0.627	0.561
−0.105	−0.357	−1.384	0.360	−0.992	−0.116	−1.698	−2.832	−1.108	−2.357
−1.339	1.827	−0.959	0.424	0.969	−1.141	−1.041	0.362	−1.726	1.956
1.041	0.535	0.731	1.377	0.983	−1.330	1.620	−1.040	0.524	−0.281
0.279	−2.056	0.717	−0.873	−1.096	−1.396	1.047	0.089	−0.573	0.932
−1.805	−2.008	−1.633	0.542	0.250	−0.166	0.032	0.079	0.471	−1.029
−1.186	1.180	1.114	0.882	1.265	−0.202	0.151	−0.376	−0.310	0.479
0.658	−1.141	1.151	−1.210	−0.927	0.425	0.290	−0.902	0.610	2.709
−0.439	0.358	−1.939	0.891	−0.227	0.602	0.873	−0.437	−0.220	−0.057
−1.399	−0.230	0.385	−0.649	−0.577	0.237	−0.289	0.513	0.738	−0.300
0.199	0.208	−1.083	−0.219	−0.291	1.221	1.119	0.004	−2.015	−0.594
0.159	0.272	−0.313	0.084	−2.828	−0.439	−0.792	−1.275	−0.623	−1.047
2.273	0.606	0.606	−0.747	0.247	1.291	0.063	−1.793	−0.699	−1.347
0.041	−0.307	0.121	0.790	−0.584	0.541	0.484	−0.986	0.481	0.996
−1.132	−2.098	0.921	0.145	0.446	−1.661	1.045	−1.363	−0.586	−1.023
0.768	0.079	−1.473	0.034	−2.127	0.665	0.084	−0.880	−0.579	0.551
0.375	−1.658	−0.851	0.234	−0.656	0.340	−0.086	−0.158	−0.120	0.418
−0.513	−0.344	0.210	−0.735	1.041	0.008	0.427	−0.831	0.191	0.074
0.292	−0.521	1.266	−1.206	−0.899	0.110	−0.528	−0.813	0.071	0.524
1.026	2.990	−0.574	−0.491	−1.114	1.297	−1.433	−1.345	−3.001	0.479
−1.334	1.278	−0.568	−0.109	−0.515	−0.566	2.923	0.500	0.359	0.326
−0.287	−0.144	−0.254	0.574	−0.451	−1.181	−1.190	−0.318	−0.094	1.114
0.161	−0.886	−0.921	−0.509	1.410	−0.518	0.192	−0.432	1.501	1.068
−1.346	0.193	−1.202	0.394	−1.045	0.843	0.942	1.045	0.031	0.772
1.250	−0.199	−0.288	1.810	1.378	0.584	1.216	0.733	0.402	0.226
0.630	−0.537	0.782	0.060	0.499	−0.431	1.705	1.164	0.884	−0.298
0.375	−1.941	0.247	−0.491	−0.665	−0.135	−0.145	−0.498	0.457	1.064
−1.420	0.489	−1.711	−1.186	0.754	−0.732	−0.066	1.006	−0.798	0.162
−0.151	−0.243	−0.430	−0.762	0.298	1.049	1.810	2.885	−0.768	−0.129
−0.309	0.531	0.416	−1.541	1.456	2.040	−0.124	0.196	0.023	−1.204
0.424	−0.444	0.593	0.993	−0.106	0.116	0.484	−1.272	1.066	1.097
0.593	0.658	−1.127	−1.407	−1.579	−1.616	1.458	1.262	0.736	−0.916
0.862	−0.885	−0.142	−0.504	0.532	1.381	0.022	−0.281	−0.342	1.222
0.235	−0.628	−0.023	−0.463	−0.899	−0.394	−0.538	1.707	−0.188	−1.153
−0.853	0.402	0.777	0.833	0.410	−0.349	−1.094	0.580	1.395	1.298

RANDOM NORMAL NUMBERS, $\mu = 0$, $\sigma = 1$

11	12	13	14	15	16	17	18	19	20
−1.329	−0.238	−0.838	−0.988	−0.445	0.964	−0.266	−0.322	−1.726	2.252
1.284	−0.229	1.058	0.090	0.050	0.523	0.016	0.277	1.639	0.554
0.619	0.628	0.005	0.973	−0.058	0.150	−0.635	−0.917	0.313	−1.203
0.699	−0.269	0.722	−0.994	−0.807	−1.203	1.163	1.244	1.306	−1.210
0.101	0.202	−0.150	0.731	0.420	0.116	−0.496	−0.037	−2.466	0.794
−1.381	0.301	0.522	0.233	0.791	−1.017	−0.182	0.926	−1.096	1.001
−0.574	1.366	−1.843	0.746	0.890	0.824	−1.249	−0.806	−0.240	0.217
0.096	0.210	1.091	0.990	0.900	−0.837	−1.097	−1.238	0.030	−0.311
1.389	−0.236	0.094	3.282	0.295	−0.416	0.313	0.720	0.007	0.354
1.249	0.706	1.453	0.366	−2.654	−1.400	0.212	0.307	−1.145	0.639
0.756	−0.397	−1.772	−0.257	1.120	1.188	−0.527	0.709	0.479	0.317
−0.860	0.412	−0.327	0.178	0.524	−0.672	−0.831	0.758	0.131	0.771
−0.778	−0.979	0.236	−1.033	1.497	−0.661	0.906	1.169	−1.582	1.303
0.037	0.062	0.426	1.220	0.471	0.784	−0.719	0.465	1.559	−1.326
2.619	−0.440	0.477	1.063	0.320	1.406	−0.701	−0.128	0.518	−0.676
−0.420	−0.287	−0.050	−0.481	1.521	−1.367	0.609	0.292	0.048	0.592
1.048	0.220	1.121	−1.789	−1.211	−0.871	−0.740	0.513	−0.558	−0.395
1.000	−0.638	1.261	0.510	−0.150	0.034	0.054	−0.055	0.639	−0.825
0.170	−1.131	−0.985	0.102	−0.939	−1.457	1.766	1.087	−1.275	2.362
0.389	0.435	0.171	0.891	1.158	1.041	1.048	−0.324	−0.404	1.060
−0.305	0.838	−2.019	−0.540	0.905	1.195	−1.190	0.106	0.571	0.298
−0.321	−0.039	1.799	−1.032	−2.225	−0.148	0.758	−0.862	0.158	−0.726
1.900	1.572	−0.244	−1.721	1.130	0.495	−0.484	0.014	−0.778	−1.483
−0.778	−0.288	−0.224	−1.324	−0.072	0.890	−0.410	0.752	0.376	−0.224
0.617	−1.718	−0.183	−0.100	1.719	0.696	−1.339	−0.614	1.071	−0.386
−1.430	−0.953	0.770	−0.007	−1.872	1.075	−0.913	−1.168	1.775	0.238
0.267	−0.048	0.972	0.734	−1.408	−1.955	−0.848	2.002	0.232	−1.273
0.078	0.500	0.300	1.000	1.170	0.005	1.175	0.000	1.000	0.000
−1.235	−1.168	0.325	1.421	2.652	−0.486	−1.253	0.270	−1.103	0.118
−0.258	0.638	2.309	0.741	−0.161	−0.679	0.336	1.973	0.370	−2.277
0.243	0.629	−1.516	−0.157	0.693	1.710	0.800	−0.265	1.218	0.655
−0.292	−1.455	−1.451	1.492	−0.713	0.821	−0.031	−0.780	1.330	0.977
−0.505	0.389	0.544	−0.042	1.615	−1.440	−0.989	−0.580	0.156	0.052
0.397	−0.287	1.712	0.289	−0.904	0.259	−0.600	−1.635	−0.009	−0.799
−0.605	−0.470	0.007	0.721	−1.117	0.635	0.592	−1.362	−1.441	0.672
1.360	0.182	−1.476	−0.599	−0.875	0.292	−0.700	0.058	−0.340	−0.639
0.480	−0.699	1.615	−0.225	1.014	−1.370	−1.097	0.294	0.309	−1.389
−0.027	−0.487	−1.000	−0.015	0.119	−1.990	−0.687	−1.964	−0.366	1.759
−1.482	−0.815	−0.121	1.884	−0.185	0.601	0.793	0.430	−1.181	0.426
−1.256	−0.567	−0.994	1.011	−1.071	−0.623	−0.420	−0.309	1.362	0.863
−1.132	2.039	1.934	−0.222	0.386	1.100	0.284	1.597	−1.718	−0.560
−0.780	−0.239	−0.497	−0.434	−0.284	−0.241	−0.333	1.348	−0.478	−0.169
−0.859	−0.215	0.241	1.471	0.389	−0.952	0.245	0.781	1.093	−0.240
0.447	1.479	0.067	0.426	−0.370	−0.675	−0.972	0.225	0.815	0.389
0.269	0.735	−0.066	−0.271	−1.439	1.036	−0.306	−1.439	−0.122	−0.336
0.097	−1.883	−0.218	0.202	−0.357	0.019	1.631	1.400	0.223	−0.793
−0.686	1.596	−0.286	0.722	0.655	−0.275	1.245	−1.504	0.066	−1.280
0.957	0.057	−1.153	0.701	−0.280	1.747	−0.745	1.338	−1.421	0.386
−0.976	−1.789	−0.696	−1.799	−0.354	0.071	2.355	0.135	−0.598	1.883
0.274	0.226	−0.909	−0.572	0.181	1.115	0.406	0.453	−1.218	−0.115

RANDOM NORMAL NUMBERS, $\mu = 0$, $\sigma = 1$

21	22	23	24	25	26	27	28	29	30
−1.752	−0.329	−1.256	0.318	1.531	0.349	−0.958	−0.059	0.415	−1.084
−0.291	0.085	1.701	−1.087	−0.443	−0.292	0.248	−0.539	−1.382	0.318
−0.933	0.130	0.634	0.899	1.409	−0.883	−0.095	0.229	0.129	0.367
−0.450	−0.244	0.072	1.028	1.730	−0.056	−1.488	−0.078	−2.361	−0.992
0.512	−0.882	0.490	−1.304	−0.266	0.757	−0.361	0.194	−1.078	0.529
−0.702	0.472	0.429	−0.664	−0.592	1.443	−1.515	−1.209	−1.043	0.278
0.284	0.039	−0.518	1.351	1.473	0.889	0.300	0.339	−0.206	1.392
−0.509	1.420	−0.782	−0.429	−1.266	0.627	−1.165	0.819	−0.261	0.409
−1.776	−1.033	1.977	0.014	0.702	−0.435	−0.816	1.131	0.656	0.061
−0.044	1.807	0.342	−2.510	1.071	−1.220	−0.060	−0.764	0.079	−0.964
0.263	−0.578	1.612	−0.148	−0.383	−1.007	−0.414	0.638	−0.186	0.507
0.986	0.439	−0.192	−0.132	0.167	0.883	−0.400	−1.440	−0.385	−1.414
−0.441	−0.852	−1.446	−0.605	−0.348	1.018	0.963	−0.004	2.504	−0.847
−0.866	0.489	0.097	0.379	0.192	−0.842	0.065	1.420	0.426	−1.191
−1.215	0.675	1.621	0.394	−1.447	2.199	−0.321	−0.540	−0.037	0.185
−0.475	−1.210	0.183	0.526	0.495	1.297	−1.613	1.241	−1.016	−0.090
1.200	0.131	2.502	0.344	−1.060	−0.909	−1.695	−0.666	−0.838	−0.866
−0.498	−1.202	−0.057	−1.354	−1.441	−1.590	0.987	0.441	0.637	−1.116
−0.743	0.894	−0.028	1.119	−0.598	0.279	2.241	0.830	0.267	−0.156
0.779	−0.780	−0.954	0.705	−0.361	−0.734	1.365	1.297	−0.142	−1.387
−0.206	−0.195	1.017	−1.167	−0.079	−0.452	0.058	−1.068	−0.394	−0.406
−0.092	−0.927	−0.439	0.256	0.503	0.338	1.511	−0.465	−0.118	−0.454
−1.222	−1.582	1.786	−0.517	−1.080	−0.409	−0.474	−1.890	0.247	0.575
0.068	0.075	−1.383	−0.084	0.159	1.276	1.141	0.186	−0.973	−0.266
0.183	1.600	−0.335	1.553	0.889	0.896	−0.035	0.461	0.486	1.246
−0.811	−2.904	0.618	0.588	0.533	0.803	−0.696	0.690	0.820	0.557
−1.010	1.149	1.033	0.336	1.306	0.835	1.523	0.296	−0.426	0.004
1.453	1.210	−0.043	0.220	−0.256	−1.161	−2.030	−0.046	0.243	1.082
0.759	−0.838	−0.877	−0.177	1.183	−0.218	−3.154	−0.963	−0.822	−1.114
0.287	0.278	−0.454	0.897	−0.122	0.013	0.346	0.921	0.238	−0.586
−0.669	0.035	−2.077	1.077	0.525	−0.154	−1.036	0.015	−0.220	0.882
0.392	0.106	−1.430	−0.204	−0.326	0.825	−0.432	−0.094	−1.566	0.679
−0.337	0.199	−0.160	0.625	−0.891	−1.464	−0.318	1.297	0.932	−0.032
0.369	−1.990	−1.190	0.666	−1.614	0.082	0.922	−0.139	−0.833	0.091
−1.694	0.710	−0.655	−0.546	1.654	0.134	0.466	0.033	−0.039	0.838
0.985	0.340	0.276	0.911	−0.170	−0.551	1.000	−0.838	0.275	−0.304
−1.063	−0.594	−1.526	−0.787	0.873	−0.405	−1.324	0.162	−0.163	−2.716
0.033	−1.527	1.422	0.308	0.845	−0.151	0.741	0.064	1.212	0.823
0.597	0.362	−3.760	1.159	0.874	−0.794	−0.915	1.215	1.627	−1.248
−1.601	−0.570	0.133	−0.660	1.485	0.682	−0.898	0.686	0.658	0.346
−0.266	−1.309	0.597	0.989	0.934	1.079	−0.656	−0.999	−0.036	−0.537
0.901	1.531	−0.889	−1.019	0.084	1.531	−0.144	−1.920	0.678	−0.402
−1.433	−1.008	−0.990	0.090	0.940	0.207	−0.745	0.638	1.469	1.214
1.327	0.763	−1.724	−0.709	−1.100	−1.346	−0.946	−0.157	0.522	−1.264
−0.248	0.788	−0.577	0.122	−0.536	0.293	1.207	−2.243	1.642	1.353
−0.401	−0.679	0.921	0.476	1.121	−0.864	0.128	−0.551	−0.872	1.511
0.344	−0.324	0.686	−1.487	−0.126	0.803	−0.961	0.183	−0.358	−0.184
0.441	−0.372	−1.336	0.062	1.506	−0.315	−0.112	−0.452	1.594	−0.264
0.824	0.040	−1.734	0.251	0.054	−0.379	1.298	−0.126	0.104	−0.529
1.385	1.320	−0.509	−0.381	−1.671	−0.524	−0.805	1.348	0.676	0.799

RANDOM NORMAL NUMBERS, $\mu = 0$, $\sigma = 1$

31	32	33	34	35	36	37	38	39	40
1.556	0.119	−0.078	0.164	−0.455	0.077	−0.043	−0.299	0.249	−0.182
0.647	1.029	1.186	0.887	1.204	−0.657	0.644	−0.410	−0.652	−0.165
0.329	0.407	1.169	−2.072	1.661	0.891	0.233	−1.628	−0.762	−0.717
−1.188	1.171	−1.170	−0.291	0.863	−0.045	−0.205	0.574	−0.926	1.407
−0.917	−0.616	−1.589	1.184	0.266	0.559	−1.833	−0.572	−0.648	−1.090
0.414	0.469	−0.182	0.397	1.649	1.198	0.067	−1.526	−0.081	−0.192
0.107	−0.187	1.343	0.472	−0.112	1.182	0.548	2.748	0.249	0.154
−0.497	1.907	0.191	0.136	−0.475	0.458	0.183	−1.640	−0.058	1.278
0.501	0.083	−0.321	1.133	1.126	−0.299	1.299	1.617	1.581	2.455
−1.382	−0.738	1.225	1.564	−0.363	−0.548	1.070	0.390	−1.398	0.524
−0.590	0.699	−0.162	−0.011	1.049	−0.689	1.225	0.339	−0.539	−0.445
−1.125	1.111	−1.065	0.534	0.102	0.425	−1.026	0.695	−0.057	0.795
0.849	0.169	−0.351	0.584	2.177	0.009	−0.696	−0.426	−0.692	−1.638
−1.233	−0.585	0.306	0.773	1.304	−1.304	0.282	−1.705	0.187	−0.880
0.104	−0.468	0.185	0.498	−0.624	−0.322	−0.875	1.478	−0.691	−0.281
0.261	−1.883	−0.181	1.675	−0.324	−1.029	−0.185	0.004	−0.101	−1.187
−0.007	1.280	0.568	−1.270	1.405	1.731	2.072	1.686	0.728	−0.417
0.794	−0.111	0.040	−0.536	−0.976	2.192	1.609	−0.190	−0.279	−1.611
0.431	−2.300	−1.081	−1.370	2.943	0.653	−2.523	0.756	0.886	−0.983
−0.149	1.294	−0.580	0.482	−1.449	−1.067	1.996	−0.274	0.721	0.490
−0.216	−1.647	1.043	0.481	−0.011	−0.587	−0.916	−1.016	−1.040	−1.117
1.604	−0.851	−0.317	−0.686	−0.008	1.939	0.078	−0.465	0.533	0.652
−0.212	0.005	0.535	0.837	0.362	1.103	0.219	0.488	1.332	−0.200
0.007	−0.076	1.484	0.455	−0.207	−0.554	1.120	0.913	−0.681	1.751
−0.217	0.937	0.860	0.323	1.321	−0.492	−1.386	−0.003	−0.230	0.539
−0.649	0.300	−0.698	0.900	0.569	0.842	0.804	1.025	0.603	−1.546
−1.541	0.193	2.047	−0.552	1.190	−0.087	2.062	−2.173	−0.791	−0.520
0.274	−0.530	0.112	0.385	0.656	0.436	0.882	0.312	−2.265	−0.218
0.876	−1.498	−0.128	−0.387	−1.259	−0.856	−0.353	0.714	0.863	1.169
−0.859	−1.083	1.288	−0.078	−0.081	0.210	0.572	1.194	−1.118	−1.543
−0.015	−0.567	0.113	2.127	−0.719	3.256	−0.721	−0.663	−0.779	−0.930
−1.529	−0.231	1.223	0.300	−0.995	−0.651	0.505	0.138	−0.064	1.341
0.278	−0.058	−2.740	−0.296	−1.180	0.574	1.452	0.846	−0.243	−1.208
1.428	0.322	2.302	−0.852	0.782	−1.322	−0.092	−0.546	0.560	−1.430
0.770	−1.874	0.347	0.994	−0.485	−1.179	0.048	−1.324	1.061	0.449
−0.303	−0.629	0.764	0.013	−1.192	−0.475	−1.085	−0.880	1.738	−1.225
−0.263	−2.105	0.509	−0.645	1.362	0.504	−0.755	1.274	1.448	0.604
0.997	−1.187	−0.242	0.121	2.510	−1.935	0.350	0.073	0.458	−0.446
−0.063	−0.475	−1.802	−0.476	0.193	−1.199	0.339	0.364	−0.684	1.353
−0.168	1.904	−0.485	−0.032	−0.554	0.056	−0.710	−0.778	0.722	−0.024
0.366	−0.491	0.301	−0.008	−0.894	−0.945	0.384	−1.748	−1.118	0.394
0.436	−0.464	0.539	0.942	−0.458	0.445	−1.883	1.228	1.113	−0.218
0.597	−1.471	−0.434	0.705	−0.788	0.575	0.086	0.504	1.445	−0.513
−0.805	−0.624	1.344	0.649	−1.124	0.680	−0.986	1.845	−1.152	−0.393
1.681	−1.910	0.440	0.067	−1.502	−0.755	−0.989	−0.054	−2.320	0.474
−0.007	−0.459	1.940	0.220	−1.259	−1.729	0.137	−0.520	−0.412	2.847
0.209	−0.633	0.299	0.174	1.975	−0.271	0.119	−0.199	0.007	2.315
1.254	1.672	−1.186	−1.310	0.474	0.878	−0.725	−0.191	0.642	−1.212
−1.016	−0.697	0.017	−0.263	−0.047	−1.294	−0.339	2.257	−0.078	−0.049
−1.169	−0.355	1.086	−0.199	0.031	0.396	−0.143	1.572	0.276	0.027

RANDOM NORMAL NUMBERS, $\mu = 0$, $\sigma = 1$

41	42	43	44	45	46	47	48	49	50
−0.856	−0.063	0.787	−2.052	−1.192	−0.831	1.623	1.135	0.759	−0.189
−0.276	−1.110	0.752	−1.378	−0.583	0.360	0.365	1.587	0.621	1.344
0.379	−0.440	0.858	1.453	−1.356	0.503	−1.134	1.950	−1.816	−0.283
1.468	0.131	0.047	0.355	0.162	−1.491	−0.739	−1.182	−0.533	−0.497
−1.805	−0.772	1.286	−0.636	−1.312	−1.045	1.559	−0.871	−0.102	−0.123
2.285	0.554	0.418	−0.577	−1.489	−1.255	0.092	−0.597	−1.051	−0.980
−0.602	0.399	1.121	−1.026	0.087	1.018	−1.437	0.661	0.091	−0.637
0.229	−0.584	0.705	0.124	0.341	1.320	−0.824	−1.541	−0.163	2.329
1.382	−1.454	1.537	−1.299	0.363	−0.356	−0.025	0.294	2.194	−0.395
0.978	0.109	1.434	−1.094	−0.265	−0.857	−1.421	−1.773	0.570	−0.053
−0.678	−2.335	1.202	−1.697	0.547	−0.201	−0.373	−1.363	−0.081	0.958
−0.366	−1.084	−0.626	0.798	1.706	−1.160	−0.838	1.462	0.636	0.570
−1.074	−1.379	0.086	−0.331	−0.288	−0.309	−1.527	−0.408	0.183	0.856
−0.600	−0.096	0.696	0.446	1.417	−2.140	0.599	−0.157	1.485	1.387
0.918	1.163	−1.445	0.759	0.878	−1.781	−0.056	−2.141	−0.234	0.975
−0.791	−0.528	0.946	1.673	−0.680	−0.784	1.494	−0.086	−1.071	−1.196
0.598	−0.352	0.719	−0.341	0.056	−1.041	1.429	0.235	0.314	−1.693
0.567	−1.156	−0.125	−0.534	0.711	−0.511	0.187	−0.644	−1.090	−1.281
0.963	0.052	0.037	0.637	−1.335	0.055	0.010	−0.860	−0.621	0.713
0.489	−0.209	1.659	0.054	1.635	0.169	0.794	−1.550	1.845	−0.388
−1.627	−0.017	0.699	0.661	−0.073	0.188	1.183	−1.054	−1.615	−0.765
−1.096	1.215	0.320	0.738	1.865	−1.169	−0.667	−0.674	−0.062	1.378
−2.532	1.031	−0.799	1.665	−2.756	−0.151	−0.704	0.602	−0.672	1.264
0.024	−1.183	−0.927	−0.629	0.204	−0.825	0.496	2.543	0.262	−0.785
0.192	0.125	0.373	−0.931	−0.079	0.186	−0.306	0.621	−0.292	1.131
−1.324	−1.229	−0.648	−0.430	0.811	0.868	0.787	1.845	−0.374	−0.651
−0.726	−0.746	1.572	−1.420	1.509	−0.361	−0.310	−3.117	1.637	0.642
−1.618	1.082	−0.319	0.300	1.524	−0.418	−1.712	0.358	−1.032	0.537
1.695	0.843	2.049	0.388	−0.297	1.077	−0.462	0.655	0.940	−0.354
0.790	0.605	−3.077	1.009	−0.906	−1.004	0.693	−1.098	1.300	0.549
1.792	−0.895	−0.136	−1.765	1.077	0.418	−0.150	0.808	0.697	0.435
0.771	−0.741	−0.492	−0.770	−0.458	−0.021	1.385	−1.225	−0.066	−1.471
−1.438	0.423	−1.211	0.723	−0.731	0.883	−2.109	−2.455	−0.210	1.644
−0.294	1.266	−1.994	−0.730	0.545	0.397	1.069	−0.383	−0.097	−0.985
−1.966	0.909	0.400	0.685	−0.800	1.759	0.268	1.387	−0.414	1.615
0.999	1.587	1.423	0.937	−0.943	0.090	1.185	−1.204	0.300	−1.354
0.581	0.481	−2.400	0.000	0.231	0.079	−2.842	−0.846	−0.508	−0.516
0.370	−1.452	−0.580	−1.462	−0.972	1.116	−0.994	0.374	−3.336	−0.058
0.834	−1.227	−0.709	−1.039	−0.014	−0.383	−0.512	−0.347	0.881	−0.638
−0.376	−0.813	0.660	−1.029	−0.137	0.371	0.376	0.968	1.338	−0.786
−1.621	0.815	−0.544	−0.376	−0.852	0.436	1.562	0.815	−1.048	0.188
0.163	−0.161	2.501	−0.265	−0.285	1.934	1.070	0.215	−0.876	0.073
1.786	−0.538	−0.437	0.324	0.105	−0.421	−0.410	−0.947	0.700	−1.006
2.140	1.218	−0.351	−0.068	0.254	0.448	−1.461	0.784	0.317	1.013
0.064	0.410	0.368	0.419	−0.982	1.371	0.100	−0.505	0.856	0.890
0.789	−0.131	1.330	0.506	−0.645	−1.414	2.426	1.389	−0.169	−0.194
−0.011	−0.372	−0.699	2.382	−1.395	−0.467	1.256	−0.585	−1.359	−1.804
−0.463	0.003	−1.470	1.493	0.960	0.364	−1.267	−0.007	0.616	0.624
−1.210	−0.669	0.009	1.284	−0.617	0.355	−0.589	−0.243	−0.015	−0.712
−1.157	0.481	0.560	1.287	1.129	−0.126	0.006	1.532	1.328	0.980

RANDOM NORMAL NUMBERS, $\mu = 0$, $\sigma = 1$

51	52	53	54	55	56	57	58	59	60
0.240	1.774	0.210	−1.471	1.167	−1.114	0.182	−0.485	−0.318	1.156
0.627	−0.758	−0.930	1.641	0.162	−0.874	−0.235	0.203	−0.724	−0.155
−0.594	0.098	0.158	−0.722	1.385	−0.985	−1.707	0.175	0.449	0.654
1.082	−0.753	−1.944	−1.964	−2.131	−2.796	−1.286	0.807	−0.122	0.527
0.060	−0.014	1.577	−0.814	−0.633	0.275	−0.087	0.517	0.474	−1.432
−0.013	0.402	−0.086	−0.394	0.292	−2.862	−1.660	−1.658	1.610	−2.205
1.586	−0.833	1.444	−0.615	−1.157	−0.220	−0.517	−1.668	−2.036	−0.850
−0.405	−1.315	−1.355	−1.331	1.394	−0.381	−0.729	−0.447	−0.906	0.622
−0.329	1.701	0.427	0.627	−0.271	−0.971	−1.010	1.182	−0.143	0.844
0.992	0.708	−0.115	−1.630	0.596	0.499	−0.862	0.508	0.474	−0.974
0.296	−0.390	2.047	−0.363	0.724	0.788	−0.089	0.930	−0.497	0.058
−2.069	−1.422	−0.948	−1.742	−1.173	0.215	0.661	0.842	−0.984	−0.577
−0.211	−1.727	−0.277	1.592	−0.707	0.327	−0.527	0.912	0.571	−0.525
−0.467	1.848	−0.263	−0.862	0.706	−0.533	0.626	−0.200	−2.221	0.368
1.284	0.412	1.512	0.328	0.203	−1.231	−1.480	−0.400	−0.491	0.913
0.821	−1.503	−1.066	1.624	1.345	0.440	−1.416	0.301	−0.355	0.106
1.056	1.224	0.281	−0.098	1.868	−0.395	0.610	−1.173	−1.449	1.171
1.090	−0.790	0.882	1.687	−0.009	−2.053	−0.030	−0.421	1.253	−0.081
0.574	0.129	1.203	0.280	1.438	−2.052	−0.443	0.522	0.468	−1.211
−0.531	2.155	0.334	0.898	−1.114	0.243	1.026	0.391	−0.011	−0.024
0.896	0.181	−0.941	−0.511	0.648	−0.710	−0.181	−1.417	−0.585	0.087
0.042	0.579	−0.316	0.394	1.133	−0.305	−0.683	−1.318	−0.050	0.993
2.328	0.213	0.534	0.241	0.275	0.060	0.727	1.459	0.174	1.072
0.486	−0.558	0.426	0.728	−0.360	−0.068	0.058	1.471	−0.051	0.337
−0.304	−0.309	0.646	0.309	−1.320	0.311	−1.407	−0.011	0.387	0.128
−2.319	−0.129	0.866	−0.424	0.236	0.419	−1.359	−1.088	−0.045	1.096
1.098	−0.875	0.659	−1.086	−0.424	−1.462	0.743	−0.787	1.472	1.677
0.000	0.110	1.205	0.545	−0.140	1.244	1.104	0.140	0.058	1.245
−0.207	−0.746	1.681	0.137	0.104	−0.491	−0.935	0.671	−0.448	−0.129
0.333	−1.386	1.840	1.089	0.837	−1.642	−0.273	−0.798	0.067	0.334
1.190	−0.547	−1.016	0.540	−0.993	0.443	−0.190	1.019	−1.021	−1.276
−1.416	−0.749	0.325	0.846	2.417	−0.479	−0.655	−1.326	−1.952	1.234
0.622	0.661	0.028	1.302	−0.032	−0.157	1.470	−0.766	0.697	−0.303
−1.134	0.499	0.538	0.564	−2.392	−1.398	0.010	1.874	1.386	0.000
0.725	−0.242	0.281	1.355	−0.036	0.204	−0.345	0.395	−0.753	1.645
−0.210	0.611	−0.219	0.450	0.308	0.993	−0.146	0.225	−1.496	0.246
0.219	0.302	0.000	−0.437	−2.127	0.883	−0.599	−1.516	0.826	1.242
−1.098	−0.252	−2.480	−0.973	0.712	−1.430	−0.167	−1.237	0.750	−0.763
0.144	0.489	−0.637	1.990	0.411	−0.563	0.027	1.278	2.105	−1.130
−1.738	−1.295	0.431	−0.503	2.327	−0.007	−1.293	−1.206	−0.066	1.370
−0.487	−0.097	−1.361	−0.340	0.204	0.938	−0.148	−1.099	−0.252	−0.384
−0.636	−0.626	1.967	1.677	−0.331	−0.440	−1.440	1.281	1.070	−1.167
−1.464	−1.493	0.945	0.180	−0.672	−0.035	−0.293	−0.905	0.196	−1.122
0.561	−0.375	−0.657	1.304	0.833	−1.159	1.501	1.265	0.438	−0.437
−0.525	−0.017	1.815	0.789	−1.908	−0.353	1.383	−1.208	−1.135	1.082
0.980	−0.111	−0.804	−1.078	−1.930	0.171	−1.318	2.377	−0.303	1.062
0.501	0.835	−0.518	−1.034	−1.493	0.712	0.421	−1.165	0.782	−1.484
1.081	−1.176	−0.542	0.321	0.688	0.670	−0.771	−0.090	−0.611	−0.813
−0.148	−1.203	−1.553	1.244	0.826	0.077	0.128	−0.772	1.683	0.318
0.096	−0.286	0.362	0.888	0.551	1.782	0.335	2.083	0.350	0.260

RANDOM NORMAL NUMBERS, $\mu = 0$, $\sigma = 1$

61	62	63	64	65	66	67	68	69	70
0.052	1.504	−1.350	−1.124	−0.521	0.515	0.839	0.778	0.438	−0.550
−0.315	−0.865	0.851	0.127	−0.379	1.640	−0.441	0.717	0.670	−0.301
0.938	−0.055	0.947	1.275	1.557	−1.484	−1.137	0.398	1.333	1.988
0.497	0.502	0.385	−0.467	2.468	−1.810	−1.438	0.283	1.740	0.420
2.308	−0.399	−1.798	0.018	0.780	1.030	0.806	−0.408	−0.547	−0.280
1.815	0.101	−0.561	0.236	0.166	0.227	−0.309	0.056	0.610	0.732
−0.421	0.432	0.586	1.059	0.278	−1.672	1.859	1.433	−0.919	−1.770
0.008	0.555	−1.310	−1.440	−0.142	−0.295	−0.630	−0.911	0.133	−0.308
1.191	−0.114	1.039	1.083	0.185	−0.492	0.419	−0.433	−1.019	−2.260
1.299	1.918	0.318	1.348	0.935	1.250	−0.175	−0.828	−0.336	0.726
0.012	−0.739	−1.181	−0.645	−0.736	1.801	−0.209	−0.389	0.867	−0.555
−0.586	−0.044	−0.983	0.332	0.371	−0.072	−1.212	1.047	−1.930	0.812
−0.122	1.515	0.338	−1.040	−0.008	0.467	−0.600	0.923	1.126	−0.752
0.879	0.516	−0.920	2.121	0.674	1.481	0.660	−0.986	1.644	−2.159
0.435	1.149	−0.065	1.391	0.707	0.548	−0.490	−1.139	0.249	−0.933
0.645	0.878	−0.904	0.896	−1.284	0.237	−0.378	−0.510	−1.123	−0.129
−0.514	−1.017	0.529	0.973	−1.202	0.005	−0.644	−0.167	−0.664	0.167
0.242	−0.427	−0.727	−1.150	−1.092	−0.736	0.925	−0.050	−0.200	−0.770
0.443	0.445	−1.287	−1.463	−0.650	0.412	−2.714	−0.903	−0.341	0.957
0.273	0.203	0.423	1.423	0.508	1.058	−0.828	0.143	−1.059	0.345
0.255	1.036	1.471	0.476	0.592	−0.658	0.677	0.155	1.068	−0.759
0.858	−0.370	0.522	−1.890	−0.389	0.609	1.210	0.489	−0.006	0.834
0.097	−1.709	1.790	−0.929	0.405	0.024	−0.036	0.580	−0.642	−1.121
0.520	0.889	−0.540	0.266	−0.354	0.524	−0.788	−0.497	−0.973	1.481
−0.311	−1.772	−0.496	1.275	−0.904	0.147	1.497	0.657	−0.469	−0.783
−0.604	0.857	−0.695	0.397	0.296	−0.285	0.191	0.158	1.672	1.190
−0.001	0.287	−0.868	−0.013	−1.576	−0.168	0.047	−0.159	0.086	−1.077
1.160	0.989	0.205	0.937	−0.099	−1.281	−0.276	0.845	0.752	0.663
1.579	−0.303	−1.174	−0.960	−0.470	−0.556	−0.689	1.535	−0.711	−0.743
−0.615	−0.154	0.008	1.353	−0.381	1.137	0.022	0.175	0.586	2.941
1.578	1.529	−0.294	−1.301	0.614	0.099	−0.700	−0.003	1.052	1.643
0.626	−0.447	−1.261	−2.029	0.182	−1.176	0.083	1.868	0.872	0.965
−0.493	−0.020	0.920	1.473	1.873	−0.289	0.410	0.394	0.881	0.054
−0.217	0.342	1.423	0.364	−0.119	0.509	−2.266	0.189	0.149	1.041
−0.792	0.347	−1.367	−0.632	−1.238	−0.136	−0.352	−0.157	−1.163	1.305
0.568	−0.226	0.391	−0.074	−0.312	0.400	1.583	0.481	−1.048	0.759
0.051	0.549	−2.192	1.257	−1.460	0.363	0.127	−1.020	−1.192	0.449
−0.891	0.490	0.279	0.372	−0.578	−0.836	2.285	−0.448	0.720	0.510
0.622	−0.126	−0.637	1.255	−0.354	0.032	−1.076	0.352	0.103	−0.496
0.623	0.819	−0.489	0.354	−0.943	−0.694	0.248	0.092	−0.673	−1.428
−1.208	−1.038	0.140	−0.762	−0.854	−0.249	2.431	0.067	−0.317	−0.874
−0.487	−2.117	0.195	2.154	1.041	−1.314	−0.785	−0.414	−0.695	2.310
0.522	0.314	−1.003	0.134	−1.748	−0.107	0.459	1.550	1.118	−1.004
0.838	0.613	0.227	0.308	−0.757	0.912	2.272	0.556	−0.041	0.008
−1.534	−0.407	1.202	1.251	−0.891	−1.588	−2.380	0.059	0.682	−0.878
−0.099	2.391	1.067	−2.060	−0.464	−0.103	3.486	1.121	0.632	−1.626
0.070	1.465	−0.080	−0.526	−1.090	−1.002	0.132	1.504	0.050	−0.393
0.115	−0.601	1.751	1.956	−0.196	0.400	−0.522	0.571	−0.101	−2.160
0.252	−0.329	−0.586	−0.118	−0.242	−0.521	0.818	−0.167	−0.469	0.430
0.017	0.185	0.377	1.883	−0.443	−0.039	−1.244	−0.820	−1.171	0.104

RANDOM NORMAL NUMBERS, $\mu = 0$, $\sigma = 1$

71	72	73	74	75	76	77	78	79	80
2.988	0.423	−1.261	−1.893	0.187	−0.412	−0.228	0.002	−0.384	−1.032
0.760	0.995	−0.256	−0.505	0.750	−0.654	0.647	0.613	0.086	−0.118
−0.650	−0.927	−1.071	−0.796	1.130	−1.042	−0.181	−1.020	1.648	−1.327
−0.394	−0.452	0.893	1.410	1.133	0.319	0.537	−0.789	0.078	−0.062
−1.168	1.902	0.206	0.303	1.413	2.012	0.278	−0.566	−0.900	0.200
1.343	−0.377	−0.131	−0.585	0.053	0.137	−1.371	−0.175	−0.878	0.118
−0.733	−1.921	0.471	−1.394	−0.885	−0.523	0.553	0.344	−0.775	1.545
−0.172	−0.575	0.066	−0.310	1.795	−1.148	0.772	−1.063	0.818	0.302
1.457	0.862	1.677	−0.507	−1.691	−0.034	0.270	0.075	−0.554	1.420
−0.087	0.744	1.829	1.203	−0.436	−0.618	−0.200	−1.134	−1.352	−0.098
−0.092	1.043	−0.255	0.189	0.270	−1.034	−0.571	−0.336	−0.742	2.141
0.441	−0.379	−1.757	0.608	0.527	−0.338	−1.995	0.573	−0.034	−0.056
0.073	−0.250	0.531	−0.695	1.402	−0.462	−0.938	1.130	1.453	−0.106
0.637	0.276	−0.013	1.968	−0.205	0.486	0.727	1.416	0.963	1.349
−0.792	−1.778	1.284	−0.452	0.602	0.668	0.516	−0.210	0.040	−0.103
−1.223	1.561	−2.099	1.419	0.223	−0.482	1.098	0.513	0.418	−1.686
−0.407	1.587	0.335	−2.475	−0.284	1.567	−0.248	−0.759	1.792	−2.319
−0.462	−0.193	−0.012	−1.208	2.151	1.336	−1.968	−1.767	−0.374	0.783
1.457	0.883	1.001	−0.169	0.836	−1.236	1.632	−0.142	−0.222	0.340
−1.918	−1.246	−0.209	0.780	−0.330	−2.953	−0.447	−0.094	1.344	−0.196
−0.126	1.094	−1.206	−1.426	1.474	−1.080	0.000	0.764	1.476	−0.016
−0.306	−0.847	0.639	−0.262	−0.427	0.391	−1.298	−1.013	2.024	−0.539
0.477	1.595	−0.762	0.424	0.799	0.312	1.151	−1.095	1.199	−0.765
0.369	−0.709	1.283	−0.007	−1.440	−0.782	0.061	1.427	1.656	0.974
−0.579	0.606	−0.866	−0.715	−0.301	−0.180	0.188	0.668	−1.091	1.476
−0.418	−0.588	0.919	−0.083	1.084	0.944	0.253	−1.833	1.305	0.171
0.128	−0.834	0.009	0.742	0.539	−0.948	−1.055	−0.689	−0.338	1.091
−0.201	0.235	−0.971	−1.696	1.119	0.272	0.635	−0.792	−1.355	1.291
−1.024	1.212	−1.100	−0.348	1.741	0.035	1.268	0.192	0.729	−0.467
−0.378	1.026	0.093	0.468	−0.967	0.675	0.807	−2.109	−1.214	0.559
1.232	−0.815	0.608	1.429	−0.748	0.201	0.400	−1.230	−0.398	−0.674
1.793	−0.581	−1.076	0.512	−0.442	−1.488	−0.580	0.172	−0.891	0.311
0.766	0.310	−0.070	0.624	−0.389	1.035	−0.101	−0.926	0.816	−1.048
−0.606	−1.224	1.465	0.012	1.061	0.491	−1.023	1.948	0.866	−0.737
0.106	−2.715	0.363	0.343	−0.159	2.672	1.110	0.731	−1.012	−0.889
−0.060	0.444	1.596	−0.630	0.362	−0.306	1.163	−0.974	0.486	−0.373
2.081	1.161	−1.167	0.021	0.053	−0.094	0.381	−0.628	−2.581	−1.243
−1.727	−1.266	0.088	0.936	0.368	0.648	−0.799	1.115	−0.968	−2.588
0.001	1.364	1.677	0.644	1.505	0.440	−0.329	0.498	0.869	−0.965
−1.114	−0.239	−0.409	−0.334	−0.605	0.501	−1.921	−0.470	2.354	−0.660
0.189	−0.547	−1.758	−0.295	−0.279	−0.515	−1.053	0.553	−0.297	0.496
−0.065	−0.023	−0.267	−0.247	1.318	0.904	−0.712	−1.152	−0.543	0.176
−1.742	−0.599	0.430	−0.615	1.165	0.084	2.017	−1.207	2.614	1.490
0.732	0.188	2.343	0.526	−0.812	0.389	1.036	−0.023	0.229	−2.262
−1.490	0.014	0.167	1.422	0.015	0.069	0.133	0.897	−1.678	0.323
1.507	−0.571	−0.724	1.741	−0.152	−0.147	−0.158	−0.076	0.652	0.447
0.513	0.168	−0.076	−0.171	0.428	0.205	−0.865	0.107	1.023	0.077
−0.834	−1.121	1.441	0.492	0.559	1.724	−1.659	0.245	1.354	−0.041
0.258	1.880	−0.536	1.246	−0.188	0.746	1.097	0.258	1.547	1.238
−0.818	0.273	0.159	−0.765	0.526	1.281	1.154	−0.687	−0.793	0.795

RANDOM NORMAL NUMBERS, $\mu = 0$, $\sigma = 1$

81	82	83	84	85	86	87	88	89	90
−0.713	−0.541	−0.571	−0.807	−1.560	1.000	0.140	−0.549	0.887	2.237
−0.117	0.530	−1.599	−1.602	0.412	−1.450	−1.217	1.074	−1.021	−0.424
1.187	−1.523	1.437	0.051	1.237	−0.798	1.616	−0.823	−1.207	1.258
−0.182	−0.186	0.517	1.438	0.831	−1.319	−0.539	−0.192	0.150	2.127
1.964	−0.629	−0.944	−0.028	0.948	1.005	0.242	−0.432	−0.329	0.113
0.230	1.523	1.658	0.753	0.724	0.183	−0.147	0.505	0.448	−0.053
0.839	−0.849	−0.145	−1.843	−1.276	0.481	−0.142	−0.534	0.403	0.370
−0.801	0.343	−1.822	0.447	−0.931	−0.824	−0.484	0.864	−1.069	0.860
−0.124	0.727	1.654	−0.182	−1.381	−1.146	−0.572	0.159	0.186	1.221
−0.088	0.032	−0.564	0.654	1.141	−0.056	−0.343	0.067	−0.267	−0.219
0.912	−1.114	−1.035	−1.070	−0.297	1.195	0.030	0.022	0.406	−0.414
1.397	−0.473	0.433	0.023	−1.204	1.254	0.551	−1.012	−0.789	0.906
−0.652	−0.029	0.064	0.511	1.117	−0.465	0.523	−0.083	0.386	0.259
1.236	−0.457	−1.354	−0.898	−0.270	−1.837	1.641	−0.657	−0.753	−1.686
−0.498	1.302	0.816	−0.936	1.404	0.555	2.450	−0.789	−0.120	0.505
−0.005	2.174	1.893	−1.361	−0.991	0.508	−0.823	0.918	0.524	0.488
0.115	−1.373	−0.900	−1.010	0.624	0.946	0.312	−1.384	0.224	2.343
0.167	0.254	1.219	1.153	−0.510	−0.007	−0.285	−0.631	−0.356	0.254
0.976	1.158	−0.469	1.099	0.509	−1.324	−0.102	−0.296	−0.907	0.449
0.653	−0.366	0.450	−2.653	−0.592	−0.510	0.983	0.023	−0.881	0.876
−0.150	−0.088	0.457	−0.448	0.605	0.668	−0.613	0.261	0.023	−0.050
0.060	0.276	0.229	−1.527	−0.316	−0.834	−1.652	−0.387	0.632	0.895
−0.678	0.547	0.243	−2.183	−0.368	1.158	−0.996	−0.705	−0.314	1.464
2.139	0.395	−0.376	−0.175	0.406	0.309	−1.021	−0.460	−0.217	0.307
0.091	1.793	0.822	0.054	0.573	−0.729	−0.517	0.589	1.927	0.940
−0.003	0.344	1.242	−1.105	0.234	−1.222	−0.474	1.831	0.124	−0.840
−0.965	0.268	−1.543	0.690	0.917	2.017	−0.297	1.087	0.371	1.495
−0.076	−0.495	−0.103	0.646	2.427	−2.172	0.660	−1.541	−0.852	0.583
−0.365	−3.305	0.805	−0.418	−1.201	0.623	−0.223	0.109	0.205	−0.663
0.578	0.145	−1.438	1.122	−1.406	1.172	0.272	−2.245	1.207	1.227
−0.398	−0.304	0.529	−0.514	−0.681	−0.366	0.338	0.801	−0.301	−0.790
−0.951	−1.483	−0.613	−0.171	−0.459	1.231	−1.232	−0.497	−0.779	0.247
1.025	−0.039	−0.721	0.813	1.203	0.245	0.402	1.541	0.691	−1.420
−0.958	0.791	0.948	0.222	−0.704	−0.375	−0.246	−0.682	−0.871	0.056
1.097	−1.428	1.402	−1.425	−0.877	0.536	0.988	2.529	0.768	−1.321
0.377	2.240	0.854	−1.158	0.066	−1.222	0.821	−1.602	−0.760	−0.871
1.729	0.073	1.022	0.891	0.659	−1.040	0.251	−0.710	−1.734	−0.038
−1.329	−0.381	−0.515	1.484	−0.430	−0.466	−0.167	−0.788	−0.660	0.003
−0.132	0.391	2.205	−1.165	0.200	0.415	−0.765	0.239	−1.182	1.135
0.336	0.657	−0.805	0.150	−0.938	1.057	−1.090	1.604	−0.598	−0.760
0.124	−1.812	1.750	0.270	−0.114	0.517	−0.226	0.127	0.129	−0.751
−0.036	0.365	0.766	0.877	−0.804	−0.140	0.182	−0.483	−0.376	−0.564
−0.609	−0.019	−0.992	−1.193	−0.516	0.517	1.677	0.839	−1.134	0.675
−0.894	0.318	0.607	−0.865	0.526	−0.971	1.365	0.319	1.804	1.740
−0.357	−0.802	0.635	−0.491	−1.110	0.785	−0.042	−1.042	−0.572	0.243
−0.258	−0.383	−1.013	0.001	−1.673	0.561	−1.054	−0.106	−0.760	−1.009
2.245	−0.431	−0.496	0.796	0.193	1.202	−0.429	−0.217	0.333	−0.643
1.956	0.477	0.812	−0.117	0.606	−0.330	0.425	−0.232	0.802	0.656
1.358	0.139	0.199	−0.475	−0.120	0.184	−0.020	−1.326	0.517	−1.708
0.656	1.081	0.180	0.145	0.376	−1.363	−0.491	0.352	−1.477	1.280

RANDOM NORMAL NUMBERS, $\mu = 0$, $\sigma = 1$

91	92	93	94	95	96	97	98	99	100
−0.181	0.583	−1.478	−0.181	0.281	−0.559	1.985	−1.122	−1.106	1.441
1.549	−1.183	−2.089	−1.997	−0.343	1.275	0.676	−0.212	1.252	0.163
0.978	−1.067	−2.640	0.134	0.328	−0.052	−0.030	−0.273	−0.570	1.026
−0.596	−0.420	−0.318	−0.057	−0.695	−1.148	0.333	−0.531	−2.037	−1.587
−0.440	0.032	0.163	1.029	0.079	1.148	0.762	−1.961	−0.674	−0.486
0.443	−1.100	0.728	−2.397	−0.543	0.872	−0.568	0.980	−0.174	0.728
−2.401	−1.375	−1.332	−2.177	−2.064	−0.245	−0.039	0.585	1.344	1.386
0.311	0.322	−0.158	0.359	0.103	0.371	0.735	0.011	2.091	0.490
−1.209	0.241	−1.488	−0.667	−1.772	−0.197	0.741	−1.303	−1.149	2.251
0.575	−1.227	−1.674	1.400	0.289	0.005	0.185	−1.072	0.431	−1.096
−0.190	0.272	1.216	0.227	1.358	0.215	−2.306	−1.301	−0.597	−1.401
−0.817	−0.769	−0.470	−0.633	0.187	−0.517	−0.888	−1.712	1.774	−0.162
0.265	−0.676	0.244	1.897	−0.629	−0.206	−1.419	1.049	0.266	−0.438
−0.221	0.678	2.149	1.486	−1.361	1.402	−0.028	0.493	0.744	0.195
−0.436	0.358	−0.602	0.107	0.085	0.573	0.529	1.577	0.239	1.898
−0.010	0.475	0.655	0.659	−0.029	−0.029	0.126	−1.335	−1.261	2.036
−0.244	1.654	1.335	−0.610	0.617	0.642	0.371	0.241	0.001	−1.799
−0.932	−1.275	−1.134	−1.246	−1.508	0.949	1.743	−0.271	−1.333	−1.875
−0.199	−1.285	−0.387	0.191	0.726	−0.151	0.064	−0.803	−0.062	0.780
−0.251	−0.431	−0.831	0.036	−0.464	−1.089	0.284	−0.451	1.693	1.004
1.074	−1.323	−1.659	−0.186	−0.612	1.612	−2.159	−1.210	0.596	−1.421
1.518	2.101	0.397	0.516	−1.169	−1.821	1.346	2.435	1.165	−0.428
0.035	−0.206	1.117	−0.241	−0.963	−0.099	0.412	−1.344	0.411	0.583
1.360	−0.380	0.031	1.066	0.893	0.431	−0.081	0.099	0.500	−2.441
0.115	−0.211	1.471	0.332	0.750	0.652	−0.812	1.383	−0.355	−0.638
0.082	−0.309	−0.355	−0.402	0.774	0.150	0.015	2.539	−0.756	−1.049
−1.492	0.259	0.323	0.697	−0.509	0.968	−0.053	1.033	−0.220	−2.322
−0.203	0.548	1.494	1.185	0.083	−1.196	−0.749	−1.105	1.324	0.689
1.857	−0.167	−1.531	1.551	0.848	0.120	0.415	−0.317	1.446	1.002
0.669	−1.017	−2.437	−0.558	−0.657	0.940	0.985	0.483	−0.361	0.095
0.128	1.463	−0.436	−0.239	−1.443	0.732	0.168	−0.144	−0.392	0.989
1.879	−2.456	0.029	0.429	0.618	−1.683	−2.262	0.034	−0.002	1.914
0.680	0.050	0.100	1.050	−1.020	0.407	−0.205	−0.224	−0.434	0.253
−0.631	0.225	−0.951	1.072	−0.285	−1.731	−0.427	−1.446	−0.873	0.619
−1.273	0.723	0.201	0.505	−0.370	−0.421	−0.015	−0.463	0.288	1.734
−0.643	−1.485	0.403	0.003	−0.243	0.000	0.964	−0.703	0.844	−0.686
−0.435	−2.162	−0.169	−1.311	−1.639	0.193	2.692	−1.994	0.326	0.562
−1.706	0.119	−1.566	0.637	−1.948	−1.068	0.935	0.738	0.650	0.491
−0.498	1.640	0.384	−0.945	−1.272	0.945	−1.013	−0.913	−0.469	2.250
−0.065	−0.005	0.618	−0.523	−0.055	1.071	0.758	−0.736	−0.959	0.598
0.190	−1.020	−1.104	0.936	−0.029	−1.004	−0.657	1.270	−0.060	−0.809
0.879	−0.642	1.155	−0.523	−0.757	−1.027	0.985	−1.222	1.078	0.163
0.559	1.094	1.587	−0.384	−1.701	0.418	0.327	0.669	0.019	0.782
−0.261	1.234	−0.505	−0.664	−0.446	−0.747	0.427	−0.369	0.089	−1.302
3.136	1.120	−0.591	2.515	−2.853	1.375	2.421	0.672	1.817	−0.067
−1.307	−0.586	−0.311	−0.026	1.633	−1.340	−1.209	0.110	−0.126	−0.288
1.455	1.099	−1.225	−0.817	0.667	−0.212	0.684	0.349	−1.161	−2.432
−0.443	−0.415	−0.660	0.098	0.435	−0.846	−0.375	−0.410	−1.747	−0.790
−0.326	0.798	0.349	0.524	0.690	−0.520	−0.522	0.602	−0.193	−0.535
−1.027	−1.459	−0.840	−1.637	−0.462	0.607	−0.760	1.342	−1.916	0.424

XII.6 RANDOM NORMAL NUMBERS, $\mu = 2$, $\sigma = 1$

01	02	03	04	05	06	07	08	09	10
2.422	0.130	2.232	1.700	1.903	0.725	2.031	0.515	−0.684	2.788
0.694	2.556	1.868	1.263	2.115	1.516	1.972	3.627	1.482	3.263
1.875	2.273	0.655	2.299	0.055	1.955	−0.147	2.168	2.193	1.879
1.017	0.757	1.288	1.322	2.080	2.170	1.502	2.953	0.171	1.951
2.453	4.199	1.403	2.017	3.496	0.165	2.556	1.003	1.973	2.159
2.274	1.767	1.564	2.412	2.207	0.475	2.656	1.579	0.394	1.225
3.000	1.618	1.530	2.224	2.881	2.715	3.103	1.941	2.179	3.748
2.510	2.256	1.146	5.177	1.931	1.693	1.021	3.337	2.137	1.839
1.233	2.085	2.251	1.578	3.796	3.017	2.863	2.514	1.615	1.548
3.075	1.730	2.427	2.990	1.680	3.250	3.050	3.243	1.846	1.798
1.344	−0.095	2.166	4.116	2.500	1.939	1.567	3.047	1.385	−0.831
1.246	3.860	1.253	1.876	4.373	1.993	1.262	2.319	2.488	2.406
0.889	2.299	2.458	1.790	1.048	2.302	0.138	2.383	1.170	2.204
1.154	1.401	1.935	3.106	1.548	−0.096	2.153	2.333	1.761	3.728
3.031	1.048	0.719	1.474	2.779	0.292	2.341	2.707	1.741	2.353
0.534	1.155	1.705	1.662	0.457	0.602	1.365	2.663	3.755	1.900
2.230	3.096	0.045	3.639	0.680	0.970	1.593	2.117	2.395	1.935
2.355	1.761	1.816	1.822	1.434	2.259	3.788	3.280	1.317	2.940
1.461	0.947	0.717	2.923	2.133	2.526	2.687	2.144	1.692	1.469
3.034	1.778	2.122	2.025	3.008	1.447	−0.305	2.452	1.726	0.870
2.761	0.473	3.726	1.893	2.455	1.633	1.654	3.006	3.523	2.317
1.961	0.965	1.481	1.402	2.106	2.214	1.727	3.670	3.795	2.258
2.639	4.010	1.915	1.713	1.484	1.443	1.444	2.394	1.688	0.793
1.349	2.225	0.644	1.404	2.583	2.149	2.359	2.274	1.432	1.610
2.959	2.797	4.635	3.268	2.889	2.349	0.933	3.403	2.206	−0.214
2.440	2.919	1.455	0.695	1.466	1.124	1.257	1.265	0.096	3.412
3.078	3.279	0.352	2.583	1.690	0.729	2.072	1.332	1.158	1.827
1.736	1.968	0.011	2.418	1.026	1.342	2.103	1.792	2.175	1.646
3.275	3.147	2.800	2.172	0.004	1.763	3.801	2.510	2.517	−0.117
2.579	2.297	2.030	2.725	3.721	2.545	1.631	−0.346	−0.011	1.961
2.549	3.546	2.805	1.250	0.769	2.238	2.284	3.722	2.085	2.653
2.954	1.990	1.249	1.028	3.241	1.926	3.056	1.732	2.116	1.825
1.442	2.542	2.557	1.741	0.630	2.117	1.662	2.237	−0.046	3.132
4.039	2.030	2.859	3.538	2.424	2.169	3.643	3.290	2.742	1.336
2.127	0.288	2.921	0.175	1.670	3.151	1.443	0.935	1.125	2.872
1.102	2.536	1.476	2.980	0.416	1.784	2.521	1.867	1.709	1.558
2.938	2.112	1.350	2.115	1.164	1.761	1.350	1.798	3.160	2.593
2.975	2.681	0.721	1.291	2.276	2.131	2.187	2.752	1.380	0.676
1.386	1.712	1.692	2.844	1.559	0.418	3.020	0.785	1.962	3.184
2.834	1.485	0.632	0.872	0.735	1.934	1.221	2.544	1.797	1.410
3.346	1.147	1.766	1.862	2.595	1.524	3.499	2.652	2.139	2.533
2.243	3.881	2.846	2.670	3.377	1.380	4.183	0.883	1.373	1.992
2.705	2.661	1.521	1.290	2.280	1.638	0.884	2.636	2.077	1.012
2.760	1.182	1.152	3.074	1.073	2.917	2.150	2.866	1.688	1.684
2.086	1.250	1.577	2.871	2.985	2.585	2.897	2.398	0.999	1.764
0.802	1.421	4.793	0.268	2.838	2.227	3.331	2.395	2.064	2.916
4.165	2.014	0.616	1.929	0.641	2.304	1.263	2.125	0.908	1.768
2.291	2.549	0.851	1.856	2.452	3.282	0.978	2.255	1.683	1.926
1.428	4.194	2.262	2.957	1.991	2.759	1.553	3.538	1.272	3.417
2.051	2.455	2.759	2.267	2.794	4.106	2.373	1.401	2.562	2.502

RANDOM NORMAL NUMBERS, $\mu = 2$, $\sigma = 1$

11	12	13	14	15	16	17	18	19	20
1.911	0.626	2.289	1.628	1.638	2.676	0.900	1.685	1.605	1.366
3.196	2.979	2.447	2.099	1.273	2.733	2.653	2.219	1.318	3.129
0.398	2.304	1.019	0.363	1.286	2.428	0.677	1.684	1.267	0.651
1.228	2.134	0.300	1.785	2.547	1.566	2.545	2.428	1.702	2.276
1.190	3.020	0.954	2.907	2.916	1.279	3.403	2.698	1.629	1.448
0.953	2.127	1.723	2.302	1.474	0.826	1.644	2.035	2.359	2.930
1.479	1.956	1.280	1.722	0.938	0.922	2.734	3.484	1.659	2.789
1.509	0.952	1.258	−0.864	1.620	1.789	2.931	2.616	1.622	1.566
0.627	2.404	0.571	2.940	2.705	1.709	2.404	1.456	2.486	2.869
1.923	2.765	2.422	1.725	1.009	2.372	1.925	1.083	3.314	1.961
2.760	2.633	3.011	2.277	1.539	0.873	2.379	2.610	1.635	−0.625
2.009	3.204	1.114	2.269	0.912	0.831	2.485	2.076	1.230	3.607
0.876	1.124	2.137	1.448	1.236	1.699	1.408	1.454	2.018	1.514
1.430	1.920	2.969	1.518	1.543	1.509	4.071	3.444	0.907	2.478
3.422	2.307	2.919	1.833	1.792	3.090	2.212	0.814	1.661	0.865
3.304	1.292	1.863	2.785	1.666	0.323	2.384	3.133	3.393	2.814
2.329	2.671	3.353	1.166	1.016	3.036	2.024	1.439	2.203	1.128
1.402	1.964	1.505	1.746	1.912	1.202	0.595	0.527	1.881	3.456
2.274	1.209	1.450	2.241	1.678	1.565	2.746	2.149	1.829	1.520
1.205	0.531	2.975	3.024	3.357	2.558	1.450	2.192	1.665	3.373
2.462	1.328	1.301	3.312	1.959	2.010	2.482	1.530	1.909	3.171
0.227	3.166	1.989	2.976	2.188	1.399	1.407	2.610	1.903	0.624
2.142	2.926	1.634	1.940	0.785	2.331	1.663	0.847	2.533	1.166
2.558	0.903	0.082	1.299	2.366	2.554	1.948	1.055	1.559	1.787
0.818	3.174	0.123	−1.149	1.606	2.118	−0.044	0.022	0.866	2.336
3.083	2.287	2.379	2.909	2.520	0.708	1.600	0.790	1.751	2.480
2.517	1.470	2.621	0.880	1.931	1.495	1.943	1.868	2.048	3.879
2.594	1.571	1.218	2.346	2.267	0.946	2.840	1.753	2.237	0.687
0.411	0.760	1.114	1.842	1.756	3.951	2.110	2.251	2.116	1.042
2.853	3.054	2.421	2.418	1.542	2.070	0.641	0.753	1.040	0.702
1.262	−0.591	1.320	2.049	2.705	3.826	3.272	1.054	2.494	2.050
0.540	1.678	2.534	1.944	1.939	2.544	1.582	1.333	1.895	1.746
2.381	2.968	1.656	3.152	1.730	3.927	3.183	3.211	3.765	2.035
2.225	1.420	1.334	1.923	1.664	1.939	0.680	2.785	1.569	1.701
1.953	2.779	2.584	2.228	0.221	1.378	1.381	2.209	2.979	2.906
3.413	2.229	2.976	2.535	3.589	0.615	3.425	1.187	2.748	0.906
1.610	2.376	2.086	0.610	2.532	3.083	1.332	1.776	0.407	0.721
0.984	2.243	2.939	1.704	2.277	1.026	1.879	0.405	1.003	0.755
1.808	2.362	1.717	0.831	2.160	0.546	2.686	1.924	1.756	1.829
−0.766	3.529	2.361	0.955	2.148	1.104	0.541	1.460	1.840	1.579
2.643	2.051	1.384	2.229	2.952	2.203	0.765	4.381	1.611	1.936
1.952	2.752	3.588	2.481	1.911	3.753	1.428	3.223	1.873	2.034
2.590	2.306	3.280	1.664	2.281	1.443	2.024	2.126	3.250	1.384
0.622	2.617	1.969	2.231	−0.079	0.768	2.547	1.365	1.163	1.280
0.433	−0.560	3.292	1.987	1.065	2.766	1.425	0.846	2.520	0.981
3.146	3.323	1.713	1.887	2.010	1.277	0.491	2.489	1.503	1.974
4.021	1.744	0.598	2.954	2.633	1.960	1.539	2.393	4.012	3.356
1.188	0.450	2.958	1.177	1.482	1.090	1.671	3.021	0.386	3.560
1.211	2.575	0.158	3.124	3.632	2.647	3.029	3.526	2.237	0.671
3.750	2.362	1.407	0.642	1.274	1.632	2.378	2.601	0.003	1.261

RANDOM NORMAL NUMBERS, $\mu = 2$, $\sigma = 1$

21	22	23	24	25	26	27	28	29	30
1.707	2.089	1.315	0.278	3.045	2.968	1.396	1.534	2.365	2.746
1.113	1.779	1.935	0.971	4.024	0.847	1.382	2.342	2.110	0.316
1.847	0.547	3.697	1.250	1.586	2.036	2.924	0.585	0.456	2.859
2.713	2.761	1.664	2.461	2.158	3.453	2.078	1.113	1.769	1.263
0.676	0.432	2.667	2.515	1.369	3.196	2.979	2.447	2.099	1.273
2.167	1.828	2.867	1.178	2.078	1.500	2.622	2.341	1.504	2.468
3.445	3.323	2.558	1.789	1.595	1.191	1.175	2.872	1.257	1.062
1.284	3.180	3.315	1.210	1.842	3.384	2.942	2.550	0.727	1.736
2.135	2.590	2.533	1.635	1.983	0.614	0.377	−0.663	0.427	2.445
2.944	2.043	2.220	1.987	2.859	3.029	2.091	1.052	1.532	1.956
3.654	2.333	1.468	3.126	1.241	2.936	1.557	2.020	1.423	2.701
0.821	1.542	2.365	2.199	3.479	3.111	−0.107	1.644	1.337	1.442
2.483	2.583	2.075	1.026	0.668	2.281	1.566	1.255	2.020	1.135
0.715	1.384	2.080	2.542	2.368	0.019	2.906	2.325	2.175	5.197
4.638	2.662	1.012	2.941	1.336	0.574	3.034	2.937	2.553	0.174
2.327	2.152	3.057	2.077	2.321	0.861	2.892	1.394	−0.556	1.459
−0.082	0.676	3.038	2.470	1.394	2.131	1.262	3.207	1.810	0.322
2.051	1.576	2.087	3.030	2.030	2.827	2.183	1.182	1.507	−0.042
2.438	0.924	1.699	0.477	2.449	2.540	1.620	2.509	2.347	3.022
2.284	2.159	2.975	3.268	0.484	1.862	1.676	1.449	2.475	2.556
0.872	0.474	2.213	3.602	3 244	3.078	1.376	2.612	2.421	1.014
2.236	1.963	1.839	1.598	2.195	2.680	2.228	1.107	−0.661	1.041
2.425	2.412	1.500	2.278	2.328	2.102	2.087	3.098	2.697	0.765
1.511	2.431	1.434	1.558	1.020	2.864	0.871	2.523	1.878	1.370
1.600	2.040	2.993	0.873	0.568	2.703	2.578	1.515	3.627	2.097
3.076	1.939	0.682	3.085	2.877	2.696	−0.771	2.560	1.954	0.999
2.593	1.610	2.800	2.456	0.226	3.575	1.435	2.170	1.165	3.506
1.362	2.727	2.145	2.023	0.509	0.336	2.045	0.375	1.010	2.316
1.603	2.783	0.682	2.108	2.031	0.854	2.028	2.357	0.722	1.562
1.908	1.635	2.009	1.203	1.775	2.868	1.949	1.391	1.151	1.352
3.486	0.507	2.322	1.204	2.434	1.720	1.804	2.235	2.439	1.492
2.029	1.352	3.629	2.076	1.587	0.891	3.029	1.242	0.014	4.019
2.894	1.688	0.657	1.800	2.943	1.373	1.269	3.411	1.316	2.405
0.965	−0.028	1.904	2.241	2.563	1.149	2.375	1.386	1.562	2.882
2.191	2.133	2.676	0.229	2.319	1.114	3.197	2.588	3.163	2.423
2.115	2.418	2.741	1.839	2.416	1.452	0.319	0.853	2.774	0.929
1.120	2.126	0.773	0.798	3.436	2.374	2.173	−0.333	2.004	1.765
3.524	0.008	3.260	1.109	4.111	2.474	2.482	2.416	0.832	4.059
0.103	2.774	2.056	2.463	0.383	−0.962	2.458	2.388	1.556	1.088
1.573	2.519	2.153	3.188	1.618	2.477	2.185	1.851	0.498	2.066
1.138	3.032	2.390	2.436	2.655	1.484	2.378	3.166	2.531	2.082
2.665	2.960	2.518	1.940	0.026	2.570	2.703	2.592	3.094	1.862
1.397	1.859	2.208	2.559	1.749	0.624	0.074	1.398	0.996	2.910
1.875	2.250	0.183	2.214	1.356	4.282	2.370	3.006	1.413	2.412
3.195	2.671	1.918	3.305	3.722	1.372	2.564	2.106	1.871	1.792
1.464	2.055	3.045	2.367	1.992	0.919	3.006	2.713	4.049	4.618
3.328	1.781	2.565	1.304	2.041	1.597	0.225	2.309	−0.558	2.504
2.804	3.606	1.858	3.028	2.456	1.730	1.430	3.405	0.474	2.222
2.590	1.641	3.857	2.582	2.594	1.933	3.341	1.002	2.704	1.341
2.980	0.601	1.595	2.248	2.381	1.911	0.626	2.289	1.628	1.638

RANDOM NORMAL NUMBERS, $\mu = 2, \sigma = 1$

31	32	33	34	35	36	37	38	39	40
3.355	0.073	3.139	2.472	1.825	0.296	1.685	3.401	1.820	1.428
1.086	1.955	2.529	2.503	1.687	1.754	4.138	2.394	0.303	3.776
2.367	1.525	2.625	1.789	0.991	4.127	0.915	3.023	1.377	3.435
0.248	0.749	3.697	4.166	2.544	1.620	3.217	1.083	1.907	2.951
1.694	0.258	1.836	1.953	1.853	3.590	3.604	1.907	1.995	2.468
1.546	1.255	2.856	3.221	2.397	−0.010	2.169	2.781	3.001	2.536
1.266	2.089	2.974	1.305	2.376	−0.475	1.792	1.546	0.583	1.214
0.713	2.473	1.381	1.750	1.064	3.744	2.470	1.004	2.155	2.332
−0.001	1.600	2.166	0.561	0.898	2.587	0.580	−0.461	0.954	1.364
3.406	2.207	2.110	1.522	3.923	1.379	3.613	3.379	2.716	2.796
1.432	1.651	1.584	3.649	2.485	2.820	2.948	2.626	1.763	3.329
1.541	1.154	4.311	2.354	2.257	1.262	2.304	2.178	1.657	2.120
2.216	3.505	−0.056	1.332	0.980	1.675	1.850	2.487	2.051	1.433
1.602	2.225	2.949	3.945	3.753	3.855	2.769	0.760	2.095	1.419
2.211	1.804	2.642	0.975	1.646	2.552	2.291	1.277	2.341	−0.219
3.006	2.279	1.097	3.473	0.919	2.535	2.459	3.934	1.826	1.587
2.520	2.468	2.156	2.438	1.625	1.604	1.628	1.139	2.608	2.643
2.666	4.058	2.805	3.069	0.945	2.533	2.761	1.140	2.604	1.627
2.852	0.570	3.920	1.572	2.924	2.135	1.558	2.604	2.191	2.529
2.014	2.825	3.502	2.006	1.879	3.304	1.538	0.906	3.125	1.009
1.540	0.444	1.541	1.850	1.793	2.284	1.890	3.091	2.293	2.491
1.190	2.087	2.159	1.157	2.314	1.753	0.722	2.447	2.124	2.927
0.741	3.411	1.689	1.945	0.286	3.288	1.390	0.240	1.448	2.768
2.169	1.937	2.261	0.766	2.075	0.457	2.031	0.831	−0.009	4.316
0.979	1.935	2.232	1.812	3.290	2.031	3.222	2.520	4.105	0.705
1.405	0.166	0.137	3.246	4.142	2.808	2.526	2.687	−0.627	2.023
0.923	2.287	1.164	0.732	0.736	0.892	2.633	2.107	1.260	0.615
1.529	3.188	2.153	3.828	3.610	1.654	2.596	0.957	1.479	1.497
0.781	3.562	3.633	0.880	0.832	2.068	2.103	3.360	1.686	1.538
2.153	2.125	1.930	3.161	2.931	1.941	3.108	1.732	4.296	1.830
3.204	3.945	0.682	4.165	2.419	0.565	1.637	1.931	1.092	2.482
2.154	1.889	1.391	1.690	1.356	2.560	1.784	1.041	2.808	0.576
3.391	2.602	2.496	2.177	1.564	1.781	0.302	2.499	1.501	1.410
3.266	2.051	1.958	0.979	2.454	1.438	2.098	3.208	2.374	2.710
1.842	0.513	1.736	2.878	1.893	1.614	2.775	1.060	1.508	1.197
2.799	0.757	0.625	3.336	2.268	1.418	1.616	2.363	0.751	2.138
0.104	3.564	0.681	1.231	2.527	0.172	1.331	0.991	3.570	1.382
2.232	3.514	−0.433	2.932	3.245	2.778	2.196	−0.326	1.034	1.889
4.201	3.351	1.761	1.957	1.342	3.575	3.216	1.335	1.527	0.812
1.046	1.646	1.363	1.051	4.600	3.209	3.041	3.234	2.034	0.682
2.874	1.663	2.591	1.396	1.052	1.068	2.226	3.048	1.906	2.755
1.389	2.966	2.846	2.410	1.663	3.620	2.151	2.036	3.733	1.462
−0.144	1.641	1.693	1.599	2.704	3.083	1.387	0.593	1.191	2.707
2.177	0.829	2.094	1.737	1.625	1.766	1.415	2.238	0.549	1.887
2.595	2.094	2.851	1.175	0.425	2.242	1.477	3.237	2.614	1.226
1.655	3.804	0.607	1.958	4.251	1.457	3.369	2.077	1.511	1.458
2.601	2.255	1.787	1.136	2.912	3.060	2.562	3.137	3.248	1.382
2.308	2.422	3.081	2.185	1.963	3.855	2.389	4.057	2.428	3.054
1.196	4.160	2.841	1.550	0.919	1.884	1.911	1.386	2.607	1.625
0.843	1.330	1.678	2.198	1.398	0.709	1.810	2.269	4.242	0.777

RANDOM NORMAL NUMBERS, $\mu = 2$, $\sigma = 1$

41	42	43	44	45	46	47	48	49	50
1.017	2.773	3.278	2.557	1.003	4.181	0.946	3.464	1.945	2.929
0.723	0.781	1.546	1.649	2.723	4.542	1.819	0.511	2.580	3.707
1.681	1.200	0.335	3.391	2.382	3.080	0.685	1.924	1.085	1.459
0.622	0.742	2.495	1.860	1.145	2.040	2.103	−0.256	0.976	2.414
1.815	2.061	2.092	2.089	2.281	2.377	1.821	1.760	2.515	1.898
4.334	1.662	0.044	1.363	0.681	2.111	2.443	1.603	1.803	2.149
0.863	2.642	5.436	0.332	2.847	1.466	3.031	1.571	3.024	1.988
2.414	1.988	2.666	0.867	1.589	2.192	3.027	2.257	1.868	1.927
1.505	2.364	0.762	1.955	1.888	1.845	3.180	2.618	1.730	1.603
3.048	2.037	2.759	2.609	−0.042	1.215	1.292	1.582	1.522	2.097
2.347	4.816	1.535	1.367	0.385	2.013	2.557	2.041	3.070	1.934
2.637	2.563	1.892	2.131	0.191	2.484	1.788	2.762	2.166	1.211
4.176	2.393	1.075	3.911	0.959	2.438	3.201	1.810	2.049	3.476
0.814	1.055	0.395	2.185	1.741	2.742	2.228	2.151	1.997	3.302
2.972	3.710	4.682	4.813	0.468	2.311	2.382	0.810	0.155	1.685
3.210	2.294	1.751	2.719	3.103	2.459	3.656	4.862	3.724	3.457
4.647	2.777	2.450	4.247	3.151	0.197	3.602	1.754	1.739	2.646
2.398	2.318	1.071	4.416	1.063	1.568	3.057	0.985	3.425	1.924
2.846	1.300	1.631	2.344	1.073	1.049	2.743	0.365	1.949	0.378
2.654	1.044	4.907	3.688	2.752	2.365	2.083	1.669	2.538	2.617
2.522	2.231	1.380	1.734	2.419	1.313	2.226	2.524	2.073	3.032
0.711	1.460	1.175	2.244	0.929	−0.091	1.096	2.061	3.099	2.186
3.372	3.769	0.942	3.646	2.481	1.554	3.715	1.193	1.956	1.735
2.854	1.464	3.607	2.428	1.384	1.977	1.504	0.492	2.102	2.624
1.851	0.855	2.913	2.684	3.043	2.595	1.803	1.303	0.233	−0.429
0.851	0.943	2.635	1.671	0.778	2.899	2.145	2.747	1.342	2.313
2.348	2.970	1.982	3.217	1.025	2.626	2.164	2.568	1.080	2.814
2.284	2.458	3.307	0.374	1.370	2.631	−0.649	1.111	1.296	2.403
0.983	2.360	1.880	4.331	3.672	−0.018	3.053	2.068	2.051	2.506
3.603	1.047	1.433	3.600	2.465	2.472	1.190	3.504	2.205	0.793
1.809	3.479	1.013	3.249	3.934	1.432	2.893	1.707	3.498	1.429
1.277	2.925	2.783	1.597	2.619	2.000	1.513	2.888	1.421	0.639
0.303	3.879	2.063	2.132	2.682	2.316	1.718	2.201	4.431	3.085
2.498	3.072	3.567	2.302	3.157	1.860	2.802	2.098	0.902	1.945
−0.542	0.666	3.987	2.668	2.360	2.762	1.351	2.835	2.972	1.796
1.640	2.193	0.976	1.777	1.383	3.100	1.663	1.609	2.503	1.596
2.248	1.911	0.620	2.295	1.884	3.421	1.086	2.085	1.861	−0.191
1.900	0.623	3.047	1.127	−0.199	3.653	0.976	−0.088	−0.966	2.626
1.536	0.718	−0.513	2.675	3.145	1.838	1.609	0.857	1.854	3.839
2.503	3.434	2.290	2.397	1.162	1.932	2.626	0.816	1.229	1.753
1.142	1.628	1.783	2.148	−0.105	3.072	2.312	3.666	2.784	2.102
1.877	3.107	0.960	1.363	1.139	1.135	2.370	4.245	3.284	0.188
3.632	2.586	1.531	1.613	1.645	0.963	4.596	1.979	2.649	1.435
4.072	0.554	1.319	2.224	1.879	1.806	1.606	3.049	0.099	2.996
1.564	1.624	1.014	1.414	1.796	1.244	1.712	2.319	2.166	2.727
2.876	0.772	−0.646	1.254	3.797	1.827	2.039	4.280	2.208	1.842
2.833	3.289	1.977	1.568	2.582	0.198	1.190	2.708	3.264	2.876
1.108	2.332	1.546	0.872	4.085	2.583	3.384	3.934	3.073	1.029
2.644	1.766	1.846	3.098	2.757	3.840	2.353	3.384	2.716	2.435
2.105	1.828	1.899	0.854	2.878	1.569	4.151	0.821	2.818	2.038

XII.7 RANDOM NORMAL NUMBERS, $\mu = 0$, $\sigma = 2$

01	02	03	04	05	06	07	08	09	10
−0.221	−0.540	−0.701	5.511	−2.404	−0.987	−0.158	−0.578	−1.893	0.854
−2.454	−2.816	0.580	−1.068	1.010	1.209	2.234	3.224	3.750	1.285
0.089	0.418	−0.421	2.448	−0.279	1.916	−3.166	−0.773	−0.818	−1.411
0.931	1.345	3.164	0.019	0.767	0.439	−3.412	−0.982	0.520	−0.473
0.361	0.794	0.120	−0.347	2.785	0.980	1.003	−1.796	−1.778	−0.783
−0.559	−2.111	−3.396	4.236	2.764	−1.990	−0.060	−2.488	−0.503	−4.406
−4.816	−1.369	1.856	0.383	0.016	−2.144	−0.187	−1.561	1.441	−2.246
0.784	0.607	0.663	−0.764	−1.395	1.738	−2.055	2.962	−1.616	1.326
2.576	−3.024	0.191	1.084	−3.698	−3.031	−0.517	−0.179	0.681	−0.719
−1.232	1.234	−0.046	1.338	1.726	1.448	2.216	−1.662	2.188	2.308
2.129	−1.936	3.381	1.319	−3.131	−1.037	1.191	1.449	0.690	−0.251
−2.753	1.049	1.616	1.232	2.910	0.389	−3.766	2.044	1.459	−0.002
0.071	1.869	−5.827	0.866	−1.191	2.508	1.552	−1.052	1.914	−0.274
0.507	0.595	−0.202	−0.775	−1.732	−2.771	0.049	5.221	3.059	0.015
0.384	−1.574	1.414	−0.789	−1.263	−0.470	0.020	1.489	0.497	1.316
1.688	4.311	2.305	−5.632	1.776	1.540	0.208	0.611	0.810	−1.241
−0.045	−1.563	3.687	−0.160	−0.101	1.838	1.590	1.222	0.377	2.069
2.516	−1.339	0.956	−1.285	0.301	3.739	−3.320	0.183	0.993	−4.678
0.536	1.965	−0.580	−0.307	1.564	0.163	−2.239	−2.460	−2.003	−1.609
0.775	1.427	−0.626	−1.134	−3.109	1.652	2.331	−0.188	2.137	−1.316
0.964	−3.740	1.995	−1.349	−1.068	−0.172	1.907	5.515	0.863	−1.018
2.597	2.328	−0.722	3.057	1.632	0.655	0.972	1.401	1.840	4.508
−1.340	−2.859	0.903	−0.001	−2.810	0.345	1.997	0.356	1.915	0.501
−1.097	0.798	−1.057	3.880	2.321	−1.677	−3.746	−1.125	−1.090	−1.972
−0.977	0.225	−0.004	−0.513	3.613	1.030	2.349	−1.278	−1.301	−5.159
2.421	−1.732	2.170	0.451	1.013	−0.912	0.615	−0.532	1.453	−2.155
0.921	−0.932	−2.511	−0.164	0.154	−0.004	0.516	2.240	−0.020	4.432
−1.854	−3.192	−3.033	0.007	3.709	0.500	−0.150	0.904	−2.018	−0.718
2.457	−0.566	−1.439	0.194	1.440	−1.568	−2.407	−1.356	0.849	0.801
1.143	0.212	4.088	−0.832	−0.361	0.303	−2.984	1.378	−0.649	−2.399
1.184	1.622	−1.896	0.026	−2.163	−1.683	3.778	3.585	−3.853	2.352
3.842	1.179	−0.987	0.498	2.348	3.263	1.924	−4.421	−0.680	2.129
1.930	0.114	−6.145	0.737	−0.353	2.478	−2.104	0.020	−2.250	−1.096
−0.174	−0.403	−1.539	1.740	−1.293	−1.922	1.228	1.433	−2.659	2.923
3.017	2.409	1.876	4.534	−0.539	−1.534	−0.847	−0.107	0.796	−1.257
2.632	−2.417	0.136	−1.155	4.277	−1.035	−0.968	−0.400	1.393	−0.858
−1.589	−2.199	0.776	0.821	3.237	4.810	1.012	−4.102	1.088	1.958
−1.308	0.561	−0.882	4.041	1.923	−0.717	0.599	1.705	0.241	2.677
−1.881	−1.808	−2.767	0.426	0.234	−4.060	1.036	−1.657	0.471	1.753
2.869	4.397	1.986	−2.123	−0.065	−0.705	−0.968	−2.265	−1.979	−1.114
0.252	−1.324	0.302	2.426	0.710	−1.454	−0.319	2.277	−0.971	−3.217
−0.833	1.653	−2.738	2.856	−0.789	−0.873	−0.809	−1.538	−1.334	2.289
0.276	0.020	−0.162	−1.720	0.048	0.401	−2.073	2.430	2.776	1.174
0.742	3.058	1.994	3.090	0.170	−0.789	−2.526	−0.980	−1.331	−1.834
0.770	1.419	4.391	1.502	−2.856	−3.648	−1.179	1.556	3.176	2.613
−2.208	1.766	−0.282	3.051	−1.734	−0.032	1.234	−0.626	1.052	−3.146
−1.161	−0.803	5.530	2.219	−0.371	1.372	−1.649	−2.059	1.456	0.677
−4.276	−0.196	−1.456	0.139	0.094	2.367	−1.902	1.123	−1.222	0.323
−1.615	−0.140	0.697	−0.647	1.289	1.416	0.811	0.523	1.406	−1.022
−3.831	−0.105	−2.271	−3.207	0.539	−1.010	2.646	−1.985	0.347	0.712

RANDOM NORMAL NUMBERS, $\mu = 0$, $\sigma = 2$

11	12	13	14	15	16	17	18	19	20
−0.686	0.678	−0.150	−0.334	5.096	0.708	0.403	1.538	1.217	−2.456
0.106	−0.018	2.558	−0.049	−1.061	−0.574	−0.510	−1.036	−0.168	2.516
−0.638	3.191	−4.587	−0.499	−0.510	−1.521	1.325	−1.355	−1.036	−3.305
−3.088	−0.998	0.883	2.230	0.603	0.906	−2.303	0.152	1.423	2.706
1.017	−2.496	−4.981	1.769	−0.252	3.018	2.764	1.105	−1.527	−1.187
0.132	−1.520	−1.748	−3.513	0.878	−0.483	−0.354	−1.103	−2.178	2.192
1.217	−2.380	−0.017	−0.072	−2.066	0.251	0.035	1.641	−1.298	2.070
0.540	−3.950	1.287	−0.771	−2.946	−1.181	−2.286	−1.561	0.420	−0.746
−0.395	−1.421	−2.163	0.270	−1.257	5.610	0.287	−1.138	−0.979	−2.224
−3.279	−2.813	1.125	−3.982	−0.102	0.576	−0.531	−0.695	−3.385	−1.045
3.510	3.235	2.623	−2.582	1.274	2.440	0.824	1.983	−0.770	2.489
−0.408	1.922	2.351	−0.146	−0.039	−0.648	−3.041	0.522	−1.659	−0.515
−2.434	1.297	2.813	−0.651	3.409	0.108	1.716	−1.801	0.344	0.923
0.541	0.820	−0.254	2.851	−3.027	1.553	2.218	1.758	1.003	−1.148
−0.813	1.562	2.116	−4.375	−2.289	1.593	0.163	−1.991	0.355	1.364
−0.238	−0.450	0.364	0.677	−0.711	−1.661	1.071	0.682	0.347	0.113
−1.214	−5.369	3.300	0.461	3.197	−0.368	−3.190	2.868	−0.943	0.931
3.521	1.655	2.373	1.993	−1.096	1.875	−1.143	−3.658	2.664	0.378
−1.075	−3.475	−2.069	−0.971	−0.909	−1.796	−0.760	−1.794	−1.576	3.863
−1.213	−1.760	0.397	−0.323	2.659	0.666	−4.368	2.704	1.160	−1.377
0.408	2.865	3.666	−0.433	−1.798	−1.434	−3.688	2.261	−1.084	0.722
−1.809	−2.890	−3.537	−2.701	0.656	0.684	0.905	1.953	2.720	−0.263
−1.633	0.283	−3.937	−0.224	−0.549	0.016	−1.265	−1.650	−1.506	0.504
−1.181	2.578	0.568	0.286	1.152	−0.929	−3.335	0.020	1.171	1.366
0.374	1.225	−0.213	−1.951	0.126	−1.551	−0.147	0.605	2.450	−1.514
−1.828	−3.459	2.624	2.605	0.698	−0.984	−2.289	−3.389	1.647	−2.592
−3.073	1.381	6.111	0.458	−0.792	−0.785	−1.254	2.784	−0.248	−0.965
−0.817	−1.048	−0.603	−0.647	−2.140	1.970	1.612	−2.050	1.962	−3.520
−0.778	−2.697	2.431	−2.011	2.810	0.010	1.830	−1.425	1.425	−2.506
1.866	0.259	−1.360	2.165	1.845	−0.326	2.054	−0.825	5.348	−0.384
0.715	−0.981	−0.126	0.263	−0.692	−3.790	−3.119	−0.547	−1.450	−0.791
0.802	−0.906	−0.726	0.071	3.693	−0.409	1.536	−0.907	3.216	−3.096
−0.363	0.030	−2.423	−0.517	−4.567	1.092	−1.194	0.253	−2.816	0.766
2.878	−2.689	0.797	0.820	0.764	0.366	−0.891	−0.122	0.196	1.052
−2.245	1.324	0.101	0.431	−2.152	0.779	−0.708	0.028	1.317	−1.259
−0.286	0.390	1.204	−4.414	−0.164	−3.724	0.207	1.835	0.334	0.660
−1.434	−0.736	−0.040	0.213	0.215	−0.565	0.915	−0.022	0.487	−0.487
0.004	−1.773	−0.480	0.768	−0.837	−0.513	0.828	4.563	1.298	2.837
1.299	−1.915	0.346	1.037	−2.953	−1.968	−1.704	1.639	2.802	−2.965
−1.694	1.993	1.021	−2.152	0.679	−0.763	0.577	2.860	0.329	−2.702
−0.506	0.328	−2.091	−0.238	2.582	−0.429	1.647	−1.048	−1.367	1.054
0.527	−3.033	−0.893	−0.776	−0.383	−0.708	−0.482	−2.686	1.369	1.040
3.815	−1.282	1.877	−1.177	0.000	−0.059	0.754	0.529	−0.522	2.073
1.838	−0.569	3.556	−0.956	−2.106	0.371	1.806	0.449	−0.867	2.664
0.810	3.394	1.224	−4.428	4.645	−0.644	−2.579	−2.198	2.683	1.338
4.048	−0.706	1.326	2.187	0.611	2.962	−2.137	−0.657	−3.539	−1.526
1.619	−1.214	−0.860	−0.625	−2.534	0.519	−2.539	0.737	−0.622	−0.146
1.732	−3.199	2.104	1.752	0.087	−0.333	3.943	0.037	0.135	1.756
−1.580	−3.456	2.934	0.580	1.665	2.331	−1.413	−1.558	2.144	1.876
1.176	−0.195	0.127	0.060	−3.145	−0.001	0.219	−1.803	−5.255	1.524

RANDOM NORMAL NUMBERS, $\mu = 0$, $\sigma = 2$

21	22	23	24	25	26	27	28	29	30
−0.625	−1.119	0.772	−1.479	0.164	3.051	0.297	1.904	2.864	3.093
1.375	1.994	1.004	−3.128	−1.517	−2.916	2.196	3.544	−1.858	−1.021
−1.835	0.393	−1.426	−0.469	−0.009	−2.366	0.408	−0.669	−0.266	−0.907
0.764	−2.796	−1.932	−1.144	−4.177	−2.150	4.163	1.003	−1.088	−0.346
−0.913	−4.834	2.310	−0.154	−2.007	−1.741	−3.570	1.361	−0.219	−1.424
−4.228	0.846	−0.794	−1.756	2.621	0.128	−1.369	2.090	−4.471	0.440
−2.724	2.694	−0.585	1.094	2.116	−1.176	0.180	1.438	1.260	−1.730
4.168	−0.764	−0.791	−2.517	−2.103	0.901	0.141	1.796	−4.435	1.711
3.286	2.374	1.605	−0.951	−1.308	−0.903	1.562	3.537	3.340	−1.417
0.197	0.212	1.303	−0.289	1.441	−2.913	−0.606	−1.302	1.281	0.147
0.713	−1.532	−4.409	−2.502	−1.488	1.696	−2.390	0.517	−2.406	−0.457
0.925	−2.267	2.010	−1.381	−2.057	0.988	−0.024	−2.096	0.116	1.383
−3.312	1.604	0.955	−0.184	0.074	−0.714	2.059	−2.293	0.899	−0.837
0.320	−2.893	−1.005	1.527	−0.990	1.930	−1.512	1.333	3.188	−1.555
0.619	−1.545	1.543	−0.207	−0.586	2.409	−2.454	−0.738	−0.060	−1.533
0.119	−0.542	−2.461	−2.475	−1.265	−3.598	0.983	−1.702	−1.735	−4.773
1.814	−0.053	−0.063	−2.921	2.076	−0.535	2.585	−3.066	−0.771	1.553
−2.068	0.648	2.066	0.610	−0.681	0.845	1.349	0.515	−1.106	−3.860
−1.881	−2.033	1.704	1.161	0.316	1.623	−3.370	−0.261	−3.559	−0.647
−2.125	0.620	−0.838	2.278	0.230	2.962	1.925	−2.209	−0.676	0.859
2.054	−2.290	2.264	1.598	2.064	−1.129	−1.381	−1.149	−0.488	0.568
−2.516	−2.190	−0.629	2.361	1.734	0.607	0.935	1.275	3.125	−0.224
−0.143	−1.222	1.061	−2.668	−4.419	0.569	0.259	−0.027	1.989	4.602
−0.007	0.017	−0.811	−0.166	0.850	0.565	0.184	−2.887	1.101	0.192
−1.749	0.231	−2.380	−3.177	−1.077	4.460	0.494	1.941	−0.106	0.015
1.300	−0.289	−2.657	−0.160	−0.490	−0.329	1.602	−1.110	4.204	2.552
0.588	−1.072	0.935	−0.164	0.113	1.139	−0.923	−0.953	0.001	−0.033
1.719	−1.183	−1.051	−0.944	0.734	1.965	2.121	2.213	3.826	−2.004
0.726	1.867	0.624	2.066	−2.792	−2.507	−0.816	−0.569	0.002	−1.934
2.369	−0.361	2.216	−1.500	−0.350	−1.063	−3.979	−3.626	−1.326	−0.488
1.790	−0.290	2.601	6.261	−0.622	−0.534	0.477	0.075	0.167	−2.351
1.801	−2.408	0.408	−2.039	0.175	3.839	3.096	−0.001	2.912	−0.560
0.392	1.600	−0.940	−0.160	−0.885	−1.083	−3.503	1.814	−0.563	−2.682
−4.113	−3.018	0.523	−1.915	−0.722	−2.769	0.210	−0.381	−0.724	−2.013
−0.393	−0.828	−0.102	−2.457	1.702	2.257	−2.473	−1.459	−1.385	−3.669
0.688	−0.214	2.741	2.906	−0.778	1.158	0.713	0.815	−0.670	0.144
1.957	1.104	3.540	2.726	−0.028	−0.181	−1.477	−4.434	0.457	0.057
1.823	−1.371	−4.951	3.333	0.248	1.691	2.311	−2.996	1.573	2.319
−0.277	0.346	−1.354	3.170	0.268	0.773	1.242	3.542	0.940	−0.535
−0.484	1.447	−0.512	−1.379	−0.808	1.014	2.103	0.005	−2.122	0.843
3.209	−1.924	−0.833	1.158	3.203	−0.040	−0.880	−2.217	0.007	0.022
1.834	2.064	−0.319	2.672	1.281	4.921	0.819	0.634	−4.961	−0.739
−1.618	0.705	0.220	−0.177	−0.117	−4.699	2.210	0.035	2.403	−0.816
2.553	1.710	−2.844	−4.619	−4.328	0.459	−2.373	−1.069	2.792	1.942
−1.665	1.627	1.072	−0.902	1.336	3.850	−0.804	1.254	−2.493	−1.101
−0.468	2.177	1.703	1.897	1.139	−1.606	−1.139	−1.435	5.162	−0.146
−1.296	−0.646	0.193	0.534	−0.863	−3.178	2.461	−1.275	0.731	2.983
−3.086	−0.115	2.325	0.088	4.652	2.833	−0.054	−0.670	−2.313	−1.956
−1.324	0.102	0.665	0.878	−1.760	−1.038	0.685	−1.034	0.380	−0.463
1.936	2.264	0.379	4.480	−3.841	−3.992	−3.565	2.558	−0.906	−0.432

RANDOM NORMAL NUMBERS, $\mu = 0$, $\sigma = 2$

31	32	33	34	35	36	37	38	39	40
−0.660	−0.996	−0.264	−1.823	0.818	−0.410	−1.786	2.399	1.986	0.242
1.785	−0.471	0.082	−3.006	−2.286	−0.222	0.388	−0.110	−0.358	−0.333
0.880	0.224	2.561	2.165	2.974	2.516	−4.148	−0.241	−1.318	−0.677
1.021	3.100	−1.783	−2.063	−2.176	1.959	0.248	0.597	1.394	0.612
−2.420	5.579	2.351	1.601	1.045	−2.857	1.400	3.411	−0.239	−2.323
−2.542	−3.145	−2.432	−0.444	−1.276	−3.342	3.479	2.630	−0.405	1.845
−2.437	0.104	1.110	0.008	−2.173	2.294	−0.529	1.723	−1.609	2.119
3.280	−1.213	−3.063	3.637	−0.038	0.217	−0.790	−1.412	−0.055	−0.612
0.502	−0.767	−1.569	0.386	−1.990	−0.062	3.319	−2.448	−0.445	0.059
−1.684	0.290	3.179	0.158	3.562	−1.929	−1.170	1.179	0.110	3.655
0.023	1.652	3.049	−1.410	−1.447	−0.638	−2.483	2.386	−0.331	1.215
−2.741	−2.313	−2.069	−1.305	−0.934	−7.769	2.654	−1.032	1.489	0.671
−0.746	2.099	−3.225	1.533	−1.741	−1.922	0.895	−2.974	−0.828	1.734
−0.934	−4.158	−3.297	−2.859	−4.026	2.722	−1.268	0.991	−1.196	−0.458
−1.574	0.097	2.122	−3.279	−0.820	0.483	2.196	0.642	−1.488	0.374
1.261	−0.663	0.616	−2.801	1.065	4.845	0.418	−0.226	1.897	3.554
2.030	1.692	0.265	0.511	−1.959	0.247	−1.381	−2.625	0.695	−2.248
−4.452	0.900	−1.646	0.573	0.973	−0.350	2.649	4.114	2.497	0.287
−0.075	−2.069	−0.574	0.001	−0.784	−1.235	−3.191	2.128	1.168	−0.742
0.369	0.919	−2.760	1.878	−5.001	−1.670	0.913	−2.853	0.002	1.885
1.360	−2.214	−2.175	0.193	3.298	−0.103	2.226	0.164	−2.429	−0.580
−3.271	2.845	−0.102	−0.822	−3.646	0.361	−3.188	−1.031	1.846	−1.622
−0.908	−3.907	1.407	0.078	1.324	0.276	−2.805	0.604	1.632	2.413
−1.323	2.717	−0.083	−1.645	1.103	−1.539	−0.173	2.429	−0.343	0.011
1.095	−0.871	1.636	2.345	−3.127	0.500	1.250	−0.072	−3.248	2.603
−1.907	−0.869	−4.388	−0.114	1.890	0.218	0.510	−0.768	−2.610	3.635
1.508	−0.333	−2.433	1.237	−1.733	−2.826	−3.761	−1.125	0.720	−0.832
2.937	1.887	−0.430	−5.194	4.716	−2.950	−0.393	−1.111	0.008	−0.186
−4.706	−1.302	−2.011	−0.124	−2.037	0.140	1.392	−1.869	−2.249	−0.075
5.019	−3.900	1.300	−0.034	−1.679	−0.621	0.285	1.197	−0.871	−1.240
−0.910	−0.495	0.074	3.144	−2.631	−3.152	0.192	−1.073	0.646	4.381
1.304	−1.010	−0.739	−1.028	2.886	−1.418	1.314	0.779	−2.139	0.173
0.371	−5.663	−0.017	−1.551	−3.508	1.305	−0.819	−0.199	−0.331	−0.358
−2.039	−3.961	0.679	2.451	−2.802	1.449	−0.964	−1.170	0.891	1.560
−0.911	1.904	0.062	−2.375	−1.548	−0.361	2.692	3.772	2.005	3.718
−1.720	0.871	3.594	0.889	0.162	0.112	−0.053	−2.597	−1.310	−2.234
−4.091	0.430	2.222	−0.141	0.506	2.751	−0.472	−1.141	1.671	−0.920
−1.797	−1.272	1.847	0.039	0.689	−0.080	1.457	−3.856	1.332	−2.898
−0.719	0.829	2.570	1.107	−0.314	−3.750	1.041	−1.657	−0.233	1.417
−1.890	3.240	1.877	2.552	3.389	0.215	1.979	−0.895	−1.996	0.611
−1.952	−1.276	−2.754	−0.049	−2.916	3.820	0.381	1.337	2.211	3.456
0.502	1.812	−0.577	0.551	−0.257	0.883	4.377	−4.180	−2.266	−0.100
1.971	2.333	−0.945	2.618	2.953	−1.997	1.491	−0.082	2.617	0.749
0.561	−1.506	4.127	0.933	−1.930	0.460	−0.008	0.352	−1.274	0.271
−1.409	−0.638	2.757	0.461	1.331	2.030	−0.846	−1.035	−1.580	−0.772
−2.066	0.218	0.070	−3.420	0.089	−0.084	4.944	−4.285	0.200	0.276
−2.734	3.622	−0.300	1.648	1.328	0.479	−0.498	1.997	2.203	2.792
−1.434	1.441	0.258	−1.893	−2.925	−1.753	0.272	0.747	−0.999	−0.155
−0.071	−4.344	−2.763	4.371	1.547	2.588	2.914	0.261	3.381	5.445
4.574	1.751	3.420	−1.383	0.966	−2.731	3.444	1.410	2.740	−2.011

RANDOM NORMAL NUMBERS, $\mu = 0$, $\sigma = 2$

41	42	43	44	45	46	47	48	49	50
−1.739	0.276	1.761	0.092	0.820	1.772	−3.258	0.707	−0.578	−1.611
−1.776	−1.482	1.399	1.031	−0.546	−0.204	2.591	2.129	1.615	0.919
−1.894	0.388	1.023	−1.493	1.513	1.003	2.547	−2.443	−1.855	2.898
−2.042	1.064	−2.399	−0.333	−2.141	−1.022	−2.976	−0.485	0.073	−0.891
0.287	0.120	−2.013	0.598	0.001	3.454	2.077	−1.966	−4.187	0.452
0.739	−4.324	0.088	1.124	0.610	0.368	0.953	−0.141	−0.441	3.163
0.749	0.597	2.194	−0.771	1.063	0.246	0.465	−3.122	−1.995	3.015
−1.111	−2.558	0.146	−0.590	−3.278	2.649	−1.299	−1.809	3.938	−1.766
−0.347	2.324	0.083	−0.152	−3.563	−1.062	0.901	0.882	0.865	0.581
−0.105	1.781	−0.775	−0.726	−3.211	−1.200	−2.688	1.639	−0.945	−1.022
1.968	2.056	−4.124	−1.126	−2.798	−1.150	−1.632	−3.405	1.182	1.985
1.614	−1.436	−4.649	−1.168	2.549	0.522	−0.616	2.009	−0.465	1.362
−1.671	−0.907	−0.459	2.880	2.640	−0.751	−2.414	−1.195	−2.334	−0.240
−1.328	0.335	−0.049	−1.903	0.225	−0.140	−1.121	0.820	0.282	0.635
−0.623	−0.823	1.655	1.997	−3.841	3.318	1.035	1.056	2.112	2.166
−2.292	−1.662	2.136	−0.223	1.372	−3.612	−0.276	−4.097	−0.419	−0.017
3.146	1.248	0.090	−1.069	−0.022	1.017	−1.157	1.803	−1.585	−1.526
1.553	−1.369	0.044	0.606	−1.734	−1.443	−3.016	−0.977	3.150	0.264
−3.179	3.510	−2.299	0.371	1.071	−1.044	−1.352	1.740	1.936	0.242
1.701	−0.455	2.119	−1.716	−2.857	−0.991	−1.621	2.934	3.487	0.754
−2.088	1.495	2.961	−2.029	−0.072	−0.664	0.992	1.659	0.834	−2.175
−3.757	0.316	0.763	−3.035	0.907	−3.804	−3.403	3.689	0.901	−2.386
−1.177	−1.422	−4.712	0.235	−1.048	−2.627	0.794	−1.473	2.598	−0.364
−1.380	−1.661	−1.714	−1.396	0.477	1.750	−2.458	−5.077	−0.194	1.093
−0.852	0.562	−0.199	0.802	0.494	−0.294	0.205	0.260	−2.616	4.117
2.591	1.323	0.458	4.020	−1.907	−0.065	−2.786	0.137	0.446	4.368
−2.240	2.744	0.551	−3.005	−2.677	4.492	2.928	0.061	−0.216	2.566
−1.488	−0.163	−0.187	2.081	−0.993	1.160	1.301	−2.236	1.586	0.011
0.622	−0.988	−0.956	−0.484	−0.648	−3.467	−3.778	1.181	1.740	0.092
−0.949	−2.527	−1.934	1.318	0.422	3.848	0.050	−1.448	0.278	3.041
−4.952	0.019	1.793	0.881	0.282	0.621	1.202	−0.373	3.665	3.386
−0.751	3.342	0.909	0.821	1.983	−0.533	−1.273	−2.214	−0.774	−1.210
0.618	−0.688	−2.960	−5.252	−0.543	0.104	−0.468	−3.139	0.594	−1.302
2.371	0.160	1.715	0.319	1.387	5.138	3.883	−1.869	−0.899	−1.019
−1.184	0.047	1.453	−0.889	−1.292	0.197	−0.302	−1.497	−1.838	−0.940
−0.287	2.329	2.028	−1.765	1.669	−1.024	1.600	0.454	3.098	2.275
1.764	−2.839	−1.942	0.008	4.001	0.083	−1.631	2.968	−0.146	−2.079
1.149	−1.571	1.296	1.510	−0.599	0.083	−0.688	6.017	0.012	−1.451
2.984	−1.432	−0.960	−2.124	1.353	0.934	0.666	3.096	2.905	−1.472
−1.701	−0.004	2.710	0.573	2.424	−0.119	−1.410	3.413	−3.588	0.047
−2.333	0.912	−0.773	−2.016	2.253	2.784	3.764	0.559	4.791	1.288
−0.214	2.787	0.095	−3.174	1.460	0.411	0.922	−0.474	3.113	−1.067
1.214	0.785	−2.686	1.909	−1.747	−4.551	0.589	−0.573	−1.364	−2.583
0.878	0.097	1.650	1.437	−1.643	−2.608	1.122	0.538	0.664	−0.323
−0.105	−0.297	3.821	2.105	2.021	−1.922	1.472	0.042	1.403	1.465
−0.593	0.136	0.910	−0.549	−1.472	3.214	−2.273	3.458	1.436	0.500
2.198	2.325	−1.229	−0.276	1.560	−0.482	−0.482	0.455	−0.181	1.417
1.160	0.139	0.997	−0.082	−0.689	0.995	−5.301	0.998	3.413	−1.797
3.024	−1.561	0.982	−1.244	1.407	−0.063	−1.176	2.355	2.006	−4.833
0.955	0.174	−0.401	2.472	0.584	3.811	1.115	0.951	−2.136	−2.324

XII.8 ORTHOGONAL POLYNOMIALS

In fitting a curvilinear model of the form

$$y_i = \beta_0 + \beta_1 x_i + \beta_2 x_i^2 + \cdots + \beta_p x_i^p + e_i\ , \quad i = 1, 2, \ldots, n,$$

it is convenient computationally to fit the model using orthogonal polynomials. Here one fits the model

$$y_i = \alpha_0 \xi_0(x) + \alpha_1 \xi_1(x) + \cdots + \alpha_p \xi_p(x) + e_i$$

where the $\xi_j(x)$ are orthogonal polynomials in x of the jth degree, namely, the Tchebycheff polynomials. The least-squares estimators $\hat{\alpha}_j$ of the α_j are given by

$$\hat{\alpha}_j = \frac{\sum_i y_i \xi_j(x_i)}{\sum_i [\xi_j(x_i)]^2} .$$

The estimators $\hat{\alpha}_j$ for any $j \le n - 1$ are independent normal variates with means α_j for $j \le p$ and 0 for $j > p$ and with variances $\frac{\sigma^2}{\sum_i [\xi_j(x_i)]^2}$. A mean-square estimate of σ^2 is provided by the error sum of squares

$$s^2 = \left\{ \sum_{i=1}^{n} y_i^2 - \sum_{j=0}^{p} \hat{\alpha}_j^2 \left(\sum_{i=1}^{n} \left[\xi_j(x_i) \right]^2 \right) \right\} \Big/ (n - p - 1) .$$

Thus the ratios $\frac{(\alpha_j - \hat{\alpha}_j)\sqrt{\sum_i [\xi_j(x_i)]^2}}{s}$ with $\hat{\alpha}_j = 0$ for $j > p$ is distributed as Student's t-distribution.

This table provides values of $\xi_j(x_i)$ for various values of n and j. To avoid fractional values and to reduce the size of the integers, the table is arranged so that the highest power of x_i in $\xi_j(x_i)$ has a coefficient λ_j. The two values at the bottom of each column are the values $D_j = \sum_{i=1}^{n} [\xi_j(x_i)]^2$ and λ_j.

ORTHOGONAL POLYNOMIALS

n = 3

	ξ_1'	ξ_2'
	−1	+1
	0	−2
	+1	+1
D	2	6
λ	1	3

n = 4

	ξ_1'	ξ_2'	ξ_3'
	−3	+1	−1
	−1	−1	+3
	+1	−1	−3
	+3	+1	+1
D	20	4	20
λ	2	1	$\frac{10}{3}$

n = 5

	ξ_1'	ξ_2'	ξ_3'	ξ_4'
	−2	+2	−1	+1
	−1	−1	+2	−4
	0	−2	0	+6
	+1	−1	−2	−4
	+2	+2	+1	+1
D	10	14	10	70
λ	1	1	$\frac{5}{6}$	$\frac{35}{12}$

n = 6

	ξ_1'	ξ_2'	ξ_3'	ξ_4'	ξ_5'
	−5	+5	−5	+1	−1
	−3	−1	+7	−3	+5
	−1	−4	+4	+2	−10
	+1	−4	−4	+2	+10
	+3	−1	−7	−3	−5
	+5	+5	+5	+1	+1
D	70	84	180	28	252
λ	2	$\frac{3}{2}$	$\frac{5}{3}$	$\frac{7}{12}$	$\frac{21}{10}$

n = 7

	ξ_1'	ξ_2'	ξ_3'	ξ_4'	ξ_5'
	−3	+5	−1	+3	−1
	−2	0	+1	−7	+4
	−1	−3	+1	+1	−5
	0	−4	0	+6	0
	+1	−3	−1	+1	+5
	+2	0	−1	−7	−4
	+3	+5	+1	+3	+1
D	28	84	6	154	84
λ	1	1	$\frac{1}{6}$	$\frac{7}{12}$	$\frac{7}{20}$

n = 8

	ξ_1'	ξ_2'	ξ_3'	ξ_4'	ξ_5'
	−7	+7	−7	+7	−7
	−5	+1	+5	−13	+23
	−3	−3	+7	−3	−17
	−1	−5	+3	+9	−15
	+1	−5	−3	+9	+15
	+3	−3	−7	−3	+17
	+5	+1	−5	−13	−23
	+7	+7	+7	+7	+7
D	168	168	264	616	2184
λ	2	1	$\frac{2}{3}$	$\frac{7}{12}$	$\frac{7}{10}$

n = 9

	ξ_1'	ξ_2'	ξ_3'	ξ_4'	ξ_5'
	0	−20	0	+18	0
	+1	−17	−9	+9	+9
	+2	−8	−13	−11	+4
	+3	+7	−7	−21	−11
	+4	+28	+14	+14	+4
D	60	2,772	990	2,002	468
λ	1	3	$\frac{5}{6}$	$\frac{7}{12}$	$\frac{3}{20}$

n = 10

	ξ_1'	ξ_2'	ξ_3'	ξ_4'	ξ_5'
	+1	−4	−12	+18	+6
	+3	−3	−31	+3	+11
	+5	−1	−35	−17	+1
	+7	+2	−14	−22	−14
	+9	+6	+42	+18	+6
D	330	132	8,580	2,860	780
λ	2	$\frac{1}{2}$	$\frac{5}{3}$	$\frac{5}{12}$	$\frac{1}{10}$

n = 11

	ξ_1'	ξ_2'	ξ_3'	ξ_4'	ξ_5'
	0	−10	0	+6	0
	+1	−9	−14	+4	+4
	+2	−6	−23	−1	+4
	+3	−1	−22	−6	−1
	+4	+6	−6	−6	−6
	+5	+15	+30	+6	+3
D	110	858	4,290	286	156
λ	1	1	$\frac{5}{6}$	$\frac{1}{12}$	$\frac{1}{40}$

n = 12

	ξ_1'	ξ_2'	ξ_3'	ξ_4'	ξ_5'
	+1	−35	−7	+28	+20
	+3	−29	−19	+12	+44
	+5	−17	−25	−13	+29
	+7	+1	−21	−33	−21
	+9	+25	−3	−27	−57
	+11	+55	+33	+33	+33
D	572	12,012	5,148	8,008	15,912
λ	2	3	$\frac{2}{3}$	$\frac{7}{24}$	$\frac{3}{20}$

n = 13

	ξ_1'	ξ_2'	ξ_3'	ξ_4'	ξ_5'
	0	−14	0	+84	0
	+1	−13	−4	+64	+20
	+2	−10	−7	+11	+26
	+3	−5	−8	−54	+11
	+4	+2	−6	−96	−18
	+5	+11	0	−66	−33
	+6	+22	+11	+99	+22
D	182	2,002	572	68,068	6,188
λ	1	1	$\frac{1}{6}$	$\frac{7}{12}$	$\frac{7}{120}$

n = 14

	ξ_1'	ξ_2'	ξ_3'	ξ_4'	ξ_5'
	+1	−8	−24	+108	+60
	+3	−7	−67	+63	+145
	+5	−5	−95	−13	+139
	+7	−2	−98	−92	+28
	+9	+2	−66	−132	−132
	+11	+7	+11	−77	−187
	+13	+13	+143	+143	+143
D	910	728	97,240	136,136	235,144
λ	2	$\frac{1}{2}$	$\frac{5}{3}$	$\frac{7}{12}$	$\frac{7}{30}$

n = 15

	ξ_1'	ξ_2'	ξ_3'	ξ_4'	ξ_5'
	0	−56	0	+756	0
	+1	−53	−27	+621	+675
	+2	−44	−49	+251	+1000
	+3	−29	−61	−249	+751
	+4	−8	−58	−704	−44
	+5	+19	−35	−869	−979
	+6	+52	+13	−429	−1144
	+7	+91	+91	+1001	+1001
D	280	37,128	39,780	6,466,460	10,581,480
λ	1	3	$\frac{5}{6}$	$\frac{35}{12}$	$\frac{21}{20}$

n = 16

	ξ_1'	ξ_2'	ξ_3'	ξ_4'	ξ_5'
	+1	−21	−63	+189	+45
	+3	−19	−179	+129	+115
	+5	−15	−265	+23	+131
	+7	−9	−301	−101	+77
	+9	−1	−267	−201	−33
	+11	+9	−143	−221	−143
	+13	+21	+91	−91	−143
	+15	+35	+455	+273	+143
D	1,360	5,712	1,007,760	470,288	201,552
λ	2	1	$\frac{10}{3}$	$\frac{7}{12}$	$\frac{1}{10}$

ORTHOGONAL POLYNOMIALS

17

	ξ'_1	ξ'_2	ξ'_3	ξ'_4	ξ'_5
	0	−24	0	+36	0
	+1	−23	−7	+31	+55
	+2	−20	−13	+17	+88
	+3	−15	−17	−3	+83
	+4	−8	−18	−24	+36
	+5	+1	−15	−39	−39
	+6	+12	−7	−39	−104
	+7	+25	+7	−13	−91
	+8	+40	+28	+52	+104
D	408	7,752	3,876	16,796	100,776
λ	1	1	$\frac{1}{6}$	$\frac{1}{12}$	$\frac{1}{20}$

18

	ξ'_1	ξ'_2	ξ'_3	ξ'_4	ξ'_5
	+1	−40	−8	+44	+220
	+3	−37	−23	+33	+583
	+5	−31	−35	+13	+733
	+7	−22	−42	−12	+588
	+9	−10	−42	−36	+156
	+11	+5	−33	−51	−429
	+13	+23	−13	−47	−871
	+15	+44	+20	−12	−676
	+17	+68	+68	+68	+884
D	1,938	23,256	23,256	28,424	6,953,544
λ	2	$\frac{3}{2}$	$\frac{1}{3}$	$\frac{1}{12}$	$\frac{3}{10}$

19

	ξ'_1	ξ'_2	ξ'_3	ξ'_4	ξ'_5
	0	−30	0	+396	0
	+1	−29	−44	+352	+44
	+2	−26	−83	+227	+74
	+3	−21	−112	+42	+79
	+4	−14	−126	−168	+54
	+5	−5	−120	−354	+3
	+6	+6	−89	−453	−58
	+7	+19	−28	−388	−98
	+8	+34	+68	−68	−68
	+9	+51	+204	+612	+102
D	570	13,566	213,180	2,288,132	89,148
λ	1	1	$\frac{5}{6}$	$\frac{7}{12}$	$\frac{1}{40}$

20

	ξ'_1	ξ'_2	ξ'_3	ξ'_4	ξ'_5
	+1	−33	−99	+1188	+396
	+3	−31	−287	+948	+1076
	+5	−27	−445	+503	+1441
	+7	−21	−553	−77	+1351
	+9	−13	−591	−687	+771
	+11	−3	−539	−1187	−187
	+13	+9	−377	−1402	−1222
	+15	+23	−85	−1122	−1802
	+17	+39	+357	−102	−1122
	+19	+57	+969	+1938	+1938
D	2,660	17,556	4,903,140	22,881,320	31,201,800
λ	2	1	$\frac{10}{3}$	$\frac{35}{24}$	$\frac{7}{20}$

21

	ξ'_1	ξ'_2	ξ'_3	ξ'_4	ξ'_5
	0	−110	0	+594	0
	+1	−107	−54	+540	+1404
	+2	−98	−103	+385	+2444
	+3	−83	−142	+150	+2819
	+4	−62	−166	−130	+2354
	+5	−35	−170	−406	+1063
	+6	−2	−149	−615	−788
	+7	+37	−98	−680	−2618
	+8	+82	−12	−510	−3468
	+9	+133	+114	0	−1938
	+10	+190	+285	+969	+3876
D	770	201,894	432,630	5,720,330	121,687,020
λ	1	3	$\frac{5}{6}$	$\frac{7}{12}$	$\frac{21}{40}$

22

	ξ'_1	ξ'_2	ξ'_3	ξ'_4	ξ'_5
	+1	−20	−12	+702	+390
	+3	−19	−35	+585	+1079
	+5	−17	−55	+365	+1509
	+7	−14	−70	+70	+1554
	+9	−10	−78	−258	+1158
	+11	−5	−77	−563	+363
	+13	+1	−65	−775	−663
	+15	+8	−40	−810	−1598
	+17	+16	0	−570	−1938
	+19	+25	+57	+57	−969
	+21	+35	+133	+1197	+2261
D	3,542	7,084	96,140	8,748,740	40,562,340
λ	2	$\frac{1}{2}$	$\frac{1}{3}$	$\frac{7}{12}$	$\frac{7}{30}$

ORTHOGONAL POLYNOMIALS

	23					24				
	ξ_1'	ξ_2'	ξ_3'	ξ_4'	ξ_5'	ξ_1'	ξ_2'	ξ_3'	ξ_4'	ξ_5'
	0	−44	0	+858	0	+1	−143	−143	+143	+715
	+1	−43	−13	+793	+65	+3	−137	−419	+123	+2005
	+2	−40	−25	+605	+116	+5	−125	−665	+85	+2893
	+3	−35	−35	+315	+141	+7	−107	−861	+33	+3171
	+4	−28	−42	−42	+132	+9	−83	−987	−27	+2721
	+5	−19	−45	−417	+87	+11	−53	−1023	−87	+1551
	+6	−8	−43	−747	+12	+13	−17	−949	−137	−169
	+7	+5	−35	−955	−77	+15	+25	−745	−165	−2071
	+8	+20	−20	−950	−152	+17	+73	−391	−157	−3553
	+9	+37	+3	−627	−171	+19	+127	+133	−97	−3743
	+10	+56	+35	+133	−76	+21	+187	+847	+33	−1463
	+11	+77	+77	+1463	+209	+23	+253	+1771	+253	+4807
D	1,012	35,420	32,890	13,123,110	340,860	4,600	394,680	17,760,600	394,680	177,928,920
λ	1	1	$\frac{1}{6}$	$\frac{7}{12}$	$\frac{1}{60}$	2	3	$\frac{10}{3}$	$\frac{1}{12}$	$\frac{3}{10}$

	25					26				
	ξ_1'	ξ_2'	ξ_3'	ξ_4'	ξ_5'	ξ_1'	ξ_2'	ξ_3'	ξ_4'	ξ_5'
	0	−52	0	+858	0	+1	−28	−84	+1386	+330
	+1	−51	−77	+803	+275	+3	−27	−247	+1221	+935
	+2	−48	−149	+643	+500	+5	−25	−395	+905	+1381
	+3	−43	−211	+393	+631	+7	−22	−518	+466	+1582
	+4	−36	−258	+78	+636	+9	−18	−606	−54	+1482
	+5	−27	−285	−267	+501	+11	−13	−649	−590	+1067
	+6	−16	−287	−597	+236	+13	−7	−637	−1099	+377
	+7	−3	−259	−857	−119	+15	0	−560	−1470	−482
	+8	+12	−196	−982	−488	+17	+8	−408	−1614	−1326
	+9	+29	−93	−897	−753	+19	+17	−171	−1419	−1881
	+10	+48	+55	517	748	+21	+27	+161	−759	−1771
	+11	+69	+253	+253	−253	+23	+38	+598	+506	−506
	+12	+92	+506	+1518	+1012	+25	+50	+1150	+2530	+2530
D	1,300	53,820	1,480,050	14,307,150	7,803,900	5,850	16,380	7,803,900	40,060,020	48,384,180
λ	1	1	$\frac{5}{6}$	$\frac{5}{12}$	$\frac{1}{20}$	2	$\frac{1}{2}$	$\frac{5}{3}$	$\frac{7}{12}$	$\frac{1}{10}$

	27					28				
	ξ_1'	ξ_2'	ξ_3'	ξ_4'	ξ_5'	ξ_1'	ξ_2'	ξ_3'	ξ_4'	ξ_5'
	0	−182	0	+1638	0	+1	−65	−39	+936	+1560
	+1	−179	−18	+1548	+3960	+3	−63	−115	+840	+4456
	+2	−170	−35	+1285	+7304	+5	−59	−185	+655	+6701
	+3	−155	−50	+870	+9479	+7	−53	−245	+395	+7931
	+4	−134	−62	+338	+10058	+9	−45	−291	+81	+7887
	+5	−107	−70	−262	+8803	+11	−35	−319	−259	+6457
	+6	−74	−73	−867	+5728	+13	−23	−325	−590	+3718
	+7	−35	−70	−1400	+1162	+15	−9	−305	−870	−22
	+8	+10	−60	−1770	−4188	+17	+7	−255	−1050	−4182
	+9	+61	−42	−1872	−9174	+19	+25	−171	−1074	−7866
	+10	+118	−15	−1587	−12144	+21	+45	−49	−879	−9821
	+11	+181	+22	−782	−10879	+23	+67	+115	−395	−8395
	+12	+250	+70	+690	−2530	+25	+91	+325	+455	−1495
	+13	+325	+130	+2990	+16445	+27	+117	+585	+1755	+13455
D	1,638	712,530	101,790	56,448,210	2,032,135,560	7,308	95,004	2,103,660	19,634,160	1,354,757,040
λ	1	3	$\frac{1}{6}$	$\frac{7}{12}$	$\frac{21}{40}$	2	1	$\frac{2}{3}$	$\frac{7}{24}$	$\frac{7}{20}$

ORTHOGONAL POLYNOMIALS

	29					30				
	ξ'_1	ξ'_2	ξ'_3	ξ'_4	ξ'_5	ξ'_1	ξ'_2	ξ'_3	ξ'_4	ξ'_5
	0	−70	0	+2184	0	+1	−112	−112	+12376	+1768
	+1	−69	−104	+2080	+1768	+3	−109	−331	+11271	+5083
	+2	−66	−203	+1775	+3298	+5	−103	−535	+9131	+7753
	+3	−61	−292	+1290	+4373	+7	−94	−714	+6096	+9408
	+4	−54	−366	+660	+4818	+9	−82	−858	+2376	+9768
	+5	−45	−420	−66	+4521	+11	−67	−957	−1749	+8679
	+6	−34	−449	−825	+3454	+13	−49	−1001	−5929	+6149
	+7	−21	−448	−1540	+1695	+15	−28	−980	−9744	+2384
	+8	−6	−412	−2120	−556	+17	−4	−884	−12704	−2176
	+9	+11	−336	+2460	−2946	+19	+23	−703	−14249	−6821
	+10	+30	−215	−2441	−4958	+21	+53	−427	−13749	−10535
	+11	+51	−44	−1930	−5885	+23	+86	−46	−10504	−11960
	+12	+74	+182	−780	−4810	+25	+122	+450	−3744	−9360
	+13	+99	+468	+1170	−585	+27	+161	+1071	+7371	−585
	+14	+126	+819	+4095	+8190	+29	+203	+1827	+23751	+16965
D	2,030	113,274	4,207,320	107,987,880	500,671,080	8,990	302,064	21,360,240	3,671,587,920	2,145,733,200
λ	1	1	$\frac{5}{6}$	$\frac{7}{12}$	$\frac{7}{40}$	2	$\frac{3}{2}$	$\frac{5}{3}$	$\frac{35}{12}$	$\frac{3}{10}$

	31					32				
	ξ'_1	ξ'_2	ξ'_3	ξ'_4	ξ'_5	ξ'_1	ξ'_2	ξ'_3	ξ'_4	ξ'_5
	+0	−80	0	+408	0	+1	−85	−51	+459	+255
	+1	−79	−119	+391	+221	+3	−83	−151	+423	+737
	+2	−76	−233	+341	+416	+5	−79	−245	+353	+1137
	+3	−71	−337	+261	+561	+7	−73	−329	+253	+1407
	+4	−64	−426	+156	+636	+9	−65	−399	+129	+1509
	+5	−55	−495	+33	+627	+11	−55	−451	−11	+1419
	+6	−44	−539	−99	+528	+13	−43	−481	−157	+1131
	+7	−31	−553	−229	+343	+15	−29	−485	−297	+661
	+8	−16	−532	−344	+88	+17	−13	−459	−417	+51
	+9	+1	−471	−429	−207	+19	+5	−399	−501	−627
	+10	+20	−365	−467	−496	+21	+25	−301	−531	−1267
	+11	+41	−209	−439	−715	+23	+47	−161	−487	−1725
	+12	+64	+2	−324	−780	+25	+71	+25	−347	−1815
	+13	+89	+273	−99	−585	+27	+97	+261	−87	−1305
	+14	+116	+609	+261	0	+29	+125	+551	+319	+87
	+15	+145	+1015	+783	+1131	+31	+155	+899	+899	+2697
D	2,480	158,224	6,724,520	4,034,712	9,536,592	10,912	185,504	5,379,616	5,379,616	54,285,216
λ	1	1	$\frac{5}{6}$	$\frac{1}{12}$	$\frac{1}{60}$	2	1	$\frac{2}{3}$	$\frac{1}{12}$	$\frac{1}{30}$

ORTHOGONAL POLYNOMIALS

33					34				
ξ'_1	ξ'_2	ξ'_3	ξ'_4	ξ'_5	ξ'_1	ξ'_2	ξ'_3	ξ'_4	ξ'_5
0	−272	0	+3672	0	1	−48	−144	+4104	+6840
+1	−269	−27	+3537	+2565	3	−47	−427	+3819	+19855
+2	−260	−53	+3139	+4864	5	−45	−695	+3263	+30917
+3	−245	−77	+2499	+6649	7	−42	−938	+2464	+38864
+4	−224	−98	+1652	+7708	9	−38	−1146	+1464	+42744
+5	−197	−115	+647	+7883	11	−33	−1309	+319	+41899
+6	−164	−127	−453	+7088	13	−27	−1417	−901	+36049
+7	−125	−133	−1571	+5327	15	−20	−1460	−2112	+25376
+8	−80	−132	−2616	+2712	17	−12	−1428	−3216	+10608
+9	−29	−123	−3483	−519	19	−3	−1311	−4101	−6897
+10	+28	−105	−4053	−3984	21	+7	−1099	−4641	−25067
+11	+91	−77	−4193	−7139	23	+18	−782	−4696	−41032
+12	+160	−38	−3756	−9260	25	+30	−350	−4112	−51040
+13	+235	+13	−2581	−9425	27	+43	+207	−2721	−50373
+14	+316	+77	−493	−6496	29	+57	+899	−341	−33263
+15	+403	+155	+2697	+899	31	+72	+1736	+3224	+7192
+16	+496	+248	+7192	+14384	33	+88	+2728	+8184	+79112
D 2,992	1,947,792	417,384	348,330,136	1,547,128,656	13,090	62,832	51,477,360	456,432,592	46,929,569,232
λ 1	3	$\frac{1}{6}$	$\frac{7}{12}$	$\frac{3}{20}$	2	$\frac{1}{2}$	$\frac{5}{3}$	$\frac{7}{12}$	$\frac{7}{10}$

	35				
	ξ'_1	ξ'_2	ξ'_3	ξ'_4	ξ'_5
	0	102	0	[illegible]	0
	1	−101	−152	+22496	+3800
	2	−98	−299	+20251	+7250
	3	−93	−436	+16626	+10021
	4	−86	−558	+11796	+11826
	5	−77	−660	+6006	+12441
	6	−66	−737	−429	+11726
	7	−53	−784	−7124	+9646
	8	−38	−796	−13624	+6292
	9	−21	−768	−19404	+1902
	10	−2	−695	−23869	−3118
	11	+19	−572	−26354	−8173
	12	+42	−394	−26124	−12458
	13	+67	−156	−22374	−14937
	14	+94	+147	−14229	−14322
	15	+123	+520	−744	−9052
	16	+154	+968	+19096	+2728
	17	+187	+1496	+46376	+23188
D	3,570	290,598	15,775,320	14,834,059,240	4,045,652,520
λ	1	1	$\frac{5}{6}$	$\frac{35}{12}$	$\frac{7}{40}$

ORTHOGONAL POLYNOMIALS

	36				
	ξ_1'	ξ_2'	ξ_3'	ξ_4'	ξ_5'
	1	−323	−323	+2584	+12920
	3	−317	−959	+2424	+37640
	5	−305	−1565	+2111	+59063
	7	−287	−2121	+1659	+75201
	9	−263	−2607	+1089	+84381
	11	−233	−3003	+429	+85371
	13	−197	−3289	−286	+77506
	15	−155	−3445	−1014	+60814
	17	−107	−3451	−1706	+36142
	19	−53	−3287	−2306	+5282
	21	+7	−2933	−2751	−28903
	23	+73	−2369	−2971	−62353
	25	+145	−1575	−2889	−89685
	27	+223	−531	−2421	−104067
	29	+307	+783	−1476	−97092
	31	+397	+2387	+44	−58652
	33	+493	+4301	+2244	+23188
	35	+595	+6545	+5236	+162316
D	15,540	3,011,652	307,618,740	191,407,216	199,046,103,984
λ	2	3	$\frac{10}{3}$	$\frac{7}{24}$	$\frac{21}{20}$

	37					38				
ξ_1'	ξ_2'	ξ_3'	ξ_4'	ξ_5'	ξ_1'	ξ_2'	ξ_3'	ξ_4'	ξ_5'	
0	−114	0	+5814	0	1	−60	−36	+918	+1530	
1	−113	−34	+5644	+680	3	−59	−107	+867	+4471	
2	−110	−67	+5141	+1304	5	−57	−175	+767	+7061	
3	−105	−98	+4326	+1819	7	−54	−238	+622	+9086	
4	−98	−126	+3234	+2178	9	−50	−294	+438	+10362	
5	−89	−150	+1914	+2343	11	−45	−341	+223	+10747	
6	−78	−169	+429	+2288	13	−39	−377	−13	+10153	
7	−65	−182	−1144	+2002	15	−32	−400	−258	+8558	
8	−50	−188	−2714	+1492	17	−24	−408	−498	+6018	
9	−33	−186	−4176	+786	19	−15	−399	−717	+2679	
10	−14	−175	−5411	−64	21	−5	−371	−897	−1211	
11	+7	−154	−6286	−979	23	+6	−322	−1018	−5290	
12	+30	−122	−6654	−1850	25	+18	−250	−1058	−9070	
13	+55	−78	−6354	−2535	27	+31	−153	−993	−11925	
14	+82	−21	−5211	−2856	29	+45	−29	−797	−13079	
15	+111	+50	−3036	−2596	31	+60	+124	−442	−11594	
16	+142	+136	+374	−1496	33	+76	+308	+102	−6358	
17	+175	+238	+5236	+748	35	+93	+525	+867	+3927	
18	+210	+357	+11781	+4488	37	+111	+777	+1887	+20757	
D 4,218	383,838	932,178	980,961,982	152,877,192	18,278	109,668	4,496,388	25,479,532	3,286,859,628	
λ 1	1	$\frac{1}{6}$	$\frac{7}{12}$	$\frac{1}{40}$	2	$\frac{1}{2}$	$\frac{1}{3}$	$\frac{1}{12}$	$\frac{1}{10}$	

ORTHOGONAL POLYNOMIALS

39

	ξ_1'	ξ_2'	ξ_3'	ξ_4'	ξ_5'
	0	−380	0	+1026	0
	1	−377	−189	+999	+5049
	2	−368	−373	+919	+9724
	3	−353	−547	+789	+13669
	4	−332	−706	+614	+16564
	5	−305	−845	+401	+18143
	6	−272	−959	+159	+18212
	7	−233	−1043	−101	+16667
	8	−188	−1092	−366	+13512
	9	−137	−1101	−621	+8877
	10	−80	−1065	−849	+3036
	11	−17	−979	−1031	−3575
	12	+52	−838	−1146	−10340
	13	+127	−637	−1171	−16445
	14	+208	−371	−1081	−20860
	15	+295	−35	−849	−22321
	16	+388	+376	−446	−19312
	17	+487	+867	+159	−10047
	18	+592	+1443	+999	+7548
	19	+703	+2109	+2109	+35853
D	4,940	4,496,388	33,722,910	32,224,114	9,860,578,884
λ	1	3	$\frac{5}{6}$	$\frac{1}{12}$	$\frac{3}{20}$

40

	ξ_1'	ξ_2'	ξ_3'	ξ_4'	ξ_5'
	1	−133	−399	+39501	+627
	3	−131	−1187	+37521	+1837
	5	−127	−1945	+33631	+2917
	7	−121	−2653	+27971	+3787
	9	−113	−3291	+20751	+4377
	11	−103	−3839	+12251	+4631
	13	−91	−4277	+2821	+4511
	15	−77	−4585	−7119	+4001
	17	−61	−4743	−17079	+3111
	19	−43	−4731	−26499	+1881
	21	−23	−4529	−34749	+385
	23	−1	−4117	−41129	−1265
	25	+23	−3475	−44869	−2915
	27	+49	−2583	−45129	−4365
	29	+77	−1421	−40999	−5365
	31	+107	+31	−31499	−5611
	33	+139	+1793	−15579	−4741
	35	+173	+3885	+7881	−2331
	37	+209	+6327	+40071	+2109
	39	+247	+9139	+82251	+9139
D	21,320	567,112	644,482,280	49,625,135,560	644,482,280
λ	2	1	$\frac{10}{3}$	$\frac{35}{12}$	$\frac{1}{30}$

ORTHOGONAL POLYNOMIALS

41					
	ξ_1'	ξ_2'	ξ_3'	ξ_4'	ξ_5'
	0	−140	0	+8778	0
	1	−139	−209	+8569	+4807
	2	−136	−413	+7949	+9292
	3	−131	−607	+6939	+13147
	4	−124	−786	+5574	+16092
	5	−115	−945	+3903	+17889
	6	−104	−1079	+1989	+18356
	7	−91	−1183	−91	+17381
	8	−76	−1252	−2246	+14936
	9	−59	−1281	−4371	+11091
	10	−40	−1265	−6347	+6028
	11	−19	−1199	−8041	+55
	12	+4	−1078	−9306	−6380
	13	+29	−897	−9981	−12675
	14	+56	−651	−9891	−18060
	15	+85	−335	−8847	−21583
	16	+116	+56	−6646	−22096
	17	+149	+527	−3071	−18241
	18	+184	+1083	+2109	−8436
	19	+221	+1729	+9139	+9139
	20	+260	+2470	+18278	+36556
D	5,740	641,732	47,900,710	2,481,256,778	10,376,164,708
λ	1	1	$\frac{5}{6}$	$\frac{7}{12}$	$\frac{7}{60}$

42					
	ξ_1'	ξ_2'	ξ_3'	ξ_4'	ξ_5'
	1	−220	−44	+9614	+48070
	3	−217	−131	+9177	+141151
	5	−211	−215	+8317	+225181
	7	−202	−294	+7062	+294546
	9	−190	−366	+5454	+344262
	11	−175	−429	+3549	+370227
	13	−157	−481	+1417	+369473
	15	−136	−520	−858	+340418
	17	−112	−544	−3178	+283118
	19	−85	−551	−5431	+199519
	21	−55	−539	−7491	+93709
	23	−22	−506	−9218	−27830
	25	+14	−450	−10458	−155970
	27	+53	−369	−11043	−278685
	29	+95	−261	−10791	−380799
	31	+140	−124	−9506	−443734
	33	+188	+44	−6978	−445258
	35	+239	+245	−2983	−359233
	37	+293	+481	+2717	−155363
	39	+350	+754	+10374	+201058
	41	+410	+1066	+20254	+749398
D	24,682	1,629,012	9,075,924	3,084,805,724	4,389,117,671,484
λ	2	$\frac{3}{2}$	$\frac{1}{3}$	$\frac{7}{12}$	$\frac{21}{10}$

ORTHOGONAL POLYNOMIALS

	43				
	ξ'_1	ξ'_2	ξ'_3	ξ'_4	ξ'_5
	0	−154	0	+10626	0
	1	−153	−46	+10396	+8740
	2	−150	−91	+9713	+16948
	3	−145	−134	+8598	+24113
	4	−138	−174	+7086	+29766
	5	−129	−210	+5226	+33501
	6	−118	−241	+3081	+34996
	7	−105	−266	+728	+34034
	8	−90	−284	−1742	+30524
	9	−73	−294	−4224	+24522
	10	−54	−295	−6599	+16252
	11	−33	−286	−8734	+6127
	12	−10	−266	−10482	−5230
	13	+15	−234	−11682	−16965
	14	+42	−189	−12159	−27972
	15	+71	−130	−11724	−36872
	16	+102	−56	−10174	−41992
	17	+135	+34	−7292	−41344
	18	+170	+141	−2847	−32604
	19	+207	+266	+3406	−13091
	20	+246	+410	+11726	+20254
	21	+287	+574	+22386	+70889
D	6,622	814,506	2,676,234	3,815,417,606	39,541,600,644
λ	1	1	$\frac{1}{6}$	$\frac{7}{12}$	$\frac{7}{40}$

	44				
	ξ'_1	ξ'_2	ξ'_3	ξ'_4	ξ'_5
	1	−161	−483	+5796	+1380
	3	−159	−1439	+5556	+4060
	5	−155	−2365	+5083	+6503
	7	−149	−3241	+4391	+8561
	9	−141	−4047	+3501	+10101
	11	−131	−4763	+2441	+11011
	13	−119	−5369	+1246	+11206
	15	−105	−5845	−42	+10634
	17	−89	−6171	−1374	+9282
	19	−71	−6327	−2694	+7182
	21	−51	−6293	−3939	+4417
	23	−29	−6049	−5039	+1127
	25	−5	−5575	−5917	−2485
	27	+21	−4851	−6489	−6147
	29	+49	−3857	−6664	−9512
	31	+79	−2573	−6344	−12152
	33	+111	−979	−5424	−13552
	35	+145	+945	−3792	−13104
	37	+181	+3219	−1329	−10101
	39	+219	+5863	+2091	−3731
	41	+259	+8897	+6601	+6929
	43	+301	+12341	+12341	+22919
D	28,380	913,836	1,257,829,980	1,173,974,648	4,162,273,752
λ	2	1	$\frac{10}{3}$	$\frac{7}{24}$	$\frac{1}{20}$

ORTHOGONAL POLYNOMIALS

45

	ξ'_1	ξ'_2	ξ'_3	ξ'_4	ξ'_5
	0	−506	0	+9108	0
	1	−503	−252	+8928	+4500
	2	−494	−499	+8393	+8750
	3	−479	−736	+7518	+12509
	4	−458	−958	+6328	+15554
	5	−431	−1160	+4858	+17689
	6	−398	−1337	+3153	+18754
	7	−359	−1484	+1268	+18634
	8	−314	−1596	−732	+17268
	9	−263	−1668	−2772	+14658
	10	−206	−1695	−4767	+10878
	11	−143	−1672	−6622	+6083
	12	−74	−1594	−8232	+518
	13	+1	−1456	−9482	−5473
	14	+82	−1253	−10247	−11438
	15	+169	−980	−10392	−16808
	16	+262	−632	−9772	−20888
	17	+361	−204	−8232	−22848
	18	+466	+309	−5607	−21714
	19	+577	+912	−1722	−16359
	20	+694	+1610	+3608	−5494
	21	+817	+2408	+10578	−12341
	22	+946	+3311	+19393	+38786
D	7,590	9,203,634	92,036,340	2,934,936,620	12,006,558,900
λ	1	3	$\frac{5}{6}$	$\frac{5}{12}$	$\frac{3}{40}$

46

	ξ'_2	ξ'_3	ξ'_4	ξ'_5
	−88	−264	+1980	+3300
	−87	−787	+1905	+9725
	−85	−1295	+1757	+15631
	−82	−1778	+1540	+20692
	−78	−2226	+1260	+24612
	−73	−2629	+925	+27137
	−67	−2977	+545	+28067
	−60	−3260	+132	−27268
	−52	−3468	−300	+24684
	−43	−3591	−735	+20349
	−33	−3619	−1155	+14399
	−22	−3542	−1540	+7084
	−10	−3350	−1868	−1220
	+3	−3033	−2115	−9999
	+17	−2581	−2255	−18589
	+32	−1984	−2260	−26164
	+48	−1232	−2100	−31724
	+65	−315	−1743	−34083
	+83	+777	−1155	−31857
	+102	+2054	−300	−23452
	+122	+3526	+860	−7052
	+143	+5203	+2365	+19393
	+165	+7095	+4257	+58179
D	285,384	429,502,920	143,167,640	27,214,866,840
λ	$\frac{1}{2}$	$\frac{5}{3}$	$\frac{1}{12}$	$\frac{1}{10}$

ORTHOGONAL POLYNOMIALS

47	ξ_2'	ξ_3'	ξ_4'	ξ_5'
	−184	0	+15180	0
	−183	−55	+14905	+3575
	−180	−109	+14087	+6968
	−175	−161	+12747	+10003
	−168	−210	+10920	+12516
	−159	−255	+8655	+14361
	−148	−295	+6015	+15416
	−135	−329	+3077	+15589
	−120	−356	−68	+14824
	−103	−375	−3315	+13107
	−84	−385	−6545	+10472
	−63	−385	−9625	+7007
	−40	−374	−12408	+2860
	−15	−351	−14733	−1755
	+12	−315	−16425	−6552
	+41	−265	−17295	−11167
	+72	−200	−17140	−15152
	+105	−119	−15743	−17969
	+140	−21	−12873	−18984
	+177	+95	−8285	−17461
	+216	+230	−1720	−12556
	+257	+385	+7095	−3311
	+300	+561	+18447	+11352
	+345	+759	+32637	+32637
D	1,271,256	4,994,220	8,518,474,580	8,629,104,120
λ	1	$\frac{1}{6}$	$\frac{7}{12}$	$\frac{1}{20}$

48	ξ_2'	ξ_3'	ξ_4'	ξ_5'
	575	115	+16445	+82225
	−569	−343	+15873	+242671
	−557	−565	+14743	+391231
	−539	−777	+13083	+520401
	−515	−975	+10935	+623307
	−485	−1155	+8355	+693957
	−449	−1313	+5413	+727493
	−407	−1445	+2193	+720443
	−359	−1547	−1207	+670973
	−305	−1615	−4675	+579139
	−245	−1645	−8085	+447139
	−179	−1633	−11297	+279565
	−107	−1575	−14157	+83655
	−29	−1467	−16497	−130455
	+55	−1305	−18135	−349479
	+145	−1085	−18875	−556729
	+241	−803	−18507	−731863
	+343	−455	−16807	−850633
	+451	−37	−13537	−884633
	+565	+455	−8445	−801047
	+685	+1025	−1265	−562397
	+811	+1677	+8283	−126291
	+943	+2415	+20493	+554829
	+1081	+3243	+35673	+1533939
D	12,712,560	92,620,080	10,301,411,120	19,208,385,771,120
λ	3	$\frac{2}{3}$	$\frac{7}{12}$	$\frac{21}{10}$

ORTHOGONAL POLYNOMIALS

	49			
	ξ_2'	ξ_3'	ξ_4'	ξ_5'
	−200	0	+17940	0
	−199	−299	+17641	+9867
	−196	−593	+16751	+19272
	−191	−877	+15291	+27767
	−184	−1146	+13296	+34932
	−175	−1395	+10815	+40389
	−164	−1619	+7911	+43816
	−151	−1813	+4661	+44961
	−136	−1972	+1156	+43656
	−119	−2091	−2499	+39831
	−100	−2165	−6185	+33528
	−79	−2189	−9769	+24915
	−56	−2158	−13104	+14300
	−31	−2067	−16029	+2145
	−4	−1911	−18369	−10920
	+25	−1685	−19935	−24083
	+56	−1384	−20524	−36336
	+89	−1003	−19919	−46461
	+124	−537	−17889	−53016
	+161	+19	−14189	−54321
	+200	+670	−8560	−48444
	+241	+1421	−729	−33187
	+284	+2277	+9591	−6072
	+329	+3243	+22701	+35673
	+376	+4324	+38916	+95128
D	1,566,040	167,230,700	12,408,517,940	74,451,107,640
λ	1	$\frac{5}{6}$	$\frac{7}{12}$	$\frac{7}{60}$

ORTHOGONAL POLYNOMIALS

	50			
	ξ'_2	ξ'_3	ξ'_4	ξ'_5
	−104	−312	+96876	+10764
	−103	−931	+93771	+31809
	−101	−1535	+87631	+51419
	−98	−2114	+78596	+68684
	−94	−2658	+66876	+82764
	−89	−3157	+52751	+92917
	−83	−3601	+36571	−98527
	−76	−3980	+18756	−99132
	−68	−4284	−204	+94452
	−59	−4503	−19749	+84417
	−49	−4627	−39249	+69195
	−38	−4646	−58004	+49220
	−26	−4550	−75244	+25220
	−13	−4329	−90129	−1755
	+1	−3973	−101749	−30305
	+16	−3472	−109124	−58652
	+32	−2816	−111204	−84612
	+49	−1995	−106869	−105567
	+67	−999	−94929	−118437
	+86	+182	−74124	−119652
	+106	+1558	−43124	−105124
	+127	+3139	−529	−70219
	+149	+4935	+55131	−9729
	+172	+6956	+125396	+82156
	+196	+9212	+211876	+211876
D	433,160	770,715,400	372,255,538,200	372,255,538,200
λ	$\frac{1}{2}$	$\frac{5}{3}$	$\frac{35}{12}$	$\frac{7}{30}$

XII.9 PERCENTAGE POINTS OF PEARSON CURVES

A system of frequency curves, defined by the solutions of the differential equation

$$\frac{dy}{dx} = \frac{y(x + a)}{b_0 + b_1 x + b_2 x^2}$$

was presented by Karl Pearson, and hence has been known as the Pearson distributions, or Pearson curves.

The parameters a, b_0, b_1, and b_2 determine and are determined by the first four moments of a Pearson curve; thus the shape of such a curve is specified completely by $\sqrt{\beta_1}$, β_2, and the information that it is a Pearson curve, where

$$\beta_1 = \frac{\mu_3^2}{\mu_2^3},$$ where μ_i represents the ith population moment around the mean,

and

$$\beta_2 = \frac{\mu_4}{\mu_2^2} \; .$$

This table gives upper and lower percentage points for the Pearson curves. Generally, to obtain the percentage points, a solution for x_α must be obtained from the integral equation

$$\alpha = \int_{l_2}^{x} f(x)\, dx \; ,$$

where $f(x)$ is a particular Pearson distribution, l_2 is the lower limit of x, and α is a given probability level. Then in the body of the tables are the values of

$$X_\alpha = \frac{x_\alpha - \mu}{\sigma}$$

for $\alpha = 0.005, 0.01, 0.025, 0.05, 0.95, 0.975, 0.99$, and 0.995. The ranges of β_1 and β_2 have been extended so as to have $0 \leq \beta_1 \leq 1.8$ and $1.2 \leq \beta_2 \leq 6.6$. This extension also allows coverage of the J and U-shaped curves.

The tables are presented assuming that $\mu_3 > 0$, i.e., the distributions are assumed to be positively skewed (long tail at right). The upper percentage points ($\alpha > 0.50$) are positive and the lower percentage points ($\alpha < 0.50$) are negative.

If $\mu_3 < 0$, the roles of the tables must be interchanged. That is to say, if $\mu_3 < 0$ and the lower percentage points are desired, i.e., $\alpha < 0.50$, obtain the value desired from the tabled upper percentage points, attaching a negative sign; and if $\mu_3 < 0$ and the upper percentage points are desired, i.e., $\alpha > 0.50$, then read the desired value from the tabled lower percentage points, attaching a positive sign.

PERCENTAGE POINTS OF PEARSON CURVES

Upper 5% points of the standardized deviate $(x_\alpha - \mu)/\sigma$, $(\alpha = 0.95)$.

β_2 \ β_1	0.00	0.01	0.03	0.05	0.10	0.15	0.20	0.30	0.40	0.50	0.60	0.70
1.2	1.1547	1.2056	1.2326	1.2458	1.2579							
1.4	1.3191	1.3781	1.4106	1.4271	1.4438	1.4436	1.4348	1.4042				
1.6	1.4638	1.5249	1.5618	1.5832	1.6128	1.6249	1.6258	1.6031	1.5604			
1.8	1.5588	1.6151	1.6517	1.6751	1.7138	1.7390	1.7558	1.7687	1.7546	1.7153	1.6598	1.6005
2.0	1.6108	1.6602	1.6941	1.7168	1.7576	1.7881	1.8129	1.8503	1.8721	1.8748	1.8538	1.8078
2.2	1.6361	1.6793	1.7100	1.7310	1.7702	1.8011	1.8279	1.8741	1.9127	1.9426	1.9606	1.9609
2.4	1.6467	1.6849	1.7126	1.7318	1.7682	1.7977	1.8238	1.8709	1.9138	1.9535	1.9888	2.0174
2.6	1.6495	1.6837	1.7088	1.7263	1.7600	1.7874	1.8119	1.8569	1.8991	1.9400	1.9799	2.0181
2.8	1.6483	1.6792	1.7021	1.7183	1.7493	1.7746	1.7975	1.8394	1.8792	1.9183	1.9574	1.9968
3.0	1.6449	1.6733	1.6944	1.7093	1.7380	1.7616	1.7827	1.8216	1.8585	1.8949	1.9317	1.9690
3.2						1.7488	1.7686	1.8046	1.8388	1.8724	1.9064	1.9410
3.4								1.7890	1.8207	1.8517	1.8830	1.9148
3.6									1.8041	1.8330	1.8618	1.8911
3.8										1.8160	1.8428	1.8698
4.0											1.8258	1.8508
4.2												1.8338

β_2 \ β_1	0.80	0.90	1.00	1.10	1.20	1.30	1.40	1.50	1.60	1.70	1.80
2.0	1.7453	1.6803									
2.2	1.9377	1.8886	1.8221	1.7532							
2.4	2.0350	2.0354	2.0119	1.9614	1.8924	1.8210					
2.6	2.0531	2.0822	2.1007	2.1022	2.0792	2.0285	1.9580	1.8847			
2.8	2.0360	2.0743	2.1100	2.1402	2.1602	2.1632	2.1415	2.0910	2.0197	1.9451	
3.0	2.0073	2.0464	2.0859	2.1249	2.1618	2.1935	2.2152	2.2200	2.1997	2.1499	2.0782
3.2	1.9767	2.0136	2.0518	2.0912	2.1314	2.1715	2.2096	2.2429	2.2665	2.2732	2.2547
3.4	1.9476	1.9816	2.0170	2.0540	2.0926	2.1325	2.1736	2.2147	2.2543	2.2893	2.3148
3.6	1.9211	1.9523	1.9847	2.0185	2.0541	2.0913	2.1304	2.1711	2.2130	2.2554	2.2965
3.8	1.8975	1.9259	1.9555	1.9864	2.0187	2.0526	2.0884	2.1261	2.1658	2.2073	2.2503
4.0	1.8763	1.9026	1.9296	1.9577	1.9871	2.0179	2.0503	2.0846	2.1207	2.1589	2.1993
4.2	1.8575	1.8817	1.9067	1.9324	1.9592	1.9872	2.0166	2.0475	2.0801	2.1146	2.1511
4.4	1.8407	1.8631	1.8861	1.9100	1.9345	1.9601	1.9868	2.0148	2.0443	2.0753	2.1082
4.6		1.8466	1.8679	1.8899	1.9126	1.9361	1.9606	1.9861	2.0128	2.0409	2.0704
4.8			1.8517	1.8722	1.8932	1.9148	1.9374	1.9608	1.9852	2.0107	2.0374
5.0				1.8562	1.8758	1.8959	1.9166	1.9383	1.9607	1.9840	2.0084
5.2					1.8602	1.8790	1.8983	1.9184	1.9389	1.9606	1.9828
5.4						1.8637	1.8817	1.9003	1.9197	1.9396	1.9602
5.6							1.8670	1.8844	1.9023	1.9203	1.9399
5.8							1.8531	1.8699	1.8867	1.9040	1.9217
6.0								1.8567	1.8725	1.8887	1.9054
6.2									1.8596	1.8749	1.8906
6.4										1.8623	1.8771
6.6											1.8647

PERCENTAGE POINTS OF PEARSON CURVES

Lower 5% points of the standardized deviate $(x_\alpha - \mu)/\sigma$, ($\alpha = 0.05$). Note that for positive skewness, i.e., $\mu_3 > 0$, the deviates in this table are negative.

β_2 \ β_1	0.00	0.01	0.03	0.05	0.10	0.15	0.20	0.30	0.40	0.50	0.60	0.70
1.2	1.1547	1.0899	1.0355	0.9954								
1.4	1.3191	1.2450	1.1828	1.1368	1.0477	0.9771	0.9170					
1.6	1.4639	1.3899	1.3270	1.2794	1.1839	1.1055	1.0380	0.9254	0.8331			
1.8	1.5588	1.4936	1.4384	1.3960	1.3078	1.2312	1.1614	1.0389	0.9365	0.8497	0.7746	
2.0	1.6108	1.5556	1.5097	1.4746	1.4007	1.3342	1.2710	1.1516	1.0433	0.9483	0.8656	0.7934
2.2	1.6361	1.5893	1.5513	1.5226	1.4622	1.4074	1.3544	1.2494	1.1463	1.0485	0.9595	0.8806
2.4	1.6467	1.6064	1.5743	1.5504	1.5006	1.4559	1.4124	1.3247	1.2342	1.1427	1.0534	0.9699
2.6	1.6495	1.6141	1.5864	1.5659	1.5241	1.4870	1.4511	1.3786	1.3025	1.2223	1.1397	1.0576
2.8	1.6483	1.6165	1.5921	1.5742	1.5382	1.5067	1.4766	1.4162	1.3526	1.2845	1.2121	1.1367
3.0	1.6449	1.6160	1.5940	1.5781	1.5464	1.5192	1.4933	1.4422	1.3887	1.3313	1.2693	1.2030
3.2						1.5264	1.5043	1.4602	1.4145	1.3658	1.3130	1.2558
3.4								1.4727	1.4331	1.3912	1.3460	1.2969
3.6									1.4466	1.4100	1.3709	1.3285
3.8										1.4241	1.3900	1.3528
4.0											1.4042	1.3716
4.2												1.3862

β_2 \ β_1	0.80	0.90	1.00	1.10	1.20	1.30	1.40	1.50	1.60	1.70	1.80
2.2	0.8107	0.7484									
2.4	0.8944	0.8267	0.7659	0.7109							
2.6	0.9792	0.9068	0.8412	0.7820	0.7282	0.6788					
2.8	1.0608	0.9872	0.9179	0.8545	0.7966	0.7440	0.6956	0.6509			
3.0	1.1337	1.0632	0.9938	0.9277	0.8663	0.8100	0.7584	0.7110	0.6672		
3.2	1.1947	1.1304	1.0646	0.9993	0.9362	0.8769	0.8222	0.7716	0.7251	0.6820	0.6419
3.4	1.2437	1.1868	1.1269	1.0653	1.0036	0.9435	0.8863	0.8332	0.7836	0.7380	0.6957
3.6	1.2824	1.2326	1.1793	1.1232	1.0652	1.0069	0.9496	0.8946	0.8427	0.7946	0.7498
3.8	1.3127	1.2692	1.2222	1.1720	1.1192	1.0646	1.0093	0.9546	0.9017	0.8514	0.8046
4.0	1.3363	1.2982	1.2569	1.2124	1.1650	1.1151	1.0634	1.0109	0.9587	0.9078	0.8591
4.2	1.3550	1.3212	1.2848	1.2454	1.2031	1.1581	1.1108	1.0617	1.0117	0.9618	0.9129
4.4	1.3698	1.3400	1.3072	1.2722	1.2346	1.1943	1.1514	1.1064	1.0596	1.0120	0.9642
4.6		1.3545	1.3254	1.2938	1.2605	1.2244	1.1857	1.1448	1.1018	1.0572	1.0117
4.8			1.3403	1.3121	1.2819	1.2494	1.2145	1.1775	1.1383	1.0971	1.0545
5.0				1.3268	1.2995	1.2701	1.2387	1.2052	1.1695	1.1318	1.0924
5.2					1.3142	1.2876	1.2591	1.2286	1.1962	1.1618	1.1255
5.4						1.3022	1.2762	1.2484	1.2189	1.1875	1.1542
5.6							1.2907	1.2653	1.2383	1.2092	1.1790
5.8							1.3030	1.2797	1.2549	1.2285	1.2005
6.0								1.2920	1.2691	1.2448	1.2190
6.2									1.2814	1.2589	1.2351
6.4										1.2711	1.2490
6.6											1.2612

PERCENTAGE POINTS OF PEARSON CURVES

Upper 2.5% points of the standardized variate $(x_\alpha - \mu)/\sigma$, $(\alpha = 0.975)$.

β_2 \ β_1	0.00	0.01	0.03	0.05	0.10	0.15	0.20	0.30	0.40	0.50	0.60	0.70
1.2	1.1547	1.2056	1.2326	1.2458	1.2579							
1.4	1.3223	1.3823	1.4144	1.4303	1.4453	1.4440	1.4348	1.4042				
1.6	1.4955	1.5631	1.6012	1.6214	1.6439	1.6472	1.6397	1.6060	1.5604			
1.8	1.6454	1.7149	1.7567	1.7809	1.8146	1.8295	1.8330	1.8157	1.7746	1.7195	1.6598	1.6005
2.0	1.7567	1.8233	1.8657	1.8918	1.9331	1.9581	1.9735	1.9833	1.9691	1.9330	1.8785	1.8131
2.2	1.8332	1.8953	1.9363	1.9626	2.0071	2.0377	2.0605	2.0902	2.1024	2.0968	2.0723	2.0279
2.4	1.8847	1.9422	1.9811	2.0066	2.0516	2.0842	2.1106	2.1511	2.1793	2.1959	2.1997	2.1881
2.6	1.9197	1.9727	2.0094	2.0338	2.0778	2.1108	2.1383	2.1834	2.2197	2.2485	2.2695	2.2813
2.8	1.9434	1.9928	2.0273	2.0507	2.0930	2.1254	2.1529	2.1995	2.2391	2.2735	2.3032	2.3277
3.0	1.9600	2.0060	2.0387	2.0609	2.1016	2.1330	2.1600	2.2062	2.2466	2.2832	2.3167	2.3471
3.2						2.1362	2.1623	2.2076	2.2476	2.2845	2.3192	2.3420
3.4								2.2060	2.2450	2.2813	2.3159	2.3492
3.6									2.2404	2.2758	2.3096	2.3424
3.8										2.2690	2.3018	2.3338
4.0											2.2935	2.3243
4.2												2.3147

β_2 \ β_1	0.80	0.90	1.00	1.10	1.20	1.30	1.40	1.50	1.60	1.70	1.80
2.0	1.7455	1.6803									
2.2	1.9664	1.8949	1.8223	1.7532							
2.4	2.1586	2.1098	2.0441	1.9687	1.8928	1.8210					
2.6	2.2813	2.2667	2.2344	2.1829	2.1145	2.0366	1.9584	1.8847			
2.8	2.3456	2.3551	2.3532	2.3368	2.3028	2.2496	2.1795	2.0998	2.0201	1.9451	
3.0	2.3741	2.3966	2.4130	2.4212	2.4183	2.4009	2.3658	2.3115	2.2402	2.1594	2.0787
3.2	2.3829	2.4115	2.4371	2.4580	2.4743	2.4819	2.4783	2.4003	2.4245	2.3695	2.2975
3.4	2.3814	2.4124	2.4421	2.4698	2.4947	2.5158	2.5311	2.5383	2.5345	2.5161	2.4799
3.6	2.3745	2.4061	2.4371	2.4672	2.4963	2.5236	2.5483	2.5692	2.5843	2.5915	2.5874
3.8	2.3653	2.3964	2.4273	2.4580	2.4883	2.5181	2.5468	2.5740	2.5987	2.6195	2.6347
4.0	2.3548	2.3851	2.4153	2.4456	2.4759	2.5061	2.5363	2.5657	2.5946	2.6218	2.6465
4.2	2.3441	2.3734	2.4027	2.4321	2.4616	2.4914	2.5214	2.5514	2.5814	2.6111	2.6400
4.4	2.3336	2.3617	2.3900	2.4183	2.4468	2.4757	2.5050	2.5345	2.5644	2.5945	2.6244
4.6			2.3776	2.4047	2.4323	2.4600	2.4882	2.5168	2.5460	2.5755	2.6054
4.8			2.3657	2.3918	2.4182	2.4448	2.4720	2.4996	2.5276	2.5561	2.5851
5.0				2.3797	2.4050	2.4304	2.4565	2.4829	2.5098	2.5371	2.5651
5.2					2.3925	2.4170	2.4418	2.4673	2.4928	2.5190	2.5458
5.4						2.4043	2.4281	2.4523	2.4769	2.5019	2.5275
5.6							2.4152	2.4385	2.4621	2.4859	2.5100
5.8							2.4033	2.4256	2.4482	2.4711	2.4941
6.0								2.4136	2.4352	2.4573	2.4795
6.2									2.4232	2.4444	2.4659
6.4										2.4324	2.4530
6.6											2.4410

PERCENTAGE POINTS OF PEARSON CURVES

Lower 2.5% points of the standardized deviate $(x_\alpha - \mu)/\sigma$, $(\alpha = 0.025)$. Note: If $\mu_3 > 0$, the variates in this table are negative.

β_2 \ β_1	0.00	0.01	0.03	0.05	0.10	0.15	0.20	0.30	0.40	0.50	0.60	0.70
1.2	1.1547	1.0899	1.0355	0.9954								
1.4	1.3223	1.2461	1.1835	1.1371	1.0477	0.9771	0.9170					
1.6	1.4955	1.4115	1.3409	1.2886	1.1870	1.1064	1.0381	0.9254	0.8331			
1.8	1.6454	1.5615	1.4906	1.4372	1.3304	1.2426	1.1665	1.0396	0.9365	0.8497		
2.0	1.7567	1.6785	1.6129	1.5631	1.4613	1.3744	1.2962	1.1595	1.0448	0.9483	0.8656	0.7934
2.2	1.8332	1.7625	1.7037	1.6593	1.5677	1.4879	1.4139	1.2782	1.1572	1.0514	0.9600	0.8806
2.4	1.8847	1.8210	1.7688	1.7295	1.6488	1.5779	1.5114	1.3852	1.2665	1.1568	1.0581	0.9710
2.6	1.9197	1.8616	1.8149	1.7801	1.7089	1.6465	1.5878	1.4746	1.3645	1.2579	1.1571	1.0644
2.8	1.9434	1.8903	1.8481	1.8167	1.7533	1.6983	1.6464	1.5463	1.4471	1.3482	1.2508	1.1573
3.0	1.9600	1.9109	1.8722	1.8437	1.7866	1.7374	1.6914	1.6027	1.5143	1.4248	1.3344	1.2445
3.2						1.7674	1.7260	1.6469	1.5682	1.4880	1.4057	1.3222
3.4								1.6818	1.6112	1.5394	1.4653	1.3890
3.6									1.6458	1.5811	1.5144	1.4452
3.8										1.6152	1.5548	1.4922
4.0											1.5883	1.5313
4.2												1.5640

β_2 \ β_1	0.80	0.90	1.00	1.10	1.20	1.30	1.40	1.50	1.60	1.70	1.80
2.2	0.8107	0.7484									
2.4	0.8944	0.8267	0.7659	0.7109							
2.6	0.9811	0.9072	0.8412	0.7820	0.7282	0.6788					
2.8	1.0700	0.9903	0.9189	0.8545	0.7966	0.7440	0.6956				
3.0	1.1573	1.0747	0.9985	0.9292	0.8666	0.8100	0.7584	0.7110	0.6672		
3.2	1.2386	1.1568	1.0786	1.0055	0.9385	0.8776	0.8222	0.7716	0.7251	0.6820	0.6419
3.4	1.3112	1.2329	1.1558	1.0815	1.0115	0.9467	0.8874	0.8332	0.7836	0.7380	0.6957
3.6	1.3738	1.3009	1.2272	1.1544	1.0837	1.0166	0.9540	0.8962	0.8433	0.7946	0.7498
3.8	1.4272	1.3600	1.2911	1.2215	1.1524	1.0851	1.0207	0.9602	0.9040	0.8524	0.8046
4.0	1.4722	1.4106	1.3470	1.2818	1.2158	1.1501	1.0858	1.0240	0.9655	0.9109	0.8603
4.2	1.5100	1.4537	1.3952	1.3348	1.2728	1.2100	1.1474	1.0858	1.0264	0.9699	0.9169
4.4	1.5420	1.4900	1.4366	1.3806	1.3231	1.2640	1.2041	1.1443	1.0853	1.0282	0.9736
4.6			1.4721	1.4200	1.3671	1.3118	1.2555	1.1982	1.1409	1.0844	1.0293
4.8			1.5026	1.4549	1.4055	1.3541	1.3012	1.2470	1.1922	1.1372	1.0829
5.0				1.4847	1.4389	1.3905	1.3417	1.2908	1.2387	1.1861	1.1333
5.2					1.4679	1.4235	1.3773	1.3297	1.2808	1.2306	1.1800
5.4						1.4519	1.4089	1.3643	1.3183	1.2710	1.2227
5.6							1.4366	1.3948	1.3517	1.3073	1.2612
5.8							1.4611	1.4220	1.3814	1.3395	1.2959
6.0								1.4460	1.4079	1.3685	1.3277
6.2									1.4315	1.3943	1.3559
6.4										1.4176	1.3812
6.6											1.4041

PERCENTAGE POINTS OF PEARSON CURVES

Upper 1% points of the standardized deviate $(x_\alpha - \mu)/\sigma$, $(\alpha = 0.99)$.

β_2 \ β_1	0.00	0.01	0.03	0.05	0.10	0.15	0.20	0.30	0.40	0.50	0.60	0.70
1.2	1.1547	1.2056	1.2326	1.2458								
1.4	1.3229	1.3831	1.4151	1.4308	1.4453	1.4440	1.4348					
1.6	1.5079	1.5786	1.6169	1.6359	1.6543	1.6535	1.6428	1.6063	1.5604			
1.8	1.6974	1.7764	1.8208	1.8444	1.8713	1.8762	1.8688	1.8320	1.7791	1.7200	1.6598	
2.0	1.8687	1.9511	1.9999	2.0274	2.0644	2.0794	2.0815	2.0601	2.0145	1.9532	1.8841	1.8137
2.2	2.0097	2.0918	2.1425	2.1726	2.2175	2.2418	2.2541	2.2548	2.2304	2.1855	2.1238	2.0507
2.4	2.1207	2.2004	2.2512	2.2826	2.3323	2.3632	2.3835	2.4030	2.4009	2.3798	2.3408	2.2848
2.6	2.2067	2.2833	2.3333	2.3649	2.4172	2.4521	2.4775	2.5103	2.5253	2.5249	2.5096	2.4785
2.8	2.2737	2.3469	2.3957	2.4270	2.4803	2.5174	2.5459	2.5872	2.6136	2.6280	2.6308	2.6215
3.0	2.3263	2.3963	2.4436	2.4744	2.5278	2.5659	2.5961	2.6424	2.6763	2.7003	2.7155	2.7217
3.2						2.6025	2.6336	2.6829	2.7211	2.7513	2.7745	2.7911
3.4								2.7129	2.7536	2.7875	2.8158	2.8390
3.6									2.7775	2.8137	2.8450	2.8723
3.8										2.8327	2.8659	2.8957
4.0											2.8809	2.9122
4.2												2.9237

β_2 \ β_1	0.80	0.90	1.00	1.10	1.20	1.30	1.40	1.50	1.60	1.70	1.80
2.0	1.7455										
2.2	1.9727	1.8956	1.8223								
2.4	2.2144	2.1344	2.0508	1.9694	1.8928						
2.6	2.4315	2.3690	2.2932	2.2087	2.1215	2.0373	1.9584				
2.8	2.5991	2.5621	2.5101	2.4432	2.3637	2.2762	2.1867	2.1006	2.0201		
3.0	2.7183	2.7037	2.6767	2.6358	2.5801	2.5101	2.4281	2.3386	2.2476	2.1602	2.0787
3.2	2.8005	2.8021	2.7945	2.7763	2.7461	2.7022	2.6439	2.5716	2.4877	2.9369	2.3049
3.4	2.8569	2.8692	2.8751	2.8734	2.8630	2.8421	2.8094	2.7631	2.7028	2.6287	2.5435
3.6	2.8957	2.9149	2.9295	2.9388	2.9421	2.9383	2.9257	2.9028	2.8679	2.8198	2.7577
3.8	2.9225	2.9459	2.9662	2.9827	2.9952	3.0026	2.0040	2.9983	2.9838	2.9592	2.9227
4.0	2.9409	2.9672	2.9910	3.0121	3.0303	3.0449	3.0559	3.0616	3.0616	3.0543	3.0384
4.2	2.9537	2.9818	3.0077	3.0318	3.0536	3.0731	3.0898	3.1032	3.1126	3.1171	3.1159
4.4	2.9623	2.9912	3.0186	3.0444	3.0686	3.0911	3.1118	3.1299	3.1455	3.1579	3.1661
4.6			3.0255	3.0525	3.0783	3.1023	3.1255	3.1468	3.1662	3.1836	3.1982
4.8			3.0301	3.0575	3.0837	3.1090	3.1334	3.1568	3.1789	3.1995	3.2179
5.0				3.0601	3.0869	3.1123	3.1377	3.1623	3.1859	3.2084	3.2296
5.2					3.0876	3.1140	3.1400	3.1647	3.1894	3.2128	3.2356
5.4						3.1138	3.1395	3.1647	3.1896	3.2138	3.2379
5.6							3.1381	3.1636	3.1885	3.2131	3.2372
5.8							3.1356	3.1611	3.1860	3.2110	3.2349
6.0								3.1583	3.1830	3.2073	3.2320
6.2									3.1789	3.2033	3.2278
6.4										3.1991	3.2231
6.6											3.2179

PERCENTAGE POINTS OF PEARSON CURVES

Lower 1% points of the standardized variate $(x_\alpha - \mu)/\sigma$, $(\alpha = 0.01)$. Note: If $\mu_3 > 0$, the deviates in this table are negative.

$\beta_2 \backslash \beta_1$	0.00	0.01	0.03	0.05	0.10	0.15	0.20	0.30	0.40	0.50	0.60	0.70
1.2	1.1547	1.0899	1.0355	0.9954								
1.4	1.3229	1.2468	1.1835	1.1371	1.0477	0.9771	0.9170					
1.6	1.5079	1.4192	1.3453	1.2912	1.1876	1.1064	1.0381	0.9254	0.8331			
1.8	1.6974	1.5996	1.5176	1.4569	1.3393	1.2462	1.1678	1.0396	0.9365	0.8497		
2.0	1.8687	1.7685	1.6842	1.6212	1.4963	1.3946	1.3070	1.1617	1.0451	0.9483	0.8656	0.7934
2.2	2.0097	1.9121	1.8304	1.7689	1.6450	1.5413	1.4494	1.2915	1.1609	1.0521	0.9600	0.8806
2.4	2.1207	2.0279	1.9509	1.8929	1.7753	1.6751	1.5844	1.4226	1.2825	1.1621	1.0594	0.9712
2.6	2.2067	2.1193	2.0475	1.9936	1.8842	1.7904	1.7042	1.5466	1.4042	1.2766	1.1642	1.0665
2.8	2.2737	2.1915	2.1244	2.0745	1.9734	1.8866	1.8065	1.6576	1.5190	1.3901	1.2722	1.1665
3.0	2.3263	2.2488	2.1861	2.1397	2.0461	1.9660	1.8920	1.7535	1.6223	1.4968	1.3783	1.2684
3.2						2.0314	1.9631	1.8350	1.7124	1.5934	1.4782	1.3681
3.4								1.9037	1.7900	1.6785	1.5688	1.4617
3.6									1.8562	1.7522	1.6492	1.5470
3.8										1.8159	1.7196	1.6232
4.0											1.7809	1.6899
4.2												1.7495

$\beta_2 \backslash \beta_1$	0.80	0.90	1.00	1.10	1.20	1.30	1.40	1.50	1.60	1.70	1.80
2.2	0.8107	0.7484									
2.4	0.8944	0.8267	0.7659	0.7109							
2.6	0.9816	0.9072	0.8412	0.7820	0.7282						
2.8	1.0731	0.9912	0.9189	0.8545	0.7966	0.7440	0.6956				
3.0	1.1684	1.0790	0.9998	0.9295	0.8666	0.8100	0.7584	0.7110	0.6672		
3.2	1.2648	1.1699	1.0842	1.0075	0.9391	0.8776	0.8222	0.7716	0.7251	0.6820	0.6419
3.4	1.3586	1.2612	1.1709	1.0885	1.0143	0.9477	0.8876	0.8332	0.7836	0.7380	0.6957
3.6	1.4467	1.3497	1.2574	1.1713	1.0921	1.0202	0.9552	0.8966	0.8433	0.7946	0.7498
3.8	1.5274	1.4329	1.3411	1.2534	1.1710	1.0948	1.0252	0.9619	0.9046	0.8524	0.8046
4.0	1.5997	1.5092	1.4199	1.3327	1.2492	1.1703	1.0969	1.0294	0.9678	0.9119	0.8606
4.2	1.6640	1.5781	1.4923	1.4074	1.3245	1.2446	1.1690	1.0982	1.0329	0.9729	0.9181
4.4	1.7208	1.6394	1.5580	1.4763	1.3954	1.3162	1.2399	1.1672	1.0989	1.0355	0.9772
4.6			1.6171	1.5390	1.4611	1.3838	1.3081	1.2347	1.1649	1.0990	1.0376
4.8			1.6699	1.5958	1.5213	1.4466	1.3725	1.2999	1.2296	1.1622	1.0986
5.0				1.6469	1.5757	1.5034	1.4325	1.3614	1.2916	1.2240	1.1591
5.2					1.6251	1.5567	1.4879	1.4185	1.3507	1.2836	1.2183
5.4						1.6045	1.5386	1.4720	1.4059	1.3400	1.2754
5.6							1.5848	1.5211	1.4569	1.3930	1.3295
5.8							1.6268	1.5658	1.5043	1.4424	1.3806
6.0								1.6068	1.5477	1.4880	1.4282
6.2									1.5875	1.5302	1.4724
6.4										1.5690	1.5133
6.6											1.5511

PERCENTAGE POINTS OF PEARSON CURVES

Upper 0.5% points of the standardized deviate $(x_\alpha - \mu)/\sigma$, (α = .095).

β_2 \ β_1	0.00	0.01	0.03	0.05	0.10	0.15	0.20	0.30	0.40	0.50	0.60	0.70
1.2	1.1547	1.2056	1.2326	1.2458								
1.4	1.3229	1.3831	1.4151	1.4308	1.4453	1.4440	1.4348					
1.6	1.5105	1.5820	1.6202	1.6388	1.6561	1.6543	1.6432	1.6063	1.5604			
1.8	1.7147	1.7974	1.8426	1.8655	1.8888	1.8893	1.8778	1.8350	1.7796	1.7200	1.6598	
2.0	1.9175	2.0079	2.0594	2.0870	2.1197	2.1278	2.1219	2.0844	2.0259	1.9569	1.8847	1.8137
2.2	2.1006	2.1946	2.2502	2.2818	2.3242	2.3420	2.3456	2.3250	2.2784	2.2133	2.1366	2.0547
2.4	2.2562	2.3506	2.4084	2.4426	2.4928	2.5192	2.5322	2.5319	2.5052	2.4577	2.3928	2.3145
2.6	2.3846	2.4776	2.5362	2.5719	2.6273	2.6603	2.6810	2.6981	2.6914	2.6652	2.6212	2.5607
2.8	2.4896	2.5805	2.6389	2.6753	2.7340	2.7715	2.7976	2.8280	2.8377	2.8304	2.8072	2.7687
3.0	2.5758	2.6639	2.7217	2.7583	2.8188	2.8594	2.8893	2.9292	2.9509	2.9580	2.9521	2.9333
3.2						2.9294	2.9620	3.0084	3.0386	3.0566	3.0636	3.0601
3.4								3.0712	3.1075	3.1329	3.1492	3.1570
3.6									3.1618	3.1928	3.2157	3.2317
3.8										3.2397	3.2680	3.2898
4.0											3.3092	3.3352
4.2												3.3711

β_2 \ β_1	0.80	0.90	1.00	1.10	1.20	1.30	1.40	1.50	1.60	1.70	1.80
2.0	1.7455										
2.2	1.9733	1.8956	1.8223								
2.4	2.2278	2.1385	2.0515	1.9694	1.8928						
2.6	2.4858	2.3996	2.3069	2.2129	2.1222	2.0373	1.9584				
2.8	2.7151	2.6466	2.5653	2.4741	2.3774	2.2804	2.1875	2.1006			
3.0	2.9010	2.8550	2.7950	2.7213	2.6356	2.5409	2.4415	2.3426	2.2483	2.1602	
3.2	3.0456	3.0197	2.9815	2.9300	2.8655	2.7879	2.6990	2.6019	2.5008	2.4007	2.3056
3.4	3.1561	3.1460	3.1258	3.0949	3.0522	2.9971	2.9289	2.8484	2.7572	2.6583	2.5562
3.6	3.2406	3.2421	3.2360	3.2213	3.1972	3.1624	3.1163	3.0579	2.9869	2.9041	2.8111
3.8	3.3055	3.3158	3.3200	3.3173	3.3072	3.2890	3.2617	3.2239	3.1748	3.1138	3.0406
4.0	3.3565	3.3726	3.3841	3.3902	3.3909	3.3848	3.3717	3.3510	3.3208	3.2805	3.2291
4.2	3.3962	3.4173	3.4339	3.4464	3.4346	3.4579	3.4556	3.4468	3.4318	3.4083	3.3759
4.4	3.4279	3.4513	3.4724	3.4899	3.5038	3.5137	3.5192	3.5202	3.5155	3.5051	3.4875
4.6			3.5031	3.5241	3.5419	3.5564	3.5677	3.5756	3.5793	3.5782	3.5718
4.8			3.5275	3.5510	3.5714	3.5900	3.6053	3.6183	3.6277	3.6335	3.6354
5.0				3.5721	3.5948	3.6156	3.6342	3.6512	3.6647	3.6760	3.6840
5.2					3.6136	3.6364	3.6569	3.6764	3.6937	3.7084	3.7206
5.4						3.6524	3.6755	3.6969	3.7155	3.7328	3.7493
5.6							3.6900	3.7116	3.7333	3.7528	3.7709
5.8							3.7008	3.7245	3.7467	3.7681	3.7873
6.0								3.7341	3.7572	3.7796	3.8010
6.2									3.7645	3.7885	3.8111
6.4										3.7959	3.8183
6.6											3.8247

PERCENTAGE POINTS OF PEARSON CURVES

Lower 0.5% points of the standardized deviate $(x_\alpha - \mu)/\sigma$, $(\alpha = 0.005)$. Note: If $\mu_3 > 0$, the variates in this table are negative.

β_2 \ β_1	0.00	0.01	0.03	0.05	0.10	0.15	0.20	0.30	0.40	0.50	0.60	0.70
1.2	1.1547	1.0899	1.0355	0.9954								
1.4	1.3229	1.2468	1.1835	1.1371	1.0477	0.9771	0.9170					
1.6	1.5105	1.4206	1.3459	1.2915	1.1876	1.1064	1.0381	0.9254	0.8331			
1.8	1.7147	1.6113	1.5252	1.4620	1.3411	1.2468	1.1680	1.0396	0.9365	0.8497		
2.0	1.9175	1.8057	1.7120	1.6426	1.5075	1.4001	1.3096	1.1621	1.0451	0.9483	0.8656	0.7934
2.2	1.1006	1.9864	1.8906	1.8190	1.6770	1.5612	1.4613	1.2949	1.1615	1.0521	0.9600	0.8806
2.4	2.2562	2.1437	2.0496	1.9791	1.8375	1.7195	1.6152	1.4356	1.2869	1.1632	1.0596	0.9712
2.6	2.3846	2.2758	2.1854	2.1176	1.9809	1.8654	1.7616	1.5774	1.4185	1.2820	1.1658	1.0668
2.8	2.4896	2.3851	2.2990	2.2348	2.1050	1.9946	1.8943	1.7126	1.5502	1.4056	1.2787	1.1687
3.0	2.5758	2.4758	2.3939	2.3330	2.2105	2.1062	2.0110	1.8362	1.6760	1.5287	1.3952	1.2760
3.2						2.2017	2.1120	1.9460	1.7915	1.6462	1.5107	1.3860
3.4								2.0422	1.8951	1.7547	1.6210	1.4947
3.6									1.9869	1.8528	1.7232	1.5986
3.8										1.9400	1.8161	1.6952
4.0											1.8997	1.7836
4.2												1.8634

β_2 \ β_1	0.80	0.90	1.00	1.10	1.20	1.30	1.40	1.50	1.60	1.70	1.80
2.2	0.8107	0.7484									
2.4	0.8944	0.8267	0.7659	0.7109							
2.6	0.9816	0.9072	0.8412	0.7820	0.7282						
2.8	1.0736	0.9912	0.9189	0.8545	0.7966	0.7440	0.6956				
3.0	1.1713	1.0799	1.0000	0.9295	0.8666	0.8100	0.7584	0.7110	0.6672		
3.2	1.2735	1.1735	1.0854	1.0079	0.9391	0.8776	0.8222	0.7716	0.7251	0.6820	0.6419
3.4	1.3776	1.2710	1.1752	1.0901	1.0148	0.9477	0.8876	0.8332	0.7836	0.7380	0.6957
3.6	1.4803	1.3697	1.2682	1.1763	1.0941	1.0208	0.9554	0.8966	0.8433	0.7946	0.7498
3.8	1.5783	1.4667	1.3619	1.2650	1.1768	1.0974	1.0261	0.9623	0.9046	0.8524	0.8046
4.0	1.6700	1.5596	1.4538	1.3542	1.2616	1.1768	1.0999	1.0306	0.9682	0.9119	0.8606
4.2	1.7540	1.6465	1.5420	1.4416	1.3465	1.2578	1.1761	1.1017	1.0343	0.9734	0.9183
4.4	1.8305	1.7263	1.6246	1.5254	1.4296	1.3388	1.2536	1.1749	1.1029	1.0373	0.9779
4.6			1.7014	1.6041	1.5094	1.4180	1.3309	1.2491	1.1732	1.1034	1.0397
4.8			1.7718	1.6774	1.5848	1.4941	1.4064	1.3230	1.2443	1.1710	1.1034
5.0				1.7453	1.6550	1.5661	1.4793	1.3953	1.3150	1.2391	1.1684
5.2					1.7202	1.6336	1.5483	1.4648	1.3842	1.3070	1.2338
5.4						1.6964	1.6132	1.5312	1.4509	1.3731	1.2987
5.6							1.6737	1.5935	1.5144	1.4373	1.3624
5.8							1.7298	1.6519	1.5746	1.4984	1.4238
6.0								1.7061	1.6309	1.5563	1.4827
6.2									1.6836	1.6108	1.5385
6.4										1.6618	1.5912
6.6											1.6408

XIII. Miscellaneous Mathematical Tables

XIII.1 MISCELLANEOUS CONSTANTS

π CONSTANTS

π = 3.14159 26535 89793 23846 26433 83279 50288 41971 69399 37511
$1/\pi$ = 0.31830 98861 83790 67153 77675 26745 02872 40689 19291 48091
π^2 = 9.86960 44010 89358 61883 44909 99876 15113 53136 99407 24079
$\log_e \pi$ = 1.14472 98858 49400 17414 34273 51353 05871 16472 94812 91531
$\log_{10} \pi$ = 0.49714 98726 94133 85435 12682 88290 89887 36516 78324 38044
$\log_{10} \sqrt{2\pi}$ = 0.39908 99341 79057 52478 25035 91507 69595 02099 34102 92127

LOGARITHMIC CONSTANTS

e = 2.71828 18284 59045 23536 02874 71352 66249 77572 47093 69996
$1/e$ = 0.36787 94411 71442 32159 55237 70161 46086 74458 11131 03176
e^2 = 7.38905 60989 30650 22723 04274 60575 00781 31803 15570 55184
$M = \log_{10} e$ = 0.43429 44819 03251 82765 11289 18916 60508 22943 97005 80366
$1/M = \log_e 10$ = 2.30258 50929 94045 68401 79914 54684 36420 76011 01488 62877
$\log_{10} M$ = 9.63778 43113 00536 78912 29674 98565 − 10

MISCELLANEOUS π AND e CONSTANTS

π^e = 22.45915 77183 61045 47342 71522
e^π = 23.14069 26327 79269 00572 90864
$e^{-\pi}$ = 0.04321 39182 63772 24977 44177
$e^{\frac{1}{2}\pi}$ = 4.81047 73809 65351 65547 30357
$i^i = e^{-\frac{1}{2}\pi}$ = 0.20787 95763 50761 90854 69556

NUMERICAL CONSTANTS

$\sqrt{2}$ = 1.41421 35623 73095 04880 16887 24209 69807 85696 71875 37694
$\sqrt[3]{2}$ = 1.25992 10498 94873 16476 72106 07278 22835 05702 51464 70150
$\log_e 2$ = 0.69314 71805 59945 30941 72321 21458 17656 80755 00134 36025
$\log_{10} 2$ = 0.30102 99956 63981 19521 37388 94724 49302 67681 89881 46210
$\sqrt{3}$ = 1.73205 08075 68877 29352 74463 41505 87236 69428 05253 81038
$\sqrt[3]{3}$ = 1.44224 95703 07408 38232 16383 10780 10958 83918 69253 49935
$\log_e 3$ = 1.09861 22886 68109 69139 52452 36922 52570 46474 90557 82274
$\log_{10} 3$ = 0.47712 12547 19662 43729 50279 03255 11530 92001 28864 19069

MISCELLANEOUS

Euler's Constant γ = 0.57721 56649 01532 86061
$\log_e \gamma$ = −0.54953 93129 81644 82234
Golden Ratio ϕ = 1.61803 39887 49894 84820 45868 34365 63811 77203 09180

XIII.2 NUMERICAL CONSTANTS

NUMBERS CONTAINING π

	Number	Logarithm		Number	Logarithm
π	3.1415 927	0.4971 499	$\pi/180$	0.0174 533	8.2418 774 − 10
2π	6.2831 853	0.7981 799	$180/\pi$	57.2957 795	1.7581 226
3π	9.4247 780	0.9742 711	$4\pi^2$	39.4784 176	1.5963 597
4π	12.5663 706	1.0992 099	$1/\pi^2$	0.1013 212	9.0057 003 − 10
8π	25.1327 412	1.4002 399	$1/(2\pi^2)$	0.0506 606	8.7046 703 − 10
$\pi/2$	1.5707 963	0.1961 199	$1/(4\pi^2)$	0.0253 303	8.4036 403 − 10
$\pi/3$	1.0471 976	0.0200 286	$\sqrt{\pi}$	1.7724 539	0.2485 749
$\pi/4$	0.7853 982	9.8950 899 − 10	$\sqrt{\pi/4}$ or	0.8862 269	9.9475 449 − 10
$\pi/6$	0.5235 988	9.7189 986 − 10	$\sqrt{\pi}/2$		
$\pi/8$	0.3926 991	9.5940 599 − 10	$\sqrt{\pi}/4$	0.4431 135	9.6465 149 − 10
$2\pi/3$	2.0943 951	0.3210 586	$\sqrt{\pi/2}$	1.2533 141	0.0980 599
$4\pi/3$	4.1887 902	0.6220 886	$\sqrt{2/\pi}$	0.7978 846	9.9019 401 − 10
$1/\pi$	0.3183 099	9.5028 501 − 10	π^3	31.0062 767	1.4914 496
$2/\pi$	0.6366 198	9.8038 801 − 10	$\sqrt[3]{\pi}$	1.4645 919	0.1657 166
$4/\pi$	1.2732 395	0.1049 101	$1/\sqrt[3]{\pi}$	0.6827 841	9.8342 834 − 10
$1/(2\pi)$	0.1591 549	9.2018 201 − 10	$\sqrt[3]{\pi^2}$	2.1450 294	0.3314 332
$1/(4\pi)$	0.0795 775	8.9007 901 − 10	$1/\sqrt{\pi}$	0.5641 896	9.7514 251 − 10
$1/(6\pi)$	0.0530 516	8.7246 989 − 10	$1/\sqrt{2\pi}$	0.3989 423	9.6009 101 − 10
$1/(8\pi)$	0.0397 887	8.5997 601 − 10	$2/\sqrt{\pi}$	1.1283 792	0.0524 551
π^2	9.8696 044	0.9942 997			
$2\pi^2$	19.7392 088	1.2953 297			

CHANGE OF BASE

$$\log_a x = \log_b x / \log_b a$$

$$\log_{10} x = \log_e x / \log_e 10 \qquad \log_e x = \log_{10} x / \log_{10} e$$

$$\log_e x = \frac{1}{M} \log_{10} x = 2.30258\ 50930 \log_{10} x \qquad \log_{10} x = M \log_e x = 0.43429\ 44819 \log_e x$$

XIII.3 RADIANS TO DEGREES, MINUTES, AND SECONDS*

Radians	1.0	0.1	0.01	0.001	0.0001
1	57° 17′ 44.8″	5° 43′ 46.5″	0° 34′ 22.6″	0° 03′ 26.3″	0° 00′ 20.6″
2	114° 35′ 29.6″	11° 27′ 33.0″	1° 08′ 45.3″	0° 06′ 52.5″	0° 00′ 41.3″
3	171° 53′ 14.4″	17° 11′ 19.4″	1° 43′ 07.9″	0° 10′ 18.8″	0° 01′ 01.9″
4	229° 10′ 59.2″	22° 55′ 05.9″	2° 17′ 30.6″	0° 13′ 45.1″	0° 01′ 22.5″
5	286° 28′ 44.0″	28° 38′ 52.4″	2° 51′ 53.2″	0° 17′ 11.3″	0° 01′ 43.1″
6	343° 46′ 28.8″	34° 22′ 38.9″	3° 26′ 15.9″	0° 20′ 37.6″	0° 02′ 03.8″
7	401° 04′ 13.6″	40° 06′ 25.4″	4° 00′ 38.5″	0° 24′ 03.9″	0° 02′ 24.4″
8	458° 21′ 58.4″	45° 50′ 11.8″	4° 35′ 01.2″	0° 27′ 30.1″	0° 02′ 45.0″
9	515° 39′ 43.3″	51° 33′ 58.3″	5° 09′ 23.8″	0° 30′ 56.4″	0° 03′ 05.6″

* If 3.214 is desired in degrees, minutes and seconds it is obtained as follows:

3	=	171° 53′ 14.4″
.2	=	11° 27′ 33.0″
.01	=	0° 34′ 22.6″
.004	=	0° 13′ 45.1″
3.214	=	184° 8′ 55.1″

XIII.4 NATURAL FUNCTIONS FOR ANGLES IN RADIANS

Rad.	Sin	Tan	Cot	Cos	Rad.	Sin	Tan	Cot	Cos
.00	.00000	.00000	∞	1.00000	**.50**	.47943	.54630	1.8305	.87758
01	.01000	.01000	99.997	0.99995	.51	.48818	.55936	1.7878	.87274
.02	.02000	.02000	49.993	.99980	.52	.49688	.57256	1.7465	.86782
.03	.03000	.03001	33.323	.99955	.53	.50553	.58592	1.7067	.86281
.04	.03999	.04002	24.987	.99920	.54	.51414	.59943	1.6683	.85771
.05	.04998	.05004	19.983	.99875	.55	.52269	.61311	1.6310	.85252
.06	.05996	.06007	16.647	.99820	.56	.53119	.62695	1.5950	.84726
.07	.06994	.07011	14.262	.99755	.57	.53963	.64097	1.5601	.84190
.08	.07991	.08017	12.473	.99680	.58	.54802	.65517	1.5263	.83646
.09	.08988	.09024	11.081	.99595	.59	.55636	.66956	1.4935	.83094
.10	.09983	.10033	9.9666	.99500	**.60**	.56464	.68414	1.4617	.82534
.11	.10978	.11045	9.0542	.99396	.61	.57287	.69892	1.4308	.81965
.12	.11971	.12058	8.2933	.99281	.62	.58104	.71391	1.4007	.81388
.13	.12963	.13074	7.6489	.99156	.63	.58914	.72911	1.3715	.80803
.14	.13954	.14092	7.0961	.99022	.64	.59720	.74454	1.3431	.80210
.15	.14944	.15114	6.6166	.98877	.65	.60519	.76020	1.3154	.79608
.16	.15932	.16138	6.1966	.98723	.66	.61312	.77610	1.2885	.78999
.17	.16918	.17166	5.8256	.98558	.67	.62099	.79225	1.2622	.78382
.18	.17903	.18197	5.4954	.98384	.68	.62879	.80866	1.2366	.77757
.19	.18886	.19232	5.1997	.98200	.69	.63654	.82534	1.2116	.77125
.20	.19867	.20271	4.9332	.98007	**.70**	.64422	.84229	1.1872	.76484
.21	.20846	.21314	4.6917	.97803	.71	.65183	.85953	1.1634	.75836
.22	.21823	.22362	4.4719	.97590	.72	.65938	.87707	1.1402	.75181
.23	.22798	.23414	4.2709	.97367	.73	.66687	.89492	1.1174	.74517
.24	.23770	.24472	4.0864	.97134	.74	.67429	.91309	1.0952	.73847
.25	.24740	.25534	3.9163	.96891	.75	.68164	.93160	1.0734	.73169
.26	.25708	.26602	3.7591	.96639	.76	.68892	.95045	1.0521	.72484
.27	.26673	.27676	3.6133	.96377	.77	.69614	.96967	1.0313	.71791
.28	.27636	.28755	3.4776	.96106	.78	.70328	.98926	1.0109	.71091
.29	.28595	.29841	3.3511	.95824	.79	.71035	1.0092	.99084	.70385
.30	.29552	.30934	3.2327	.95534	**.80**	.71736	1.0296	.97121	.69671
.31	.30506	.32033	3.1218	.95233	.81	.72429	1.0505	.95197	.68950
.32	.31457	.33139	3.0176	.94924	.82	.73115	1.0717	.93309	.68222
.33	.32404	.34252	2.9195	.94604	.83	.73793	1.0934	.91455	.67488
.34	.33349	.35374	2.8270	.94275	.84	.74464	1.1156	.89635	.66746
.35	.34290	.36503	2.7395	.93937	.85	.75128	1.1383	.87848	.65998
.36	.35227	.37640	2.6567	.93590	.86	.75784	1.1616	.86091	.65244
.37	.36162	.38786	2.5782	.93233	.87	.76433	1.1853	.84365	.64483
.38	.37092	.39941	2.5037	.92866	.88	.77074	1.2097	.82668	.63715
.39	.38019	.41105	2.4328	.92491	.89	.77707	1.2346	.80998	.62941
.40	.38942	.42279	2.3652	.92106	**.90**	.78333	1.2602	.79355	.62161
.41	.39861	.43463	2.3008	.91712	.91	.78950	1.2864	.77738	.61375
.42	.40776	.44657	2.2393	.91309	.92	.79560	1.3133	.76146	.60582
.43	.41687	.45862	2.1804	.90897	.93	.80162	1.3409	.74578	.59783
.44	.42594	.47078	2.1241	.90475	.94	.80756	1.3692	.73034	.58979
.45	.43497	.48306	2.0702	.90045	.95	.81342	1.3984	.71511	.58168
.46	.44395	.49545	2.0184	.89605	.96	.81919	1.4284	.70010	.57352
.47	.45289	.50797	1.9686	.89157	.97	.82489	1.4592	.68531	.56530
.48	.46178	.52061	1.9208	.88699	.98	.83050	1.4910	.67071	.55702
.49	.47063	.53339	1.8748	.88233	.99	.83603	1.5237	.65631	.54869
.50	.47943	.54630	1.8305	.87758	**1.00**	.84147	1.5574	.64209	.54030
Rad.	Sin	Tan	Cot	Cos	Rad.	Sin	Tan	Cot	Cos

NATURAL FUNCTIONS FOR ANGLES IN RADIANS

Rad.	Sin	Tan	Cot	Cos	Rad.	Sin	Tan	Cot	Cos
1.00	.84147	1.5574	.64209	.54030	**1.50**	.99749	14.101	.07091	.07074
1.01	.84683	1.5922	.62806	.53186	1.51	.99815	16.428	.06087	.06076
1.02	.85211	1.6281	.61420	.52337	1.52	.99871	19.670	.05084	.05077
1.03	.85730	1.6652	.60051	.51482	1.53	.99917	24.498	.04082	.04079
1.04	.86240	1.7036	.58699	.50622	1.54	.99953	32.461	.03081	.03079
1.05	.86742	1.7433	.57362	.49757	1.55	.99978	48.078	.02080	.02079
1.06	.87236	1.7844	.56040	.48887	1.56	.99994	92.621	.01080	.01080
1.07	.87720	1.8270	.54734	.48012	1.57	1.00000	1255.8	.00080	.00080
1.08	.88196	1.8712	.53441	.47133	1.58	.99996	−108.65	−.00920	−.00920
1.09	.88663	1.9171	.52162	.46249	1.59	.99982	−52.067	−.01921	−.01920
1.10	.89121	1.9648	.50897	.45360	**1.60**	.99957	−34.233	−.02921	−.02920
1.11	.89570	2.0143	.49644	.44466	1.61	.99923	−25.495	−.03922	−.03919
1.12	.90010	2.0660	.48404	.43568	1.62	.99879	−20.307	−.04924	−.04918
1.13	.90441	2.1198	.47175	.42666	1.63	.99825	−16.871	−.05927	−.05917
1.14	.90863	2.1759	.45959	.41759	1.64	.99761	−14.427	−.06931	−.06915
1.15	.91276	2.2345	.44753	.40849	1.65	.99687	−12.599	−.07937	−.07912
1.16	.91680	2.2958	.43558	.39934	1.66	.99602	−11.181	−.08944	−.08909
1.17	.92075	2.3600	.42373	.39015	1.67	.99508	−10.047	−.09953	−.09904
1.18	.92461	2.4273	.41199	.38092	1.68	.99404	− 9.1208	−.10964	−.10899
1.19	.92837	2.4979	.40034	.37166	1.69	.99290	− 8.3492	−.11977	−.11892
1.20	.93204	2.5722	.38878	.36236	**1.70**	99166	− 7.6966	−.12993	−.12884
1.21	.93562	2.6503	.37731	.35302	1.71	.99033	− 7.1373	−.14011	−.13875
1.22	.93910	2.7328	.36593	.34365	1.72	.98889	− 6.6524	−.15032	−.14865
1.23	.94249	2.8198	.35463	.33424	1.73	.98735	− 6.2281	−.16056	−.15853
1.24	.94578	2.9119	.34341	.32480	1.74	.98572	− 5.8535	−.17084	−.16840
1.25	.94898	3.0096	.33227	.31532	1.75	.98399	− 5.5204	−.18115	−.17825
1.26	.95209	3.1133	.32121	.30582	1.76	.98215	− 5.2221	−.19149	−.18808
1.27	.95510	3.2236	.31021	.29628	1.77	.98022	− 4.9534	−.20188	−.19789
1.28	.95802	3.3413	.29928	.28672	1.78	.97820	− 4.7101	−.21231	−.20768
1.29	.96084	3.4672	.28842	.27712	1.79	.97607	− 4.4887	−.22278	−.21745
1.30	.96356	3.6021	.27762	.26750	**1.80**	.97385	− 4.2863	−.23330	−.22720
1.31	.96618	3.7471	.26687	.25785	1.81	.97153	− 4.1005	−.24387	−.23693
1.32	.96872	3.9033	.25619	.24818	1.82	.96911	− 3.9294	−.25449	−.24663
1.33	.97115	4.0723	.24556	.23848	1.83	.96659	− 3.7712	−.26517	−.25631
1.34	.97348	4.2556	.23408	.22875	1.84	.96398	− 3.6245	−.27590	−.26596
1.35	.97572	4.4552	.22446	.21901	1.85	.96128	− 3.4881	−.28669	−.27559
1.36	.97786	4.6734	.21398	.20924	1.86	.95847	− 3.3608	−.29755	−.28519
1.37	.97991	4.9131	.20354	.19945	1.87	.95557	− 2.2419	−.30846	−.29476
1.38	.98185	5.1774	.19315	.18964	1.88	.95258	− 3.1304	−.31945	−.30430
1.39	.98370	5.4707	.18279	.17981	1.89	.94949	− 3.0257	−.33051	−.31381
1.40	.98545	5.7979	.17248	.16997	**1.90**	.94630	− 2.9271	−.34164	−.32329
1.41	.98710	6.1654	.16220	.16010	1.91	.94302	− 2.8341	−.35284	−.33274
1.42	.98865	6.5811	.15195	.15023	1.92	.93965	− 2.7463	−.36413	−.34215
1.43	.99010	7.0555	.14173	.14033	1.93	.93618	− 2.6632	−.37549	−.35153
1.44	.99146	7.6018	.13155	042	1.94	.93262	− 2.5843	−.38695	−.36087
1.45	.99271	8.2381	.12139	.12050	1.95	.92896	− 2.5095	−.39849	−.37018
1.46	.99387	8.9886	.11125	.11057	1.96	.92521	− 2.4383	−.41012	−.37945
1.47	.99492	9.8874	.10114	.10063	1.97	.92137	− 2.3705	−.42185	−.38868
1.48	.99588	10.983	.09105	.09067	1.98	.91744	− 2.3058	−.43368	−.39788
1.49	.99674	12.350	.08097	.08071	1.99	.91341	− 2.2441	−.44562	−.40703
1.50	.99749	14.101	.07091	.07074	**2.00**	.90930	− 2.1850	−.45766	−.41615
Rad.	Sin	Tan	Cot	Cos	Rad.	Sin	Tan	Cot	Cos

XIII.5 SQUARES, CUBES AND ROOTS

Roots of numbers other than those given directly may be found by the following relations: $\sqrt{100n} = 10\sqrt{n}$; $\sqrt{1000n} = 10\sqrt{10n}$; $\sqrt{\frac{1}{10}n} = \frac{1}{10}\sqrt{10n}$; $\sqrt{\frac{1}{100}n} = \frac{1}{10}\sqrt{n}$; $\sqrt{\frac{1}{1000}n} = \frac{1}{100}\sqrt{10n}$; $\sqrt[3]{1000n} = 10\sqrt[3]{n}$; $\sqrt[3]{10{,}000n} = 10\sqrt[3]{10n}$; $\sqrt[3]{100{,}000n} = 10\sqrt[3]{100n}$; $\sqrt[3]{\frac{1}{10}n} = \frac{1}{10}\sqrt[3]{100n}$; $\sqrt[3]{\frac{1}{100}n} = \frac{1}{10}\sqrt[3]{10n}$; $\sqrt[3]{\frac{1}{1000}n} = \frac{1}{10}\sqrt[3]{n}$.

n	n^2	$\sqrt{n}$	$\sqrt{10n}$	n^3	$\sqrt[3]{n}$	$\sqrt[3]{10n}$	$\sqrt[3]{100n}$
1	1	1.000 000	3.162 278	1	1.000 000	2.154 435	4.641 589
2	4	1.414 214	4.472 136	8	1.259 921	2.714 418	5.848 035
3	9	1.732 051	5.477 226	27	1.442 250	3.107 233	6.694 330
4	16	2.000 000	6.324 555	64	1.587 401	3.419 952	7.368 063
5	25	2.236 068	7.071 068	125	1.709 976	3.684 031	7.937 005
6	36	2.449 490	7.745 967	216	1.817 121	3.914 868	8.434 327
7	49	2.645 751	8.366 600	343	1.912 931	4.121 285	8.879 040
8	64	2.828 427	8.944 272	512	2.000 000	4.308 869	9.283 178
9	81	3.000 000	9.486 833	729	2.080 084	4.481 405	9.654 894
10	100	3.162 278	10.00000	1 000	2.154 435	4.641 589	10.00000
11	121	3.316 625	10.48809	1 331	2.223 980	4.791 420	10.32280
12	144	3.464 102	10.95445	1 728	2.289 428	4.932 424	10.62659
13	169	3.605 551	11.40175	2 197	2.351 335	5.065 797	10.91393
14	196	3.741 657	11.83216	2 744	2.410 142	5.192 494	11.18689
15	225	3.872 983	12.24745	3 375	2.466 212	5.313 293	11.44714
16	256	4.000 000	12.64911	4 096	2.519 842	5.428 835	11.69607
17	289	4.123 106	13.03840	4 913	2.571 282	5.539 658	11.93483
18	324	4.242 641	13.41641	5 832	2.620 741	5.646 216	12.16440
19	361	4.358 899	13.78405	6 859	2.668 402	5.748 897	12.38562
20	400	4.472 136	14.14214	8 000	2.714 418	5.848 035	12.59921
21	441	4.582 576	14.49138	9 261	2.758 924	5.943 922	12.80579
22	484	4.690 416	14.83240	10 648	2.802 039	6.036 811	13.00591
23	529	4.795 832	15.16575	12 167	2.843 867	6.126 926	13.20006
24	576	4.898 979	15.49193	13 824	2.884 499	6.214 465	13.38866
25	625	5.000 000	15.81139	15 625	2.924 018	6.299 605	13.57209
26	676	5.099 020	16.12452	17 576	2.962 496	6.382 504	13.75069
27	729	5.196 152	16.43168	19 683	3.000 000	6.463 304	13.92477
28	784	5.291 503	16.73320	21 952	3.036 589	6.542 133	14.09460
29	841	5.385 165	17.02939	24 389	3.072 317	6.619 106	14.26043
30	900	5.477 226	17.32051	27 000	3.107 233	6.694 330	14.42250
31	961	5.567 764	17.60682	29 791	3.141 381	6.767 899	14.58100
32	1 024	5.656 854	17.88854	32 768	3.174 802	6.839 904	14.73613
33	1 089	5.744 563	18.16590	35 937	3.207 534	6.910 423	14.88806
34	1 156	5.830 952	18.43909	39 304	3.239 612	6.979 532	15.03695
35	1 225	5.916 080	18.70829	42 875	3.271 066	7.047 299	15.18294
36	1 296	6.000 000	18.97367	46 656	3.301 927	7.113 787	15.32619
37	1 369	6.082 763	19.23538	50 653	3.332 222	7.179 054	15.46680
38	1 444	6.164 414	19.49359	54 872	3.361 975	7.243 156	15.60491
39	1 521	6.244 998	19.74842	59 319	3.391 211	7.306 144	15.74061
40	1 600	6.324 555	20.00000	64 000	3.419 952	7.368 063	15.87401
41	1 681	6.403 124	20.24846	68 921	3.448 217	7.428 959	16.00521
42	1 764	6.480 741	20.49390	74 088	3.476 027	7.488 872	16.13429
43	1 849	6.557 439	20.73644	79 507	3.503 398	7.547 842	16.26133
44	1 936	6.633 250	20.97618	85 184	3.530 348	7.605 905	16.38643
45	2 025	6.708 204	21.21320	91 125	3.556 893	7.663 094	16.50964
46	2 116	6.782 330	21.44761	97 336	3.583 048	7.719 443	16.63103
47	2 209	6.855 655	21.67948	103 823	3.608 826	7.774 980	16.75069
48	2 304	6.928 203	21.90890	110 592	3.634 241	7.829 735	16.86865
49	2 401	7.000 000	22.13594	117 649	3.659 306	7.883 735	16.98499

SQUARES, CUBES AND ROOTS

n	n^2	$\sqrt{n}$	$\sqrt{10n}$	n^3	$\sqrt[3]{n}$	$\sqrt[3]{10n}$	$\sqrt[3]{100n}$
50	2 500	7.071 068	22.36068	125 000	3.684 031	7.937 005	17.09976
51	2 601	7.141 428	22.58318	132 651	3.708 430	7.989 570	17.21301
52	2 704	7.211 103	22.80351	140 608	3.732 511	8.041 452	17.32478
53	2 809	7.280 110	23.02173	148 877	3.756 286	8.092 672	17.43513
54	2 916	7.348 469	23.23790	157 464	3.779 763	8.143 253	17.54411
55	3 025	7.416 198	23.45208	166 375	3.802 952	8.193 213	17.65174
56	3 136	7.483 315	23.66432	175 616	3.825 862	8.242 571	17.75808
57	3 249	7.549 834	23.87467	185 193	3.848 501	8.291 344	17.86316
58	3 364	7.615 773	24.08319	195 112	3.870 877	8.339 551	17.96702
59	3 481	7.681 146	24.28992	205 379	3.892 996	8.387 207	18.06969
60	3 600	7.745 967	24.49490	216 000	3.914 868	8.434 327	18.17121
61	3 721	7.810 250	24.69818	226 981	3.936 497	8.480 926	18.27160
62	3 844	7.874 008	24.89980	238 328	3.957 892	8.527 019	18.37091
63	3 969	7.937 254	25.09980	250 047	3.979 057	8.572 619	18.46915
64	4 096	8.000 000	25.29822	262 144	4.000 000	8.617 739	18.56636
65	4 225	8.062 258	25.49510	274 625	4.020 726	8.662 391	18.66256
66	4 356	8.124 038	25.69047	287 496	4.041 240	8.706 588	18.75777
67	4 489	8.185 353	25.88436	300 763	4.061 548	8.750 340	18.85204
68	4 624	8.246 211	26.07681	314 432	4.081 655	8.793 659	18.94536
69	4 761	8.306 624	26.26785	328 509	4.101 566	8.836 556	19.03778
70	4 900	8.366 600	26.45751	343 000	4.121 285	8.879 040	19.12931
71	5 041	8.426 150	26.64583	357 911	4.140 818	8.921 121	19.21997
72	5 184	8.485 281	26.83282	373 248	4.160 168	8.962 809	19.30979
73	5 329	8.544 004	27.01851	389 017	4.179 339	9.004 113	19.39877
74	5 476	8.602 325	27.20294	405 224	4.198 336	9.045 042	19.48695
75	5 625	8.660 254	27.38613	421 875	4.217 163	9.085 603	19.57434
76	5 776	8.717 798	27.56810	438 976	4.235 824	9.125 805	19.66095
77	5 929	8.774 964	27.74887	456 533	4.254 321	9.165 656	19.74681
78	6 084	8.831 761	27.92848	474 552	4.272 659	9.205 164	19.83192
79	6 241	8.888 194	28.10694	493 039	4.290 840	9.244 335	19.91632
80	6 400	8.944 272	28.28427	512 000	4.308 869	9.283 178	20.00000
81	6 561	9.000 000	28.46050	531 441	4.326 749	9.321 698	20.08299
82	0 724	9.055 385	28.03504	551 308	4.344 481	9.359 902	20.16530
83	6 889	9.110 434	28.80972	571 787	4.362 071	9.397 796	20.24694
84	7 056	9.165 151	28.98275	592 704	4.379 519	9.435 388	20.32793
85	7 225	9.219 544	29.15476	614 125	4.396 830	9.472 682	20.40828
86	7 396	9.273 618	29.32576	636 056	4.414 005	9.509 685	20.48800
87	7 569	9.327 379	29.49576	658 503	4.431 048	9.546 403	20.56710
88	7 744	9.380 832	29.66479	681 472	4.447 960	9.582 840	20.64560
89	7 921	9.433 981	29.83287	704 969	4.464 745	9.619 002	20.72351
90	8 100	9.486 833	30.00000	729 000	4.481 405	9.654 894	20.80084
91	8 281	9.539 392	30.16621	753 571	4.497 941	9.690 521	20.87759
92	8 464	9.591 663	30.33150	778 688	4.514 357	9.725 888	20.95379
93	8 649	9.643 651	30.49590	804 357	4.530 655	9.761 000	21.02944
94	8 836	9.695 360	30.65942	830 584	4.546 836	9.795 861	21.10454
95	9 025	9.746 794	30.82207	857 375	4.562 903	9.830 476	21.17912
96	9 216	9.797 959	30.98387	884 736	4.578 857	9.864 848	21.25317
97	9 409	9.848 858	31.14482	912 673	4.594 701	9.898 983	21.32671
98	9 604	9.899 495	31.30495	941 192	4.610 436	9.932 884	21.39975
99	9 801	9.949 874	31.46427	970 299	4.626 065	9.966 555	21.47229
100	10 000	10.00000	31.62278	1 000 000	4.641 589	10.00000	21.54435
101	10 201	10.04988	31.78050	1 030 301	4.657 010	10.03322	21.61592
102	10 404	10.09950	31.93744	1 061 208	4.672 329	10.06623	21.68703
103	10 609	10.14889	32.09361	1 092 727	4.687 548	10.09902	21.75767
104	10 816	10.19804	32.24903	1 124 864	4.702 669	10.13159	21.82786
105	11 025	10.24695	32.40370	1 157 625	4.717 694	10.16396	21.89760
106	11 236	10.29563	32.55764	1 191 016	4.732 623	10.19613	21.96689
107	11 449	10.34408	32.71085	1 225 043	4.747 459	10.22809	22.03575
108	11 664	10.39230	32.86335	1 259 712	4.762 203	10.25986	22.10419
109	11 881	10.44031	33.01515	1 295 029	4.776 856	10.29142	22.17220

SQUARES, CUBES AND ROOTS

n	n^2	$\sqrt{n}$	$\sqrt{10n}$	n^3	$\sqrt[3]{n}$	$\sqrt[3]{10n}$	$\sqrt[3]{100n}$
110	12 100	10.48809	33.16625	1 331 000	4.791 420	10.32280	22.23980
111	12 321	10.53565	33.31666	1 367 631	4.805 896	10.35399	22.30699
112	12 544	10.58301	33.46640	1 404 928	4.820 285	10.38499	22.37378
113	12 769	10.63015	33.61547	1 442 897	4.834 588	10.41580	22.44017
114	12 996	10.67708	33.76389	1 481 544	4.848 808	10.44644	22.50617
115	13 225	10.72381	33.91165	1 520 875	4.862 944	10.47690	22.57179
116	13 456	10.77033	34.05877	1 560 896	4.876 999	10.50718	22.63702
117	13 689	10.81665	34.20526	1 601 613	4.890 973	10.53728	22.70189
118	13 924	10.86278	34.35113	1 643 032	4.904 868	10.56722	22.76638
119	14 161	10.90871	34.49638	1 685 159	4.918 685	10.59699	22.83051
120	14 400	10.95445	34.64102	1 728 000	4.932 424	10.62659	22.89428
121	14 641	11.00000	34.78505	1 771 561	4.946 087	10.65602	22.95770
122	14 884	11.04536	34.92850	1 815 848	4.959 676	10.68530	23.02078
123	15 129	11.09054	35 07136	1 860 867	4.973 190	10.71441	23.08350
124	15 376	11.13553	35 21363	1 906 624	4.986 631	10.74337	23.14589
125	15 625	11.18034	35.35534	1 953 125	5.000 000	10.77217	23.20794
126	15 876	11.22497	35.49648	2 000 376	5.013 298	10.80082	23.26967
127	16 129	11.26943	35.63706	2 048 383	5.026 526	10.82932	23.33107
128	16 384	11.31371	35.77709	2 097 152	5.039 684	10.85767	23.39214
129	16 641	11.35782	35.91657	2 146 689	5.052 774	10.88587	23.45290
130	16 900	11.40175	36.05551	2 197 000	5.065 797	10.91393	23.51335
131	17 161	11.44552	36.19392	2 248 091	5.078 753	10.94184	23.57348
132	17 424	11.48913	36.33180	2 299 968	5.091 643	10.96961	23.63332
133	17 689	11.53256	36.46917	2 352 637	5.104 469	10.99724	23.69285
134	17 956	11.57584	36.60601	2 406 104	5.117 230	11.02474	23.75208
135	18 225	11.61895	36.74235	2 460 375	5.129 928	11.05209	23.81102
136	18 496	11.66190	36.87818	2 515 456	5.142 563	11.07932	23.86966
137	18 769	11.70470	37.01351	2 571 353	5.155 137	11.10641	23.92803
138	19 044	11.74734	37.14835	2 628 072	5.167 649	11.13336	23.98610
139	19 321	11.78983	37.28270	2 685 619	5.180 101	11.16019	24.04390
140	19 600	11.83216	37.41657	2 744 000	5.192 494	11.18689	24.10142
141	19 881	11.87434	37.54997	2 803 221	5.204 828	11.21346	24.15867
142	20 164	11.91638	37.68289	2 863 288	5.217 103	11.23991	24.21565
143	20 449	11.95826	37.81534	2 924 207	5.229 322	11.26623	24.27236
144	20 736	12.00000	37.94733	2 985 984	5.241 483	11.29243	24.32881
145	21 025	12.04159	38.07887	3 048 625	5.253 588	11.31851	24.38499
146	21 316	12.08305	38.20995	3 112 136	5.265 637	11.34447	24.44092
147	21 609	12.12436	38.34058	3 176 523	5.277 632	11.37031	24.49660
148	21 904	12.16553	38.47077	3 241 792	5.289 572	11.39604	24.55202
149	22 201	12.20656	38.60052	3 307 949	5.301 459	11.42165	24.60719
150	22 500	12.24745	38.72983	3 375 000	5.313 293	11.44714	24.66212
151	22 801	12.28821	38.85872	3 442 951	5.325 074	11.47252	24.71680
152	23 104	12.32883	38.98718	3 511 808	5.336 803	11.49779	24.77125
153	23 409	12.36932	39.11521	3 581 577	5.348 481	11.52295	24.82545
154	23 716	12.40967	39.24283	3 652 264	5.360 108	11.54800	24.87942
155	24 025	12.44990	39.37004	3 723 875	5.371 685	11.57295	24.93315
156	24 336	12.49000	39.49684	3 796 416	5.383 213	11.59778	24.98666
157	24 649	12.52996	39.62323	3 869 893	5.394 691	11.62251	25.03994
158	24 964	12.56981	39.74921	3 944 312	5.406 120	11.64713	25.09299
159	25 281	12.60952	39.87480	4 019 679	5.417 502	11.67165	25.14581
160	25 600	12.64911	40.00000	4 096 000	5.428 835	11.69607	25.19842
161	25 921	12.68858	40.12481	4 173 281	5.440 122	11.72039	25.25081
162	26 244	12.72792	40.24922	4 251 528	5.451 362	11.74460	25.30298
163	26 569	12.76715	40.37326	4 330 747	5.462 556	11.76872	25.35494
164	26 896	12.80625	40.49691	4 410 944	5.473 704	11.79274	25.40668
165	27 225	12.84523	40.62019	4 492 125	5.484 807	11.81666	25.45822
166	27 556	12.88410	40.74310	4 574 296	5.495 865	11.84048	25.50954
167	27 889	12.92285	40.86563	4 657 463	5.506 878	11.86421	25.56067
168	28 224	12.96148	40.98780	4 741 632	5.517 848	11.88784	25.61158
169	28 561	13.00000	41.10961	4 826 809	5.528 775	11.91138	25.66230

SQUARES, CUBES AND ROOTS

n	n^2	$\sqrt{n}$	$\sqrt{10n}$	n^3	$\sqrt[3]{n}$	$\sqrt[3]{10n}$	$\sqrt[3]{100n}$
170	28 900	13.03840	41.23106	4 913 000	5.539 658	11.93483	25.71282
171	29 241	13.07670	41.35215	5 000 211	5.550 499	11.95819	25.76313
172	29 584	13.11488	41.47288	5 088 448	5.561 298	11.98145	25.81326
173	29 929	13.15295	41.59327	5 177 717	5.572 055	12.00463	25.86319
174	30 276	13.19091	41.71331	5 268 024	5.582 770	12.02771	25.91292
175	30 625	13.22876	41.83300	5 359 375	5.593 445	12.05071	25.96247
176	30 976	13.26650	41.95235	5 451 776	5.604 079	12.07362	26.01183
177	31 329	13.30413	42.07137	5 545 233	5.614 672	12.09645	26.06100
178	31 684	13.34166	42.19005	5 639 752	5.625 226	12.11918	26.10999
179	32 041	13.37909	42.30839	5 735 339	5.635 741	12.14184	26.15879
180	32 400	13.41641	42.42641	5 832 000	5.646 216	12.16440	26.20741
181	32 761	13.45362	42.54409	5 929 741	5.656 653	12.18689	26.25586
182	33 124	13.49074	42.66146	6 028 568	5.667 051	12.20929	26.30412
183	33 489	13.52775	42.77850	6 128 487	5.677 411	12.23161	26.35221
184	33 856	13.56466	42.89522	6 229 504	5.687 734	12.25385	26.40012
185	34 225	13.60147	43.01163	6 331 625	5.698 019	12.27601	26.44786
186	34 596	13.63818	43.12772	6 434 856	5.708 267	12.29809	26.49543
187	34 969	13.67479	43.24350	6 539 203	5.718 479	12.32009	26.54283
188	35 344	13.71131	43.35897	6 644 672	5.728 654	12.34201	26.59006
189	35 721	13.74773	43.47413	6 751 269	5.738 794	12.36386	26.63712
190	36 100	13.78405	43.58899	6 859 000	5.748 897	12.38562	26.68402
191	36 481	13.82027	43.70355	6 967 871	5.758 965	12.40731	26.73075
192	36 864	13.85641	43.81780	7 077 888	5.768 998	12.42893	26.77732
193	37 249	13.89244	43.93177	7 189 057	5.778 997	12.45047	26.82373
194	37 636	13.92839	44.04543	7 301 384	5.788 960	12.47194	26.86997
195	38 025	13.96424	44.15880	7 414 875	5.798 890	12.49333	26.91606
196	38 416	14.00000	44.27189	7 529 536	5.808 786	12.51465	26.96199
197	38 809	14.03567	44.38468	7 645 373	5.818 648	12.53590	27.00777
198	39 204	14.07125	44.49719	7 762 392	5.828 477	12.55707	27.05339
199	39 601	14.10674	44.60942	7 880 599	5.838 272	12.57818	27.09886
200	40 000	14.14214	44.72136	8 000 000	5.848 035	12.59921	27.14418
201	40 401	14.17745	44.83302	8 120 601	5.857 766	12.62017	27.18934
202	40 804	14.21267	44.94441	8 242 408	5.867 464	12.64107	27.23436
203	41 209	14.24781	45.05552	8 365 427	5.877 131	12.66189	27.27922
204	41 616	14.28286	45.16636	8 489 664	5.886 765	12.68265	27.32394
205	42 025	14.31782	45.27693	8 615 125	5.896 369	12.70334	27.36852
206	42 436	14.35270	45.38722	8 741 816	5.905 941	12.72396	27.41295
207	42 849	14.38749	45.49725	8 869 743	5.915 482	12.74452	27.45723
208	43 264	14.42221	45.60702	8 998 912	5.924 992	12.76501	27.50138
209	43 681	14.45683	45.71652	9 129 329	5.934 472	12.78543	27.54538
210	44 100	14.49138	45.82576	9 261 000	5.943 922	12.80579	27.58924
211	44 521	14.52584	45.93474	9 393 931	5.953 342	12.82609	27.63296
212	44 944	14.56022	46.04346	9 528 128	5.962 732	12.84632	27.67655
213	45 369	14.59452	46.15192	9 663 597	5.972 093	12.86648	27.72000
214	45 796	14.62874	46.26013	9 800 344	5.981 424	12.88659	27.76331
215	46 225	14.66288	46.36809	9 938 375	5.990 726	12.90663	27.80649
216	46 656	14.69694	46.47580	10 077 696	6.000 000	12.92661	27.84953
217	47 089	14.73092	46.58326	10 218 313	6.009 245	12.94653	27.89244
218	47 524	14.76482	46.69047	10 360 232	6.018 462	12.96638	27.93522
219	47 961	14.79865	46.79744	10 503 459	6.027 650	12.98618	27.97787
220	48 400	14.83240	46.90416	10 648 000	6.036 811	13.00591	28.02039
221	48 841	14.86607	47.01064	10 793 861	6.045 944	13.02559	28.06278
222	49 284	14.89966	47.11688	10 941 048	6.055 049	13.04521	28.10505
223	49 729	14.93318	47.22288	11 089 567	6.064 127	13.06477	28.14718
224	50 176	14.96663	47.32864	11 239 424	6.073 178	13.08427	28.18919
225	50 625	15.00000	47.43416	11 390 625	6.082 202	13.10371	28.23108
226	51 076	15.03330	47.53946	11 543 176	6.091 199	13.12309	28.27284
227	51 529	15.06652	47.64452	11 697 083	6.100 170	13.14242	28.31448
228	51 984	15.09967	47.74935	11 852 352	6.109 115	13.16169	28.35600
229	52 441	15.13275	47.85394	12 008 989	6.118 033	13.18090	28.39739

SQUARES, CUBES AND ROOTS

n	n^2	$\sqrt{n}$	$\sqrt{10n}$	n^3	$\sqrt[3]{n}$	$\sqrt[3]{10n}$	$\sqrt[3]{100n}$
230	52 900	15.16575	47.95832	12 167 000	6.126 926	13.20006	28.43867
231	53 361	15.19868	48.06246	12 326 391	6.135 792	13.21916	28.47983
232	53 824	15.23155	48.16638	12 487 168	6.144 634	13.23821	28.52086
233	54 289	15.26434	48.27007	12 649 337	6.153 449	13.25721	28.56178
234	54 756	15.29706	48.37355	12 812 904	6.162 240	13.27614	28.60259
235	55 225	15.32971	48.47680	12 977 875	6.171 006	13.29503	28.64327
236	55 696	15.36229	48.57983	13 144 256	6.179 747	13.31386	28.68384
237	56 169	15.39480	48.68265	13 312 053	6.188 463	13.33264	28.72430
238	56 644	15.42725	48.78524	13 481 272	6.197 154	13.35136	28.76464
239	57 121	15.45962	48.88763	13 651 919	6.205 822	13.37004	28.80487
240	57 600	15.49193	48.98979	13 824 000	6.214 465	13.38866	28.84499
241	58 081	15.52417	49.09175	13 997 521	6.223 084	13.40723	28.88500
242	58 564	15.55635	49.19350	14 172 488	6.231 680	13.42575	28.92489
243	59 049	15.58846	49.29503	14 348 907	6.240 251	13.44421	28.96468
244	59 536	15.62050	49.39636	14 526 784	6.248 800	13.46263	29.00436
245	60 025	15.65248	49.49747	14 706 125	6.257 325	13.48100	29.04393
246	60 516	15.68439	49.59839	14 886 936	6.265 827	13.49931	29.08339
247	61 009	15.71623	49.69909	15 069 223	6.274 305	13.51758	29.12275
248	61 504	15.74802	49.79960	15 252 992	6.282 761	13.53580	29.16199
249	62 001	15.77973	49.89990	15 438 249	6.291 195	13.55397	29.20114
250	62 500	15.81139	50.00000	15 625 000	6.299 605	13.57209	29.24018
251	63 001	15.84298	50.09990	15 813 251	6.307 994	13.59016	29.27911
252	63 504	15.87451	50.19960	16 003 008	6.316 360	13.60818	29.31794
253	64 009	15.90597	50.29911	16 194 277	6.324 704	13.62616	29.35667
254	64 516	15.93738	50.39841	16 387 064	6.333 026	13.64409	29.39530
255	65 025	15.96872	50.49752	16 581 375	6.341 326	13.66197	29.43383
256	65 536	16.00000	50.59644	16 777 216	6.349 604	13.67981	29.47225
257	66 049	16.03122	50.69517	16 974 593	6.357 861	13.69760	29.51058
258	66 564	16.06238	50.79370	17 173 512	6.366 097	13.71534	29.54880
259	67 081	16.09348	50.89204	17 373 979	6.374 311	13.73304	29.58693
260	67 600	16.12452	50.99020	17 576 000	6.382 504	13.75069	29.62496
261	68 121	16.15549	51.08816	17 779 581	6.390 677	13.76830	29.66289
262	68 644	16.18641	51.18594	17 984 728	6.398 828	13.78586	29.70073
263	69 169	16.21727	51.28353	18 191 447	6.406 959	13.80337	29.73847
264	69 696	16.24808	51.38093	18 399 744	6.415 069	13.82085	29.77611
265	70 225	16.27882	51.47815	18 609 625	6.423 158	13.83828	29.81366
266	70 756	16.30951	51.57519	18 821 096	6.431 228	13.85566	29.85111
267	71 289	16.34013	51.67204	19 034 163	6.439 277	13.87300	29.88847
268	71 824	16.37071	51.76872	19 248 832	6.447 306	13.89030	29.92574
269	72 361	16.40122	51.86521	19 465 109	6.455 315	13.90755	29.96292
270	72 900	16.43168	51.96152	19 683 000	6.463 304	13.92477	30.00000
271	73 441	16.46208	52.05766	19 902 511	6.471 274	13.94194	30.03699
272	73 984	16.49242	52.15362	20 123 648	6.479 224	13.95906	30.07389
273	74 529	16.52271	52.24940	20 346 417	6.487 154	13.97615	30.11070
274	75 076	16.55295	52.34501	20 570 824	6.495 065	13.99319	30.14742
275	75 625	16.58312	52.44044	20 796 875	6.502 957	14.01020	30.18405
276	76 176	16.61325	52.53570	21 024 576	6.510 830	14.02716	30.22060
277	76 729	16.64332	52.63079	21 253 933	6.518 684	14.04408	30.25705
278	77 284	16.67333	52.72571	21 484 952	6.526 519	14.06096	30.29342
279	77 841	16.70329	52.82045	21 717 639	6.534 335	14.07780	30.32970
280	78 400	16.73320	52.91503	21 952 000	6.542 133	14.09460	30.36589
281	78 961	16.76305	53.00943	22 188 041	6.549 912	14.11136	30.40200
282	79 524	16.79286	53.10367	22 425 768	6.557 672	14.12808	30.43802
283	80 089	16.82260	53.19774	22 665 187	6.565 414	14.14476	30.47395
284	80 656	16.85230	53.29165	22 906 304	6.573 138	14.16140	30.50981
285	81 225	16.88194	53.38539	23 149 125	6.580 844	14.17800	30.54557
286	81 796	16.91153	53.47897	23 393 656	6.588 532	14.19456	30.58126
287	82 369	16.94107	53.57238	23 639 903	6.596 202	14.21109	30.61686
288	82 944	16.97056	53.66563	23 887 872	6.603 854	14.22757	30.65238
289	83 521	17.00000	53.75872	24 137 569	6.611 489	14.24402	30.68781

SQUARES, CUBES AND ROOTS

n	n^2	$\sqrt{n}$	$\sqrt{10n}$	n^3	$\sqrt[3]{n}$	$\sqrt[3]{10n}$	$\sqrt[3]{100n}$
290	84 100	17.02939	53.85165	24 389 000	6.619 106	14.26043	30.72317
291	84 681	17.05872	53.94442	24 642 171	6.626 705	14.27680	30.75844
292	85 264	17.08801	54.03702	24 897 088	6.634 287	14.29314	30.79363
293	85 849	17.11724	54.12947	25 153 757	6.641 852	14.30944	30.82875
294	86 436	17.14643	54.22177	25 412 184	6.649 400	14.32570	30.86378
295	87 025	17.17556	54.31390	25 672 375	6.656 930	14.34192	30.89873
296	87 616	17.20465	54.40588	25 934 336	6.664 444	14.35811	30.93361
297	88 209	17.23369	54.49771	26 198 073	6.671 940	14.37426	30.96840
298	88 804	17.26268	54.58938	26 463 592	6.679 420	14.39037	31.00312
299	89 401	17.29162	54.68089	26 730 899	6.686 883	14.40645	31.03776
300	90 000	17.32051	54.77226	27 000 000	6.694 330	14.42250	31.07233
301	90 601	17.34935	54.86347	27 270 901	6.701 759	14.43850	31.10681
302	91 204	17.37815	54.95453	27 543 608	6.709 173	14.45447	31.14122
303	91 809	17.40690	55.04544	27 818 127	6.716 570	14.47041	31.17556
304	92 416	17.43560	55.13620	28 094 464	6.723 951	14.48631	31.20982
305	93 025	17.46425	55.22681	28 372 625	6.731 315	14.50218	31.24400
306	93 636	17.49286	55.31727	28 652 616	6.738 664	14.51801	31.27811
307	94 249	17.52142	55.40758	28 934 443	6.745 997	14.53381	31.31214
308	94 864	17.54993	55.49775	29 218 112	6.753 313	14.54957	31.34610
309	95 481	17.57840	55.58777	29 503 629	6.760 614	14.56530	31.37999
310	96 100	17.60682	55.67764	29 791 000	6.767 899	14.58100	31.41381
311	96 721	17.63519	55.76737	30 080 231	6.775 169	14.59666	31.44755
312	97 344	17.66352	55.85696	30 371 328	6.782 423	14.61229	31.48122
313	97 969	17.69181	55.94640	30 664 297	6.789 661	14.62788	31.51482
314	98 596	17.72005	56.03570	30 959 144	6.796 884	14.64344	31.54834
315	99 225	17.74824	56.12486	31 255 875	6.804 092	14.65807	31.58180
316	99 856	17.77639	56.21388	31 554 496	6.811 285	14.67447	31.61518
317	100 489	17.80449	56.30275	31 855 013	6.818 462	14.68993	31.64850
318	101 124	17.83255	56.39149	32 157 432	6.825 624	14.70536	31.68174
319	101 761	17.86057	56.48008	32 461 759	6.832 771	14.72076	31.71492
320	102 400	17.88854	56.56854	32 768 000	6.839 904	14.73613	31.74802
321	103 041	17.91647	56.65686	33 076 161	6.847 021	14.75146	31.78106
322	103 684	17.94436	56.74504	33 386 248	6.854 124	14.76676	31.81403
323	104 329	17.97220	56.83309	33 698 267	6.861 212	14.78203	31.84693
324	104 976	18.00000	56.92100	34 012 224	6.868 285	14.79727	31.87976
325	105 625	18.02776	57.00877	34 328 125	6.875 344	14.81248	31.91252
326	106 276	18.05547	57.09641	34 645 976	6.882 389	14.82766	31.94522
327	106 929	18.08314	57.18391	34 965 783	6.889 419	14.84280	31.97785
328	107 584	18.11077	57.27128	35 287 552	6.896 434	14.85792	32.01041
329	108 241	18.13836	57.35852	35 611 289	6.903 436	14.87300	32.04291
330	108 900	18.16590	57.44563	35 937 000	6.910 423	14.88806	32.07534
331	109 561	18.19341	57.53260	36 264 691	6.917 396	14.90308	32.10771
332	110 224	18.22087	57.61944	36 594 368	6.924 356	14.91807	32.14001
333	110 889	18.24829	57.70615	36 926 037	6.931 301	14.93303	32.17225
334	111 556	18.27567	57.79273	37 259 704	6.938 232	14.94797	32.20442
335	112 225	18.30301	57.87918	37 595 375	6.945 150	14.96287	32.23653
336	112 896	18.33030	57.96551	37 933 056	6.952 053	14.97774	32.26857
337	113 569	18.35756	58.05170	38 272 753	6.958 943	14.99259	32.30055
338	114 244	18.38478	58.13777	38 614 472	6.965 820	15.00740	32.33247
339	114 921	18.41195	58.22371	38 958 219	6.972 683	15.02219	32.36433
340	115 600	18.43909	58.30952	39 304 000	6.979 532	15.03695	32.39612
341	116 281	18.46619	58.39521	39 651 821	6.986 368	15.05167	32.42785
342	116 964	18.49324	58.48077	40 001 688	6.993 191	15.06637	32.45952
343	117 649	18.52026	58.56620	40 353 607	7.000 000	15.08104	32.49112
344	118 336	18.54724	58.65151	40 707 584	7.006 796	15.09568	32.52267
345	119 025	18.57418	58.73670	41 063 625	7.013 579	15.11030	32.55415
346	119 716	18.60108	58.82176	41 421 736	7.020 349	15.12488	32.58557
347	120 409	18.62794	58.90671	41 781 923	7.027 106	15.13944	32.61694
348	121 104	18.65476	58.99152	42 144 192	7.033 850	15.15397	32.64824
349	121 801	18.68154	59.07622	42 508 549	7.040 581	15.16847	32.67948

SQUARES, CUBES AND ROOTS

n	n^2	$\sqrt{n}$	$\sqrt{10n}$	n^3	$\sqrt[3]{n}$	$\sqrt[3]{10n}$	$\sqrt[3]{100n}$
350	122 500	18.70829	59.16080	42 875 000	7.047 299	15.18294	32.71066
351	123 201	18.73499	59.24525	43 243 551	7.054 004	15.19739	32.74179
352	123 904	18.76166	59.32959	43 614 208	7.060 697	15.21181	32.77285
353	124 609	18.78829	59.41380	43 986 977	7.067 377	15.22620	32.80386
354	125 316	18.81489	59.49790	44 361 864	7.074 044	15.24057	32.83480
355	126 025	18.84144	59.58188	44 738 875	7.080 699	15.25490	32.86569
356	126 736	18.86796	59.66574	45 118 016	7.087 341	15.26921	32.89652
357	127 449	18.89444	59.74948	45 499 293	7.093 971	15.28350	32.92730
358	128 164	18.92089	59.83310	45 882 712	7.100 588	15.29775	32.95801
359	128 881	18.94730	59.91661	46 268 279	7.107 194	15.31198	32.98867
360	129 600	18.97367	60.00000	46 656 000	7.113 787	15.32619	33.01927
361	130 321	19.00000	60.08328	47 045 881	7.120 367	15.34037	33.04982
362	131 044	19.02630	60.16644	47 437 928	7.126 936	15.35452	33.08031
363	131 769	19.05256	60.24948	47 832 147	7.133 492	15.36864	33.11074
364	132 496	19.07878	60.33241	48 228 544	7.140 037	15.38274	33.14112
365	133 225	19.10497	60.41523	48 627 125	7.146 569	15.39682	33.17144
366	133 956	19.13113	60.49793	49 027 896	7.153 090	15.41087	33.20170
367	134 689	19.15724	60.58052	49 430 863	7.159 599	15.42489	33.23191
368	135 424	19.18333	60.66300	49 836 032	7.166 096	15.43889	33.26207
369	136 161	19.20937	60.74537	50 243 409	7.172 581	15.45286	33.29217
370	136 900	19.23538	60.82763	50 653 000	7.179 054	15.46680	33.32222
371	137 641	19.26136	60.90977	51 064 811	7.185 516	15.48073	33.35221
372	138 384	19.28730	60.99180	51 478 848	7.191 966	15.49462	33.38215
373	139 129	19.31321	61.07373	51 895 117	7.198 405	15.50849	33.41204
374	139 876	19.33908	61.15554	52 313 624	7.204 832	15.52234	33.44187
375	140 625	19.36492	61.23724	52 734 375	7.211 248	15.53616	33.47165
376	141 376	19.39072	61.31884	53 157 376	7.217 652	15.54996	33.50137
377	142 129	19.41649	61.40033	53 582 633	7.224 045	15.56373	33.53105
378	142 884	19.44222	61.48170	54 010 152	7.230 427	15.57748	33.56067
379	143 641	19.46792	61.56298	54 439 939	7.236 797	15.59121	33.59024
380	144 400	19.49359	61.64414	54 872 000	7.243 156	15.60491	33.61975
381	145 161	19.51922	61.72520	55 306 341	7.249 505	15.61858	33.64922
382	145 924	19.54482	61.80615	55 742 968	7.255 842	15.63224	33.67863
383	146 689	19.57039	61.88699	56 181 887	7.262 167	15.64587	33.70800
384	147 456	19.59592	61.96773	56 623 104	7.268 482	15.65947	33.73731
385	148 225	19.62142	62.04837	57 066 625	7.274 786	15.67305	33.76657
386	148 996	19.64688	62.12890	57 512 456	7.281 079	15.68661	33.79578
387	149 769	19.67232	62.20932	57 960 603	7.287 362	15.70014	33.82494
388	150 544	19.69772	62.28965	58 411 072	7.293 633	15.71366	33.85405
389	151 321	19.72308	62.36986	58 863 869	7.299 894	15.72714	33.88310
390	152 100	19.74842	62.44998	59 319 000	7.306 144	15.74061	33.91211
391	152 881	19.77372	62.52999	59 776 471	7.312 383	15.75405	33.94107
392	153 664	19.79899	62.60990	60 236 288	7.318 611	15.76747	33.96999
393	154 449	19.82423	62.68971	60 698 457	7.324 829	15.78087	33.99885
394	155 236	19.84943	62.76942	61 162 984	7.331 037	15.79424	34.02766
395	156 025	19.87461	62.84903	61 629 875	7.337 234	15.80759	34.05642
396	156 816	19.89975	62.92853	62 099 136	7.343 420	15.82092	34.08514
397	157 609	19.92486	63.00794	62 570 773	7.349 597	15.83423	34.11381
398	158 404	19.94994	63.08724	63 044 792	7.355 762	15.84751	34.14242
399	159 201	19.97498	63.16645	63 521 199	7.361 918	15.86077	34.17100
400	160 000	20.00000	63.24555	64 000 000	7.368 063	15.87401	34.19952
401	160 801	20.02498	63.32456	64 481 201	7.374 198	15.88723	34.22799
402	161 604	20.04994	63.40347	64 964 808	7.380 323	15.90042	34.25642
403	162 409	20.07486	63.48228	65 450 827	7.386 437	15.91360	34.28480
404	163 216	20.09975	63.56099	65 939 264	7.392 542	15.92675	34.31314
405	164 025	20.12461	63.63961	66 430 125	7.398 636	15.93988	34.34143
406	164 836	20.14944	63.71813	66 923 416	7.404 721	15.95299	34.36967
407	165 649	20.17424	63.79655	67 419 143	7.410 795	15.96607	34.39786
408	166 464	20.19901	63.87488	67 917 312	7.416 860	15.97914	34.42601
409	167 281	20.22375	63.95311	68 417 929	7.422 914	15.99218	34.45412

SQUARES, CUBES AND ROOTS

n	n^2	$\sqrt{n}$	$\sqrt{10n}$	n^3	$\sqrt[3]{n}$	$\sqrt[3]{10n}$	$\sqrt[3]{100n}$
410	168 100	20.24846	64.03124	68 921 000	7.428 959	16.00521	34.48217
411	168 921	20.27313	64.10928	69 426 531	7.434 994	16.01821	34.51018
412	169 744	20.29778	64.18723	69 934 528	7.441 019	16.03119	34.53815
413	170 569	20.32240	64.26508	70 444 997	7.447 034	16.04415	34.56607
414	171 396	20.34699	64.34283	70 957 944	7.453 040	16.05709	34.59395
415	172 225	20.37155	64.42049	71 473 375	7.459 036	16.07001	34.62178
416	173 056	20.39608	64.49806	71 991 296	7.465 022	16.08290	34.64956
417	173 889	20.42058	64.57554	72 511 713	7.470 999	16.09578	34.67731
418	174 724	20.44505	64.65292	73 034 632	7.476 966	16.10864	34.70500
419	175 561	20.46949	64.73021	73 560 059	7.482 924	16.12147	34.73266
420	176 400	20.49390	64.80741	74 088 000	7.488 872	16.13429	34.76027
421	177 241	20.51828	64.88451	74 618 461	7.494 811	16.14708	34.78783
422	178 084	20.54264	64.96153	75 151 448	7.500 741	16.15986	34.81535
423	178 929	20.56696	65.03845	75 686 967	7.506 661	16.17261	34.84283
424	179 776	20.59126	65.11528	76 225 024	7.512 572	16.18534	34.87027
425	180 625	20.61553	65.19202	76 765 625	7.518 473	16.19806	34.89766
426	181 476	20.63977	65.26868	77 308 776	7.524 365	16.21075	34.92501
427	182 329	20.66398	65.34524	77 854 483	7.530 248	16.22343	34.95232
428	183 184	20.68816	65.42171	78 402 752	7.536 122	16.23608	34.97958
429	184 041	20.71232	65.49809	78 953 589	7.541 987	16.24872	35.00680
430	184 900	20.73644	65.57439	79 507 000	7.547 842	16.26133	35.03398
431	185 761	20.76054	65.65059	80 062 991	7.553 680	16.27393	35.06112
432	186 624	20.78461	65.72671	80 621 568	7.559 526	16.28651	35.08821
433	187 489	20.80865	65.80274	81 182 737	7.565 355	16.29906	35.11527
434	188 356	20.83267	65.87868	81 746 504	7.571 174	16.31160	35.14228
435	189 225	20.85665	65.95453	82 312 875	7.576 985	16.32419	35.16925
436	190 096	20.88061	66.03030	82 881 856	7.582 787	16.33662	35.19618
437	190 969	20.90454	66.10598	83 453 453	7.588 579	16.34910	35.22307
438	191 844	20.92845	66.18157	84 027 672	7.594 363	16.36156	35.24991
439	192 721	20.95233	66.25708	84 604 519	7.600 139	16.37400	35.27672
440	193 600	20.97618	66.33250	85 184 000	7.605 905	16.38643	35.30348
441	194 481	21.00000	66.40783	85 766 121	7.611 663	16.39883	35.33021
442	195 364	21.02380	66.48308	86 350 888	7.617 412	16.41122	35.35689
443	196 249	21.04757	66.55825	86 938 307	7.623 152	16.42358	35.38354
444	197 136	21.07131	66.63332	87 528 384	7.628 884	16.43593	35.41014
445	198 025	21.09502	66.70832	88 121 125	7.634 607	16.44826	35.43671
446	198 916	21.11871	66.78323	88 716 536	7.640 321	16.46057	35.46323
447	199 809	21.14237	66.85806	89 314 623	7.646 027	16.47287	35.48971
448	200 704	21.16601	66.93280	89 915 392	7.651 725	16.48514	35.51616
449	201 601	21.18962	67.00746	90 518 849	7.657 414	16.49740	35.54257
450	202 500	21.21320	67.08204	91 125 000	7.663 094	16.50964	35.56893
451	203 401	21.23676	67.15653	91 733 851	7.668 766	16.52186	35.59526
452	204 304	21.26029	67.23095	92 345 408	7.674 430	16.53406	35.62155
453	205 209	21.28380	67.30527	92 959 677	7.680 086	16.54624	35.64780
454	206 116	21.30728	67.37952	93 576 664	7.685 733	16.55841	35.67401
455	207 025	21.33073	67.45369	94 196 375	7.691 372	16.57056	35.70018
456	207 936	21.35416	67.52777	94 818 816	7.697 002	16.58269	35.72632
457	208 849	21.37756	67.60178	95 443 993	7.702 625	16.59480	35.75242
458	209 764	21.40093	67.67570	96 071 912	7.708 239	16.60690	35.77848
459	210 681	21.42429	67.74954	96 702 579	7.713 845	16.61897	35.80450
460	211 600	21.44761	67.82330	97 336 000	7.719 443	16.63103	35.83048
461	212 521	21.47091	67.89698	97 972 181	7.725 032	16.64308	35.85642
462	213 444	21.49419	67.97058	98 611 128	7.730 614	16.65510	35.88233
463	214 369	21.51743	68.04410	99 252 847	7.736 188	16.66711	35.90820
464	215 296	21.54066	68.11755	99 897 344	7.741 753	16.67910	35.93404
465	216 225	21.56386	68.19091	100 544 625	7.747 311	16.69108	35.95983
466	217 156	21.58703	68.26419	101 194 696	7.752 861	16.70303	35.98559
467	218 089	21.61018	68.33740	101 847 563	7.758 402	16.71497	36.01131
468	219 024	21.63331	68.41053	102 503 232	7.763 936	16.72689	36.03700
469	219 961	21.65641	68.48357	103 161 709	7.769 462	16.73880	36.06265

SQUARES, CUBES AND ROOTS

n	n^2	$\sqrt{n}$	$\sqrt{10n}$	n^3	$\sqrt[3]{n}$	$\sqrt[3]{10n}$	$\sqrt[3]{100n}$
470	220 900	21.67948	68.55655	103 823 000	7.774 980	16.75069	36.08826
471	221 841	21.70253	68.62944	104 487 111	7.780 490	16.76256	36.11384
472	222 784	21.72556	68.70226	105 154 048	7.785 993	16.77441	36.13938
473	223 729	21.74856	68.77500	105 823 817	7.791 488	16.78625	36.16488
474	224 676	21.77154	68.84766	106 496 424	7.796 975	16.79807	36.19035
475	225 625	21.79449	68.92024	107 171 875	7.802 454	16.80988	36.21578
476	226 576	21.81742	68.99275	107 850 176	7.807 925	16.82167	36.24118
477	227 529	21.84033	69.06519	108 531 333	7.813 389	16.83344	36.26654
478	228 484	21.86321	69.13754	109 215 352	7.818 846	16.84519	36.29187
479	229 441	21.88607	69.20983	109 902 239	7.824 294	16.85693	36.31716
480	230 400	21.90890	69.28203	110 592 000	7.829 735	16.86865	36.34241
481	231 361	21.93171	69.35416	111 284 641	7.835 169	16.88036	36.36763
482	232 324	21.95450	69.42622	111 980 168	7.840 595	16.89205	36.39282
483	233 289	21.97726	69.49820	112 678 587	7.846 013	16.90372	36.41797
484	234 256	22.00000	69.57011	113 379 904	7.851 424	16.91538	36.44308
485	235 225	22.02272	69.64194	114 084 125	7.856 828	16.92702	36.46817
486	236 196	22.04541	69.71370	114 791 256	7.862 224	16.93865	36.49321
487	237 169	22.06808	69.78539	115 501 303	7.867 613	16.95026	36.51822
488	238 144	22.09072	69.85700	116 214 272	7.872 994	16.96185	36.54320
489	239 121	22.11334	69.92853	116 930 169	7.878 368	16.97343	36.56815
490	240 100	22.13594	70.00000	117 649 000	7.883 735	16.98499	36.59306
491	241 081	22.15852	70.07139	118 370 771	7.889 095	16.99654	36.61793
492	242 064	22.18107	70.14271	119 095 488	7.894 447	17.00807	36.64278
493	243 049	22.20360	70.21396	119 823 157	7.899 792	17.01959	36.66758
494	244 036	22.22611	70.28513	120 553 784	7.905 129	17.03108	36.69236
495	245 025	22.24860	70.35624	121 287 375	7.910 460	17.04257	36.71710
496	246 016	22.27106	70.42727	122 023 936	7.915 783	17.05404	36.74181
497	247 009	22.29350	70.49823	122 763 473	7.921 099	17.06549	36.76649
498	248 004	22.31591	70.56912	123 505 992	7.926 408	17.07693	36.79113
499	249 001	22.33831	70.63993	124 251 499	7.931 710	17.08835	36.81574
500	250 000	22.36068	70.71068	125 000 000	7.937 005	17.09976	36.84031
501	251 001	22.38303	70.78135	125 751 501	7.942 293	17.11115	36.86486
502	252 004	22.40536	70.85196	126 506 008	7.947 574	17.12253	36.88937
503	253 009	22.42766	70.92249	127 263 527	7.952 848	17.13389	36.91385
504	254 016	22.44994	70.99296	128 024 064	7.958 114	17.14524	36.93830
505	255 025	22.47221	71.06335	128 787 625	7.963 374	17.15657	36.96271
506	256 036	22.49444	71.13368	129 554 216	7.968 627	17.16789	36.98709
507	257 049	22.51666	71.20393	130 323 843	7.973 873	17.17919	37.01144
508	258 064	22.53886	71.27412	131 096 512	7.979 112	17.19048	37.03576
509	259 081	22.56103	71.34424	131 872 229	7.984 344	17.20175	37.06004
510	260 100	22.58318	71.41428	132 651 000	7.989 570	17.21301	37.08430
511	261 121	22.60531	71.48426	133 432 831	7.994 788	17.22425	37.10852
512	262 144	22.62742	71.55418	134 217 728	8.000 000	17.23548	37.13271
513	263 169	22.64950	71.62402	135 005 697	8.005 205	17.24669	37.15687
514	264 196	22.67157	71.69379	135 796 744	8.010 403	17.25789	37.18100
515	265 225	22.69361	71.76350	136 590 875	8.015 595	17.26908	37.20509
516	266 256	22.71563	71.83314	137 388 096	8.020 779	17.28025	37.22916
517	267 289	22.73763	71.90271	138 188 413	8.025 957	17.29140	37.25319
518	268 324	22.75961	71.97222	138 991 832	8.031 129	17.30254	37.27720
519	269 361	22.78157	72.04165	139 798 359	8.036 293	17.31367	37.30117
520	270 400	22.80351	72.11103	140 608 000	8.041 452	17.32478	37.32511
521	271 441	22.82542	72.18033	141 420 761	8.046 603	17.33588	37.34902
522	272 484	22.84732	72.24957	142 236 648	8.051 748	17.34696	37.37290
523	273 529	22.86919	72.31874	143 055 667	8.056 886	17.35804	37.39675
524	274 576	22.89105	72.38784	143 877 824	8.062 018	17.36909	37.42057
525	275 625	22.91288	72.45688	144 703 125	8.067 143	17.38013	37.44436
526	276 676	22.93469	72.52586	145 531 576	8.072 262	17.39116	37.46812
527	277 729	22.95648	72.59477	146 363 183	8.077 374	17.40218	37.49185
528	278 784	22.97825	72.66361	147 197 952	8.082 480	17.41318	37.51555
529	279 841	23.00000	72.73239	148 035 889	8.087 579	17.42416	37.53922

SQUARES, CUBES AND ROOTS

n	n^2	$\sqrt{n}$	$\sqrt{10n}$	n^3	$\sqrt[3]{n}$	$\sqrt[3]{10n}$	$\sqrt[3]{100n}$
530	280 900	23.02173	72.80110	148 877 000	8.092 672	17.43513	37.56286
531	281 961	23.04344	72.86975	149 721 291	8.097 759	17.44609	37.58647
532	283 024	23.06513	72.93833	150 568 768	8.102 839	17.45704	37.61005
533	284 089	23.08679	73.00685	151 419 437	8.107 913	17.46797	37.63360
534	285 156	23.10844	73.07530	152 273 304	8.112 980	17.47889	37.65712
535	286 225	23.13007	73.14369	153 130 375	8.118 041	17.48979	37.68061
536	287 296	23.15167	73.21202	153 990 656	8.123 096	17.50068	37.70407
537	288 369	23.17326	73.28028	154 854 153	8.128 145	17.51156	37.72751
538	289 444	23.19483	73.34848	155 720 872	8.133 187	17.52242	37.75091
539	290 521	23.21637	73.41662	156 590 819	8.138 223	17.53327	37.77429
540	291 600	23.23790	73.48469	157 464 000	8.143 253	17.54411	37.79763
541	292 681	23.25941	73.55270	158 340 421	8.148 276	17.55493	37.82095
542	293 764	23.28089	73.62065	159 220 088	8.153 294	17.56574	37.84424
543	294 849	23.30236	73.68853	160 103 007	8.158 305	17.57654	37.86750
544	295 936	23.32381	73.75636	160 989 184	8.163 310	17.58732	37.89073
545	297 025	23.34524	73.82412	161 878 625	8.168 309	17.59809	37.91393
546	298 116	23.36664	73.89181	162 771 336	8.173 302	17.60885	37.93711
547	299 209	23.38803	73.95945	163 667 323	8.178 289	17.61959	37.96025
548	300 304	23.40940	74.02702	164 566 592	8.183 269	17.63032	37.98337
549	301 401	23.43075	74.09453	165 469 149	8.188 244	17.64104	38.00646
550	302 500	23.45208	74.16198	166 375 000	8.193 213	17.65174	38.02952
551	303 601	23.47339	74.22937	167 284 151	8.198 175	17.66243	38.05256
552	304 704	23.49468	74.29670	168 196 608	8.203 132	17.67311	38.07557
553	305 809	23.51595	74.36397	169 112 377	8.208 082	17.68378	38.09854
554	306 916	23.53720	74.43118	170 031 464	8.213 027	17.69443	38.12149
555	308 025	23.55844	74.49832	170 953 875	8.217 966	17.70507	38.14442
556	309 136	23.57965	74.56541	171 879 616	8.222 899	17.71570	38.16731
557	310 249	23.60085	74.63243	172 808 693	8.227 825	17.72631	38.19018
558	311 364	23.62202	74.69940	173 741 112	8.232 746	17.73691	38.21302
559	312 481	23.64318	74.76630	174 676 879	8.237 661	17.74750	38.23584
560	313 600	23.66432	74.83315	175 616 000	8.242 571	17.75808	38.25862
561	314 721	23.68544	74.89993	176 558 481	8.247 474	17.76864	38.28138
562	315 844	23.70654	74.96666	177 504 328	8.252 372	17.77920	38.30412
563	316 969	23.72762	75.03333	178 453 547	8.257 263	17.78973	38.32682
564	318 096	23.74868	75.09993	179 406 144	8.262 149	17.80026	38.34950
565	319 225	23.76973	75.16648	180 362 125	8.267 029	17.81077	38.37215
566	320 356	23.79075	75.23297	181 321 496	8.271 904	17.82128	38.39478
567	321 489	23.81176	75.29940	182 284 263	8.276 773	17.83177	38.41737
568	322 624	23.83275	75.36577	183 250 432	8.281 635	17.84224	38.43995
569	323 761	23.85372	75.43209	184 220 009	8.286 493	17.85271	38.46249
570	324 900	23.87467	75.49834	185 193 000	8.291 344	17.86316	38.48501
571	326 041	23.89561	75.56454	186 169 411	8.296 190	17.87360	38.50750
572	327 184	23.91652	75.63068	187 149 248	8.301 031	17.88403	38.52997
573	328 329	23.93742	75.69676	188 132 517	8.305 865	17.89444	38.55241
574	329 476	23.95830	75.76279	189 119 224	8.310 694	17.90485	38.57482
575	330 625	23.97916	75.82875	190 109 375	8.315 517	17.91524	38.59721
576	331 776	24.00000	75.89466	191 102 976	8.320 335	17.92562	38.61958
577	332 929	24.02082	75.96052	192 100 033	8.325 148	17.93599	38.64191
578	334 084	24.04163	76.02631	193 100 552	8.329 954	17.94634	38.66422
579	335 241	24.06242	76.09205	194 104 539	8.334 755	17.95669	38.68651
580	336 400	24.08319	76.15773	195 112 000	8.339 551	17.96702	38.70877
581	337 561	24.10394	76.22336	196 122 941	8.344 341	17.97734	38.73100
582	338 724	24.12468	76.28892	197 137 368	8.349 126	17.98765	38.75321
583	339 889	24.14539	76.35444	198 155 287	8.353 905	17.99794	38.77539
584	341 056	24.16609	76.41989	199 176 704	8.358 678	18.00823	38.79755
585	342 225	24.18677	76.48529	200 201 625	8.363 447	18.01850	38.81968
586	343 396	24.20744	76.55064	201 230 056	8.368 209	18.02876	38.84179
587	344 569	24.22808	76.61593	202 262 003	8.372 967	18.03901	38.86387
588	345 744	24.24871	76.68116	203 297 472	8.377 719	18.04925	38.88593
589	346 921	24.26932	76.74634	204 336 469	8.382 465	18.05947	38.90796

SQUARES, CUBES AND ROOTS

n	n^2	$\sqrt{n}$	$\sqrt{10n}$	n^3	$\sqrt[3]{n}$	$\sqrt[3]{10n}$	$\sqrt[3]{100n}$
590	348 100	24.28992	76.81146	205 379 000	8.387 207	18.06969	38.92996
591	349 281	24.31049	76.87652	206 425 071	8.391 942	18.07989	38.95195
592	350 464	24.33105	76.94154	207 474 688	8.396 673	18.09008	38.97390
593	351 649	24.35159	77.00649	208 527 857	8.401 398	18.10026	38.99584
594	352 836	24.37212	77.07140	209 584 584	8.406 118	18.11043	39.01774
595	354 025	24.39262	77.13624	210 644 875	8.410 833	18.12059	39.03963
596	355 216	24.41311	77.20104	211 708 736	8.415 542	18.13074	39.06149
597	356 409	24.43358	77.26578	212 776 173	8.420 246	18.14087	39.08332
598	357 604	24.45404	77.33046	213 847 192	8.424 945	18.15099	39.10513
599	358 801	24.47448	77.39509	214 921 799	8.429 638	18.16111	39.12692
600	360 000	24.49490	77.45967	216 000 000	8.434 327	18.17121	39.14868
601	361 201	24.51530	77.52419	217 081 801	8.439 010	18.18130	39.17041
602	362 404	24.53569	77.58866	218 167 208	8.443 688	18.19137	39.19213
603	363 609	24.55606	77.65307	219 256 227	8.448 361	18.20144	39.21382
604	364 816	24.57641	77.71744	220 348 864	8.453 028	18.21150	39.23548
605	366 025	24.59675	77.78175	221 445 125	8.457 691	18.22154	39.25712
606	367 236	24.61707	77.84600	222 545 016	8.462 348	18.23158	39.27874
607	368 449	24.63737	77.91020	223 648 543	8.467 000	18.24160	39.30033
608	369 664	24.65766	77.97435	224 755 712	8.471 647	18.25161	39.32190
609	370 881	24.67793	78.03845	225 866 529	8.476 289	18.26161	39.34345
610	372 100	24.69818	78.10250	226 981 000	8.480 926	18.27160	39.36497
611	373 321	24.71841	78.16649	228 099 131	8.485 558	18.28158	39.38647
612	374 544	24.73863	78.23043	229 220 928	8.490 185	18.29155	39.40795
613	375 769	24.75884	78.29432	230 346 397	8.494 807	18.30151	39.42940
614	376 996	24.77902	78.35815	231 475 544	8.499 423	18.31145	39.45083
615	378 225	24.79919	78.42194	232 608 375	8.504 035	18.32139	39.47223
616	379 456	24.81935	78.48567	233 744 896	8.508 642	18.33131	39.49362
617	380 689	24.83948	78.54935	234 885 113	8.513 243	18.34123	39.51498
618	381 924	24.85961	78.61298	236 029 032	8.517 840	18.35113	39.53631
619	383 161	24.87971	78.67655	237 176 659	8.522 432	18.36102	39.55763
620	384 400	24.89980	78.74008	238 328 000	8.527 019	18.37091	39.57892
621	385 641	24.91987	78.80355	239 483 061	8.531 601	18.38078	39.60018
622	386 884	24.93993	78.86698	240 641 848	8.536 178	18.39064	39.62143
623	388 129	24.95997	78.93035	241 804 367	8.540 750	18.40049	39.64265
624	389 376	24.97999	78.99367	242 970 624	8.545 317	18.41033	39.66385
625	390 625	25.00000	79.05694	244 140 625	8.549 880	18.42016	39.68503
626	391 876	25.01999	79.12016	245 314 376	8.554 437	18.42998	39.70618
627	393 129	25.03997	79.18333	246 491 883	8.558 990	18.43978	39.72731
628	394 384	25.05993	79.24645	247 673 152	8.563 538	18.44958	39.74842
629	395 641	25.07987	79.30952	248 858 189	8.568 081	18.45937	39.76951
630	396 900	25.09980	79.37254	250 047 000	8.572 619	18.46915	39.79057
631	398 161	25.11971	79.43551	251 239 591	8.577 152	18.47891	39.81161
632	399 424	25.13961	79.49843	252 435 968	8.581 681	18.48867	39.83263
633	400 689	25.15949	79.56130	253 636 137	8.586 205	18.49842	39.85363
634	401 956	25.17936	79.62412	254 840 104	8.590 724	18.50815	39.87461
635	403 225	25.19921	79.68689	256 047 875	8.595 238	18.51788	39.89556
636	404 496	25.21904	79.74961	257 259 456	8.599 748	18.52759	39.91649
637	405 769	25.23886	79.81228	258 474 853	8.604 252	18.53730	39.93740
638	407 044	25.25866	79.87490	259 694 072	8.608 753	18.54700	39.95829
639	408 321	25.27845	79.93748	260 917 119	8.613 248	18.55668	39.97916
640	409 600	25.29822	80.00000	262 144 000	8.617 739	18.56636	40.00000
641	410 881	25.31798	80.06248	263 374 721	8.622 225	18.57602	40.02082
642	412 164	25.33772	80.12490	264 609 288	8.626 706	18.58568	40.04162
643	413 449	25.35744	80.18728	265 847 707	8.631 183	18.59532	40.06240
644	414 736	25.37716	80.24961	267 089 984	8.635 655	18.60495	40.08316
645	416 025	25.39685	80.31189	268 336 125	8.640 123	18.61458	40.10390
646	417 316	25.41653	80.37413	269 586 136	8.644 585	18.62419	40.12461
647	418 609	25.43619	80.43631	270 840 023	8.649 044	18.63380	40.14530
648	419 904	25.45584	80.49845	272 097 792	8.653 497	18.64340	40.16598
649	421 201	25.47548	80.56054	273 359 449	8.657 947	18.65298	40.18663

SQUARES, CUBES AND ROOTS

n	n^2	$\sqrt{n}$	$\sqrt{10n}$	n^3	$\sqrt[3]{n}$	$\sqrt[3]{10n}$	$\sqrt[3]{100n}$
650	422 500	25.49510	80.62258	274 625 000	8.662 391	18.66256	40.20726
651	423 801	25.51470	80.68457	275 894 451	8.666 831	18.67212	40.22787
652	425 104	25.53429	80.74652	277 167 808	8.671 266	18.68168	40.24845
653	426 409	25.55386	80.80842	278 445 077	8.675 697	18.69122	40.26902
654	427 716	25.57342	80.87027	279 726 264	8.680 124	18.70076	40.28957
655	429 025	25.59297	80.93207	281 011 375	8.684 546	18.71029	40.31009
656	430 336	25.61250	80.99383	282 300 416	8.688 963	18.71980	40.33059
657	431 649	25.63201	81.05554	283 593 393	8.693 376	18.72931	40.35108
658	432 964	25.65151	81.11720	284 890 312	8.697 784	18.73881	40.37154
659	434 281	25.67100	81.17881	286 191 179	8.702 188	18.74830	40.39198
660	435 600	25.69047	81.24038	287 496 000	8.706 588	18.75777	40.41240
661	436 921	25.70992	81.30191	288 804 781	8.710 983	18.76724	40.43280
662	438 244	25.72936	81.36338	290 117 528	8.715 373	18.77670	40.45318
663	439 569	25.74879	81.42481	291 434 247	8.719 760	18.78615	40.47354
664	440 896	25.76820	81.48620	292 754 944	8.724 141	18.79559	40.49388
665	442 225	25.78759	81.54753	294 079 625	8.728 519	18.80502	40.51420
666	443 556	25.80698	81.60882	295 408 296	8.732 892	18.81444	40.53449
667	444 889	25.82634	81.67007	296 740 963	8.737 260	18.82386	40.55477
668	446 224	25.84570	81.73127	298 077 632	8.741 625	18.83326	40.57503
669	447 561	25.86503	81.79242	299 418 309	8.745 985	18.84265	40.59526
670	448 900	25.88436	81.85353	300 763 000	8.750 340	18.85204	40.61548
671	450 241	25.90367	81.91459	302 111 711	8.754 691	18.86141	40.63568
672	451 584	25.92296	81.97561	303 464 448	8.759 038	18.87078	40.65585
673	452 929	25.94224	82.03658	304 821 217	8.763 381	18.88013	40.67601
674	454 276	25.96151	82.09750	306 182 024	8.767 719	18.88948	40.69615
675	455 625	25.98076	82.15838	307 546 875	8.772 053	18.89882	40.71626
676	456 976	26.00000	82.21922	308 915 776	8.776 383	18.90814	40.73636
677	458 329	26.01922	82.28001	310 288 733	8.780 708	18.91746	40.75644
678	459 684	26.03843	82.34076	311 665 752	8.785 030	18.92677	40.77650
679	461 041	26.05763	82.40146	313 046 839	8.789 347	18.93607	40.79653
680	462 400	26.07681	82.46211	314 432 000	8.793 659	18.94536	40.81655
681	463 761	26.09598	82.52272	315 821 241	8.797 968	18.95465	40.83655
682	465 124	26.11513	82.58329	317 214 568	8.802 272	18.96392	40.85653
683	466 489	26.13427	82.64381	318 611 987	8.806 572	18.97318	40.87649
684	467 856	26.15339	82.70429	320 013 504	8.810 868	18.98244	40.89643
685	469 225	26.17250	82.76473	321 419 125	8.815 160	18.99169	40.91635
686	470 596	26.19160	82.82512	322 828 856	8.819 447	19.00092	40.93625
687	471 969	26.21068	82.88546	324 242 703	8.823 731	19.01015	40.95613
688	473 344	26.22975	82.94577	325 660 672	8.828 010	19.01937	40.97599
689	474 721	26.24881	83.00602	327 082 769	8.832 285	19.02858	40.99584
690	476 100	26.26785	83.06624	328 509 000	8.836 556	19.03778	41.01566
691	477 481	26.28688	83.12641	329 939 371	8.840 823	19.04698	41.03546
692	478 864	26.30589	83.18654	331 373 888	8.845 085	19.05616	41.05525
693	480 249	26.32489	83.24662	332 812 557	8.849 344	19.06533	41.07502
694	481 636	26.34388	83.30666	334 255 384	8.853 599	19.07450	41.09476
695	483 025	26.36285	83.36666	335 702 375	8.857 849	19.08366	41.11449
696	484 416	26.38181	83.42661	337 153 536	8.862 095	19.09281	41.13420
697	485 809	26.40076	83.48653	338 608 873	8.866 338	19.10195	41.15389
698	487 204	26.41969	83.54639	340 068 392	8.870 576	19.11108	41.17357
699	488 601	26.43861	83.60622	341 532 099	8.874 810	19.12020	41.19322
700	490 000	26.45751	83.66600	343 000 000	8.879 040	19.12931	41.21285
701	491 401	26.47640	83.72574	344 472 101	8.883 266	19.13842	41.23247
702	492 804	26.49528	83.78544	345 948 408	8.887 488	19.14751	41.25207
703	494 209	26.51415	83.84510	347 428 927	8.891 706	19.15660	41.27164
704	495 616	26.53300	83.90471	348 913 664	8.895 920	19.16568	41.29120
705	497 025	26.55184	83.96428	350 402 625	8.900 130	19.17475	41.31075
706	498 436	26.57066	84.02381	351 895 816	8.904 337	19.18381	41.33027
707	499 849	26.58947	84.08329	353 393 243	8.908 539	19.19286	41.34977
708	501 264	26.60827	84.14274	354 894 912	8.912 737	19.20191	41.36926
709	502 681	26.62705	84.20214	356 400 829	8.916 931	19.21095	41.38873

SQUARES, CUBES AND ROOTS

n	n^2	$\sqrt{n}$	$\sqrt{10n}$	n^3	$\sqrt[3]{n}$	$\sqrt[3]{10n}$	$\sqrt[3]{100n}$
710	504 100	26.64583	84.26150	357 911 000	8.921 121	19.21997	41.40818
711	505 521	26.66458	84.32082	359 425 431	8.925 308	19.22899	41.42761
712	506 944	26.68333	84.38009	360 944 128	8.929 490	19.23800	41.44702
713	508 369	26.70206	84.43933	362 467 097	8.933 669	19.24701	41.46642
714	509 796	26.72078	84.49852	363 994 344	8.937 843	19.25600	41.48579
715	511 225	26.73948	84.55767	365 525 875	8.942 014	19.26499	41.50515
716	512 656	26.75818	84.61678	367 061 696	8.946 181	19.27396	41.52449
717	514 089	26.77686	84.67585	368 601 813	8.950 344	19.28293	41.54382
718	515 524	26.79552	84.73488	370 146 232	8.954 503	19.29189	41.56312
719	516 961	26.81418	84.79387	371 694 959	8.958 658	19.30084	41.58241
720	518 400	26.83282	84.85281	373 248 000	8.962 809	19.30979	41.60168
721	519 841	26.85144	84.91172	374 805 361	8.966 957	19.31872	41.62093
722	521 284	26.87006	84.97058	376 367 048	8 971 101	19.32765	41.64016
723	522 729	26.88866	85.02941	377 933 067	8.975 241	19.33657	41.65938
724	524 176	26.90725	85.08819	379 503 424	8.979 377	19.34548	41.67857
725	525 625	26.92582	85.14693	381 078 125	8.983 509	19.35438	41.69775
726	527 076	26.94439	85.20563	382 657 176	8.987 637	19.36328	41.71692
727	528 529	26.96294	85.26429	384 240 583	8.991 762	19.37216	41.73606
728	529 984	26.98148	85.32292	385 828 352	8.995 883	19.38104	41.75519
729	531 441	27.00000	85.38150	387 420 489	9.000 000	19.38991	41.77430
730	532 900	27.01851	85.44004	389 017 000	9.004 113	19.39877	41.79339
731	534 361	27.03701	85.49854	390 617 891	9.008 223	19.40763	41.81247
732	535 824	27.05550	85 55700	392 223 168	9.012 329	19.41647	41.83152
733	537 289	27.07397	85.61542	393 832 837	9.016 431	19.42531	41.85056
734	538 756	27.09243	85.67380	395 446 904	9.020 529	19.43414	41.86959
735	540 225	27.11088	85.73214	397 065 375	9.024 624	19.44296	41.88859
736	541 696	27.12932	85.79044	398 688 256	9.028 715	19.45178	41.90758
737	543 169	27.14774	85.84870	400 315 553	9.032 802	19.46058	41.92655
738	544 644	27.16616	85.90693	401 947 272	9.036 886	19.46938	41.94551
739	546 121	27.18455	85.96511	403 583 419	9.040 966	19.47817	41.96444
740	547 600	27.20294	86.02325	405 224 000	9.045 042	19.48695	41.98336
741	549 081	27.22132	86.08136	406 869 021	9.049 114	19.49573	42.00227
742	550 564	27.23968	86.13942	408 518 488	9.053 183	19.50449	42.02115
743	552 049	27.25803	86.19745	410 172 407	9.057 248	19.51325	42.04002
744	553 536	27.27636	86.25543	411 830 784	9.061 310	19.52200	42.05887
745	555 025	27 29469	86.31338	413 493 625	9.065 368	19.53074	42.07771
746	556 516	27.31300	86.37129	415 160 936	9.069 422	19.53948	42.09653
747	558 009	27.33130	86.42916	416 832 723	9.073 473	19.54820	42.11533
748	559 504	27.34959	86.48699	418 508 992	9.077 520	19 55692	42.13411
749	561 001	27.36786	86.54479	420 189 749	9.081 563	19.56563	42.15288
750	562 500	27.38613	86.60254	421 875 000	9.085 603	19.57434	42.17163
751	564 001	27.40438	86.66026	423 564 751	9.089 639	19.58303	42.19037
752	565 504	27.42262	86.71793	425 259 008	9.093 672	19.59172	42.20909
753	567 009	27.44085	86.77557	426 957 777	9.097 701	19.60040	42.22779
754	568 516	27.45906	86.83317	428 661 064	9.101 727	19.60908	42.24647
755	570 025	27.47726	86.89074	430 368 875	9.105 748	19.61774	42.26514
756	571 536	27.49545	86.94826	432 081 216	9.109 767	19.62640	42.28379
757	573 049	27.51363	87.00575	433 798 093	9.113 782	19.63505	42.30243
758	574 564	27.53180	87.06320	435 519 512	9.117 793	19.64369	42.32105
759	576 081	27.54995	87.12061	437 245 479	9.121 801	19.65232	42.33965
760	577 600	27.56810	87.17798	438 976 000	9.125 805	19.66095	42.35824
761	579 121	27.58623	87.23531	440 711 081	9.129 806	19.66957	42.37681
762	580 644	27.60435	87.29261	442 450 728	9.133 803	19.67818	42.39536
763	582 169	27.62245	87.34987	444 194 947	9.137 797	19.68679	42.41390
764	583 696	27.64055	87.40709	445 943 744	9.141 787	19.69538	42.43242
765	585 225	27.65863	87.46428	447 697 125	9.145 774	19.70397	42.45092
766	586 756	27.67671	87.52143	449 455 096	9.149 758	19.71256	42.46941
767	588 289	27.69476	87.57854	451 217 663	9.153 738	19.72113	42.48789
768	589 824	27.71281	87.63561	452 984 832	9.157 714	19.72970	42.50634
769	591 361	27.73085	87.69265	454 756 609	9.161 687	19.73826	42.52478

SQUARES, CUBES AND ROOTS

n	n^2	$\sqrt{n}$	$\sqrt{10n}$	n^3	$\sqrt[3]{n}$	$\sqrt[3]{10n}$	$\sqrt[3]{100n}$
770	592 900	27.74887	87.74964	456 533 000	9.165 656	19.74681	42.54321
771	594 441	27.76689	87.80661	458 314 011	9.169 623	19.75535	42.56162
772	595 984	27.78489	87.86353	460 099 648	9.173 585	19.76389	42.58001
773	597 529	27.80288	87.92042	461 889 917	9.177 544	19.77242	42.59839
774	599 076	27.82086	87.97727	463 684 824	9.181 500	19.78094	42.61675
775	600 625	27.83882	88.03408	465 484 375	9.185 453	19.78946	42.63509
776	602 176	27.85678	88.09086	467 288 576	9.189 402	19.79797	42.65342
777	603 729	27.87472	88.14760	469 097 433	9.193 347	19.80647	42.67174
778	605 284	27.89265	88.20431	470 910 952	9.197 290	19.81496	42.69004
779	606 841	27.91057	88.26098	472 729 139	9.201 229	19.82345	42.70832
780	608 400	27.92848	88.31761	474 552 000	9.205 164	19.83192	42.72659
781	609 961	27.94638	88.37420	476 379 541	9.209 096	19.84040	42.74484
782	611 524	27.96426	88.43076	478 211 768	9.213 025	19.84886	42.76307
783	613 089	27.98214	88.48729	480 048 687	9.216 950	19.85732	42.78129
784	614 656	28.00000	88.54377	481 890 304	9.220 873	19.86577	42.79950
785	616 225	28.01785	88.60023	483 736 625	9.224 791	19.87421	42.81769
786	617 796	28.03569	88.65664	485 587 656	9.228 707	19.88265	42.83586
787	619 369	28.05352	88.71302	487 443 403	9.232 619	19.89107	42.85402
788	620 944	28.07134	88.76936	489 303 872	9.236 528	19.89950	42.87216
789	622 521	28.08914	88.82567	491 169 069	9.240 433	19.90791	42.89029
790	624 100	28.10694	88.88194	493 039 000	9.244 335	19.91632	42.90840
791	625 681	28.12472	88.93818	494 913 671	9.248 234	19.92472	42.92650
792	627 264	28.14249	88.99438	496 793 088	9.252 130	19.93311	42.94458
793	628 849	28.16026	89.05055	498 677 257	9.256 022	19.94150	42.96265
794	630 436	28.17801	89.10668	500 566 184	9.259 911	19.94987	42.98070
795	632 025	28.19574	89.16277	502 459 875	9.263 797	19.95825	42.99874
796	633 616	28.21347	89.21883	504 358 336	9.267 680	19.96661	43.01676
797	635 209	28.23119	89.27486	506 261 573	9.271 559	19.97497	43.03477
798	636 804	28.24889	89.33085	508 169 592	9.275 435	19.98332	43.05276
799	638 401	28.26659	89.38680	510 082 399	9.279 308	19.99166	43.07073
800	640 000	28.28427	89.44272	512 000 000	9.283 178	20.00000	43.08869
801	641 601	28.30194	89.49860	513 922 401	9.287 044	20.00833	43.10664
802	643 204	28.31960	89.55445	515 849 608	9.290 907	20.01665	43.12457
803	644 809	28.33725	89.61027	517 781 627	9.294 767	20.02497	43.14249
804	646 416	28.35489	89.66605	519 718 464	9.298 624	20.03328	43.16039
805	648 025	28.37252	89.72179	521 660 125	9.302 477	20.04158	43.17828
806	649 636	28.39014	89.77750	523 606 616	9.306 328	20.04988	43.19615
807	651 249	28.40775	89.83318	525 557 943	9.310 175	20.05816	43.21400
808	652 864	28.42534	89.88882	527 514 112	9.314 019	20.06645	43.23185
809	654 481	28.44293	89.94443	529 475 129	9.317 860	20.07472	43.24967
810	656 100	28.46050	90.00000	531 441 000	9.321 698	20.08299	43.26749
811	657 721	28.47806	90.05554	533 411 731	9.325 532	20.09125	43.28529
812	659 344	28.49561	90.11104	535 387 328	9.329 363	20.09950	43.30307
813	660 969	28.51315	90.16651	537 367 797	9.333 192	20.10775	43.32084
814	662 596	28.53069	90.22195	539 353 144	9.337 017	20.11599	43.33859
815	664 225	28.54820	90.27735	541 343 375	9.340 839	20.12423	43.35633
816	665 856	28.56571	90.33272	543 338 496	9.344 657	20.13245	43.37406
817	667 489	28.58321	90.38805	545 338 513	9.348 473	20.14067	43.39177
818	669 124	28.60070	90.44335	547 343 432	9.352 286	20.14889	43.40947
819	670 761	28.61818	90.49862	549 353 259	9.356 095	20.15710	43.42715
820	672 400	28.63564	90.55385	551 368 000	9.359 902	20.16530	43.44481
821	674 041	28.65310	90.60905	553 387 661	9.363 705	20.17349	43.46247
822	675 684	28.67054	90.66422	555 412 248	9.367 505	20.18168	43.48011
823	677 329	28.68798	90.71935	557 441 767	9.371 302	20.18986	43.49773
824	678 976	28.70540	90.77445	559 476 224	9.375 096	20.19803	43.51534
825	680 625	28.72281	90.82951	561 515 625	9.378 887	20.20620	43.53294
826	682 276	28.74022	90.88454	563 559 976	9.382 675	20.21436	43.55052
827	683 929	28.75761	90.93954	565 609 283	9.386 460	20.22252	43.56809
828	685 584	28.77499	90.99451	567 663 552	9.390 242	20.23066	43.58564
829	687 241	28.79236	91.04944	569 722 789	9.394 021	20.23880	43.60318

SQUARES, CUBES AND ROOTS

n	n^2	$\sqrt{n}$	$\sqrt{10n}$	n^3	$\sqrt[3]{n}$	$\sqrt[3]{10n}$	$\sqrt[3]{100n}$
830	688 900	28.80972	91.10434	571 787 000	9.397 796	20.24694	43.62071
831	690 561	28.82707	91.15920	573 856 191	9.401 569	20.25507	43.63822
832	692 224	28.84441	91.21403	575 930 368	9.405 339	20.26319	43.65572
833	693 889	28.86174	91.26883	578 009 537	9.409 105	20.27130	43.67320
834	695 556	28.87906	91.32360	580 093 704	9.412 869	20.27941	43.69067
835	697 225	28.89637	91.37833	582 182 875	9.416 630	20.28751	43.70812
836	698 896	28.91366	91.43304	584 277 056	9.420 387	20.29561	43.72556
837	700 569	28.93095	91.48770	586 376 253	9.424 142	20.30370	43.74299
838	702 244	28.94823	91.54234	588 480 472	9.427 894	20.31178	43.76041
839	703 921	28.96550	91.59694	590 589 719	9.431 642	20.31986	43.77781
840	705 600	28.98275	91.65151	592 704 000	9.435 388	20.32793	43.79519
841	707 281	29.00000	91.70605	594 823 321	9.439 131	20.33599	43.81256
842	708 964	29.01724	91.76056	596 947 688	9.442 870	20.34405	43.82992
843	710 649	29.03446	91.81503	599 077 107	9.446 607	20.35210	43.84727
844	712 336	29.05168	91.86947	601 211 584	9.450 341	20.36014	43.86460
845	714 025	29.06888	91.92388	603 351 125	9.454 072	20.36818	43.88191
846	715 716	29.08608	91.97826	605 495 736	9.457 800	20.37621	43.89922
847	717 409	29.10326	92.03260	607 645 423	9.461 525	20.38424	43.91651
848	719 104	29.12044	92.08692	609 800 192	9.465 247	20.39226	43.93378
849	720 801	29.13760	92.14120	611 960 049	9.468 966	20.40027	43.95105
850	722 500	29.15476	92.19544	614 125 000	9.472 682	20.40828	43.96830
851	724 201	29.17190	92.24966	616 295 051	9.476 396	20.41628	43.98553
852	725 904	29.18904	92.30385	618 470 208	9.480 106	20.42427	44.00275
853	727 609	29.20616	92.35800	620 650 477	9.483 814	20.43226	44.01996
854	729 316	29.22328	92.41212	622 835 864	9.487 518	20.44024	44.03716
855	731 025	29.24038	92.46621	625 026 375	9.491 220	20.44821	44.05434
856	732 736	29.25748	92.52027	627 222 016	9.494 919	20.45618	44.07151
857	734 449	29.27456	92.57429	629 422 793	9.498 615	20.46415	44.08866
858	736 164	29.29164	92.62829	631 628 712	9.502 308	20.47210	44.10581
859	737 881	29.30870	92.68225	633 839 779	9.505 998	20.48005	44.12293
860	739 600	29.32576	92.73618	636 056 000	9.509 685	20.48800	44.14005
861	741 321	29.34280	92.79009	638 277 381	9.513 370	20.49593	44.15715
862	743 044	29.35984	92.84396	640 503 928	9.517 052	20.50387	44.17424
863	744 769	29.37686	92.89779	642 735 647	9.520 730	20.51179	44.19132
864	746 496	29.39388	92.95160	644 972 544	9.524 406	20.51971	44.20838
865	748 225	29.41088	93.00538	647 214 625	9.528 079	20.52762	44.22543
866	749 956	29.42788	93.05912	649 461 896	9.531 750	20.53553	44.24246
867	751 689	29.44486	93.11283	651 714 363	9.535 417	20.54343	44.25949
868	753 424	29.46184	93.16652	653 972 032	9.539 082	20.55133	44.27650
869	755 161	29.47881	93.22017	656 234 909	9.542 744	20.55922	44.29349
870	756 900	29.49576	93.27379	658 503 000	9.546 403	20.56710	44.31048
871	758 641	29.51271	93.32738	660 776 311	9.550 059	20.57498	44.32745
872	760 384	29.52965	93.38094	663 054 848	9.553 712	20.58285	44.34440
873	762 129	29.54657	93.43447	665 338 617	9.557 363	20.59071	44.36135
874	763 876	29.56349	93.48797	667 627 624	9.561 011	20.59857	44.37828
875	765 625	29.58040	93.54143	669 921 875	9.564 656	20.60643	44.39520
876	767 376	29.59730	93.59487	672 221 376	9.568 298	20.61427	44.41211
877	769 129	29.61419	93.64828	674 526 133	9.571 938	20.62211	44.42900
878	770 884	29.63106	93.70165	676 836 152	9.575 574	20.62995	44.44588
879	772 641	29.64793	93.75500	679 151 439	9.579 208	20.63778	44.46275
880	774 400	29.66479	93.80832	681 472 000	9.582 840	20.64560	44.47960
881	776 161	29.68164	93.86160	683 797 841	9.586 468	20.65342	44.49644
882	777 924	29.69848	93.91486	686 128 968	9.590 094	20.66123	44.51327
883	779 689	29.71532	93.96808	688 465 387	9.593 717	20.66904	44.53009
884	781 456	29.73214	94.02127	690 807 104	9.597 337	20.67684	44.54689
885	783 225	29.74895	94.07444	693 154 125	9.600 955	20.68463	44.56368
886	784 996	29.76575	94.12757	695 506 456	9.604 570	20.69242	44.58046
887	786 769	29.78255	94.18068	697 864 103	9.608 182	20.70020	44.59723
888	788 544	29.79933	94.23375	700 227 072	9.611 791	20.70798	44.61398
889	790 321	29.81610	94.28680	702 595 369	9.615 398	20.71575	44.63072

SQUARES, CUBES AND ROOTS

n	n^2	$\sqrt{n}$	$\sqrt{10n}$	n^3	$\sqrt[3]{n}$	$\sqrt[3]{10n}$	$\sqrt[3]{100n}$
890	792 100	29.83287	94.33981	704 969 000	9.619 002	20.72351	44.64745
891	793 881	29.84962	94.39280	707 347 971	9.622 603	20.73127	44.66417
892	795 664	29.86637	94.44575	709 732 288	9.626 202	20.73902	44.68087
893	797 449	29.88311	94.49868	712 121 957	9.629 797	20.74677	44.69756
894	799 236	29.89983	94.55157	714 516 984	9.633 391	20.75451	44.71424
895	801 025	29.91655	94.60444	716 917 375	9.636 981	20.76225	44.73090
896	802 816	29.93326	94.65728	719 323 136	9.640 569	20.76998	44.74756
897	804 609	29.94996	94.71008	721 734 273	9.644 154	20.77770	44.76420
898	806 404	29.96665	94.76286	724 150 792	9.647 737	20.78542	44.78083
899	808 201	29.98333	94.81561	726 572 699	9.651 317	20.79313	44.79744
900	810 000	30.00000	94.86833	729 000 000	9.654 894	20.80084	44.81405
901	811 801	30.01666	94.92102	731 432 701	9.658 468	20.80854	44.83064
902	813 604	30.03331	94.97368	733 870 808	9.662 040	20.81623	44.84722
903	815 409	30.04996	95.02631	736 314 327	9.665 610	20.82392	44.86379
904	817 216	30.06659	95.07891	738 763 264	9.669 176	20.83161	44.88034
905	819 025	30.08322	95.13149	741 217 625	9.672 740	20.83929	44.89688
906	820 836	30.09983	95.18403	743 677 416	9.676 302	20.84696	44.91341
907	822 649	30.11644	95.23655	746 142 643	9.679 860	20.85463	44.92993
908	824 464	30.13304	95.28903	748 613 312	9.683 417	20.86229	44.94644
909	826 281	30.14963	95.34149	751 089 429	9.686 970	20.86994	44.96293
910	828 100	30.16621	95.39392	753 571 000	9.690 521	20.87759	44.97941
911	829 921	30.18278	95.44632	756 058 031	9.694 069	20.88524	44.99588
912	831 744	30.19934	95.49869	758 550 528	9.697 615	20.89288	45.01234
913	833 569	30.21589	95.55103	761 048 497	9.701 158	20.90051	45.02879
914	835 396	30.23243	95.60335	763 551 944	9.704 699	20.90814	45.04522
915	837 225	30.24897	95.65563	766 060 875	9.708 237	20.91576	45.06164
916	839 056	30.26549	95.70789	768 575 296	9.711 772	20.92338	45.07805
917	840 889	30.28201	95.76012	771 095 213	9.715 305	20.93099	45.09445
918	842 724	30.29851	95.81232	773 620 632	9.718 835	20.93860	45.11084
919	844 561	30.31501	95.86449	776 151 559	9.722 363	20.94620	45.12721
920	846 400	30.33150	95.91663	778 688 000	9.725 888	20.95379	45.14357
921	848 241	30.34798	95.96874	781 229 961	9.729 411	20.96138	45.15992
922	850 084	30.36445	96.02083	783 777 448	9.732 931	20.96896	45.17626
923	851 929	30.38092	96.07289	786 330 467	9.736 448	20.97654	45.19259
924	853 776	30.39737	96.12492	788 889 024	9.739 963	20.98411	45.20891
925	855 625	30.41381	96.17692	791 453 125	9.743 476	20.99168	45.22521
926	857 476	30.43025	96.22889	794 022 776	9.746 986	20.99924	45.24150
927	859 329	30.44667	96.28084	796 597 983	9.750 493	21.00680	45.25778
928	861 184	30.46309	96.33276	799 178 752	9.753 998	21.01435	45.27405
929	863 041	30.47950	96.38465	801 765 089	9.757 500	21.02190	45.29030
930	864 900	30.49590	96.43651	804 357 000	9.761 000	21.02944	45.30655
931	866 761	30.51229	96.48834	806 954 491	9.764 497	21.03697	45.32278
932	868 624	30.52868	96.54015	809 557 568	9.767 992	21.04450	45.33900
933	870 489	30.54505	96.59193	812 166 237	9.771 485	21.05203	45.35521
934	872 356	30.56141	96.64368	814 780 504	9.774 974	21.05954	45.37141
935	874 225	30.57777	96.69540	817 400 375	9.778 462	21.06706	45.38760
936	876 096	30.59412	96.74709	820 025 856	9.781 946	21.07456	45.40377
937	877 969	30.61046	96.79876	822 656 953	9.785 429	21.08207	45.41994
938	879 844	30.62679	96.85040	825 293 672	9.788 909	21.08956	45.43609
939	881 721	30.64311	96.90201	827 936 019	9.792 386	21.09706	45.45223
940	883 600	30.65942	96.95360	830 584 000	9.795 861	21.10454	45.46836
941	885 481	30.67572	97.00515	833 237 621	9.799 334	21.11202	45.48448
942	887 364	30.69202	97.05668	835 896 888	9.802 804	21.11950	45.50058
943	889 249	30.70831	97.10819	838 561 807	9.806 271	21.12697	45.51668
944	891 136	30.72458	97.15966	841 232 384	9.809 736	21.13444	45.53276
945	893 025	30.74085	97.21111	843 908 625	9.813 199	21.14190	45.54883
946	894 916	30.75711	97.26253	846 590 536	9.816 659	21.14935	45.56490
947	896 809	30.77337	97.31393	849 278 123	9.820 117	21.15680	45.58095
948	898 704	30.78961	97.36529	851 971 392	9.823 572	21.16424	45.59698
949	900 601	30.80584	97.41663	854 670 349	9.827 025	21.17168	45.61301

SQUARES, CUBES AND ROOTS

n	n^2	$\sqrt{n}$	$\sqrt{10n}$	n^3	$\sqrt[3]{n}$	$\sqrt[3]{10n}$	$\sqrt[3]{100n}$
950	902 500	30.82207	97.46794	857 375 000	9.830 476	21.17912	45.62903
951	904 401	30.83829	97.51923	860 085 351	9.833 924	21.18655	45.64503
952	906 304	30.85450	97.57049	862 801 408	9.837 369	21.19397	45.66102
953	908 209	30.87070	97.62172	865 523 177	9.840 813	21.20139	45.67701
954	910 116	30.88689	97.67292	868 250 664	9.844 254	21.20880	45.69298
955	912 025	30.90307	97.72410	870 983 875	9.847 692	21.21621	45.70894
956	913 936	30.91925	97.77525	873 722 816	9.851 128	21.22361	45.72489
957	915 849	30.93542	97.82638	876 467 493	9.854 562	21.23101	45.74082
958	917 764	30.95158	97.87747	879 217 912	9.857 993	21.23840	45.75675
959	919 681	30.96773	97.92855	881 974 079	9.861 422	21.24579	45.77267
960	921 600	30.98387	97.97959	884 736 000	9.864 848	21.25317	45.78857
961	923 521	31.00000	98.03061	887 503 681	9.868 272	21.26055	45.80446
962	925 444	31.01612	98.08160	890 277 128	9.871 694	21.26792	45.82035
963	927 369	31.03224	98.13256	893 056 347	9.875 113	21.27529	45.83622
964	929 296	31.04835	98.18350	895 841 344	9.878 530	21.28265	45.85208
965	931 225	31.06445	98.23441	898 632 125	9.881 945	21.29001	45.86793
966	933 156	31.08054	98.28530	901 428 696	9.885 357	21.29736	45.88376
967	935 089	31.09662	98.33616	904 231 063	9.888 767	21.30470	45.89959
968	937 024	31.11270	98.38699	907 039 232	9.892 175	21.31204	45.91541
969	938 961	31.12876	98.43780	909 853 209	9.895 580	21.31938	45.93121
970	940 900	31.14482	98.48858	912 673 000	9.898 983	21.32671	45.94701
971	942 841	31.16087	98.53933	915 498 611	9.902 384	21.33404	45.96279
972	944 784	31.17691	98.59006	918 330 048	9.905 782	21.34136	45.97857
973	946 729	31.19295	98.64076	921 167 317	9.909 178	21.34868	45.99433
974	948 676	31.20897	98.69144	924 010 424	9.912 571	21.35599	46.01008
975	950 625	31.22499	98.74209	926 859 375	9.915 962	21.36329	46.02582
976	952 576	31.24100	98.79271	929 714 176	9.919 351	21.37059	46.04155
977	954 529	31.25700	98.84331	932 574 833	9.922 738	21.37789	46.05727
978	956 484	31.27299	98.89388	935 441 352	9.926 122	21.38518	46.07298
979	958 441	31.28898	98.94443	938 313 739	9.929 504	21.39247	46.08868
980	960 400	31.30495	98.99495	941 192 000	9.932 884	21.39975	46.10436
981	962 361	31.32092	99.04544	944 076 141	9.936 261	21.40703	46.12004
982	964 324	31.33688	99.09591	946 966 168	9.939 636	21.41430	46.13571
983	966 289	31.35283	99.14636	949 862 087	9.943 009	21.42156	46.15136
984	968 256	31.36877	99.19677	952 763 904	9.946 380	21.42883	46.16700
985	970 225	31.38471	99.24717	955 671 625	9.949 748	21.43608	46.18264
986	972 196	31.40064	99.29753	958 585 256	9.953 114	21.44333	46.19826
987	974 169	31.41656	99.34787	961 504 803	9.956 478	21.45058	46.21387
988	976 144	31.43247	99.39819	964 430 272	9.959 839	21.45782	46.22948
989	978 121	31.44837	99.44848	967 361 669	9.963 198	21.46506	46.24507
990	980 100	31.46427	99.49874	970 299 000	9.966 555	21.47229	46.26065
991	982 081	31.48015	99.54898	973 242 271	9.969 910	21.47952	46.27622
992	984 064	31.49603	99.59920	976 191 488	9.973 262	21.48674	46.29178
993	986 049	31.51190	99.64939	979 146 657	9.976 612	21.49396	46.30733
994	988 036	31.52777	99.69955	982 107 784	9.979 960	21.50117	46.32287
995	990 025	31.54362	99.74969	985 074 875	9.983 305	21.50838	46.33840
996	992 016	31.55947	99.79980	988 047 936	9.986 649	21.51558	46.35392
997	994 009	31.57531	99.84989	991 026 973	9.989 990	21.52278	46.36943
998	996 004	31.59114	99.89995	994 011 992	9.993 329	21.52997	46.38492
999	998 001	31.60696	99.94999	997 002 999	9.996 666	21.53716	46.40041
1000	1 000 000	31.62278	100.00000	1 000 000 000	10.000 000	21.54435	46.41589

XIII.6 EXPONENTIAL FUNCTIONS

Values of e^x, log e^x and e^{-x} where e is the base of the natural system of logarithms 2.71828 . . . and x has values from 0 to 10. Facilitating the solution of exponential equations, these tables also serve as a table of natural or Naperian antilogarithms. For instance, if the logarithm or exponent $x = 3.26$, the corresponding number or value of e^x is 26.050. Its reciprocal e^{-x} is .038388.

EXPONENTIAL FUNCTIONS

x	e^x	$\text{Log}_{10}(e^x)$	e^{-x}	x	e^x	$\text{Log}_{10}(e^x)$	e^{-x}
0.00	1.0000	0.00000	1.000000	**0.50**	1.6487	0.21715	0.606531
0.01	1.0101	.00434	0.990050	0.51	1.6653	.22149	.600496
0.02	1.0202	.00869	.980199	0.52	1.6820	.22583	.594521
0.03	1.0305	.01303	.970446	0.53	1.6989	.23018	.588605
0.04	1.0408	.01737	.960789	0.54	1.7160	.23452	.582748
0.05	1.0513	0.02171	0.951229	**0.55**	1.7333	0.23886	0.576950
0.06	1.0618	.02606	.941765	0.56	1.7507	.24320	.571209
0.07	1.0725	.03040	.932394	0.57	1.7683	.24755	.565525
0.08	1.0833	.03474	.923116	0.58	1.7860	.25189	.559898
0.09	1.0942	.03909	.913931	0.59	1.8040	.25623	.554327
0.10	1.1052	0.04343	0.904837	**0.60**	1.8221	0.26058	0.548812
0.11	1.1163	.04777	.895834	0.61	1.8404	.26492	.543351
0.12	1.1275	.05212	.886920	0.62	1.8589	.26926	.537944
0.13	1.1388	.05646	.878095	0.63	1.8776	.27361	.532592
0.14	1.1503	.06080	.869358	0.64	1.8965	.27795	.527292
0.15	1.1618	0.06514	0.860708	**0.65**	1.9155	0.28229	0.522046
0.16	1.1735	.06949	.852144	0.66	1.9348	.28663	.516851
0.17	1.1853	.07383	.843665	0.67	1.9542	.29098	.511709
0.18	1.1972	.07817	.835270	0.68	1.9739	.29532	.506617
0.19	1.2092	.08252	.826959	0.69	1.9937	.29966	.501576
0.20	1.2214	0.08686	0.818731	**0.70**	2.0138	0.30401	0.496585
0.21	1.2337	.09120	.810584	0.71	2.0340	.30835	.491644
0.22	1.2461	.09554	.802519	0.72	2.0544	.31269	.486752
0.23	1.2586	.09989	.794534	0.73	2.0751	.31703	.481909
0.24	1.2712	.10423	.786628	0.74	2.0959	.32138	.477114
0.25	1.2840	0.10857	0.778801	**0.75**	2.1170	0.32572	0.472367
0.26	1.2969	.11292	.771052	0.76	2.1383	.33006	.467666
0.27	1.3100	.11726	.763379	0.77	2.1598	.33441	.463013
0.28	1.3231	.12160	.755784	0.78	2.1815	.33875	.458406
0.29	1.3364	.12595	.748264	0.79	2.2034	.34309	.453845
0.30	1.3499	0.13029	0.740818	**0.80**	2.2255	0.34744	0.449329
0.31	1.3634	.13463	.733447	0.81	2.2479	.35178	.444858
0.32	1.3771	.13897	.726149	0.82	2.2705	.35612	.440432
0.33	1.3910	.14332	.718924	0.83	2.2933	.36046	.436049
0.34	1.4049	.14766	.711770	0.84	2.3164	.36481	.431711
0.35	1.4191	0.15200	0.704688	**0.85**	2.3396	0.36915	0.427415
0.36	1.4333	.15635	.697676	0.86	2.3632	.37349	.423162
0.37	1.4477	.16069	.690734	0.87	2.3869	.37784	.418952
0.38	1.4623	.16503	.683861	0.88	2.4109	.38218	.414783
0.39	1.4770	.16937	.677057	0.89	2.4351	.38652	.410656
0.40	1.4918	0.17372	0.670320	**0.90**	2.4596	0.39087	0.406570
0.41	1.5068	.17806	.663650	0.91	2.4843	.39521	.402524
0.42	1.5220	.18240	.657047	0.92	2.5093	.39955	.398519
0.43	1.5373	.18675	.650509	0.93	2.5345	.40389	.394554
0.44	1.5527	.19109	.644036	0.94	2.5600	.40824	.390628
0.45	1.5683	0.19543	0.637628	**0.95**	2.5857	0.41258	0.386741
0.46	1.5841	.19978	.631284	0.96	2.6117	.41692	.382893
0.47	1.6000	.20412	.625002	0.97	2.6379	.42127	.379083
0.48	1.6161	.20846	.618783	0.98	2.6645	.42561	.375311
0.49	1.6323	.21280	.612626	0.99	2.6912	.42995	.371577
0.50	1.6487	0.21715	0.606531	**1.00**	2.7183	0.43429	0.367879

EXPONENTIAL FUNCTIONS

x	e^x	$\text{Log}_{10}(e^x)$	e^{-x}	x	e^x	$\text{Log}_{10}(e^x)$	e^{-x}
1.00	2.7183	0.43429	0.367879	**1.50**	4.4817	0.65144	0.223130
1.01	2.7456	.43864	.364219	1.51	4.5267	.65578	.220910
1.02	2.7732	.44298	.360595	1.52	4.5722	.66013	.218712
1.03	2.8011	.44732	.357007	1.53	4.6182	.66447	.216536
1.04	2.8292	.45167	.353455	1.54	4.6646	.66881	.214381
1.05	2.8577	0.45601	0.349938	**1.55**	4.7115	0.67316	0.212248
1.06	2.8864	.46035	.346456	1.56	4.7588	.67750	.210136
1.07	2.9154	.46470	.343009	1.57	4.8066	.68184	.208045
1.08	2.9447	.46904	.339596	1.58	4.8550	.68619	.205975
1.09	2.9743	.47338	.336216	1.59	4.9037	.69053	.203926
1.10	3.0042	0.47772	0.332871	**1.60**	4.9530	0.69487	0.201897
1.11	3.0344	.48207	.329559	1.61	5.0028	.69921	.199888
1.12	3.0649	.48641	.326280	1.62	5.0531	.70356	.197899
1.13	3.0957	.49075	.323033	1.63	5.1039	.70790	.195930
1.14	3.1268	.49510	.319819	1.64	5.1552	.71224	.193980
1.15	3.1582	0.49944	0.316637	**1.65**	5.2070	0.71659	0.192050
1.16	3.1899	.50378	.313486	1.66	5.2593	.72093	.190139
1.17	3.2220	.50812	.310367	1.67	5.3122	.72527	.188247
1.18	3.2544	.51247	.307279	1.68	5.3656	.72961	.186374
1.19	3.2871	.51681	.304221	1.69	5.4195	.73396	.184520
1.20	3.3201	0.52115	0.301194	**1.70**	5.4739	0.73830	0.182684
1.21	3.3535	.52550	.298197	1.71	5.5290	.74264	.180866
1.22	3.3872	.52984	.295230	1.72	5.5845	.74699	.179066
1.23	3.4212	.53418	.292293	1.73	5.6407	.75133	.177284
1.24	3.4556	.53853	.289384	1 74	5.6973	75567	175520
1.25	3.4903	0.54287	0.286505	**1.75**	5.7546	0.76002	0.173774
1.26	3.5254	.54721	.283654	1.76	5.8124	.76436	.172045
1.27	3.5609	.55155	.280832	1.77	5.8709	.76870	170333
1.28	3.5966	.55590	.278037	1.78	5.9299	.77304	168638
1.29	3.6328	.56024	.275271	1.79	5.9895	.77739	.166960
1.30	3.6693	0.56458	0.272532	**1.80**	6.0496	0.78173	0.165299
1.31	3.7062	.56893	.269820	1.81	6.1104	.78607	.163654
1.32	3.7434	.57327	.267135	1.82	6.1719	.79042	.162026
1.33	3.7810	.57761	.264477	1.83	6.2339	.79476	.160414
1.34	3.8190	.58195	.261846	1.84	6.2965	79910	.158817
1.35	3.8574	0.58630	0.259240	**1.85**	6.3598	0.80344	0.157237
1.36	3.8962	.59064	.256661	1.86	6.4237	.80779	.155673
1.37	3.9354	.59498	.254107	1.87	6.4883	.81213	.154124
1.38	3.9749	.59933	.251579	1.88	6.5535	.81647	.152590
1.39	4.0149	.60367	.249075	1.89	6.6194	.82082	.151072
1.40	4.0552	0.60801	0.246597	**1.90**	6.6859	0.82516	0.149569
1.41	4.0960	.61236	.244143	1.91	6.7531	.82950	.148080
1.42	4.1371	.61670	.241714	1.92	6.8210	.83385	.146607
1.43	4.1787	.62104	.239309	1.93	6.8895	.83819	.145148
1.44	4.2207	.62538	.236928	1.94	6.9588	.84253	.143704
1.45	4.2631	0.62973	0.234570	**1.95**	7.0287	0.84687	0.142274
1.46	4.3060	.63407	.232236	1.96	7.0993	.85122	.140858
1.47	4.3492	.63841	.229925	1.97	7.1707	.85556	.139457
1.48	4.3929	.64276	.227638	1.98	7.2427	.85990	.138069
1.49	4.4371	.64710	.225373	1.99	7.3155	.86425	.136695
1.50	4.4817	0.65144	0.223130	**2.00**	7.3891	0.86859	0.135335

EXPONENTIAL FUNCTIONS

x	e^x	$\text{Log}_{10}(e^x)$	e^{-x}	x	e^x	$\text{Log}_{10}(e^x)$	e^{-x}
2.00	7.3891	0.86859	0.135335	**2.50**	12.182	1.08574	0.082085
2.01	7.4633	.87293	.133989	2.51	12.305	1.09008	.081268
2.02	7.5383	.87727	.132655	2.52	12.429	1.09442	.080460
2.03	7.6141	.88162	.131336	2.53	12.554	1.09877	.079659
2.04	7.6906	.88596	.130029	2.54	12.680	1.10311	.078866
2.05	7.7679	0.89030	0.128735	**2.55**	12.807	1.10745	0.078082
2.06	7.8460	.89465	.127454	2.56	12.936	1.11179	.077305
2.07	7.9248	.89899	.126186	2.57	13.066	1.11614	.076536
2.08	8.0045	.90333	.124930	2.58	13.197	1.12048	.075774
2.09	8.0849	.90768	.123687	2.59	13.330	1.12482	.075020
2.10	8.1662	0.91202	0.122456	**2.60**	13.464	1.12917	0.074274
2.11	8.2482	.91636	.121238	2.61	13.599	1.13351	.073535
2.12	8.3311	.92070	.120032	2.62	13.736	1.13785	.072803
2.13	8.4149	.92505	.118837	2.63	13.874	1.14219	.072078
2.14	8.4994	.92939	.117655	2.64	14.013	1.14654	.071361
2.15	8.5849	0.93373	0.116484	**2.65**	14.154	1.15088	0.070651
2.16	8.6711	.93808	.115325	2.66	14.296	1.15522	.069948
2.17	8.7583	.94242	.114178	2.67	14.440	1.15957	.069252
2.18	8.8463	.94676	.113042	2.68	14.585	1.16391	.068563
2.19	8.9352	.95110	.111917	2.69	14.732	1.16825	.067881
2.20	9.0250	0.95545	0.110803	**2.70**	14.880	1.17260	0.067206
2.21	9.1157	.95979	.109701	2.71	15.029	1.17694	.066537
2.22	9.2073	.96413	.108609	2.72	15.180	1.18128	.065875
2.23	9.2999	.96848	.107528	2.73	15.333	1.18562	.065219
2.24	9.3933	.97282	.106459	2.74	15.487	1.18997	.064570
2.25	9.4877	0.97716	0.105399	**2.75**	15.643	1.19431	0.063928
2.26	9.5831	.98151	.104350	2.76	15.800	1.19865	.063292
2.27	9.6794	.98585	.103312	2.77	15.959	1.20300	.062662
2.28	9.7767	.99019	.102284	2.78	16.119	1.20734	.062039
2.29	9.8749	.99453	.101266	2.79	16.281	1.21168	.061421
2.30	9.9742	0.99888	0.100259	**2.80**	16.445	1.21602	0.060810
2.31	10.074	1.00322	.099261	2.81	16.610	1.22037	.060205
2.32	10.176	1.00756	.098274	2.82	16.777	1.22471	.059606
2.33	10.278	1.01191	.097296	2.83	16.945	1.22905	.059013
2.34	10.381	1.01625	.096328	2.84	17.116	1.23340	.058426
2.35	10.486	1.02059	0.095369	**2.85**	17.288	1.23774	0.057844
2.36	10.591	1.02493	.094420	2.86	17.462	1.24208	.057269
2.37	10.697	1.02928	.093481	2.87	17.637	1.24643	.056699
2.38	10.805	1.03362	.092551	2.88	17.814	1.25077	.056135
2.39	10.913	1.03796	.091630	2.89	17.993	1.25511	.055576
2.40	11.023	1.04231	0.090718	**2.90**	18.174	1.25945	0.055023
2.41	11.134	1.04665	.089815	2.91	18.357	1.26380	.054476
2.42	11.246	1.05099	.088922	2.92	18.541	1.26814	.053934
2.43	11.359	1.05534	.088037	2.93	18.728	1.27248	.053397
2.44	11.473	1.05968	.087161	2.94	18.916	1.27683	.052866
2.45	11.588	1.06402	0.086294	**2.95**	19.106	1.28117	0.052340
2.46	11.705	1.06836	.085435	2.96	19.298	1.28551	.051819
2.47	11.822	1.07271	.084585	2.97	19.492	1.28985	.051303
2.48	11.941	1.07705	.083743	2.98	19.688	1.29420	.050793
2.49	12.061	1.08139	.082910	2.99	19.886	1.29854	.050287
2.50	12.182	1.08574	0.082085	**3.00**	20.086	1.30288	0.049787

EXPONENTIAL FUNCTIONS

x	e^x	$\text{Log}_{10}(e^x)$	e^{-x}	x	e^x	$\text{Log}_{10}(e^x)$	e^{-x}
3.00	20.086	1.30288	0.049787	**3.50**	33.115	1.52003	0.030197
3.01	20.287	1.30723	.049292	3.51	33.448	1.52437	.029897
3.02	20.491	1.31157	.048801	3.52	33.784	1.52872	.029599
3.03	20.697	1.31591	.048316	3.53	34.124	1.53306	.029305
3.04	20.905	1.32026	.047835	3.54	34.467	1.53740	.029013
3.05	21.115	1.32460	0.047359	**3.55**	34.813	1.54175	0.028725
3.06	21.328	1.32894	.046888	3.56	35.163	1.54609	.028439
3.07	21.542	1.33328	.046421	3.57	35.517	1.55043	.028156
3.08	21.758	1.33763	.045959	3.58	35.874	1.55477	.027876
3.09	21.977	1.34197	.045502	3.59	36.234	1.55912	.027598
3.10	22.198	1.34631	0.045049	**3.60**	36.598	1.56346	0.027324
3.11	22.421	1.35066	.044601	3.61	36.966	1.56780	.027052
3.12	22.646	1.35500	.044157	3.62	37.338	1.57215	.026783
3.13	22.874	1.35934	.043718	3.63	37.713	1.57649	.026516
3.14	23.104	1.36368	.043283	3.64	38.092	1.58083	.026252
3.15	23.336	1.36803	0.042852	**3.65**	38.475	1.58517	0.025991
3.16	23.571	1.37237	.042426	3.66	38.861	1.58952	.025733
3.17	23.807	1.37671	.042004	3.67	39.252	1.59386	.025476
3.18	24.047	1.38106	.041586	3.68	39.646	1.59820	.025223
3.19	24.288	1.38540	.041172	3.69	40.045	1.60255	.024972
3.20	24.533	1.38974	0.040762	**3.70**	40.447	1.60689	0.024724
3.21	24.779	1.39409	.040357	3.71	40.854	1.61123	.024478
3.22	25.028	1.39843	.039955	3.72	41.264	1.61558	.024234
3.23	25.280	1.40277	.039557	3.73	41.679	1.61992	.023993
3.24	25.534	1.40711	.039164	3.74	42.098	1.62426	.023754
3.25	25.790	1.41146	0.038774	**3.75**	42.521	1.62860	0.023518
3.26	26.050	1.41580	.038388	3.76	42.948	1.63295	.023284
3.27	26.311	1.42014	.038006	3.77	43.380	1.63729	.023052
3.28	26.576	1.42449	.037628	3.78	43.816	1.64163	.022823
3.29	26.843	1.42883	.037254	3.79	44.256	1.64598	.022596
3.30	27.113	1.43317	0.036883	**3.80**	44.701	1.65032	0.022371
3.31	27.385	1.43751	.036516	3.81	45.150	1.65466	.022148
3.32	27.660	1.44186	.036153	3.82	45.604	1.65900	.021928
3.33	27.938	1.44620	.035703	3.83	[illegible]	[illegible]	.021710
3.34	28.219	1.45054	.035437	3.84	46.525	1.66769	.021494
3.35	28.503	1.45489	0.035084	**3.85**	46.993	1.67203	0.021280
3.36	28.789	1.45923	.034735	3.86	47.465	1.67638	.021068
3.37	29.079	1.46357	.034390	3.87	47.942	1.68072	.020858
3.38	29.371	1.46792	.034047	3.88	48.424	1.68506	.020651
3.39	29.666	1.47226	.033709	3.89	48.911	1.68941	.020445
3.40	29.964	1.47000	0.033373	**3.90**	49.402	1.69375	0.020242
3.41	30.265	1.48094	.033041	3.91	49.899	1.69809	.020041
3.42	30.569	1.48529	.032712	3.92	50.400	1.70243	.019841
3.43	30.877	1.48963	.032387	3.93	50.907	1.70678	.019644
3.44	31.187	1.49397	.032065	3.94	51.419	1.71112	.019448
3.45	31.500	1.49832	0.031746	**3.95**	51.935	1.71546	0.019255
3.46	31.817	1.50266	.031430	3.96	52.457	1.71981	.019063
3.47	32.137	1.50700	.031117	3.97	52.985	1.72415	.018873
3.48	32.460	1.51134	.030807	3.98	53.517	1.72849	.018686
3.49	32.786	1.51569	.030501	3.99	54.055	1.73283	.018500
3.50	33.115	1.52003	0.030197	**4.00**	54.598	1.73718	0.018316

EXPONENTIAL FUNCTIONS

x	e^x	$\text{Log}_{10}(e^x)$	e^{-x}	x	e^x	$\text{Log}_{10}(e^x)$	e^{-x}
4.00	54.598	1.73718	0.018316	**4.50**	90.017	1.95433	0.011109
4.01	55.147	1.74152	.018133	4.51	90.922	1.95867	.010998
4.02	55.701	1.74586	.017953	4.52	91.836	1.96301	.010889
4.03	56.261	1.75021	.017774	4.53	92.759	1.96735	.010781
4.04	56.826	1.75455	.017597	4.54	93.691	1.97170	.010673
4.05	57.397	1.75889	0.017422	**4.55**	94.632	1.97604	0.010567
4.06	57.974	1.76324	.017249	4.56	95.583	1.98038	.010462
4.07	58.557	1.76758	.017077	4.57	96.544	1.98473	.010358
4.08	59.145	1.77192	.016907	4.58	97.514	1.98907	.010255
4.09	59.740	1.77626	.016739	4.59	98.494	1.99341	.010153
4.10	60.340	1.78061	0.016573	**4.60**	99.484	1.99775	0.010052
4.11	60.947	1.78495	.016408	4.61	100.48	2.00210	.009952
4.12	61.559	1.78929	.016245	4.62	101.49	2.00644	.009853
4.13	62.178	1.79364	.016083	4.63	102.51	2.01078	.009755
4.14	62.803	1.79798	.015923	4.64	103.54	2.01513	.009658
4.15	63.434	1.80232	0.015764	**4.65**	104.58	2.01947	0.009562
4.16	64.072	1.80667	.015608	4.66	105.64	2.02381	.009466
4.17	64.715	1.81101	.015452	4.67	106.70	2.02816	.009372
4.18	65.366	1.81535	.015299	4.68	107.77	2.03250	.009279
4.19	66.023	1.81969	.015146	4.69	108.85	2.03684	.009187
4.20	66.686	1.82404	0.014996	**4.70**	109.95	2.04118	0.009095
4.21	67.357	1.82838	.014846	4.71	111.05	2.04553	.009005
4.22	68.033	1.83272	.014699	4.72	112.17	2.04987	.008915
4.23	68.717	1.83707	.014552	4.73	113.30	2.05421	.008826
4.24	69.408	1.84141	.014408	4.74	114.43	2.05856	.008739
4.25	70.105	1.84575	0.014264	**4.75**	115.58	2.06290	0.008652
4.26	70.810	1.85009	.014122	4.76	116.75	2.06724	.008566
4.27	71.522	1.85444	.013982	4.77	117.92	2.07158	.008480
4.28	72.240	1.85878	.013843	4.78	119.10	2.07593	.008396
4.29	72.966	1.86312	.013705	4.79	120.30	2.08027	.008312
4.30	73.700	1.86747	0.013569	**4.80**	121.51	2.08461	0.008230
4.31	74.440	1.87181	.013434	4.81	122.73	2.08896	.008148
4.32	75.189	1.87615	.013300	4.82	123.97	2.09330	.008067
4.33	75.944	1.88050	.013168	4.83	125.21	2.09764	.007987
4.34	76.708	1.88484	.013037	4.84	126.47	2.10199	.007907
4.35	77.478	1.88918	0.012907	**4.85**	127.74	2.10633	0.007828
4.36	78.257	1.89352	.012778	4.86	129.02	2.11067	.007750
4.37	79.044	1.89787	.012651	4.87	130.32	2.11501	.007673
4.38	79.838	1.90221	.012525	4.88	131.63	2.11936	.007597
4.39	80.640	1.90655	.012401	4.89	132.95	2.12370	.007521
4.40	81.451	1.91090	0.012277	**4.90**	134.29	2.12804	0.007447
4.41	82.269	1.91524	.012155	4.91	135.64	2.13239	.007372
4.42	83.096	1.91958	.012034	4.92	137.00	2.13673	.007299
4.43	83.931	1.92392	.011914	4.93	138.38	2.14107	.007227
4.44	84.775	1.92827	.011796	4.94	139.77	2.14541	.007155
4.45	85.627	1.93261	0.011679	**4.95**	141.17	2.14976	0.007083
4.46	86.488	1.93695	.011562	4.96	142.59	2.15410	.007013
4.47	87.357	1.94130	.011447	4.97	144.03	2.15844	.006943
4.48	88.235	1.94564	.011333	4.98	145.47	2.16279	.006874
4.49	89.121	1.94998	.011221	4.99	146.94	2.16713	.006806
4.50	90.017	1.95433	0.011109	**5.00**	148.41	2.17147	0.006738

EXPONENTIAL FUNCTIONS

x	e^x	$\mathrm{Log}_{10}(e^x)$	e^{-x}	x	e^x	$\mathrm{Log}_{10}(e^x)$	e^{-x}
5.00	148.41	2.17147	0.006738	**5.50**	244.69	2.38862	0.0040868
5.01	149.90	2.17582	.006671	5.55	257.24	2.41033	.0038875
5.02	151.41	2.18016	.006605	5.60	270.43	2.43205	.0036979
5.03	152.93	2.18450	.006539	5.65	284.29	2.45376	.0035175
5.04	154.47	2.18884	.006474	5.70	298.87	2.47548	.0033460
5.05	156.02	2.19319	0.006409	**5.75**	314.19	2.49719	0.0031828
5.06	157.59	2.19753	.006346	5.80	330.30	2.51891	.0030276
5.07	159.17	2.20187	.006282	5.85	347.23	2.54062	.0028799
5.08	160.77	2.20622	.006220	5.90	365.04	2.56234	.0027394
5.09	162.39	2.21056	.006158	5.95	383.75	2.58405	.0026058
5.10	164.02	2.21400	0.006097	**6.00**	403.43	2.60577	0.0024788
5.11	165.67	2.21924	.006036	6.05	424.11	2.62748	.0023579
5.12	167.34	2.22359	.005976	6.10	445.86	2.64920	.0022429
5.13	169.02	2.22793	.005917	6.15	468.72	2.67091	.0021335
5.14	170.72	2.23227	.005858	6.20	492.75	2.69263	.0020294
5.15	172.43	2.23662	0.005799	**6.25**	518.01	2.71434	0.0019305
5.16	174.16	2.24096	.005742	6.30	544.57	2.73606	.0018363
5.17	175.91	2.24530	.005685	6.35	572.49	2.75777	.0017467
5.18	177.68	2.24965	.005628	6.40	601.85	2.77948	.0016616
5.19	179.47	2.25399	.005572	6.45	632.70	2.80120	.0015805
5.20	181.27	2.25833	0.005517	**6.50**	665.14	2.82291	0.0015034
5.21	183.09	2.26267	.005462	6.55	699.24	2.84463	.0014301
5.22	184.93	2.26702	.005407	6.60	735.10	2.86634	.0013604
5.23	186.79	2.27136	.005354	6.65	772.78	2.88806	.0012940
5.24	188.67	2.27570	.005300	6.70	812.41	2.90977	.0012309
5.25	190.57	2.28005	0.005248	**6.75**	854.06	2.93149	0.0011709
5.26	192.48	2.28439	.005195	6.80	897.85	2.95320	.0011138
5.27	194.42	2.28873	.005144	6.85	943.88	2.97492	.0010595
5.28	196.37	2.29307	.005092	6.90	992.27	2.99663	.0010078
5.29	198.34	2.29742	.005042	6.95	1043.1	3.01835	.0009586
5.30	200.34	2.30176	0.004992	**7.00**	1096.6	3.04006	0.0009119
5.31	202.35	2.30610	.004942	7.05	1152.9	3.06178	.0008674
5.32	204.38	2.31045	.004893	7.10	1212.0	3.08349	.0008251
5.33	206.44	2.31479	.004844	7.15	1274.1	3.10521	.0007849
5.34	208.51	2.31913	.004796	7.20	1339.4	3.12692	.0007466
5.35	210.61	2.32348	0.004748	**7.25**	1408.1	3.14863	0.0007102
5.36	212.72	2.32782	.004701	7.30	1480.3	3.17035	.0006755
5.37	214.86	2.33216	.004654	7.35	1556.2	3.19206	.0006426
5.38	217.02	2.33650	.004608	7.40	1636.0	3.21378	.0006113
5.39	219.20	2.34085	.004562	7.45	1719.9	3.23549	.0005814
5.40	221.41	2.34519	0.004517	**7.50**	1808.0	3.25721	0.0005531
5.41	223.63	2.34953	.004472	7.55	1900.7	3.27892	.0005261
5.42	225.88	2.35388	.004427	7.60	1998.2	3.30064	.0005005
5.43	228.15	2.35822	.004383	7.65	2100.6	3.32235	.0004760
5.44	230.44	2.36256	.004339	7.70	2208.3	3.34407	.0004528
5.45	232.76	2.36690	0.004296	**7.75**	2321.6	3.36578	0.0004307
5.46	235.10	2.37125	.004254	7.80	2440.6	3.38750	.0004097
5.47	237.46	2.37559	.004211	7.85	2565.7	3.40921	.0003898
5.48	239.85	2.37993	.004169	7.90	2697.3	3.43093	.0003707
5.49	242.26	2.38428	.004128	7.95	2835.6	3.45264	.0003527
5.50	244.69	2.38862	0.004087	**8.00**	2981.0	3.47436	0.0003355

EXPONENTIAL FUNCTIONS

x	e^x	$\text{Log}_{10}(e^x)$	e^{-x}	x	e^x	$\text{Log}_{10}(e^x)$	e^{-x}
8.00	2981.0	3.47436	0.0003355	**9.00**	8103.1	3.90865	0.0001234
8.05	3133.8	3.49607	.0003191	9.05	8518.5	3.93037	.0001174
8.10	3294.5	3.51779	.0003035	9.10	8955.3	3.95208	.0001117
8.15	3463.4	3.53950	.0002887	9.15	9414.4	3.97379	.0001062
8.20	3641.0	3.56121	.0002747	9.20	9897.1	3.99551	.0001010
8.25	3827.6	3.58293	0.0002613	**9.25**	10405	4.01722	0.0000961
8.30	4023.9	3.60464	.0002485	9.30	10938	4.03894	.0000914
8.35	4230.2	3.62636	.0002364	9.35	11499	4.06065	.0000870
8.40	4447.1	3.64807	.0002249	9.40	12088	4.08237	.0000827
8.45	4675.1	3.66979	.0002139	9.45	12708	4.10408	.0000787
8.50	4914.8	3.69150	0.0002035	**9.50**	13360	4.12580	0.0000749
8.55	5166.8	3.71322	.0001935	9.55	14045	4.14751	.0000712
8.60	5431.7	3.73493	.0001841	9.60	14765	4.16923	.0000677
8.65	5710.1	3.75665	.0001751	9.65	15522	4.19094	.0000644
8.70	6002.9	3.77836	.0001666	9.70	16318	4.21266	.0000613
8.75	6310.7	3.80008	0.0001585	**9.75**	17154	4.23437	0.0000583
8.80	6634.2	3.82179	.0001507	9.80	18034	4.25609	.0000555
8.85	6974.4	3.84351	.0001434	9.85	18958	4.27780	.0000527
8.90	7332.0	3.86522	.0001364	9.90	19930	4.29952	.0000502
8.95	7707.9	3.88694	.0001297	9.95	20952	4.32123	0.0000477
9.00	8103.1	3.90865	0.0001234	10.00	22026	4.34294	0.0000454

XIII.7 SIX-PLACE LOGARITHMS: 100–150

N	0	1	2	3	4	5	6	7	8	9
100	00 0000	0434	0868	1301	1734	2166	2598	3029	3461	3891
01	4321	4751	5181	5609	6038	6466	6894	7321	7748	8174
02	00 8600	9026	9451	9876	*0300	*0724	*1147	*1570	*1993	*2415
03	01 2837	3259	3680	4100	4521	4940	5360	5779	6197	6616
04	01 7033	7451	7868	8284	8700	9116	9532	9947	*0361	*0775
05	02 1189	1603	2016	2428	2841	3252	3664	4075	4486	4896
06	5306	5715	6125	6533	6942	7350	7757	8164	8571	8978
07	02 9384	9789	*0195	*0600	*1004	*1408	*1812	*2216	*2619	*3021
08	03 3424	3826	4227	4628	5029	5430	5830	6230	6629	7028
09	03 7426	7825	8223	8620	9017	9414	9811	*0207	*0602	*0998
110	04 1393	1787	2182	2576	2969	3362	3755	4148	4540	4932
11	5323	5714	6105	6495	6885	7275	7664	8053	8442	8830
12	04 9218	9606	9993	*0380	*0766	*1153	*1538	*1924	*2309	*2694
13	05 3078	3463	3846	4230	4613	4996	5378	5760	6142	6524
14	05 6905	7286	7666	8046	8426	8805	9185	9563	9942	*0320
15	06 0698	1075	1452	1829	2206	2582	2958	3333	3709	4083
16	4458	4832	5206	5580	5953	6326	6699	7071	7443	7815
17	06 8186	8557	8928	9298	9668	*0038	*0407	*0776	*1145	*1514
18	07 1882	2250	2617	2985	3352	3718	4085	4451	4816	5182
19	5547	5912	6276	6640	7004	7368	7731	8094	8457	8819
120	07 9181	9543	9904	*0266	*0626	*0987	*1347	*1707	*2067	*2426
21	08 2785	3144	3503	3861	4219	4576	4934	5291	5647	6004
22	6360	6716	7071	7426	7781	8136	8490	8845	9198	9552
23	08 9905	*0258	*0611	*0963	*1315	*1667	*2018	*2370	*2721	*3071
24	09 3422	3772	4122	4471	4820	5169	5518	5866	6215	6562
25	09 6910	7257	7604	7951	8298	8644	8990	9335	9681	*0026
26	10 0371	0715	1059	1403	1747	2091	2434	2777	3119	3462
27	3804	4146	4487	4828	5169	5510	5851	6191	6531	6871
28	10 7210	7549	7888	8227	8565	8903	9241	9579	9916	*0253
29	11 0590	0926	1263	1599	1934	2270	2605	2940	3275	3609
130	3943	4277	4611	4944	5278	5611	5943	6276	6608	6940
31	11 7271	7603	7934	8265	8595	8926	9256	9586	9915	*0245
32	12 0574	0903	1231	1560	1888	2216	2544	2871	3198	3525
33	3852	4178	4504	4830	5156	5481	5806	6131	6456	6781
34	12 7105	7429	7753	8076	8399	8722	9045	9368	9690	*0012
35	13 0334	0655	0977	1298	1619	1939	2260	2580	2900	3219
36	3539	3858	4177	4496	4814	5133	5451	5769	6086	6403
37	6721	7037	7354	7671	7989	8303	8618	8934	9249	9564
38	13 9879	*0194	*0508	*0822	*1136	*1450	*1763	*2076	*2380	*2702
39	14 3015	3327	3639	3851	4263	4574	4885	5196	5507	5818
140	6128	6438	6748	7058	7367	7676	7985	8294	8603	8911
41	14 9219	9527	9835	*0142	*0449	*0756	*1063	*1370	*1676	*1982
42	15 2288	2594	2900	3205	3510	3815	4120	4424	4728	5032
43	5336	5640	5943	6246	6549	6852	7154	7457	7759	8061
44	15 8362	8664	8965	9266	9567	9868	*0168	*0469	*0769	*1068
45	16 1368	1667	1967	2266	2564	2863	3161	3460	3758	4055
46	4353	4650	4947	5244	5541	5838	6134	6430	6726	7022
47	16 7317	7613	7908	8203	8497	8792	9086	9380	9674	9968
48	17 0262	0555	0848	1141	1434	1726	2019	2311	2603	2895
49	3186	3478	3769	4060	4351	4641	4932	5222	5512	5802
150	17 6091	6381	6670	6959	7248	7536	7825	8113	8401	8689
N	0	1	2	3	4	5	6	7	8	9

SIX-PLACE LOGARITHMS: 150–200

N	0	1	2	3	4	5	6	7	8	9
150	17 6091	6381	6670	6959	7248	7536	7825	8113	8401	8689
51	17 8977	9264	9552	9839	*0126	*0413	*0699	*0986	*1272	*1558
52	18 1844	2129	2415	2700	2985	3270	3555	3839	4123	4407
53	4691	4975	5259	5542	5825	6108	6391	6674	6956	7239
54	18 7521	7803	8084	8366	8647	8928	9209	9490	9771	*0051
55	19 0332	0612	0892	1171	1451	1730	2010	2289	2567	2846
56	3125	3403	3681	3959	4237	4514	4792	5069	5346	5623
57	5900	6176	6453	6829	7005	7281	7556	7832	8107	8382
58	19 8657	8932	9206	9481	9755	*0029	*0303	*0577	*0850	*1124
59	20 1397	1670	1943	2216	2488	2761	3033	3305	3577	3848
160	4120	4391	4663	4934	5204	5475	5746	6016	6286	6556
61	6826	7096	7365	7634	7904	8173	8441	8710	8979	9247
62	20 9515	9783	*0051	*0319	*0586	*0853	*1121	*1388	*1654	*1921
63	21 2188	2454	2720	2986	3252	3518	3783	4049	4314	4579
64	4844	5109	5373	5638	5902	6166	6430	6694	6957	7221
65	21 7484	7747	8010	8273	8536	8798	9060	9323	9585	9846
66	22 0108	0370	0631	0892	1153	1414	1675	1936	2196	2456
67	2716	2976	3236	3496	3755	4015	4274	4533	4792	5051
68	5309	5568	5826	6084	6342	6600	6858	7115	7372	7630
69	22 7887	8144	8400	8657	8913	9170	9426	9682	9938	*0193
170	23 0449	0704	0960	1215	1470	1724	1979	2234	2488	2742
71	2996	3250	3504	3757	4011	4264	4517	4770	5023	5276
72	5528	5781	6033	6285	6537	6789	7041	7292	7544	7795
73	23 8046	8297	8548	8799	9049	9299	9550	9800	*0050	*0300
74	24 0549	0799	1048	1297	1546	1795	2044	2293	2541	2790
75	3038	3286	3534	3782	4030	4277	4525	4772	5019	5266
76	5513	5759	6006	6252	6499	6745	6991	7237	7482	7728
77	24 7973	8219	8464	8709	8954	9198	9443	9687	9932	*0176
78	25 0420	0664	0908	1151	1395	1638	1881	2125	2368	2610
79	2853	3096	3338	3580	3822	4064	4306	4548	4790	5031
180	5273	5514	5755	5996	6237	6477	6718	6958	7198	7439
81	25 7679	7918	8158	8398	8637	8877	9116	9355	9594	9833
82	26 0071	0310	0548	0787	1025	1263	1501	1739	1976	2214
83	2451	2688	2925	3162	3399	3636	3873	4109	4346	4582
84	4818	5054	5290	5525	5761	5996	6232	6467	6702	6937
85	7172	7406	7641	7875	8110	8344	8578	8812	9046	9279
86	26 9513	9746	9980	*0213	*0446	*0679	*0912	*1144	*1377	*1609
87	27 1842	2074	2306	2538	2770	3001	3233	3464	3696	3927
88	4158	4389	4620	4850	5081	5311	5542	5772	6002	6232
89	6462	6692	6921	7151	7380	7609	7838	8067	8296	8525
190	27 8754	8982	9211	9439	9667	9895	*0123	*0351	*0578	*0806
91	28 1033	1261	1488	1715	1942	2169	2396	2622	2849	3075
92	3301	3527	3753	3979	4205	4431	4656	4882	5107	5332
93	5557	5782	6007	6232	6456	6681	6905	7130	7354	7578
94	28 7802	8026	8249	8473	8696	8920	9143	9366	9589	9812
95	29 0035	0257	0480	0702	0925	1147	1369	1591	1813	2034
96	2256	2478	2699	2920	3141	3363	3584	3804	4025	4246
97	4466	4687	4907	5127	5347	5567	5787	6007	6226	6446
98	6665	6884	7104	7323	7542	7761	7979	8198	8416	8635
99	29 8853	9071	9289	9507	9725	9943	*0161	*0378	*0595	*0813
200	30 1030	1247	1464	1681	1898	2114	2331	2547	2764	2980
N	**0**	**1**	**2**	**3**	**4**	**5**	**6**	**7**	**8**	**9**

SIX-PLACE LOGARITHMS: 200–250

N	0	1	2	3	4	5	6	7	8	9
200	30 1030	1247	1464	1681	1898	2114	2331	2547	2764	2980
01	3196	3412	3628	3844	4059	4275	4491	4706	4921	5136
02	5351	5566	5781	5996	6211	6425	6639	6854	7068	7282
03	7496	7710	7924	8137	8351	8564	8778	8991	9204	9417
04	30 9630	9843	*0056	*0268	*0481	*0693	*0906	*1118	*1330	*1542
05	31 1754	1966	2177	2389	2600	2812	3023	3234	3445	3656
06	3867	4078	4289	4499	4710	920	5130	5340	5551	5760
07	5970	6180	6390	6599	6809	7018	7227	7436	7646	7854
08	31 8063	8272	8481	8689	8898	9106	9314	9522	9730	9938
09	32 0146	0354	0562	0769	0977	1184	1391	1598	1805	2012
210	2219	2426	2633	2839	3046	3252	3458	3665	3871	4077
11	4282	4488	4694	4899	5105	5310	5516	5721	5926	6131
12	6336	6541	6745	6950	7155	7359	7563	7767	7972	8176
13	32 8380	8583	8787	8991	9194	9398	9601	9805	*0008	*0211
14	33 0414	0617	0819	1022	1225	1427	1630	1832	2034	2236
15	2438	2640	2842	3044	3246	3447	3649	3850	4051	4253
16	4454	4655	4856	5057	5257	5458	5658	5859	6059	6260
17	6460	6660	6860	7060	7260	7459	7659	7858	8058	8257
18	33 8456	8656	8855	9054	9253	9451	9650	9849	*0047	*0246
19	34 0444	0642	0841	1039	1237	1435	1632	1830	2028	2225
220	2423	2620	2817	3014	3212	3409	3606	3802	3999	4196
21	4392	4589	4785	4981	5178	5374	5570	5766	5962	6157
22	6353	6549	6744	6939	7135	7330	7525	7720	7915	8110
23	34 8305	8500	8694	8889	9083	9278	9472	9666	9860	*0054
24	35 0248	0442	0636	0829	1023	1216	1410	1603	1796	1989
25	2183	2375	2568	2761	2954	3147	3339	3532	3724	3916
26	4108	4301	4493	4685	4876	5068	5260	5452	5643	5834
27	6026	6217	6408	6599	6790	6981	7172	7363	7554	7744
28	7935	8125	8316	8506	8696	8886	9076	9266	9456	9646
29	35 9835	*0025	*0215	*0404	*0593	*0783	*0972	*1161	*1350	*1539
230	36 1728	1917	2105	2294	2482	2671	2859	3048	3236	3424
31	3612	3800	3988	4176	4363	4551	4739	4926	5113	5301
32	5488	5675	5862	6049	6236	6423	6610	6796	6983	7169
33	7356	7542	7729	7915	8101	8287	8473	8659	8845	9030
34	36 9216	9401	9587	9772	9958	*0143	*0328	*0513	*0698	*0883
35	37 1068	1253	1437	1622	1806	1991	2175	2360	2544	2728
36	2912	3096	3280	3464	3647	3831	4015	4198	4382	4565
37	4748	4932	5115	5298	5481	5664	5846	6029	6212	6394
38	6577	6759	6942	7124	7306	7488	7670	7852	8034	8216
39	37 8398	8580	8761	8943	9124	9306	9487	9668	9849	*0030
240	38 0211	0392	0573	0754	0934	1115	1296	1476	1656	1837
41	2017	2197	2377	2557	2737	2917	3097	3277	3456	3636
42	3815	3995	4174	4353	4533	4712	4891	5070	5249	5428
43	5606	5785	5964	6142	6321	6499	6677	6856	7034	7212
44	7390	7568	7746	7924	8101	8279	8456	8634	8811	8989
45	38 9166	9343	9520	9698	9875	*0051	*0228	*0405	*0582	*0759
46	39 0935	1112	1288	1464	1641	1817	1993	2169	2345	2521
47	2697	2873	3048	3224	3400	3575	3751	3926	4101	4277
48	4452	4627	4802	4977	5152	5326	5501	5676	5850	6025
49	6199	6374	6548	6722	6896	7071	7245	7419	7592	7766
250	39 7940	8114	8287	8461	8634	8808	8981	9154	9328	9501
N	**0**	**1**	**2**	**3**	**4**	**5**	**6**	**7**	**8**	**9**

SIX-PLACE LOGARITHMS: 250–300

N	0	1	2	3	4	5	6	7	8	9
250	39 7940	8114	8287	8461	8634	8808	8981	9154	9328	9501
51	39 9674	9847	*0020	*0192	*0365	*0538	*0711	*0883	*1056	*1228
52	40 1401	1573	1745	1917	2089	2261	2433	2605	2777	2949
53	3121	3292	3464	3635	3807	3978	4149	4320	4492	4663
54	4834	5005	5176	5346	5517	5688	5858	6029	6199	6370
55	6540	6710	6881	7051	7221	7391	7561	7731	7901	8070
56	8240	8410	8579	8749	8918	9087	9257	9426	9595	9764
57	40 9933	*0102	*0271	*0440	*0609	*0777	*0946	*1114	*1283	*1451
58	41 1620	1788	1956	2124	2293	2461	2629	2796	2964	3132
59	3300	3467	3635	3803	3970	4137	4305	4472	4639	4806
260	4973	5140	5307	5474	5641	5808	5974	6141	6308	6474
61	6641	6807	6973	7139	7306	7472	7638	7804	7970	8135
62	8301	8467	8633	8798	8964	9129	9295	9460	9625	9791
63	41 9956	*0121	*0286	*0451	*0616	*0781	*0945	*1110	*1275	*1439
64	42 1604	1768	1933	2097	2261	2426	2590	2754	2918	3082
65	3246	3410	3574	3737	3901	4065	4228	4392	4555	4718
66	4882	5045	5208	5371	5534	5697	5860	6023	6186	6349
67	6511	6674	6836	6999	7161	7324	7486	7648	7811	7973
68	8135	8297	8459	8621	8783	8944	9106	9268	9429	9591
69	42 9752	9914	*0075	*0236	*0398	*0559	*0720	*0881	*1042	*1203
270	43 1364	1525	1685	1846	2007	2167	2328	2488	2649	2809
71	2969	3130	3290	3450	3610	3770	3930	4090	4249	4409
72	4569	4729	4888	5048	5207	5367	5526	5685	5844	6004
73	6163	6322	6481	6640	6799	6957	7116	7275	7433	7592
74	7751	7909	8067	8226	8384	8542	8701	8859	9017	9175
75	43 9333	9491	9648	9806	9964	*0122	*0279	*0437	*0594	*0752
76	44 0909	1066	1224	1381	1538	1695	1852	2009	2166	2323
77	2480	2637	2793	2950	3106	3263	3419	3576	3732	3889
78	4045	4201	4357	4513	4669	4825	4981	5137	5293	5449
79	5604	5760	5915	6071	6226	6382	6537	6692	6848	7003
280	7158	7313	7468	7623	7778	7933	8088	8242	8397	8552
81	44 8706	8861	9015	9170	9324	9478	9633	9787	9941	*0095
82	45 0249	0403	0557	0711	0865	1018	1172	1326	1479	1633
83	1786	1940	2093	2247	2400	2553	2706	2859	3012	3165
84	3318	3471	3624	3777	3930	4082	4235	4387	4540	4692
85	4845	4997	5150	5302	5454	5606	5758	5910	6062	6214
86	6366	6518	6670	6821	6973	7125	7276	7428	7579	7731
87	7882	8033	8184	8336	8487	8638	8789	8940	9091	9242
88	45 9392	9543	9694	9845	9995	*0146	*0296	*0447	*0597	*0748
89	46 0898	1048	1198	1348	1499	1649	1799	1948	2098	2248
290	2398	2548	2697	2847	2997	3146	3296	3445	3594	3744
91	3893	4042	4191	4340	4490	4639	4788	4936	5085	5234
92	5383	5532	5680	5829	5977	6126	6274	6423	6571	6719
93	6868	7016	7164	7312	7460	7608	7756	7904	8052	8200
94	8347	8495	8643	8790	8938	9085	9233	9380	9527	9675
95	46 9822	9969	*0116	*0263	*0410	*0557	*0704	*0851	*0998	*1145
96	47 1292	1438	1585	1732	1878	2025	2171	2318	2464	2610
97	2756	2903	3049	3195	3341	3487	3633	3779	3925	4071
98	4216	4362	4508	4653	4799	4944	5090	5235	5381	5526
99	5671	5816	5962	6107	6252	6397	6542	6687	6832	6976
300	47 7121	7266	7411	7555	7700	7844	7989	8133	8278	8422
N	**0**	**1**	**2**	**3**	**4**	**5**	**6**	**7**	**8**	**9**

SIX-PLACE LOGARITHMS: 300–350

N	0	1	2	3	4	5	6	7	8	9
300	47 7121	7266	7411	7555	7700	7844	7989	8133	8278	8422
01	47 8566	8711	8855	8999	9143	9287	9431	9575	9719	9863
02	48 0007	0151	0294	0438	0582	0725	0869	1012	1156	1299
03	1443	1586	1729	1872	2016	2159	2302	2445	2588	2731
04	2874	3016	3159	3302	3445	3587	3730	3872	4015	4157
05	4300	4442	4585	4727	4869	5011	5153	5295	5437	5579
06	5721	5863	6005	6147	6289	6430	6572	6714	6855	6997
07	7138	7280	7421	7563	7704	7845	7986	8127	8269	8410
08	8551	8692	8833	8974	9114	9255	9396	9537	9677	9818
09	48 9958	*0099	*0239	*0380	*0520	*0661	*0801	*0941	*1081	*1222
310	49 1362	1502	1642	1782	1922	2062	2201	2341	2481	2621
11	2760	2900	3040	3179	3319	3458	3597	3737	3876	4015
12	4155	4294	4433	4572	4711	4850	4989	5128	5267	5406
13	5544	5683	5822	5960	6099	6238	6376	6515	6653	6791
14	6930	7068	7206	7344	7483	7621	7759	7897	8035	8173
15	8311	8448	8586	8724	8862	8999	9137	9275	9412	9550
16	49 9687	9824	9962	*0099	*0236	*0374	*0511	*0648	*0785	*0922
17	50 1059	1196	1333	1470	1607	1744	1880	2017	2154	2291
18	2427	2564	2700	2837	2973	3109	3246	3382	3518	3655
19	3791	3927	4063	4199	4335	4471	4607	4743	4878	5014
320	5150	5286	5421	5557	5693	5828	5964	6099	6234	6370
21	6505	6640	6776	6911	7046	7181	7316	7451	7586	7721
22	7856	7991	8126	8260	8395	8530	8664	8799	8934	9068
23	50 9203	9337	9471	9606	9740	9874	*0009	*0143	*0277	*0411
24	51 0545	0679	0813	0947	1081	1215	1349	1482	1616	1750
25	1883	2017	2151	2284	2418	2551	2684	2818	2951	3084
26	3218	3351	3484	3617	3750	3883	4016	4149	4282	4415
27	4548	4681	4813	4946	5079	5211	5344	5476	5609	5741
28	5874	6006	6139	6271	6403	6535	6668	6800	6932	7064
29	7196	7329	7460	7592	7724	7855	7987	8119	8251	8382
330	8514	8646	8777	8909	9040	9171	9303	9434	9566	9697
31	51 9828	9959	*0090	*0221	*0353	*0484	*0615	*0745	*0876	*1007
32	52 1138	1269	1400	1530	1661	1792	1922	2053	2183	2314
33	2444	2575	2705	2835	2966	3096	3226	3356	3486	3616
34	3746	3876	4006	4136	4266	4396	4526	4656	4785	4915
35	5045	5174	5304	5434	5563	5693	5822	5951	6081	6210
36	6339	6469	6598	6727	6856	6985	7114	7243	7372	7501
37	7630	7759	7888	8016	8145	8274	8402	8531	8660	8788
38	52 8917	9045	9174	9312	9430	9559	9687	9815	9943	*0072
39	53 0200	0328	0456	0584	0712	0840	0968	1096	1223	1351
340	1479	1607	1734	1862	1990	2117	2245	2372	2500	2627
41	2754	2882	3009	3136	3264	3391	3518	3645	3772	3899
42	4026	4153	4280	4407	4534	4661	4787	4914	5041	5167
43	5294	5421	5547	5674	5800	5927	6053	6180	6306	6432
44	6558	6685	6811	6937	7063	7189	7315	7441	7567	7693
45	7819	7945	8071	8197	8322	8448	8574	8699	8825	8951
46	53 9076	9202	9327	9452	9578	9703	9829	9954	*0079	*0204
47	54 0329	0455	0580	0705	0830	0955	1080	1205	1330	1454
48	1579	1704	1829	1953	2078	2203	2327	2452	2576	2701
49	2825	2950	3074	3199	3323	3447	3571	3696	3820	3944
350	54 4068	4192	4316	4440	4564	4688	4812	4936	5060	5183
N	0	1	2	3	4	5	6	7	8	9

SIX-PLACE LOGARITHMS: 350–400

N	0	1	2	3	4	5	6	7	8	9
350	54 4068	4192	4316	4440	4564	4688	4812	4936	5060	5183
51	5307	5431	5555	5678	5802	5925	6049	6172	6296	6419
52	6543	6666	6789	6913	7036	7159	7282	7405	7529	7652
53	7775	7898	8021	8144	8267	8389	8512	8635	8758	8881
54	54 9003	9126	9249	9371	9494	9616	9739	9861	9984	*0106
55	55 0228	0351	0473	0595	0717	0840	0962	1084	1206	1328
56	1450	1572	1694	1816	1938	2060	2181	2303	2425	2547
57	2668	2790	2911	3033	3155	3276	3398	3519	3640	3762
58	3883	4004	4126	4247	4368	4489	4610	4731	4852	4973
59	5094	5215	5336	5457	5578	5699	5820	5940	6061	6182
360	6303	6423	6544	6664	6785	6905	7026	7146	7267	7387
61	7507	7627	7748	7868	7988	8108	8228	8349	8469	8589
62	8709	8829	8948	9068	9188	9308	9428	9548	9667	9787
63	55 9907	*0026	*0146	*0265	*0385	*0504	*0624	*0743	*0863	*0982
64	56 1101	1221	1340	1459	1578	1698	1817	1936	2055	2174
65	2293	2412	2531	2650	2769	2887	3006	3125	3244	3362
66	3481	3600	3718	3837	3955	4074	4192	4311	4429	4548
67	4666	4784	4903	5021	5139	5257	5376	5494	5612	5730
68	5848	5966	6084	6202	6320	6437	6555	6673	6791	6909
69	7026	7144	7262	7379	7497	7614	7732	7849	7967	8084
370	8202	8319	8436	8554	8671	8788	8905	9023	9140	9257
71	56 9374	9491	9608	9725	9842	9959	*0076	*0193	*0309	*0426
72	57 0543	0660	0776	0893	1010	1126	1243	1359	1476	1592
73	1709	1825	1942	2058	2174	2291	2407	2523	2639	2755
74	2872	2988	3104	3220	3336	3452	3568	3684	3800	3915
75	4031	4147	4263	4379	4494	4610	4726	4841	4957	5072
76	5188	5303	5419	5534	5650	5765	5880	5996	6111	6226
77	6341	6457	6572	6687	6802	6917	7032	7147	7262	7377
78	7492	7607	7722	7836	7951	8066	8181	8295	8410	8525
79	8639	8754	8868	8983	9097	9212	9326	9441	9555	9669
380	57 9784	9898	*0012	*0126	*0241	*0355	*0469	*0583	*0697	*0811
81	58 0925	1039	1153	1267	1381	1495	1608	1722	1836	1950
82	2063	2177	2291	2404	2518	2631	2745	2858	2972	3085
83	3199	3312	3426	3539	3652	3765	3879	3992	4105	4218
84	4331	4444	4557	4670	4783	4896	5009	5122	5235	5348
85	5461	5574	5686	5799	5912	6024	6137	6250	6362	6475
86	6587	6700	6812	6925	7037	7149	7262	7374	7486	7599
87	7711	7823	7935	8047	8160	8272	8384	8496	8608	8720
88	8832	8944	9056	9167	9279	9391	9503	9615	9726	9838
89	58 9950	*0061	*0173	*0284	*0396	*0507	*0619	*0730	*0842	*0953
390	59 1065	1176	1287	1399	1510	1621	1732	1843	1955	2066
91	2177	2288	2399	2510	2621	2732	2843	2954	3064	3175
92	3286	3397	3508	3618	3729	3840	3950	4061	4171	4282
93	4393	4503	4614	4724	4834	4945	5055	5165	5276	5386
94	5496	5606	5717	5827	5937	6047	6157	6267	6377	6487
95	6597	6707	6817	6927	7037	7146	7256	7366	7476	7586
96	7695	7805	7914	8024	8134	8243	8353	8462	8572	8681
97	8791	8900	9009	9119	9228	9337	9446	9556	9665	9774
98	9883	9992	*0101	*0210	*0319	*0428	*0537	*0646	*0755	*0864
99	60 0973	1082	1191	1299	1408	1517	1625	1734	1843	1951
400	60 2060	2169	2277	2386	2494	2603	2711	2819	2928	3036
N	**0**	**1**	**2**	**3**	**4**	**5**	**6**	**7**	**8**	**9**

SIX-PLACE LOGARITHMS: 400–450

N	0	1	2	3	4	5	6	7	8	9
400	60 2060	2169	2277	2386	2494	2603	2711	2819	2928	3036
01	3144	3253	3361	3469	3577	3686	3794	3902	4010	4118
02	4226	4334	4442	4550	5658	4766	4874	4982	5089	5197
03	5305	5413	5521	5628	5736	5844	5951	6059	6166	6274
04	6381	6489	6596	6704	6811	6919	7026	7133	7241	7348
05	7455	7562	7669	7777	7884	7991	8098	8205	8312	8419
06	8526	8633	8740	8847	8954	9061	9167	9274	9381	9488
07	60 9594	9701	9808	9914	*0021	*0128	*0234	*0341	*0447	*0554
08	61 0660	0767	0873	0979	1086	1192	1298	1405	1511	1617
09	1723	1829	1936	2042	2148	2254	2360	2466	2572	2678
410	2784	2890	2996	3102	3207	3313	3419	3525	3630	3736
11	3842	3947	4053	4159	4264	4370	4475	4581	4686	4792
12	4897	5003	5108	5213	5319	5425	5529	5634	5740	5845
13	5950	6055	6160	6265	6370	6476	6581	6686	6790	6895
14	7000	7105	7210	7315	7420	7525	7629	7734	7839	7943
15	8048	8153	8257	8362	8466	8571	8676	8780	8884	8989
16	61 9093	9198	9302	9406	9511	9615	9719	9824	9928	*0032
17	62 0136	0240	0344	0448	0552	0656	0760	0864	0968	1072
18	1176	1280	1384	1488	1592	1695	1799	1903	2007	2110
19	2214	2318	2421	2525	2628	2732	2835	2939	3042	3146
420	3249	3353	3456	3559	3663	3766	3869	3973	4076	4179
21	4282	4385	4488	4591	4695	4798	4901	5004	5107	5210
22	5312	5415	5518	5621	5724	5827	5929	6032	6135	6238
23	6340	6443	6546	6648	6751	6853	6956	7058	7161	7263
24	7366	7468	7571	7673	7775	7878	7980	8082	8185	8287
25	8389	8491	8593	8695	8797	8900	9002	9104	9206	9308
26	62 9410	9512	9613	9715	9817	9919	*0021	*0123	*0224	*0326
27	63 0428	0530	0631	0733	0835	0936	1038	1139	1241	1342
28	1444	1545	1647	1748	1849	1951	2052	2153	2255	2356
29	2457	2559	2660	2761	2862	2963	3064	3165	3266	3367
430	3468	3569	3670	3771	3872	3973	4074	4175	4276	4376
31	4477	4578	4679	4779	4880	4981	5081	5182	5283	5383
32	5484	5584	5685	5785	5886	5986	6087	6187	6287	6388
33	6488	6588	6688	6789	6889	6989	7089	7189	7290	7390
34	7490	7590	7690	7790	7890	7990	8090	8190	8290	8389
35	8489	8589	8689	8789	8888	8988	9088	9188	9287	9387
36	63 9486	9586	9686	9785	9885	9984	*0084	*0183	*0283	* 382
37	64 0481	0581	0680	0779	0879	0978	1077	1177	1276	1375
38	1474	1573	1672	1771	1871	1970	2069	2168	2267	2366
39	2465	2563	2662	2761	2860	2959	3058	3156	3255	3354
440	3453	3551	3650	3749	3847	3946	4044	4143	4242	4340
41	4439	4537	4636	4734	4832	4931	5029	5127	5226	5324
42	5422	5521	5619	5717	5815	5913	6011	6110	6208	6306
43	6404	6502	6600	6698	6796	6894	6992	7089	7187	7285
44	7383	7481	7579	7676	7774	7872	7969	8067	8165	8262
45	8360	8458	8555	8653	8750	8848	8945	9043	9140	9237
46	64 9335	9432	9530	9627	9724	9821	9919	*0016	*0113	*0210
47	65 0308	0405	0502	0599	0696	0793	0890	0987	1084	1181
48	1278	1375	1472	1569	1666	1762	1859	1956	2053	2150
49	2246	2343	2440	2536	2633	2730	2826	2923	3019	3116
450	65 3213	3309	3405	3502	3598	3695	3791	3888	3984	4080
N	**0**	**1**	**2**	**3**	**4**	**5**	**6**	**7**	**8**	**9**

SIX-PLACE LOGARITHMS: 450–500

N	0	1	2	3	4	5	6	7	8	9
450	65 3213	3309	3405	3502	3598	3695	3791	3888	3984	4080
51	4177	4273	4369	4465	4562	4658	4754	4850	4946	5042
52	5138	5235	5331	5427	5523	5619	5715	5810	5906	6002
53	6098	6194	6290	6386	6482	6577	6673	6769	6864	6960
54	7056	7152	7247	7343	7438	7534	7629	7725	7820	7916
55	8011	8017	8202	8298	8393	8488	8584	8679	8774	8870
56	8965	9060	9155	9250	9346	9441	9536	9631	9726	8921
57	65 9916	*0011	*0106	*0201	*0296	*0391	*0486	*0581	*0676	*0771
58	66 0865	0960	1055	1150	1245	1339	1434	1529	1623	1718
59	1813	1907	2002	2096	2191	2286	2380	2475	2569	2663
460	2758	2852	2947	3041	3135	3230	3324	3418	3512	3607
61	3701	3795	3889	3983	4078	4172	4266	4360	4454	4548
62	4642	4736	4830	4924	5018	5112	5206	5200	5393	5487
63	5581	5675	5769	5862	5956	6050	6143	6237	6331	6424
64	6518	6612	6705	6799	6892	6986	7079	7173	7266	7360
65	7453	7546	7640	7733	7826	7920	8013	8106	8199	8293
66	8386	8479	8572	8665	8759	8852	8945	9038	9131	9224
67	66 9317	9410	9503	9506	9689	9782	9875	9967	*0060	*0153
68	67 0246	0339	0431	0524	0617	0710	0802	0895	0988	1080
69	1173	1265	1358	1451	1543	1636	1728	1821	1913	2005
470	2098	2190	2283	2375	2467	2560	2652	2744	2836	2929
71	3021	3113	3205	3207	3390	3482	3574	3666	3758	3850
72	3942	4034	4126	4218	4310	4402	4494	4586	4677	4769
73	4861	4953	5045	5137	5228	5320	5412	5503	5595	5687
74	5778	5870	5962	6053	6145	6236	6328	6419	6511	6602
75	6694	6785	6876	6968	7059	7151	7242	7333	7424	7516
76	7607	7698	7789	7881	7972	8063	8154	8245	8336	8427
77	8518	8609	8700	8791	8882	8973	9064	9155	9246	9337
78	67 9428	9519	9610	9700	9791	9882	9973	*0063	*0154	*0245
79	68 0336	0426	0517	0607	0698	0789	0879	0970	1060	1151
480	1241	1332	1422	1513	1603	1693	1784	1874	1964	2055
81	2145	2235	2326	2416	2506	2596	2686	2777	2867	2957
82	3047	3137	3227	3317	3407	3497	3587	3677	3767	3857
83	3947	4037	4127	4217	4307	4396	4486	4576	4666	4756
84	4845	4935	5025	5114	5204	5294	5383	5473	5563	5652
85	5742	5831	5921	6010	6100	6189	6279	6368	6458	6547
86	6636	6726	6815	6904	6994	7083	7172	7261	7351	7440
87	7529	7618	7707	7796	7886	7975	8064	8153	8242	8331
88	8420	8509	8598	8687	8776	8865	8953	9042	9131	9220
89	68 9309	9398	9486	9575	9664	9753	9841	9930	*0019	*0107
490	69 0196	0285	0373	0462	0550	0639	0728	0816	0905	0993
91	1081	1170	1258	1347	1435	1524	1612	1700	1789	1877
92	1965	2053	2142	2230	2318	2406	2494	2583	2671	2759
93	2847	2935	3023	3111	3199	3287	3375	3463	3551	3639
94	3727	3815	3903	3991	4078	4166	4254	4342	4430	4517
95	4605	4693	4781	4868	4956	5044	5131	5219	5307	5394
96	5482	5569	5657	5744	5832	5919	6007	6094	6182	6269
97	6356	6444	6531	6618	6706	6793	6880	6968	7055	7142
98	7229	7317	7404	7491	7578	7665	7752	7839	7926	8014
99	8101	8188	8275	8362	8449	8535	8622	8709	8796	8883
500	69 8970	9051	9144	9231	9317	9404	9491	9578	9664	9751
N	**0**	**1**	**2**	**3**	**4**	**5**	**6**	**7**	**8**	**9**

SIX-PLACE LOGARITHMS: 500–550

N	0	1	2	3	4	5	6	7	8	9
500	69 8970	9057	9144	9231	9317	9404	9491	9578	9664	9751
01	69 9838	9924	*0011	*0098	*0184	*0271	*0358	*0444	*0531	*0617
02	70 0704	0790	0877	0963	1050	1136	1222	1309	1395	1482
03	1568	1654	1741	1827	1913	1999	2086	2172	2258	3244
04	2431	2517	2603	2689	2775	2861	2947	3033	3119	3205
05	3291	3377	3463	3549	3635	3721	3807	3893	3979	4065
06	4151	4236	4322	4408	4494	4579	4665	4751	4837	4922
07	5008	5094	5179	5265	5350	5463	5522	5607	5693	5778
08	5864	5949	6035	6120	6206	6291	6376	6462	6547	6632
09	6718	6803	6888	6974	7059	7144	7229	7315	7400	7485
510	7570	7655	7740	7826	7911	7996	8081	8166	8251	8336
11	8421	8506	8591	8676	8761	8846	8931	9015	9100	9185
12	70 9270	9355	9440	9524	9609	9694	9779	9863	9948	*0033
13	71 0117	0202	0287	0371	0456	0540	0625	0710	0794	0879
14	0963	1048	1132	1217	1301	1385	1470	1554	1639	1723
15	1807	1892	1976	2060	2144	2229	2313	2397	2481	2566
16	2650	2734	2818	2902	2986	3070	3154	3238	3323	3407
17	3491	3575	3659	3742	3826	3910	3994	4078	4162	4246
18	4330	4414	4497	4581	4665	4749	4833	4916	5000	5084
19	5167	5251	5335	5418	5502	5586	5669	5753	5836	5920
520	6003	6087	6170	6254	6337	6421	6504	6588	6671	6754
21	6838	6921	7004	7088	7171	7254	7338	7421	7504	7587
22	7671	7754	7837	7920	8003	8086	8169	8253	8336	8419
23	8502	8585	8668	8751	8834	9817	9000	9083	9165	9248
24	71 9331	9414	9497	9580	9663	9745	9828	9911	9994	*0077
25	72 0159	0242	0325	0407	0490	0573	0655	0738	0821	0903
26	0986	1068	1151	1233	1316	1398	1481	1563	1646	1728
27	1811	1893	1975	2058	2140	2222	2305	2387	2469	2552
28	2634	2716	2798	2881	2963	3045	3127	3209	3291	3374
29	3456	3538	3620	3702	3784	3866	3948	4030	4112	4194
530	4276	4358	4440	4522	4604	4685	4767	4849	4931	5013
31	5095	5176	5258	5340	5422	5503	5585	5667	5748	5830
32	5912	5993	6075	6156	6238	6320	6401	6483	6564	6646
33	6727	6809	6890	6972	7053	7134	7216	7297	7379	7460
34	7541	7623	7704	7785	7866	7948	8029	8110	8191	8273
35	8354	8435	8516	8597	8678	8759	8841	8922	9003	9084
36	9165	9246	9327	9408	9489	9570	9651	9732	9813	9893
37	72 9974	*0055	*0136	*0217	*0298	*0378	*0459	*0540	*0621	*0702
38	73 0782	0863	0944	1024	1105	1186	1266	1347	1428	1508
39	1589	1669	1750	1830	1911	1991	2072	2152	2233	2313
540	2394	2474	2555	2635	2715	2796	2876	2956	3037	3117
41	3197	3278	3358	3438	3518	3598	3679	3759	3839	3919
42	3999	4079	4160	4240	4320	4400	4480	4560	4640	4720
43	4800	4880	4960	5040	5120	4200	5279	5359	5439	5519
44	5599	5679	5759	5838	5918	5998	6078	6157	6237	6317
45	6397	6476	6556	6635	6715	6795	6874	6954	7034	7113
46	7193	7272	7352	7431	7511	7590	7670	7749	7829	7908
47	7987	8067	8146	8225	8305	8384	8463	8543	8622	8701
48	8781	8860	8939	9018	9097	9177	9256	9335	9414	9493
49	73 9572	9651	9731	9810	9889	9968	*0047	*0126	*0205	*0284
550	74 0363	0442	0521	0600	0678	0757	0836	0915	0994	1073
N	0	1	2	3	4	5	6	7	8	9

SIX-PLACE LOGARITHMS: 550–600

N	0	1	2	3	4	5	6	7	8	9
550	74 0363	0442	0521	0600	0678	0757	0836	0915	0994	1073
51	1152	1230	1309	1388	1467	1546	1624	1703	1782	1800
52	1939	2018	2096	2175	2254	2332	2411	2489	2568	2647
53	2725	2804	2882	2961	3039	3118	3196	3275	3353	3431
54	3510	3588	3667	3745	3823	3902	3980	4058	4136	4215
55	4293	4371	4449	4528	4606	4684	4762	4840	4919	4997
56	5075	5153	5231	5309	5387	5465	5543	5621	5699	5777
57	5855	5933	6011	6089	6167	6245	6323	6401	6479	6556
58	6634	6712	6790	6868	6945	7023	7101	7179	7256	7334
59	7412	7489	7567	7645	7722	7800	7878	7955	8033	8110
560	8188	8266	8343	8421	8498	8576	8653	8731	8808	8885
61	8963	9040	9118	9195	9272	9350	9427	9504	9582	9659
62	74 9736	9814	9891	9968	*0045	*0123	*0200	*0277	*0354	*0431
63	75 0508	0586	0663	0740	0817	0894	0971	1048	1125	1202
64	1279	1356	1433	1510	1587	1664	1741	1818	1895	1972
65	2048	2125	2202	2279	2356	2433	2509	2586	2663	2740
66	2816	2893	2970	3047	3123	3200	3277	3353	3430	3506
67	3583	3660	3736	3813	3889	3966	4042	4119	4195	4272
68	4348	4425	4501	4578	4654	4730	4807	4883	4960	5036
69	5112	5189	5265	5341	5417	5494	5570	5646	5722	5799
570	5875	5951	6027	6103	6180	6256	6332	6408	6484	6560
71	6636	6712	6788	6864	6940	7016	7092	7168	7244	7320
72	7396	7472	7548	7624	7700	7775	7851	7927	8003	8079
73	8155	8230	8306	8382	8458	8533	8609	8685	8761	8836
74	8912	8988	9063	9139	9214	9290	9366	9441	9517	9592
75	75 9668	9743	9819	9894	9970	*0045	*0121	*0196	*0272	*0347
76	76 0422	0498	0573	0649	0724	0799	0875	0950	1025	1101
77	1176	1251	1326	1402	1477	1552	1627	1702	1778	1853
78	1928	2003	2078	2153	2228	2303	2378	2453	2529	2604
79	2679	2754	2829	2904	2978	3053	3128	3203	3278	3353
580	3428	3503	3578	3653	3727	3802	3877	3952	4027	4101
81	4176	4251	4326	4400	4475	4550	4624	4699	4774	4848
82	4923	4998	5072	5147	5221	5296	5370	5445	5520	5594
83	5669	5743	5818	5892	5966	6041	6115	6190	6264	6338
84	6413	6487	6562	6636	6710	6785	6859	6933	7007	7082
85	7156	7230	7304	7379	7453	7527	7601	7675	7749	7823
86	7898	7972	8046	8120	8194	8268	8342	8416	8490	8564
87	8638	8712	8786	8860	8934	9008	9082	9156	9230	9303
88	76 9377	9451	9525	9599	9673	9746	9820	9894	9968	*0042
89	77 0115	0189	0263	0336	0410	0484	0557	0631	0705	0778
590	0852	0926	0999	1073	1146	1220	1293	1367	1440	1514
91	1587	1661	1734	1808	1881	1955	2028	2102	2175	2248
92	2322	2395	2468	2542	2615	2688	2762	2835	2908	2981
93	3055	3128	3201	3274	3348	3421	3494	3567	3640	3713
94	3786	3860	3933	4006	4079	4152	4225	4298	4371	4444
95	4517	4590	4663	4736	4809	4882	4955	5028	5100	5173
96	5246	5319	5392	5465	5538	5610	5683	5756	5829	5902
97	5974	6047	6120	6193	6265	6338	6411	6483	6556	6629
98	6701	6774	6846	6919	6992	7064	7137	7209	7282	7354
99	7427	7499	7572	7644	7717	7789	7862	7934	8006	8079
600	77 8151	8224	8296	8368	8441	8513	8585	8658	8730	8802
N	**0**	**1**	**2**	**3**	**4**	**5**	**6**	**7**	**8**	**9**

SIX-PLACE LOGARITHMS: 600–650

N	0	1	2	3	4	5	6	7	8	9
600	77 8151	8224	8296	8368	8441	8513	8585	8658	8730	8802
01	8874	8947	9019	9091	9163	9236	9308	9380	9452	9524
02	77 9596	9669	9741	9813	9885	9957	*0029	*0101	*0173	*0245
03	78 0317	0389	0461	0533	0605	0677	0749	0821	0893	0965
04	1037	1109	1181	1253	1324	1396	1468	1540	1612	1684
05	1755	1827	1899	1971	2042	2114	2186	2258	2329	2401
06	2473	2544	2616	2688	2759	2831	2902	2974	3046	3117
07	3189	3260	3332	3403	3475	3546	3618	3689	3761	3832
08	3904	3975	4046	4118	4189	4261	4332	4403	4475	4546
09	4617	4689	4760	4831	4902	4974	5045	5116	5187	5259
610	5330	5401	5472	5543	5615	5686	5757	5828	5899	5970
11	6041	6112	6183	6254	6325	6396	6467	6538	6609	6680
12	6751	6822	6893	6964	7035	7106	7177	7248	7319	7390
13	7460	7531	7602	7673	7744	7815	7885	7956	8027	8098
14	8168	8239	8310	8381	8451	8522	8593	8663	8734	8804
15	8875	8946	9016	9087	9157	9228	9299	9369	9440	9510
16	78 9581	9651	9722	9762	9863	9933	*0004	*0074	*0144	*0215
17	79 0285	0356	0426	0496	0567	0637	0707	0778	0848	0918
18	0988	1059	1129	1199	1269	1340	1410	1480	1550	1620
19	1691	1761	1831	1901	1971	2041	2111	2181	2252	2322
620	2392	2462	2532	2602	2672	2742	2812	2882	2952	3022
21	3092	3162	3231	3301	3371	3441	3511	3581	3651	3721
22	3790	3860	3930	4000	4070	4139	4209	4279	4349	4418
23	4488	4558	4627	4697	4767	4836	4906	4976	5045	5115
24	5185	5254	5324	5393	5463	5532	5602	5672	5741	5811
25	5880	5949	6019	6088	6158	6227	6297	6366	6436	6505
26	6574	6644	6713	6782	6852	6921	6990	7060	7129	7198
27	7268	7337	7406	7475	7545	7614	7683	7752	7821	7890
28	7960	8029	8098	8167	8236	8305	8374	8443	8513	8582
29	8651	8720	8789	8858	8927	8996	9065	9134	9203	9272
630	79 9341	9409	9478	9547	9616	9685	9754	9823	9892	9961
31	80 0029	0098	0167	0236	0305	0373	0442	0511	0580	0648
32	0717	0786	0854	0923	0992	1061	1129	1198	1266	1335
33	1404	1472	1541	1609	1678	1747	1815	1884	1952	2021
34	2089	2158	2226	2295	2363	2432	2500	2568	2637	2705
35	2774	2842	2910	2979	3047	3116	3184	3252	3321	3389
36	3457	3525	3594	3662	3730	3798	3867	3935	4003	4071
37	4139	4208	4276	4344	4412	4480	4548	4616	4685	4753
38	4821	4889	4957	5025	5093	5161	5229	5297	5365	5433
39	5501	5569	5637	5705	5773	5841	5908	5976	6044	6112
640	6180	6248	6316	6384	6451	6519	6587	6655	6723	6790
41	6858	6926	6994	7061	7129	7197	7264	7332	7400	7467
42	7537	7603	7670	7738	7806	7873	7941	8008	8076	8143
43	8211	8279	8346	8414	8481	8549	8616	8684	8751	8818
44	8886	8953	9021	9088	9156	9223	9290	9358	9425	9492
45	80 9560	9627	9694	9762	9829	9896	9964	*0031	*0098	*0165
46	81 0233	0300	0367	0434	0501	0569	0636	0703	0770	0837
47	0904	0971	1039	1106	1173	1240	1307	1374	1441	1508
48	1575	1642	1709	1776	1843	1910	1977	2044	2111	2178
49	2245	2312	2379	2445	2512	2579	2646	2713	2780	2847
650	81 2913	2980	3047	3114	3181	3247	3314	3381	3448	3514
N	**0**	**1**	**2**	**3**	**4**	**5**	**6**	**7**	**8**	**9**

SIX-PLACE LOGARITHMS: 650–700

N	0	1	2	3	4	5	6	7	8	9
650	81 2913	2980	3047	3114	3181	3247	3314	3381	3448	3514
51	3581	3648	3714	3781	3848	3914	3981	4048	4114	4181
52	4248	4314	4381	4447	4514	4581	4647	4714	4780	4847
53	4913	4980	5046	5113	5179	5246	5312	5378	5445	5511
54	5578	5644	5711	5777	5843	5910	5976	6042	6109	6175
55	6241	6308	6374	6440	6506	6573	6639	6705	6771	6838
56	6904	6970	7036	7102	7169	7235	7301	7367	7433	7499
57	7565	7631	7698	7764	7830	7896	7962	8028	8094	8160
58	8226	8292	8358	8424	8490	8556	8622	8688	8754	8820
59	8885	8951	9017	9083	9149	9215	9281	9346	9412	9478
660	81 9544	9610	9676	9741	9807	9873	9939	*0004	*0070	*0136
61	82 0201	0267	0333	0399	0464	0530	0595	0661	0727	0792
62	0858	0924	0989	1055	1120	1186	1251	1317	1382	1448
63	1514	1579	1645	1710	1775	1841	1906	1972	2037	2103
64	2168	2233	2299	2364	2430	2495	2560	2626	2691	2756
65	2822	2887	2952	3018	3083	3148	3213	3279	3344	3409
66	3474	3539	3605	3670	3735	3800	3865	3930	3996	4061
67	4126	4191	4256	4321	4386	4451	4516	4581	4646	4711
68	4776	4841	4906	4971	5036	5101	5166	5231	5296	5361
69	5426	5491	5556	5621	5686	5751	5815	5880	5945	6010
670	6075	6140	6204	6269	6334	6399	6464	6528	6593	6658
71	6723	6787	6852	6917	6981	7046	7111	7175	7240	7305
72	7369	7434	7499	7563	7628	7692	7757	7821	7886	7951
73	8015	8080	8144	8209	8273	8338	8402	8467	8531	8595
74	8660	8724	8789	8853	8918	8982	9046	9111	9175	9239
75	9304	9368	9432	9497	9561	9625	9690	9754	9818	9882
76	82 9947	*0011	*0075	*0139	*0204	*0268	*0332	*0396	*0460	*0525
77	83 0589	0653	0717	0781	0845	0909	0973	1037	1102	1166
78	1230	1294	1358	1422	1486	1550	1614	1678	1742	1806
79	1870	1934	1998	2062	2126	2189	2253	2317	2381	2445
680	2509	2573	2637	2700	2764	2828	2892	2956	3020	3083
81	3147	3211	3275	3338	3402	3466	3530	3593	3657	3721
82	3784	3848	3912	3975	4039	4103	4166	4230	4294	4357
83	4421	4484	4548	4611	4675	4739	4802	4866	4929	4993
84	5056	5120	5183	5247	5310	5373	5437	5500	5564	5627
85	5691	5754	5817	5881	5944	6007	6071	6134	6197	6261
86	6324	6387	6451	6514	6577	6641	6704	6767	6830	6894
87	6957	7020	7083	7146	7210	7273	7336	7399	7462	7525
88	7588	7652	7715	7778	7841	7904	7967	8030	8093	8156
89	8219	8282	8345	8408	8471	8534	8597	8660	8723	8786
690	8849	8912	8975	9038	9101	9164	9227	9289	9352	9415
91	83 9478	9541	9604	9667	9729	9792	9855	9918	9981	*0043
92	84 0106	0169	0232	0294	0357	0420	0482	0545	0608	0671
93	0733	0796	0859	0921	0984	1046	1109	1172	1234	1297
94	1359	1422	1485	1547	1610	1672	1735	1797	1860	1922
95	1985	2047	2110	2172	2235	2297	2360	2422	2484	2547
96	2609	2672	2734	2796	2859	2921	2983	3046	3108	3170
97	3233	3295	3357	3420	3482	3544	3606	3669	3731	3793
98	3855	3918	3980	4042	4104	4166	4229	4291	4353	4415
99	4477	4539	4601	4664	4726	4788	4850	4912	4974	5036
700	84 5098	5160	5222	5284	5346	5408	5470	5532	5594	5656
N	**0**	**1**	**2**	**3**	**4**	**5**	**6**	**7**	**8**	**9**

SIX-PLACE LOGARITHMS: 700–750

N	0	1	2	3	4	5	6	7	8	9
700	84 5098	5160	5222	5284	5346	5408	5470	5532	5594	5656
01	5718	5780	5842	5904	5966	6028	6090	6151	6213	6275
02	6337	6399	6461	6523	6585	6646	6708	6770	6832	6894
03	6955	7017	7079	7141	7202	7264	7326	7388	7449	7511
04	7573	7634	7696	7758	7819	7881	7943	8004	8066	8128
05	8189	8251	8312	8374	8435	8497	8559	8620	8682	8743
06	8805	8866	8928	8989	9051	9112	9174	9235	9297	9358
07	84 9419	9481	9542	9604	9665	9726	9788	9849	9911	9972
08	85 0033	0095	0156	0217	0279	0340	0401	0462	0524	0585
09	0646	0707	0769	0830	0891	0952	1014	1075	1136	1197
710	1258	1320	1381	1442	1503	1564	1625	1686	1747	1809
11	1870	1931	1992	2053	2114	2175	2236	2297	2358	2419
12	2480	2541	2602	2663	2724	2785	2846	2907	2968	3029
13	3090	3150	3211	3272	3333	3394	3455	3516	3577	3637
14	3698	3759	3820	3881	3941	4002	4063	4124	4185	4245
15	4306	4367	4428	4488	4549	4610	4670	4731	4792	4852
16	4913	4974	5034	5095	5156	5216	5277	5337	5398	5459
17	5519	5580	5640	5701	5761	5822	5882	5943	6003	6064
18	6124	6185	6245	6306	6366	6427	6487	6548	6608	6668
19	6729	6789	6850	6910	6970	7031	7091	7152	7212	7272
720	7332	7393	7453	7513	7574	7634	7694	7755	7815	7875
21	7935	7995	8056	8116	8176	8236	8297	8357	8417	8477
22	8537	8597	8657	8718	8778	8838	8898	8958	9018	9078
23	9138	9198	9258	9318	9379	9439	9499	9559	9619	9679
24	85 9739	9799	9859	9918	9978	*0038	*0098	*0158	*0218	*0278
25	86 0338	0398	0458	0518	0578	0637	0697	0757	0817	0877
26	0937	0996	1056	1116	1176	1236	1295	1355	1415	1475
27	1534	1594	1654	1714	1773	1833	1893	1952	2012	2072
28	2131	2191	2251	2310	2370	2430	2489	2549	2608	2668
29	2728	2787	2847	2906	2966	3025	3085	3144	3204	3263
730	3323	3382	3442	3501	3561	3620	3680	3739	3799	3858
31	3917	3977	4036	4096	4155	4214	4274	4333	4392	4452
32	4511	4570	4630	4689	4748	4808	4867	4926	4985	5045
33	5104	5163	5222	5282	5341	5400	5459	5519	5578	5637
34	5696	5755	5814	5874	5933	5992	6051	6110	6169	6228
35	6287	6346	6405	6465	6524	6583	6642	6701	6760	6819
36	6878	6937	6996	7055	7114	7173	7232	7291	7350	7409
37	7467	7526	7585	7644	7703	7762	7821	7880	7939	7998
38	8056	8115	8174	8233	8292	8350	8409	8468	8527	8586
39	8644	8703	8762	8821	8879	8938	8997	9056	9114	9173
740	9232	9290	9349	9408	9466	9525	9584	9642	9701	9760
41	86 9818	9877	9935	9994	*0053	*0111	*0170	*0228	*0287	*0345
42	87 0404	0462	0521	0579	0638	0696	0755	0813	0872	0930
43	0989	1047	1106	1164	1223	1281	1339	1398	1456	1515
44	1573	1631	1690	1748	1806	1865	1923	1981	2040	2098
45	2156	2215	2273	2331	2389	2448	2506	2564	2622	2681
46	2739	2797	2855	2913	2972	3030	3088	3146	3204	3262
47	3321	3379	3437	3495	3553	3611	3669	3727	3785	3844
48	3902	3960	4018	4076	4134	4192	4250	4308	4366	4424
49	4482	4540	4598	4656	4714	4772	4830	4888	4945	5003
750	87 5061	5119	5177	5235	5293	5351	5409	5466	5524	5582
N	**0**	**1**	**2**	**3**	**4**	**5**	**6**	**7**	**8**	**9**

SIX-PLACE LOGARITHMS: 750–800

N	0	1	2	3	4	5	6	7	8	9
750	87 5061	5119	5177	5235	5293	5351	5409	5466	5524	5582
51	5640	5698	5756	5813	5871	5929	5987	6045	6102	6160
52	6218	6276	6333	6391	6449	6507	6564	6622	6680	6737
53	6795	6853	6910	6968	7026	7083	7141	7199	7256	7314
54	7371	7429	7487	7544	7602	7659	7717	7774	7832	7889
55	7947	8004	8062	8119	8177	8234	8292	8349	8407	8464
56	8522	8579	8637	8694	8752	8809	8866	8924	8981	9039
57	9096	9153	9211	9268	9325	9383	9440	9497	9555	9612
58	87 9669	9726	9784	9841	9898	9956	*0013	*0070	*0127	*0185
59	88 0242	0299	0356	0413	0417	0528	0585	0642	0699	0756
760	0814	0871	0928	0985	1042	1099	1156	1213	1271	1328
61	1385	1442	1499	1556	1613	1670	1727	1784	1841	1898
62	1955	2012	2069	2126	2183	2240	2297	2354	2411	2468
63	2525	2581	2638	2695	2752	2809	2866	2923	2980	3037
64	3093	3150	3207	3264	3321	3377	3434	3491	3548	3605
65	3661	3718	3775	3832	3888	3945	4002	4059	4115	4172
66	4229	4285	4342	4399	4455	4512	4569	4625	4682	4739
67	4795	4852	4909	4965	5022	5078	5135	5192	5248	5305
68	5361	5418	5474	5531	5587	5644	5700	5757	5813	5870
69	5926	5983	6039	6096	6152	6209	6265	6321	6378	6434
770	6491	6547	6604	6660	6716	6773	6829	6885	6942	6998
71	7054	7111	7167	7223	7280	7336	7392	7449	7505	7561
72	7617	7674	7730	7786	7842	7898	7955	8011	8067	8123
73	8179	8236	8292	8348	8404	8460	8516	8573	8629	8685
74	8741	8797	8853	8909	8965	9021	9077	9134	9190	9246
75	9302	9358	9414	9470	9526	9582	9638	9694	9750	9806
76	88 9862	9918	9974	*0030	*0086	*0141	*0197	*0253	*0309	*0365
77	89 0421	0477	0533	0589	0645	0700	0756	0812	0868	0924
78	0980	1035	1091	1147	1203	1259	1314	1370	1426	1482
79	1537	1593	1649	1705	1760	1816	1872	1928	1983	2039
780	2095	2150	2206	2262	2317	2373	2429	2484	2540	2595
81	2651	2707	2762	2818	2873	2929	2985	3040	3096	3151
82	3207	3262	3318	3373	3429	3484	3540	3595	3651	3706
83	3762	3817	3873	3928	3984	4039	4094	4150	4205	4261
84	4316	4371	4427	4482	4538	4593	4648	4704	4759	4814
85	4870	4925	4980	5036	5091	5146	5201	5257	5312	5367
86	5423	5478	5533	5588	5644	5699	5754	5809	5864	5920
87	5975	6030	6085	6140	6195	6251	6306	6361	6416	6471
88	6526	6581	6636	6692	6747	6802	6857	6912	6967	7022
89	7077	7132	7187	7242	7297	7352	7407	7462	7517	7572
790	7627	7682	7737	7792	7847	7902	7957	8012	8067	8122
91	8176	8231	8286	8341	8396	8451	8506	8561	8615	8670
92	8725	8780	8835	8890	8944	8999	9054	9109	9164	9218
93	9273	9328	9383	9437	9492	9547	9602	9656	9711	9766
94	89 9821	9875	9930	9985	*0039	*0094	*0149	*0203	*0258	*0312
95	90 0367	0422	0476	0531	0586	0640	0695	0749	0804	0859
96	0913	0968	1022	1077	1131	1186	1240	1295	1349	1404
97	1458	1513	1567	1622	1676	1731	1785	1840	1894	1948
98	2003	2057	2112	2166	2221	2275	2329	2384	2438	2492
99	2547	2601	2655	2710	2764	2818	2873	2927	2981	3036
800	90 3090	3144	3199	3253	3307	3361	3416	3470	3524	3578
N	**0**	**1**	**2**	**3**	**4**	**5**	**6**	**7**	**8**	**9**

SIX-PLACE LOGARITHMS: 800–850

N	0	1	2	3	4	5	6	7	8	9
800	90 3090	3144	3199	3253	3307	3361	3416	3470	3524	3578
01	3633	3687	3741	3795	3849	3904	3958	4012	4066	4120
02	4174	4229	4283	4337	4391	4445	4499	4553	4607	4661
03	4716	4770	4824	4878	4932	4986	5040	5094	5148	5202
04	5256	5310	5364	5418	5472	5526	5580	5634	5688	5742
05	5796	5850	5904	5958	6012	6066	6119	6173	6227	6281
06	6335	6389	6443	6497	6551	6604	6658	6712	6766	6820
07	6874	6927	6981	7035	7089	7143	7196	7250	7304	7358
08	7411	7465	7519	7573	7626	7680	7734	7787	7841	7895
09	7949	8002	8056	8110	8163	8217	8270	8324	8378	8431
810	8485	8539	8592	8646	8699	8753	8807	8860	8914	8967
11	9021	9074	9128	9181	9235	9289	9342	9396	9449	9503
12	90 9556	9610	9663	9716	9770	9823	9877	9930	9984	*0037
13	91 0091	0144	0197	0251	0304	0358	0411	0464	0518	0571
14	0624	0678	0731	0784	0838	0891	0944	0998	1051	1104
15	1158	1211	1264	1317	1371	1424	1477	1530	1584	1637
16	1690	1743	1797	1850	1903	1956	2009	2063	2116	2169
17	2222	2275	2328	2381	2435	2488	2541	2594	2647	2700
18	2753	2806	2859	2913	2966	3019	3072	3125	3178	3231
19	3284	3337	3390	3443	3496	3549	3602	3655	3708	3761
820	3814	3867	3920	3973	4026	4079	4132	4184	4237	4290
21	4343	4396	4449	4502	4555	4608	4660	4713	4766	4819
22	4872	4925	4977	5030	5083	5136	5189	5241	5294	5347
23	5400	5453	5505	5558	5611	5664	5716	5769	5822	5875
24	5927	5980	6033	6085	6138	6191	6243	6296	6349	6401
25	6454	6507	6559	6612	6664	6717	6770	6822	6875	6927
26	6980	7033	7085	7138	7190	7243	7295	7348	7400	7453
27	7506	7558	7611	7663	7716	7768	7820	7873	7925	7978
28	8030	8083	8135	8188	8240	8293	8345	8397	8450	8502
29	8555	8607	8659	8712	8764	8816	8869	8921	8973	9026
830	9078	9130	9183	9235	9287	9340	9392	9444	9496	9549
31	91 9601	9653	9706	9758	9810	9862	9914	9967	*0019	*0071
32	92 0123	0176	0228	0280	0332	0384	0436	0489	0541	0593
33	0645	0697	0749	0801	0853	0906	0958	1010	1062	1114
34	1166	1218	1270	1322	1374	1426	1478	1530	1582	1634
35	1686	1738	1790	1842	1894	1946	1998	2050	2102	2154
36	2206	2258	2310	2362	2414	2466	2518	2570	2622	2674
37	2725	2777	2829	2881	2933	2985	3037	3089	3140	3192
38	3244	3296	3348	3399	3451	3503	3555	3607	3658	3710
39	3762	3814	3865	3917	3969	4021	4072	4124	4176	4228
840	4279	4331	4383	4434	4486	4538	4589	4641	4693	4744
41	4796	4848	4899	4951	5003	5054	5106	5157	5209	5261
42	5312	5364	5415	5467	5518	5570	5621	5673	5725	5776
43	5828	5879	5931	5982	6034	6085	6137	6188	6240	6291
44	6342	6394	6445	6497	6548	6600	6651	6702	6754	6805
45	6857	6908	6959	7011	7062	7114	7165	7216	7268	7319
46	7370	7422	7473	7524	7576	7627	7678	7730	7781	7832
47	7883	7935	7986	8037	8088	8140	8191	8242	8293	8345
48	8396	8447	8498	8549	8601	8652	8703	8754	8805	8857
49	8908	8959	9010	9061	9112	9163	9215	9266	9317	9368
850	92 9419	9470	9521	9572	9623	9674	9725	9776	9827	9879
N	0	1	2	3	4	5	6	7	8	9

SIX-PLACE LOGARITHMS: 850–900

N	0	1	2	3	4	5	6	7	8	9
850	92 9419	9470	9521	9572	9623	9674	9725	9776	9827	9879
51	92 9930	9981	*0032	*0083	*0134	*0185	*0236	*0287	*0338	*0389
52	93 0440	0491	0542	0592	0643	0694	0745	0796	0847	0898
53	0949	1000	1051	1102	1153	1204	1254	1305	1356	1407
54	1458	1509	1560	1610	1661	1712	1763	1814	1865	1915
55	1966	2017	2068	2118	2169	2220	2271	2322	2372	2423
56	2474	2524	2575	2626	2677	2727	2778	2829	2879	2930
57	2981	3031	3082	3133	3183	3234	3285	3335	3386	3437
58	3487	3538	3589	3639	3690	3740	3791	3841	3892	3943
59	3993	4044	4094	4145	4195	4246	4296	4347	4397	4448
860	4498	4549	4599	4650	4700	4751	4801	4852	4902	4953
61	5003	5054	5104	5154	5205	5255	5306	5356	5406	5457
62	5507	5558	5608	5658	5709	5759	5809	5860	5910	5960
63	6011	6061	6111	6162	6212	6262	6313	6363	6413	6463
64	6514	6564	6614	6665	6715	6765	6815	6865	6916	6966
65	7016	7066	7117	7167	7217	7267	7317	7367	7418	7468
66	7518	7568	7618	7668	7718	7769	7819	7869	7919	7969
67	8019	8069	8119	8169	8219	8269	8320	8370	8420	8470
68	8520	8570	8620	8670	8720	8770	8820	8870	8920	8970
69	9020	9070	9120	9170	9220	9270	9320	9369	9419	9469
870	93 9519	9569	9619	9669	9719	9769	9819	9869	9918	9968
71	94 0018	0068	0118	0168	0218	0267	0317	0367	0417	0467
72	0516	9566	0616	0666	0716	0765	0815	0865	0915	0964
73	1014	1064	1114	1163	1213	1263	1313	1362	1412	1462
74	1511	1561	1611	1660	1710	1760	1809	1859	1909	1958
75	2008	2058	2107	2157	2207	2256	2306	2355	2405	2455
76	2504	2554	2603	2653	2702	2752	2801	2851	2901	2950
77	3000	3049	3099	3148	3198	3247	3297	3346	3396	3445
78	3495	3544	3593	3643	3692	3742	3791	3841	3890	3939
79	3989	4038	4088	4137	4186	4236	4285	4335	4384	4433
880	4483	4532	4581	4631	4680	4729	4779	4828	4877	4927
81	4976	5025	5074	5124	5173	5222	5272	5321	5370	5419
82	5469	5518	5567	5616	5665	5715	5764	5813	5862	5912
83	5961	6010	6059	6108	6157	6207	6256	6305	6354	6403
84	6452	6501	6551	6600	6649	6698	6747	6796	6845	6894
85	6943	6992	7041	7090	7140	7189	7238	7287	7336	7385
86	7434	7483	7532	7581	7630	7679	7728	7777	7826	7875
87	7924	7973	8022	8070	8119	8168	8217	8266	8315	8364
88	8413	8462	8511	8560	8609	8657	8706	8755	8804	8853
89	8902	8951	8999	9048	9097	9146	9195	9244	9292	9341
890	9390	9439	9488	9536	9585	9634	9683	9731	9780	9829
91	94 9878	9926	9975	*0024	*0073	*0121	*0170	*0219	*0267	*0316
92	95 0365	0414	0462	0511	0560	0608	0657	0706	0754	0803
93	0851	0900	0949	0997	1046	1095	1143	1192	1240	1289
94	1338	1386	1435	1483	1532	1580	1629	1677	1726	1775
95	1823	1872	1920	1969	2017	2066	2114	2163	2211	2260
96	2308	2356	2405	2453	2502	2550	2599	2647	2696	2744
97	2792	2841	2889	2938	2986	3034	3083	3131	3180	3228
98	3276	3325	3373	3421	3470	3518	3566	3615	3663	3711
99	3760	3808	3856	3905	3953	4001	4049	4098	4146	4194
900	95 4243	4291	4339	4387	4435	4484	4532	4580	4628	4677
N	**0**	**1**	**2**	**3**	**4**	**5**	**6**	**7**	**8**	**9**

SIX-PLACE LOGARITHMS: 900–950

N	0	1	2	3	4	5	6	7	8	9
900	95 4243	4291	4339	4387	4435	4484	4532	4580	4628	4677
01	4725	4773	4821	4869	4918	4966	5014	5062	5110	5158
02	5207	5255	5303	5351	5399	5447	5495	5543	5592	5640
03	5688	5736	5784	5832	5880	5928	5976	6024	6072	6120
04	6168	6216	6265	6313	6361	6409	6457	6505	6553	6601
05	6649	6697	6745	6793	6840	6888	6936	6984	7032	7080
06	7128	7176	7224	7272	7320	7368	7416	7464	7512	7559
07	7607	7655	7703	7751	7799	7847	7894	7942	7990	8038
08	8086	8134	8181	8229	8277	8325	8373	8421	8468	8516
09	8564	8612	8659	8707	8755	8803	8850	8898	8946	8994
910	9041	9089	9137	9185	9232	9280	9328	9375	9423	9471
11	9518	9566	9614	9661	9709	9757	9804	9852	9900	9947
12	95 9995	*0042	*0090	*0138	*0185	*0233	*0280	*0328	*0376	*0423
13	96 0471	0518	0566	0613	0661	0709	0756	0804	0851	0899
14	0946	0994	1041	1089	1136	1184	1231	1279	1326	1374
15	1421	1469	1516	1563	1611	1658	1706	1753	1801	1848
16	1895	1943	1990	2038	2085	2132	2180	2227	2275	2322
17	2369	2417	2464	2511	2559	2606	2653	2701	2748	2795
18	2843	2890	2937	2985	3032	3079	3126	3174	3221	3268
19	3316	3363	3410	3457	3504	3552	3599	3646	3693	3741
920	3788	3835	3882	3929	3977	4024	4071	4118	4165	4212
21	4260	4307	4354	4401	4448	4495	4542	4590	4637	4684
22	4731	4778	4825	4872	4919	4966	5013	5061	5108	5155
23	5202	5249	5296	5343	5390	5437	5484	5531	5578	5625
24	5672	5719	5766	5813	5860	5907	5954	6001	6048	6095
25	6142	6189	6236	6283	6329	6376	6423	6470	6517	6564
26	6611	6658	6705	6752	6799	6845	6892	6939	6986	7033
27	7080	7127	7173	7220	7267	7314	7361	7408	7454	7501
28	7548	7595	7642	7688	7735	7782	7829	7875	7922	7969
29	8016	8062	8109	8156	8203	8249	8296	8343	8390	8436
930	8483	8530	8576	8623	8670	8716	8763	8810	8856	8903
31	8950	8996	9043	9090	9136	9183	9229	9276	9323	9369
32	9416	9463	9509	9556	9602	9649	9695	9742	9789	9835
33	96 9882	9928	9975	*0021	*0068	*0114	*0161	*0207	*0254	*0300
34	97 0347	0393	0440	0486	0533	0579	0626	0672	0719	0765
35	0812	0858	0904	0951	0997	1044	1090	1137	1183	1229
36	1276	1322	1369	1415	1461	1508	1554	1601	1647	1693
37	1740	1786	1832	1879	1925	1971	2018	2064	2110	2157
38	2203	2249	2295	2342	2388	2434	2481	2527	2573	2619
39	2666	2712	2758	2804	2851	2897	2943	2989	3035	3082
940	3128	3174	3220	3266	3313	3359	3405	3451	3497	3543
41	3590	3636	3682	3728	3774	3820	3866	3913	3959	4005
42	4051	4097	4143	4189	4235	4281	4327	4374	4420	4466
43	4512	4558	4604	4650	4696	4742	4788	4834	4880	4926
44	4972	5018	5064	5110	5156	5202	5248	5294	5340	5386
45	5432	5478	5524	5570	5616	5662	5707	5753	5799	5845
46	5891	5937	5983	6029	6075	6121	6167	6212	6258	6304
47	6350	6396	6442	6488	6533	6579	6625	6671	6717	6763
48	6808	6854	6900	6946	6992	7037	7083	7129	7175	7220
49	7266	7312	7358	7403	7449	7495	7541	7586	7632	7678
950	97 7724	7769	7815	7861	7906	7952	7998	8043	8089	8135
N	0	1	2	3	4	5	6	7	8	9

SIX-PLACE LOGARITHMS: 950–1000

N	0	1	2	3	4	5	6	7	8	9
950	97 7724	7769	7815	7861	7906	7952	7998	8043	8089	8135
51	8181	8226	8272	8317	8363	8409	8454	8500	8546	8591
52	8637	8683	8728	8774	8819	8865	8911	8956	9002	9047
53	9093	9138	9184	9230	9275	9321	9366	9412	9457	9503
54	97 9548	9594	9639	9685	9730	9776	9821	9867	9912	9958
55	98 0003	0049	0094	0140	0185	0231	0276	0322	0367	0412
56	0458	0503	0549	0594	0640	0685	0730	0776	0821	0867
57	0912	0957	1003	1048	1093	1139	1184	1229	1275	1320
58	1366	1411	1456	1501	1547	1592	1637	1683	1728	1773
59	1819	1864	1909	1954	2000	2045	2090	2135	2181	2226
960	2271	2316	2362	2407	2452	2497	2543	2588	2633	2678
61	2723	2769	2814	2859	2904	2949	2994	3040	3085	3130
62	3175	3220	3265	3310	3356	3401	3446	3491	3536	3581
63	3626	3671	3716	3762	3807	3852	3897	3942	3987	4032
64	4077	4122	4167	4212	4257	4302	4347	4392	4437	4482
65	4527	4572	4617	4662	4707	4752	4797	4842	4887	4932
66	4977	5022	5067	5112	5157	5202	5247	5292	5337	5382
67	5426	5471	5516	5561	5606	5651	5696	5741	5786	5830
68	5875	5920	5965	6010	6055	6100	6144	6189	6234	6279
69	6324	6369	6413	6458	6503	6548	6593	6637	6682	6727
970	6772	6817	6861	6906	6951	6996	7040	7085	7130	7175
71	7219	7264	7309	7353	7398	7443	7488	7532	7577	7622
72	7666	7711	7756	7800	7845	7890	7934	7979	8024	8068
73	8113	8157	8202	8247	8291	8336	8381	8425	8470	8514
74	8559	8604	8648	8693	8737	8782	8826	8871	8916	8960
75	9005	9049	9094	9138	9183	9227	9272	9316	9361	9405
76	9450	9494	9539	9583	9628	9672	9717	9761	9806	9850
77	98 9895	9939	9983	*0028	*0072	*0117	*0161	*0206	*0250	*0294
78	99 0339	0383	0428	0472	0516	0561	0605	0650	0694	0738
79	0783	0827	0871	0916	0960	1004	1049	1093	1137	1182
980	1226	1270	1315	1359	1403	1448	1492	1536	1580	1625
81	1669	1713	1758	1802	1846	1890	1935	1979	2023	2067
82	2111	2156	2200	2244	2288	2333	2377	2421	2465	2509
83	2554	2598	2642	2686	2730	2774	2819	2863	2907	2951
84	2995	3039	3083	3127	3172	3216	3260	3304	3348	3392
85	3436	3480	3524	3568	3613	3657	3701	3745	3789	3833
86	3877	3921	3965	4009	4053	4097	4141	4185	4229	4273
87	4317	4361	4405	4449	4493	4537	4581	4625	4669	4713
88	4757	4801	4845	4889	4933	4977	5021	5065	5108	5152
89	5196	5240	5284	5328	5372	5416	5460	5504	5547	5591
990	5635	5679	5723	5767	5811	5854	5898	5942	5986	6030
91	6074	6117	6161	6205	6249	6293	6337	6380	6424	6468
92	6512	6555	6599	6643	6687	6731	6774	6818	6862	6906
93	6949	6993	7037	7080	7124	7168	7212	7255	7299	7343
94	7386	7430	7474	7517	7561	7605	7648	7692	7736	7779
95	7823	7868	7910	7954	7998	8041	8085	8129	8172	8216
96	8259	8303	8347	8390	8434	8477	8521	8564	8608	8651
97	8695	9738	8782	8826	8869	8913	8956	9000	9043	9087
98	9131	9174	9218	9261	9305	9348	9392	9435	9479	9522
99	99 9565	9609	9652	9696	9739	9783	9826	9870	9913	9957
1000	00 0000	0043	0087	0130	0174	0217	0260	0304	0347	0391
N	**0**	**1**	**2**	**3**	**4**	**5**	**6**	**7**	**8**	**9**

SIX-PLACE LOGARITHMS: 1000–1050

N	0	1	2	3	4	5	6	7	8	9
1000	000 0000	0434	0869	1303	1737	2171	2605	3039	3473	3907
1001	4341	4775	5208	5642	6076	6510	6943	7377	7810	8244
1002	8677	9111	9544	9977	*0411	*0844	*1277	*1710	*2143	*2576
1003	001 3009	3442	3875	4308	4741	5174	5607	6039	6472	6905
1004	7337	7770	8202	8635	9067	9499	9932	*0364	*0796	*1228
1005	002 1661	2093	2525	2957	3389	3821	4253	4685	5116	5548
1006	5980	6411	6843	7275	7706	8138	8569	9001	9432	9863
1007	003 0295	0726	1157	1588	2019	2451	2882	3313	3744	4174
1008	4605	5036	5467	5898	6328	6759	7190	7620	8051	8481
1009	8912	9342	9772	*0203	*0633	*1063	*1493	*1924	*2354	*2784
1010	004 3214	3644	4074	4504	4933	5363	5793	6223	6652	7082
1011	7512	7941	8371	8800	9229	9659	*0088	*0517	*0947	*1376
1012	005 1805	2234	2663	3092	3521	3950	4379	4808	5237	5666
1013	6094	6523	6952	7380	7809	8238	8666	9094	9523	9951
1014	006 0380	0808	1236	1664	2092	2521	2949	3377	3805	4233
1015	4660	5088	5516	5944	6372	6799	7227	7655	8082	8510
1016	8937	9365	9792	*0219	*0647	*1074	*1501	*1928	*2355	*2782
1017	007 3210	3637	4064	4490	4917	5344	5771	6198	6624	7051
1018	7478	7904	8331	8757	9184	9610	*0037	*0463	*0889	*1316
1019	008 1742	2168	2594	3020	3446	3872	4298	4724	5150	5576
1020	6002	6427	6853	7279	7704	8130	8556	8981	9407	9832
1021	009 0257	0683	1108	1533	1959	2384	2809	3234	3659	4084
1022	4509	4934	5359	5784	6208	6633	7058	7483	7907	8332
1023	8756	9181	9605	*0030	*0454	*0878	*1303	*1727	*2151	*2575
1024	010 3000	3424	3848	4272	4696	5120	5544	5967	6391	6815
1025	7239	7662	8086	8510	8933	9357	9780	*0204	*0627	*1050
1026	011 1474	1897	2320	2743	3166	3590	4013	4436	4859	5282
1027	5704	6127	6550	6973	7396	7818	8241	8664	9086	9509
1028	9931	*0354	*0776	*1198	*1621	*2043	*2465	*2887	*3310	*3732
1029	012 4154	4576	4998	5420	5842	6264	6685	7107	7529	7951
1030	8372	8794	9215	9637	*0059	*0480	*0901	*1323	*1744	*2165
1031	013 2587	3008	3429	3850	4271	4692	5113	5534	5955	6376
1032	6797	7218	7639	8059	8480	8901	9321	9742	*0162	*0583
1033	014 1003	1424	1844	2264	2685	3105	3525	3945	4365	4785
1034	5205	5625	6045	6465	6885	7305	7725	8144	8564	8984
1035	9403	9823	*0243	*0662	*1082	*1501	*1920	*2340	*2759	*3178
1036	015 3598	4017	4436	4855	5274	5693	6112	6531	6950	7369
1037	7788	8206	8625	9044	9462	9881	*0300	*0718	*1137	*1555
1038	016 1974	2392	2810	3229	3647	4065	4483	4901	5319	5737
1039	6155	6573	6991	7409	7827	8245	8663	9080	9498	9916
1040	017 0333	0751	1168	1586	2003	2421	2838	3256	3673	4090
1041	4507	4924	5342	5759	6176	6593	7010	7427	7844	8260
1042	8677	9094	9511	9927	*0344	*0761	*1177	*1594	*2010	*2427
1043	018 2843	3259	3676	4092	4508	4925	5341	5757	6173	6589
1044	7005	7421	7837	8253	8669	9084	9500	9916	*0332	*0747
1045	019 1163	1578	1994	2410	2825	3240	3656	4071	4486	4902
1046	5317	5732	6147	6562	6977	7392	7807	8222	8637	9052
1047	9467	9882	*0296	*0711	*1126	*1540	*1955	*2369	*2784	*3198
1048	020 3613	4027	4442	4856	5270	5684	6099	6513	6927	7341
1049	7755	8169	8583	8997	9411	9824	*0238	*0652	*1066	*1479
1050	021 1893	2307	2720	3134	3547	3961	4374	4787	5201	5614
N	**0**	**1**	**2**	**3**	**4**	**5**	**6**	**7**	**8**	**9**

SIX-PLACE LOGARITHMS: 1050–1100

N	0	1	2	3	4	5	6	7	8	9
1050	021 1893	2307	2720	3134	3547	3961	4374	4787	5201	5614
1051	6027	6440	6854	7267	7680	8093	8506	8919	9332	9745
1052	022 0157	0570	0983	1396	1808	2221	2634	3046	3459	3871
1053	4284	4696	5109	5521	5933	6345	6758	7170	7582	7994
1054	8406	8818	9230	9642	*0054	*0466	*0878	*1289	*1701	*2113
1055	023 2525	2936	3348	3759	4171	4582	4994	5405	5817	6228
1056	6639	7050	7462	7873	8284	8695	9106	9517	9928	*0339
1057	024 0750	1161	1572	1982	2393	2804	3214	3625	4036	4446
1058	4857	5267	5678	6088	6498	6909	7319	7729	8139	8549
1059	8960	9370	9780	*0190	*0600	*1010	*1419	*1829	*2239	*2649
1060	025 3059	3468	3878	4288	4697	5107	5516	5926	6335	6744
1061	7154	7563	7972	8382	8791	9200	9609	*0018	*0427	*0836
1062	026 1245	1654	2063	2472	2881	3289	3698	4107	4515	4924
1063	5333	5741	6150	6558	6967	7375	7783	8192	8600	9008
1064	9416	9824	*0233	*0641	*1049	*1457	*1865	*2273	*2680	*3088
1065	027 3496	3904	4312	4719	5127	5535	5942	6350	6757	7165
1066	7572	7979	8387	8794	9201	9609	*0016	*0423	*0830	*1237
1067	028 1644	2051	2458	2865	3272	3679	4086	4492	4899	5306
1068	5713	6119	6526	6932	7339	7745	8152	8558	8964	9371
1069	9777	*0183	*0590	*0996	*1402	*1808	*2214	*2620	*3026	*3432
1070	029 3838	4244	4649	5055	5461	5867	6272	6678	7084	7489
1071	7895	8300	8706	9111	9516	9922	*0327	*0732	*1138	*1543
1072	030 1948	2353	2758	3163	3568	3973	4378	4783	5188	5592
1073	5997	6402	6807	7211	7616	8020	8425	8830	9234	9638
1074	031 0043	0447	0851	1256	1660	2064	2468	2872	3277	3681
1075	4085	4489	4893	5296	5700	6104	6508	6912	7315	7719
1076	8123	8526	8930	9333	9737	*0140	*0544	*0947	*1350	*1754
1077	032 2157	2560	2963	3367	3770	4173	4576	4979	5382	5785
1078	6188	6590	6993	7396	7799	8201	8604	9007	9409	9812
1079	033 0214	0617	1019	1422	1824	2226	2629	3031	3433	3835
1080	4238	4640	5042	5444	5846	6248	6650	7052	7453	7855
1081	8257	8659	9060	9462	9864	*0265	*0667	*1068	*1470	*1871
1082	034 2273	2674	3075	3477	3878	4279	4680	5081	5482	5884
1083	6285	6686	7087	7487	7888	8289	8690	9091	9491	9892
1084	035 0293	0693	1094	1495	1895	2296	2696	3096	3497	3897
1085	4297	4698	5098	5498	5898	6298	6698	7098	7498	7898
1086	8298	8698	9098	9498	9898	*0297	*0697	*1097	*1496	*1896
1087	036 2295	2695	3094	3494	3893	4293	4692	5091	5491	5890
1088	6289	6688	7087	7486	7885	8284	8683	9082	9481	9880
1089	037 0279	0678	1076	1475	1874	2272	2671	3070	3468	3867
1090	4265	4663	5062	5460	5858	6257	6655	7053	7451	7849
1091	8248	8646	9044	9442	9839	*0237	*0635	*1033	*1431	*1829
1092	038 2226	2624	3022	3419	3817	4214	4612	5009	5407	5804
1093	6202	6599	6996	7393	7791	8188	8585	8982	9379	9776
1094	039 0173	0570	0967	1364	1761	2158	2554	2951	3348	3745
1095	4141	4538	4934	5331	5727	6124	6520	6917	7313	7709
1096	8106	8502	8898	9294	9690	*0086	*0482	*0878	*1274	*1670
1097	040 2066	2462	2858	3254	3650	4045	4441	4837	5232	5628
1098	6023	6419	6814	7210	7605	8001	8396	8791	9187	9582
1099	9977	*0372	*0767	*1162	*1557	*1952	*2347	*2742	*3137	*3532
1100	041 3927	4322	4716	5111	5506	5900	6295	6690	7084	7479
N	**0**	**1**	**2**	**3**	**4**	**5**	**6**	**7**	**8**	**9**

SIX-PLACE LOGARITHMS: 1100–1150

N	0	1	2	3	4	5	6	7	8	9
1100	041 3927	4322	4716	5111	5506	5900	6295	6690	7084	7479
1101	7873	8268	8662	9056	9451	9845	*0239	*0633	*1028	*1422
1102	042 1816	2210	2604	2998	3392	3786	4180	4574	4968	5361
1103	5755	6149	6543	6936	7330	7723	8117	8510	8904	9297
1104	9691	*0084	*0477	*0871	*1264	*1657	*2050	*2444	*2837	*3230
1105	043 3623	4016	4409	4802	5195	5587	5980	6373	6766	7159
1106	7551	7944	8337	8729	9122	9514	9907	*0299	*0692	*1084
1107	044 1476	1869	2261	2653	3045	3437	3829	4222	4614	5006
1108	5398	5790	6181	6573	6965	7357	7749	8140	8532	8924
1109	9315	9707	*0099	*0490	*0882	*1273	*1664	*2056	*2447	*2839
1110	045 3230	3621	4012	4403	4795	5186	5577	5968	6359	6750
1111	7141	7531	7922	8313	8704	9095	9485	9876	*0267	*0657
1112	046 1048	1438	1829	2219	2610	3000	3391	3781	4171	4561
1113	4952	5342	5732	6122	6512	6902	7292	7682	8072	8462
1114	8852	9242	9632	*0021	*0411	*0801	*1190	*1580	*1970	*2359
1115	047 2749	3138	3528	3917	4306	4696	5085	5474	5864	6253
1116	6642	7031	7420	7809	8198	8587	8976	9365	9754	*0143
1117	048 0532	0921	1309	1698	2087	2475	2864	3253	3641	4030
1118	4418	4806	5195	5583	5972	6360	6748	7136	7525	7913
1119	8301	8689	9077	9465	9853	*0241	*0629	*1017	*1405	*1792
1120	049 2180	2568	2956	3343	3731	4119	4506	4894	5281	5669
1121	6056	6444	6831	7218	7606	7993	8380	8767	9154	9541
1122	9929	*0316	*0703	*1090	*1477	*1863	*2250	*2637	*3024	*3411
1123	050 3798	4184	4571	4958	5344	5731	6117	6504	6890	7277
1124	7663	8049	8436	8822	9208	9595	9981	*0367	*0753	*1139
1125	051 1525	1911	2297	2683	3069	3455	3841	4227	4612	4998
1126	5384	5770	6155	6541	6926	7312	7697	8083	8468	8854
1127	9239	9624	*0010	*0395	*0780	*1166	*1551	*1936	*2321	*2706
1128	052 3091	3476	3861	4246	4631	5016	5400	5785	6170	6555
1129	6939	7324	7700	8093	8478	8862	9247	9631	*0016	*0400
1130	053 0784	1169	1553	1937	2321	2706	3090	3474	3858	4242
1131	4626	5010	5394	5778	6162	6546	6929	7313	7697	8081
1132	8464	8848	9232	9615	9999	*0382	*0766	*1149	*1532	*1916
1133	054 2299	2682	3066	3449	3832	4215	4598	4981	5365	5748
1134	6131	6514	6896	7279	7662	8045	8428	8811	9193	9576
1135	9959	*0341	*0724	*1106	*1489	*1871	*2254	*2636	*3019	*3401
1136	055 3783	4166	4548	4930	5312	5694	6077	6459	6841	7223
1137	7605	7987	8369	8750	9132	9514	9896	*0278	*0659	*1041
1138	056 1423	1804	2186	2567	2949	3330	3712	4093	4475	4856
1139	5237	5619	6000	6381	6762	7143	7524	7905	8287	8668
1140	9049	9429	9810	*0191	*0572	*0953	*1334	*1714	*2095	*2476
1141	057 2856	3237	3618	3998	4379	4759	5140	5520	5900	6281
1142	6661	7041	7422	7802	8182	8562	8942	9322	9702	*0082
1143	058 0462	0842	1222	1602	1982	2362	2741	3121	3501	3881
1144	4260	4640	5019	5399	5778	6158	6537	6917	7296	7676
1145	8055	8434	8813	9193	9572	9951	*0330	*0709	*1088	*1467
1146	059 1846	2225	2604	2983	3362	3741	4119	4498	4877	5256
1147	5634	6013	6391	6770	7148	7527	7905	8284	8662	9041
1148	9419	9797	*0175	*0554	*0932	*1310	*1688	*2066	*2444	*2822
1149	060 3200	3578	3956	4334	4712	5090	5468	5845	6223	6601
1150	6978	7356	7734	8111	8489	8866	9244	9621	9999	*0376
N	**0**	**1**	**2**	**3**	**4**	**5**	**6**	**7**	**8**	**9**

SIX-PLACE LOGARITHMS: 1150–1200

N	0	1	2	3	4	5	6	7	8	9
1150	060 6978	7356	7734	8111	8489	8866	9244	9621	9999	*0376
1151	061 0753	1131	1508	1885	2262	2639	3017	3394	3771	4148
1152	4525	4902	5279	5656	6032	6409	6786	7163	7540	7916
1153	8293	8670	9046	9423	9799	*0176	*0552	*0929	*1305	*1682
1154	062 2058	2434	2811	3187	3563	3939	4316	4692	5068	5444
1155	5820	6196	6572	6948	7324	7699	8075	8451	8827	9203
1156	9578	9954	*0330	*0705	*1081	*1456	*1832	*2207	*2583	*2958
1157	063 3334	3709	4084	4460	4835	5210	5585	5960	6335	6711
1158	7086	7461	7836	8211	8585	8960	9335	9710	*0085	*0460
1159	064 0834	1209	1584	1958	2333	2708	3082	3457	3831	4205
1160	4580	4954	5329	5703	6077	6451	6826	7200	7574	7948
1161	8322	8696	9070	9444	9818	*0192	*0566	*0940	*1314	*1688
1162	065 2061	2435	2809	3182	3556	3930	4303	4677	5050	5424
1163	5797	6171	6544	6917	7291	7664	8037	8410	8784	9157
1164	9530	9903	*0276	*0649	*1022	*1395	*1768	*2141	*2514	*2886
1165	066 3259	3632	4005	4377	4750	5123	5495	5868	6241	6613
1166	6986	7358	7730	8103	8475	8847	9220	9592	9964	*0336
1167	067 0709	1081	1453	1825	2197	2569	2941	3313	3685	4057
1168	4428	4800	5172	5544	5915	6287	6659	7030	7402	7774
1169	8145	8517	8888	9259	9631	*0002	*0374	*0745	*1116	*1487
1170	068 1859	2230	2601	2972	3343	3714	4085	4456	4827	5198
1171	5569	5940	6311	6681	7052	7423	7794	8164	8535	8906
1172	9276	9647	*0017	*0388	*0758	*1129	*1499	*1869	*2240	*2610
1173	069 2980	3350	3721	4091	4461	4831	5201	5571	5941	6311
1174	6681	7051	7421	7791	8160	8530	8900	9270	9639	*0009
1175	070 0379	0748	1118	1487	1857	2226	2596	2965	3335	3704
1176	4073	4442	4812	5181	5550	5919	6288	6658	7027	7396
1177	7765	8134	8503	8871	9240	9609	9978	*0347	*0715	*1084
1178	071 1453	1822	2190	2559	2927	3296	3664	4033	4401	4770
1179	5138	5506	5875	6243	6611	6979	7348	7716	8084	8452
1180	8820	9188	9556	9924	*0292	*0660	*1028	*1396	*1763	*2131
1181	072 2499	2867	3234	3602	3970	4337	4705	5072	5440	5807
1182	6175	6542	6910	7277	7644	8011	8379	8746	9113	9480
1183	9847	*0215	*0582	*0949	*1316	*1683	*2050	*2416	*2783	*3150
1184	073 3517	3884	4251	4617	4984	5351	5717	6084	6450	6817
1185	7184	7550	7916	8283	8649	9016	9382	9748	*0114	*0481
1186	074 0847	1213	1579	1945	2311	2677	3043	3409	3775	4141
1187	4507	4873	5239	5605	5970	6336	6702	7068	7433	7799
1188	8164	8530	8895	9261	9626	9992	*0357	*0723	*1088	*1453
1189	075 1819	2184	2549	2914	3279	3644	4010	4375	4740	5105
1190	5470	5835	6199	6564	6929	7294	7659	8024	8388	8753
1191	9118	9482	9847	*0211	*0576	*0940	*1305	*1669	*2034	*2398
1192	076 2763	3127	3491	3855	4220	4584	4948	5312	5676	6040
1193	6404	6768	7132	7496	7860	8224	8588	8952	9316	9680
1194	077 0043	0407	0771	1134	1498	1862	2225	2589	2952	3316
1195	3679	4042	4406	4769	5133	5496	5859	6222	6585	6949
1196	7312	7675	8038	8401	8764	9127	9490	9853	*0216	*0579
1197	078 0942	1304	1667	2030	2393	2755	3118	3480	3843	4206
1198	4568	4931	5293	5656	6018	6380	6743	7105	7467	7830
1199	8192	8554	8916	9278	9640	*0003	*0365	*0727	*1089	*1451
1200	079 1812	2174	2536	2898	3260	3622	3983	4345	4707	5068
N	**0**	**1**	**2**	**3**	**4**	**5**	**6**	**7**	**8**	**9**

XIII.8 NATURAL OR NAPERIAN LOGARITHMS

0.000–0.499

N	0	1	2	3	4	5	6	7	8	9
0.00	−∞	−6‡ .90776	−6 .21461	−5 .80914	−5 .52146	−5 .29832	−5 .11600	−4 .96185	−4 .82831	−4 .71053
.01	−4.60517	.50986	.42285	.34281	.26870	.19971	.13517	.07454	.01738	*.96332
.02	−3.91202	.86323	.81671	.77226	.72970	.68888	.64966	.61192	.57555	.54046
.03	.50656	.47377	.44202	.41125	.38139	.35241	.32424	.29684	.27017	.24419
.04	.21888	.19418	.17009	.14656	.12357	.10109	.07911	.05761	.03655	.01593
.05	−2.99573	.97593	.95651	.93746	.91877	.90042	.88240	.86470	.84731	.83022
.06	.81341	.79688	.78062	.76462	.74887	.73337	.71810	.70306	.68825	.67365
.07	.65926	.64508	.63109	.61730	.60369	.59027	.57702	.56395	.55105	.53831
.08	.52573	.51331	.50104	.48891	.47694	.46510	.45341	.44185	.43042	.41912
.09	.40795	.39690	.38597	.37516	.36446	.35388	.34341	.33304	.32279	.31264
0.10	−2.30259	.29263	.28278	.27303	.26336	.25379	.24432	.23493	.22562	.21641
.11	.20727	.19823	.18926	.18037	.17156	.16282	.15417	.14558	.13707	.12863
.12	.12026	.11196	.10373	.09557	.08747	.07944	.07147	.06357	.05573	.04794
.13	.04022	.03256	.02495	.01741	.00992	.00248	*.99510	*.98777	*.98050	*.97328
.14	−1.96611	.95900	.95193	.94491	.93794	.93102	.92415	.91732	.91054	.90381
.15	.89712	.89048	.88387	.87732	.87080	.86433	.85790	.85151	.84516	.83885
.16	.83258	.82635	.82016	.81401	.80789	.80181	.79577	.78976	.78379	.77786
.17	.77196	.76609	.76026	.75446	.74870	.74297	.73727	.73161	.72597	.72037
.18	.71480	.70926	.70375	.69827	.69282	.68740	.68201	.67665	.67131	.66601
.19	.66073	.65548	.65026	.64507	.63990	.63476	.62964	.62455	.61949	.61445
0.20	−1.60944	.60445	.59949	.59455	.58964	.58475	.57988	.57504	.57022	.56542
.21	.56065	.55590	.55117	.54646	.54178	.53712	.53248	.52786	.52326	.51868
.22	.51413	.50959	.50508	.50058	.49611	.49165	.48722	.48281	.47841	.47403
.23	.46968	.46534	.46102	.45672	.45243	.44817	.44392	.43970	.43548	.43129
.24	.42712	.42296	.41882	.41469	.41059	.40650	.40242	.39837	.39433	.39030
.25	.38629	.38230	.37833	.37437	.37042	.36649	.36258	.35868	.35480	.35093
.26	.34707	.34323	.33941	.33560	.33181	.32803	.32426	.32051	.31677	.31304
.27	.30933	.30564	.30195	.29828	.29463	.29098	.28735	.28374	.28013	.27654
.28	.27297	.26940	.26585	.26231	.25878	.25527	.25176	.24827	.24479	.24133
.29	.23787	.23443	.23100	.22758	.22418	.22078	.21740	.21402	.21066	.20731
0.30	−1.20397	.20065	.19733	.19402	.19073	.18744	.18417	.18091	.17766	.17441
.31	.17118	.16796	.16475	.16155	.15836	.15518	.15201	.14885	.14570	.14256
.32	.13943	.13631	.13320	.13010	.12701	.12393	.12086	.11780	.11474	.11170
.33	.10866	.10564	.10262	.09961	.09661	.09362	.09064	.08767	.08471	.08176
.34	.07881	.07587	.07294	.07002	.06711	.06421	.06132	.05843	.05555	.05268
.35	−1.04982	.04697	.04412	.04129	.03846	.03564	.03282	.03002	.02722	.02443
.36	.02165	.01888	.01611	.01335	.01060	.00786	.00512	.00239	*.99967	*.99696
.37	−0.99425	.99155	.98886	.98618	.98350	.98083	.97817	.97551	.97286	.97022
.38	.96758	.96496	.96233	.95972	.95711	.95451	.95192	.94933	.94675	.94418
.39	.94161	.93905	.93649	.93395	.93140	.92887	.92634	.92382	.92130	.91879
0.40	−0.91629	.91379	.91130	.90882	.90634	.90387	.90140	.89894	.89649	.89404
.41	.89160	.88916	.88673	.88431	.88189	.87948	.87707	.87467	.87227	.86988
.42	.86750	.86512	.86275	.86038	.85802	.85567	.85332	.85097	.84863	.84630
.43	.84397	.84165	.83933	.83702	.83471	.83241	.83011	.82782	.82554	.82326
.44	.82098	.81871	.81645	.81419	.81193	.80968	.80744	.80520	.80296	.80073
.45	.79851	.79629	.79407	.79186	.78966	.78746	.78526	.78307	.78089	.77871
.46	.77653	.77436	.77219	.77003	.76787	.76572	.76357	.76143	.75929	.75715
.47	.75502	.75290	.75078	.74866	.74655	.74444	.74234	.74024	.73814	.73605
.48	.73397	.73189	.72981	.72774	.72567	.72361	.72155	.71949	.71744	.71539
.49	.71335	.71131	.70928	.70725	.70522	.70320	.70118	.69917	.69716	.69515

‡ Note that the whole number values are given above the decimal values for the first line. In the second and following lines they are given at the left. All decimal values are negative on this page.

NATURAL OR NAPERIAN LOGARITHMS

0.500–0.999

N	0	1	2	3	4	5	6	7	8	9
0.50	−0.69315	.69115	.68916	.68717	.68518	.68320	.68122	.67924	.67727	.67531
.51	.67334	.67139	.66943	.66748	.66553	.66359	.66165	.65971	.65778	.65585
.52	.65393	.65201	.65009	.64817	.64626	.64436	.64245	.64055	.63866	.63677
.53	.63488	.63299	.63111	.62923	.62736	.62549	.62362	.62176	.61990	.61804
.54	.61619	.61434	.61249	.61065	.60881	.60697	.60514	.60331	.60148	.59966
.55	.59784	.59602	.59421	.59240	.59059	.58879	.58699	.58519	.58340	.58161
.56	.57982	.57803	.57625	.57448	.57270	.57093	.56916	.56740	.56563	.56387
.57	.56212	.56037	.55862	.55687	.55513	.55339	.55165	.54991	.54818	.54645
.58	.54473	.54300	.54128	.53957	.53785	.53614	.53444	.53273	.53103	.52933
.59	.52763	.52594	.52425	.52256	.52088	.51919	.51751	.51584	.51416	.51249
0.60	−0.51083	.50916	.50750	.50584	.50418	.50253	.50088	.49923	.49758	.49594
.61	.49430	.49266	.49102	.48939	.48776	.48613	.48451	.48289	.48127	.47965
.62	.47804	.47642	.47482	.47321	.47160	.47000	.46840	.46681	.46522	.46362
.63	.46204	.46045	.45887	.45728	.45571	.45413	.45256	.45099	.44942	.44785
.64	.44629	.44473	.44317	.44161	.44006	.43850	.43696	.43541	.43386	.43232
.65	.43078	.42925	.42771	.42618	.42465	.42312	.42159	.42007	.41855	.41703
.66	.41552	.41400	.41249	.41098	.40947	.40797	.40647	.40497	.40347	.40197
.67	.40048	.39899	.39750	.39601	.39453	.39304	.39156	.39008	.38861	.38713
.68	.38566	.38419	.38273	.38126	.37980	.37834	.37688	.37542	.37397	.37251
.69	.37106	.36962	.36817	.36673	.36528	.36384	.36241	.36097	.35954	.35810
0.70	−0.35667	.35525	.35382	.35240	.35098	.34956	.34814	.34672	.34531	.34390
.71	.34249	.34108	.33968	.33827	.33687	.33547	.33408	.33268	.33129	.32989
.72	.32850	.32712	.32573	.32435	.32296	.32158	.32021	.31883	.31745	.31608
.73	.31471	.31334	.31197	.31061	.30925	.30788	.30653	.30517	.30381	.30246
.74	.30111	.29975	.29841	.29706	.29571	.29437	.29303	.29169	.29035	.28902
.75	.28768	.28635	.28502	.28369	.28236	.28104	.27971	.27839	.27707	.27575
.76	.27444	.27312	.27181	.27050	.26919	.26788	.26657	.26527	.26397	.26266
.77	.26136	.26007	.25877	.25748	.25618	.25489	.25360	.25231	.25103	.24974
.78	.24846	.24718	.24590	.24462	.24335	.24207	.24080	.23953	.23826	.23699
.79	.23572	.23446	.23319	.23193	.23067	.22941	.22816	.22690	.22565	.22439
0.80	−0.22314	.22189	.22065	.21940	.21816	.21691	.21567	.21443	.21319	.21196
.81	.21072	.20949	.20825	.20702	.20579	.20457	.20334	.20212	.20089	.19967
.82	.19845	.19723	.19601	.19480	.19358	.19237	.19116	.18995	.18874	.18754
.83	.18633	.18513	.18392	.18272	.18152	.18032	.17913	.17793	.17674	.17554
.84	.17435	.17316	.17198	.17079	.16960	.16842	.16724	.16605	.16487	.16370
.85	−0.16252	.16134	.16017	.15900	.15782	.15665	.15548	.15432	.15315	.15199
.86	.15082	.14966	.14850	.14734	.14618	.14503	.14387	.14272	.14156	.14041
.87	.13926	.13811	.13697	.13582	.13467	.13353	.13239	.13125	.13011	.12897
.88	.12783	.12670	.12556	.12443	.12330	.12217	.12104	.11991	.11878	.11766
.89	.11653	.11541	.11429	.11317	.11205	.11093	.10981	.10870	.10759	.10647
0.90	−0.10536	.10425	.10314	.10203	.10093	.09982	.09872	.09761	.09651	.09541
.91	.09431	.09321	.09212	.09102	.08992	.08883	.08774	.08665	.08556	.08447
.92	.08338	.08230	.08121	.08013	.07904	.07796	.07688	.07580	.07472	.07365
.93	.07257	.07150	.07042	.06935	.06828	.06721	.06614	.06507	.06401	.06294
.94	.06188	.06081	.05975	.05869	.05763	.05657	.05551	.05446	.05340	.05235
.95	.05129	.05024	.04919	.04814	.04709	.04604	.04500	.04395	.04291	.04186
.96	.04082	.03978	.03874	.03770	.03666	.03563	.03459	.03356	.03252	.03149
.97	.03046	.02943	.02840	.02737	.02634	.02532	.02429	.02327	.02225	.02122
.98	.02020	.01918	.01816	.01715	.01613	.01511	.01410	.01309	.01207	.01106
.99	.01005	.00904	.00803	.00702	.00602	.00501	.00401	.00300	.00200	.00100

NATURAL OR NAPERIAN LOGARITHMS

To find the natural logarithm of a number which is 1/10, 1/100, 1/1000, etc. of a number whose logarithm is given, subtract from the given logarithm $\log_e 10$, $2 \log_e 10$, $3 \log_e 10$, etc.

To find the natural logarithm of a number which is 10, 100, 1000, etc. times a number whose logarithm is given, add to the given logarithm $\log_e 10$, $2 \log_e 10$, $3 \log_e 10$, etc.

$\log_e 10$ =	2.30258 50930	$6 \log_e 10$ =	13.81551 05580
$2 \log_e 10$ =	4.60517 01860	$7 \log_e 10$ =	16.11809 56510
$3 \log_e 10$ =	6.90775 52790	$8 \log_e 10$ =	18.42068 07440
$4 \log_e 10$ =	9.21034 03720	$9 \log_e 10$ =	20.72326 58369
$5 \log_e 10$ =	11.51292 54650	$10 \log_e 10$ =	23.02585 09299

See preceding table for logarithms for numbers between 0.000 and 0.999.

1.00–4.99

N	0	1	2	3	4	5	6	7	8	9
1.0	0.00000	.00995	.01980	.02956	.03922	.04879	.05827	.06766	.07696	.08618
.1	.09531	.10436	.11333	.12222	.13103	.13976	.14842	.15700	.16551	.17395
.2	.18232	.19062	.19885	.20701	.21511	.22314	.23111	.23902	.24686	.25464
.3	.26236	.27003	.27763	.28518	.29267	.30010	.30748	.31481	.32208	.32930
.4	.33647	.34359	.35066	.35767	.36464	.37156	.37844	.38526	.39204	.39878
.5	.40547	.41211	.41871	.42527	.43178	.43825	.44469	.45108	.45742	.46373
.6	.47000	.47623	.48243	.48858	.49470	.50078	.50682	.51282	.51879	.52473
.7	.53063	.53649	.54232	.54812	.55389	.55962	.56531	.57098	.57661	.58222
.8	.58779	.59333	.59884	.60432	.60977	.61519	.62058	.62594	.63127	.63658
.9	.64185	.64710	.65233	.65752	.66269	.66783	.67294	.67803	.68310	.68813
2.0	0.69315	.69813	.70310	.70804	.71295	.71784	.72271	.72755	.73237	.73716
.1	.74194	.74669	.75142	.75612	.76081	.76547	.77011	.77473	.77932	.78390
.2	.78846	.79299	.79751	.80200	.80648	.81093	.81536	.81978	.82418	.82855
.3	.83291	.83725	.84157	.84587	.85015	.85442	.85866	.86289	.86710	.87129
.4	.87547	.87963	.88377	.88789	.89200	.89609	.90016	.90422	.90826	.91228
.5	.91629	.92028	.92426	.92822	.93216	.93609	.94001	.94391	.94779	.95166
.6	.95551	.95935	.96317	.96698	.97078	.97456	.97833	.98208	.98582	.98954
.7	.99325	.99695	*.00063	*.00430	*.00796	*.01160	*.01523	*.01885	*.02245	*.02604
.8	1.02962	.03318	.03674	.04028	.04380	.04732	.05082	.05431	.05779	.06126
.9	.06471	.06815	.07158	.07500	.07841	.08181	.08519	.08856	.09192	.09527
3.0	1.09861	.10194	.10526	.10856	.11186	.11514	.11841	.12168	.12493	.12817
.1	.13140	.13462	.13783	.14103	.14422	.14740	.15057	.15373	.15688	.16002
.2	.16315	.16627	.16938	.17248	.17557	.17865	.18173	.18479	.18784	.19089
.3	.19392	.19695	.19996	.20297	.20507	.20896	.21194	.21491	.21788	.22083
.4	.22378	.22671	.22964	.23256	.23547	.23837	.24127	.24415	.24703	.24990
.5	.25276	.25562	.25846	.26130	.26413	.26695	.26976	.27257	.27536	.27815
.6	.28093	.28371	.28647	.28923	.29198	.29473	.29746	.30019	.30291	.30563
.7	.30833	.31103	.31372	.31641	.31909	.32176	.32442	.32708	.32972	.33237
.8	.33500	.33763	.34025	.34286	.34547	.34807	.35067	.35325	.35584	.35841
.9	.36098	.36354	.36609	.36864	.37118	.37372	.37624	.37877	.38128	.38379
4.0	1.38629	.38879	.39128	.39377	.39624	.39872	.40118	.40364	.40610	.40854
.1	.41099	.41342	.41585	.41828	.42070	.42311	.42552	.42792	.43031	.43270
.2	.43508	.43746	.43984	.44220	.44456	.44692	.44927	.45161	.45395	.45629
.3	.45862	.46094	.46326	.46557	.46787	.47018	.47247	.47476	.47705	.47933
.4	.48160	.48387	.48614	.48840	.49065	.49290	.49515	.49739	.49962	.50185
.5	.50408	.50630	.50851	.51072	.51293	.51513	.51732	.51951	.52170	.52388
.6	.52606	.52823	.53039	.53256	.53471	.53687	.53902	.54116	.54330	.54543
.7	.54756	.54969	.55181	.55393	.55604	.55814	.56025	.56235	.56444	.56653
.8	.56862	.57070	.57277	.57485	.57691	.57898	.58104	.58309	.58515	.58719
.9	.58924	.59127	.59331	.59534	.59737	.59939	.60141	.60342	.60543	.60744

NATURAL OR NAPERIAN LOGARITHMS

5.00–9.99

N	0	1	2	3	4	5	6	7	8	9
5.0	1.60944	.61144	.61343	.61542	.61741	.61939	.62137	.62334	.62531	.62728
.1	.62924	.63120	.63315	.63511	.63705	.63900	.64094	.64287	.64481	.64673
.2	.64866	.65058	.65250	.65441	.65632	.65823	.66013	.66203	.66393	.66582
.3	.66771	.66959	.67147	.67335	.67523	.67710	.67896	.68083	.68269	.68455
.4	.68640	.68825	.69010	.69194	.69378	.69562	.69745	.69928	.70111	.70293
.5	.70475	.70656	.70838	.71019	.71199	.71380	.71560	.71740	.71919	.72098
.6	.72277	.72455	.72633	.72811	.72988	.73166	.73342	.73519	.73695	.73871
.7	.74047	.74222	.74397	.74572	.74746	.74920	.75094	.75267	.75440	.75613
.8	.75786	.75958	.76130	.76302	.76473	.76644	.76815	.76985	.77156	.77326
.9	.77495	.77665	.77834	.78002	.78171	.78339	.78507	.78675	.78842	.79009
6.0	1.79176	.79342	.79509	.79675	.79840	.80006	.80171	.80336	.80500	.80665
.1	.80829	.80993	.81156	.81319	.81482	.81645	.81808	.81970	.82132	.82294
.2	.82455	.82616	.82777	.82938	.83098	.83258	.83418	.83578	.83737	.83896
.3	.84055	.84214	.84372	.84530	.84688	.84845	.85003	.85160	.85317	.85473
.4	.85630	.85786	.85942	.86097	.86253	.86408	.86563	.86718	.86872	.87026
.5	.87180	.87334	.87487	.87641	.87794	.87947	.88099	.88251	.88403	.88555
.6	.88707	.88858	.89010	.89160	.89311	.89462	.89612	.89762	.89912	.90061
.7	.90211	.90360	.90509	.90658	.90806	.90954	.91102	.91250	.91398	.91545
.8	.91692	.91839	.91986	.92132	.92279	.92425	.92571	.92716	.92862	.93007
.9	.93152	.93297	.93442	.93586	.93730	.93874	.94018	.94162	.94305	.94448
7.0	1.94591	.94734	.94876	.95019	.95161	.95303	.95445	.95586	.95727	.95869
.1	.96009	.96150	.96291	.96431	.96571	.96711	.96851	.96991	.97130	.97269
.2	.97408	.97547	.97685	.97824	.97962	.98100	.98238	.98376	.98513	.98650
.3	.98787	.98924	.99061	.99198	.99334	.99470	.99606	.99742	.99877	*.00013
.4	2.00148	.00283	.00418	.00553	.00687	.00821	.00956	.01089	.01223	.01357
.5	.01490	.01624	.01757	.01890	.02022	.02155	.02287	.02419	.02551	.02683
.6	.02815	.02946	.03078	.03209	.03340	.03471	.03601	.03732	.03862	.03992
.7	.04122	.04252	.04381	.04511	.04640	.04769	.04898	.05027	.05156	.05284
.8	.05412	.05540	.05668	.05796	.05924	.06051	.06179	.06306	.06433	.06560
.9	.06686	.06813	.06939	.07065	.07191	.07317	.07443	.07568	.07694	.07819
8.0	2.07944	.08069	.08194	.08318	.08443	.08567	.08691	.08815	.08939	.09063
.1	.09186	.09310	.09433	.09556	.09679	.09802	.09924	.10047	.10169	.10291
.2	.10413	.10535	.10657	.10779	.10900	.11021	.11142	.11263	.11384	.11505
.3	.11626	.11746	.11866	.11986	.12106	.12226	.12346	.12465	.12585	.12704
.4	.12823	.12942	.13061	.13180	.13298	.13417	.13535	.13653	.13771	.13889
.5	.14007	.14124	.14242	.14359	.14476	.14593	.14710	.14827	.14943	.15060
.6	.15176	.15292	.15409	.15524	.15640	.15756	.15871	.15987	.16102	.16217
.7	.16332	.16447	.16562	.16677	.16791	.16905	.17020	.17134	.17248	.17361
.8	.17475	.17589	.17702	.17816	.17929	.18042	.18155	.18267	.18380	.18493
.9	.18605	.18717	.18830	.18942	.19054	.19165	.19277	.19389	.19500	.19611
9.0	2.19722	.19834	.19944	.20055	.20166	.20276	.20387	.20497	.20607	.20717
.1	.20827	.20937	.21047	.21157	.21266	.21375	.21485	.21594	.21703	.21812
.2	.21920	.22029	.22138	.22246	.22354	.22462	.22570	.22678	.22786	.22894
.3	.23001	.23109	.23216	.23324	.23431	.23538	.23645	.23751	.23858	.23965
.4	.24071	.24177	.24284	.24390	.24496	.24601	.24707	.24813	.24918	.25024
.5	.25129	.25234	.25339	.25444	.25549	.25654	.25759	.25863	.25968	.26072
.6	.26176	.26280	.26384	.26488	.26592	.26696	.26799	.26903	.27006	.27109
.7	.27213	.27316	.27419	.27521	.27624	.27727	.27829	.27932	.28034	.28136
.8	.28238	.28340	.28442	.28544	.28646	.28747	.28849	.28950	.29051	.29152
.9	.29253	.29354	.29455	.29556	.29657	.29757	.29858	.29958	.30058	.30158

NATURAL OR NAPERIAN LOGARITHMS

Constants

$\log_e 10 = 2.30258\ 50930$	$6 \log_e 10 = 13.81551\ 05580$
$2 \log_e 10 = 4.60517\ 01860$	$7 \log_e 10 = 16.11809\ 56510$
$3 \log_e 10 = 6.90775\ 52790$	$8 \log_e 10 = 18.42068\ 07440$
$4 \log_e 10 = 9.21034\ 03720$	$9 \log_e 10 = 20.72326\ 58369$
$5 \log_e 10 = 11.51292\ 54650$	$10 \log_e 10 = 23.02585\ 09299$

10.0–49.9

N	0	1	2	3	4	5	6	7	8	9
10.	2.30259	.31254	.32239	.33214	.34181	.35138	.36085	.37024	.37955	.38876
11.	.39790	.40695	.41591	.42480	.43361	.44235	.45101	.45959	.46810	.47654
12.	.48491	.49321	.50144	.50960	.51770	.52573	.53370	.54160	.54945	.55723
13.	.56495	.57261	.58022	.58776	.59525	.60269	.61007	.61740	.62467	.63189
14.	.63906	.64617	.65324	.66026	.66723	.67415	.68102	.68785	.69463	.70136
15.	.70805	.71469	.72130	.72785	.73437	.74084	.74727	.75366	.76001	.76632
16.	.77259	.77882	.78501	.79117	.79728	.80336	.80940	.81541	.82138	.82731
17.	.83321	.83908	.84491	.85071	.85647	.86220	.86790	.87356	.87920	.88480
18.	.89037	.89591	.90142	.90690	.91235	.91777	.92316	.92852	.93386	.93916
19.	.94444	.94969	.95491	.96011	.96527	.97041	.97553	.98062	.98568	.99072
20.	2.99573	*.00072	*.00568	*.01062	*.01553	*.02042	*.02529	*.03013	*.03495	*.03975
21.	3.04452	.04927	.05400	.05871	.06339	.06805	.07269	.07731	.08191	.08649
22.	.09104	.09558	.10009	.10459	.10906	.11352	.11795	.12236	.12676	.13114
23.	.13549	.13983	.14415	.14845	.15274	.15700	.16125	.16548	.16969	.17388
24.	.17805	.18221	.18635	.19048	.19458	.19867	.20275	.20680	.21084	.21487
25.	.21888	.22287	.22684	.23080	.23475	.23868	.24259	.24649	.25037	.25424
26.	.25810	.26194	.26576	.26957	.27336	.27714	.28091	.28466	.28840	.29213
27.	.29584	.29953	.30322	.30689	.31054	.31419	.31782	.32143	.32504	.32863
28.	.33220	.33577	.33932	.34286	.34639	.34990	.35341	.35690	.36038	.36384
29.	.36730	.37074	.37417	.37759	.38099	.38439	.38777	.39115	.39451	.39786
30.	3.40120	.40453	.40784	.41115	.41444	.41773	.42100	.42426	.42751	.43076
31.	.43399	.43721	.44042	.44362	.44681	.44999	.45316	.45632	.45947	.46261
32.	.46574	.46886	.47197	.47507	.47816	.48124	.48431	.48738	.49043	.49347
33.	.49651	.49953	.50255	.50556	.50856	.51155	.51453	.51750	.52046	.52342
34.	.52636	.52930	.53223	.53515	.53806	.54096	.54385	.54674	.54962	.55249
35.	.55535	.55820	.56105	.56388	.56671	.56953	.57235	.57515	.57795	.58074
36.	.58352	.58629	.58906	.59182	.59457	.59731	.60005	.60278	.60550	.60821
37.	.61092	.61362	.61631	.61899	.62167	.62434	.62700	.62966	.63231	.63495
38.	.63759	.64021	.64284	.64545	.64806	.65066	.65325	.65584	.65842	.66099
39.	.66356	.66612	.66868	.67122	.67377	.67630	.67883	.68135	.68387	.68638
40.	3.68888	.69138	.69387	.69635	.69883	.70130	.70377	.70623	.70868	.71113
41.	.71357	.71601	.71844	.72086	.72328	.72569	.72810	.73050	.73290	.73529
42.	.73767	.74005	.74242	.74479	.74715	.74950	.75185	.75420	.75654	.75887
43.	.76120	.76352	.76584	.76815	.77046	.77276	.77506	.77735	.77963	.78191
44.	.78419	.78646	.78872	.79098	.79324	.79549	.79773	.79997	.80221	.80444
45.	.80666	.80888	.81110	.81331	.81551	.81771	.81991	.82210	.82428	.82647
46.	.82864	.83081	.83298	.83514	.83730	.83945	.84160	.84374	.84588	.84802
47.	.85015	.85227	.85439	.85651	.85862	.86073	.86283	.86493	.86703	.86912
48.	.87120	.87328	.87536	.87743	.87950	.88156	.88362	.88568	.88773	.88978
49.	.89182	.89386	.89589	.89792	.89995	.90197	.90399	.90600	.90801	.91002

NATURAL OR NAPERIAN LOGARITHMS

50.0–99.9

N	0	1	2	3	4	5	6	7	8	9
50.	3.91202	.91402	.91602	.91801	.91999	.92197	.92395	.92593	.92790	.92986
51.	.93183	.93378	.93574	.93769	.93964	.94158	.94352	.94546	.94739	.94932
52.	.95124	.95316	.95508	.95700	.95891	.96081	.96272	.96462	.96651	.96840
53.	.97029	.97218	.97406	.97594	.97781	.97968	.98155	.98341	.98527	.98713
54.	.98898	.99083	.99268	.99452	.99636	.99820	*.00003	*.00186	*.00369	*.00551
55.	4.00733	.00915	.01096	.01277	.01458	.01638	.01818	.01998	.02177	.02356
56.	.02535	.02714	.02892	.03069	.03247	.03424	.03601	.03777	.03954	.04130
57.	.04305	.04480	.04655	.04830	.05004	.05178	.05352	.05526	.05699	.05872
58.	.06044	.06217	.06389	.06560	.06732	.06903	.07073	.07244	.07414	.07584
59.	.07754	.07923	.08092	.08261	.08429	.08598	.08766	.08933	.09101	.09268
60.	4.09434	.09601	.09767	.09933	.10099	.10264	.10429	.10594	.10759	.10923
61.	.11087	.11251	.11415	.11578	.11741	.11904	.12066	.12228	.12390	.12552
62.	.12713	.12875	.13036	.13196	.13357	.13517	.13677	.13836	.13996	.14155
63.	.14313	.14472	.14630	.14789	.14946	.15104	.15261	.15418	.15575	.15732
64.	.15888	.16044	.16200	.16356	.16511	.16667	.16821	.16976	.17131	.17285
65.	.17439	.17592	.17746	.17899	.18052	.18205	.18358	.18510	.18662	.18814
66.	.18965	.19117	.19268	.19419	.19570	.19720	.19870	.20020	.20170	.20320
67.	.20469	.20618	.20767	.20916	.21065	.21213	.21361	.21509	.21656	.21804
68.	.21951	.22098	.22244	.22391	.22537	.22683	.22829	.22975	.23120	.23266
69.	.23411	.23555	.23700	.23844	.23989	.24133	.24276	.24420	.24563	.24707
70.	4.24850	.24992	.25135	.25277	.25419	.25561	.25703	.25845	.25986	.26127
71.	.26268	.26409	.26549	.26690	.26830	.26970	.27110	.27249	.27388	.27528
72.	.27667	.27805	.27944	.28082	.28221	.28359	.28496	.28634	.28772	.28909
73.	.29046	.29183	.29320	.29456	.29592	.29729	.29865	.30000	.30136	.30271
74.	.30407	.30542	.30676	.30811	.30946	.31080	.31214	.31348	.31482	.31615
75.	.31749	.31882	.32015	.32149	.32281	.32413	.32546	.32678	.32810	.32942
76.	.33073	.33205	.33336	.33467	.33598	.33729	.33860	.33990	.34120	.34251
77.	.34381	.34510	.34640	.34769	.34899	.35028	.35157	.35286	.35414	.35543
78.	.35671	.35800	.35927	.36055	.36182	.36310	.36437	.36564	.36691	.36818
79.	.36945	.37071	.37198	.37324	.37450	.37576	.37701	.37827	.37952	.38078
80.	4.38203	.38328	.38452	.38577	.38701	.38826	.38950	.39074	.39198	.39321
81.	.39445	.39568	.39692	.39815	.39938	.40060	.40183	.40305	.40428	.40550
82.	.40672	.40794	.40916	.41037	.41159	.41280	.41401	.41522	.41643	.41764
83.	.41884	.42004	.42125	.42245	.42365	.42485	.42604	.42724	.42843	.42963
84.	.43082	.43201	.43319	.43438	.43557	.43675	.43793	.43912	.44030	.44147
85.	.44265	.44383	.44500	.44617	.44735	.44852	.44969	.45085	.45202	.45318
86.	.45435	.45551	.45667	.45783	.45899	.46014	.46130	.46245	.46361	.46476
87.	.46591	.46706	.46820	.46935	.47050	.47164	.47278	.47392	.47506	.47620
88.	.47734	.47847	.47961	.48074	.48187	.48300	.48413	.48526	.48639	.48751
89.	.48864	.48976	.49088	.49200	.49312	.49424	.49536	.49647	.49758	.49870
90.	4.49981	.50092	.50203	.50314	.50424	.50535	.50645	.50756	.50866	.50976
91.	.51086	.51196	.51305	.51415	.51525	.51634	.51743	.51852	.51961	.52070
92.	.52179	.52287	.52396	.52504	.52613	.52721	.52829	.52937	.53045	.53152
93.	.53260	.53367	.53475	.53582	.53689	.53796	.53903	.54010	.54116	.54223
94.	.54329	.54436	.54542	.54648	.54754	.54860	.54966	.55071	.55177	.55282
95.	.55388	.55493	.55598	.55703	.55808	.55913	.56017	.56122	.56226	.56331
96.	.56435	.56539	.56643	.56747	.56851	.56954	.57058	.57161	.57265	.57368
97.	.57471	.57574	.57677	.57780	.57883	.57985	.58088	.58190	.58292	.58395
98.	.58497	.58599	.58701	.58802	.58904	.59006	.59107	.59208	.59310	.59411
99.	.59512	.59613	.59714	.59815	.59915	.60016	.60116	.60217	.60317	.60417

NATURAL OR NAPERIAN LOGARITHMS

0–499

N	0	1	2	3	4	5	6	7	8	9
0	− ∞	0.00000	0.69315	1.09861	.38629	.60944	.79176	.94591	*.07944	*.19722
1	2.30259	.39790	.48491	.56495	.63906	.70805	.77259	.83321	.89037	.94444
2	.99573	*.04452	*.09104	*.13549	*.17805	*.21888	*.25810	*.29584	*.33220	*.36730
3	3.40120	.43399	.46574	.49651	.52636	.55535	.58352	.61092	.63759	.66356
4	.68888	.71357	.73767	.76120	.78419	.80666	.82864	.85015	.87120	.89182
5	.91202	.93183	.95124	.97029	.98898	*.00733	*.02535	*.04305	*.06044	*.07754
6	4.09434	.11087	.12713	.14313	.15888	.17439	.18965	.20469	.21951	.23411
7	.24850	.26268	.27667	.29046	.30407	.31749	.33073	.34381	.35671	.36945
8	.38203	.39445	.40672	.41884	.43082	.44265	.45435	.46591	.47734	.48864
9	.49981	.51086	.52179	.53260	.54329	.55388	.56435	.57471	.58497	.59512
10	4.60517	.61512	.62497	.63473	.64439	.65396	.66344	.67283	.68213	.69135
11	.70048	.70953	.71850	.72739	.73620	.74493	.75359	.76217	.77068	.77912
12	.78749	.79579	.80402	.81218	.82028	.82831	.83628	.84419	.85203	.85981
13	.86753	.87520	.88280	.89035	.89784	.90527	.91265	.91998	.92725	.93447
14	.94164	.94876	.95583	.96284	.96981	.97673	.98361	.99043	.99721	*.00395
15	5.01064	.01728	.02388	.03044	.03695	.04343	.04986	.05625	.06260	.06890
16	.07517	.08140	.08760	.09375	.09987	.10595	.11199	.11799	.12396	.12990
17	.13580	.14166	.14740	.15320	.15906	.16479	.17048	.17615	.18178	.18739
18	.19296	.19850	.20401	.20949	.21494	.22036	.22575	.23111	.23644	.24175
19	.24702	.25227	.25750	.26269	.26786	.27300	.27811	.28320	.28827	.29330
20	5.29832	.30330	.30827	.31321	.31812	.32301	.32788	.33272	.33754	.34233
21	.34711	.35186	.35659	.36129	.36598	.37064	.37528	.37990	.38450	.38907
22	.39363	.39816	.40268	.40717	.41165	.41610	.42053	.42495	.42935	.43372
23	.43808	.44242	.44674	.45104	.45532	.45959	.46383	.46806	.47227	.47646
24	.48064	.48480	.48894	.49306	.49717	.50126	.50533	.50939	.51343	.51745
25	.52146	.52545	.52943	.53339	.53733	.54126	.54518	.54908	.55296	.55683
26	.56068	.56452	.56834	.57215	.57595	.57973	.58350	.58725	.59099	.59471
27	.59842	.60212	.60580	.60947	.61313	.61677	.62040	.62402	.62762	.63121
28	.63479	.63835	.64191	.64545	.64897	.65249	.65599	.65948	.66296	.66643
29	.66988	.67332	.67675	.68017	.68358	.68698	.69036	.69373	.69709	.70044
30	5.70378	.70711	.71043	.71373	.71703	.72031	.72359	.72685	.73010	.73334
31	.73657	.73979	.74300	.74620	.74939	.75257	.75574	.75890	.76205	.76519
32	.76832	.77144	.77455	.77765	.78074	.78383	.78690	.78996	.79301	.79606
33	.79909	.80212	.80513	.80814	.81114	.81413	.81711	.82008	.82305	.82600
34	.82895	.83188	.83481	.83773	.84064	.84354	.84644	.84932	.85220	.85507
35	.85793	.86079	.86363	.86647	.86930	.87212	.87493	.87774	.88053	.88332
36	.88610	.88888	.89164	.89440	.89715	.89990	.90263	.90536	.90808	.91080
37	.91350	.91620	.91889	.92158	.92426	.92693	.92959	.93225	.93489	.93754
38	.94017	.94280	.94542	.94803	.95064	.95324	.95584	.95842	.96101	.96358
39	.96615	.96871	.97126	.97381	.97635	.97889	.98141	.98394	.98645	.98896
40	5.99146	.99396	.99645	.99894	*.00141	*.00389	*.00635	*.00881	*.01127	*.01372
41	6.01616	.01859	.02102	.02345	.02587	.02828	.03069	.03309	.03548	.03787
42	.04025	.04263	.04501	.04737	.04973	.05209	.05444	.05678	.05912	.06146
43	.06379	.06611	.06843	.07074	.07304	.07535	.07764	.07993	.08222	.08450
44	.08677	.08904	.09131	.09357	.09582	09807	.10032	.10256	.10479	.10702
45	.10925	.11147	.11368	.11589	.11810	.12030	.12249	.12468	.12687	.12905
46	.13123	.13340	.13556	.13773	.13988	.14204	.14419	.14633	.14847	.15060
47	.15273	.15486	.15698	.15910	.16121	.16331	.16542	.16752	.16961	.17170
48	.17379	.17587	.17794	.18002	.18208	.18415	.18621	.18826	.19032	.19236
49	.19441	.19644	.19848	.20051	.20254	.20456	.20658	.20859	.21060	.21261

NATURAL OR NAPERIAN LOGARITHMS

500–999

N	0	1	2	3	4	5	6	7	8	9
50	6.21461	.21661	.21860	.22059	.22258	.22456	.22654	.22851	.23048	.23245
51	.23441	.23637	.23832	.24028	.24222	.24417	.24611	.24804	.24998	.25190
52	.25383	.25575	.25767	.25958	.26149	.26340	.26530	.26720	.26910	.27099
53	.27288	.27476	.27664	.27852	.28040	.28227	.28413	.28600	.28786	.28972
54	.29157	.29342	.29527	.29711	.29895	.30079	.30262	.30445	.30628	.30810
55	.30992	.31173	.31355	.31536	.31716	.31897	.32077	.32257	.32436	.32615
56	.32794	.32972	.33150	.33328	.33505	.33683	.33859	.34036	.34212	.34388
57	.34564	.34739	.34914	.35089	.35263	.35437	.35611	.35784	.35957	.36130
58	.36303	.36475	.36647	.36819	.36990	.37161	.37332	.37502	.37673	.37843
59	.38012	.38182	.38351	.38519	.38688	.38856	.39024	.39192	.39359	.39526
60	6.39693	.39859	.40026	.40192	.40357	.40523	.40688	.40853	.41017	.41182
61	.41346	.41510	.41673	.41836	.41999	.42162	.42325	.42487	.42649	.42811
62	.42972	.43133	.43294	.43455	.43615	.43775	.43935	.44095	.44254	.44413
63	.44572	.44731	.44889	.45047	.45205	.45362	.45520	.45677	.45834	.45990
64	.46147	.46303	.46459	.46614	.46770	.46925	.47080	.47235	.47389	.47543
65	.47697	.47851	.48004	.48158	.48311	.48464	.48616	.48768	.48920	.49072
66	.49224	.49375	.49527	.49677	.49828	.49979	.50129	.50279	.50429	.50578
67	.50728	.50877	.51026	.51175	.51323	.51471	.51619	.51767	.51915	.52062
68	.52209	.52356	.52503	.52649	.52796	.52942	.53088	.53233	.53379	.53524
69	.53669	.53814	.53959	.54103	.54247	.54391	.54535	.54679	.54822	.54965
70	6.55108	.55251	.55393	.55536	.55678	.55820	.55962	.56103	.56244	.56386
71	.56526	.56667	.56808	.56948	.57088	.57228	.57368	.57508	.57647	.57786
72	.57925	.58064	.58203	.58341	.58479	.58617	.58755	.58893	.59030	.59167
73	.59304	.59441	.59578	.59715	.59851	.59987	.60123	.60259	.60394	.60530
74	.60665	.60800	.60935	.61070	.61204	.61338	.61473	.61607	.61740	.61874
75	.62007	.62141	.62274	.62407	.62539	.62672	.62804	.62936	.63068	.63200
76	.63332	.63463	.63595	.63726	.63857	.63988	.64118	.64249	.64379	.64509
77	.64639	.64769	.64898	.65028	.65157	.65286	.65415	.65544	.65673	.65801
78	.65929	.66058	.66185	.66313	.66441	.66568	.66696	.66823	.66950	.67077
79	.67203	.67330	.67456	.67582	.67708	.67834	.67960	.68085	.68211	.68336
80	6.68461	.68586	.68711	.68835	.68960	.69084	.69208	.69332	.69456	.69580
81	.69703	.69827	.69950	.70073	.70196	.70319	.70441	.70564	.70686	.70808
82	.70930	.71052	.71174	.71296	.71417	.71538	.71659	.71780	.71901	.72022
83	.72143	.72263	.72383	.72503	.72623	.72743	.72863	.72982	.73102	.73221
84	.73340	.73459	.73578	.73697	.73815	.73934	.74052	.74170	.74288	.74406
85	.74524	.74641	.74759	.74876	.74993	.75110	.75227	.75344	.75460	.75577
86	.75693	.75809	.75926	.76041	.76157	.76273	.76388	.76504	.76619	.76734
87	.76849	.76964	.77079	.77194	.77308	.77422	.77537	.77651	.77765	.77878
88	.77992	.78106	.78219	.78333	.78446	.78559	.78672	.78784	.78897	.79010
89	.79122	.79234	.79347	.79459	.79571	.79682	.79794	.79906	.80017	.80128
90	6.80239	.80351	.80461	.80572	.80683	.80793	.80904	.81014	.81124	.81235
91	.81344	.81454	.81564	.81674	.81783	.81892	.82002	.82111	.82220	.82329
92	.82437	.82546	.82655	.82763	.82871	.82979	.83087	.83195	.83303	.83411
93	.83518	.83626	.83733	.83841	.83948	.84055	.84162	.84268	.84375	.84482
94	.84588	.84694	.84801	.84907	.85013	.85118	.85224	.85330	.85435	.85541
95	.85646	.85751	.85857	.85961	.86066	.86171	.86276	.86380	.86485	.86589
96	.86693	.86797	.86901	.87005	.87109	.87213	.87316	.87420	.87523	.87626
97	.87730	.87833	.87936	.88038	.88141	.88244	.88346	.88449	.88551	.88653
98	.88755	.88857	.88959	.89061	.89163	.89264	.89366	.89467	.89568	.89669
99	.89770	.89871	.89972	.90073	.90174	.90274	.90375	.90475	.90575	.90675

XIII.9 FACTORIALS AND THEIR LOGARITHMS

The product $n \times (n - 1) \times (n - 2) \times \cdots \times 1$ is called factorial n, expressed as $n!$ or $\underline{|n}$. For example: factorial $5 = 5 \times 4 \times 3 \times 2 \times 1 = 120$. Factorials are very often met with in series. For purposes of computation in such cases the table giving the values of the factorials and of their logarithms for numbers from 1 to 100 is provided. The values of the factorials are expressed exponentially to 5 significant figures.

FACTORIALS AND THEIR LOGARITHMS

n	$n!$	log $n!$	n	$n!$	log $n!$
			50	3.0414×10^{64}	64.48307
1	1.0000	0.00000	51	1.5511×10^{66}	66.19065
2	2.0000	0.30103	52	8.0658×10^{67}	67.90665
3	6.0000	0.77815	53	4.2749×10^{69}	69.63092
4	2.4000×10	1.38021	54	2.3084×10^{71}	71.36332
5	1.2000×10^{2}	2.07918	**55**	1.2696×10^{73}	73.10368
6	7.2000×10^{2}	2.85733	56	7.1100×10^{74}	74.85187
7	5.0400×10^{3}	3.70243	57	4.0527×10^{76}	76.60774
8	4.0320×10^{4}	4.60552	58	2.3506×10^{78}	78.37117
9	3.6288×10^{5}	5.55976	59	1.3868×10^{80}	80.14202
10	3.6288×10^{6}	6.55976	**60**	8.3210×10^{81}	81.92017
11	3.9917×10^{7}	7.60116	61	5.0758×10^{83}	83.70550
12	4.7900×10^{8}	8.68034	62	3.1470×10^{85}	85.49790
13	6.2270×10^{9}	9.79428	63	1.9826×10^{87}	87.29724
14	8.7178×10^{10}	10.94041	64	1.2689×10^{89}	89.10342
15	1.3077×10^{12}	12.11650	**65**	8.2477×10^{90}	90.91633
16	2.0923×10^{13}	13.32062	66	5.4435×10^{92}	92.73587
17	3.5569×10^{14}	14.55107	67	3.6471×10^{94}	94.56195
18	6.4024×10^{15}	15.80634	68	2.4800×10^{96}	96.39446
19	1.2165×10^{17}	17.08509	69	1.7112×10^{98}	98.23331
20	2.4329×10^{18}	18.38612	**70**	1.1979×10^{100}	100.07841
21	5.1091×10^{19}	19.70834	71	8.5048×10^{101}	101.92966
22	1.1240×10^{21}	21.05077	72	6.1234×10^{103}	103.78700
23	2.5852×10^{22}	22.41249	73	4.4701×10^{105}	105.65032
24	6.2045×10^{23}	23.79271	74	3.3079×10^{107}	107.51955
25	1.5511×10^{25}	25.19065	**75**	2.4809×10^{109}	109.39461
26	4.0329×10^{26}	26.60562	76	1.8855×10^{111}	111.27543
27	1.0889×10^{28}	28.03698	77	1.4518×10^{113}	113.16192
28	3.0489×10^{29}	29.48414	78	1.1324×10^{115}	115.05401
29	8.8418×10^{30}	30.94654	79	8.9462×10^{116}	116.95164
30	2.6525×10^{32}	32.42366	**80**	7.1569×10^{118}	118.85473
31	8.2228×10^{33}	33.91502	81	5.7971×10^{120}	120.76321
32	2.6313×10^{35}	35.42017	82	4.7536×10^{122}	122.67703
33	8.6833×10^{36}	36.93869	83	3.9455×10^{124}	124.59610
34	2.9523×10^{38}	38.47016	84	3.3142×10^{126}	126.52038
35	1.0333×10^{40}	40.01423	**85**	2.8171×10^{128}	128.44980
36	3.7199×10^{41}	41.57054	86	2.4227×10^{130}	130.38430
37	1.3764×10^{43}	43.13874	87	2.1078×10^{132}	132.32382
38	5.2302×10^{44}	44.71852	88	1.8548×10^{134}	134.26830
39	2.0398×10^{46}	46.30959	89	1.6508×10^{136}	136.21769
40	8.1592×10^{47}	47.91165	**90**	1.4857×10^{138}	138.17194
41	3.3453×10^{49}	49.52443	91	1.3520×10^{140}	140.13098
42	1.4050×10^{51}	51.14768	92	1.2438×10^{142}	142.09477
43	6.0415×10^{52}	52.78115	93	1.1568×10^{144}	144.06325
44	2.6583×10^{54}	54.42460	94	1.0874×10^{146}	146.03638
45	1.1962×10^{56}	56.07781	**95**	1.0330×10^{148}	148.01410
46	5.5026×10^{57}	57.74057	96	9.9168×10^{149}	149.99637
47	2.5862×10^{59}	59.41267	97	9.6193×10^{151}	151.98314
48	1.2414×10^{61}	61.09391	98	9.4269×10^{153}	153.97437
49	6.0828×10^{62}	62.78410	99	9.3326×10^{155}	155.97000
50	3.0414×10^{64}	64.48307	**100**	9.3326×10^{157}	157.97000

$$n! = \frac{n}{e}\sqrt{2\pi n} + h; \; n = 1, 2, 3, \ldots \quad \left[0 < \frac{h}{n!} < \frac{1}{12n}\right]$$

$$\lim_{n\to\infty} \frac{n!e^n}{n^{n+\frac{1}{2}}} = \sqrt{2\pi} \qquad \lim_{n\to\infty} \frac{(n!)^{\frac{1}{n}}}{n} = \frac{1}{e}$$

XIII.10 RECIPROCALS OF FACTORIALS AND THEIR LOGARITHMS

n	$1/n!$	$\log (1/n!)$	n	$1/n!$	$\log (1/n!)$
1	1.	.00000	51	$.64470 \times 10^{-66}$	$\overline{67}.80934$
2	0.5	$\overline{1}.69897$	52	$.12398 \times 10^{-67}$	$\overline{68}.09335$
3	.16667	$\overline{1}.22185$	53	$.23392 \times 10^{-69}$	$\overline{70}.36908$
*4	$.41667 \times 10^{-1}$	$\overline{2}.61979$	54	$.45282 \times 10^{-71}$	$\overline{72}.63668$
5	$.83333 \times 10^{-2}$	$\overline{3}.92082$	55	$.78765 \times 10^{-73}$	$\overline{74}.89632$
6	$.13389 \times 10^{-2}$	$\overline{3}.14267$	56	$.14065 \times 10^{-74}$	$\overline{75}.14813$
7	$.19841 \times 10^{-3}$	$\overline{4}.29757$	57	$.24675 \times 10^{-76}$	$\overline{77}.39226$
8	$.24802 \times 10^{-4}$	$\overline{5}.39448$	58	$.42542 \times 10^{-78}$	$\overline{79}.62883$
9	$.27557 \times 10^{-5}$	$\overline{6}.44024$	59	$.72108 \times 10^{-80}$	$\overline{81}.85798$
10	$.27557 \times 10^{-6}$	$\overline{7}.44024$	60	$.12018 \times 10^{-81}$	$\overline{82}.07983$
11	$.25052 \times 10^{-7}$	$\overline{8}.39884$	61	$.19701 \times 10^{-83}$	$\overline{84}.29450$
12	$.20877 \times 10^{-8}$	$\overline{9}.31966$	62	$.31776 \times 10^{-85}$	$\overline{86}.50210$
13	$.16059 \times 10^{-9}$	$\overline{10}.20572$	63	$.50439 \times 10^{-87}$	$\overline{88}.70276$
14	$.11471 \times 10^{-10}$	$\overline{11}.05959$	64	$.78808 \times 10^{-89}$	$\overline{90}.89658$
15	$.76472 \times 10^{-12}$	$\overline{13}.88350$	65	$.12125 \times 10^{-90}$	$\overline{91}.08367$
16	$.47795 \times 10^{-13}$	$\overline{14}.67938$	66	$.18371 \times 10^{-92}$	$\overline{93}.26413$
17	$.28115 \times 10^{-14}$	$\overline{15}.44893$	67	$.27419 \times 10^{-94}$	$\overline{95}.43805$
18	$.15619 \times 10^{-15}$	$\overline{16}.19365$	68	$.40323 \times 10^{-96}$	$\overline{97}.60554$
19	$.82206 \times 10^{-17}$	$\overline{18}.91491$	69	$.58439 \times 10^{-98}$	$\overline{99}.76668$
20	$.41103 \times 10^{-18}$	$\overline{19}.61388$	70	$.83479 \times 10^{-100}$	$\overline{101}.92159$
21	$.19573 \times 10^{-19}$	$\overline{20}.29165$	71	$.11758 \times 10^{-101}$	$\overline{102}.07034$
22	$.88968 \times 10^{-21}$	$\overline{22}.94923$	72	$.16331 \times 10^{-103}$	$\overline{104}.21300$
23	$.38682 \times 10^{-22}$	$\overline{23}.58751$	73	$.22371 \times 10^{-105}$	$\overline{106}.34968$
24	$.16117 \times 10^{-23}$	$\overline{24}.20728$	74	$.30231 \times 10^{-107}$	$\overline{108}.48045$
25	$.64470 \times 10^{-25}$	$\overline{26}.80935$	75	$.40308 \times 10^{-109}$	$\overline{110}.60538$
26	$.24796 \times 10^{-26}$	$\overline{27}.39438$	76	$.53036 \times 10^{-111}$	$\overline{112}.72457$
27	$.91836 \times 10^{-28}$	$\overline{29}.96302$	77	$.68880 \times 10^{-113}$	$\overline{114}.83808$
28	$.32799 \times 10^{-29}$	$\overline{30}.51586$	78	$.88308 \times 10^{-115}$	$\overline{116}.94599$
29	$.11310 \times 10^{-30}$	$\overline{31}.05346$	79	$.11178 \times 10^{-116}$	$\overline{117}.04836$
30	$.37644 \times 10^{-32}$	$\overline{33}.57634$	80	$.13973 \times 10^{-118}$	$\overline{119}.14527$
31	$.12161 \times 10^{-33}$	$\overline{34}.08498$	81	$.17250 \times 10^{-120}$	$\overline{121}.23679$
32	$.38004 \times 10^{-35}$	$\overline{36}.57983$	82	$.21037 \times 10^{-122}$	$\overline{123}.32297$
33	$.11516 \times 10^{-36}$	$\overline{37}.06131$	83	$.25345 \times 10^{-124}$	$\overline{125}.40390$
34	$.33872 \times 10^{-38}$	$\overline{39}.52984$	84	$.30173 \times 10^{-126}$	$\overline{127}.47962$
35	$.96775 \times 10^{-40}$	$\overline{41}.98577$	85	$.35497 \times 10^{-128}$	$\overline{129}.55020$
36	$.26882 \times 10^{-41}$	$\overline{42}.42946$	86	$.41276 \times 10^{-130}$	$\overline{131}.61570$
37	$.72653 \times 10^{-43}$	$\overline{44}.86126$	87	$.47443 \times 10^{-132}$	$\overline{133}.67618$
38	$.19120 \times 10^{-44}$	$\overline{45}.28148$	88	$.53914 \times 10^{-134}$	$\overline{135}.73170$
39	$.49024 \times 10^{-46}$	$\overline{47}.69041$	89	$.60577 \times 10^{-136}$	$\overline{137}.78231$
40	$.12256 \times 10^{-47}$	$\overline{48}.08835$	90	$.67308 \times 10^{-138}$	$\overline{139}.82806$
41	$.29893 \times 10^{-49}$	$\overline{50}.47557$	91	$.73964 \times 10^{-140}$	$\overline{141}.86902$
42	$.71174 \times 10^{-51}$	$\overline{52}.85232$	92	$.80399 \times 10^{-142}$	$\overline{143}.90523$
43	$.16552 \times 10^{-52}$	$\overline{53}.21885$	93	$.86445 \times 10^{-144}$	$\overline{145}.93675$
44	$.37618 \times 10^{-54}$	$\overline{55}.57540$	94	$.91962 \times 10^{-146}$	$\overline{147}.96362$
45	$.83598 \times 10^{-56}$	$\overline{57}.92219$	95	$.96805 \times 10^{-148}$	$\overline{149}.98590$
46	$.18173 \times 10^{-57}$	$\overline{58}.25943$	96	$.10084 \times 10^{-149}$	$\overline{150}.00363$
47	$.38667 \times 10^{-59}$	$\overline{60}.58733$	97	$.10396 \times 10^{-151}$	$\overline{152}.01686$
48	$.80554 \times 10^{-61}$	$\overline{62}.90609$	98	$.10608 \times 10^{-153}$	$\overline{154}.02563$
49	$.16440 \times 10^{-62}$	$\overline{63}.21590$	99	$.10715 \times 10^{-155}$	$\overline{156}.03000$
50	$.32880 \times 10^{-64}$	$\overline{65}.51693$	100	$.10715 \times 10^{-157}$	$\overline{158}.03000$

* For example $\log \frac{1}{4!} = \overline{2}.61979 = .61979 - 2 = 8.61979 - 10.$

XIII.11 POWERS OF NUMBERS

n	n^4	n^5	n^6	n^7	n^8	n^9
1	1	1	1	1	1	1
2	16	32	64	128	256	512
3	81	243	729	2187	6561	19683
4	256	1024	4096	16384	65536	262144
5	625	3125	15625	78125	390625	1953125
6	1296	7776	46656	279936	1679616	10077696
7	2401	16807	117649	823543	5764801	40353607
8	4096	32768	262144	2097152	16777216	134217728
9	6561	59049	531441	4782969	43046721	387420489
					$\times 10^8$	$\times 10^9$
10	10000	100000	1000000	10000000	1.000000	1.000000
11	14641	161051	1771561	19487171	2.143589	2.357948
12	20736	248832	2985984	35831808	4.299817	5.159780
13	28561	371293	4826809	62748517	8.157307	10.604499
14	38416	537824	7529536	105413504	14.757891	20.661047
15	50625	759375	11390625	170859375	25.628906	38.443359
16	65536	1048576	16777216	268435456	42.949673	68.719477
17	83521	1419857	24137569	410338673	69.757574	118.587876
18	104976	1889568	34012224	612220032	110.199606	198.359291
19	130321	2476099	47045881	893871739	169.835630	322.687697
				$\times 10^9$	$\times 10^{10}$	$\times 10^{11}$
20	160000	3200000	64000000	1.280000	2.560000	5.120000
21	194481	4084101	85766121	1.801089	3.782286	7.942800
22	234256	5153632	113379904	2.494358	5.487587	12.072692
23	279841	6436343	148035889	3.404825	7.831099	18.011527
24	331776	7962624	191102976	4.586471	11.007531	26.418075
25	390625	9765625	244140625	6.103516	15.258789	38.146973
26	456976	11881376	308915776	8.031810	20.882706	54.295037
27	531441	14348907	387420489	10.460353	28.242954	76.255975
28	614656	17210368	481890304	13.492929	37.780200	105.784559
29	707281	20511149	594823321	17.249876	50.024641	145.071460
			$\times 10^8$	$\times 10^{10}$	$\times 10^{11}$	$\times 10^{13}$
30	810000	24300000	7.290000	2.187000	6.561000	1.968300
31	923521	28629151	8.875037	2.751261	8.528910	2.643962
32	1048576	33554432	10.737418	3.435974	10.995116	3.518437
33	1185921	39135393	12.914680	4.261844	14.064086	4.641148
34	1336336	45435424	15.448044	5.252335	17.857939	6.071699
35	1500625	52521875	18.382656	6.433930	22.518754	7.881564
36	1679616	60466176	21.767823	7.836416	28.211099	10.155996
37	1874161	69343957	25.657264	9.493188	35.124795	12.996174
38	2085136	79235168	30.109364	11.441558	43.477921	16.521610
39	2313441	90224199	35.187438	13.723101	53.520093	20.872836
			$\times 10^9$	$\times 10^{10}$	$\times 10^{12}$	$\times 10^{14}$
40	2560000	102400000	4.096000	16.384000	6.553600	2.621440
41	2825761	115856201	4.750104	19.475427	7.984925	3.273819
42	3111696	130691232	5.489032	23.053933	9.682652	4.066714
43	3418801	147008443	6.321363	27.181861	11.688200	5.025926
44	3748096	164916224	7.256314	31.927781	14.048224	6.181218
45	4100625	184528125	8.303766	37.366945	16.815125	7.566806
46	4477456	205962976	9.474297	43.581766	20.047612	9.221902
47	4879681	229345007	10.779215	50.662312	23.811287	11.191305
48	5308416	254803968	12.230590	58.706834	28.179280	13.526055
49	5764801	282475249	13.841287	67.822307	33.232931	16.284136
50	6250000	312500000	15.625000	78.125000	39.062500	19.531250

POWERS OF NUMBERS

n	n^4	n^5	n^6	n^7	n^8	n^9
			$\times 10^9$	$\times 10^{11}$	$\times 10^{13}$	$\times 10^{14}$
50	6250000	312500000	15.625000	7.812500	3.906250	19.531250
51	6765201	345025251	17.596288	8.974107	4.576794	23.341652
52	7311616	380204032	19.770610	10.280717	5.345973	27.799059
53	7890481	418195493	22.164361	11.747111	6.225969	32.997636
54	8503056	459165024	24.794911	13.389252	7.230196	39.043059
55	9150625	503284375	27.680641	15.224352	8.373394	46.053666
56	9834496	550731776	30.840979	17.270948	9.671731	54.161695
57	10556001	601692057	34.296447	19.548975	11.142916	63.514619
58	11316496	656356768	38.068693	22.079842	12.806308	74.276588
59	12117361	714924299	42.180534	24.886515	14.683044	86.629958
		$\times 10^8$	$\times 10^{10}$	$\times 10^{11}$	$\times 10^{13}$	$\times 10^{16}$
60	12960000	7.776000	4.665600	27.993600	16.796160	1.007770
61	13845841	8.445963	5.152037	31.427428	19.170731	1.169415
62	14776336	9.161328	5.680024	35.216146	21.834011	1.353709
63	15752961	9.924365	6.252350	39.389806	24.815578	1.563381
64	16777216	10.737418	6.871948	43.980465	28.147498	1.801440
65	17850625	11.602906	7.541889	49.022279	31.864481	2.071191
66	18974736	12.523326	8.265395	54.551607	36.004061	2.376268
67	20151121	13.501251	9.045838	60.607116	40.606768	2.720653
68	21381376	14.539336	9.886748	67.229888	45.716324	3.108710
69	22667121	15.640313	10.791816	74.463533	51.379837	3.545209
		$\times 10^8$	$\times 10^{10}$	$\times 10^{12}$	$\times 10^{14}$	$\times 10^{16}$
70	24010000	16.807000	11.764900	8.235430	5.764801	4.035361
71	25411681	18.042294	12.810028	9.095120	6.457535	4.584850
72	26873856	19.349176	13.931407	10.030613	7.222041	5.199870
73	28398241	20.730716	15.133423	11.047399	8.064601	5.887159
74	29986576	22.190066	16.420649	12.151280	8.991947	6.654041
75	31640625	23.730469	17.797852	13.348389	10.011292	7.508469
76	33362176	25.355254	19.269993	14.645195	11.130348	8.459064
77	35153041	27.067842	20.842238	16.048523	12.357363	9.515169
78	37015056	28.871744	22.519960	17.565569	13.701144	10.686892
79	38950081	30.770564	24.308746	19.203909	15.171088	11.985160
		$\times 10^8$	$\times 10^{10}$	$\times 10^{12}$	$\times 10^{14}$	$\times 10^{16}$
80	40960000	32.768000	26.214400	20.971520	16.777216	13.421773
81	43046721	34.867844	28.242954	22.876792	18.530202	15.009464
82	45212176	37.073984	30.400667	24.928547	20.441409	16.761955
83	47458321	39.390406	32.694037	27.136051	22.522922	18.694026
84	49787136	41.821194	35.129803	29.509035	24.787589	20.821575
85	52200625	44.370531	37.714952	32.057709	27.249053	23.161695
86	54700816	47.042702	40.456724	34.792782	29.921793	25.732742
87	57289761	49.842092	43.362620	37.725479	32.821167	28.554415
88	59969536	52.773192	46.440409	40.867560	35.963452	31.647838
89	62742241	55.840594	49.698129	44.231335	39.365888	35.035640
		$\times 10^9$	$\times 10^{11}$	$\times 10^{13}$	$\times 10^{15}$	$\times 10^{17}$
90	65610000	5.904900	5.314410	4.782969	4.304672	3.874205
91	68574961	6.240321	5.678693	5.167610	4.702525	4.279298
92	71639296	6.590815	6.063550	5.578466	5.132189	4.721614
93	74805201	6.956884	6.469902	6.017009	5.595818	5.204111
94	78074896	7.339040	6.898698	6.484776	6.095689	5.729948
95	81450625	7.737809	7.350919	6.983373	6.634204	6.302494
96	84934656	8.153727	7.827578	7.514475	7.213896	6.925340
97	88529281	8.587340	8.329720	8.079828	7.837434	7.602311
98	92236816	9.039208	8.858424	8.681255	8.507630	8.337478
99	96059601	9.509900	9.414801	9.320653	9.227447	9.135172
100	100000000	10.000000	10.000000	10.000000	10.000000	10.000000

XIII.12 SUMS OF POWERS OF INTEGERS, $\sum_{k=1}^{n} k^m$

$(m = 1, 2, 3, 4)$; $1 \leq n \leq 40$

n	Σk	Σk^2	Σk^3	Σk^4
1	1	1	1	1
2	3	5	9	17
3	6	14	36	98
4	10	30	100	354
5	15	55	225	979
6	21	91	441	2275
7	28	140	784	4676
8	36	204	1296	8772
9	45	285	2025	15333
10	55	385	3025	25333
11	66	506	4356	39974
12	78	650	6084	60710
13	91	819	8281	89271
14	105	1015	11025	127687
15	120	1240	14400	178312
16	136	1496	18496	243848
17	153	1785	23409	327369
18	171	2109	29241	432345
19	190	2470	36100	562666
20	210	2870	44100	722666
21	231	3311	53361	917147
22	253	3795	64009	1151403
23	276	4324	76176	1431244
24	300	4900	90000	1763020
25	325	5525	105625	2153645
26	351	6201	123201	2610621
27	378	6930	142884	3142062
28	406	7714	164836	3756718
29	435	8555	189225	4463999
30	465	9455	216225	5273999
31	496	10416	246016	6197520
32	528	11440	278784	7246096
33	561	12529	314721	8432017
34	595	13685	354025	9768353
35	630	14910	396900	11268978
36	666	16206	443556	12948594
37	703	17575	494209	14822755
38	741	19019	549081	16907891
39	780	20540	608400	19221332
40	820	22140	672400	21781332

SUMS OF POWERS OF THE FIRST n INTEGERS

$$\sum_{k=1}^{n} k = 1 + 2 + 3 + \cdots + n = \frac{n(n+1)}{2}$$

$$\sum_{k=1}^{n} k^2 = 1^2 + 2^2 + 3^2 + \cdots + n^2 = \frac{n(n+1)(2n+1)}{6}$$

$$\sum_{k=1}^{n} k^3 = \frac{n^2(n+1)^2}{4}$$

$$\sum_{k=1}^{n} k^4 = \frac{n}{30}(n+1)(2n+1)(3n^2+3n-1).$$

$$\sum_{k=1}^{n} k^5 = \frac{n^2}{12}(n+1)^2(2n^2+2n-1).$$

$$\sum_{k=1}^{n} k^6 = \frac{n}{42}(n+1)(2n+1)(3n^4+6n^3-3n+1).$$

$$\sum_{k=1}^{n} k^7 = \frac{n^2}{24}(n+1)^2(3n^4+6n^3-n^2-4n+2).$$

$$\sum_{k=1}^{n} k^8 = \frac{n}{90}(n+1)(2n+1)(5n^6+15n^5+5n^4-15n^3-n^2+9n-3).$$

$$\sum_{k=1}^{n} k^9 = \frac{n^2}{20}(n+1)^2(2n^6+6n^5+n^4-8n^3+n^2+6n-3).$$

$$\sum_{k=1}^{n} k^{10} = \frac{n}{66}(n+1)(2n+1)(3n^8+12n^7+8n^6-18n^5 - 10n^4+24n^3+2n^2-15n+5).$$

XIII.13 INTEGRALS

ELEMENTARY FORMS

1. $\int a\,dx = ax$

2. $\int a \cdot f(x)dx = a \int f(x)dx$

3. $\int \phi(y)\,dx = \int \frac{\phi(y)}{y'}\,dy,\qquad \text{where } y' = dy/dx$

4. $\int (u + v)\,dx = \int u\,dx + \int v\,dx$, where u and v are any functions of x

5. $\int u\,dv = u \int dv - \int v\,du = uv - \int v\,du$

6. $\int u \frac{dv}{dx}\,dx = uv - \int v \frac{du}{dx}\,dx$

7. $\int x^n\,dx = \frac{x^{n+1}}{n+1},\qquad \text{except } n = -1$

8. $\int \frac{f'(x)\,dx}{f(x)} = \log f(x),\qquad (df(x) = f'(x)\,dx)$

9. $\int \frac{dx}{x} = \log x$

10. $\int \frac{f'(x)\,dx}{2\sqrt{f(x)}} = \sqrt{f(x)},\qquad (df(x) = f'(x)\,dx)$

11. $\int e^x\,dx = e^x$

12. $\int e^{ax}\,dx = e^{ax}/a$

13. $\int b^{ax}\,dx = \frac{b^{ax}}{a \log b}$

14. $\int \log x\,dx = x \log x - x$

15. $\int a^x \log a\,dx = a^x$

16. $\int \frac{dx}{a^2 + x^2} = \frac{1}{a} \tan^{-1} \frac{x}{a}$

17. $$\int \frac{dx}{a^2 - x^2} = \begin{cases} \dfrac{1}{a} \tanh^{-1} \dfrac{x}{a} \\ \text{or} \\ \dfrac{1}{2a} \log \dfrac{a + x}{a - x}, \end{cases} \qquad (a^2 > x^2)$$

INTEGRALS

18. $$\int \frac{dx}{x^2 - a^2} = \begin{cases} -\frac{1}{a}\coth^{-1}\frac{x}{a} \\ \text{or} \\ \frac{1}{2a}\log\frac{x-a}{x+a}, \quad (x^2 > a^2) \end{cases}$$

19. $$\int \frac{dx}{\sqrt{a^2 - x^2}} = \begin{cases} \sin^{-1}\frac{x}{a} \\ \text{or} \\ -\cos^{-1}\frac{x}{a}, \quad (a > 0) \end{cases}$$

20. $$\int \frac{dx}{\sqrt{x^2 \pm a^2}} = \log(x + \sqrt{x^2 \pm a^2})$$

21. $$\int \frac{dx}{x\sqrt{x^2 - a^2}} = \frac{1}{a}\sec^{-1}\frac{x}{a}$$

22. $$\int \frac{dx}{x\sqrt{a^2 \pm x^2}} = -\frac{1}{a}\log\left(\frac{a + \sqrt{a^2 \pm x^2}}{x}\right)$$

23. $$\int \frac{dx}{x\sqrt{a + bx}} = \begin{cases} \frac{2}{\sqrt{-a}}\tan^{-1}\sqrt{\frac{a+bx}{-a}}, \quad (a < 0) \\ \text{or} \\ \frac{-2}{\sqrt{a}}\tanh^{-1}\sqrt{\frac{a+bx}{a}} \\ \text{or} \\ \frac{1}{\sqrt{a}}\log\frac{\sqrt{a+bx} - \sqrt{a}}{\sqrt{a+bx} + \sqrt{a}} \end{cases}$$

FORMS CONTAINING $(a + bx)$

For forms containing $a + bx$, but not listed in the table, the substitution $u = \frac{a + bx}{x}$ may prove helpful.

24. $$\int (a + bx)^n\,dx = \frac{(a + bx)^{n+1}}{(n + 1)b}, \quad (n \neq -1)$$

25. $$\int x(a + bx)^n\,dx$$
$$= \frac{1}{b^2(n + 2)}(a + bx)^{n+2} - \frac{a}{b^2(n + 1)}(a + bx)^{n+1}, \quad (n \neq -1, -2)$$

26. $$\int x^2(a + bx)^n\,dx = \frac{1}{b^3}\left[\frac{(a + bx)^{n+3}}{n + 3} - 2a\frac{(a + bx)^{n+2}}{n + 2} + a^2\frac{(a + bx)^{n+1}}{n + 1}\right]$$

27. $$\int x^m(a + bx)^n\,dx = \frac{x^{m+1}(a + bx)^n}{m + n + 1} + \frac{an}{m + n + 1}\int x^m(a + bx)^{n-1}\,dx$$

INTEGRALS

28. $$\int x^m(a+bx)^n\,dx = \begin{cases} \dfrac{1}{a(n+1)}\left[-x^{m+1}(a+bx)^{n+1} + (m+n+2)\displaystyle\int x^m(a+bx)^{n+1}\,dx\right] \\ \text{or} \\ \dfrac{1}{b(m+n+1)}\left[x^m(a+bx)^{n+1} - ma\displaystyle\int x^{m-1}(a+bx)^n\,dx\right] \end{cases}$$

29. $$\int \frac{dx}{a+bx} = \frac{1}{b}\log(a+bx)$$

30. $$\int \frac{dx}{(a+bx)^2} = -\frac{1}{b(a+bx)}$$

31. $$\int \frac{dx}{(a+bx)^3} = -\frac{1}{2b(a+bx)^2}$$

32. $$\int \frac{xdx}{a+bx} = \begin{cases} \dfrac{1}{b^2}[a+bx-a\log(a+bx)] \\ \text{or} \\ \dfrac{x}{b}-\dfrac{a}{b^2}\log(a+bx) \end{cases}$$

33. $$\int \frac{xdx}{(a+bx)^2} = \frac{1}{b^2}\left[\log(a+bx)+\frac{a}{a+bx}\right]$$

34. $$\int \frac{xdx}{(a+bx)^3} = \frac{1}{b^2}\left[-\frac{1}{a+bx}+\frac{a}{2(a+bx)^2}\right]$$

35. $$\int \frac{xdx}{(a+bx)^n} = \frac{1}{b^2}\left[\frac{-1}{(n-2)(a+bx)^{n-2}}+\frac{a}{(n-1)(a+bx)^{n-1}}\right], \quad n \neq 1, 2$$

36. $$\int \frac{x^2dx}{a+bx} = \frac{1}{b^3}\left[\frac{1}{2}(a+bx)^2-2a(a+bx)+a^2\log(a+bx)\right]$$

37. $$\int \frac{x^2\,dx}{(a+bx)^2} = \frac{1}{b^3}\left[a+bx-2a\log(a+bx)-\frac{a^2}{a+bx}\right]$$

38. $$\int \frac{x^2\,dx}{(a+bx)^3} = \frac{1}{b^3}\left[\log(a+bx)+\frac{2a}{a+bx}-\frac{a^2}{2(a+bx)^2}\right]$$

39. $$\int \frac{x^2\,dx}{(a+bx)^n} = \frac{1}{b^3}\left[\frac{1}{(n-3)(a+bx)^{n-3}} + \frac{2a}{(n-2)(a+bx)^{n-2}} - \frac{a^2}{(n-1)(a+bx)^{n-1}}\right], \quad n \neq 1, 2, 3$$

40. $$\int \frac{dx}{x(a+bx)} = -\frac{1}{a}\log\frac{a+bx}{x}$$

41. $$\int \frac{dx}{x(a+bx)^2} = \frac{1}{a(a+bx)}-\frac{1}{a^2}\log\frac{a+bx}{x}$$

INTEGRALS

42. $$\int \frac{dx}{x(a+bx)^3} = \frac{1}{a^3}\left[\frac{1}{2}\left(\frac{2a+bx}{a+bx}\right)^2 + \log\frac{x}{a+bx}\right]$$

43. $$\int \frac{dx}{x^2(a+bx)} = -\frac{1}{ax} + \frac{b}{a^2}\log\frac{a+bx}{x}$$

44. $$\int \frac{dx}{x^3(a+bx)} = \frac{2bx-a}{2a^2x^2} + \frac{b^2}{a^3}\log\frac{x}{a+bx}$$

45. $$\int \frac{dx}{x^2(a+bx)^2} = -\frac{a+2bx}{a^2x(a+bx)} + \frac{2b}{a^3}\log\frac{a+bx}{x}$$

FORMS CONTAINING $c^2 \pm x^2$, $x^2 - c^2$

46. $$\int \frac{dx}{c^2+x^2} = \frac{1}{c}\tan^{-1}\frac{x}{c}$$

47. $$\int \frac{dx}{ax^2+c} = \frac{1}{\sqrt{ac}}\tan^{-1}\left(x\sqrt{\frac{a}{c}}\right), \qquad (a, c > 0)$$

48. $$\int \frac{dx}{c^2-x^2} = \frac{1}{2c}\log\frac{c+x}{c-x}, \qquad (c^2 > x^2)$$

49. $$\int \frac{dx}{ax^2+c} = \begin{cases} \dfrac{1}{2\sqrt{-ac}}\log\dfrac{x\sqrt{a}-\sqrt{c}}{x\sqrt{a}+\sqrt{c}}, & (a > 0, c < 0) \\ \text{or} & \\ \dfrac{1}{2\sqrt{-ac}}\log\dfrac{\sqrt{c}+2\sqrt{-a}}{\sqrt{c}-x\sqrt{-a}}, & (a < 0, c > 0) \end{cases}$$

50. $$\int \frac{dx}{x^2-c^2} = \frac{1}{2c}\log\frac{x-c}{x+c}, \qquad (x^2 > c^2)$$

FORMS CONTAINING $a + bx$ AND $a' + b'x$

51. $$\int \frac{dx}{(a+bx)(a'+b'x)} = \frac{1}{ab'-a'b}\cdot\log\left(\frac{a'+b'x}{a+bx}\right)$$

52. $$\int \frac{x\,dx}{(a+bx)(a'+b'x)} = \frac{1}{ab'-a'b}\left[\frac{a}{b}\log(a+bx) - \frac{a'}{b'}\log(a'+b'x)\right]$$

53. $$\int \frac{dx}{(a+bx)^2(a'+b'x)} = \frac{1}{ab'-a'b}\left(\frac{1}{a+bx} + \frac{b'}{ab'-a'b}\log\frac{a'+b'x}{a+bx}\right)$$

54. $$\int \frac{x\,dx}{(a+bx)^2(a'+b'x)} = \frac{-a}{b(ab'-a'b)(a+bx)} - \frac{a'}{(ab'-a'b)^2}\log\frac{a'+b'x}{a+bx}$$

55. $$\int \frac{x^2\,dx}{(a+bx)^2(a'+b'x)}$$
$$= \frac{a^2}{b^2(ab'-a'b)(a+bx)} + \frac{1}{(ab'-a'b)^2}\left[\frac{a'^2}{b'}\log(a'+b'x) + \frac{a(ab'-2a'b)}{b^2}\log(a+bx)\right]$$

INTEGRALS

56. $$\int \frac{dx}{(a+bx)^n(a'+b'x)^m} = \frac{1}{(m-1)(ab'-a'b)}\left[\frac{-1}{(a+bx)^{n-1}(a'+b'x)^{m-1}} - (m+n-2)b\int \frac{dx}{(a+bx)^n(a'+b'x)^{m-1}}\right]$$

57. $$\int \frac{a+bx}{a'+b'x}\,dx = \frac{bx}{b'} + \frac{ab'-a'b}{b'^2}\log(a'+b'x)$$

58. $$\int \frac{(a+bx)^m dx}{(a'+b'x)^n} = \begin{cases} -\dfrac{1}{(n-1)(ab'-a'b)}\left[\dfrac{(a+bx)^{m+1}}{(a'+b'x)^{n-1}} + b(n-m-2)\displaystyle\int \frac{(a+bx)^m\,dx}{(a'+b'x)^{n-1}}\right] \\ \text{or} \\ -\dfrac{1}{b'(n-m-1)}\left[\dfrac{(a+bx)^m}{(a'+b'x)^{n-1}} + m(ab'-a'b)\displaystyle\int \frac{(a+bx)^{m-1}\,dx}{(a'+b'x)^n}\right] \\ \text{or} \\ \dfrac{-1}{(n-1)b'}\left[\dfrac{(a+bx)^m}{(a'+b'x)^{n-1}} - mb\displaystyle\int \frac{(a+bx)^{m-1}\,dx}{(a'+b'x)^{n-1}}\right] \end{cases}$$

FORMS CONTAINING $\sqrt{a+bx} = \sqrt{u}$ AND $\sqrt{a'+b'x} = \sqrt{v}$ WITH $k = ab' - a'b$

In integrals 59–66, if $k = 0$, then $v = \frac{a'}{a}u$, and formulas starting with 112 should be used in place of these.

59. $$\int \sqrt{uv}\,dx = \frac{k+2bv}{4bb'}\sqrt{uv} - \frac{k^2}{8bb'}\int \frac{dx}{\sqrt{uv}}$$

60. $$\int \frac{dx}{v\sqrt{u}} = \begin{cases} \dfrac{1}{\sqrt{kb'}}\log\dfrac{b'\sqrt{u}-\sqrt{kb'}}{b'\sqrt{u}+\sqrt{kb'}} \\ \text{or} \\ \dfrac{2}{\sqrt{-kb'}}\tan^{-1}\dfrac{b'\sqrt{u}}{\sqrt{-kb'}} \end{cases}$$

61. $$\int \frac{dx}{\sqrt{uv}} = \begin{cases} \dfrac{2}{\sqrt{bb'}}\tanh^{-1}\dfrac{\sqrt{bb'uv}}{bv}, & (v > 0) \\ \text{or} \\ \dfrac{1}{\sqrt{bb'}}\log\dfrac{bv+\sqrt{bb'uv}}{bv-\sqrt{bb'uv}}, & (bv > 0) \\ \text{or} \\ \dfrac{1}{\sqrt{bb'}}\log\dfrac{(bv+\sqrt{bb'uv})^2}{|v|}, & (bv > 0) \\ \text{or} \\ \dfrac{2}{\sqrt{-bb'}}\tan^{-1}\dfrac{\sqrt{-bb'uv}}{bv}, & (bb' < 0) \end{cases}$$

62. $$\int \frac{x\,dx}{\sqrt{uv}} = \frac{\sqrt{uv}}{bb'} - \frac{ab'+a'b}{2bb'}\int \frac{dx}{\sqrt{uv}}$$

INTEGRALS

63. $\int \frac{dx}{v\sqrt{uv}} = \frac{2\sqrt{uv}}{kv}$ or $= \frac{-2\sqrt{u}}{k\sqrt{v}}, \quad (v > 0)$

64. $\int \frac{\sqrt{v}}{\sqrt{u}}\,dx = \int \frac{v\,dx}{\sqrt{uv}}$ or $= \frac{\sqrt{uv}}{b} - \frac{k}{2b}\int \frac{dx}{\sqrt{uv}}, \quad (v > 0)$

65. $\int v^m \sqrt{u}\,dx = \frac{1}{(2m+3)b'}\left(2v^{m+1}\sqrt{u} + k\int \frac{v^m\,dx}{\sqrt{u}}\right)$

66. $\int \frac{dx}{v^m\sqrt{u}} = -\frac{1}{(m-1)k}\left(\frac{\sqrt{u}}{v^{m-1}} + \left(m - \frac{3}{2}\right)b\int \frac{dx}{v^{m-1}\sqrt{u}}\right)$

FORMS CONTAINING $(a + bx^n)$

67. $\int \frac{dx}{a + bx^2} = \frac{1}{\sqrt{ab}}\tan^{-1}\frac{x\sqrt{ab}}{a}$

68. $\int \frac{dx}{a + bx^2} = \begin{cases} \frac{1}{2\sqrt{-ab}}\log\frac{a + x\sqrt{-ab}}{a - x\sqrt{-ab}}, \\ \text{or} \\ \frac{1}{\sqrt{-ab}}\tanh^{-1}\frac{x\sqrt{-ab}}{a}, \qquad (ab < 0) \end{cases}$

69. $\int \frac{dx}{a^2 + b^2x^2} = \frac{1}{ab}\tan^{-1}\frac{bx}{a}$

70. $\int \frac{xdx}{a + bx^2} = \frac{1}{2b}\log\left(x^2 + \frac{a}{b}\right)$

71. $\int \frac{xdx}{a^2 + b^2x^2} = \frac{1}{2b^2}\log(a^2 + b^2x^2)$

72. $\int \frac{x^2\,dx}{a + bx^2} = \frac{x}{b} - \frac{a}{b}\int \frac{dx}{a + bx^2}$

73. $\int \frac{dx}{(a + bx^2)^2} = \frac{x}{2a(a + bx^2)} + \frac{1}{2a}\int \frac{dx}{a + bx^2}$

74. $\int \frac{dx}{(x^2 + a^2)^2} = \frac{1}{2a^3}\tan^{-1}\frac{x}{a} + \frac{x}{2a^2(x^2 + a^2)}$

75. $\int \frac{dx}{(a^2 - b^2x^2)^2} = \frac{1}{2ab}\log\frac{a + bx}{a - bx}$

76. $\int \frac{dx}{(x^2 - a^2)^2} = -\frac{x}{2a^2(x^2 - a^2)} + \frac{1}{4a^3}\log\frac{a + x}{a - x}$

77. $\int \frac{dx}{(a + bx^2)^{m+1}} = \frac{1}{2ma}\frac{x}{(a + bx^2)^m} + \frac{2m - 1}{2ma}\int \frac{dx}{(a + bx^2)^m}$

78. $\frac{xdx}{(a + bx^2)^{m+1}} = \frac{1}{2}\int \frac{dz}{(a + bz)^{m+1}}, \quad [z = x^2]$

79. $\int \frac{x^2\,dx}{(a + bx^2)^{m+1}} = \frac{-x}{2mb(a + bx^2)^m} + \frac{1}{2mb}\int \frac{dx}{(a + bx^2)^m}$

INTEGRALS

80. $\int \frac{dx}{x(a+bx^2)} = \frac{1}{2a}\log\frac{x^2}{a+bx^2}$

81. $\int \frac{dx}{x^2(a+bx^2)} = -\frac{1}{ax} - \frac{b}{a}\int\frac{dx}{a+bx^2}$

82. $\int \frac{dx}{x(a+bx^2)^{m+1}} = \frac{1}{2am(a+bx^2)^m} + \frac{1}{a}\int\frac{dx}{x(a+bx^2)^m}, \qquad (m \neq 0)$

83. $\int \frac{dx}{x^2(a+bx^2)^{m+1}} = \frac{1}{a}\int\frac{dx}{x^2(a+bx^2)^m} - \frac{b}{a}\int\frac{dx}{(a+bx^2)^{m+1}}$

84. $\int \frac{dx}{a+bx^3} = \frac{k}{3a}\left[\frac{1}{2}\log\frac{(k+x)^2}{k^2-kx+x^2} + \sqrt{3}\tan^{-1}\frac{2x-k}{k\sqrt{3}}\right], \qquad (bk^3 = a)$

85. $\int \frac{xdx}{a+bx^3} = \frac{1}{3bk}\left[\frac{1}{2}\log\frac{k^2-kx+x^2}{(k+x)^2} + \sqrt{3}\tan^{-1}\frac{2x-k}{k\sqrt{3}}\right], \qquad (bk^3 = a)$

86. $\int \frac{dx}{x(a+bx^n)} = \frac{1}{an}\log\frac{x^n}{a+bx^n}.$

87. $\int \frac{dx}{(a+bx^n)^{m+1}} = \frac{1}{a}\int\frac{dx}{(a+bx^n)^m} - \frac{b}{a}\int\frac{x^n\,dx}{(a+bx^n)^{m+1}}$

88. $\int \frac{x^m\,dx}{(a+bx^n)^{p+1}} = \frac{1}{b}\int\frac{x^{m-n}\,dx}{(a+bx^n)^p} - \frac{a}{b}\int\frac{x^{m-n}\,dx}{(a+bx^n)^{p+1}}$

89. $\int \frac{dx}{x^m(a+bx^n)^{p+1}} = \frac{1}{a}\int\frac{dx}{x^m(a+bx^n)^p} - \frac{b}{a}\int\frac{dx}{x^{m-n}(a+bx^n)^{p+1}}$

90. $\int x^m(a+bx^n)^p\,dx$

$$= \frac{x^{m-n+1}(a+bx^n)^{p+1}}{b(np+m+1)} - \frac{a(m-n+1)}{b(np+m+1)}\int x^{m-n}(a+bx^n)^p\,dx$$

91. $\int x^m(a+bx^n)^p\,dx = \frac{x^{m+1}(a+bx^n)^p}{np+m+1} + \frac{anp}{np+m+1}\int x^m(a+bx^n)^{p-1}\,dx$

92. $\int x^{m-1}(a+bx^n)^p\,dx$

$$= \frac{1}{b(m+np)}\left[x^{m-n}(a+bx^n)^{p+1} - (m-n)a\int x^{m-n-1}(a+bx^n)^p\,dx\right]$$

93. $\int x^{m-1}(a+bx^n)^p\,dx$

$$= \frac{1}{m+np}\left[x^m(a+bx^n)^p + npa\int x^{m-1}(a+bx^n)^{p-1}\,dx\right]$$

94. $\int x^{m-1}(a+bx^n)^p\,dx$

$$= \frac{1}{ma}\left[x^m(a+bx^n)^{p+1} - (m+np+n)b\int x^{m+n-1}(a+bx^n)^p\,dx\right]$$

95. $\int x^{m-1}(a + bx^n)^p\,dx$

$$= \frac{1}{an(p+1)}\left[-x^m(a + bx^n)^{p+1} + (m + np + n)\int x^{m-1}(a + bx^n)^{p+1}\,dx\right]$$

FORMS CONTAINING $(a + bx + cx^2)$

$X = a + bx + cx^2$ and $q = 4ac - b^2$

For integrals 96–111, if $q = 0$, then $X = c\left(x + \frac{b}{2c}\right)^2$, and formulas starting with 24 should be used in place of these.

96. $\int \frac{dx}{X} = \frac{2}{\sqrt{q}}\tan^{-1}\frac{2cx + b}{\sqrt{q}}$

97. $\int \frac{dx}{X} = \frac{-2}{\sqrt{-q}}\tanh^{-1}\frac{2cx + b}{\sqrt{-q}}$

98. $\int \frac{dx}{X} = \frac{1}{\sqrt{-q}}\log\frac{2cx + b - \sqrt{-q}}{2cx + b + \sqrt{-q}}$

99. $\int \frac{dx}{X^2} = \frac{2cx + b}{qX} + \frac{2c}{q}\int\frac{dx}{X}$

100. $\int \frac{dx}{X^3} = \frac{2cx + b}{q}\left(\frac{1}{2X^2} + \frac{3c}{qX}\right) + \frac{6c^2}{q^2}\int\frac{dx}{X}$

101. $$\int \frac{dx}{X^{n+1}} = \begin{cases} \dfrac{2cx + b}{nqX^n} + \dfrac{2(2n-1)c}{qn}\displaystyle\int\frac{dx}{X^n} \\ \text{or} \\ \dfrac{(2n)!}{(n!)^2}\left(\dfrac{c}{q}\right)^n\left[\dfrac{2cx + b}{q}\displaystyle\sum_{r=1}^{n}\left(\dfrac{q}{cX}\right)^r\left(\dfrac{(r-1)!r!}{(2r)!}\right) + \displaystyle\int\frac{dx}{X}\right] \end{cases}$$

102. $\int \frac{x\,dx}{X} = \frac{1}{2c}\log X - \frac{b}{2c}\int\frac{dx}{X}$

103. $\int \frac{x\,dx}{X^2} = -\frac{bx + 2a}{qX} - \frac{b}{q}\int\frac{dx}{X}$

104. $\int \frac{x\,dx}{X^{n+1}} = -\frac{2a + bx}{nqX^n} - \frac{b(2n-1)}{nq}\int\frac{dx}{X^n}$

105. $\int \frac{x^2}{X}\,dx = \frac{x}{c} - \frac{b}{2c^2}\log X + \frac{b^2 - 2ac}{2c^2}\int\frac{dx}{X}$

106. $\int \frac{x^2}{X^2}\,dx = \frac{(b^2 - 2ac)x + ab}{cqX} + \frac{2a}{q}\int\frac{dx}{X}$

107. $$\int \frac{x^m\,dx}{X^{n+1}} = -\frac{x^{m-1}}{(2n - m + 1)cX^n} - \frac{n - m + 1}{2n - m + 1}\cdot\frac{b}{c}\int\frac{x^{m-1}\,dx}{X^{n+1}} + \frac{m - 1}{2n - m + 1}\cdot\frac{a}{c}\int\frac{x^{m-2}\,dx}{X^{n+1}}$$

INTEGRALS

108. $\int \frac{dx}{xX} = \frac{1}{2a} \log \frac{x^2}{X} - \frac{b}{2a} \int \frac{dx}{X}$

109. $\int \frac{dx}{x^2X} = \frac{b}{2a^2} \log \frac{X}{x^2} - \frac{1}{ax} + \left(\frac{b^2}{2a^2} - \frac{c}{a}\right) \int \frac{dx}{X}$

110. $\int \frac{dx}{xX^n} = \frac{1}{2a(n-1)X^{n-1}} - \frac{b}{2a} \int \frac{dx}{X^n} + \frac{1}{a} \int \frac{dx}{xX^{n-1}}$

111. $\int \frac{dx}{x^m X^{n+1}} = -\frac{1}{(m-1)ax^{m-1}X^n} - \frac{n+m-1}{m-1} \frac{b}{a} \int \frac{dx}{x^{m-1}X^{n+1}}$

$$- \frac{2n+m-1}{m-1} \cdot \frac{c}{a} \int \frac{dx}{x^{m-2}X^{n+1}}$$

FORMS CONTAINING $\sqrt{a+bx}$

112. $\int \sqrt{a+bx}\, dx = \frac{2}{3b} \sqrt{(a+bx)^3}$

113. $\int x\sqrt{a+bx}\, dx = -\frac{2(2a-3bx)\sqrt{(a+bx)^3}}{15b^2}$

114. $\int x^2\sqrt{a+bx}\, dx = \frac{2(8a^2-12abx+15b^2x^2)\sqrt{(a+bx)^3}}{105b^3}$

115. $\int x^m \sqrt{a+bx}\, dx$

$$= \frac{2}{b(2m+3)} \left[x^m \sqrt{(a+bx)^3} - ma \int x^{m-1}\sqrt{a+bx}\, dx\right]$$

116. $\int \frac{\sqrt{a+bx}}{x} dx = 2\sqrt{a+bx} + a \int \frac{dx}{x\sqrt{a+bx}}$

(see No. 123 and No. 124)

117. $\int \frac{\sqrt{a+bx}}{x^2} dx = -\frac{\sqrt{a+bx}}{x} + \frac{b}{2} \int \frac{dx}{x\sqrt{a+bx}}$

(see No. 123 and No. 124)

118. $\int \frac{\sqrt{a+bx}}{x^m} = -\frac{1}{(m-1)a}\left[\frac{\sqrt{(a+bx)^3}}{x^{m-1}}\right.$

$$\left. + \frac{(2m-5)b}{2} \int \frac{\sqrt{a+bx}\, dx}{x^{m-1}}\right], \qquad (m \neq 1)$$

119. $\int \frac{dx}{\sqrt{a+bx}} = \frac{2\sqrt{a+bx}}{b}$

120. $\int \frac{xdx}{\sqrt{a+bx}} = -\frac{2(2a-bx)}{3b^2}\sqrt{a+bx}$

121. $\int \frac{x^2\, dx}{\sqrt{a+bx}} = \frac{2(8a^2-4abx+3b^2x^2)}{15b^3}\sqrt{a+bx}$

INTEGRALS

122. $$\int \frac{x^m\,dx}{\sqrt{a+bx}} = \frac{2x^m\sqrt{a+bx}}{(2m+1)b} - \frac{2ma}{(2m+1)b}\int \frac{x^{m-1}\,dx}{\sqrt{a+bx}}$$

123. $$\int \frac{dx}{x\sqrt{a+bx}} = \frac{1}{\sqrt{a}}\log\left(\frac{\sqrt{a+bx}-\sqrt{a}}{\sqrt{a+bx}+\sqrt{a}}\right) \qquad a > 0$$

124. $$\int \frac{dx}{x\sqrt{a+bx}} = \frac{-2}{\sqrt{a}}\tanh^{-1}\sqrt{\frac{a+bx}{a}} \qquad a > 0$$

(123, 124: See #23 for $a < 0$)

125. $$\int \frac{dx}{x^2\sqrt{a+bx}} = -\frac{\sqrt{a+bx}}{ax} - \frac{b}{2a}\int \frac{dx}{x\sqrt{a+bx}}$$

126. $$\int \frac{dx}{x^n\sqrt{a+bx}} = \begin{cases} -\dfrac{\sqrt{a+bx}}{(n-1)ax^{n-1}} - \dfrac{(2n-3)b}{(2n-2)a}\displaystyle\int \frac{dx}{x^{n-1}\sqrt{a+bx}} \\ \text{or} \\ \dfrac{(2n-2)!}{[(n-1)!]^2}\left[\dfrac{4\sqrt{a+bx}}{b}\displaystyle\sum_{r=1}^{n}\frac{r!(r-1)!}{x^r(2r)!} \right. \\ \left. + \left(\dfrac{-b}{4a}\right)^{n-1}\displaystyle\int \frac{dx}{x\sqrt{a+bx}}\right] \end{cases}$$

127. $$\int (a+bx)^{\pm\frac{n}{2}}\,dx = \frac{2(a+bx)^{\frac{2\pm n}{2}}}{b(2\pm n)}$$

128. $$\int x(a+bx)^{\pm\frac{n}{2}}\,dx = \frac{2}{b^2}\left[\frac{(a+bx)^{\frac{4\pm n}{2}}}{4\pm n} - \frac{a(a+bx)^{\frac{2\pm n}{2}}}{2\pm n}\right]$$

129. $$\int \frac{dx}{x(a+bx)^{\frac{m}{2}}} = \frac{1}{a}\int \frac{dx}{x(a+bx)^{\frac{m-2}{2}}} - \frac{b}{a}\int \frac{dx}{(a+bx)^{\frac{m}{2}}}$$

130. $$\int \frac{(a+bx)^{\frac{n}{2}}\,dx}{x} = b\int (a+bx)^{\frac{n-2}{2}}\,dx + a\int \frac{(a+bx)^{\frac{n-2}{2}}}{x}\,dx$$

131. $$\int f(x,\sqrt{a+bx})\,dx = \frac{2}{b}\int f\left(\frac{z^2-a}{b}, z\right), zdz \qquad (z^2 = a+bx)$$

FORMS CONTAINING $\sqrt{x^2 \pm a^2}$

132. $$\int \sqrt{x^2 \pm a^2}\,dx = \tfrac{1}{2}[x\sqrt{x^2 \pm a^2} \pm a^2 \log(x + \sqrt{x^2 \pm a^2})]$$

133. $$\int \frac{dx}{\sqrt{x^2 \pm a^2}} = \log(x + \sqrt{x^2 \pm a^2})$$

134. $$\int \frac{dx}{x\sqrt{x^2 - a^2}} = \frac{1}{a}\sec^{-1}\frac{x}{a}$$

135. $$\int \frac{dx}{x\sqrt{x^2 + a^2}} = -\frac{1}{a}\log\left(\frac{a + \sqrt{x^2 + a^2}}{x}\right)$$

INTEGRALS

136. $$\int \frac{\sqrt{x^2+a^2}}{x}\,dx = \sqrt{x^2+a^2} - a\log\left(\frac{a+\sqrt{x^2+a^2}}{x}\right)$$

137. $$\int \frac{\sqrt{x^2-a^2}}{x}\,dx = \sqrt{x^2-a^2} - a\sec^{-1}\frac{x}{a}$$

138. $$\int \frac{x\,dx}{\sqrt{x^2\pm a^2}} = \sqrt{x^2\pm a^2}$$

139. $$\int x\sqrt{x^2\pm a^2}\,dx = \tfrac{1}{3}\sqrt{(x^2\pm a^2)^3}$$

140. $$\int \sqrt{(x^2\pm a^2)^3}\,dx = \frac{1}{4}\left[x\sqrt{(x^2\pm a^2)^3} \pm \frac{3a^2x}{2}\sqrt{x^2\pm a^2} + \frac{3a^4}{2}\log\left(x+\sqrt{x^2\pm a^2}\right)\right]$$

141. $$\int \frac{dx}{\sqrt{(x^2\pm a^2)^3}} = \frac{\pm x}{a^2\sqrt{x^2\pm a^2}}$$

142. $$\int \frac{x\,dx}{\sqrt{(x^2\pm a^2)^3}} = \frac{-1}{\sqrt{x^2\pm a^2}}$$

143. $$\int x\sqrt{(x^2\pm a^2)^3}\,dx = \tfrac{1}{5}\sqrt{(x^2\pm a^2)^5}$$

144. $$\int x^2\sqrt{x^2\pm a^2}\,dx = \frac{x}{4}\sqrt{(x^2\pm a^2)^3} \mp \frac{a^2}{8}x\sqrt{x^2\pm a^2} - \frac{a^4}{8}\log\left(x+\sqrt{x^2\pm a^2}\right)$$

145. $$\int x^3\sqrt{x^2+a^2}\,dx = \left(\tfrac{1}{5}x^2 - \tfrac{2}{15}a^2\right)\sqrt{(a^2+x^2)^3}$$

146. $$\int x^3\sqrt{x^2-a^2}\,dx = \frac{1}{5}\sqrt{(x^2-a^2)^5} + \frac{a^2}{3}\sqrt{(x^2-a^2)^3}$$

147. $$\int \frac{x^2dx}{\sqrt{x^2\pm a^2}} = \frac{x}{2}\sqrt{x^2\pm a^2} \mp \frac{a^2}{2}\log\left(x+\sqrt{x^2\pm a^2}\right)$$

148. $$\int \frac{x^3\,dx}{\sqrt{x^2\pm a^2}} = \frac{1}{3}\sqrt{(x^2\pm a^2)^3} \mp a^2\sqrt{x^2\pm a^2}$$

149. $$\int \frac{dx}{x^2\sqrt{x^2\pm a^2}} = \mp\frac{\sqrt{x^2\pm a^2}}{a^2x}$$

150. $$\int \frac{dx}{x^3\sqrt{x^2+a^2}} = -\frac{\sqrt{x^2+a^2}}{2a^2x^2} + \frac{1}{2a^3}\log\frac{a+\sqrt{x^2+a^2}}{x}$$

151. $$\int \frac{dx}{x^3\sqrt{x^2-a^2}} = \frac{\sqrt{x^2-a^2}}{2a^2x^2} + \frac{1}{2a^3}\sec^{-1}\frac{x}{a}$$

INTEGRALS

152. $$\int x^2 \sqrt{(x^2 \pm a^2)^3}\, dx = \frac{x}{6}\sqrt{(x^2 \pm a^2)^5} \mp \frac{a^2 x}{24}\sqrt{(x^2 \pm a^2)^3} - \frac{a^4 x}{16}\sqrt{x^2 \pm a^2} \mp \frac{a^6}{16}\log\left(x + \sqrt{x^2 \pm a^2}\right)$$

153. $$\int x^3 \sqrt{(x^2 \pm a^2)^3}\, dx = \frac{1}{7}\sqrt{(x^2 \pm a^2)^7} \mp \frac{a^2}{5}\sqrt{(x^2 \pm a^2)^5}$$

154. $$\int \frac{\sqrt{x^2 \pm a^2}\, dx}{x^2} = -\frac{\sqrt{x^2 \pm a^2}}{x} + \log\left(x + \sqrt{x^2 \pm a^2}\right)$$

155. $$\int \frac{\sqrt{x^2 + a^2}}{x^3}\, dx = -\frac{\sqrt{x^2 + a^2}}{2x^2} - \frac{1}{2a}\log\frac{a + \sqrt{x^2 + a^2}}{x}$$

156. $$\int \frac{\sqrt{x^2 - a^2}}{x^3}\, dx = -\frac{\sqrt{x^2 - a^2}}{2x^2} + \frac{1}{2a}\sec^{-1}\frac{x}{a}$$

157. $$\int \frac{x^2\, dx}{\sqrt{(x^2 + a^2)^3}} = \frac{-x}{\sqrt{x^2 \pm a^2}} + \log\left(x + \sqrt{x^2 \pm a^2}\right)$$

158. $$\int \frac{x^3\, dx}{\sqrt{(x^2 \pm a^2)^3}} = \sqrt{x^2 \pm a^2} \pm \frac{a^2}{\sqrt{x^2 \pm a^2}}$$

159. $$\int \frac{dx}{x\sqrt{(x^2 + a^2)^3}} = \frac{1}{a^2\sqrt{x^2 + a^2}} - \frac{1}{a^3}\log\frac{a + \sqrt{x^2 + a^2}}{x}$$

160. $$\int \frac{dx}{x\sqrt{(x^2 - a^2)^3}} = -\frac{1}{a^2\sqrt{x^2 - a^2}} - \frac{1}{a^3}\sec^{-1}\frac{x}{a}$$

161. $$\int \frac{dx}{x^2\sqrt{(x^2 \pm a^2)^3}} = -\frac{1}{a^4}\left[\frac{\sqrt{x^2 \pm a^2}}{x} + \frac{x}{\sqrt{x^2 \pm a^2}}\right]$$

162. $$\int \frac{dx}{x^3\sqrt{(x^2 + a^2)^3}} = -\frac{1}{2a^2x^2\sqrt{x^2 + a^3}} - \frac{3}{2a^4\sqrt{x^2 + a^2}} + \frac{3}{2a^5}\log\frac{a + \sqrt{x^2 + a^2}}{x}$$

163. $$\int \frac{dx}{x^3\sqrt{(x^2 - a^2)^3}} = \frac{1}{2a^2x^2\sqrt{x^2 - a^2}} - \frac{3}{2a^4\sqrt{x^2 - a^2}} - \frac{3}{2a^5}\sec^{-1}\frac{x}{a}$$

164. $$\int f\left(x, \sqrt{x^2 + a^2}\right) dx = a\int f(a\tan u, a\sec u)\sec^2 u\, du, \qquad (x = a\tan u)$$

165. $$\int f\left(x, \sqrt{x^2 - a^2}\right) dx = a\int f(a\sec u, a\tan u)\sec u\tan u\, du, \qquad (x = a\sec u)$$

INTEGRALS

FORMS CONTAINING $\sqrt{a^2 - x^2}$

166. $\int \sqrt{a^2 - x^2}\,dx = \frac{1}{2}\left[x\sqrt{a^2 - x^2} + a^2 \sin^{-1}\frac{x}{a}\right], \qquad (a > 0)$

167. $\int \frac{dx}{\sqrt{a^2 - x^2}} = \begin{cases} \sin^{-1}\frac{x}{a} \\ \text{or} \\ -\cos^{-1}\frac{x}{a}, \qquad (a > 0) \end{cases}$

168. $\int \frac{dx}{x\sqrt{a^2 - x^2}} = -\frac{1}{a}\log\left(\frac{a + \sqrt{a^2 - x^2}}{x}\right)$

169. $\int \frac{\sqrt{a^2 - x^2}}{x}\,dx = \sqrt{a^2 - x^2} - a\log\left(\frac{a + \sqrt{a^2 - x^2}}{x}\right)$

170. $\int \frac{x\,dx}{\sqrt{a^2 - x^2}} = -\sqrt{a^2 - x^2}$

171. $\int x\sqrt{a^2 - x^2}\,dx = -\frac{1}{3}\sqrt{(a^2 - x^2)^3}$

172. $\int \sqrt{(a^2 - x^2)^3}\,dx$

$$= \frac{1}{4}\left[x\sqrt{(a^2 - x^2)^3} + \frac{3a^2x}{2}\sqrt{a^2 - x^2} + \frac{3a^4}{2}\sin^{-1}\frac{x}{a}\right], \qquad (a > 0)$$

173. $\int \frac{dx}{\sqrt{(a^2 - x^2)^3}} = \frac{x}{a^2\sqrt{a^2 - x^2}}$

174. $\int \frac{x\,dx}{\sqrt{(a^2 - x^2)^3}} = \frac{1}{\sqrt{a^2 - x^2}}$

175. $\int x\sqrt{(a^2 - x^2)^3}\,dx = -\frac{1}{5}\sqrt{(a^2 - x^2)^5}$

176. $\int x^2\sqrt{a^2 - x^2}\,dx = -\frac{x}{4}\sqrt{(a^2 - x^2)^3} + \frac{a^2}{8}\left(x\sqrt{a^2 - x^2} + a^2\sin^{-1}\frac{x}{a}\right),$

$(a > 0)$

177. $\int x^3\sqrt{a^2 - x^2}\,dx = (-\frac{1}{5}x^2 - \frac{2}{15}a^2)\sqrt{(a^2 - x^2)^3}$

178. $\int x^2\sqrt{(a^2 - x^2)^3}\,dx = -\frac{1}{6}x\sqrt{(a^2 - x^2)^5} + \frac{a^2x}{24}\sqrt{(a^2 - x^2)^3}$

$$+ \frac{a^4x}{16}\sqrt{a^2 - x^2} + \frac{a^6}{16}\sin^{-1}\frac{x}{a}, \qquad (a > 0)$$

179. $\int x^3\sqrt{(a^2 - x^2)^3}\,dx = \frac{1}{7}\sqrt{(a^2 - x^2)^7} - \frac{a^2}{5}\sqrt{(a^2 - x^2)^5}$

180. $\int \frac{x^2\,dx}{\sqrt{a^2 - x^2}} = -\frac{x}{2}\sqrt{a^2 - x^2} + \frac{a^2}{2}\sin^{-1}\frac{x}{a}, \qquad (a > 0)$

INTEGRALS

181. $$\int \frac{dx}{x^2\sqrt{a^2-x^2}} = -\frac{\sqrt{a^2-x^2}}{a^2x}$$

182. $$\int \frac{\sqrt{a^2-x^2}}{x^2}\,dx = -\frac{\sqrt{a^2-x^2}}{x} - \sin^{-1}\frac{x}{a}, \qquad (a > 0)$$

183. $$\int \frac{\sqrt{a^2-x^2}}{x^3}\,dx = -\frac{\sqrt{a^2-x^2}}{2x^2} + \frac{1}{2a}\log\frac{a+\sqrt{a^2-x^2}}{x}$$

184. $$\int \frac{x^2\,dx}{\sqrt{(a^2-x^2)^3}} = \frac{x}{\sqrt{a^2-x^2}} - \sin^{-1}\frac{x}{a}, \qquad (a > 0)$$

185. $$\int \frac{x^3\,dx}{\sqrt{a^2-x^2}} = -\frac{2}{3}(a^2-x^2)^{\frac{3}{2}} - x^2(a^2-x^2)^{\frac{1}{2}}$$

186. $$\int \frac{x^3\,dx}{\sqrt{(a^2-x^2)^3}} = 2(a^2-x^2)^{\frac{1}{2}} + \frac{x^2}{(a^2-x^2)^{\frac{1}{2}}}$$

187. $$\int \frac{dx}{x^3\sqrt{a^2-x^2}} = -\frac{\sqrt{a^2-x^2}}{2a^2x^2} - \frac{1}{2a^3}\log\frac{a+\sqrt{a^2-x^2}}{x}$$

188. $$\int \frac{dx}{x\sqrt{(a^2-x^2)^3}} = \frac{1}{a^2\sqrt{a^2-x^2}} + \frac{1}{a^3}\log\frac{a+\sqrt{a^2-x^2}}{x}$$

189. $$\int \frac{dx}{x^2\sqrt{(a^2-x^2)^3}} = \frac{1}{a^4}\left[-\frac{\sqrt{a^2-x^2}}{x} + \frac{x}{\sqrt{a^2-x^2}}\right]$$

190. $$\int \frac{dx}{x^3\sqrt{(a^2-x^2)^3}} = -\frac{1}{2a^2x^2\sqrt{a^2-x^2}} + \frac{3}{2a^4\sqrt{a^2-x^2}} - \frac{3}{2a^5}\log\frac{a+\sqrt{a^2-x^2}}{x}$$

191. $$\int \frac{\sqrt{a^2-x^2}}{b^2+x^2}\,dx = \frac{\sqrt{a^2+b^2}}{b}\sin^{-1}\frac{x\sqrt{a^2+b^2}}{a\sqrt{x^2+b^2}} - \sin^{-1}\frac{x}{a}, \qquad (a, b > 0)$$

192. $$\int f(x, \sqrt{a^2-x^2})\,dx = a\int f(a\sin u, a\cos u)\cos u\,du, \qquad (x = a\sin u)$$

FORMS CONTAINING $\sqrt{a+bx+cx^2}$

$$X = a + bx + cx^2,\ q = 4\,ac - b^2, \text{ and } k = \frac{4c}{q}$$

For integrals 193–219, when $q = 0$, then $X = c\left(x + \frac{b}{2c}\right)^2$ and formulas starting with 24 should be used.

193. $$\int \frac{dx}{\sqrt{X}} = \frac{1}{\sqrt{c}}\log\left(\sqrt{X} + x\sqrt{c} + \frac{b}{2\sqrt{c}}\right) \qquad \text{if } c > 0$$

194. $$\int \frac{dx}{\sqrt{X}} = \frac{1}{\sqrt{c}}\sinh^{-1}\left(\frac{2cx+b}{\sqrt{4ac-b^2}}\right) \qquad \text{if } c > 0$$

INTEGRALS

195. $\int \frac{dx}{\sqrt{X}} = \frac{1}{\sqrt{-c}} \sin^{-1}\left(\frac{-2cx - b}{\sqrt{b^2 - 4ac}}\right) \qquad \text{if } c < 0$

196. $\int \frac{dx}{X\sqrt{X}} = \frac{2(2cx + b)}{q\sqrt{X}}$

197. $\int \frac{dx}{X^2\sqrt{X}} = \frac{2(2cx + b)}{3q\sqrt{X}}\left(\frac{1}{X} + 2k\right)$

198. $$\int \frac{dx}{X^n\sqrt{X}} = \begin{cases} \dfrac{2(2cx + b)\sqrt{X}}{(2n - 1)qX^n} + \dfrac{2k(n - 1)}{2n - 1}\displaystyle\int \frac{dx}{X^{n-1}\sqrt{X}} \\ \text{or} \\ \dfrac{(2cx + b)(n!)(n - 1)!4^n k^{n-1}}{q[(2n)!]\sqrt{X}} \displaystyle\sum_{r=0}^{n-1} \frac{(2r)!}{(4kX)^r(r!)^2} \end{cases}$$

199. $\int \sqrt{X}\,dx = \frac{(2cx + b)\sqrt{X}}{4c} + \frac{1}{2k}\int \frac{dx}{\sqrt{X}}$

200. $\int X\sqrt{X}\,dx = \frac{(2cx + b)\sqrt{X}}{8c}\left(X + \frac{3}{2k}\right) + \frac{3}{8k^2}\int \frac{dx}{\sqrt{X}}$

201. $\int X^2\sqrt{X}\,dx = \frac{(2cx + b)\sqrt{X}}{12c}\left(X^2 + \frac{5X}{4k} + \frac{15}{8k^2}\right) + \frac{5}{16k^3}\int \frac{dx}{\sqrt{X}}$

202. $$\int X^n\sqrt{X}\,dx = \begin{cases} \dfrac{(2cx + b)X^n\sqrt{X}}{4(n + 1)c} + \dfrac{2n + 1}{2(n + 1)k}\displaystyle\int \frac{X^n\,dx}{\sqrt{X}} \\ \text{or} \\ \dfrac{(2n + 2)!}{[(n + 1)!]^2(4k)^{n+1}}\left[\dfrac{k(2c + b)\sqrt{X}}{c}\displaystyle\sum_{r=0}^{n} \frac{r!(r + 1)!(4kX)^r}{(2r + 2)!} \right. \\ \qquad\qquad\left. + \displaystyle\int \frac{dx}{X}\right] \end{cases}$$

203. $\int \frac{x\,dx}{\sqrt{X}} = \frac{\sqrt{X}}{c} - \frac{b}{2c}\int \frac{dx}{\sqrt{X}}$

204. $\int \frac{x\,dx}{X\sqrt{X}} = -\frac{2(bx + 2a)}{q\sqrt{X}}$

205. $\int \frac{x\,dx}{X^n\sqrt{X}} = -\frac{\sqrt{X}}{(2n - 1)cX^n} - \frac{b}{2c}\int \frac{dx}{X^n\sqrt{X}}$

206. $\int \frac{x^2\,dx}{\sqrt{X}} = \left(\frac{x}{2c} - \frac{3b}{4c^2}\right)\sqrt{X} + \frac{3b^2 - 4ac}{8c^2}\int \frac{dx}{\sqrt{X}}$

207. $\int \frac{x^2\,dx}{X\sqrt{X}} = \frac{(2b^2 - 4ac)x + 2ab}{cq\sqrt{X}} + \frac{1}{c}\int \frac{dx}{\sqrt{X}}$

208. $\int \frac{x^2\,dx}{X^n\sqrt{X}} = \frac{(2b^2 - 4ac)x + 2ab}{(2n - 1)cqX^{n-1}\sqrt{X}} + \frac{4ac + (2n - 3)b^2}{(2n - 1)cq}\int \frac{dx}{X^{n-1}\sqrt{X}}$

INTEGRALS

209. $\int \frac{x^3\,dx}{\sqrt{X}} = \left(\frac{x^2}{3c} - \frac{5bx}{12c^2} + \frac{5b^2}{8c^3} - \frac{2a}{3c^2}\right)\sqrt{X} + \left(\frac{3ab}{4c^2} - \frac{5b^3}{16c^3}\right)\int \frac{dx}{\sqrt{X}}$

210. $\int x\sqrt{X}\,dx = \frac{X\sqrt{X}}{3c} - \frac{b}{2c}\int \sqrt{X}\,dx$

211. $\int xX\sqrt{X}\,dx = \frac{X^2\sqrt{X}}{5c} - \frac{b}{2c}\int X\sqrt{X}\,dx$

212. $\int \frac{xX^n\,dx}{\sqrt{X}} = \frac{X^n\sqrt{X}}{(2n+1)c} - \frac{b}{2c}\int \frac{X^n\,dx}{\sqrt{X}}$

213. $\int x^2\sqrt{X}\,dx = \left(x - \frac{5b}{6c}\right)\frac{X\sqrt{X}}{4c} + \frac{5b^2 - 4ac}{16c^2}\int \sqrt{X}\,dx$

214. $\int \frac{dx}{x\sqrt{X}} = -\frac{1}{\sqrt{a}}\log\left(\frac{\sqrt{X}+\sqrt{a}}{x} + \frac{b}{2\sqrt{a}}\right), \qquad (a > 0)$

215. $\int \frac{dx}{x\sqrt{X}} = \frac{1}{\sqrt{-a}}\sin^{-1}\left(\frac{bx + 2a}{x\sqrt{b^2 - 4ac}}\right), \qquad (a < 0)$

216. $\int \frac{dx}{x\sqrt{X}} = -\frac{2\sqrt{X}}{bx}, \qquad (a = 0)$

217. $\int \frac{dx}{x^2\sqrt{X}} = -\frac{\sqrt{X}}{ax} - \frac{b}{2a}\int \frac{dx}{x\sqrt{X}}$

218. $\int \frac{\sqrt{X}\,dx}{x} = \sqrt{X} + \frac{b}{2}\int \frac{dx}{\sqrt{X}} + a\int \frac{dx}{x\sqrt{X}}$

219. $\int \frac{\sqrt{X}\,dx}{x^2} = -\frac{\sqrt{X}}{x} + \frac{b}{2}\int \frac{dx}{x\sqrt{X}} + c\int \frac{dx}{\sqrt{X}}$

FORMS INVOLVING $\sqrt{2ax - x^2}$

220. $\int \sqrt{2ax - x^2}\,dx = \frac{1}{2}\left[(x-a)\sqrt{2ax - x^2} + a^2\sin^{-1}\frac{x-a}{a}\right], \qquad (a > 0)$

221. $\int \frac{dx}{\sqrt{2ax - x^2}} = \begin{cases} \cos^{-1}\frac{a-x}{|a|} \text{ or } \sin^{-1}\frac{x-a}{|a|} \text{ for all } a \\ \text{or} \\ 2\sin^{-1}\sqrt{\frac{x}{2a}}, \qquad (a > 0) \end{cases}$

222. $\int x^n\sqrt{2ax - x^2}\,dx$

$$= -\frac{x^{n-1}(2ax - x^2)^{3/2}}{n+2} + \frac{(2n+1)a}{n+2}\int x^{n-1}\sqrt{2ax - x^2}\,dx, \qquad (n \neq -2)$$

223. $\int \frac{\sqrt{2ax - x^2}}{x^n}\,dx = \frac{(2ax - x^2)^{3/2}}{(3-2n)ax^n} + \frac{n-3}{(2n-3)a}\int \frac{\sqrt{2ax - x^2}}{x^{n-1}}\,dx, \qquad \left(n \neq \frac{3}{2}\right)$

INTEGRALS

224. $\int \frac{x^n\,dx}{\sqrt{2ax - x^2}} = \frac{-x^{n-1}\sqrt{2ax - x^2}}{n} + \frac{a(2n-1)}{n}\int \frac{x^{n-1}}{\sqrt{2ax - x^2}}\,dx, \quad (n \neq 0)$

225. $\int \frac{dx}{x^n\sqrt{2ax - x^2}} = \frac{\sqrt{2ax - x^2}}{a(1-2n)x^n} + \frac{n-1}{(2n-1)a}\int \frac{dx}{x^{n-1}\sqrt{2ax - x^2}}, \quad \left(n \neq \frac{1}{2}\right)$

226. $\int \frac{dx}{(2ax - x^2)^{\frac{3}{2}}} = \frac{x - a}{a^2\sqrt{2ax - x^2}}$

227. $\int \frac{x\,dx}{(2ax - x^2)^{\frac{3}{2}}} = \frac{x}{a\sqrt{2ax - x^2}}$

228. $\int \frac{dx}{\sqrt{2ax + x^2}} = \log\left(x + a + \sqrt{2ax + x^2}\right)$

MISCELLANEOUS ALGEBRAIC FORMS

229. $\int \sqrt{ax^2 + c}\,dx = \begin{cases} \frac{x}{2}\sqrt{ax^2 + c} + \frac{c}{2\sqrt{a}}\log\left(x\sqrt{a} + \sqrt{ax^2 + c}\right), & (a > 0) \\ \text{or} & \\ \frac{x}{2}\sqrt{ax^2 + c} + \frac{c}{2\sqrt{-a}}\sin^{-1}\left(x\sqrt{\frac{-a}{c}}\right), & (a < 0) \end{cases}$

230. $\int \frac{dx}{\sqrt{a + bx}\cdot\sqrt{a' + b'x}} = \begin{cases} \frac{2}{\sqrt{bb'}}\tanh^{-1}\frac{\sqrt{bb'uv}}{bv}, & (v > 0) \\ \text{or} & \\ \frac{1}{\sqrt{bb'}}\log\frac{bv + \sqrt{bb'uv}}{bv - \sqrt{bb'uv}}, & (bv > 0) \\ \text{or} & \\ \frac{1}{\sqrt{bb'}}\log\left(bv + \sqrt{bb'uv}\right)^2, & (bv > 0) \\ \text{or} & \\ \frac{2}{\sqrt{-bb'}}\tan^{-1}\frac{\sqrt{-bb'uv}}{bv}, & (bb' < 0) \end{cases}$

231. $\int \sqrt{\frac{1 + x}{1 - x}}\,dx = \sin^{-1} x - \sqrt{1 - x^2}$

232. $\int \frac{dx}{\sqrt{a \pm 2bx + cx^2}}$

$= \frac{1}{\sqrt{c}}\log\left(\pm b + cx + \sqrt{c}\sqrt{a \pm 2bx + cx^2}\right), \quad (b^2 - 4ac \neq 0)$

233. $\int \frac{dx}{\sqrt{a \pm 2bx - cx^2}} = \frac{1}{\sqrt{c}}\sin^{-1}\frac{cx \mp b}{\sqrt{b^2 + ac}}$

234. $\int \frac{x\,dx}{\sqrt{a \pm 2bx + cx^2}} = \frac{1}{c}\sqrt{a \pm 2bx + cx^2}$

$\mp \frac{b}{\sqrt{c^3}}\log\left(\pm b + cx + \sqrt{c}\sqrt{a \pm 2bx + cx^2}\right), \quad (b^2 - 4ac \neq 0)$

INTEGRALS

235. $\int \frac{x\,dx}{\sqrt{a \pm 2bx - cx^2}} = -\frac{1}{c}\sqrt{a \pm 2bx - cx^2} \pm \frac{b}{\sqrt{c^3}} \sin^{-1} \frac{cx \mp b}{\sqrt{b^2 + ac}}$

FORMS INVOLVING TRIGONOMETRIC FUNCTIONS

***236.** $\int \sin x\,dx = -\cos x$

237. $\int \cos x\,dx = \sin x$

238. $\int \tan x\,dx = -\log \cos x = \log \sec x$

239. $\int \cot x\,dx = \log \sin x = -\log \csc x$

240. $\int \sec x\,dx = \log(\sec x + \tan x) = \log \tan\left(\frac{\pi}{4} + \frac{x}{2}\right)$

241. $\int \csc x\,dx = \log(\csc x - \cot x) = \log \tan \frac{x}{2}$

242. $\int \sin^2 x\,dx = -\frac{1}{2}\cos x \sin x + \frac{1}{2}x = \frac{1}{2}x - \frac{1}{4}\sin 2x$

243. $\int \sin^3 x\,dx = -\frac{1}{3}\cos x(\sin^2 x + 2)$

244. $\int \sin^n x\,dx = -\frac{\sin^{n-1} x \cos x}{n} + \frac{n-1}{n}\int \sin^{n-2} x\,dx$

245. $\int \cos^2 x\,dx = \frac{1}{2}\sin x \cos x + \frac{1}{2}x = \frac{1}{2}x + \frac{1}{4}\sin 2x$

246. $\int \cos^3 x\,dx = \frac{1}{3}\sin x(\cos^2 x + 2)$

247. $\int \cos^n x\,dx = \frac{1}{n}\cos^{n-1} x \sin x + \frac{n-1}{n}\int \cos^{n-2} x\,dx$

***248.** $\int \sin\frac{x}{a}\,dx = -a\cos\frac{x}{a}$

249. $\int \cos\frac{x}{a}\,dx = a\sin\frac{x}{a}$

* Usually formulas like 248 are omitted from tables if 236 is given since it is easily attainable from it by a simple transformation. If the argument x in 236 is everywhere replaced by $\frac{x}{a}$ it becomes $\int \sin\left(\frac{x}{a}\right) d\left(\frac{x}{a}\right) = -\cos\left(\frac{x}{a}\right)$ or $\frac{1}{a}\int \sin\left(\frac{x}{a}\right) dx = -\cos\left(\frac{x}{a}\right)$ from which follows 248. Similarily if argument x is everywhere replaced by ax in 236, it becomes $\int \sin(ax)d(ax) = -\cos(ax)$ or $a\int \sin(ax)\,dx = -\cos(ax)$ from which follows an integral formula $\int \sin(ax)\,dx = -\frac{1}{a}\cos(ax)$, a formula not contained in these tables. This fact should be borne in mind as one uses these tables from 236 onward.

INTEGRALS

250. $\int \sin(a+bx)\,dx = -\frac{1}{b}\cos(a+bx)$

251. $\int \cos(a+bx)\,dx = \frac{1}{b}\sin(a+bx)$

252. $$\int \frac{dx}{\sin x} = \begin{cases} \int \csc x\,dx = \log(\csc x - \cot x) \\ \text{or} \\ -\frac{1}{2}\log\frac{1+\cos x}{1-\cos x} = \log\tan\frac{x}{2} \end{cases}$$

253. $$\int \frac{dx}{\cos x} = \begin{cases} \int \sec x\,dx = \log(\sec x + \tan x) \\ \text{or} \\ \frac{1}{2}\log\left(\frac{1+\sin x}{1-\sin x}\right) = \log\tan\left(\frac{\pi}{4}+\frac{x}{2}\right) \end{cases}$$

254. $\int \frac{dx}{\cos^2 x} = \int \sec^2 x\,dx = \tan x$

255. $\int \frac{dx}{\cos^n x} = \frac{1}{n-1}\cdot\frac{\sin x}{\cos^{n-1} x} + \frac{n-2}{n-1}\int\frac{dx}{\cos^{n-2} x}$

256. $\int \frac{dx}{1 \pm \sin x} = \mp\tan\left(\frac{\pi}{4} \mp \frac{x}{2}\right)$

257. $\int \frac{dx}{1+\cos x} = \tan\frac{x}{2}$

258. $\int \frac{dx}{1-\cos x} = -\cot\frac{x}{2}$

259. $$\int \frac{dx}{a+b\sin x} = \begin{cases} \frac{2}{\sqrt{a^2-b^2}}\tan^{-1}\frac{a\tan\frac{1}{2}x+b}{\sqrt{a^2-b^2}} \\ \text{or} \\ \frac{1}{\sqrt{b^2-a^2}}\log\frac{a\tan\frac{1}{2}x+b-\sqrt{b^2-a^2}}{a\tan\frac{1}{2}x+b+\sqrt{b^2-a^2}} \end{cases}$$

260. $$\int \frac{dx}{a+b\cos x} = \begin{cases} \frac{2}{\sqrt{a^2-b^2}}\tan^{-1}\frac{\sqrt{a^2-b^2}\tan\frac{1}{2}x}{a+b} \\ \text{or} \\ \frac{1}{\sqrt{b^2-a^2}}\log\left(\frac{\sqrt{b^2-a^2}\tan\frac{1}{2}x+a+b}{\sqrt{b^2-a^2}\tan\frac{1}{2}x-a-b}\right) \end{cases}$$

INTEGRALS

261. $\displaystyle\int \frac{dx}{a + b\sin x + c\cos x}$

$$= \begin{cases} \dfrac{1}{\sqrt{b^2 + c^2 - a^2}} \log \dfrac{b - \sqrt{b^2 + c^2 - a^2} + (a - c)\tan\frac{x}{2}}{b + \sqrt{b^2 + c^2 - a^2} + (a - c)\tan\frac{x}{2}}, & \text{if } a^2 < b^2 + c^2,\ a \neq c \\ \text{or} & \\ \dfrac{2}{\sqrt{a^2 - b^2 - c^2}} \tan^{-1} \dfrac{b + (a - c)\tan\frac{x}{2}}{\sqrt{a^2 - b^2 - c^2}}, & \text{if } a^2 > b^2 + c^2,\ a \neq c \\ \text{or} & \\ \dfrac{1}{a}\left[\dfrac{a - (b + c)\cos x - (b - c)\sin x}{a - (b - c)\cos x + (b + c)\sin x}\right], & \text{if } a^2 = b^2 + c^2,\ a \neq c \end{cases}$$

262. $\displaystyle\int \frac{\sin^2 x\,dx}{a + b\cos^2 x} = \frac{1}{b}\sqrt{\frac{a + b}{a}} \tan^{-1}\left(\sqrt{\frac{a}{a + b}} \tan x\right) - \frac{x}{b},$

$[ab > 0, \text{ or } |a| > |b|]$

263. $\displaystyle\int \frac{dx}{a^2\cos^2 x + b^2\sin^2 x} = \frac{1}{ab}\tan^{-1}\left(\frac{b\tan x}{a}\right)$

264. $\displaystyle\int \sqrt{1 - \cos x}\,dx = \pm 2\sqrt{2}\cos\frac{x}{2},$

[use + when $(4k - 2)\pi < x \leq 4k\pi$, otherwise −; k an integer]

265. $\displaystyle\int \sqrt{1 + \cos x}\,dx = \pm 2\sqrt{2}\sin\frac{x}{2},$

[use + when $(4k - 1)\pi < x \leq (4k + 1)\pi$, otherwise −; k an integer]

266. $\displaystyle\int \sqrt{1 + \sin x}\,dx = \pm 2\left(\sin\frac{x}{2} - \cos\frac{x}{2}\right),$

[use + if $(8k - 1)\frac{\pi}{2} < x \leq (8k + 3)\frac{\pi}{2}$, otherwise −; k an integer]

267. $\displaystyle\int \sqrt{1 - \sin x}\,dx = \pm 2\left(\sin\frac{x}{2} + \cos\frac{x}{2}\right),$

[use + if $(8k - 3)\frac{\pi}{2} < x \leq (8k + 1)\frac{\pi}{2}$, otherwise −; k an integer]

268. $\displaystyle\int \frac{dx}{\sqrt{1 - \cos x}} = \pm\sqrt{2}\log\tan\frac{x}{4},$

[use + if $4k\pi < x < (4k + 2)\pi$, otherwise −; k an integer]

269. $\displaystyle\int \frac{dx}{\sqrt{1 + \cos x}} = \pm\sqrt{2}\log\tan\left(\frac{x + \pi}{4}\right),$

[use + if $(4k - 1)\pi < x < (4k + 1)\pi$, otherwise −; k an integer]

270. $\displaystyle\int \frac{dx}{\sqrt{1 - \sin x}} = \pm\sqrt{2}\log\tan\left(\frac{x}{4} - \frac{\pi}{8}\right)$

[use + if $(8k + 1)\frac{\pi}{2} < x < (8k + 5)\frac{\pi}{2}$, otherwise −; k an integer]

INTEGRALS

271. $\int \frac{dx}{\sqrt{1+\sin x}} = \pm\sqrt{2}\log\tan\left(\frac{x}{4}+\frac{\pi}{8}\right),$

[use + if $(8k-1)\frac{\pi}{2} < x < (8k+3)\frac{\pi}{2}$, otherwise −; k an integer]

272. $\int \sin mx \sin nx\, dx = \frac{\sin(m-n)x}{2(m-n)} - \frac{\sin(m+n)x}{2(m+n)},\qquad [m^2 \neq n^2]$

273. $\int x\sin^2 x\, dx = \frac{x^2}{4} - \frac{x\sin 2x}{4} - \frac{\cos 2x}{8}$

274. $\int x^2\sin^2 x\, dx = \frac{x^3}{6} - \left(\frac{x^2}{4}-\frac{1}{8}\right)\sin 2x - \frac{x\cos 2x}{4}$

275. $\int x\sin^3 x\, dx = \frac{x\cos 3x}{12} - \frac{\sin 3x}{36} - \frac{3}{4}x\cos x + \frac{3}{4}\sin x$

276. $\int \sin^4 x\, dx = \frac{3x}{8} - \frac{\sin 2x}{4} + \frac{\sin 4x}{32}$

277. $\int \cos mx\cos nx\, dx = \frac{\sin(m-n)x}{2(m-n)} + \frac{\sin(m+n)x}{2(m+n)},\qquad [m^2 \neq n^2]$

278. $\int x\cos^2 x\, dx = \frac{x^2}{4} + \frac{x\sin 2x}{4} + \frac{\cos 2x}{8}$

279. $\int x^2\cos^2 x\, dx = \frac{x^3}{6} + \left(\frac{x^2}{4}-\frac{1}{8}\right)\sin 2x + \frac{x\cos 2x}{4}$

280. $\int x\cos^3 x\, dx = \frac{x\sin 3x}{12} + \frac{\cos 3x}{36} + \frac{3}{4}x\sin x + \frac{3}{4}\cos x$

281. $\int \cos^4 x\, dx = \frac{3x}{8} + \frac{\sin 2x}{4} + \frac{\sin 4x}{32}$

282. $\int \frac{\sin x\, dx}{x^m} = -\frac{\sin x}{(m-1)x^{m-1}} + \frac{1}{m-1}\int \frac{\cos x\, dx}{x^{m-1}}$

283. $\int \frac{\cos x\, dx}{x^m} = -\frac{\cos x}{(m-1)x^{m-1}} - \frac{1}{m-1}\int \frac{\sin x\, dx}{x^{m-1}}$

284. $\int \tan^3 x\, dx = \frac{1}{2}\tan^2 x + \log\cos x$

285. $\int \tan^4 x\, dx = \frac{1}{3}\tan^3 x - \tan x + x$

286. $\int \cot^3 x\, dx = -\frac{1}{2}\cot^2 x - \log\sin x$

287. $\int \cot^4 x\, dx = -\frac{1}{3}\cot^3 x + \cot x + x$

288. $\int \cot^n x\, dx = -\frac{\cot^{n-1} x}{n-1} - \int \cot^{n-2} x\, dx,\qquad [n \neq 1]$

INTEGRALS

289. $\int \sin x \cos x\, dx = \frac{1}{2}\sin^2 x$

290. $\int \sin mx \cos nx\, dx = -\frac{\cos(m-n)x}{2(m-n)} - \frac{\cos(m+n)x}{2(m+n)}, \quad (m^2 \neq n^2)$

291. $\int \sin^2 x \cos^2 x\, dx = -\frac{1}{8}(\frac{1}{4}\sin 4x - x)$

292. $\int \sin x \cos^m x\, dx = -\frac{\cos^{m+1} x}{m+1}$

293. $\int \sin^m x \cos x\, dx = \frac{\sin^{m+1} x}{m+1}$

294. $\int \cos^m x \sin^n x\, dx = \frac{\cos^{m-1} x \sin^{n+1} x}{m+n} + \frac{m-1}{m+n}\int \cos^{m-2} x \sin^n x\, dx, \quad (m \neq -n)$

295. $\int \cos^m x \sin^n x\, dx = -\frac{\sin^{n-1} x \cos^{m+1} x}{m+n} + \frac{n-1}{m+n}\int \cos^m x \sin^{n-2} x\, dx, \quad (m \neq -n)$

296. $\int \frac{\cos^m x\, dx}{\sin^n x} = -\frac{\cos^{m+1} x}{(n-1)\sin^{n-1} x} - \frac{m-n+2}{n-1}\int \frac{\cos^m x\, dx}{\sin^{n-2} x}$

297. $\int \frac{\cos^m x\, dx}{\sin^n x} = \frac{\cos^{m-1} x}{(m-n)\sin^{n-1} x} + \frac{m-1}{m-n}\int \frac{\cos^{m-2} x\, dx}{\sin^n x}, \quad (m \neq n)$

298. $\int \frac{\sin^m x\, dx}{\cos^n x} = -\int \frac{\cos^m\left(\frac{\pi}{2} - x\right) d\left(\frac{\pi}{2} - x\right)}{\sin^n\left(\frac{\pi}{2} - x\right)}$

299. $\int \frac{\sin x\, dx}{\cos^2 x} = \frac{1}{\cos x} = \sec x$

300. $\int \frac{\sin^2 x\, dx}{\cos x} = -\sin x + \log \tan\left(\frac{\pi}{4} + \frac{x}{2}\right)$

301. $\int \frac{\cos x\, dx}{\sin^2 x} = \frac{-1}{\sin x} = -\operatorname{cosec} x$

302. $\int \frac{dx}{\sin x \cos x} = \log \tan x$

303. $\int \frac{dx}{\sin x \cos^2 x} = \frac{1}{\cos x} + \log \tan \frac{x}{2}$

304. $\int \frac{dx}{\sin x \cos^n x} = \frac{1}{(n-1)\cos^{n-1} x} + \int \frac{dx}{\sin x \cos^{n-2} x}, \quad (n \neq 1)$

305. $\int \frac{dx}{\sin^2 x \cos x} = -\frac{1}{\sin x} + \log \tan\left(\frac{\pi}{4} + \frac{x}{2}\right)$

306. $\int \frac{dx}{\sin^2 x \cos^2 x} = -2 \cot 2x$

INTEGRALS

307. $$\int \frac{dx}{\sin^m x \cos^n x} = -\frac{1}{m-1}\cdot\frac{1}{\sin^{m-1} x\cdot\cos^{n-1} x} + \frac{m+n-2}{m-1}\int\frac{dx}{\sin^{m-2} x\cdot\cos^n x}$$

308. $$\int \frac{dx}{\sin^m x} = -\frac{1}{m-1}\cdot\frac{\cos x}{\sin^{m-1} x} + \frac{m-2}{m-1}\int\frac{dx}{\sin^{m-2} x}$$

309. $$\int \frac{dx}{\sin^2 x} = -\cot x$$

310. $$\int \tan^2 x\,dx = \tan x - x$$

311. $$\int \tan^n x\,dx = \frac{\tan^{n-1} x}{n-1} - \int \tan^{n-2} x\,dx, \quad (n \neq 1)$$

312. $$\int \cot^2 x\,dx = -\cot x - x$$

313. $$\int \cot^n x\,dx = -\frac{\cot^{n-1} x}{n-1} - \int \cot^{n-2} x\,dx$$

314. $$\int \sec^2 x\,dx = \tan x$$

315. $$\int \sec^n x\,dx = \int\frac{dx}{\cos^n x} = \frac{1}{n-1}\frac{\sin x}{\cos^{n-1} x} + \frac{n-2}{n-1}\int\frac{dx}{\cos^{n-2} x}$$

316. $$\int \csc^2 x\,dx = -\cot x$$

317. $$\int \csc^n x\,dx = \int\frac{dx}{\sin^n x} = -\frac{1}{n-1}\frac{\cos x}{\sin^{n-1} x} + \frac{n-2}{n-1}\int\frac{dx}{\sin^{n-2} x}$$

318. $$\int x\sin x\,dx = \sin x - x\cos x$$

***319.** $$\int x\sin(ax)\,dx = \frac{1}{a^2}\sin(ax) - \frac{x}{a}\cos(ax)$$

320. $$\int x^2\sin x\,dx = 2x\sin x - (x^2-2)\cos x$$

321. $$\int x^2\sin(ax)\,dx = \frac{2x}{a^2}\sin(ax) - \frac{a^2x^2-2}{a^3}\cos(ax)$$

* Formulas of this character produce others where a is everywhere replaced by a^{-1}. For example 319 produces

$$\int x\sin(a^{-1}x)\,dx = \frac{1}{(a^{-1})^2}\sin(a^{-1}x) - \frac{x}{(a^{-1})}\cos(a^{-1}x)$$

which gives

$$\int x\sin\left(\frac{x}{a}\right)dx = a^2\sin\left(\frac{x}{a}\right) - ax\cos\left(\frac{x}{a}\right)$$

INTEGRALS

322. $\int x^3 \sin x \, dx = (3x^2 - 6) \sin x - (x^3 - 6x) \cos x$

323. $\int x^3 \sin (ax) \, dx = \frac{3a^2x^2 - 6}{a^4} \sin (ax) - \frac{a^2x^3 - 6^x}{a^3} \cos (ax)$

324. $\int x^m \sin x \, dx = -x^m \cos x + m \int x^{m-1} \cos x \, dx$

325. $\int x^m \sin (ax) \, dx = -\frac{1}{a} x^m \cos (ax) + \frac{m}{a} \int x^{m-1} \cos (ax) \, dx,$ (*m* pos. integer)

326. $\int x \cos x \, dx = \cos x + x \sin x$

327. $\int x \cos (ax) \, dx = \frac{1}{a^2} \cos (ax) + \frac{x}{a} \sin (ax)$

328. $\int x^2 \cos x \, dx = 2x \cos x + (x^2 - 2) \sin x$

329. $\int x^2 \cos (ax) \, dx = \frac{2x \cos (ax)}{a^2} + \frac{a^2x^2 - 2}{a^3} \sin (ax)$

330. $\int x^3 \cos x \, dx = (3x^2 - 6) \cos x + (x^3 - 6x) \sin x$

331. $\int x^3 \cos (ax) \, dx = \frac{(3a^2x^2 - 6) \cos (ax)}{a^4} + \frac{a^2x^3 - 6x}{a^3} \sin (ax)$

332. $\int x^m \cos x \, dx = x^m \sin x - m \int x^{m-1} \sin x \, dx$

333. $\int x^m \cos (ax) \, dx = \frac{1}{a} x^m \sin (ax) - \frac{m}{a} \int x^{m-1} \sin (ax) \, dx,$ (*m* pos. integer)

334. $\int \frac{\sin x}{x} \, dx = x - \frac{x^3}{3 \cdot 3!} + \frac{x^5}{5 \cdot 5!} - \frac{x^7}{7 \cdot 7!} + \frac{x^9}{9 \cdot 9!} \cdots$

335. $\int \frac{\sin (ax)}{x} \, dx = \frac{a}{x} - \frac{a^3x^3}{3 \cdot 3!} + \frac{a^5x^5}{5 \cdot 5!} - \frac{a^7x^7}{7 \cdot 7!} + \frac{a^9x^9}{9 \cdot 9!} + - \cdots$

336. $\int \frac{\cos x}{x} \, dx = \log x - \frac{x^2}{2 \cdot 2!} + \frac{x^4}{4 \cdot 4!} - \frac{x^6}{6 \cdot 6!} + \frac{x^8}{8 \cdot 8!} \cdots$

337. $\int \frac{\cos (ax)}{x} \, dx = \log x - \frac{a^2x^2}{2 \cdot 2!} + \frac{a^4x^4}{4 \cdot 4!} - \frac{a^6x^6}{6 \cdot 6!} + \frac{a^8x^8}{8 \cdot 8!} - + \cdots$

FORMS INVOLVING INVERSE TRIGONOMETRIC FUNCTIONS

338. $\int \sin^{-1} x \, dx = x \sin^{-1} x + \sqrt{1 - x^2}$

339. $\int \cos^{-1} x \, dx = x \cos^{-1} x - \sqrt{1 - x^2}$

INTEGRALS

340. $\int \tan^{-1} x\, dx = x \tan^{-1} x - \frac{1}{2} \log (1 + x^2)$

341. $\int \cot^{-1} x\, dx = x \cot^{-1} x + \frac{1}{2} \log (1 + x^2)$

342. $\int \sec^{-1} x\, dx = x \sec^{-1} x - \log (x + \sqrt{x^2 - 1})$

343. $\int \csc^{-1} x\, dx = x \csc^{-1} x + \log (x + \sqrt{x^2 - 1})$

344. $\int \text{vers}^{-1} x\, dx = (x - 1)\ \text{vers}^{-1} x + \sqrt{2x - x^2}$

345. $\int \sin^{-1} \frac{x}{a}\, dx = x \sin^{-1} \frac{x}{a} + \sqrt{a^2 - x^2}, \qquad (a > 0)$

346. $\int \cos^{-1} \frac{x}{a}\, dx = x \cos^{-1} \frac{x}{a} - \sqrt{a^2 - x^2}, \qquad (a > 0)$

347. $\int \tan^{-1} \frac{x}{a}\, dx = x \tan^{-1} \frac{x}{a} - \frac{a}{2} \log (a^2 + x^2)$

348. $\int \cot^{-1} \frac{x}{a}\, dx = x \cot^{-1} \frac{x}{a} + \frac{a}{2} \log (a^2 + x^2)$

349. $\int (\sin^{-1} x)^2\, dx = x (\sin^{-1} x)^2 - 2x + 2 \sqrt{1 - x^2}\, (\sin^{-1} x)$

350. $\int (\cos^{-1} x)^2\, dx = x (\cos^{-1} x)^2 - 2x - 2 \sqrt{1 - x^2}\, (\cos^{-1} x)$

351. $\int x \sin^{-1} x\, dx = \frac{1}{4}[(2x^2 - 1) \sin^{-1} x + x \sqrt{1 - x^2}]$

352. $\int x \sin^{-1} (ax)\, dx = \frac{1}{4a^2} [(2a^2x^2 - 1) \sin^{-1} (ax) + ax \sqrt{1 - a^2x^2}]$

353. $\int x \cos^{-1} x\, dx = \frac{1}{4}[(2x^2 - 1) \cos^{-1} x - x \sqrt{1 - x^2}]$

354. $\int x \cos^{-1} (ax)\, dx = \frac{1}{4a^2} [(2a^2x^2 - 1) \cos^{-1} (ax) - ax \sqrt{1 - a^2x^2}]$

355. $\int x^n \sin^{-1} x\, dx = \frac{x^{n+1} \sin^{-1} x}{n + 1} - \frac{1}{n + 1} \int \frac{x^{n+1}\, dx}{\sqrt{1 - x^2}}$

356. $\int x^n \sin^{-1} (ax)\, dx = \frac{x^{n+1}}{n + 1} \sin^{-1} (ax) - \frac{a}{n + 1} \int \frac{x^{n+1}}{\sqrt{1 - a^2x^2}}, \qquad (n \neq -1)$

357. $\int x^n \cos^{-1} x\, dx = \frac{x^{n+1} \cos^{-1} x}{n + 1} + \frac{1}{n + 1} \int \frac{x^{n+1}\, dx}{\sqrt{1 - x^2}}$

358. $\int x^n \cos^{-1} (ax)\, dx = \frac{x^{n+1}}{n + 1} \cos^{-1} (ax) + \frac{a}{n + 1} \int \frac{x^{n+1}}{\sqrt{1 - a^2x^2}}, \qquad (n \neq -1)$

INTEGRALS

359. $$\int x \tan^{-1} x\, dx = \frac{1}{2}(1 + x^2) \tan^{-1} x - \frac{x}{2}$$

360. $$\int x^n \tan^{-1}(ax)\, dx = \frac{x^{n+1}}{n+1} \tan^{-1}(ax) - \frac{a}{n+1} \int \frac{x^{n+1}\, dx}{1 + a^2x^2}, \qquad (n \neq -1)$$

361. $$\int x \cot^{-1} x\, dx = \frac{1}{2}(1 + x^2) \cot^{-1} x + \frac{x}{2}$$

362. $$\int x^n \cot^{-1} x\, dx = \frac{x^{n+1}}{n+1} \cot^{-1} x + \frac{1}{n+1} \int \frac{x^{n+1}}{1 + x^2}\, dx$$

363. $$\int \frac{\sin^{-1} x\, dx}{x^2} = \log\left(\frac{1 - \sqrt{1 - x^2}}{x}\right) - \frac{\sin^{-1} x}{x}$$

364. $$\int \frac{\sin^{-1}(ax)}{x^2}\, dx = a \log\left(\frac{1 - \sqrt{1 - a^2x^2}}{x}\right) - \frac{\sin^{-1}(ax)}{x}$$

365. $$\int \frac{\cos^{-1}(ax)}{x}\, dx = \frac{\pi}{2} \log x - ax - \frac{1}{2 \cdot 3 \cdot 3}(ax)^3 - \frac{1 \cdot 3}{2 \cdot 4 \cdot 5 \cdot 5}(ax)^5 - \frac{1 \cdot 3 \cdot 5}{2 \cdot 4 \cdot 6 \cdot 7 \cdot 7}(ax)^7$$

366. $$\int \frac{\cos^{-1}(ax)}{x^2} = -\frac{1}{x} \cos^{-1}(ax) + a \log \frac{1 + \sqrt{1 - a^2x^2}}{x}$$

367. $$\int \frac{\tan^{-1} x\, dx}{x^2} = \log x - \frac{1}{2} \log(1 + x^2) - \frac{\tan^{-1} x}{x}$$

368. $$\int \frac{\tan^{-1}(ax)}{x^2} = \frac{1}{x} \tan^{-1}(ax) - \frac{a}{2} \log \frac{1 + a^2x^2}{x^2}$$

FORMS INVOLVING TRIGONOMETRIC SUBSTITUTIONS

369. $$\int f(\sin x)\, dx = 2 \int f\left(\frac{2z}{1 + z^2}\right) \cdot \frac{dz}{1 + z^2}, \qquad \left(z = \tan \frac{x}{2}\right)$$

370. $$\int f(\cos x)\, dx = 2 \int f\left(\frac{1 - z^2}{1 + z^2}\right) \frac{dz}{1 + z^2}, \qquad \left(z = \tan \frac{x}{2}\right)$$

371. $$\int f(\sin x)\, dx = \int f(u) \frac{du}{\sqrt{1 - u^2}}, \qquad (u = \sin x)$$

372. $$\int f(\cos x)\, dx = -\int f(u) \frac{du}{\sqrt{1 - u^2}}, \qquad (u = \cos x)$$

373. $$\int f(\sin x, \cos x)\, dx = \int f(u, \sqrt{1 - u^2}) \frac{du}{\sqrt{1 - u^2}}, \qquad (u = \sin x)$$

374. $$\int f(\sin x, \cos x)\, dx = 2 \int f\left(\frac{2z}{1 + z^2}, \frac{1 - z^2}{1 + z^2}\right) \frac{dz}{1 + z^2}, \qquad \left(z = \tan \frac{x}{2}\right)$$

---

375. $$\int \frac{dx}{a + b \tan x} = \frac{1}{a^2 + b^2}[ax + b \log(a \cos x + b \sin x)]$$

INTEGRALS

376. $$\int \frac{dx}{a + b\cot x} = \frac{1}{a^2 + b^2}[ax - b\log(a\sin x + b\cos x)]$$

LOGARITHMIC FORMS

377. $$\int \log x\, dx = x\log x - x$$

378. $$\int x\log x\, dx = \frac{x^2}{2}\log x - \frac{x^2}{4}$$

379. $$\int x^2\log x\, dx = \frac{x^3}{3}\log x - \frac{x^3}{9}$$

380. $$\int (\log X)\, dx = \begin{cases} \left(x + \frac{b}{2c}\right)\log X - 2x + \frac{\sqrt{4ac - b^2}}{c}\tan^{-1}\frac{2cx + b}{\sqrt{4ac - b^2}}, & (b^2 - 4ac < 0) \\ \text{or} & \\ \left(x + \frac{b}{2c}\right)\log X - 2x + \frac{\sqrt{b^2 - 4ac}}{c}\tanh^{-1}\frac{2cx + b}{\sqrt{b^2 - 4ac}}, & (b^2 - 4ac > 0) \\ \text{and} & \\ X = a + bx + cx^2 & \end{cases}$$

381. $$\int x^p\log(ax)\, dx = \frac{x^{p+1}}{p + 1}\log(ax) - \frac{x^{p+1}}{(p + 1)^2}, \qquad (p \neq -1)$$

382. $$\int x^n\log X\, dx = \frac{x^{n+1}}{n + 1}\log X - \frac{2c}{n + 1}\int \frac{x^{n+2}}{X}\, dx - \frac{b}{n + 1}\int \frac{x^{n+1}}{X}\, dx$$
where $X = a + bx + cx^2$

383. $$\int (\log x)^2\, dx = x(\log x)^2 - 2x\log x + 2x$$

384. $$\int (\log x)^n\, dx = x(\log x)^n - n\int (\log x)^{n-1}\, dx, \qquad (n \neq -1)$$

385. $$\int \frac{(\log x)^n}{x}\, dx = \frac{1}{n + 1}(\log x)^{n-1}$$

386. $$\int \frac{dx}{\log x} = \log(\log x) + \log x + \frac{(\log x)^2}{2 \cdot 2!} + \frac{(\log x)^3}{3 \cdot 3!} + \cdots$$

387. $$\int \frac{dx}{x\log x} = \log(\log x)$$

388. $$\int \frac{dx}{x(\log x)^n} = -\frac{1}{(n - 1)(\log x)^{n-1}}$$

389. $$\int \frac{x^m\, dx}{(\log x)} = -\frac{x^{m+1}}{(n - 1)(\log x)^{n-1}} + \frac{m + 1}{n - 1}\int \frac{x^m\, dx}{(\log x)^{n-1}}$$

390. $$\int x^m\log x\, dx = x^{m+1}\left[\frac{\log x}{m + 1} - \frac{1}{(m + 1)^2}\right]$$

INTEGRALS

391. $\int x^m (\log x)^n\, dx = \frac{x^{m+1}(\log x)^n}{m+1} - \frac{n}{m+1}\int x^m (\log x)^{n-1}\, dx, \qquad [m, n \neq -1]$

392. $\int \sin \log x\, dx = \frac{1}{2}x \sin \log x - \frac{1}{2}x \cos \log x$

393. $\int \cos \log x\, dx = \frac{1}{2}x \sin \log x + \frac{1}{2}x \cos \log x$

EXPONENTIAL FORMS

394. $\int e^x\, dx = e^x$

395. $\int e^{-x}\, dx = -e^{-x}$

396. $\int e^{ax}\, dx = \frac{e^{ax}}{a}$

397. $\int x\, e^{ax}\, dx = \frac{e^{ax}}{a^2}(ax - 1)$

398. $\int x^m\, e^{ax}\, dx = \begin{cases} \dfrac{x^m e^{ax}}{a} - \dfrac{m}{a}\displaystyle\int x^{m-1} e^{ax}\, dx \\ \text{or} \\ e^{ax}\displaystyle\sum_{r=0}^{m} (-1)^r \dfrac{m!\,x^{m-r}}{(m-r)!\,a^{r+1}} \end{cases}$

399. $\int \frac{e^{ax}\, dx}{x} = \log x + \frac{ax}{1!} + \frac{a^2x^2}{2 \cdot 2!} + \frac{a^3x^3}{3 \cdot 3!} + \cdots$

400. $\int \frac{e^{ax}}{x^m}\, dx = -\frac{1}{m-1}\frac{e^{ax}}{x^{m-1}} + \frac{a}{m-1}\int \frac{e^{ax}}{x^{m-1}}\, dx$

401. $\int e^{ax} \log x\, dx = \frac{e^{ax} \log x}{a} - \frac{1}{a}\int \frac{e^{ax}}{x}\, dx$

402. $\int \frac{dx}{1 + e^x} = x - \log(1 + e^x) = \log \frac{e^x}{1 + e^x}$

403. $\int \frac{dx}{a + be^{px}} = \frac{x}{a} - \frac{1}{ap}\log(a + be^{px})$

404. $\int \frac{dx}{ae^{mx} + be^{-mx}} = \frac{1}{m\sqrt{ab}}\tan^{-1}\left(e^{mx}\sqrt{\frac{a}{b}}\right), \qquad (a > 0, b > 0)$

405. $\int \frac{dx}{ae^{mx} - be^{-mx}} = \begin{cases} \dfrac{1}{2m\sqrt{ab}}\log \dfrac{\sqrt{a}e^{mx} - \sqrt{b}}{\sqrt{a}e^{mx} + \sqrt{b}} \\ \text{or} \\ \dfrac{1}{m\sqrt{ab}}\tanh^{-1}\left(\sqrt{\dfrac{a}{b}}\, e^{mx}\right) \\ \text{or} \\ -\dfrac{1}{m\sqrt{ab}}\coth^{-1}\left(\sqrt{\dfrac{a}{b}}\, e^{mx}\right), \qquad (a > 0, b > 0) \end{cases}$

INTEGRALS

406. $\int (x^x + x^{-x}) \log x \, dx = x^x + x^{-x}$

407. $\int e^{ax} \sin (bx) \, dx = \dfrac{e^{ax}[a \sin (bx) - b \cos (bx)]}{a^2 + b^2}$

408. $\int e^{ax} \sin (bx) \sin (cx) \, dx = \dfrac{e^{ax}[(b - c) \sin (b - c)x + a \cos (b - c)x]}{2[a^2 + (b - c)^2]} - \dfrac{e^{ax}[(b + c) \sin (b + c)x + a \cos (b + c)x]}{2[a^2 + (b + c)^2]}$

409. $\int e^{ax} \sin (bx) \cos (cx) \, dx = \dfrac{e^{ax}[a \sin (b - c)x - (b - c) \cos (b - c)x]}{2[a^2 + (b - c)^2]} + \dfrac{e^{ax}[a \sin (b + c)x - (b + c) \cos (b + c)x]}{2[a^2 + (b + c)^2]}$

410. $\int e^{ax} \sin (bx) \sin (bx + c) \, dx$

$$= \frac{e^{ax} \cos c}{2a} - \frac{e^{ax}[a \cos (2bx + c) + 2b \sin (2bx + c)]}{2(a^2 + 4b^2)}$$

411. $\int e^{ax} \sin (bx) \cos (bx + c) \, dx$

$$= \frac{-e^{ax} \sin c}{2a} + \frac{e^{ax}[a \sin (2bx + c) - 2b \cos (2bx + c)]}{2(a^2 + 4b^2)}$$

412. $\int e^{ax} \cos (bx) \, dx = \dfrac{e^{ax}}{a^2 + b^2} [a \cos (bx) + b \sin (bx)]$

413. $\int e^{ax} \cos (bx) \cos (cx) \, dx = \dfrac{e^{ax}[(b - c) \sin (b - c)x + a \cos (b - c)x]}{2[a^2 + (b - c)^2]} + \dfrac{e^{ax}[(b + c) \sin (b + c)x + a \cos (b + c)x]}{2[a^2 + (b + c)^2]}$

414. $\int e^{ax} \cos (bx) \cos (bx + c) \, dx$

$$= \frac{e^{ax} \cos c}{2a} + \frac{e^{ax}[a \cos (2bx + c) + 2b \sin (2bx + c)]}{2(a^2 + 4b^2)}$$

415. $\int e^{ax} \cos (bx) \sin (bx + c) \, dx$

$$= \frac{e^{ax} \sin c}{2a} + \frac{e^{ax}[a \sin (2bx + c) - 2b \cos (2bx + c)]}{2(a^2 + 4b^2)}$$

416. $\int e^{ax} \sin^n bx \, dx = \dfrac{1}{a^2 + n^2b^2} \Big[(a \sin bx - nb \cos bx) e^{ax} \sin^{n-1} bx + n(n - 1)b^2 \int e^{ax} \sin^{n-2} bx \cdot dx \Big]$

417. $\int e^{ax} \cos^n bx \, dx = \dfrac{1}{a^2 + n^2b^2} \Big[(a \cos bx + nb \sin bx) e^{ax} \cos^{n-1} bx + n(n - 1)b^2 \int e^{ax} \cos^{n-2} bx \, dx \Big]$

INTEGRALS

418. $$\int x^m e^x \sin x\,dx = \frac{1}{2} x^m e^x(\sin x - \cos x) - \frac{m}{2}\int x^{m-1}e^x \sin x\,dx + \frac{m}{2}\int x^{m-1}e^x \cos x\,dx$$

419. $$\int x^m e^{ax} \sin bx\,dx = \begin{cases} = x^m e^{ax}\dfrac{a\sin bx - b\cos bx}{a^2+b^2} - \dfrac{m}{a^2+b^2}\displaystyle\int x^{m-1}e^{ax}(a\sin bx - b\cos bx)\,dx \\ \text{or} \\ = e^{ax}\left[\dfrac{1}{\rho}x^m \sin(bx-\alpha) - \dfrac{m}{\rho^2}x^{m-1}\sin(bx-2\alpha) \pm \dfrac{m(m-1)\cdots 1}{\rho^{m+1}}\sin\{bx-(m+1)\alpha\}\right] \\ \text{where } a + b\sqrt{-1} = \rho(\cos\alpha + \sqrt{-1}\sin\alpha) \end{cases}$$

420. $$\int x^m e^x \cos x\,dx = \frac{1}{2}x^m e^x(\sin x + \cos x) - \frac{m}{2}\int x^{m-1}e^x \sin x\,dx - \frac{m}{2}\int x^{m-1}e^x \cos x\,dx$$

421. $$\int x^m\, e^{ax} \cos bx\,dx = \begin{cases} x^m e^{ax}\dfrac{a\cos bx + b\sin bx}{a^2+b^2} - \dfrac{m}{a^2+b^2}\displaystyle\int x^{m-1}e^{ax}(a\cos bx + b\sin bx)\,dx \\ \text{or} \\ e^{ax}\left[\dfrac{1}{\rho}x^m \cos(bx-\alpha) - \dfrac{m}{\rho^2}x^{m-1}\cos(bx-2\alpha) + \cdots \pm \dfrac{m(m-1)\cdots 1}{\rho^{m+1}}\cos(bx-(m+1)\alpha)\right] \\ \text{where } a + b\sqrt{-1} = \rho(\cos\alpha + \sqrt{-1}\sin\alpha) \end{cases}$$

422. $$\int e^{ax}\sin x \cos bx\,dx$$
$$= \frac{e^{ax}}{c}((a\sin x - \cos x)\cos(bx-\beta) - b\sin x \sin(bx-\beta))$$
$$\text{where } 1 + a^2 - b^2 = c\cos\beta,\ 2ab = c\sin\beta$$

423. $$\int e^{ax}\cos^m x \sin^n x\,dx$$
$$= \frac{e^{ax}\cos^{m-1}x\sin^n x\{a\cos x + (m+n)\sin x\}}{(m+n)^2+a^2} - \frac{na}{(m+n)^2+a^2}\int e^{ax}\cos^{m-1}x\sin^{n-1}x\,dx + \frac{(m-1)(m+n)}{(m+n)^2+a^2}\int e^{ax}\cos^{m-2}x\sin^n x\,dx$$

INTEGRALS

423. (Continued)

or

$$= \frac{e^{ax}\cos^m x\sin^{n-1} x\{a\sin x - (m+n)\cos x\}}{(m+n)^2+a^2} + \frac{ma}{(m+n)^2+a^2}\int e^{ax}\cos^{m-1} x\sin^{n-1} x\,dx + \frac{(n-1)(m+n)}{(m+n)^2+a^2}\int e^{ax}\cos^m x\sin^{n-2} x\,dx$$

or

$$= \frac{e^{ax}\cos^{m-1} x\sin^{n-1} x(a\sin x\cos x + m\sin^2 x - n\cos^2 x)}{(m+n)^2+a^2} + \frac{m(m-1)}{(m+n)^2+a^2}\int e^{ax}\cos^{m-2} x\sin^n x\,dx + \frac{n(n-1)}{(m+n)^2+a^2}\int e^{ax}\cos^m x\sin^{n-2} x\,dx$$

or

$$= \frac{e^{ax}\cos^{m-1} x\sin^{n-1} x(a\cos x\sin x + m\sin^2 x - \cos^2 x)}{(m+n)^2+a^2} + \frac{m(m-1)}{(m+n)^2+a^2}\int e^{ax}\cos^{m-2} x\sin^{n-2} x\,dx + \frac{(n-m)(n+m-1)}{(m+n)^2+a^2}\int e^{ax}\cos^m x\sin^{n-2} x\,dx$$

424. $$\int \frac{e^{ax}}{\sin^n x}\,dx = -\frac{e^{ax}\{a\sin x + (n-2)\cos x\}}{(n-1)(n-2)\sin^{n-1} x} + \frac{a^2+(n-2)^2}{(n-1)(n-2)}\int \frac{e^{ax}}{\sin^{n-2} x}\,dx$$

425. $$\int \frac{e^{ax}}{\cos^n x}\,dx = -\frac{e^{ax}\{a\cos x - (n-2)\sin x\}}{(n-1)(n-2)\cos^{n-1} x} + \frac{a^2+(n-2)^2}{(n-1)(n-2)}\int \frac{e^{ax}}{\cos^{n-2} x}\,dx$$

426. $$\int e^{ax}\tan^n x\,dx = e^{ax}\frac{\tan^{n-1} x}{n-1} - \frac{a}{n-1}\int e^{ax}\tan^{n-1} x\,dx - \int e^{ax}\tan^{n-2} x\,dx$$

HYPERBOLIC FORMS

427. $$\int \sinh x\,dx = \cosh x$$

428. $$\int \cosh x\,dx = \sinh x$$

429. $$\int \tanh x\,dx = \log\cosh x$$

430. $$\int \coth x\,dx = \log\sinh x$$

431. $$\int \operatorname{sech} x\,dx = \tan^{-1}(\sinh x)$$

432. $$\int \operatorname{csch} x\,dx = \log\tanh\left(\frac{x}{2}\right)$$

INTEGRALS

433. $\int x \sinh x\, dx = x \cosh x - \sinh x$

434. $\int x^n \sinh x\, dx = x^n \cosh x - n \int x^{n-1} \cosh x\, dx$

435. $\int x \cosh x\, dx = x \sinh x - \cosh x$

436. $\int x^n \cosh x\, dx = x^n \sinh x - n \int x^{n-1} \sinh x\, dx$

437. $\int \operatorname{sech} x \tanh x\, dx = -\operatorname{sech} x$

438. $\int \operatorname{csch} x \coth x\, dx = -\operatorname{csch} x$

439. $\int \sinh^2 x\, dx = \frac{\sinh 2x}{4} - \frac{x}{2}$

440. $$\int \sinh^m x \cosh^n x\, dx = \begin{cases} \frac{1}{m+n} \sinh^{m+1} x \cosh^{n-1} x \\ \qquad + \frac{n-1}{m+n} \int \sinh^m x \cosh^{n-2} x\, dx \\ \text{or} \\ \frac{1}{m+n} \sinh^{m-1} x \cosh^{n+1} x \\ \qquad - \frac{m-1}{m+n} \int \sinh^{m-2} x \cosh^n x\, dx, \quad (m+n \neq 0) \end{cases}$$

441. $$\frac{dx}{\sinh^m x \cosh^n x} = \begin{cases} -\frac{1}{(m-1)\sinh^{m-1} x \cosh^{n-1} x} \\ \qquad - \frac{m+n-2}{m-1} \int \frac{dx}{\sinh^{m-2} x \cosh^n x}, \quad (m \neq 1) \\ \text{or} \\ \frac{1}{(n-1)\sinh^{m-1} x \cosh^{n-1} x} \\ \qquad + \frac{m+n-2}{n-1} \int \frac{dx}{\sinh^m x \cosh^{n-2} x}, \quad (n \neq 1) \end{cases}$$

442. $\int \tanh^2 x\, dx = x - \tanh x$

443. $\int \tanh^n x\, dx = -\frac{\tanh^{n-1} x}{n-1} + \int \tanh^{n-2} x\, dx, \quad (n \neq 1)$

444. $\int \operatorname{sech}^2 x\, dx = \tanh x$

445. $\int \cosh^2 x\, dx = \frac{\sinh 2x}{4} + \frac{x}{2}$

446. $\int \coth^2 x\, dx = x - \coth x$

INTEGRALS

447. $\int \coth^n x\,dx = -\frac{\coth^{n-1} x}{n-1} + \int \coth^{n-2} x\,dx, \quad (n \neq 1)$

448. $\int \operatorname{csch}^2 x\,dx = -\operatorname{ctnh} x$

449. $\int \sinh mx \sinh nx\,dx = \frac{\sinh (m+n)x}{2(m+n)} - \frac{\sinh (m-n)x}{2(m-n)}, \quad (m^2 \neq n^2)$

450. $\int \cosh mx \cosh nx\,dx = \frac{\sinh (m+n)x}{2(m+n)} + \frac{\sinh (m-n)x}{2(m-n)}, \quad (m^2 \neq n^2)$

451. $\int \sinh mx \cosh nx\,dx = \frac{\cosh (m+n)x}{2(m+n)} + \frac{\cosh (m-n)x}{2(m-n)}, \quad (m^2 \neq n^2)$

452. $\int \sinh^{-1} \frac{x}{a}\,dx = x \sinh^{-1} \frac{x}{a} - \sqrt{x^2 + a^2}, \quad (a > 0)$

453. $\int x \sinh^{-1} \frac{x}{a}\,dx = \left(\frac{x^2}{2} + \frac{a^2}{4}\right) \sinh^{-1} \frac{x}{a} - \frac{x}{4}\sqrt{x^2 + a^2}, \quad (a > 0)$

454. $\int x^n \sinh^{-1} x\,dx = \frac{x^{n+1}}{n+1} \sinh^{-1} x - \frac{1}{n+1} \int \frac{x^{n+1}}{(1+x^2)^{\frac{1}{2}}}\,dx, \quad (n \neq -1)$

455. $\int \cosh^{-1} \frac{x}{a}\,dx = \begin{cases} x \cosh^{-1} \frac{x}{a} - \sqrt{x^2 - a^2}, & \left(\cosh^{-1} \frac{x}{a} > 0\right) \\ \text{or} & \\ x \cosh^{-1} \frac{x}{a} + \sqrt{x^2 - a^2}, & \left(\cosh^{-1} \frac{x}{a} < 0\right), \ (a > 0) \end{cases}$

456. $\int x \cosh^{-1} \frac{x}{a}\,dx = \frac{2x^2 - a^2}{4} \cosh^{-1} \frac{x}{a} - \frac{x}{4}(x^2 - a^2)^{\frac{1}{2}}$

457. $\int x^n \cosh^{-1} x\,dx = \frac{x^{n+1}}{n+1} \cosh^{-1} x - \frac{1}{n+1} \int \frac{x^{n+1}}{(x^2-1)^{\frac{1}{2}}}\,dx, \quad (n \neq -1)$

458. $\int \tanh^{-1} \frac{x}{a}\,dx = x \tanh^{-1} \frac{x}{a} + \frac{a}{2} \log (a^2 - x^2), \quad \left(\left|\frac{x}{a}\right| < 1\right)$

459. $\int \coth^{-1} \frac{x}{a}\,dx = x \coth^{-1} \frac{x}{a} + \frac{a}{2} \log (x^2 - a^2), \quad \left(\left|\frac{x}{a}\right| > 1\right)$

460. $\int x \tanh^{-1} \frac{x}{a}\,dx = \frac{x^2 - a^2}{2} \tanh^{-1} \frac{x}{a} + \frac{ax}{2}, \quad \left(\left|\frac{x}{a}\right| < 1\right)$

461. $\int x^n \tanh^{-1} x\,dx = \frac{x^{n+1}}{n+1} \tanh^{-1} x - \frac{1}{n+1} \int \frac{x^{n+1}}{1-x^2}\,dx, \quad (n \neq -1)$

462. $\int x \coth^{-1} \frac{x}{a}\,dx = \frac{x^2 - a^2}{2} \coth^{-1} \frac{x}{a} + \frac{ax}{2}, \quad \left(\left|\frac{x}{a}\right| > 1\right)$

463. $\int x^n \coth^{-1} x\,dx = \frac{x^{n+1}}{n+1} \coth^{-1} x + \frac{1}{n+1} \int \frac{x^{n+1}}{x^2-1}\,dx, \quad (n \neq -1)$

464. $\int \operatorname{sech}^{-1} x\,dx = x \operatorname{sech}^{-1} x + \arcsin x$

INTEGRALS

465. $\int x \operatorname{sech}^{-1} x\, dx = \frac{x^2}{2} \operatorname{sech}^{-1} x - \frac{1}{2}(1 - x^2)$

466. $\int x^n \operatorname{sech}^{-1} x\, dx = \frac{x^{n+1}}{n+1} \operatorname{sech}^{-1} x + \frac{1}{n+1} \int \frac{x^n}{(1-x^2)^{\frac{1}{2}}} dx, \qquad (n \neq -1)$

467. $\int \operatorname{csch}^{-1} x\, dx = x \operatorname{csch}^{-1} x + \sinh^{-1} x$

468. $\int x \operatorname{csch}^{-1} x\, dx = \frac{x^2}{2} \operatorname{csch}^{-1} x + \frac{1}{2}(1 + x^2)^{\frac{1}{2}}$

469. $\int x^n \operatorname{csch}^{-1} x\, dx = \frac{x^{n+1}}{n+1} \operatorname{csch}^{-1} x + \frac{1}{n+1} \int \frac{x^n}{(x^2+1)^{\frac{1}{2}}} dx, \qquad (n \neq -1)$

DEFINITE INTEGRALS

470. $\int_0^\infty x^{n-1} e^{-x}\, dx = \int_0^1 \left(\log \frac{1}{x}\right)^{n-1} dx = \frac{1}{x} \prod_{n=1}^{\infty} \frac{\left(1 + \frac{1}{n}\right)^x}{\left(1 + \frac{x}{n}\right)}$

$= \Gamma(n),\ n \neq 0, -1, -2, -3, \ldots$ (Gamma Function)

471. $\int_0^\infty t^n p^{-t}\, dt = \frac{n!}{(\log p)^{n+1}}, \qquad (n = 0, 1, 2, 3, \ldots \text{ and } p > 0)$

472. $\int_0^\infty t^{n-1} e^{-(a+1)t}\, dt = \frac{\Gamma(n)}{(a+1)^n}, \qquad (n > 0,\ a > -1)$

473. $\int_0^1 x^m \left(\log \frac{1}{x}\right)^n dx = \frac{\Gamma(n+1)}{(m+1)^{n+1}}, \qquad (m > -1,\ n > -1)$

474. $\Gamma(n)$ is finite if $n > 0$, $\Gamma(n+1) = n\Gamma(n)$

475. $\Gamma(n) \cdot \Gamma(1-n) = \frac{\pi}{\sin n\pi}$

476. $\Gamma(n) = (n-1)!$ if $n =$ integer > 0

477. $\Gamma(\frac{1}{2}) = 2 \int_0^\infty e^{-t^2}\, dt = \sqrt{\pi} = 1.7724538509 \ldots = (-\frac{1}{2})!$

478. $\Gamma\left(n + \frac{1}{2}\right) = \frac{1 \cdot 3 \cdot 5 \cdot 7 \cdots (2n-1)}{2^n} \sqrt{\pi}$, where n is an integer and > 0 (see values of $\Gamma(n)$ at end of integral table)

479. $\int_0^1 x^{m-1}(1-x)^{n-1}\, dx = B(m, n)$, (Beta function)

480. $B(m, n) = B(n, m) = \frac{\Gamma(m)\Gamma(n)}{\Gamma(m+n)}$, where m and n are any positive real numbers

481. $\int_0^1 x^{m-1}(1-x)^{n-1}\, dx = \int_0^\infty \frac{x^{m-1}\, dx}{(1+x)^{m+n}} = \frac{\Gamma(m)\Gamma(n)}{\Gamma(m+n)}$

INTEGRALS

482. $\int_a^b (x-a)^m(b-x)^n\,dx = (b-a)^{m+n+1}\dfrac{\Gamma(m+1)\cdot\Gamma(n+1)}{\Gamma(m+n+2)},$
$(m > -1, n > -1, b > a)$

483. $\int_1^\infty \dfrac{dx}{x^m} = \dfrac{1}{m-1}, \qquad [m > 1]$

484. $\int_0^\infty \dfrac{dx}{(1+x)x^p} = \pi \csc p\pi, \qquad [p < 1]$

485. $\int_0^\infty \dfrac{dx}{(1-x)x^p} = -\pi \cot p\pi, \qquad [p < 1]$

486. $\int_0^\infty \dfrac{x^{p-1}\,dx}{1+x} = \dfrac{\pi}{\sin p\pi}$
$= \mathrm{B}(p, 1-p) = \Gamma(p)\Gamma(1-p), \qquad [0 < p < 1]$

487. $\int_0^\infty \dfrac{x^{m-1}\,dx}{1+x^n} = \dfrac{\pi}{n \sin \dfrac{m\pi}{n}}, \qquad [0 < m < n]$

488. $\int_0^\infty \dfrac{x^a\,dx}{(m+x^b)^c} = m^{\frac{a+1}{b}-c}\left[\dfrac{\Gamma\left(\dfrac{a+1}{b}\right)\Gamma\left(c-\dfrac{a+1}{b}\right)}{\Gamma(c)}\right],$
$\left(a > -1, b > 0, m > 0, c > \dfrac{a+1}{b}\right)$

489. $\int_0^\infty \dfrac{dx}{(1+x)\sqrt{x}} = \pi$

490. $\int_0^\infty \dfrac{a\,dx}{a^2+x^2} = \dfrac{\pi}{2}$, if $a > 0$; 0, if $a = 0$; $-\dfrac{\pi}{2}$, if $a < 0$

491. $\int_0^a (a^2-x^2)^{\frac{n}{2}}\,dx = \dfrac{1}{2}\int_{-a}^a (a^2-x^2)^{\frac{n}{2}}\,dx = \dfrac{1\cdot 3\cdot 5\cdots n}{2\cdot 4\cdot 6\cdots(n+1)}\cdot\dfrac{\pi}{2}\cdot a^{n+1}$
$(n \text{ odd})$

492. $\int_0^a x^m(a^2-x^2)^{\frac{n}{2}}\,dx$

$$= \begin{cases} a^{m+n+1}\displaystyle\int_0^{\pi/2} (\sin^m x)(\cos^{n+1} x)\,dx \\ \text{or} \\ \dfrac{1\cdot 3\cdot 5\cdot 7\cdots(m-1)1\cdot 3\cdot 5\cdot 7\cdots n}{(m+n+1)!2^{\frac{m+n+3}{2}}}\pi a^{m+n+1}, & (n \text{ odd}, m \text{ even}) \\ \text{or} \\ \dfrac{2\cdot 4\cdot 6\cdots(m+1)}{(n+2)(n+4)\cdots(n+m+1)}a^{m+n+1}, & (n \text{ odd}, m \text{ even}) \end{cases}$$

INTEGRALS

493. $$\int_0^{\pi/2} (\sin^n x)\,dx = \begin{cases} \displaystyle\int_0^{\pi/2} (\cos^n x)\,dx \\ \text{or} \\ \dfrac{1\cdot 3\cdot 5\cdot 7\cdots(n-1)}{2\cdot 4\cdot 6\cdot 8\cdots(n)}\dfrac{\pi}{2}, & (n \text{ an even integer}, n \neq 0) \\ \text{or} \\ \dfrac{2\cdot 4\cdot 6\cdot 8\cdots(n-1)}{1\cdot 3\cdot 5\cdot 7\cdots(n)}, & (n \text{ an odd integer}, n \neq 1) \\ \text{or} \\ \dfrac{\sqrt{\pi}}{2}\dfrac{\Gamma\left(\frac{n+1}{2}\right)}{\Gamma\left(\frac{n}{2}+1\right)}, & (n > -1) \end{cases}$$

494. $$\int_0^{\infty} \frac{\sin mx\,dx}{x} = \frac{\pi}{2}, \text{ if } m > 0;\ 0, \text{ if } m = 0;\ -\frac{\pi}{2}, \text{ if } m < 0$$

495. $$\int_0^{\infty} \frac{\cos x\,dx}{x} = \infty$$

496. $$\int_0^{\infty} \frac{\tan x\,dx}{x} = \frac{\pi}{2}$$

497. $$\int_0^{\pi} \sin ax \cdot \sin bx\,dx = \int_0^{\pi} \cos ax \cdot \cos bx\,dx = 0, \qquad (a \neq b;\ a, b \text{ integers})$$

498. $$\int_0^{\pi/a} [\sin (ax)][\cos (ax)]\,dx = \int_0^{\pi} [\sin (ax)][\cos (ax)]\,dx = 0$$

499. $$\int_0^{\pi} [\sin (ax)][\cos (bx)]\,dx = \frac{2a}{a^2 - b^2}, \text{ if } a - b \text{ is odd, or zero if } a - b \text{ is even}$$

500. $$\int_0^{\infty} \frac{\sin x \cos mx\,dx}{x}$$

$$= 0, \text{ if } m < -1 \text{ or } m > 1,\ = \frac{\pi}{4}, \text{ if } m = \pm 1;\ = \frac{\pi}{2}, \text{ if } m^2 < 1$$

501. $$\int_0^{\infty} \frac{\sin ax \sin bx}{x^2}\,dx = \frac{\pi a}{2}, \qquad (a \leq b)$$

502. $$\int_0^{\pi} \sin^2 mx\,dx = \int_0^{\pi} \cos^2 mx\,dx = \frac{\pi}{2}$$

503. $$\int_0^{\infty} \frac{\sin^2 x\,dx}{x^2} = \frac{\pi}{2}$$

504. $$\int \frac{\cos mx}{1 + x^2}\,dx = \frac{\pi}{2} e^{-|m|}$$

505. $$\int_0^{\infty} \cos (x^2)\,dx = \int_0^{\infty} \sin (x^2)\,dx = \frac{1}{2}\sqrt{\frac{\pi}{2}}$$

506. $$\int_0^{\infty} \frac{\sin x\,dx}{\sqrt{x}} = \int_0^{\infty} \frac{\cos x\,dx}{\sqrt{x}} = \sqrt{\frac{\pi}{2}}$$

INTEGRALS

507. $\int_0^{\pi/2} \frac{dx}{1 + a \cos x} = \frac{\cos^{-1} a}{\sqrt{1 - a^2}}, \qquad (a < 1)$

508. $\int_0^{\infty} \frac{dx}{a + b \cos x} = \frac{\pi}{\sqrt{a^2 - b^2}}, \qquad (a > b \geq 0)$

509. $\int_0^{2\pi} \frac{dx}{1 + a \cos x} = \frac{2\pi}{\sqrt{1 - a^2}}, \qquad (a^2 < 1)$

510. $\int_0^{\infty} \frac{\cos ax - \cos bx}{x} dx = \log \frac{b}{a}$

511. $\int_0^{\pi/2} \frac{dx}{a^2 \sin^2 x + b^2 \cos^2 x} = \frac{\pi}{2ab}$

512. $\int_0^{\pi/2} \frac{dx}{(a^2 \sin^2 x + b^2 \cos^2 x)^2} = \frac{\pi(a^2 + b^2)}{4a^3b^3}, \qquad (a, b > 0)$

513. $\int_0^{\pi/2} \sin^{n-1} x \cos^{m-1} x \, dx = \frac{1}{2} \mathrm{B}\left(\frac{n}{2}, \frac{m}{2}\right), \qquad m$ and n positive integers

514. $\int_0^{\pi/2} (\sin^{2n+1} \theta) \, d\theta = \frac{2 \cdot 4 \cdot 6 \cdots (2n)}{1 \cdot 3 \cdot 5 \cdots (2n + 1)}, \qquad (n = 1, 2, 3 \ldots)$

515. $\int_0^{\pi/2} (\sin^{2n} \theta) \, d\theta = \frac{1 \cdot 3 \cdot 5 \cdots (2n - 1)}{2 \cdot 4 \cdots (2n)} \left(\frac{\pi}{2}\right), \qquad (n = 1, 2, 3 \ldots)$

516. $\int_0^{\pi/2} \sqrt{\cos \theta} \, d\theta = \frac{(2\pi)^{\frac{3}{2}}}{[\Gamma(\frac{1}{4})]^2}$

517. $\int_0^{\pi/2} (\tan^h \theta) \, d\theta = \frac{\pi}{2 \cos \left(\frac{h\pi}{2}\right)}, \qquad (0 < h < 1)$

518. $\int_0^{\infty} \frac{\tan^{-1} (ax) - \tan^{-1} (bx)}{x} dx = \frac{\pi}{2} \log \frac{a}{b}, \qquad (a, b > 0)$

519. The area enclosed by a curve defined through the equation $x^{\frac{b}{c}} + y^{\frac{b}{c}} = a^{\frac{b}{c}}$ where $a > 0$, c a positive odd integer and b a positive even integer is given by

$$\frac{\left[\Gamma\left(\frac{c}{b}\right)\right]^2}{\Gamma\left(\frac{2c}{b}\right)} \left(\frac{2ca^2}{b}\right)$$

520. $I = \iiint\limits_R x^{h-1} y^{m-1} z^{n-1} \, dv$, where R denotes the region of space bounded by the co-ordinate planes and that portion of the surface $\left(\frac{x}{a}\right)^p + \left(\frac{y}{b}\right)^q + \left(\frac{z}{c}\right)^k = 1$, which lies in the first octant and where h, m, n, p, q, k, a, b, c, denote positive real numbers is given by

INTEGRALS

520. (Continued)

$$\int_0^a x^{h-1}\,dx \int_0^{b\left[1-\left(\frac{x}{a}\right)^p\right]^{\frac{1}{q}}} y^m\,dy \int_0^{c\left[1-\left(\frac{x}{a}\right)^p-\left(\frac{y}{b}\right)^q\right]^{\frac{1}{k}}} z^{n-1}\,dz$$

$$= \frac{a^h b^m c^n}{pqk} \frac{\Gamma\left(\frac{h}{p}\right)\Gamma\left(\frac{m}{q}\right)\Gamma\left(\frac{n}{k}\right)}{\Gamma\left(\frac{h}{p}+\frac{m}{q}+\frac{n}{k}+1\right)}$$

521. $\int_0^\infty e^{-ax}\,dx = \frac{1}{a}, \qquad (a > 0)$

522. $\int_0^\infty \frac{e^{-ax}-e^{-bx}}{x}\,dx = \log\frac{b}{2}, \qquad (a, b > 0)$

523. $\int_0^\infty x^n e^{-ax}\,dx = \frac{\Gamma(n+1)}{a^{n+1}}, \qquad (n > -1, a > 0)$

$= \frac{n!}{a^{n+1}}, \qquad$ (n pos. integ., $a > 0$)

524. $\int_0^\infty e^{-a^2x^2}\,dx = \frac{1}{2a}\sqrt{\pi} = \frac{1}{2a}\Gamma\left(\frac{1}{2}\right), \qquad (a > 0)$

525. $\int_0^\infty xe^{-x^2}\,dx = \frac{1}{2}$

526. $\int_0^\infty x^2e^{-x^2}\,dx = \frac{\sqrt{\pi}}{4}$

527. $\int_0^\infty x^{2n}e^{-ax^2}\,dx = \frac{1\cdot 3\cdot 5\ \cdots\ (2n-1)}{2^{n+1}a^n}\sqrt{\frac{\pi}{a}}$

528. $\int_0^\infty x^m e^{-ax}\,dx = \frac{m!}{a^{m+1}}\left[1 - e^{-a}\sum_{r=0}^{m}\frac{a^r}{r!}\right]$

529. $\int_0^\infty e^{\left(-x^2-\frac{a^2}{x^2}\right)}\,dx = \frac{e^{-2a}\sqrt{\pi}}{2}$

530. $\int_0^\infty e^{-nx}\sqrt{x}\,dx = \frac{1}{2n}\sqrt{\frac{\pi}{n}}$

531. $\int_0^\infty \frac{e^{-nx}}{\sqrt{x}}\,dx = \sqrt{\frac{\pi}{n}}$

532. $\int_0^\infty e^{-ax}\cos mx\,dx = \frac{a}{a^2+m^2}, \qquad (a > 0)$

533. $\int_0^\infty e^{-ax}\sin mx\,dx = \frac{m}{a^2+m^2}, \qquad (a > 0)$

534. $\int_0^\infty xe^{-ax}[\sin(bx)]\,dx = \frac{2ab}{(a^2+b^2)^2}, \qquad (a > 0)$

535. $\int_0^\infty xe^{-ax}[\cos(bx)]\,dx = \frac{a^2-b^2}{(a^2+b^2)^2}, \qquad (a > 0)$

INTEGRALS

536. $\int_0^\infty x^n e^{-ax}[\sin(bx)]\,dx = \frac{n![(a-ib)^{n+1}-(a+ib)^{n+1}]}{2(a^2+b^2)^{n+1}}, \quad (i^2=-1,\ a>0)$

537. $\int_0^\infty x^n e^{-ax}[\cos(bx)]\,dx = \frac{n![(a-ib)^{n+1}+(a+ib)^{n+1}]}{2(a^2+b^2)^{n+1}}, \quad (i^2=-1,\ a>0)$

538. $\int_0^\infty \frac{e^{-ax}\sin x}{x}\,dx = \cot^{-1} a, \quad (a>0)$

539. $\int_0^\infty e^{-a^2x^2}\cos bx\,dx = \frac{\sqrt{\pi}}{2a}e^{\frac{-b^2}{4a^2}}, \quad (ab \neq 0)$

540. $\int_0^\infty e^{-t\cos\phi}t^{b-1}[\sin(t\sin\phi)\,dt = [\Gamma(b)]\sin(b\phi), \quad \left(b>0,\ -\frac{\pi}{2}<\phi<\frac{\pi}{2}\right)$

541. $\int_0^\infty e^{-t\cos\phi}t^{b-1}[\cos(t\sin\phi)]\,dt = [\Gamma(b)]\cos(b\phi), \quad \left(b>0,\ -\frac{\pi}{2}<\phi<\frac{\pi}{2}\right)$

542. $\int_0^\infty t^{b-1}\cos t\,dt = [\Gamma(b)]\cos\left(\frac{b\pi}{2}\right), \quad (0<b<1)$

543. $\int_0^\infty t^{b-1}(\sin t)\,dt = [\Gamma(b)]\sin\left(\frac{b\pi}{2}\right), \quad (0<b<1)$

544. $\int_0^1 (\log x)^n\,dx = (-1)^n \cdot n!$

545. $\int_0^1 \left(\log\frac{1}{x}\right)^{\frac{1}{2}} dx = \frac{\sqrt{\pi}}{2}$

546. $\int_0^1 \left(\log\frac{1}{x}\right)^{-\frac{1}{2}} dx = \sqrt{\pi}$

547. $\int_0^1 \left(\log\frac{1}{x}\right)^n dx = n!$

548. $\int_0^1 x\log(1-x)\,dx = -\frac{3}{4}$

549. $\int_0^1 x\log(1+x)\,dx = \frac{1}{4}$

550. $\int_0^1 \frac{\log x}{1+x}\,dx = -\frac{\pi^2}{12}$

551. $\int_0^1 \frac{\log x}{1-x}\,dx = -\frac{\pi^2}{6}$

552. $\int_0^1 \frac{\log x}{1-x^2}\,dx = -\frac{\pi^2}{8}$

553. $\int_0^1 \log\left(\frac{1+x}{1-x}\right)\cdot\frac{dx}{x} = \frac{\pi^2}{4}$

554. $\int_0^1 \frac{\log x\,dx}{\sqrt{1-x^2}} = -\frac{\pi}{2}\log 2$

INTEGRALS

555. $\int_0^1 x^m \left[\log\left(\frac{1}{x}\right)\right]^n dx = \frac{\Gamma(n+1)}{(m+1)^{n+1}}$, if $m + 1 > 0$, $n + 1 > 0$

556. $\int_0^1 \frac{(x^p - x^q)\,dx}{\log x} = \log\left(\frac{p+1}{q+1}\right)$, $(p + 1 > 0, q + 1 > 0)$

557. $\int_0^1 \frac{dx}{\sqrt{\log\left(\frac{1}{x}\right)}} = \sqrt{\pi}$

558. $\int_0^\infty \log\left(\frac{e^x + 1}{e^x - 1}\right) dx = \frac{\pi^2}{4}$

559. $\int_0^{\pi/2} \log \sin x\,dx = \int_0^{\pi/2} \log \cos x\,dx = -\frac{\pi}{2}\log 2$

560. $\int_0^{\pi/2} \log \sec x\,dx = \int_0^{\pi/2} \log \csc x\,dx = \frac{\pi}{2}\log 2$

561. $\int_0^\pi x \log \sin x\,dx = -\frac{\pi^2}{2}\log 2$

562. $\int_0^{\pi/2} \sin x \log \sin x\,dx = \log 2 - 1$

563. $\int_0^{\pi/2} \log \tan x\,dx = 0$

564. $\int_0^\pi \log(a \pm b\cos x)\,dx = \pi \log\left(\frac{a + \sqrt{a^2 - b^2}}{2}\right)$, $(a \geqq b)$

565. $\int_0^\infty \frac{dx}{\cosh ax} = \frac{\pi}{2a}$

566. $\int_0^\infty \frac{x\,dx}{\sinh ax} = \frac{\pi^2}{4a^2}$

567. $\int_0^\infty e^{-ax}\cosh bx\,dx = \frac{a}{a^2 - b^2}$, $(0 \leq |b| < a)$

568. $\int_0^\infty e^{-ax}\sinh bx\,dx = \frac{b}{a^2 - b^2}$, $(0 \leq |b| < a)$

569. $\int_{+\infty}^1 \frac{e^{-xu}}{u}\,du = \gamma + \log x - x + \frac{x^2}{2 \cdot 2!} - \frac{x^3}{3 \cdot 3!} + \frac{x^4}{4 \cdot 4!} - \cdots,$

where $\gamma = \lim_{z\to\infty}\left(1 + \frac{1}{2} + \frac{1}{3} + \cdots + \frac{1}{z} - \log z\right)$

$= 0.5772157 \cdots,$ $(0 < x < \infty)$

570. $\int_0^{\pi/2} \frac{dx}{\sqrt{1 - k^2\sin^2 x}} = \frac{\pi}{2}\left[1 + \left(\frac{1}{2}\right)^2 k^2 + \left(\frac{1 \cdot 3}{2 \cdot 4}\right)^2 k^4 + \left(\frac{1 \cdot 3 \cdot 5}{2 \cdot 4 \cdot 6}\right)^2 k^6 + \cdots\right]$, if $k^2 < 1$

INTEGRALS

571. $$\int_0^{\pi/2} \sqrt{1 - k^2 \sin^2 x}\, dx = \frac{\pi}{2}\left[1 - \left(\frac{1}{2}\right)^2 k^2 - \left(\frac{1 \cdot 3}{2 \cdot 4}\right)^2 \frac{k^4}{3} - \left(\frac{1 \cdot 3 \cdot 5}{2 \cdot 4 \cdot 6}\right)^2 \frac{k^6}{5} - \cdots\right], \text{ if } k^2 < 1$$

572. $$\int_0^\infty e^{-x} \log x\, dx = -\gamma = -0.5772157 \cdots$$

573. $$\int_0^\infty \left(\frac{1}{1 - e^{-x}} - \frac{1}{x}\right) e^{-x}\, dx = \gamma = 0.5772157 \cdots$$ [Euler's Constant]

574. $$\int_0^\infty \frac{1}{x}\left(\frac{1}{1 + x} - e^{-x}\right) dx = \gamma = 0.5772157 \cdots$$

XIII.14 GAMMA FUNCTION*

Values of $\Gamma(n) = \int_0^\infty e^{-x}x^{n-1}\,dx$; $\Gamma(n+1) = n\Gamma(n)$

n	$\Gamma(n)$	n	$\Gamma(n)$	n	$\Gamma(n)$	n	$\Gamma(n)$
1.00	1.00000	1.25	.90640	1.50	.88623	1.75	.91906
1.01	.99433	1.26	.90440	1.51	.88659	1.76	.92137
1.02	.98884	1.27	.90250	1.52	.88704	1.77	.92376
1.03	.98355	1.28	.90072	1.53	.88757	1.78	.92623
1.04	.97844	1.29	.89904	1.54	.88818	1.79	.92877
1.05	.97350	1.30	.89747	1.55	.88887	1.80	.93138
1.06	.96874	1.31	.89600	1.56	.88964	1.81	.93408
1.07	.96415	1.32	.89464	1.57	.89049	1.82	.93685
1.08	.95973	1.33	.89338	1.58	.89142	1.83	.93969
1.09	.95546	1.34	.89222	1.59	.89243	1.84	.94261
1.10	.95135	1.35	.89115	1.60	.89352	1.85	.94561
1.11	.94739	1.36	.89018	1.61	.89468	1.86	.94869
1.12	.94359	1.37	.88931	1.62	.89592	1.87	.95184
1.13	.93993	1.38	.88854	1.63	.89724	1.88	.95507
1.14	.93642	1.39	.88785	1.64	.89864	1.89	.95838
1.15	.93304	1.40	.88726	1.65	.90012	1.90	.96177
1.16	.92980	1.41	.88676	1.66	.90167	1.91	.96523
1.17	.92670	1.42	.88636	1.67	.90330	1.92	.96878
1.18	.92373	1.43	.88604	1.68	.90500	1.93	.97240
1.19	.92088	1.44	.88580	1.69	.90678	1.94	.97610
1.20	.91817	1.45	.88565	1.70	.90864	1.95	.97988
1.21	.91558	1.46	.88560	1.71	.91057	1.96	.98374
1.22	.91311	1.47	.88563	1.72	.91258	1.97	.98768
1.23	.91075	1.48	.88575	1.73	.91466	1.98	.99171
1.24	.90852	1.49	.88595	1.74	.91683	1.99	.99581
						2.00	1.00000

* For large positive values of x, $\Gamma(x)$ approximates the asymptotic series

$$x^x e^{-x}\sqrt{\frac{2\pi}{x}}\left[1 + \frac{1}{12x} + \frac{1}{288x^2} - \frac{139}{51840x^3} - \frac{571}{2488320x^4} + \cdots\right].$$

Index

(Note: Numbers in parenthesis refer to table numbers)